5.4 Intramedullary Nailing of a Proximal Humeral Fracture, 297

5.5 Open Reduction and Internal Fixation of Proximal Humeral Fractures, 298

5.6 Anterolateral Acromial Approach for Internal Fixation of Proximal Humeral Fracture (Gardner et al.; Mackenzie), 299

5.7 Open Reduction and Internal Fixation of the Humeral Shaft Through a Modified Posterior Approach (Triceps-Reflecting), 306

5.8 Minimally Invasive Plate Osteosynthesis (Apivatthakakul et al.; Tetsworth et al.), 308

5.9 Antegrade Intramedullary Nailing of Humeral Shaft Fractures, 311

5.10 Open Reduction and Internal Fixation of the Distal Humerus with Olecranon Osteotomy, 320

5.11 Open Reduction and Internal Fixation of Radial Head Fracture, 325

5.12 Stabilization of "Terrible Triad" Elbow Fracture-Dislocation (McKee et al.), 328

5.13 Internal Joint Stabilization for Elbow Instability (Orbay et al.), 332

5.14 Open Reduction and Internal Fixation of Olecranon Fracture, 337

5.15 Open Reduction and Internal Fixation of Both-Bone Forearm Fractures, 341

5.16 Closed Reduction and Percutaneous Pinning of Distal Radial Fracture (Glickel et al.), 347

5.17 External Fixation of Fracture of the Distal Radius, 349

5.18 Volar Plate Fixation of Fracture of the Distal Radius (Chung et al.), 352

5.19 Distraction Plate Fixation (Burke and Singer as Modified by Ruch et al.), 355

6. Malunited Fractures

6.1 Correction of Metatarsal Angulati

6.2 Correction of Tarsal Malunion, 3

6.3 Posterior Subtalar Arthrodesis (Ga...),

6.4 Distraction Arthrodesis (Carr et al.), 376

6.5 Resection of Lateral Prominence of Calcaneus (Kashiwagi, Modified), 377

6.6 Correction of Calcaneal Malunion Through Extensile Lateral Approach (Clare et al.), 378

6.7 Correction of Valgus Malunion of Extraarticular Calcaneal Fracture (Aly), 380

6.8 Osteotomy for Bimalleolar Fracture, 382

6.9 Correction of Diastasis of the Tibia and Fibula, 383

6.10 Supramalleolar Osteotomy, 383

6.11 Oblique Tibial Osteotomy (Sanders et al.), 386

6.12 Clamshell Osteotomy (Russell et al.), 389

6.13 Subcondylar Osteotomy and Wedge Graft for Malunion of Lateral Condyle, 393

6.14 Osteotomy and Internal Fixation of the Lateral Condyle, 393

6.15 Open Reduction and Internal Fixation, 394

6.16 Osteotomy for Femoral Malunion, 396

6.17 Osteotomy for Femoral Malunion in Children, 399

6.18 Correction of Cervicotrochanteric Malunion, 401

6.19 Osteotomy and Reorientation of Scapular Neck (Cole et al.), 404

6.20 Osteotomy and Plate Fixation, 405

6.21 Osteotomy and Elastic Intramedullary Nailing of Midshaft Clavicular Fracture (Smekal et al.), 408

6.22 Closing Wedge Valgus Osteotomy for Varus Malunion of Proximal Humerus (Benegas et al., Modified), 412

6.23 Correction of Proximal Third Humeral Malunion, 413

6.24 Correction of Radial Neck Malunion (Inhofe and Moneim, Modified), 414

6.25 Osteotomy and Fixation of Monteggia Fracture Malunion, 414

6.26 Resection of Proximal Part of Radial Shaft (Kamineni et al.), 416

6.27 Osteotomy and Plating for Forearm Malunion (Trousdale and Linscheid, Modified), 417

6.28 Correction of Forearm Malunion with Distal Radioulnar Joint Instability (Trousdale and Linscheid, Modified), 418

6.29 Drill Osteoclasis (Blackburn et al.), 418

6.30 Opening Wedge Metaphyseal Osteotomy with Bone Grafting And Internal Fixation with Plate and Screws (Fernandez), 423

6.31 Volar Osteotomy (Shea et al.), 424

6.32 Intramedullary Fixation, 426

6.33 External Fixation (Melendez), 427

6.34 Osteotomy for Intraarticular Malunion (Marx and Axelrod), 428

6.35 Radiolunate Arthrodesis (Saffar), 429

6.36 Ulnar Shortening Osteotomy (Milch), 430

6.37 Resection of the Distal Ulna (Darrach), 431

7. Delayed Union and Nonunion of Fractures

7.1 Decortication, 443

7.2 Fibular Autograft (Nonvascularized), 444

7.3 Intramedullary Fibular Strut Allograft (Humerus) (Willis et al.), 444

7.4 Resection of the Distal Fragment of the Medial Malleolus, 454

7.5 Sliding Graft, 454

7.6 Bone Graft of Medial Malleolar Nonunion (Banks), 455

7.7 Posterolateral Bone Grafting, 456

7.8 Anterior Central Bone Grafting, 456

7.9 Percutaneous Bone Marrow Injection (Connolly et al., Brinker et al.), 457

7.10 Tibial Exchange Nailing, 458

7.11 Plate Fixation and Bone Grafting of the Clavicle, 466

8. Acute Dislocations

8.1 Open Reduction and Repair of Patellar Dislocation, 474

8.2 Grafting of the Medial Patellar Retinaculum, 475

8.3 Open Reduction and Repair of the Extensor Mechanism, 475

8.4 Open Reduction of Hip Dislocation, 480

8.5 Anatomic Reconstruction of the Conoid and Trapezoid Ligaments (Mazzocca et al.), 484

8.6 Open Reduction of Radial Head Dislocation, 486

9. Old Unreduced Dislocations

9.1 Ligamentous Reconstruction for Old Unreduced Dislocation of the Proximal Tibiofibular Joint, 491

9.2 Open Reduction for Old Unreduced Dislocation of the Knee, 491

9.3 Open Reduction for Old Unreduced Dislocation of the Patella, 493

9.4 Intertrochanteric Osteotomy for Chronic Anterior Dislocation of the Hip (Aggarwal and Singh), 493

9.5 Traction and Abduction for Chronic Posterior Hip Dislocation (Gupta and Shravat), 494

坎贝尔骨科手术学
创伤与截肢

Campbell's Operative Orthopaedics

第 14 版
（影印版）

Frederick M. Azar, MD

James H. Beaty, MD

人民卫生出版社
·北 京·

图书在版编目（CIP）数据

坎贝尔骨科手术学 . 创伤与截肢：英文 /（美）弗雷德里克・M. 阿扎尔（Frederick M. Azar），（美）詹姆斯・H. 比蒂（James H. Beaty）主编 .—影印本 .—北京：人民卫生出版社，2021.12

ISBN 978-7-117-32521-9

Ⅰ. ①坎… Ⅱ. ①弗… ②詹… Ⅲ. ①骨科学 – 外科手术 – 英文②骨损伤 – 外科手术 – 英文③截肢 – 外科手术 – 英文 Ⅳ. ①R68

中国版本图书馆 CIP 数据核字（2021）第 241285 号

人卫智网	www.ipmph.com	医学教育、学术、考试、健康，购书智慧智能综合服务平台
人卫官网	www.pmph.com	人卫官方资讯发布平台

图字：01–2021–6747 号

坎贝尔骨科手术学
创伤与截肢
Kanbeier Guke Shoushuxue
Chuangshang yu Jiezhi

主　　编：Frederick M. Azar　James H. Beaty
出版发行：人民卫生出版社（中继线 010-59780011）
地　　址：北京市朝阳区潘家园南里 19 号
邮　　编：100021
E - mail：pmph @ pmph.com
购书热线：010-59787592　010-59787584　010-65264830
印　　刷：三河市宏达印刷有限公司（胜利）
经　　销：新华书店
开　　本：889×1194　1/16　印张：43
字　　数：2047 千字
版　　次：2021 年 12 月第 1 版
印　　次：2022 年 1 月第 1 次印刷
标准书号：ISBN 978-7-117-32521-9
定　　价：556.00 元

打击盗版举报电话：**010-59787491**　E-mail：**WQ @ pmph.com**
质量问题联系电话：**010-59787234**　E-mail：**zhiliang @ pmph.com**

坎贝尔骨科手术学
创伤与截肢

Campbell's Operative Orthopaedics

第 14 版
（影印版）

Frederick M. Azar, MD

Professor

Department of Orthopaedic Surgery and Biomedical Engineering University of Tennessee–Campbell Clinic

Chief of Staff, Campbell Clinic

Memphis, Tennessee

James H. Beaty, MD

Harold B. Boyd Professor and Chair

Department of Orthopaedic Surgery and Biomedical Engineering University of Tennessee–Campbell Clinic

Memphis, Tennessee

Editorial Assistance

Kay Daugherty *and* **Linda Jones**

人民卫生出版社

·北 京·

Elsevier (Singapore) Pte Ltd.
3 Killiney Road,
#08–01 Winsland House I,
Singapore 239519
Tel:（65）6349–0200; Fax:（65）6733–1817

ELSEVIER

This English Reprint of Parts XV, XVI, and VI from Campbell's Operative Orthopaedics, 14E by Frederick M. Azar and James H. Beaty was undertaken by People's Medical Publishing House and is published by arrangement with Elsevier (Singapore) Pte Ltd.

Parts XV, XVI, and VI from Campbell' s Operative Orthopaedics, 14E by Frederick M. Azar and James H. Beaty由人民卫生出版社进行影印,并根据人民卫生出版社与爱思唯尔(新加坡)私人有限公司的协议约定出版。

Notice

Practitioners and researchers must always rely on their own experience and knowledge in evaluating and using any information, methods, compounds or experiments described herein. Because of rapid advances in the medical sciences, in particular, independent verification of diagnoses and drug dosages should be made. To the fullest extent of the law, no responsibility is assumed by Elsevier, authors, editors or contributors in relation to the adaptation or for any injury and/or damage to persons or property as a matter of products liability, negligence or otherwise, or from any use or operation of any methods, products, instructions, or ideas contained in the material herein.

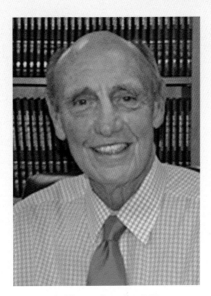

S. Terry Canale, MD

It is with humble appreciation and admiration that we dedicate this edition of *Campbell's Operative Orthopaedics* to Dr. S. Terry Canale, who served as editor or co-editor of five editions. He took great pride in this position and worked tirelessly to continue to improve "The Book." As noted by one of his co-editors, "Terry is probably the only person in the world who has read every word of multiple editions of *Campbell's Operative Orthopaedics*." He considered *Campbell's Operative Orthopaedics* an opportunity for worldwide orthopaedic education and made it a priority to ensure that each edition provided valuable and up-to-date information. His commitment to and enthusiasm for this work will continue to influence and inspire every future edition.

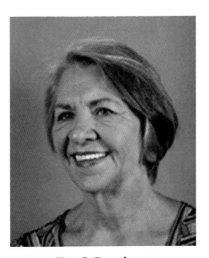

Kay C. Daugherty

It is with equal appreciation and regard that we dedicate this edition to Kay C. Daugherty, the managing editor of the last nine editions *Campbell's Operative Orthopaedics*. Over the last 40 years, she has faithfully and tirelessly edited, reshaped, and overseen all aspects of publication from manuscript preparation to proofing. She has a profound talent to put ideas and disjointed words into comprehensible text, ensuring that each revision maintains the gold standard in readability. Each edition is a testament to her dedication to excellence in writing and education. A favorite quote of Mrs. Daugherty to one of our late authors was, "I'll make a deal. I won't operate if you won't punctuate." We are grateful for her many years of continual service to the Campbell Foundation and for the publications yet to come.

CONTRIBUTORS

FREDERICK M. AZAR, MD
Professor
Director, Sports Medicine Fellowship
University of Tennessee–Campbell Clinic
Department of Orthopaedic Surgery and
    Biomedical Engineering
Chief-of-Staff, Campbell Clinic
Memphis, Tennessee

JAMES H. BEATY, MD
Harold B. Boyd Professor and Chair
University of Tennessee–Campbell Clinic
Department of Orthopaedic Surgery and
    Biomedical Engineering
Memphis, Tennessee

MICHAEL J. BEEBE, MD
Instructor
University of Tennessee–Campbell Clinic
Department of Orthopaedic Surgery and
    Biomedical Engineering
Memphis, Tennessee

CLAYTON C. BETTIN, MD
Assistant Professor
Director, Foot and Ankle Fellowship
Associate Residency Program Director
University of Tennessee–Campbell Clinic
Department of Orthopaedic Surgery and
    Biomedical Engineering
Memphis, Tennessee

TYLER J. BROLIN, MD
Assistant Professor
University of Tennessee–Campbell Clinic
Department of Orthopaedic Surgery and
    Biomedical Engineering
Memphis, Tennessee

JAMES H. CALANDRUCCIO, MD
Associate Professor
Director, Hand Fellowship
University of Tennessee–Campbell Clinic
Department of Orthopaedic Surgery and
    Biomedical Engineering
Memphis, Tennessee

DAVID L. CANNON, MD
Associate Professor
University of Tennessee–Campbell Clinic
Department of Orthopaedic Surgery and
    Biomedical Engineering
Memphis, Tennessee

KEVIN B. CLEVELAND, MD
Instructor
University of Tennessee–Campbell Clinic
Department of Orthopaedic Surgery and
    Biomedical Engineering
Memphis, Tennessee

ANDREW H. CRENSHAW JR., MD
Professor Emeritus
University of Tennessee–Campbell Clinic
Department of Orthopaedic Surgery and
    Biomedical Engineering
Memphis, Tennessee

JOHN R. CROCKARELL, MD
Professor
University of Tennessee–Campbell Clinic
Department of Orthopaedic Surgery and
    Biomedical Engineering
Memphis, Tennessee

GREGORY D. DABOV, MD
Assistant Professor
University of Tennessee–Campbell Clinic
Department of Orthopaedic Surgery and
    Biomedical Engineering
Memphis, Tennessee

MARCUS C. FORD, MD
Instructor
University of Tennessee–Campbell Clinic
Department of Orthopaedic Surgery and
    Biomedical Engineering
Memphis, Tennessee

RAYMOND J. GARDOCKI, MD
Assistant Professor
University of Tennessee–Campbell Clinic
Department of Orthopaedic Surgery and
    Biomedical Engineering
Memphis, Tennessee

BENJAMIN J. GREAR, MD
Instructor
University of Tennessee–Campbell Clinic
Department of Orthopaedic Surgery and
    Biomedical Engineering
Memphis, Tennessee

JAMES L. GUYTON, MD
Associate Professor
University of Tennessee–Campbell Clinic
Department of Orthopaedic Surgery and
    Biomedical Engineering
Memphis, Tennessee

JAMES W. HARKESS, MD
Associate Professor
University of Tennessee–Campbell Clinic
Department of Orthopaedic Surgery and
    Biomedical Engineering
Memphis, Tennessee

ROBERT K. HECK JR., MD
Associate Professor
University of Tennessee–Campbell Clinic
Department of Orthopaedic Surgery and
    Biomedical Engineering
Memphis, Tennessee

MARK T. JOBE, MD
Associate Professor
University of Tennessee–Campbell Clinic
Department of Orthopaedic Surgery and
    Biomedical Engineering
Memphis, Tennessee

DEREK M. KELLY, MD
Professor
Director, Pediatric Orthopaedic Fellowship
Director, Resident Education
University of Tennessee–Campbell Clinic
Department of Orthopaedic Surgery and
    Biomedical Engineering
Memphis, Tennessee

SANTOS F. MARTINEZ, MD
Assistant Professor
University of Tennessee–Campbell Clinic
Department of Orthopaedic Surgery and
    Biomedical Engineering
Memphis, Tennessee

ANTHONY A. MASCIOLI, MD
Assistant Professor
University of Tennessee–Campbell Clinic
Department of Orthopaedic Surgery and
    Biomedical Engineering
Memphis, Tennessee

BENJAMIN M. MAUCK, MD
Assistant Professor
Director, Hand Fellowship
University of Tennessee–Campbell Clinic
Department of Orthopaedic Surgery and
    Biomedical Engineering
Memphis, Tennessee

MARC J. MIHALKO, MD
Assistant Professor
University of Tennessee–Campbell Clinic
Department of Orthopaedic Surgery and
    Biomedical Engineering
Memphis, Tennessee

WILLIAM M. MIHALKO, MD PhD
Professor, H.R. Hyde Chair of Excellence in
    Rehabilitation Engineering
Director, Biomedical Engineering
University of Tennessee–Campbell Clinic
Department of Orthopaedic Surgery and
    Biomedical Engineering
Memphis, Tennessee

ROBERT H. MILLER III, MD
Associate Professor
University of Tennessee–Campbell Clinic
Department of Orthopaedic Surgery and
  Biomedical Engineering
Memphis, Tennessee

G. ANDREW MURPHY, MD
Associate Professor
University of Tennessee–Campbell Clinic
Department of Orthopaedic Surgery and
  Biomedical Engineering
Memphis, Tennessee

ASHLEY L. PARK, MD
Clinical Assistant Professor
University of Tennessee–Campbell Clinic
Department of Orthopaedic Surgery and
  Biomedical Engineering
Memphis, Tennessee

EDWARD A. PEREZ, MD
Associate Professor
University of Tennessee–Campbell Clinic
Department of Orthopaedic Surgery and
  Biomedical Engineering
Memphis, Tennessee

BARRY B. PHILLIPS, MD
Professor
University of Tennessee–Campbell Clinic
Department of Orthopaedic Surgery and
  Biomedical Engineering
Memphis, Tennessee

DAVID R. RICHARDSON, MD
Associate Professor
University of Tennessee–Campbell Clinic
Department of Orthopaedic Surgery and
  Biomedical Engineering
Memphis, Tennessee

MATTHEW I. RUDLOFF, MD
Assistant Professor
Co-Director, Trauma Fellowship
University of Tennessee–Campbell Clinic
Department of Orthopaedic Surgery and
  Biomedical Engineering
Memphis, Tennessee

JEFFREY R. SAWYER, MD
Professor
Co-Director, Pediatric Orthopaedic
  Fellowship
University of Tennessee–Campbell Clinic
Department of Orthopaedic Surgery and
  Biomedical Engineering
Memphis, Tennessee

BENJAMIN W. SHEFFER, MD
Assistant Professor
University of Tennessee–Campbell Clinic
Department of Orthopaedic Surgery and
  Biomedical Engineering
Memphis, Tennessee

DAVID D. SPENCE, MD
Assistant Professor
University of Tennessee–Campbell Clinic
Department of Orthopaedic Surgery and
  Biomedical Engineering
Memphis, Tennessee

NORFLEET B. THOMPSON, MD
Instructor
University of Tennessee–Campbell Clinic
Department of Orthopaedic Surgery and
  Biomedical Engineering
Memphis, Tennessee

THOMAS W. THROCKMORTON, MD
Professor
Co-Director, Sports Medicine Fellowship
University of Tennessee–Campbell Clinic
Department of Orthopaedic Surgery and
  Biomedical Engineering
Memphis, Tennessee

PATRICK C. TOY, MD
Associate Professor
University of Tennessee–Campbell Clinic
Department of Orthopaedic Surgery and
  Biomedical Engineering
Memphis, Tennessee

WILLIAM C. WARNER JR., MD
Professor
University of Tennessee–Campbell Clinic
Department of Orthopaedic Surgery and
  Biomedical Engineering
Memphis, Tennessee

JOHN C. WEINLEIN, MD
Assistant Professor
Director, Trauma Fellowship
University of Tennessee–Campbell Clinic
Department of Orthopaedic Surgery and
  Biomedical Engineering
Memphis, Tennessee

WILLIAM J. WELLER, MD
Instructor
University of Tennessee–Campbell Clinic
Department of Orthopaedic Surgery and
  Biomedical Engineering
Memphis, Tennessee

A. PAIGE WHITTLE, MD
Associate Professor
University of Tennessee–Campbell Clinic
Department of Orthopaedic Surgery and
  Biomedical Engineering
Memphis, Tennessee

KEITH D. WILLIAMS, MD
Associate Professor
University of Tennessee–Campbell Clinic
Department of Orthopaedic Surgery and
  Biomedical Engineering
Memphis, Tennessee

DEXTER H. WITTE III, MD
Clinical Assistant Professor in
  Radiology
University of Tennessee–Campbell Clinic
Department of Orthopaedic Surgery and
  Biomedical Engineering
Memphis, Tennessee

When Dr. Willis Campbell published the first edition of *Campbell's Operative Orthopaedics* in 1939, he could not have envisioned that over 80 years later it would have evolved into a four-volume text and earned the accolade of the "bible of orthopaedics" as a mainstay in orthopaedic practices and educational institutions all over the world. This expansion from some 400 pages in the first edition to over 4,500 pages in this 14th edition has not changed Dr. Campbell's original intent: "to present to the student, the general practitioner, and the surgeon the subject of orthopaedic surgery in a simple and comprehensive manner." In each edition since the first, authors and editors have worked diligently to fulfill these objectives. This would have not been possible without the hard work of our contributors who always strive to present the most up-to-date information while retaining "tried and true" techniques and tips. The scope of this text continues to expand in the hope that the information will be relevant to physicians no matter their location or resources.

As always, this edition also is the result of the collaboration of a group of "behind the scenes" individuals who are involved in the actual production process. The Campbell Foundation staff—Kay Daugherty, Linda Jones, and Tonya Priggel—contributed their considerable talents to editing often confusing and complex author contributions, searching the literature for obscure references, and, in general, "herding the cats." Special thanks to Kay and Linda who have worked on multiple editions of *Campbell's Operative Orthopaedics* (nine editions for Kay and six for Linda). They probably know more about orthopaedics than most of us, and they certainly know how to make it more understandable. Thanks, too, to the Elsevier personnel who provided guidance and assistance throughout the publication process: John Casey, Senior Project Manager; Jennifer Ehlers, Senior Content Development Specialist; and Belinda Kuhn, Senior Content Strategist.

We are especially appreciative of our spouses, Julie Azar and Terry Beaty, and our families for their patience and support as we worked through this project.

The preparation and publication of this 14th edition was fraught with difficulties because of the worldwide pandemic and social unrest, but our contributors and other personnel worked tirelessly, often in creative and innovative ways, to bring it to fruition. It is our hope that these efforts have provided a text that is informative and valuable to all orthopaedists as they continue to refine and improve methods that will ensure the best outcomes for their patients.

Frederick M. Azar, MD
James H. Beaty, MD

CONTENTS

PART **I**

FRACTURES AND DISLOCATIONS IN ADULTS

1 General Principles of Fracture Treatment 2
A. Paige Whittle

2 Fractures of the Lower Extremity 56
Matthew I. Rudloff

3 Fractures and Dislocations of the Hip 153
John C. Weinlein

4 Fractures of the Acetabulum and Pelvis 202
Michael J. Beebe

5 Fractures of the Shoulder, Arm, and Forearm 275
Edward A. Perez

6 Malunited Fractures 371
A. Paige Whittle

7 Delayed Union and Nonunion of Fractures 436
John C. Weinlein

8 Acute Dislocations 472
Anthony A. Mascioli

9 Old Unreduced Dislocations 490
Andrew H. Crenshaw Jr.

PART **II**

PERIPHERAL NERVE INJURIES OF THE UPPER AND LOWER EXTREMITIES

10 Peripheral Nerve Injuries 516
Mark T. Jobe, Santos F. Martinez, William J. Weller

PART **III**

AMPUTATIONS

11 General Principles of Amputations 568
Patrick C. Toy

12 Amputations of the Foot 586
David R. Richardson

13 Amputations of the Lower Extremity 608
Marcus C. Ford

14 Amputations of the Hip and Pelvis 621
Kevin B. Cleveland

15 Major Amputations of the Upper Extremity 630
Kevin B. Cleveland

16 Amputations of the Hand 647
James H. Calandruccio, Benjamin M. Mauck

FRACTURES AND DISLOCATIONS IN ADULTS

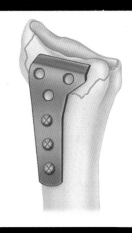

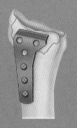

CHAPTER 1

GENERAL PRINCIPLES OF FRACTURE TREATMENT

A. Paige Whittle

CLASSIFICATION OF FRACTURES	3
CLASSIFICATION OF SOFT-TISSUE INJURIES	3
TRAUMA PRINCIPLES	7
Open fractures	8
Open fractures caused by firearms	8
Amputation versus limb salvage	10
Antibiotic treatment	10
Treatment of soft-tissue injuries	14
Debridement	15
Treatment of bone injuries	19
Fracture stabilization	19
FRACTURE HEALING (BONE REGENERATION)	20
Stimulation of fracture healing	21
Bone grafting	21
Bone graft substitutes	23
Electrical and ultrasound stimulation	27
Factors that negatively affect bone healing	27

PRINCIPLES OF SURGICAL TREATMENT	27
General indications for surgical reduction and stabilization	27
Contraindications to surgical reduction and stabilization	28
Disadvantages of surgical reduction and stabilization	28
Timing of surgical treatment	28
Lambotte's principles of surgical treatment of fractures	29
BIOMATERIALS OF FRACTURE FIXATION	29
Metals	29
Bioabsorbable materials	30
Complications	30
BIOMECHANICS OF IMPLANT DESIGN AND FRACTURE FIXATION	31
Pin and wire fixation	31
Screw fixation	31
Machine screws	33
Internal fixation screws	33
Screws fixation techniques	34
Plate and screw fixation	36

Locking plates	38
Intramedullary nail fixation	38
Types of intramedullary nails	41
Reamed versus unreamed intramedullary nailing	42
External fixation	42
Advantages	42
Disadvantages	43
Complications	43
Indications	44
Design and application of external fixators	45
REHABILITATION	49
TREATMENT OF COMPLICATIONS FROM SURGICAL TREATMENT OF FRACTURES	49
Infection	49
Gas gangrene	50
Tetanus	51
Soft-tissue complications	51
Thromboembolic complications	52
Biomechanical construct complications	52

Accidental injury is the most common cause of death in the United States in individuals between the ages of 1 and 45 (Table 1.1). In 2017 nearly 8.6 million accidental (unintentional), nonfatal falls were reported in the United States in all age groups. In adults older than 65 years of age, one in three experiences a fall that results in serious injury or death. Falls are the most common reasons for hospitalization in this older age group and account for 87% of fractures. In 2012 there were 3.2 million medically treated nonfatal fall–related injuries in seniors in the United States, with direct medical costs estimated to be $30.3 billion in 2012. These costs increased to $31.3 billion in 2015. For hip fractures alone, Medicare costs rose from over $3 billion in the 1990s to $15 billion currently. It is estimated that 300,000 hip fractures occur in the United States and 1.6 million internationally. As life expectancy increases, so will the incidence and cost of fragility fractures.

Fractures have been identified as medical problems throughout history. Most of Hippocrates' medical essays described the management of injuries, especially fractures. Knowledge of the biologic aspects of fracture care expanded greatly during the twentieth century. Patient expectations have reached unprecedented levels, and large, multinational industries have developed around the surgical and medical treatment of fractures.

The vascular supply of bone is the basis of all fracture healing. In 1932 Girdlestone warned that "there is danger inherent in the mechanical efficiency of our modern methods, danger lest the craftsman forget that union cannot be imposed but may have to be encouraged. Where bone is a plant, with its roots in soft tissues, and when its vascular connections are damaged, it often requires, not the technique of a cabinet maker, but the patient care and understanding of a gardener."

Orthopaedic surgeons are feeling the full impact of Girdlestone's prophetic words. An orthopaedic surgeon dealing with trauma must combine the knowledge of the systemic effects of trauma, including immunologic impairment, malnutrition, pulmonary and gastrointestinal dysfunction, and neurologic injury in planning both the timing and the type of surgical intervention required. The choice of fracture treatment is not a clear-cut decision because of the number of treatment options available. Each has its benefits and potential complications. A thorough knowledge of the underlying principles is essential in determining the right procedure to be done at the right time.

The goal of fracture treatment is to obtain union of the fracture in the most anatomic position compatible with maximal functional return of the extremity. Because it is impossible to intervene surgically without adding further injury to the extremity, the technique chosen should minimize additional soft-tissue damage and bone injury. An anatomic reduction obtained at the expense of total

TABLE 1.1

Most Common Causes of Death in the United States Among Individuals 25-44 Years Old

1980	2003	2017
1. Accidental injuries	1. Accidental injuries	1. Accidental injuries
2. Cancer (all types)	2. Cancer (all types)	2. Suicide
3. Heart disease	3. Heart disease	3. Cancer (all types)
4. Homicide	4. Suicide	4. Heart disease
5. Suicide	5. Homicide	5. Homicide
6. Chronic liver disease/cirrhosis	6. HIV	6. Liver disease
7. Cerebrovascular disease	7. Chronic liver disease/cirrhosis	7. Diabetes mellitus
8. Diabetes mellitus	8. Cerebrovascular disease	8. Cerebrovascular disease
9. Pneumonia and influenza	9. Diabetes mellitus	9. HIV
10. Congenital anomalies	10. Influenza and pneumonia	10. Septicemia

From the National Center for Health Statistics: Health, United States, 2018. https://www.cdc.gov/nchs/hus/contents2018.htm.

devascularization of the fracture is not a well-planned or well-executed procedure. The mechanical stresses that will be applied to the extremity and the planned fixation also must be considered. Finally, the general health status of the patient and the risks of surgery must be weighed to determine the best therapy.

Any form of fixation is at best a splinting device with a finite life span. There is a continual race between failure of fixation and healing of the bone. The problem is identifying the therapy that will result in the most predictable and acceptable fracture union with a minimal number of complications. Before attempting a complicated open reduction and internal fixation, surgeons must consider their own training and surgical ability and must be familiar with the proposed procedure. The institution in which the procedure is performed also must be considered. The environment in the operating room suite should be superior. The personnel should be familiar with the proposed technique and instrumentation, and a complete set of all instruments and implants should be readily available and well maintained. Excellent anesthesia and extensive intraoperative monitoring of the patient are necessary for safe surgical fracture management. A patient who is fully informed of the rewards and risks of the surgical methods chosen and who is willing to cooperate with required rehabilitation after surgery is vital to the success of any method of treatment.

Successful treatment of fractures depends on a thorough evaluation of the patient, not just the injured parts, as well as on the formulation of a treatment plan tailored specifically to the needs of the patient. The chosen treatment method should be the most likely to result in bone and soft-tissue healing and optimal functional recovery with the fewest complications.

CLASSIFICATION OF FRACTURES

When combined with an assessment of the surgeon's capabilities, facility, and resources, as well as an assessment of the patient profile, classification of the extent and type of fracture and its associated soft-tissue injuries allows determination of the best treatment. Analysis of the fracture pattern reveals the amount of energy imparted to the extremity and the stability of the fracture after reduction and alerts the surgeon to

higher-risk patterns of injury. Classification also allows the surgeon to monitor results and to compare treatment results with those of other surgeons and investigators; it also provides a basis for the evaluation of new treatment methods.

The extensive Orthopaedic Trauma Association (OTA) classification (Fig. 1.1) correlates the coding of the fracture with the expanded International Classification of Disease, tenth edition (ICD-10) codes for diagnosis and treatment. It incorporates well-recognized classification systems, such as the Judet, Judet, and Letournel classification of acetabular fractures, Young and Burgess' classification of pelvic fractures, Pauwels' classification of femoral neck fractures, and Neer's classification of proximal humeral injuries. Sample follow-up assessment forms were created to allow consistent postoperative evaluations. The 2007 update of the OTA classification included the AO classification. The AO alphanumeric classification was the result of an international effort by numerous individuals based on information from the AO Documentation Center and their clinical experience. This system was based on the morphologic characteristics and the location of the fracture. This AO classification system was applied to 2700 surgically treated diaphyseal fractures with correlation of the system ideology. It was specifically evaluated in 400 fractures of the tibial or fibular diaphysis. As the severity of the fracture pattern increased, the resulting impairment correlated with progression of the type and group. The 2018 revision of the OTA/AO Fracture and Dislocation Classification Compendium streamlines the information in the 2007 edition and includes the OTA open fracture classification. These classification systems are detailed and complex, and the reader is referred to the references for complete discussions.

CLASSIFICATION OF SOFT-TISSUE INJURIES

Just as the bony injury must be classified to evaluate the fracture adequately and to validate results for comparative studies, associated soft-tissue injuries also must be evaluated. Open wounds have been classified several ways. Gustilo and Anderson in 1976 described their treatment of 1025 open fractures with application of a grading system that offered

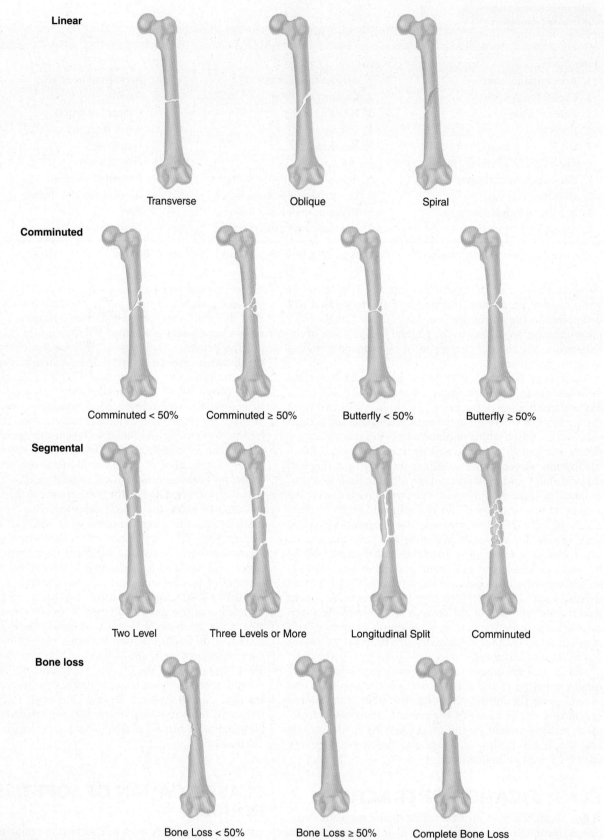

Linear

Transverse   Oblique   Spiral

Comminuted

Comminuted < 50%   Comminuted ≥ 50%   Butterfly < 50%   Butterfly ≥ 50%

Segmental

Two Level   Three Levels or More   Longitudinal Split   Comminuted

Bone loss

Bone Loss < 50%   Bone Loss ≥ 50%   Complete Bone Loss

FIGURE 1.1 Orthopaedic Trauma Association classification of long bone fractures (see text). (From Gustilo RB: *The fracture classification manual*, St. Louis, 1991, Mosby.)

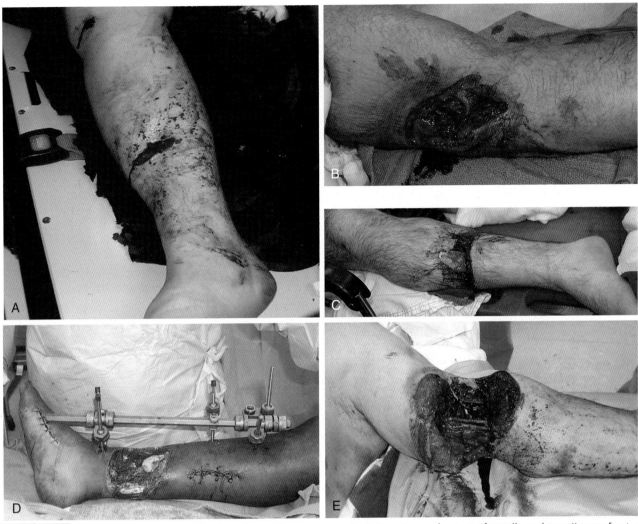

FIGURE 1.2 Gustilo-Anderson classification of open fracture wounds. **A,** Type I open fracture of patella and type II open fracture of tibial shaft. **B,** Type IIIA open fracture with extensive laceration of skin and muscles that involves almost entire leg. **C,** Type IIIA open tibial fracture with extensive periosteal stripping but without massive contamination. **D,** Type IIIB open fracture of tibia stabilized with external fixation. **E,** Type IIIC fracture of proximal third of humerus.

prognostic information about the outcome of infected fractures. In 1984, this system was modified and their results updated. The modified classification is based on the size of the wound, periosteal soft-tissue damage, periosteal stripping, and vascular injury (Fig. 1.2).

- Type I open fractures have a clean wound less than 1 cm long.
- In type II wounds the laceration is more than 1 cm long but is without extensive soft-tissue damage, skin flaps, or avulsions.
- Type IIIA open fractures have extensive soft-tissue lacerations or flaps but maintain adequate soft-tissue coverage of bone, or they result from high-energy trauma regardless of the size of the wound. This group includes segmental or severely comminuted fractures, even those with 1-cm lacerations.
- Type IIIB open fractures have extensive soft-tissue loss with periosteal stripping and bone exposure. They usually are massively contaminated.

- Type IIIC open fractures include open fractures with an arterial injury that requires repair regardless of the size of the soft-tissue wound.

This classification has prognostic significance and is discussed in greater detail later in the section on open fractures.

Other classifications include that of Tscherne and Gotzen, which is widely used in Europe. Closed fractures are divided into grades 0 through 3 (Fig. 1.3). Open fractures are divided into grades 1 through 4 (Table 1.2). This system includes soft-tissue damage and compartment syndrome, which are not included in other grading schemes. The AO-ASIF group added to their extensive fracture classification a soft-tissue classification scheme that closely follows that of Tscherne and Gotzen. This classification includes both closed and open injuries, musculotendinous injury, and neurovascular injury (Box 1.1). A number of other trauma scoring systems have been proposed, including the Trauma Score (TS), Revised Trauma Score (RTS), Injury Severity Score (ISS), Modified Abbreviated Injury Severity Scale (MISS), Pediatric Trauma

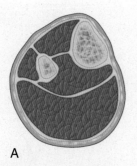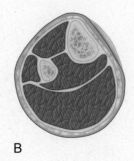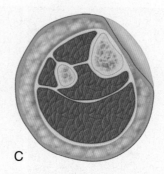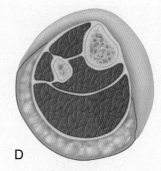

A   B   C   D

FIGURE 1.3   Grading system of soft-tissue injury in closed fractures. **A,** Grade 0: little or no soft-tissue injury. **B,** Grade 1: superficial abrasion with local contusional damage to skin or muscle. **C,** Grade 2: deep contaminated abrasion with local contusional damage to skin and muscle. **D,** Grade 3: extensive contusion or crushing of skin or destruction of muscle.

TABLE 1.2

Tscherne Classification for Open Tibial Fractures

Grade 1	Skin lacerations caused by a bone fragment from inside, little or no contusion of skin
Grade 2	Any type of skin laceration with circumscribed skin or soft-tissue contusion and moderate contamination; can occur with any type of fracture
Grade 3	Fracture must have severe soft-tissue damage, often with major vessel or nerve injury or both; all fractures accompanied by ischemia and severe bone comminution belong in this group and those associated with compartment syndrome
Grade 4	Subtotal and total amputation, defined as separation of all important anatomic structures, especially major vessels with total ischemia; remaining soft tissue may not exceed one fourth of circumference of extremity (any revascularization is grade 3)

Score (PTS), Nerve Injury, Ischemia, Soft-Tissue Injury, Skeletal Injury, Shock, and Age of Patient Score (NISSSA), and the Hanover Fracture Scale-97 (HFS-97). These classification systems attempt to quantitate the degree of soft-tissue injury in relation to the fracture and the potential for infection or other healing problems. An evaluation of the AO/OTA fracture classification system, however, found that patients with C-type fractures had significantly worse functional performance and impairment compared with patients with B-type fractures but were not significantly different from patients with A-type fractures, suggesting that the AO/OTA classification may not be a good predictor of functional performance and impairment in patients who have isolated unilateral lower extremity fractures.

In 2010 the classification committee of the OTA recommended a new classification scheme for open fractures. This new classification uses five categories of assessment: skin injury, muscle injury, arterial injury, contamination, and bone loss (Box 1.2). This provides a systemic approach to classification at the time of arrival before treatment has occurred. As with all classification systems, its complexity may make it less reproducible for general use. Its predictive ability is currently

BOX 1.1

AO-ASIF Soft-Tissue Injury Classification

Scale
1   Normal (except open fractures)
2-4 Increasing severity of lesion
5   A special situation

Skin Lesions (Closed Fractures)
IC 1 No skin lesion
IC 2 No skin laceration, but contusion
IC 3 Circumferential degloving
IC 4 Extensive, closed degloving
IC 5 Necrosis from contusion

Skin Lesions (Open Fractures)
IO 1 Skin breakage from inside out
IO 2 Skin breakage < 5 cm, edges contused
IO 3 Skin breakage > 5 cm, devitalized edges
IO 4 Full-thickness contusion, avulsion, soft-tissue defect, muscle-tendon unit injury

Muscle-Tendon Unit Injury
MT 1 No muscle injury
MT 2 Circumferential injury, one compartment only
MT 3 Considerable injury, two compartments
MT 4 Muscle defect, tendon laceration, extensive contusion
MT 5 Compartment syndrome/crush injury

Neurovascular Injury
NV 1 No neurovascular injury
NV 2 Isolated nerve injury
NV 3 Localized vascular injury
NV 4 Extensive segmental vascular injury
NV 5 Combined neurovascular injury including subtotal or complete amputation

From German G, Sherman R, Levin LS: *Decision-making in reconstructive surgery upper-extremity*, New York, 1999, Springer-Verlag.

being evaluated. Hao et al., in a retrospective review of 512 patients, found that the OTA open fracture classification was more predictive of infection, need for soft-tissue coverage, and need for amputation in patients with a long bone fracture compared to the Gustilo and Anderson classification. A cumulative OTA score of 10 or less was associated with a greater probability of successful limb salvage.

BOX 1.2

Orthopaedic Trauma Association Open Fracture Classification

Skin
1. Laceration with edges that approximate
2. Laceration with edges that do not approximate
3. Laceration associated with extensive degloving

Muscle
1. No appreciable muscle necrosis, some muscle injury with intact muscle function
2. Loss of muscle but the muscle remains functional, some localized necrosis in the zone of injury that requires excision, intact muscle-tendon unit
3. Dead muscle, loss of muscle function, partial or complete compartment excision, complete disruption of a muscle-tendon unit, muscle defect does not approximate

Arterial
1. No major vessel disruption
2. Vessel injury without distal ischemia
3. Vessel injury with distal ischemia

Contamination
1. No or minimal contamination
2. Surface contamination (not ground in).
3. Contaminant embedded in bone or deep soft tissues or high-risk environmental conditions (e.g., barnyard, fecal, dirty water)

Bone Loss
1. None
2. Bone missing or devascularized but still some contact between proximal and distal fragments
3. Segmental bone loss

From Orthopaedic Trauma Association: OTA open fracture classification (OTA-OFC), *J Orthop Trauma* 32:S106, 2018.

TRAUMA PRINCIPLES

Treatment of patients with multiple trauma requires additional resources that often are unavailable in small community hospitals. The resources of equipment and physician and nursing support personnel may not be available for acute stabilization of long bone, pelvic, and spinal fractures according to current trauma center protocols. Treatment in a level 1 or 2 trauma center has been documented to improve the care and survival of patients with multiple injuries. The length of hospital stay and cost of treatment are significantly lower in patients who are treated initially in trauma centers compared with those transferred to a trauma center from another location. The best management, in terms of quality of care and economics, of patients with multiple injuries is referral to a dedicated trauma center as soon as possible.

Since the early 1990s emphasis has been on early *total* care of multiply injured patients, including fracture stabilization. The frequency of pulmonary complications, such as adult respiratory distress syndrome, fat emboli syndrome, and pneumonia, has been correlated to the timing and type of treatment of long bone fractures. Statistically significant increases in morbidity, pulmonary complications, and length of hospital stay have been reported for patients in whom stabilization of major

fractures was delayed. A large multicenter study also reported reduced mortality when early total care was implemented.

More than half of patients with multiple injuries have fractures or dislocations or both, and the orthopaedic surgeon plays a pivotal role in the trauma team. The management of orthopaedic injuries can have a profound effect on the patient's ultimate functional recovery and may save the patient's life and limb. An example is placement of a pelvic binder in a patient with an open-book pelvic injury who remains hemodynamically unstable despite aggressive initial fluid and blood replacement. Open fractures, pelvic or acetabular injuries with associated genitourinary injuries, and extremity fractures with vascular injuries are other examples of situations in which communication and coordination among the various team members are essential.

Early stabilization of fractures of the spine, pelvis, and acetabulum, as well as other major articular fractures, is desirable to decrease pulmonary complications and other sequelae of forced recumbency, but the treatment of such fractures requires more complex surgical skills, equipment, and often neurologic monitoring. "Damage control orthopaedics" in the form of rapid immobilization of fractures with external fixation to obtain stability and recover length, while allowing full evaluation of the extremity, is now standard care. Operative treatment should not be undertaken if hemodynamic stabilization is not obtained, if potentially life-threatening conditions have not been resolved, or if laboratory and radiographic evaluations are inadequate for formulation of a satisfactory surgical plan.

Orthopaedic damage control measures can be undertaken in the emergency department or resuscitation area in special circumstances. Emergent external fixation of long bones in unstable patients may be necessary but can be complicated by pin site infections, or less frequently, deep vein thrombosis. In some patients, the fixation may be retained until fracture union. A significant decrease in the frequency of adult respiratory distress syndrome has been noted in patients with externally fixed femoral fractures compared with patients with nail fixation. In a prospective, randomized, multicenter study, inflammatory cytokines were measured in femoral fractures treated with immediate nailing and with immediate external fixation. An inflammatory response was noted with intramedullary fixation but not with external fixation. There was no difference in the clinical complications, and the total numbers studied were small. The concept of damage control in trauma surgery is presently the subject of intense evaluation. We have found this concept to be helpful in dealing with complex fractures in an emergency situation. Complications have occurred primarily in patients who never improved enough clinically to allow conversion to more definitive fixation.

Polytrauma and the resuscitation procedures often required in multiply injured patients result in the activation of cellular factors that have systemic effects, including inflammatory, immune, and hemodynamic factors that are mediated by chemicals known as cytokines. Elevation of cytokines is associated with organ dysfunction. Polytrauma also is associated with a systemic immune response syndrome, a diffuse inflammatory reaction mediated by cytokines and other chemicals in response to the massive tissue injuries. Damage control orthopaedics is a method to deal with the double insult of injury and surgery that may potentiate this response further.

An estimated 5% to 20% of patients with multiple trauma have injuries that are not recognized during the initial examination because of factors such as an altered level of consciousness or hemodynamic instability that precludes a thorough orthopaedic examination, a more apparent injury in the same extremity, and inadequate initial radiographs. Repeat orthopaedic examination after more critical injuries are stabilized should identify any missed injuries and allow early treatment. Studies have indicated that CT evaluation of the cervical spine and pelvis reveals more injuries than were apparent in the initial screening studies and on plain radiographs.

Management of a patient who has sustained multiple injuries requires very specific and reliable methods of evaluation and treatment. The Advanced Trauma Life Support system (ATLS) developed by the American College of Surgeons is the most widely used method for evaluating trauma patients. Evaluation is based on the mnemonic *ABCDE*:

Airway, which should be free and unobstructed

Breathing, which should be as normal as possible under the circumstances with normal oxygenation

Circulation, both central and peripheral; the goal is good capillary filling of all extremities and maintenance of a normal blood pressure

Disability, which includes neurologic, musculoskeletal, urologic, and reproductive injuries. These injuries, although rarely life threatening, can result in serious long-term disability.

Environment. Many of these injuries do not occur in an isolated situation and may result in contamination that can expose caregivers to disease.

From an orthopaedic standpoint, the musculoskeletal and neurologic evaluation protocols are extremely important in determining the type and extent of injury. Life- and limb-threatening musculoskeletal problems include hemorrhage from wounds and fractures, infections from open fractures, limb loss from vascular damage and compartment syndrome, and loss of function from spinal or peripheral neurologic injuries. Occult bleeding and unexplained blood loss from multiple areas, with concomitant hemodynamic instability, are major areas of concern with regard to the evaluation of circulation. Blood loss from multiple fractures, especially pelvic and long bone fractures, demands early stabilization to minimize blood loss.

The first consideration in management is the patient's general condition. Emergency measures are necessary to combat pain, hemorrhage, and shock. Hemorrhage should be controlled with pressure. Tourniquets rarely are recommended because of the potential for further nerve and limb damage. The blind use of a hemostat in a wound also is not recommended because of the risk of damage to peripheral nerves lying near the vessels. From the time of injury until the patient is ready for surgery, the wound should be protected by a sterile dressing and the extremity should be splinted to prevent additional soft-tissue injury from movement of the sharp bone fragments.

The medical history should include when and where the injury occurred. The examination should include determination of the extent and type of soft-tissue wound and the existence of any vascular or neurologic damage. Vascular injury or compartment syndrome should be treated promptly to avoid tissue ischemia, which, if present for 8 hours or more, can cause irreversible muscle and nerve damage. An experimental canine study found that irreversible muscle damage occurred with tissue pressures of 10 mm Hg less than diastolic blood pressure or within 30 mm Hg of mean arterial pressure. This study emphasized that rather than an absolute tissue pressure value, a

difference between tissue pressure and diastolic pressure of 10 to 20 mm Hg is an indication for immediate fasciotomy.

Radiographs should be made to show the extent and type of injury to the bone. The extent of soft-tissue damage sometimes cannot be determined until surgical exploration. The time since injury and the type and extent of soft-tissue damage have a direct bearing on the choice of treatment. High-velocity or high-energy trauma results in more extensive damage to both the soft tissues and the bone and carries with it a much more uncertain prognosis for healing than does low-velocity or low-energy trauma. The patient's general condition, the presence of related injuries, and numerous other factors influence the ultimate outcome and should influence treatment.

OPEN FRACTURES

Open fractures are surgical emergencies that perhaps should be thought of as incomplete amputations. Tscherne described four eras of open fracture treatment: life preservation, limb preservation, infection avoidance, and functional preservation. The first, or preantiseptic, era lasted well into the twentieth century. The era of limb preservation encompassed both world wars but was marked by a high incidence of amputations and resulting interest in artificial limb prosthetic designs. The third era lasted until the mid-1960s, during which time attention was focused on the avoidance of infection and the use of antibiotics. The fourth era (functional preservation) was characterized by aggressive wound debridement, definitive fracture stabilization with internal or external fixation, and delayed wound closure. The current fifth era is a product of rapid and high-value trauma care. Recent studies have confirmed that wound closure can be done in most open fractures (up to Gustilo-Anderson type IIIA) without significant risk and with decreased morbidity and hospital stay. Although there is general consensus that prophylactic antibiotics should be given for open fractures, there is a lack of high-quality evidence regarding the type, timing, and duration of antibiotic therapy. A systematic survey of articles published between January 2007 and January 2010 examined current practice and recommendations for antibiotic prophylaxis in the management of open fractures. Nearly 75% advocated gram-positive coverage for Gustilo types I and II open fractures, and the others recommended broad coverage. For more severe injuries, most authors recommended broad-spectrum antibiotic coverage. More than half of the articles recommended antibiotics be given as soon as possible after injury. The others proposed starting antibiotic prophylaxis within 3 hours of injury. For types I and II open fractures, 50% of the publications recommended a duration of 24 hours or less, and the rest for 48 to 72 hours. For type III open fractures, the majority proposed a duration of 2 to 3 days of antibiotic therapy. Some advocated for 72 hours total or 24 hours after wound closure. More than one third of the articles recommended that antibiotics be continued 4 to 7 days in severe open fractures. Historically, debridement and irrigation of open fractures within 6 hours after injury was considered essential to prevent infection. However, multiple current studies have shown that strict adherence to a 6-hour time frame is not necessary, although debridement should be performed as soon as the patient is stable and resources allow.

■ OPEN FRACTURES CAUSED BY FIREARMS

Evaluation of a patient with an open fracture caused by a firearm should include plain anteroposterior and lateral radiographs of the area of injury, as well as the joints above and below the injury. Arthrography may be necessary to

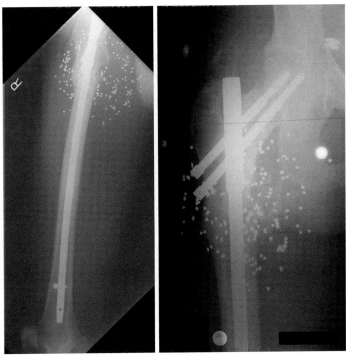

FIGURE 1.4 Low-velocity gunshot wound of femur; note minimal soft-tissue disruption.

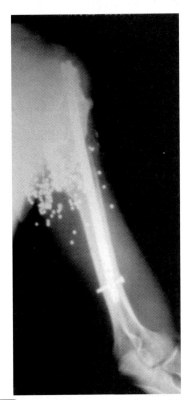

FIGURE 1.5 High-velocity gunshot wound to humerus.

identify joint penetration by a projectile. CT should be used to determine the precise location of the missile if the spine or pelvis is involved and is helpful in evaluating articular injuries. If vascular injury is suspected, angiography or arteriography may be necessary to confirm the diagnosis.

As encountered in civilian practice, firearm wounds are of three distinct types: (1) low-velocity pistol or rifle wounds, (2) high-velocity rifle wounds, and (3) close-range shotgun wounds. In low-velocity pistol or rifle wounds, soft-tissue damage usually is minimal and extensive debridement is unnecessary (Fig. 1.4). The wounds of entry and exit are small. They usually do not require closure, and only their skin edges require debridement. In low-velocity gunshot wounds, irrigation and local debridement, tetanus prophylaxis, and a single dose of a long-acting intramuscular cephalosporin have been found to be as effective as 48 hours of intravenous antibiotics, and oral and intravenous administrations of antibiotics were shown to be equally effective for prophylaxis against infection. Infection in this type of wound is rare. A proposed treatment protocol for intraarticular fractures includes 1 to 2 days of antibiotic prophylaxis for injuries in which the bullet passed through "clean" skin or clothing and 1 to 2 weeks of broad-spectrum antibiotic treatment for wounds in which the bullet penetrated lung, bowel, or grossly contaminated skin or clothing. Civilian gunshot wounds have been classified according to energy, vital structures involved, wound characteristics, fracture, and degree of contamination. This classification, however, is complex, has not been validated, and offers no guidelines for treatment.

Some gunshot wounds can be treated with outpatient oral antibiotics following a single dose of intravenous cephalosporin. Dickson et al. reported that a superficial infection occurred in only one of 41 patients (44 fractures) with Gustilo type I or II open fractures caused by low-velocity gunshot wounds who were treated with their outpatient protocol: tetanus toxoid, 0.5 mL, irrigation and local wound debridement, closed reduction (if necessary), placement of a dressing or splint, 1 g of intravenous cefazolin, and 500 mg of oral cephalexin four times daily for 7 days.

In high-velocity rifle and shotgun wounds, the damage to soft tissue and bone is massive and tissue necrosis is extensive (Fig. 1.5). These wounds should be treated in much the same manner as battle wounds. They require wide exposure and debridement of all devitalized soft tissues. These wounds should be left open for delayed primary or secondary closure depending on the nature of the wound. In close-range shotgun wounds, damage to soft tissue and bone is extensive. Unless the wound is through and through, the wadding of the shell usually is retained within it and can cause severe foreign body reactions. All wadding must be found and removed and devitalized soft tissue excised. Removing all of the lead shot is unnecessary; it seems to cause little reaction, and attempting to remove it can cause further damage to the soft tissues. However, bullets and bullet fragments should be removed from intraarticular or intrabursal locations because they can produce complications of mechanical wear, lead synovitis, and systemic lead toxicity. Systemic lead toxicity has been reported to occur as early as 2 days and as late as 40 years after intraarticular gunshot injury. These wounds also should be left open and are closed later.

Although both delayed and immediate reamed interlocked nailing have been successful in the treatment of femoral fractures, immediate nailing of femoral fractures caused by gunshots has been reported to result in shorter hospital stays, with significant decreases in hospital expenses, and no detrimental effect on clinical results compared with delayed nailing. Statically locked intramedullary nailing is currently our preferred treatment for most low-velocity and mid-velocity femoral shaft fractures, including most subtrochanteric and supracondylar fractures. Femoral fractures caused by high-velocity weapons or shotguns can be temporarily stabilized with external fixation. When wound healing is satisfactory, intramedullary nailing can be performed (approximately 2 weeks after injury). Some high-velocity fractures can be treated with immediate unreamed intramedullary nailing. Primary amputation may be required for severe soft-tissue injury that includes vascular and neurologic injury. In a series of 52 femoral fractures with arterial injuries treated at our local level 1 trauma center, limb salvage was successful in 32 (61.5%). All 22 limbs in which the femoral fractures were stabilized with intramedullary nails either initially (16 limbs) or after traction or external fixation were salvaged. Primary amputation was required in eight limbs with high-velocity injuries, secondary amputations were required in nine limbs, and three patients died of other injuries. No disruption of the anastomoses occurred in patients in whom vascular repair preceded fracture fixation (Fig. 1.6).

External fixation may be appropriate for severe (Gustilo type III) injuries. Ilizarov fixation and delayed primary closure have been reported to yield a low overall complication rate and a low infection rate in these complex fractures.

In a report of gunshot injuries to the hip, the best diagnostic test to detect joint penetration was hip aspiration followed by an arthrogram. Although selected patients were treated successfully with antibiotic therapy without arthrotomy, all transabdominal injuries required immediate arthrotomy. Bullets left in contact with joint fluid resulted in joint destruction or infection. Because all displaced femoral neck fractures treated with internal fixation had poor results, hip arthroplasty or arthrodesis was recommended for definitive management of these injuries.

■ AMPUTATION VERSUS LIMB SALVAGE

The development of sophisticated protocols for open fracture management has permitted the development of techniques that result in salvaged but nonfunctional extremities. There is concern, however, about "technique over reason" and not only the end result of a useless limb but also the physical, psychologic, financial, and social effects on the individual. Inevitable amputation often is delayed too long, with increased financial, personal, and social expenses and, more important, the attendant morbidity and possible mortality. In a study of open tibial fractures, patients who had limb salvage had more complications, more operative procedures, longer hospital stays, and higher hospital charges than patients who had early below-knee amputations. More patients with limb salvage considered themselves disabled than did those with early amputation.

Several attempts have been made to better evaluate injuries and identify injury patterns that would best be treated by early amputation. The Mangled Extremity Severity Score (MESS) is based on a four-group system: skeletal and soft-tissue injuries, shock, ischemia, and age (Table 1.3). Some studies have found that limbs with scores of 7 to 12 ultimately required amputation, whereas scores of 3 to 6 resulted in viable limbs; others have found no predictive utility of the MESS, Limb Salvage Index (LSI), or Predictive Salvage Index (PSI). A high specificity of the scores confirmed that low scores could be used to predict limb-salvage potential, but the low sensitivity failed to support the validity of the scores as predictors of amputation. These scoring systems appear to have limited usefulness and cannot be used as the sole criterion to determine whether amputation is indicated, and lower extremity injury-severity scores at or above the amputation threshold should be used with caution in determining the potential for salvaging a lower extremity with a high-energy injury.

Rajasekaran et al. proposed a scoring system for Gustilo types IIIA and IIIB open fractures of the tibia that evaluated skin coverage, skeletal structures, tendon and nerve injury, and comorbid conditions (Box 1.3). Using this system, they divided 109 type III open tibial fractures into four groups to assess the possibilities of limb salvage. Group 1 had scores of 5 or less, group 2 had scores of 6 to 10, group 3 had scores of 11 to 15, and group 4 had scores of 16 or greater. A score of 14 or greater as an indicator for amputation had a sensitivity of 98%, a specificity of 100%, a positive predictive value of 100%, and a negative predictive value of 70%. These were similar to the MESS scores of 99% sensitivity and 97% positive predictive value, but better than the 17% specificity and 50% negative predictive value. The high specificity of this new scoring system may make it a much better predictor of amputation. Currently, however, the predictive power of all extremity injury scores remains low.

■ ANTIBIOTIC TREATMENT

The treatment of an open fracture wound actually is an exercise in applied microbiology. Once the skin barrier is disrupted, bacteria enter from the local environment and attempt to attach and grow (Fig. 1.7). The greater the zone of injury and the more necrotic the tissue, the greater the potential for nutritional support of the bacteria. With impairment of circulation in the injured area, the body's immune system is compromised in its ability to use cellular and humoral defenses. A race then ensues between the bacteria to establish an infection and the body to mobilize sufficient immune mechanisms to combat the infection.

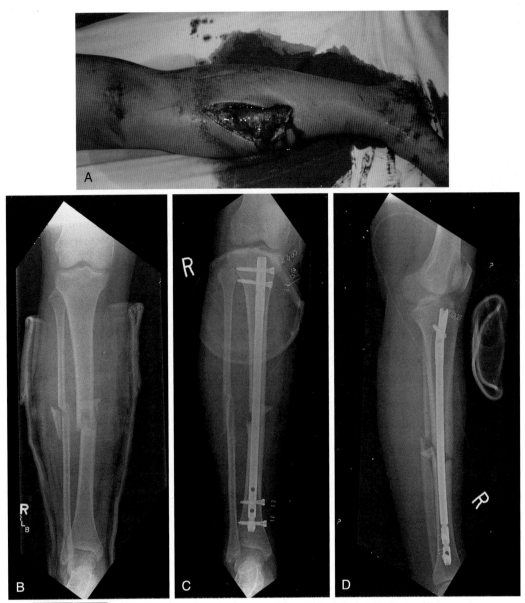

FIGURE 1.6   **A,** Open type IIIB tibial fracture with vascular injury. **B,** Radiographic appearance.
C and **D,** After fixation with locked intramedullary nail.

The virulence of the infecting organism depends on its ability to adhere to the host substrate (e.g., necrotic skin, fascia, muscle, and bone), its pathogenicity, and its offensive efforts to neutralize the host defenses by the bacteria's own humoral and mechanical factors. The foreign body reaction is now recognized as a complex interaction of bacterial glycoprotein that protects the bacteria from the phagocytic white blood cells (Fig. 1.8). After the bacteria have invaded the body, adhered to the host cellular substrate, and secreted the humoral and glycoprotein protective shield, they can then proceed with cell replication, establishing a clinical infection. Growth of the bacteria then proceeds in a logarithmic fashion until the available nutrients are exhausted, the host dies, or the host defenses successfully neutralize the infection. If the latter occurs and the host survives, the bacteria either will be eradicated or suppressed and isolated, creating chronic osteomyelitis (Fig. 1.9).

The care of open wounds generally includes postoperative systemic antibiotics. A 2004 Cochrane systematic review confirmed the benefit of antibiotics in patients with open fractures. This review showed that the administration of antibiotics after open fracture reduces the risk of infection by 59%. The data reviewed supported the conclusion that a short course of first-generation cephalosporins, begun as soon as possible after injury, significantly lowers the risk of infection when used in combination with prompt, modern orthopaedic fracture wound management. Evidence was insufficient to support other common management practices, such as prolonged courses or repeated short courses of antibiotics, the use of antibiotic coverage extending to gram-negative bacilli or clostridial species, or the use of local antibiotic therapies such as beads.

Most protocols recommend the use of a broad-spectrum antibiotic, usually a first-generation cephalosporin, with the addition of an aminoglycoside, such as tobramycin or gentamicin, for highly contaminated wounds in which there is a risk of gram-negative contamination (Gustilo type III). If there is the possibility of anaerobic organisms, such as *Clostridium,*

TABLE 1.3

Mangled Extremity Severity Score

TYPE	CHARACTERISTICS	INJURIES	POINTS
SKELETAL/SOFT-TISSUE GROUP			
1	Low energy	Stab wounds, simple closed fractures, small-caliber gunshot wounds	1
2	Medium energy	Open or multiple-level fractures, dislocations, moderate crush injuries	2
3	High energy	Shotgun blast (close range), high-velocity wounds	3
4	Massive crush	Logging, railroad, oil-rig accidents	4
SHOCK GROUP			
1	Normotensive hemodynamics	Blood pressure stable in field and in operating room	0
2	Transiently hypotensive	Blood pressure unstable in field but responsive to intravenous fluids	1
3	Prolonged hypotensive	Systolic blood pressure <90 mm Hg in field and responsive to intravenous fluid only in operating room	2
ISCHEMIA GROUP			
1	None	Pulsatile limb without signs of ischemia	0*
2	Mild	Diminished pulses without signs of ischemia	1*
3	Moderate	No pulse by Doppler, sluggish capillary refill, paresthesia, diminished motor activity	2*
4	Advanced	Pulseless, cool, paralyzed, and numb without capillary refill	3*
AGE GROUP			
1	<30 years		0
2	30-50 years		1
3	>50 years		2

*If ischemia time greater than 6 hours, add 2 points.
From Helfet DL, Howey T, Sanders R, Johansen K: Limb salvage versus amputation: preliminary results of the mangled extremity severity score, *Clin Orthop Relat Res* 256:80, 1990.

BOX 1.3

Injury Severity Score for Gustilo Types IIIA and IIIB Open Tibial Fractures

Covering Structures: Skin and Fascia
Wounds without skin loss
  Not over the fracture: 1
  Exposing the fracture: 2
Wounds with skin loss
  Not over the fracture: 3
  Over the fracture: 4
Circumferential wound with skin loss: 5

Skeletal Structures: Bone and Joints
Transverse or oblique fracture or butterfly fragment <50% circumference: 1
Large butterfly fragment >50% circumference: 2
Comminution or segmental fractures without bone loss: 3
Bone loss <4 cm: 4
Bone loss >4 cm: 5

Functional Tissues: Musculotendinous and Nerve Units
Partial injury to musculotendinous unit: 1
Complete but repairable injury to musculotendinous units: 2

Irreparable injury to musculotendinous units, partial loss of a compartment, or complete injury to posterior tibial nerve: 3
Loss of one compartment of musculotendinous units: 4
Loss of two or more compartments or subtotal amputations: 5

Comorbid Conditions: Add 2 Points for Each Condition Present
Injury leading to debridement interval >12 hours
Sewage or organic contamination or farmyard injuries
Age >65 years
Drug-dependent diabetes mellitus or cardiorespiratory diseases leading to increased anesthetic risk
Polytrauma involving chest or abdomen with injury severity score >25 or fat embolism
Hypotension with systolic blood pressure <90 mm Hg at presentation
Another major injury to the same limb or compartment syndrome

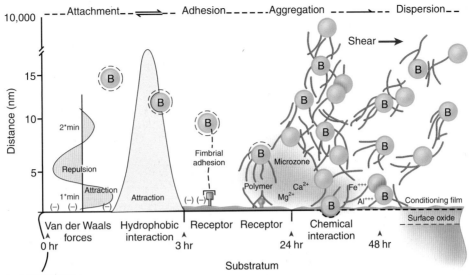

FIGURE 1.7 Molecular sequence in bacterial *(B)* attachment, adhesion, aggregation, and dispersion at substratum surface. Several possible interactions may occur depending on characteristics of bacteria and substratum system (nutrients, contaminants, macromolecules, species, and materials). (Modified from Gristina AG: Biomaterial-centered infection: microbial adhesion versus tissue integration, *Science* 237:1588, 1987.)

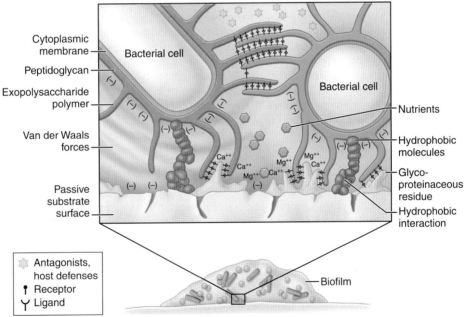

FIGURE 1.8 At specific distances, initial repelling forces of negative bacteria and substrate surface charges are overcome by attracting van der Waals forces. There also are hydrophobic interactions between molecules. Under appropriate conditions, extensive exopolysaccharide polymer develops, aiding ligand-receptor interactions and bacterial attachment and adhesion to substrate. (From Gristina AG, Oga M, Webb LX, et al: Adherent bacterial colonization in the pathogenesis of osteomyelitis, *Science* 228:990, 1985.)

high-dose penicillin is recommended. The duration of antibiotic treatment should be limited because in most series the infecting organisms are hospital acquired. Gustilo recommended administration of 2 g of cefamandole on admission and 1 g every 8 hours for 3 days only in types I and II open fractures. In type III open fractures he recommended an aminoglycoside in dosages of 3 to 5 mg/kg daily, adding penicillin, 10 to 12 million U daily, for farm injuries. Gustilo continued double antibiotic therapy for 3 days only and repeated the antibiotic regimen during wound closure, internal fixation, and bone grafting. Okike and Bhattacharyya recommended the administration of cefazolin, 1 g intravenously, every 8 hours until 24 hours after the wound is closed, with intravenous gentamicin (with weight-adjusted dosing) or levofloxacin (500 mg

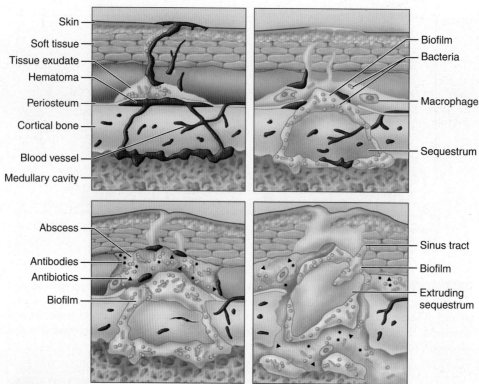

FIGURE 1.9 Sequence of pathogenesis in osteomyelitis. *Top left,* Initial trauma produces soft-tissue destruction, bone fragmentation, and contamination by bacteria. In closed wounds, contamination may occur by hematogenous seeding. *Top right,* As infection progresses, bacterial colonization occurs within protective exopolysaccharide biofilm, which is especially abundant on devitalized bone fragment, which acts as passive substratum for colonization. *Bottom left,* Host defenses are mobilized against infection but cannot penetrate biofilm. *Bottom right,* Progressive inflammation and abscess formation result in development of sinus track and in some cases ultimate extrusion of sequestrum, which is focus of resistant infection. (From Gristina AG, Barth E, Webb LX: Microbial adhesion and the pathogenesis of biomaterial-centered infections. In Gustilo RB, Gruninger RP, Tsukayama DT, editors: *Orthopaedic infection: diagnosis and treatment,* Philadelphia, 1989, Saunders.)

every 24 hours) added for type III fractures. Because of their adverse effect on healing, fluoroquinolones should not be used for antibiotic prophylaxis in patients with open fractures.

Although there is general agreement regarding the effectiveness of antibiotic treatment in open fractures, debate is ongoing about the duration, mode of administration, and type of antibiotics. A prospective, double-blind study showed a 13.9% infection rate without antibiotics compared with a 2.3% infection rate with cephalosporin treatment, but these results have been questioned, and the number of reliable studies in this area is very limited. Another study found that a once-daily, high-dose regimen of antibiotic therapy was as effective as a divided, low-dose regimen. Our current antibiotic protocol for open fractures is intravenous cefazolin 2 g every 8 hours for 24 hours after operative debridement in types I and II open fractures. In patients with cephalosporin or penicillin allergies, clindamycin 900 mg is substituted. For type III open fractures, patients receive intravenous piperacillin/tazobactam 3.375 g every 6 hours for 24 hours after operative debridement; intravenous clindamycin 900 mg every 8 hours with intravenous aztreonam 2 g every 8 hours is substituted for patients with penicillin or cephalosporin allergy. In patients with open pelvic fractures associated with bowel injury, antibiotics are continued for 48 hours. Nonoperatively treated gunshot fractures receive one dose of cefazolin 2 g or clindamycin 900 mg intravenously.

The appropriate time to obtain cultures from open wounds also is controversial. A very small number of bacteria present before debridement are believed to eventually cause infection, suggesting that bacterial cultures taken before or after debridement are essentially of no value. The most common infecting organisms appear to be gram-negative and methicillin-resistant *Staphylococcus aureus* (MRSA), which may be hospital or community acquired. We do recommend obtaining cultures when obvious clinical findings of infection are present at the second debridement. More recently, a marked improvement was noted in infection rates using cultures obtained after debridement and irrigation to determine the need for repeat formal irrigation and debridement, although there was an increased rate of return to surgery with this rationale. Early and rapid empirical administration of antibiotics as determined by wound protocols has been shown to be the most effective means of preventing infection in open fractures.

TREATMENT OF SOFT-TISSUE INJURIES

Initial treatment of open wounds before transport to a medical facility should include pressure over the wound, splinting of fractures, and placement of sterile dressings. Rapid transport to an appropriate medical center is essential because further bacterial contamination can occur with exposure of the tissue to air. A 3.5% rate of infection was found in patients who received treatment at a trauma center within 20 minutes of injury, compared with a 22% infection rate in patients who reached a trauma center by way of another hospital within 10 hours of injury.

In the emergency department, rapid evaluation of the patient's condition and immediate debridement and irrigation of the wound are essential. Debridement and irrigation have been used in the prevention of posttraumatic infections only since World War I. DePag, a Belgian surgeon, introduced the concept of debridement of devitalized tissue and delayed wound closure based on a bacteriologic evaluation of the wound. Debridement has since been combined with irrigation as a mainstay of treatment of open wounds, especially those associated with fractures.

The following steps are recommended for open injuries:

1. Treat open fractures as emergencies.
2. Perform a thorough initial evaluation to diagnose life- and limb-threatening injuries.
3. Begin appropriate antibiotic therapy in the emergency department or at the latest in the operating room and continue treatment for 2 to 3 days only.
4. Immediately debride the wound of contaminated and devitalized tissue, copiously irrigate, and perform repeat debridement within 24 to 72 hours.
5. Stabilize the fracture with the method determined at initial evaluation.
6. Leave the wound open (controversial).
7. Perform early autogenous cancellous bone grafting.
8. Rehabilitate the involved extremity aggressively.

In general, reported incidences of wound infection are 0% to 2% in type I fractures, 2% to 7% in type II fractures, 10% to 25% in all type III fractures, 7% in type IIIA fractures, 10% to 50% in type IIIB fractures, and 25% to 50% in type IIIC fractures. Amputation rates of 50% or more have been reported in type IIIC fractures.

Soft-tissue injuries associated with closed fractures may be more severe, although they are less obvious than those in open fractures. Failure to recognize these injuries and consider them in the treatment decisions can result in serious complications, ranging from delayed healing to partial- or full-thickness tissue slough and massive infection. One frequently missed injury of this type is the Morel-Lavallée syndrome, which occurs when the skin is separated from the fascia. This creates a pocket under which considerable bleeding can occur. Usually this is a subcutaneous hematoma, but the hematoma can become so large that it seriously threatens the viability of the skin above it (Fig. 1.10). This syndrome occurs frequently in patients with pelvic fractures, especially in obese individuals in whom there was a shear component to the injury. MRI and ultrasonography have been recommended to confirm the diagnosis.

Multiple treatment options have been suggested for Morel-Lavallée syndrome, including radical incision, which frequently leaves a massive wound, and less invasive methods, such as wound drainage. The primary recommendation is to treat the soft-tissue problem at the same time the fracture is stabilized. We prefer to wait and watch initially rather than to proceed with immediate decompression because of the risk of devascularizing additional skin by opening the wound. We have some experience with percutaneous aspiration, but we have noted recurrence of

the swelling. The thigh is especially at risk because of the erratic course of its blood supply (Fig. 1.11). This lesion should be treated at the time of internal fixation. Draining the hematoma with a small incision followed by application of a compression bandage has been recommended. We have used a similar drainage technique but have noted an increased incidence of infection when skin necrosis or wound breakdown occurs.

Tseng and Tornetta described good results in 19 patients with Morel-Lavallée lesions using a percutaneous technique of drainage done within 3 days of admission. In six acetabular surgeries and two pelvic ring surgeries, there was a delay of at least 24 hours before the drain was removed. Only 3 of the 19 patients had a positive culture at the time of drainage; one required exploration for persistent drainage. There were no deep infections at 6-month follow-up.

PERCUTANEOUS DRAINAGE OF A MOREL-LAVALLÉE LESION

TECHNIQUE 1.1

(TSENG AND TORNETTA)

- Position the patient to allow exposure of the involved area.
- Make a 2-cm incision over the distal aspect of the lesion.
- Make a second 2-cm incision at the superior and posterior extent of the injury.
- Determine the extent of the lesion by placing a suction tip through the lesion.
- Additional incisions may be required depending on the extent of the lesion.
- Send fluid from the lesion for culture and sensitivity.
- Drain the hematoma with suction.
- Use a plastic brush (used for canal preparation in joint replacement) to debride the loose fat.
- Wash the cavity with a pulsed lavage. Continue the lavage until the fluid is clear and no further fat debris can be removed.
- Place a medium closed suction drain in the wound to drain the entire cavity.
- Close the incisions tightly.
- Attach the drain to wall suction until the drainage is less than 30 mL in 24 hours. (This may require 8 days.)
- Continue cephalosporin or specific antibiotics intravenously for 24 hours after removal of the drain.

■ DEBRIDEMENT

Individual patient characteristics should be considered in determining the exact extent of debridement necessary, but generally the skin should be debrided until there is a bleeding edge. This should not be done under tourniquet control because the viability of the skin may not be known.

Muscle debridement should remove all nonviable muscle that is noncontractile or grossly contaminated. Completely severed tendon ends that are highly contaminated also may

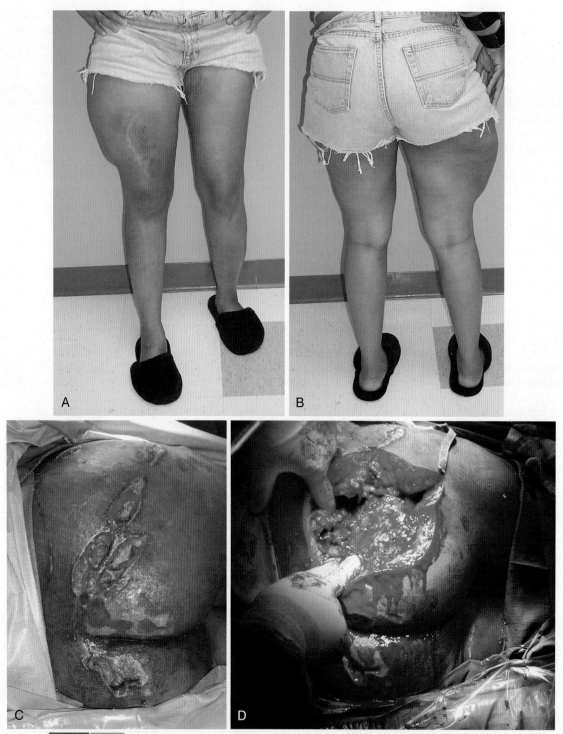

FIGURE 1.10 Morel-Lavallée lesion. **A** and **B,** Clinical appearance of large Morel-Lavallée lesion in thigh after pelvic fracture. **C,** Appearance of large Morel-Lavallée lesion in buttock. **D,** At operative exposure showing depth of lesion.

require excision, although this becomes a much more questionable practice if the musculotendinous unit is intact. Removal of contamination with preservation of the tendon itself may be possible. Care must be taken to maintain moisture around such structures because once the tendon becomes dried it is dead and excision will be necessary. Early flap placement or a sealed dressing may prevent desiccation of these delicate tissues. When dealing with muscles, the four

"C"s must be observed: consistency, color, contractility, and circulation. Normal muscle contraction should be seen when the muscle is pinched or electrically stimulated. The muscle should be of normal consistency, not waxy, fibrotic, or friable. The muscle should be a normal color of red, not brown. Good circulation should be visible within bleeding edges.

The empirical standard for timely debridement has been the "6-hour rule," although only a few studies have shown decreased infection rates when debridement was done within 6 hours, and many studies have questioned the validity of this standard. A few authors have suggested that operative debridement might be unnecessary for low-grade open fractures. We consider thorough operative debridement done as soon as possible after injury the standard of care for all open fractures, however. One recent study questioned whether surgeons were removing normal muscle at times. The surgeons' impression of muscle viability based on the four "C"s was compared with histologic analysis. In 60% of specimens, histologic analysis revealed normal muscle or mild interstitial inflammation of tissue deemed dead or borderline by the surgeon. It is unclear what would have happened to this muscle if left in situ. Until better methods of intraoperative assessment of muscle viability are available, it seems prudent to debride any questionable tissue (or return to the operating room for a second-look debridement).

After the dead, contaminated, and necrotic tissues have been removed, the next step is copious irrigation. Some experimental but few clinical studies have evaluated the efficacy of irrigation (Table 1.4). The most commonly used irrigant is normal saline, and it can be applied by bulb syringe, pouring, or low- or high-pressure lavage. Each method has its benefits. High-pressure irrigation removes more bacteria and necrotic tissue

than a bulb syringe and may be more effective when there has been massive contamination or delay in treatment. However, a decrease in new bone formation has been noted in the first week after high-pressure irrigation when compared with control sites, and contamination has been found 1 to 4 cm away from the wound after pulsatile lavage, as well as some propagation of the contamination down the bone canal. In addition, the position of the irrigation tip close to the tissue may affect the degree of cleaning. More recently, Draeger and Dhaners noted more soft-tissue damage in an in vitro experimental model in which high-pressure pulsatile lavage was used than when bulb-syringe suction was used. They also noted that the high-pressure lavage removed less contaminant than other debridement methods and postulated that the lavage may drive contaminants deeper into the tissue. Other authors also have shown increased soft-tissue damage with high-pressure lavage compared with low-pressure lavage. The current consensus seems to lean toward high-volume, low-pressure lavage repeated an adequate number of times to effect the best healing and prevention of infection.

The amount of fluid used varies with the method of application. There also is a question of whether additives to the irrigation solution are beneficial. Additives are generally of three types: antiseptics, which include among others povidone-iodine, chlorhexidine gluconate, hexachlorophene, and hydrogen peroxide; antibiotics, such as bacitracin, polymyxin, and neomycin; and surfactants, such as castile soap or benzalkonium chloride (Table 1.5). Bhandari et al. noted that the combination of low-pressure lavage and 1% liquid soap was the most effective irrigating solution for in vivo removal of bacteria. In a more recent prospective, randomized, controlled trial, Anglen compared nonsterile castile soap with bacitracin solution for the irrigation of 398 lower extremity open fractures. Anglen found no significant differences with respect to infection and bone healing, but wound healing problems were more common in the bacitracin group.

All these additives have advantages and disadvantages, but none has been shown to be clinically efficacious at this time. The FLOW study (Fluid Lavage of Open Wound) was undertaken to help clarify the conflicting recommendations regarding irrigation pressure and irrigation solutions. In an international, multicenter, blinded, randomized, controlled trial, patients with open extremity fractures were divided into six groups: high-pressure irrigation (>20 psi), low-pressure irrigation (5 to 10 psi), or very low-pressure irrigation (1 to 2 psi), with either normal saline or

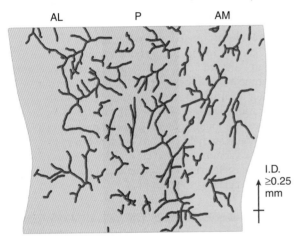

FIGURE 1.11 Tracing of thigh vessels with internal diameter (I.D.) 0.25 mm. *AL,* Anterolateral; *AM,* anteromedial; *P,* posterior. (From Cormack GC, Lamberty BGH: The blood supply of thigh skin, *Plast Reconstr Surg* 75:342, 1985.)

TABLE 1.4

Irrigation Variables

VARIABLE	EFFECT	RECOMMENDATION
Volume	In animal studies, increasing volume removes more particulate matter and bacteria, but the effect plateaus at a level dependent on the system.	Grade 1 fractures, 3 L Grade 2 fractures, 6 L Grade 3 fractures, 9 L
Pressure	Increased pressure removes more debris and bacteria; however, the highest pressure settings damage bone, delay fracture healing, and may increase risk of infection by damaging soft tissues.	Use a power irrigation system that provides a variety of settings; select a low- or middle-range setting.
Pulsation	In theory, pulsation improves removal of surface debris by means of tissue elasticity; limited studies have not confirmed the effect or have suggested decreased efficacy.	Not established

From Anglen JO: Wound irrigation in musculoskeletal injury, *J Am Acad Orthop Surg* 9:219, 2001.

TABLE 1.5				
Irrigation Additives				
CLASS	EXAMPLES	ADVANTAGES	DISADVANTAGES	RECOMMENDATION
Antiseptics	Povidone-iodine, chlorhexidine, hydrogen peroxide	Broad spectrum of activity against bacteria, fungi, viruses; kill pathogens in the wound	Toxic to host cells, may impair immune cell function and delay or weaken wound healing	Findings from animal and clinical studies are contradictory; toxicity is more clearly established than benefits; should not be used
Antibiotics	Bacitracin, polymyxin, neomycin	Bacterial or bacteriostatic activity in the wound, if in adequate concentration and duration	Cost, rare toxicity or allergic reaction, promotion of bacterial resistance	Clinical efficacy in preventing infection not proved; should not be used routinely
Surfactants	Castile soap, green soap, benzalkonium chloride	Interfere with bacterial adhesion to surfaces; emulsify and remove debris	Mild host-cell toxicities	Clinical efficacy not proved; consider use in highly contaminated wounds; first irrigations

From Anglen JO: Wound irrigation in musculoskeletal injury, *J Am Acad Orthop Surg* 9:219, 2001.

a 0.45% solution of normal saline and castile soap. Fractures of the hands, toes, and pelvis were excluded. Reoperation within 12 months for bone or wound healing problems or wound infection was chosen as the primary end point of the study. In 2447 eligible patients, there was no significant difference in reoperation among the pressure groups (13.2% high pressure, 12.7% low pressure, and 13.7% very low pressure). Reoperation was significantly higher in the soap group (14.8%) than the saline group (11.6%). The authors concluded that very low-pressure irrigation is an acceptable, low cost alternative to pressure-irrigation devices and that soap solution is not superior to saline alone.

Our protocol has been to use 9 L of gravity-flow irrigation in most cases. Additional fluid may be needed in highly contaminated fractures, whereas lesser amounts (5 to 6 L) are usually sufficient in minimally contaminated upper extremity injuries. Our previous protocol called for genitourinary irrigant as an additive; however, we are currently not placing additives in our irrigation fluid. Regardless of the type of irrigation, the most important part of wound cleansing is the surgical debridement of dead and contaminated tissue.

Controversy also surrounds the closure of wounds after irrigation. Historically, leaving the wound open has been recommended, but, with the development of powerful antibiotics and early aggressive debridement, more institutions are reporting success with *loose* closure of wounds, with or without drainage. If debridement does not result in a surgically clean wound, closure should not be done. In addition, the skin should not be closed under tension because this may result in further skin necrosis and ischemia. The proper tension has been described as a wound that can be closed with 2-0 nylon without breaking. Structures should be kept moist with occlusive dressings. The use of a "bead pouch" in which methyl methacrylate impregnated with powdered antibiotics, such as vancomycin or tobramycin, is rolled into small beads that are placed on a wire and laid in the wound has been shown to be very cost effective in control of deep infection.

Early closure of the wound has been shown to decrease the incidences of infection, malunion, and nonunion. A variety of methods can be used for wound closure, including direct suturing, split-thickness skin grafting, and free or local muscle flaps. The method chosen depends on several factors, including the size and location of the defect and associated injuries. In a multicenter study of 195 tibial fractures that required flap coverage, ASIF/OTA class C injuries that were treated with a rotational flap were 4.3 times more likely to have a wound complication requiring operative intervention than were injuries treated with a free flap.

A relatively recent innovation, vacuum-assisted closure (KCI, San Antonio, TX), has been reported to be useful in accelerating wound healing by reducing chronic edema, increasing local blood flow, and enhancing granulation tissue formation. The few reports of the use of vacuum-assisted closure in the management of orthopaedic injuries have been generally favorable, but its efficacy has not been clearly proven. The vacuum-assisted closure device usually is applied at the end of each irrigation and debridement until the wound is considered clean.

IRRIGATION AND DEBRIDEMENT OF OPEN WOUNDS

Our policy is to repeat debridement of all Gustilo type III open fractures within 24 to 72 hours of the first debridement. We also repeat debridement and irrigation of all wounds that are questionable, regardless of the Gustilo classification. Debridement and irrigation are repeated at 48-hour intervals until a clean wound is obtained. This may require removing any internal fixation or external fixation to allow complete exposure of the bone.

TECHNIQUE 1.2

- Begin the procedure by ensuring adequate personal protection, including splash guards, goggles, boots, and additional protective gloves.
- Prepare the patient and the skin and apply a sterile tourniquet if possible, but do not inflate the tourniquet.
- Wash and drape the wound as for a normal surgical procedure, but allow for a wide exposure of the involved

area (entire limb, possibly extending to the torso). Use impermeable drapes.

- Begin the debridement at the skin and proceed in an orderly fashion. Remove devitalized skin until bleeding is visible in the skin edge. Progressive removal of skin is recommended over wide margins.
- In a similar fashion, remove the subcutaneous tissue, including all contaminated tissue.
- Cut and coagulate veins.
- Preserve superficial nerves if they are intact, which is infrequent.
- Remove devitalized fat beneath the flaps down to clean, bleeding, subcutaneous tissue.
- Open the fascia to allow exposure of the muscle tendon and removal of all devitalized muscle, paying attention to the four "C"s (color, contractility, circulation, and consistency).
- Trim completely severed tendons back to viable tendon. Intact tendons should be cleaned and not excised, at least in the first debridement.
- Enlarge the wound to allow adequate debridement and exposure of the fracture. In most cases, remove devascularized bone, especially if it is highly contaminated. Remove contamination in the medullary canal by progressively removing bone with a saw or rongeur. Curettage of the medullary canal should be avoided to prevent proximal migration of the infected material.
- After all dead tissue has been removed, irrigate the wound with normal saline and an appropriate additive.
- If the wound can be closed, suture the surgically created wound first. Loosely close the remaining wound over a drain if necessary, provided there is no excessive pressure or tension on the skin. If closure is not possible, leave the wound open. Keep structures such as bone, nerve, and tendon moist. A bead pouch can be used as an impervious dressing to maintain moisture. Alternatively, a negative pressure wound therapy dressing can be placed. This type of dressing facilitates reduction of dead space and edema. A specialized sponge is used over bone or tendon.
- Whether to use internal or external fixation usually is decided after debridement is done and may influence the wound closure and dressing. We prefer to prepare and drape the patient again, discard all instruments used during the debridement, and change operating gowns and gloves before applying internal or external fixation.

POSTOPERATIVE CARE Antibiotics are continued according to the grade of wound severity (see section on open fractures).

TREATMENT OF BONE INJURIES

Small fragments of bone that are completely devoid of soft-tissue attachment and are avascular are removed. Small fragments that are grossly contaminated with foreign material probably should be removed as well because adequate cleansing is rarely possible. Removal of large avascular fragments is controversial. It generally is best to remove any avascular bone and plan on later replacement with autogenous bone grafting. Retained avascular fragments are a source of adherence for bacteria and probably are the most frequent cause of persistent infection after open fractures. When large segments of cortical bone are extruded, sterilization of these segments has been done experimentally with the use of povidone-iodine, autoclaving, and chlorhexidine-gluconate antibiotic solutions. The use of Ilizarov distraction histogenesis techniques for losses of large segments of bone also has been reported. Judgment must be exercised in this aspect of the management of open fractures. Small pieces of bone with intact periosteum and soft tissue should be retained because they may act as small grafts and stimulate fracture healing.

In addition to the contamination of open fractures, the disruption of the periosteum reduces bone vascularity and viability and adds to the difficulty in management of open fractures compared with closed fractures. More severe disruption of the soft tissue around the fracture usually produces more fracture instability and makes stabilization of the fracture more difficult.

■ FRACTURE STABILIZATION

An open fracture generally should be stabilized with the method that provides adequate stability with a minimum of further damage to the vascularity of the zone of injury and its associated soft tissues. For type I wounds, essentially any technique that is suitable for closed fracture management is satisfactory. Treatment of types II and III wounds is more controversial, with proponents of traction, external fixation, nonreamed intramedullary nailing, and occasionally plate and screw fixation. Generally, external fixation is preferred for metaphyseal-diaphyseal fractures with occasional limited internal fixation with screws. In the upper extremity, casting, external fixation, and plate and screw fixation are popular methods of stabilization. In the lower extremity, open diaphyseal femoral and tibial fractures have been treated successfully with intramedullary nailing, and results are encouraging for the use of nonreamed intramedullary nails in types I, II, and IIIA fractures.

Our experience with open femoral and tibial fractures treated at the Elvis Presley Regional Trauma Center confirms the effectiveness of unreamed intramedullary fixation of these fractures. Of 125 open femoral fractures treated with unreamed and reamed nailing, all united, and infection developed in only five (4%). Of 50 open tibial fractures (three Gustilo type I, 13 type II, 22 type IIIB, and 12 type IIIB), union was obtained in 48 (96%), infection occurred in four (8%), and malunion occurred in two (4%). Eighteen fractures (36%) required dynamization, bone grafting, or both to obtain union. For types IIIB and IIIC injuries that are salvageable, external fixation is still the primary method of treatment. As important as any other factor is the surgeon's familiarity with the surgical stabilization technique chosen, as long as further devascularization is minimized.

The method used to reduce and immobilize the fracture depends on the bone involved, the type of fracture, the efficacy of the debridement, and the patient's general condition. When it is desirable to limit further trauma from surgery, and when the fracture is stable, it can be reduced and a cast applied as for a closed fracture. The cast must be bivalved or windowed to allow inspection of the wound. External fixation allows easy evaluation of the skin and soft tissues and may be preferable even for stable fractures with unstable soft tissues, such as tibial pilon fractures. Open fractures involving the shaft of the humerus, the tibia, the fibula, or the small bones

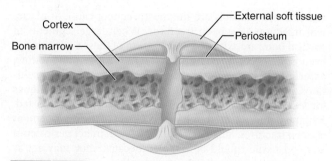

FIGURE 1.12 Tissue types that contribute to four main fracture healing responses. (Redrawn from Einhorn TA: The cell and molecular biology of fracture healing, *Clin Orthop Relat Res* 355[Suppl]:7, 1998.)

can be reduced and immobilized in this fashion. If sophisticated techniques are unavailable, skeletal traction provides enough stability and allows adequate exposure of most wounds. The more unstable a fracture, the more justified is some type of surgical stabilization or a staged stabilization.

Fractures involving joints or physes may require internal fixation to maintain alignment of the articular surfaces and physes. Usually, Kirschner wires or limited internal fixation with or without external fixation is sufficient to accomplish this purpose without introducing much foreign material. If possible, we treat the soft tissues and the wound, allow the soft tissues to heal, and then proceed with open reduction and internal fixation of intraarticular fractures through a clean surgical wound. Specific methods of fracture fixation are discussed later in this chapter.

FRACTURE HEALING (BONE REGENERATION)

The multitude of factors involved in fracture healing have been investigated in numerous clinical, biomechanical, and laboratory studies but are not yet fully defined. Understanding of the cellular and molecular pathways that govern the process of fracture healing has increased but is far from complete. Fracture healing can be considered from any of several viewpoints, including biologic, biochemical, mechanical, and clinical. A discussion of all the aspects of fracture healing is beyond the scope of this book, and the reader is referred to the excellent journal articles and textbooks devoted to this subject for more information.

Fracture healing is a complex process that requires the recruitment of appropriate cell (fibroblasts, macrophages, chondroblasts, osteoblasts, osteoclasts) and the subsequent expression of the appropriate genes (those that control matrix production and organization, growth factors, transcription factors) at the right time and in the right anatomic location. A fracture initiates a sequence of inflammation, repair, and remodeling that can restore the injured bone to its original state within a few months if each stage of this complex interdependent cascade proceeds undisturbed. *Clinical union* occurs when progressively increasing stiffness and strength provided by the mineralization process makes the fracture site stable and pain free. *Radiographic union* is present when plain radiographs show bone trabeculae or cortical bone crossing the fracture site. Radioisotope studies have shown increased activity in fracture sites long after painless function has been restored and radiographic union is present, indicating that the remodeling process continues for years.

In the inflammatory phase of fracture healing, a hematoma is formed from the blood vessels ruptured by the injury. Inflammatory cells invade the hematoma and initiate the lysosomal degradation of necrotic tissue. The hematoma may be a source of signaling molecules, such as transforming growth factor-beta (TGF-beta) and platelet-derived growth factor (PDGF), which initiate and regulate the cascades of cellular events that result in fracture healing. The reparative phase, which usually begins 4 or 5 days after injury, is characterized by the invasion of pluripotential mesenchymal cells, which differentiate into fibroblasts, chondroblasts, and osteoblasts and form a soft fracture callus. Proliferation of blood vessels (angiogenesis) within the periosteal tissues and marrow space helps route the appropriate cells to the fracture site and contributes to the formation of a bed of granulation tissue. The transition of the fracture callus to woven bone and the process of mineralization, which stiffens and strengthens the newly formed bone, signal the beginning of the remodeling phase, which may last for months or even years. The woven bone is replaced by lamellar bone, the medullary canal is restored, and the bone is restored to normal or nearly normal morphology and mechanical strength. Each of these stages overlaps the end of the stage preceding it, so fracture healing is a continuous process.

Einhorn described four distinct healing responses, characterizing them by location: bone marrow, cortex, periosteum, and external soft tissues (Fig. 1.12). He suggested that perhaps the most important response in fracture healing is that of the periosteum, where committed osteoprogenitor cells and uncommitted, undifferentiated mesenchymal cells contribute to the process by a recapitulation of embryonic intramembranous ossification and endochondral bone formation. The periosteal response has been shown to be rapid and capable of bridging gaps as large as half the diameter of the bone; it is enhanced by motion and inhibited by rigid fixation. The external soft-tissue response also depends heavily on mechanical factors and may be depressed by rigid immobilization. This response involves rapid cellular activity and the development of early bridging callus that stabilizes the fracture fragments. The type of tissue formed evolves through endochondral ossification in which undifferentiated mesenchymal cells are recruited, attach, proliferate, and eventually differentiate into cartilage-forming cells.

During the complex fracture-repair process, four basic types of new bone formation occur: osteochondral ossification, intramembranous ossification, oppositional new bone formation, and osteonal migration (creeping substitution). The type, amount, and location of bone formed can be influenced by fracture type, gap condition, fixation rigidity, loading, and biologic environment. Cells subjected to compression and low oxygen tension have been shown to differentiate into chondroblasts and cartilage, whereas those under tension and high oxygen tension differentiate into fibroblasts and produce fibrous tissue, suggesting that the type of stress applied to immature or undifferentiated tissue determines the type of bone formed (Fig. 1.13).

Uhthoff listed a number of systemic and local factors that affect fracture healing (Box 1.4) and classified them as being present at the time of injury, caused by the injury, dependent on treatment, or associated with complications. Factors identified as predictive of complications, especially infection, include the condition of the soft tissues and the level of trauma energy, as evidenced by the AO classification; body mass index of 40 or higher; and compromising comorbidities such as age 80 years or older, smoking, diabetes, malignant disease, pulmonary insufficiency, and systemic immunodeficiency. Infections were found to be almost eight times more frequent in patients with three or more compromising factors than in those with none.

We also have found that a patient's general health and habits, socioeconomic situation, and neuropsychiatric history are good predictors of the risk of complications after open fractures. Taking into consideration several patient variables, we developed a host classification (Box 1.5) that has been helpful. In a retrospective review of 87 patients with open tibial fractures, we found that complications developed in 48% of type C hosts, in 32% of type B hosts, and in 19% of type A hosts. Specifically, infections occurred in 32% of type C hosts, in 17% of type B hosts, and in 11% of type A hosts. Because the host classification can be determined at initial evaluation, it allows an earlier prediction of complications than does the Gustilo classification (which often can be definitively determined only at debridement). Used as an adjunct to the Gustilo system, host classification also can help determine at initial evaluation whether a wound can be closed after debridement.

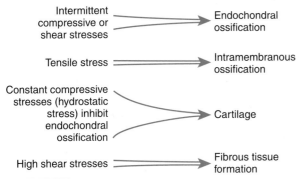

FIGURE 1.13 Hypothetical bone formation mechanism under different types of mechanical stress, as proposed by Carter et al. (From Carter DR, Beaupré GS, Giori NJ, et al: Mechanobiology of skeletal regeneration, *Clin Orthop Relat Res* 355[Suppl]:41, 1998.)

STIMULATION OF FRACTURE HEALING
■ BONE GRAFTING
▌AUTOLOGOUS BONE GRAFTS

Autologous bone grafts contain the three required components for the formation of bone: osteoconduction, osteoinduction, and cellular osteogenesis. Osteoconduction refers to the scaffolding that allows bone ingrowth. Osteoinduction is the ability to induce the production of osteoblasts. Primitive osteocytes are necessary to form osteoblasts.

BOX 1.4

Factors Influencing Fracture Healing

I. Systemic Factors
 A. Age
 B. Activity level including
  1. General immobilization
  2. Space flight
 C. Nutritional status
 D. Hormonal factors
  1. Growth hormone
  2. Corticosteroids (microvascular osteonecrosis)
  3. Others (thyroid, estrogen, androgen, calcitonin, parathyroid hormone, prostaglandins)
 E. Diseases: diabetes, anemia, neuropathies, tabes
 F. Vitamin deficiencies: A, C, D, K
 G. Drugs: nonsteroidal antiinflammatory drugs, anticoagulants, factor XIII, calcium channel blockers (verapamil), cytotoxins, diphosphonates, phenytoin, sodium fluoride, tetracycline
 H. Other substances (nicotine, alcohol)
 I. Hyperoxia
 J. Systemic growth factors
 K. Environmental temperature
 L. Central nervous system trauma
II. Local Factors
 A. Factors independent of injury, treatment, or complications
  1. Type of bone
  2. Abnormal bone
   a. Radiation necrosis
   b. Infection
   c. Tumors and other pathologic conditions
  3. Denervation

 B. Factors depending on injury
  1. Degree of local damage
   a. Compound fracture
   b. Comminution of fracture
   c. Velocity of injury
   d. Low circulatory levels of vitamin K_1
  2. Extent of disruption of vascular supply to bone, its fragments (macrovascular osteonecrosis), or soft tissues; severity of injury
  3. Type and location of fracture (one or two bones, e.g., tibia and fibula or tibia alone)
  4. Loss of bone
  5. Soft-tissue interposition
  6. Local growth factors
 C. Factors depending on treatment
  1. Extent of surgical trauma (blood supply, heat)
  2. Implant-induced altered blood flow
  3. Degree and kind of rigidity of internal or external fixation and the influence of timing
  4. Degree, duration, and direction of load-induced deformation of bone and soft tissues
  5. Extent of contact between fragments (gap, displacement, overdistraction)
  6. Factors stimulating posttraumatic osteogenesis (bone grafts, bone morphogenetic protein, electrical stimulation, surgical technique, intermittent venous stasis [Bier])
 D. Factors associated with complications
  1. Infection
  2. Venous stasis
  3. Metal allergy

From Uhthoff HK: Fracture healing. In Gustilo RB, Kyle RF, Templeman DC: *Fractures and dislocations*, St. Louis, 1993, Mosby.

Autologous grafts are obtained from multiple areas. Local bone removed at the time of arthrodesis can be reused after removing all soft tissue and then morselizing this bone into much smaller pieces. A bone mill also can be used to finely morselize this bone. This increases the number of live cells and proteins for osteoinduction.

The iliac crest is the second most common area for autograft harvest. The posterior iliac crest offers more bone for grafting than the anterior surface and can be used for morcelized bone or structural bone such as a tricortical graft. Unfortunately, bone harvest from the iliac crest is prone to complications such as donor site pain, neuromas, fracture, and heterotopic bone formation. Techniques for harvest of iliac bone grafts are described in other chapter.

The fibula can be used for a structural graft, and the ribs can be used for a structural or morcelized graft. The tibia also has been used for long corticocancellous structural grafts, but the use of these structural grafts has declined with the advent of rigid internal fixation and reliable allografts.

The harvest of femoral bone marrow using the techniques of femoral nailing and a specialized reamer/irrigator/aspirator (RIA) (Synthes) is a more recent method for obtaining significant amounts of marrow from the femur (Fig. 1.14). The RIA was developed to decrease intramedullary pressure and fat embolism during reaming, and significant decreases in intramedullary pressure and femoral vein fat have been documented with its use. In the process of doing this, the reamings and effluent are captured, and a sizable amount of marrow may be aspirated for bone grafting.

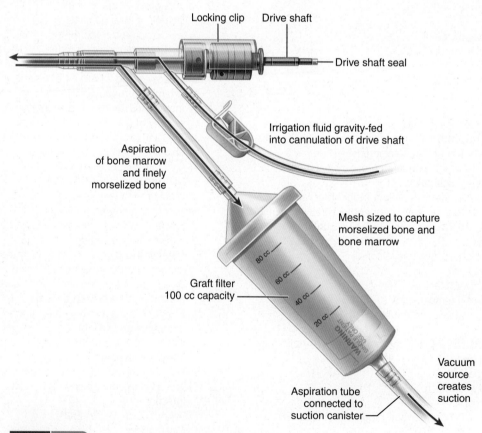

Locking clip   Drive shaft

Drive shaft seal

Irrigation fluid gravity-fed into cannulation of drive shaft

Aspiration of bone marrow and finely morselized bone

Mesh sized to capture morselized bone and bone marrow

Graft filter 100 cc capacity

Vacuum source creates suction

Aspiration tube connected to suction canister

FIGURE 1.14 Reamer, irrigator, aspirator for obtaining marrow during femoral reaming; the aspirated marrow can be used for bone grafting.

Depending on the patient and the source bone, from 25 to 90 mL of bone may be captured. These bony fragments are rich in mesenchymal stem cells. Additionally, the supernatant is rich in fibroblast growth factor (FGF)-2, insulin-like growth factor (IGF)-beta1, and latent TGF-beta1 but not bone morphogenetic protein-2 (BMP2). As a result, the RIA is a potential source for autologous bone, mesenchymal stem cells, and bone growth factors. When used as a spinal graft, however, this technique may require obtaining the graft before the spinal procedure with a different position and draping.

This technique is not without complications. Fractures of the donor bone have been reported, some requiring additional fixation. Perforation of the cortex of the reamed bone that required insertion of prophylactic intramedullary fixation also has been described. Significant blood loss from aspiration has been reported. To avoid or minimize these problems, several actions have been suggested.

- Preoperative radiographs of the donor bone should be evaluated for deformity, and the isthmus should be measured to determine the limits of reaming.
- Blood should be available to replace aspirated blood and marrow.
- The aspirator should be turned off when reaming is not being performed to avoid unnecessary blood loss.
- The donor bone should be carefully evaluated after reaming to check for perforations. A prophylactic intramedullary device should be available if a perforation is detected.
- Postoperative ambulation should be protected to prevent donor bone fracture.
- The patient's hematocrit level should be checked at the end of the procedure and over the next 24 hours to detect significant blood loss.
- Finally, patients with known metabolic bone disease such as osteoporosis or even simple osteopenia of the involved bone may not be the best candidates for this procedure.

HARVEST OF FEMORAL OR TIBIAL BONE GRAFT WITH THE RIA INSTRUMENTATION

TECHNIQUE 1.3

PREOPERATIVELY
- Select the proper tube length and assembly for the bone to be reamed.
- Confirm the reaming diameter with diaphyseal radiographic measurement (Fig. 1.15A).
- For bone harvesting, select a reamer head no larger than 1.5 mm than the measured isthmus diameter.

OPERATIVELY
- Position the patient as for a standard intramedullary nailing (supine or lateral for the femur and supine for the tibia).

- Gain access to the bone as for a standard intramedullary nailing procedure (Fig. 1.15B and C).
- Insert the guidewire (reaming wire) down to the physeal scar and confirm placement by image intensification on both anteroposterior and lateral views.
- Assemble the RIA according to the manufacturer's directions.
  - Attach the drive shaft to the RIA and cover the connection with the locking clip.
  - Attach the drive shaft seal to the proximal end of the drive shaft.
  - Attach the drive unit (reamer driver).
  - Connect the irrigation, clamped closed until irrigation begins, to the smaller port marked "I."
  - Connect the aspiration (suction) to the larger port.
  - Be sure the graft filter is on this tubing to collect the bone aspirate.
  - Connect the aspiration tube to suction.
- Slide the RIA over the guidewire (Fig. 1.15D).
- Start the irrigation and aspiration to confirm proper functioning before insertion.
- Insert the reamer into the bone (Fig. 1.15E) and confirm its position with image intensification.
- A flow of bone should be visible in the aspiration tube as the reamer is advanced under power. Never ream when there is no irrigation or aspiration.
- Ream 20 to 30 mm and then retract 50 to 80 mm to allow the irrigation fluid to fill the space (Fig. 1.15F).
- Repeat this slow advancement until resistance is felt.
- Repeat the retraction maneuver with reinsertion until the desired end point is reached on image intensification.
- The reamer can be reversed if reaming becomes difficult.
- Stop irrigating after removing the RIA from the medullary canal.
- Turn off the suction or clamp the suction tubing.
- Hold the graft filter vertically and compress the graft with a plunger; record the volume measurement.
- With the plunger inserted, invert the filter and remove the inner filter from the outer canister.
- Hold the inner filter over an appropriate container and push out the bone graft (Fig. 1.15G).
- Carefully check the donor bone for areas of weakness or reamer perforation.
- Close the wound in layers as after intramedullary nailing.

POSTOPERATIVE CARE Although cadaver studies have found that RIA does not dramatically diminish the mechanical properties of the femur and does not require postoperative weight-bearing restrictions, we prefer to protect the donor bone by having the patient use crutches and limit weight bearing until healing is confirmed on a radiograph.

■ BONE GRAFT SUBSTITUTES

Although autogenous material, such as iliac crest bone, remains the gold standard for filling bone defects caused by trauma, infection, tumor, or surgery, its use increases the morbidity of the surgical procedure, increases anesthesia time and blood loss, and often causes significant postoperative donor-site complications (e.g., pain, cosmetic defect,

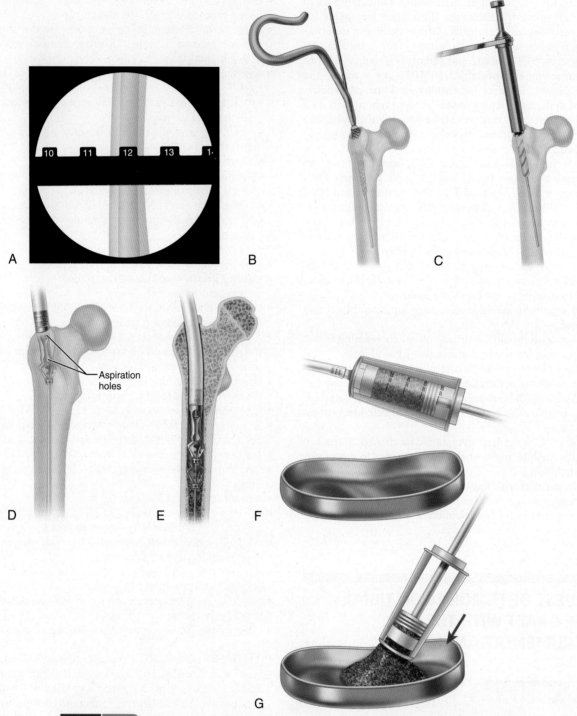

FIGURE 1.15 Harvest of femoral or tibial bone graft with RIA instrumentation (see text). **A,** Confirmation of reaming diameter. **B** and **C,** Access to and reaming of medullary canal. **D,** Insertion of reamer. **E,** Reaming of canal. **F,** Removal of graft material. **G,** Bone graft pushed out of inner filter. **SEE TECHNIQUE 1.3.**

fatigue fracture, heterotopic bone formation). The amount of autogenous bone available for grafting also is limited. Because of these limitations, a number of bone graft substitutes have been developed.

A bone graft substitute classification system proposed by Laurencin et al. divides these into five major categories:

allograft-based, factor-based, cell-based, ceramic-based, and polymer-based (Table 1.6). Allograft substitutes use allograft bone with or without other elements and can be used as structural or filler grafts. Factor-based substances include both natural and recombinant growth factors and can be used alone or in combination with other products.

TABLE 1.6

Bone Graft and Bone Graft Substitutes

CLASS	USE	EXAMPLE	PROPERTIES	CARRIER
Autograft	Use alone	ICBG	Osteoinductive Osteoconductive Osteogenic	No
Allograft	Alone or combination	Freeze-dried bone DBM	Osteoconductive Osteoinductive	Yes
Factor based	Combination required	rhBMP-7	Osteoinductive	No
Cell based	Alone or combination	Mesenchymal stem cells	Osteogenic	
Ceramic	Alone or combination	Calcium phosphate, calcium sulfate Bioactive glass	Osteoconductive	Yes
Polymer	Combination	Nondegradable and biodegradable polymers	Osteoconductive	Yes
Miscellaneous	Alone or combination	Coralline hydroxyapatite	Osteoconductive	Yes

BMP, Bone morphogenetic protein; *DBM,* demineralized bone matrix; *ICBG,* iliac crest bone graft.

TABLE 1.7

Transforming Growth Factor-Beta Family Ligands

TGF-BETA 1	TGF-BETA 2
TGF-beta 1,2,3	TGF-beta 2/1.2
TGF-beta 1.2	TGF-beta 3
TGF-beta 1/1.2	TGF-beta 5

TGF, Transforming growth factor.

Cell-based substitutes use cells to produce new bone. Ceramic-based substitutes use various ceramics as a scaffold for bone growth, and polymer-based substitutes use biodegradable polymers alone or with other materials. A miscellaneous group includes tissue from marine sources such as coral and sponge skeleton.

ALLOGRAFT-BASED BONE GRAFT SUBSTITUTES

Allograft comes in many forms and is prepared in many ways, including freeze-dried, irradiated (electron beam and gamma ray), and decalcified. Freeze-dried and irradiated forms can be used for structural support when taken from cortical bone. Some forms can be milled for special applications, such as use in intervertebral cages or morcelized as a bone extender. Demineralized bone matrix (DBM) is the decalcified form of allograft that contains the osteoinductive proteins that stimulate bone formation. It is supplied as a putty, injectable gel, paste, powder, strips, and mixtures of these. Some of these forms may be mixed with bone marrow to add osteogenic pluripotent cells. There is considerable variability in bone stimulation between different DBM products, which may be because of multiple factors, including the source (bone bank and/or donor), processing procedures, form, and carrier type. Demineralized allograft usually is mixed with a carrier such as glycerol, calcium sulfate powder, sodium hyaluronate, and gelatin. Sterilization of DBM by gamma irradiation and ethylene oxide exposure decreases the risk of disease transmission but also may decrease the osteoinductive activity of the product. All of these factors add significant variability in the efficacy of bone activation by these substances.

DBM is contraindicated in patients with severe vascular or neurologic disease, fever, uncontrolled diabetes, severe degenerative bone disease, pregnancy, hypercalcemia, renal compromise, Pott disease, or osteomyelitis or sepsis at the surgical site.

Transmission of disease from the donor is a rare but documented risk. Other complications of allografts include variable osteoinductive strength and infection of the graft. Even with rigorous donor screening and various methods of sterilization, complete removal of viral and bacterial infectious agents cannot be fully achieved. Large allografts for structural replacement have the greatest risks of disease transmission. Bacterial infections and hepatitis B and C have been reported in patients who received allografts. DBM is much less likely to transmit infection from the donor to the recipient.

GROWTH FACTOR–BASED BONE GRAFT SUBSTITUTES

Urist first discovered BMP in 1965 when he recognized its ability to induce enchondral bone formation. Since then, numerous proteins have been isolated from this group. They are part of a very large group of cytokines and metabologens grouped together as growth factors and aid in the development of multiple tissues. Most of the BMPs used today are in the bone superfamily TGF-beta. This superfamily includes the inhibin/activin family, Müllerian-inhibiting substance family, and the decapentaplegic family (Table 1.7). Most of the proteins in the TGF-beta family do not help form bone but are involved in the production, regulation, and modulation of other tissues (Table 1.8). Presently, only two proteins have been isolated, produced, and approved for use in humans. Because they are produced by the recombinant process, they are designated rhBMP-2 and rhBMP-7. Other BMPs that have been shown to have osteogenic properties are BMP-4, -6, and -9. The US Food and Drug Administration (FDA) has approved rhBMP-2 for use in anterior lumbar fusion with a titanium cage. The use of rhBMP-7 or OP-1 is limited to use under the Humanitarian Device Exemptions for revision spinal fusion by the FDA.

BMP-2 and BMP-7 are water soluble and require a carrier to remain in the operative area to be effective. They are either supplied in a carrier or added to a carrier. By choosing

TABLE 1.8

Bone Morphogenetic Proteins

	KNOWN FUNCTIONS	GENE LOCUS
BMP1	BMP1 does not belong to the TGF-beta family of proteins. It is a metalloprotease that acts on procollagen I, II, and III. It is involved in cartilage development.	Chromosome: 8 Location: 8p21
BMP2	Acts as a disulfide-linked homodimer and induces bone and cartilage formation. It is a candidate as a retinoid mediator and plays a key role in osteoblast differentiation.	Chromosome: 20 Location: 20p12
BMP3	Induces bone formation	Chromosome: 14 Location: 14p22
BMP4	Regulates the formation of teeth, limbs, and bone from mesoderm. It also plays a role in fracture repair.	Chromosome: 14 Location: 14q22-q23
BMP5	Performs functions in cartilage development	Chromosome: 6 Location: 6p12.1
BMP6	Plays a role in joint integrity in adults	Chromosome: 6 Location: 6p12.1
BMP7	Plays a key role in osteoblast differentiation. It also induces the production of SMAD1 and is key in renal development and repair.	Chromosome: 20 Location: 20q13
BMP8a	Involved in bone and cartilage development	Chromosome: 1 Location: 1p35-p32
BMP8b	Expressed in the hippocampus	Chromosome: 1 Location: 1p35-p32
BMP10	May play a role in the trabeculation of the embryonic heart	Chromosome: 2 Location: 2p14
BMP15	May play a role in oocyte and follicular development	Chromosome: X Location: Xp11.2

BMP, Bone morphogenetic protein; *TGF-beta*, transforming growth factor-beta.

a carrier that also has osteoconductive properties, the power of the inductive process is magnified. Care must be taken in choosing the carrier to avoid loss of the BMP.

Complications have been reported with the use of BMP in spinal surgery, and these are discussed in other chapter.

Other proteins that show promise in bone formation include PDGF and vascular endothelial growth factor (VEGF).

❚ CELL-BASED BONE GRAFT SUBSTITUTES

Cells may be used to stimulate or seed cells for new tissue. Presently, the most frequently used cell-based graft is autologous bone marrow. In the future, adult and embryonic stem cells, somatic stem cells such as bone marrow stromal cells, dermal stem cells, and cells in fetal cord blood may be grown for use as grafts.

Collagen in its denatured form is an osteoinductive material. The usual forms of this material are bovine (xenograft) and human type 1 collagen. It is used as a carrier for BMP. Both rhBMP-2 and rhBMP-7 use bone collagen to avoid the problem of compressibility and potential loss of the BMP found in tendon and ligament collagen.

❚ CERAMIC-BASED BONE GRAFT SUBSTITUTES

Ceramic and collagen bone substitutes can provide osteoconduction without the risk of disease transmission. Available ceramics include calcium sulfate, calcium phosphate, and bioactive glass. In addition to osteoconduction these products are osseointegrative, having the ability to form intimate bonds with the tissue. These products are brittle and may be used with other products as a carrier or for protection (such as cages). Calcium phosphate ceramics come in several varieties, including tricalcium phosphate and synthetic hydroxyapatite. These products are available as pastes, solid matrices, putties, and granules. Bioactive glass is silicate-based glass that is biologically active. Presently, it is used with polymethyl methacrylate to improve bonding. These products are not recommended for load bearing individually without modification or use with stronger products. Some may be used with DBM or as carriers for BMP.

❚ POLYMER-BASED BONE GRAFT SUBSTITUTES

Polymers available for bone graft substitutes include both natural and synthetic polymers, biodegradable and nonbiodegradable. Some nonbiodegradable natural and synthetic polymers are composites of the polymer and a ceramic and can be used in load-bearing areas. Biodegradable natural and synthetic materials include polyglycolic acid (PGA) and poly(lactic-co-glycolic) acid. The resorption of these products limits their use in load bearing.

❚ MISCELLANEOUS BONE GRAFT SUBSTITUTES

Coralline hydroxyapatite is one of the first substances used as a bone substitute. It is resorbed very slowly and can be used as a carrier for BMP. This material is strong in compression but weak in shear, limiting its use in spinal applications. When used as a filler, it also may migrate because of bone compression with healing because of its slow resorption.

Chitosan and sponge skeleton are other potential graft substitutes that appear promising but have yet to be proven reliably effective. They require close proximity to the host bone to achieve bone conduction.

■ ELECTRICAL AND ULTRASOUND STIMULATION

Electromagnetic stimulation has been used since the early 1970s in the treatment of delayed unions and nonunions, with reported success rates of 64% to 85%, but it has not been proved to be effective in the treatment of fresh fractures. Double-blind prospective studies have shown positive effects of electromagnetic stimulation on the healing of femoral and tibial osteotomies. The effects of electromagnetic stimulation on the cellular processes of fracture healing are not well understood, but in vitro exposure of osteoblasts to electromagnetic fields was found to stimulate the secretion of numerous growth factors, including BMP-2 and BMP-4, TGF-beta, and IGF-2.

Although animal and clinical studies have confirmed the ability of ultrasound to enhance fracture healing, the exact physical mechanism has not been established. Low-intensity ultrasound has been shown to increase the incorporation of calcium ions in cultures of cartilage and bone cells and to stimulate the expression of numerous genes involved in the healing process, including IGF and TGF-beta. In a murine model, exposure to ultrasound increased the formation of soft callus and resulted in earlier onset of endochondral ossification. Animal studies of fresh fractures in rats and rabbits showed a mean acceleration of the healing process by 1.5 times in the group treated with ultrasound. Clinical comparison studies have shown an approximately 40% shorter healing time in tibial and radial fractures with ultrasound treatment. Low-intensity ultrasound also has been suggested to enhance fracture healing in smokers, a group at risk for delayed union; in patients with diseases such as diabetes, vascular insufficiency, and osteoporosis; and in patients taking medications such as steroids, nonsteroidal antiinflammatory drugs (NSAIDs), or calcium channel blockers.

■ FACTORS THAT NEGATIVELY AFFECT BONE HEALING

Numerous factors have been shown to have a negative effect on bone healing. Tobacco smoking is the most notable of these factors. Clinical and animal studies have shown that smoking, previous smoking, and use of smokeless tobacco significantly delay fracture healing. Tobacco use also delays simple wound healing. Smoking may double the time for a fracture to heal and significantly increases the risk of nonunion. NSAIDs (cyclooxygenase-1 and cyclooxygenase-2) have been shown to delay or, in the case of ibuprofen, stop the bone healing cascade. These effects vary with the individual drug. The fluoroquinolone family of antibiotics has been implicated in slowing bone healing, although these drugs have been shown to be effective in the outpatient treatment of deep bone infections. Other factors include a lack of weight bearing or muscular stimulation of the fracture site and the presence of some comorbid conditions such as diabetes (Box 1.3).

PRINCIPLES OF SURGICAL TREATMENT
GENERAL INDICATIONS FOR SURGICAL REDUCTION AND STABILIZATION

Previously, orthopaedic schools of thought have fallen into one of two groups. Those who preferred nonoperative methods, such as closed reduction, casting, and traction techniques, were referred to as proponents of "conservative treatment." The second school of thought included proponents of surgical treatment of all fractures. As with most labels, these distinctions have become obsolete; all orthopaedic surgeons are members of a "conservative orthopaedic consensus" in that our goal is to conserve as much functional potential of the injured extremity as possible.

In some circumstances a complex open reduction and internal fixation of a comminuted intraarticular fracture may be the patient's only chance for regaining a functional extremity and would be conservative treatment. In contrast, an isolated, simple, closed, stable midshaft tibial or fibular fracture can be treated with casting, plating, intramedullary nailing, or external fixation, but most surgeons currently would favor a long leg walking cast followed by some type of cast bracing as the most conservative option. For that same tibial or fibular fracture with an ipsilateral femoral fracture, tibial plateau fracture, or malleolar fracture, however, surgical repair with an intramedullary nail, external fixation, or plate and screws would be considered, depending on the soft-tissue injury, the Injury Severity Score of the patient, associated upper extremity and systemic injuries, and the proximity of the adjacent fractures and their combined effect on the mobility and potential for recovery of the adjacent joints. In this situation conservative management of the tibial shaft fracture most likely would be surgical.

Rather than a listing of absolute indications for surgical reduction and stabilization, those situations are described in which the probability is high that surgical treatment will be required to obtain an optimal result:

1. Displaced intraarticular fractures suitable for surgical reduction and stabilization
2. Unstable fractures in which an appropriate trial of conservative management has failed
3. Major avulsion fractures associated with disruption of important musculotendinous units or ligamentous groups that have been shown to have a poor result with conservative treatment
4. Displaced pathologic fractures in patients not imminently terminal
5. Fractures for which conservative treatment is known to yield poor functional results, such as femoral neck fractures, Galeazzi fracture-dislocations, and Monteggia fracture-dislocations
6. Displaced physeal injuries that have a propensity for growth arrest (Salter-Harris types III and IV)
7. Fractures with compartment syndromes that require fasciotomies
8. Nonunions, especially malreduced ones, in which previous conservative or surgical treatments have failed

Fractures in which surgical reduction and stabilization have a moderate probability of resulting in improved function include the following:

1. Unstable spinal injuries, long bone fractures, and unstable pelvic fractures, especially in polytrauma patients
2. Delayed unions after an appropriate trial of conservative management
3. Impending pathologic fractures
4. Unstable open fractures
5. Fractures associated with complex soft-tissue lesions (Gustilo type IIIB open fractures, burns over fractured areas, or preexisting dermatitis)

6. Fractures in patients in whom prolonged immobilization will lead to increased systemic complications (e.g., hip and femoral fractures in elderly patients and multiple fractures in patients with injury severity scores of < 18)
7. Unstable infected fractures or unstable septic nonunions
8. Fractures associated with vascular or neurologic deficits that require surgical repair, including long bone fractures in patients with spinal cord, conus, or proximal nerve root lesions

Situations with a low probability for improvement of functional outcome after surgery include the following:

1. Cosmetic improvement of fracture deformities that do not impair function
2. Stabilization for economic considerations to allow more rapid discharge from an acute care facility without a significant functional improvement over conservative methods

CONTRAINDICATIONS TO SURGICAL REDUCTION AND STABILIZATION

Boyd, Lipinski, and Wiley stated that good surgical judgment comes from experience and that experience comes from bad surgical judgment. Just as there are no absolute indications for surgical management of a fracture, there are no absolute contraindications. However, if the possibility for a successful outcome with surgery is overshadowed by the probability of complications and failure, nonoperative treatment is recommended. Situations in which there is a high probability for failure with surgical treatment are as follows:

1. Osteoporotic bone that is too fragile to allow stabilization by internal or external fixation. In severely comminuted osteoporotic fractures of the distal humerus, or less commonly the distal femur, some surgeons have found success with arthroplasty or a tumor prosthesis.
2. Soft tissues overlying the fracture or planned surgical approach of such poor quality because of scarring, burns, active infection, or dermatitis that internal fixation would result in loss of soft-tissue coverage or exacerbation of infection; external fixation is preferred in this situation.
3. Active infection or osteomyelitis. Currently the favored treatment is external fixation combined with a biologic approach to control of the infection. Occasionally, intramedullary nail stabilization combined with biologic control of the infection has been used successfully to obtain fracture stability; these infected fractures have been treated by experts in intramedullary nailing techniques as a last resort, and this approach cannot be routinely recommended.
4. Fracture comminution to a degree that does not allow successful reconstruction. This is most commonly seen in severe intraarticular fractures in which impaction has destroyed the articular surface.
5. General medical conditions that are contraindications to anesthesia are generally contraindications to the surgical treatment of fractures.
6. Undisplaced or stable impacted fractures in acceptable position do not require surgical exposure or reduction, but they may benefit from prophylactic fixation in special circumstances (e.g., impacted or undisplaced femoral neck fractures).
7. Inadequate equipment, manpower, training, and experience

DISADVANTAGES OF SURGICAL REDUCTION AND STABILIZATION

Surgical treatment adds further trauma to any injury. The challenge is to improve the overall outcome of the injury. If open reduction is required, the technique should minimize the dangers of infection and further vascular destruction to the injured tissues to lessen the possibility of inactivating the biology of fracture repair, which leads to delayed union or nonunion. Any surgical dissection produces scar tissue to heal the incision, but the dissection in itself can cause contracture and debilitation of the musculotendinous units responsible for functional reactivation of the extremity. Surgical approaches should follow internervous planes and should avoid transection of musculotendinous units. With any surgical approach, the possibility of nerve and vascular damage is constant. Surgical treatment also involves the use of anesthesia, with all its attendant risks.

The risks of bloodborne infection to the patient and the surgical team are becoming better appreciated. Blood transfusions carry the risks of hepatitis, acquired immunodeficiency syndrome (AIDS), and immunologic reactions. The surgical team must minimize blood loss and blood contamination. The American Academy of Orthopaedic Surgeons published recommendations for the prevention of human immunodeficiency virus (HIV) transmission in the practice of orthopaedic surgery. The task force recommended that all health care providers have voluntary testing on a regular basis and that knowledge of the HIV status of individuals be pursued after proper counseling and voluntary consent of the patient. They noted that "theoretically, if patients have advanced HIV infection, the immune status might be compromised to such a degree that they are at an increased risk of nosocomial infection were surgery to be performed."

Implants or external fixation systems frequently require removal, with the attendant risks of a second surgical procedure. Refractures have been reported after implant and external fixation removal.

TIMING OF SURGICAL TREATMENT

The best time for surgical treatment after an injury depends on several factors. Surgical procedures can be divided into three categories: *emergency, urgent,* and *elective.* Injuries requiring emergency procedures include open fractures, irreducible dislocations of major joints, fractures with lacerations or deep excoriations in the operative field, spinal injuries with deteriorating neurologic deficits, fracture-dislocations that impair the vascularity of the limb or overlying soft tissues, and fractures with compartment syndromes. In these situations delays in surgery can lead to infection, neurologic damage, amputation, and possibly loss of life. Urgent procedures are those that should be done within 24 to 72 hours of injury, such as re-debridement of severe open fractures and long bone stabilization in polytrauma patients, hip fractures, and unstable fracture-dislocations. Elective operations in trauma surgery are those that can be delayed 3 or 4 days and up to 3 or 4 weeks. Injuries that can be treated with elective surgery include isolated skeletal injuries that have been initially reduced and stabilized with nonoperative techniques but will have a better outcome with surgery, such as both-bone forearm fractures, fractures with damaged soft tissues or fracture blisters overlying the planned operative approach, and intraarticular fractures that require further radiographic evaluation for adequate preoperative planning.

If open reductions are delayed for longer than 4 to 6 weeks, shortening of the musculotendinous units, lack of clearly defined tissue planes in the zone of injury, and resorption of the fracture surfaces make surgery more difficult. With delayed operations, autogenous bone grafting may be desirable, as in nonunion treatment.

LAMBOTTE'S PRINCIPLES OF SURGICAL TREATMENT OF FRACTURES

Lambotte's four principles of surgical treatment of fractures are as applicable now as they were in the 1700s. Based on these principles, the AO-ASIF formulated four treatment guidelines for fracture treatment: (1) anatomic reduction of the fracture fragments, especially in joint fractures, (2) stable internal fixation to fulfill the local biomechanical demands, (3) preservation of blood supply to the injured area of the extremity, and (4) active, pain-free mobilization of adjacent muscles and joints to prevent the development of fracture disease. These principles all have been validated by time, but the methods of applying them have been further refined.

1. *Exposure of the fracture.* With open techniques, internervous extensile planes should be used whenever possible. Limited dissection, ligamentotaxis, distractors, and fracture tables with reduction apparatus all aid the surgical exposure and decrease the degree of devascularization at the fracture. An image intensifier with image storage capability frequently allows surgical approaches without soft-tissue dissection at the fracture, as in closed intramedullary nailing techniques. However, adequate exposure allows development of a three-dimensional perspective of the fracture configuration, its attached soft tissues, and its degree of multiplanar displacement. This should be augmented by adequate preoperative planning.

2. *Reduction of the fracture.* When the anatomy and mechanics of the fracture are understood, recreating the deforming force and realigning the fracture with traction often result in reduction. This is the mainstay of closed treatment of fractures and dislocations. This maneuver depends on competence of the associated ligamentous and muscular attachments to the fracture fragments. When these musculoligamentous allies are lost, open reduction must be used. The placement and application of instruments and mechanical distractors should be planned to minimize the force required and the damage to the injured tissues at the fracture. In evaluating the adequacy of the reduction, the anatomic location and tolerance to malreduction must be considered. A weight-bearing intraarticular fracture of the femoral condyle requires an anatomic reduction, whereas a comminuted closed midshaft fracture of the femur may permit marked displacement of intermediary fragments if it is treated with an interlocking intramedullary nail. The adequacy of a diaphyseal or metaphyseal fracture reduction is measured by four criteria of decreasing importance:
   a. Alignment of the axis of the bone should be corrected in anteroposterior and mediolateral planes. Excessive deviations of alignment lead to abnormal load deformations on weight-bearing joints with the potential for posttraumatic osteoarthritis or changes in gait that may change the force transmission to other joints or to the spine.
   b. Rotation of the axis of the bone should be corrected to be as close as possible to that of the normal opposite

extremity. Malrotation is better tolerated in the upper extremity than in the lower extremity because of the shoulder's greater range of motion as compared with that of the hip. External malrotation seems better tolerated than internal malrotation in the lower extremity. Although there are no concrete guidelines for acceptable degrees of malreduction, 5 to 10 degrees of angulatory deformation and 10 to 15 degrees of rotary deformity may be functionally tolerated.
   c. Length correction is difficult when bone is lost, and up to 1 cm of shortening or lengthening is well tolerated if it does not compromise fracture regeneration biology.
   d. If alignment, rotation, and length are restored, displacement of fracture fragments is well tolerated, with so-called secondary bone healing occurring after closed treatment of fractures or after indirect reduction techniques such as closed intramedullary nailing.

3. *Provisional stabilization of the fracture.* When the fracture is acceptably reduced, provisional stabilization, usually with Kirschner wires or screws, allows radiographic confirmation of the reduction, choice of definitive fixation, and determination of the need for bone graft augmentation. If provisional fixation is not used, reduction may be lost when definitive fixation is applied. The placement of provisional stabilization requires careful preoperative planning so that it will not interfere with the placement of definitive fixation.

4. *Definitive stabilization of the fracture.* The definitive fixation must obtain the mechanical stability dictated by the preoperative plan to encourage the selected type of fracture healing. The mechanical construct (nail, plate and screws, or external fixator) must have sufficient fatigue life to support the injured extremity until bony regeneration can assume progressively higher loads. The fixation optimally should allow relatively pain-free range of motion of adjacent joints and musculotendinous units so that secondary contractures and stiffness are avoided or minimized. The fixation should permit some load sharing if it does not compromise the stability of the fixation or impair the biology of bone regeneration.

BIOMATERIALS OF FRACTURE FIXATION
METALS

In the treatment of fractures, metals are the mainstays of materials because of their strength and ductility. Since the report by Venable, Stuck, and Beach in 1937 that some metals create an electrical potential when bathed with the saline environment of the soft tissues and cause local tissue necrosis, corrosion of the metal, and resultant loosening of the implants, metals with the lowest electrolytic coefficient have been evaluated and tested, and currently most orthopaedic implants are constructed of 316 L stainless steel (composed of iron, chromium, and nickel), titanium-aluminum-vanadium alloys, or commercially pure titanium (titanium and oxygen).

A newer material, tantalum, is a trabecular metal composed of a carbon substrate with elemental tantalum deposited on the surface. This so-called tantalum porous trabecular metal forms a biologic scaffold for new bone formation. Tantalum can be fabricated in a highly porous form, which has a modulus of elasticity closer to that of bone than stainless steel or the cobalt-based alloys. Tantalum balls have been used in studies that have required bone markers; however, it has not been used in the manufacture of implants until more recently. Because of its remarkable resistance to corrosion, tantalum seems well suited to a biologic ingrowth setting, but long-term studies are needed to confirm its usefulness.

Concerns have been raised about metal sensitization from chromium and nickel. The incidence of metal sensitivity complications from internal fixation devices that actually effect a change in fracture regeneration is unknown, but it seems to be quite low.

All metals and alloys corrode in saline environments. This corrosion increases significantly with fretting wear caused by motion between metal components (plates or nails and screws). Most implants are passivated to resist corrosion. Care should be taken not to scratch implants during insertion and to avoid using dissimilar metals so as to minimize the effects of corrosion and electrolytic potentials.

BIOABSORBABLE MATERIALS

Polyglycolic acid (PGA) was the first totally synthetic bioabsorbable suture developed, followed by Vicryl, a copolymer of 92% PGA and 8% polylactic acid (PLA) and polydioxanone (PDS). PDS was the first bioabsorbable material to be made into screws. Currently, PGA, PDS, polylevolactic acid (PLLA), and racemic poly(D,L)-lactic acid (PDLLA) are the primary alpha polyesters used for bioabsorbable implants. PGA is degraded by hydrolysis primarily to pyruvic acid and is excreted as carbon dioxide and water. PDLLA is similarly hydrolyzed via the tricarboxylic acid cycle to carbon dioxide and water and excreted by respiration. PDS also is hydrolyzed, but it primarily is excreted in the urine. Biodegradable implants cannot be contoured intraoperatively because they have a high glass transition temperature: the temperature at which the compound becomes as hard as glass. The implants can be given greater tensile and flexural strength by orienting the fibers in the implant in the longitudinal axis of the implant (self-reinforcement).

These absorbable polymers are subject to creep and stress relaxation. Claes demonstrated that self-reinforced PLA (SR-PLA) and PDLLA-PLLA screws lost 20% of their compressive force within 20 minutes. In a more natural saline environment, this loss was more rapid. Similarly, because these implants are absorbable, they lose strength relatively rapidly. SR-PGA rods are at 50% strength at 2 weeks and 13% strength at 4 weeks. The slowest degradation and loss of strength is exhibited by PLLA. The biomechanical properties of these polymers also are affected by their chemical composition, manufacturing process, physical dimensions, environmental factors, and time (Box 1.6).

■ COMPLICATIONS

PGA has been implicated in aseptic inflammation and sinus track formation. PLLA has not been implicated as having this problem, possibly because of its slower degradation, which leaves less local residue to be removed by the body. Osteolysis also has been reported around PGA and is thought to be a nonspecific foreign body reaction. Severe synovitis has been reported with the use of both PGA and PLLA bioabsorbable implants to fix osteochondral lesions. This also is believed to be the result of the amount of biodegradation debris that is present; slower resorption of high-strength PLLA may avoid this problem.

The most common orthopaedic use of bioabsorbable implants is for the attachment of soft tissue to bone, as in shoulder and knee surgeries, and few reports of bioabsorbable fracture fixation are available. In a review of more than 2500 fractures fixed with bioabsorbable implants, bacterial wound infections were reported in 3.6%, nonspecific foreign body reaction in 2.3%, and failures of fixation in 3.7%. In a study of 3111 ankle fractures, infection was slightly less frequent with bioabsorbable fixation (3.2%) than with metallic fixation (4.1%). In a prospective, randomized comparison of PLA screws with stainless steel screws for fixation of displaced medial malleolar fractures, no statistically significant differences were found in operative or postoperative complications. A more recent report of absorbable plate-and-screw fixation of metacarpal fractures, however, reported foreign body reactions in four of 12 patients, all four of which required surgical debridement.

Bioabsorbable implants offer the advantages of gradual load transfer to the healing tissue, reduced need for hardware removal, and radiolucency, which facilitates postoperative radiographic evaluation. Bioabsorbable bone implants currently should be limited to applications where there is minimal load applied until healing is evident, such as periarticular fractures that are immobilized (Box 1.7). Bioabsorbable implants do dissolve, but most are not replaced by bone. Postoperative CT scans of bones with bioabsorbable implants show no bony ingrowth at the screw site after the fractures have healed. When they break off in a joint, arthropathy may result or surgery may be required

BOX 1.7

Indications for Absorbable Fixation Devices

Metatarsal osteotomies (hallux valgus)
Metacarpal and metatarsal fusions
Malleolar fractures
Osteochondritis dissecans
Fractures of the radius and olecranon
Epiphyseal fractures
Ruptures of the ulnar collateral ligament of the thumb
Arthroscopic fixation of meniscal lesions
Femoral canal occlusion for cement restriction
Drug delivery
Cell transplantation (e.g., Dermagraft)
Nerve reconstruction (e.g., Neurotube)
Adhesion prevention

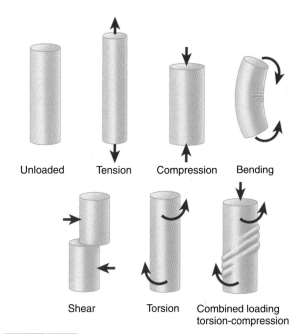

FIGURE 1.16 Various loading modes (see text). (Redrawn from Frankel VH, Nordin M: *Basic biomechanics of the skeletal system*, Philadelphia, 1980, Lea & Febiger.)

to retrieve the broken parts. Bioabsorbable implants have been used as carriers for BMP-2 and other biochemicals, and this ultimately may be the best application for this technology.

BIOMECHANICS OF IMPLANT DESIGN AND FRACTURE FIXATION

The factors usually cited in evaluating failure of bone are the type, magnitude, and rate of load and the material and structural properties of bone. Bone is an anisotropic material in that it exhibits different stress-strain relationships depending on the direction in which the stress is applied. Cancellous and cortical bone also differ because of the porosity and diameter of their respective cross sections. Cortical bone fractures in vitro when strain exceeds 2% of the original length, whereas cancellous bone does not fail until strain exceeds 7%. In analyzing fracture patterns, the mode of loading offers insight into the mechanism of injury and possible associated injuries. Loads usually are described as tension, compression, bending, shear, torsion, or a combination of these (Fig. 1.16). The mode of bone failure can predict the soft-tissue injury and stability of the fracture (Table 1.9).

Devices used to stabilize the skeleton are subjected to loading and deforming forces that rarely cause acute load-to-failure as occurs with the fracture, but these devices can fail because of fatigue if the bone does not regenerate to accommodate the load. Material properties, as noted, are expressed by stress-strain curves (Fig. 1.17), and structural properties are expressed by load deformation curves (Fig. 1.18). Structural properties of area moment of inertia and polar moment of inertia are modified to obtain the desired stiffness and strength of implants. Most implants function within the elastic deformation phase of the load deformation curve. Theoretically, there is probably an elastic range of deformation of implants that favors bone regeneration, but this range is different for direct and indirect forms of bone healing. When an intramedullary nail, plate and screws, or external fixator is used, the preoperative plan must consider the forces that the internal or external fixation will sustain and the fatigue life of the implant; this also is necessary to determine the postoperative rehabilitation program.

PIN AND WIRE FIXATION

Küntscher described the biomechanical differences between pins, rods, and nails used for fracture fixation. Pins resist

alignment changes only, rods resist deviations in alignment and translation, and nails resist changes in alignment, translation, and rotation. Kirschner wires and Steinmann pins frequently are used for both provisional and definitive fracture fixation. Because their resistance to bending loads is poor, if used alone they should be supplemented by bracing or casting. If used as definitive fixation, they usually are inserted percutaneously or with limited open reduction. To prevent thermal damage to bone and soft tissues, they should be inserted slowly with power equipment and with frequent stops of the drill. We prefer smooth wires to make their removal easier after fracture healing.

Threaded wires hold fractures in place better for temporary fixation, but the fragments must be held together during wire insertion to avoid distraction. There also is a risk of pin breakage if the cortical bone is hard. Pin or wire fixation usually is adequate for small fragments in metaphyseal and epiphyseal regions, especially in fractures of the distal foot, forearm, and hand, such as Colles fractures, and in displaced metacarpal and phalangeal fractures after closed reduction. Most frequently, pins are inserted under image intensifier control. This protects the soft tissues from further damage, theoretically permitting maximal bone regeneration; however, care must be taken that tendons and nerves are not wound around the pin during insertion. Wire fixation is used alone or in combination with other implants for definitive fixation of some metaphyseal fractures, such as in the proximal humerus, patella, and cervical spine. Notching of the wire should be avoided because it shortens the fatigue life of the implant. Rarely does wire alone provide sufficient stability for functional rehabilitation of the extremity.

SCREW FIXATION

Screws are complex tools with a four-part construction: head, shaft, thread, and tip. The head serves as an attachment for the screwdriver, which can be hexagonal, cruciate, slotted, or Phillips in design. The head also serves as the counterforce against which compression generated by the screw acts on the

TABLE 1.9

Summary of Long Bone Fracture Biomechanics

FRACTURE PATTERN	APPEARANCE	MECHANISM OF INJURY	LOCATION OF SOFT-TISSUE HINGE	ENERGY
Transverse		Bending	Concavity	Low
Spiral		Torsion	Vertical segment	Low
Oblique-transverse or butterfly		Compression + bending	Concavity or side of butterfly	Moderate
Oblique		Compression + bending	Concavity (often destroyed)	Moderate
Comminuted		Torsion variable	Destroyed	High
Metaphyseal compression		Compression	Variable	Variable

From Gozna ER, Harrington IJ: *Biomechanics of musculoskeletal injury*, Baltimore, 1982, Williams & Wilkins.

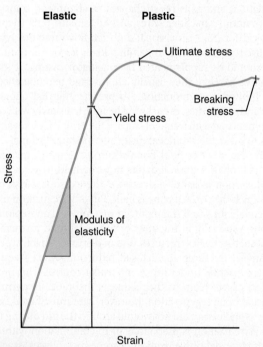

FIGURE 1.17 Stress-strain curve shows material properties in single-cycle stress until failure. Testing usually is performed in fixed sample with stress applied under tension. (From Russell TA: Biomechanical concepts of femoral intramedullary nailing, *J Int Orthop Trauma* 1:35, 1991.)

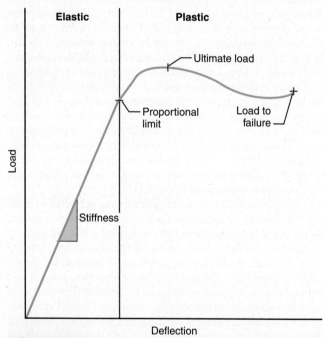

FIGURE 1.18 Load deflection curve shows material and structural properties. Note elastic phase, which is working area of intramedullary implant. (From Russell TA: Biomechanical concepts of femoral intramedullary nailing, *J Int Orthop Trauma* 1:35, 1991.)

bone. The shaft or shank is the smooth portion of the screw between the head and the threaded portion. The thread is defined by its root (or core) diameter, its thread (or outside) diameter, its pitch (or distance between adjacent threads), and its lead (or distance it advances into the bone with each

complete turn). The root area determines the resistance of the screw to pull-out forces and relates to the area of the bone at the thread interface and the root area of the tapped thread. The cross-sectional design usually is a buttress (ASIF screws) or V-thread (usually used in machine screws) (Fig. 1.19). The tip of the screw is either round (requires pretapping) or self-tapping (fluted or trocar). Clinically, if pull-out of the screw is a concern because of soft bone, a larger thread diameter may be preferred, whereas if the bone is strong and fatigue is more of a concern, a screw with a wider root diameter has a higher resistance to fatigue failure. Screws also usually are grouped into machine-type screws and ASIF screw designs. Other manufacturers now make screws and plates similar in design to those introduced by the ASIF group.

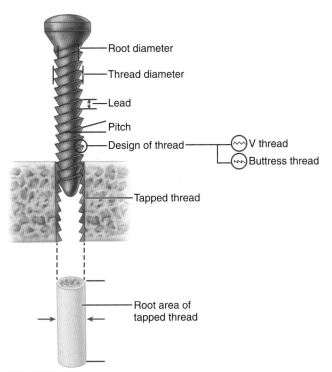

FIGURE 1.19 Design parameters of orthopaedic bone screw (see text). (From Gonza ER, Harrington IJ: *Biomechanics of musculo-skeletal injury*, Baltimore, 1982, Williams & Wilkins.)

The use of a screw to convert torque forces to compression forces across a fracture is a valuable technique. Its success requires application of the screw in a manner that allows gliding of the proximal portion of the screw in the near bone and thread purchase in the opposite cortex so that the head of the screw exerts load and forces the fracture together. Careful selection of the screw angle respective to the fracture is necessary to prevent sliding of the fracture fragments as they are compressed (Fig. 1.20). Any type of screw can be used as an interfragmentary device if the principles are maintained. Any screw that crosses a fracture line should be inserted with interfragmentary technique. Screws that attach an implant to bone are referred to as *positional* or *neutralization screws*.

■ MACHINE SCREWS

Machine screws are threaded their whole length and can either be self-tapping or require threads to be cut before insertion. Most are self-tapping; the end has a cutting flute that cuts the screw threads as the screw is inserted. Machine screws are used primarily to fasten hip compression screw devices to the shaft of the femur. The size of the hole drilled for machine screws is of critical importance. A hole that is too large will result in an insecure purchase by the threads, and a hole that is too small can result in inability to insert the screw or fragmentation of the bone as it is inserted. The drill point selected should be slightly smaller than the shank of the screw minus its thread. For a self-tapping screw, the drill point used for a hole in cortical bone should be 0.3 mm larger than that used for a hole in soft bone. Screws and drill points should be checked for proper size before surgery.

■ INTERNAL FIXATION SCREWS

Screws designed for the techniques and principles of osteosynthesis developed by the ASIF group in Switzerland are widely used. The threads are more horizontal than those of machine screws, and with rare exception these screws are not self-tapping; the drill hole must be tapped with a cutting tapper

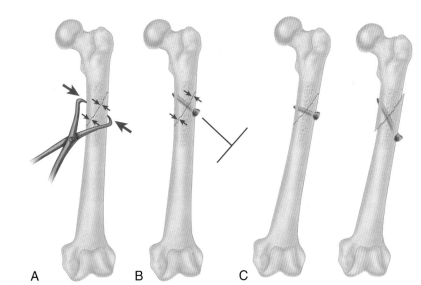

FIGURE 1.20 Principles of lag screw technique. **A,** To determine best location and inclination, forceps temporarily compress fracture. **B,** Lag screw replaces forceps in location and position (inclination). **C,** Lag screw is best positioned at right angle to fracture plane. Use of bisecting angle is correct only for fractures with less than 40 degrees of inclination. If inclination is 60 degrees, fracture is displaced because of insufficient inclination of lag screw. (Redrawn after Müller ME, Allgöwer M, Schneider R, et al: *Manual of internal fixation: techniques recommended by the AO-ASIF group*, ed 3, Berlin, 1990, Springer-Verlag.) **SEE TECHNIQUE 1.4.**

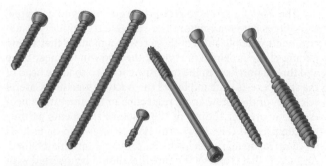

FIGURE 1.21 Examples of cancellous and cortical screws for fracture fixation. (From Bechtold JE: Biomechanics of fracture fixation devices. In Gustilo RB, Kyle RF, Templeman DC, editors: *Fractures and dislocations*, St. Louis, 1993, Mosby.)

before the screw is inserted. Cortical, cancellous, and malleolar designs are available in ASIF screws. Miniscrews for fixation of small fragments and small bones, as well as the standard cancellous and cortical screws, come in multiple lengths and diameters (Fig. 1.21). The heads of the standard cancellous and cortical screws have a hexagonal recess for a special screwdriver, whereas the smaller screws have a Phillips head.

CORTICAL SCREWS

The cortical ASIF screws are threaded their entire length and are available in the following diameters: 4.5, 3.5, 2.7, 2.4, 2.0, and 1.5 mm. The cortical screws can function as either positional or lag screws for interfragmentary compression if the hole in the near cortex is overdrilled.

CANCELLOUS SCREWS

These screws have larger threads that provide more purchase in soft cancellous bone and therefore are more frequently used in the metaphyseal areas. The cancellous screws are available in 6.5- and 4.0-mm diameters and in two thread lengths: 16 and 32 mm. They are threaded for these two lengths only, regardless of the length of the screw. The malleolar screw, a 4.5-mm screw, also is included in this group, but it is unique in that it has a self-tapping trephine tip. Selecting the proper drill size and tapping the drill hole are essential for secure purchase. Plastic and metal washers are used frequently with these types of screws for reattaching ligamentous avulsions or to increase interfragmentary compression by providing a larger surface area of the cortex for the screw head to compress against.

SELF-TAPPING, SELF-DRILLING SCREWS

Self-tapping screws are available in the same sizes as cortical screws. These screws have a small bit at the end of the screw to remove bone debris. Self-tapping screws have less pull-out strength because of their construction. These screws are best used in external fixation pins.

LOCKING SCREWS

Locking screws are self-tapping screws with a locking screw at the head. These screws require precise predrilling to allow tight fixation with a locking plate, and specialized screwdrivers are required for implantation.

SCREWS FIXATION TECHNIQUES

For transverse or short oblique fractures, screws must be combined with plates or other forms of internal fixation. Use

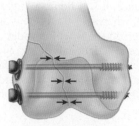

Lag screws

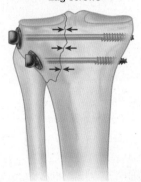

FIGURE 1.22 Lag screw insertion. To apply compression, thread must be engaged only in far fragment to pull far fragment toward near fragment and create compression across fracture site. (From Bechtold JE: Biomechanics of fracture fixation devices. In Gustilo RB, Kyle RF, Templeman DC, editors: *Fractures and dislocations*, St. Louis, 1993, Mosby.)

of interfragmentary compression techniques always is more desirable than use of a screw as a positional fixation device. If a screw is threaded its entire length, it can function only as a positional screw unless the near cortex is overdrilled so that the threads purchase only in the far cortex; then as the screw is tightened, compression across the fracture line may be produced. If the screw is threaded over only part of its length, with the portion nearer the head being unthreaded, then compression across the fracture line can be obtained without overdrilling the proximal cortex, but the threaded portion that has purchase should not cross the fracture line, or interfragmentary compression will not be possible (Fig. 1.22). If interfragmentary compression across the fracture line is desired, the following technique is recommended by the AO group.

SCREW FIXATION

TECHNIQUE 1.4

- Reduce the fracture and secure the reduction with forceps or provisional fixation by Kirschner wires.
- Plan the position of the screw so that it is inserted in the middle of the fragment, equidistant from the fracture edges and directed at a right angle to the fracture plane. If the screw is not inserted perpendicular to the fracture plane, shearing forces will be introduced as the torque forces of the screw create compression at the fracture line, resulting in displacement of the fracture reduction (see Fig. 1.20).
- Drill the near cortex with a 4.5-mm drill.

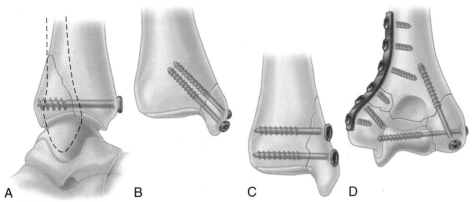

A   B   C   D

FIGURE 1.23   Intraarticular epiphyseal and metaphyseal fractures reconstructed with lag screws. **A,** Cancellous screw (6.4 mm) for posterior lip ankle fracture. **B,** Two 4-mm partially threaded small fragment cancellous bone screws used for medial malleolar fracture. **C,** Two 4-mm partially threaded small fragment cancellous bone screws used for type A fracture of medial malleolus. **D,** Two 4-mm partially threaded small fragment cancellous bone screws used for lag screw fixation of epiphysis and fixation of condyle to metaphysis of distal humerus. (Redrawn from Müller ME, Allgöwer M, Schneider R, et al: *Manual of internal fixation: techniques recommended by the AO-ASIF group*, ed 3, Berlin, 1990, Springer-Verlag.)

- Insert the drill reduction sleeve for the 3.2-mm drill and drill the far cortex with a 3.2-mm drill.
- Countersink the 4.5-mm drill hole to allow maximal contact with the head of the screw to increase load dispersion on the cortex.
- Determine the screw length with a depth gauge, insert the 4.5-mm tap, and cut threads in the hole in the far cortex; thus the screw threads will have purchase only in the far cortex.
- Insert a screw of the proper length and observe interfragmentary compression occurring by means of the lag effect as the screw is tightened. Do not remove the provisional fixation or holding forceps until the screw is fully seated.
  Interfragmentary screw fixation alone is well suited for repair of avulsion fractures, in which shear forces cause epiphyseal and metaphyseal intraarticular fractures (Fig. 1.23).

increase the surface area and help prevent the screw head from being pulled through the cortex as the screw is tightened.
- If the metaphyseal bone is firm and hard, tap for the cancellous screw as for the cortical screw, but only in the near cortex.
- Use a 2.5-mm drill and a 3.5-mm tap for the 4-mm cancellous screw, and use a 3.2-mm drill with a 6.5-mm tap for the 6.5-mm cancellous screw.
- If the bone is osteoporotic and soft, tapping may not be necessary.
- Proper selection of the length of the threaded portion of the screw is necessary if interfragmentary compression is to be accomplished. Select a length of thread that places all the threads in the far fragment and none in the near fragment so that compression can be achieved.

ASIF CANCELLOUS SCREW TECHNIQUE

The ASIF cancellous screw technique should be used for screw fixation through a plate using the 4.5-mm ASIF cortical screw. If the screw is to serve a positional function, select a 3.2-mm drill and drill through both cortices. Determine the screw length with a depth gauge; then with a 4.5-mm tapper cut the threads along the drill hole and insert a 4.5-mm cortical screw that is of the proper length. Cancellous screw insertion is similar to that of cortical screws except that the near cortex is not overdrilled; that portion of the screw nearest the head is not threaded and does not hold the near cortex.

TECHNIQUE 1.5

- When cancellous bone in which these screws are used is soft, insert a washer under the head of the screw to

Cannulated screws (Fig. 1.24) are available from several manufacturers. For small fracture fragments, the ideal provisional fixation frequently is in the same location as the desired definitive screw fixation. The major difference from conventional lag screw technique is the need to drill over the guidewire with a cannulated drill. The principles of interfragmentary lag screw fixation still must be followed with respect to planning of screw orientation, provisional fixation, and the need for all threads to purchase only in the opposite bone fragment and cortex. Figure 1.25 shows one technique and instrumentation.

Hip screws (Fig. 1.26) are used to fix various types of femoral neck fractures. Early hip screw designs, such as the Jewett nail, consisted of a nail or screw that was fixed in the femoral head and was attached to a side plate that was fixed to the femur. More recent compression hip screw designs allow sliding of the screw or nail within a barrel attached to the side plate to accommodate the inevitable collapse that occurs during fracture healing. These compression hip screws act according to a tension band principle in that the screw is loaded in tension and the bone at the fracture site is loaded

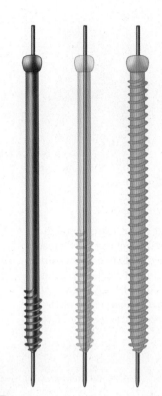

FIGURE 1.24 Various cannulated screws are available from several manufacturers.

in compression. The applied bending moment, and thus the fatigue strength, of these devices depends on the angle between the side plate and the screw or nail. Biomechanical studies have shown that higher angles with shorter moment arms result in smaller bending moments than do lower angles with longer moment arms (Fig. 1.27). Use of these devices for fixation of femoral neck fractures is discussed in chapter 2.

PLATE AND SCREW FIXATION

Plate and screw fixation of fractures has undergone continual design modifications and improvements. Pauwels first defined and applied the tension band principle in the fixation of fractures and nonunions. This engineering principle applies to the conversion of tensile forces to compression forces on the convex side of an eccentrically loaded bone. This is accomplished by placing a tension band (bone plate) across the fracture on the tension (or convex) side of the bone. Tension forces are counteracted by the tension band in this position and converted into compressive forces. If the plate is applied to the compression (or concave) side of the bone, it is likely to bend, fatigue, and fail. Therefore, a basic principle of tension band plating is that it must be applied to the tension side of the bone so that the bone itself will receive the compressive forces, and thus the tension band appliance need not be heavy and rigid (Fig. 1.28). Tension band principles also are used for some olecranon and patellar fractures with pins or screws and wires; these techniques are discussed in chapters 2 and 5. The tension band and axial compression principles frequently are combined when using plates and screws.

Although the use of axial compression in promoting union of fractures in cancellous bone is now well accepted, the effects of compression on cortical bone have been controversial. A number of compression plates have been developed and modified several times since their introduction in 1963 (Fig. 1.29).

Plates offer the benefits of anatomic reduction of the fracture with open techniques and stability for early function of musculotendinous units and joints, but they must be protected from premature weight bearing. Disadvantages of plate fixation include the risk of bone refracture after their removal, stress protection and osteoporosis beneath a plate, plate irritation, and, rarely, an immunologic reaction.

Plates neutralize deforming forces that cannot be counteracted by screws alone. Plates require contouring to maintain optimal stability of the fracture reduction. The application of the screws also is critical because incorrect placement or sequence will result in displacement or shear and loss of reduction (Fig. 1.30). For plates of any type to function, adequate screw fixation in bone is required. Usually six to eight cortices of purchase are required above and below the fracture, except with buttress plates. One of the most common mistakes is to use a plate of insufficient length. The larger the bone and the greater the stresses, the longer the plates should be. We have added cancellous bone grafts to severely comminuted fractures when the comminution involved more than one third of the circumference of the bone. Overtorquing of the screws should be avoided during insertion. Before closure of the wound, all screws should be retightened to allow time for stress relaxation of the screw-bone interface.

Specific plate designs include semitubular, one third and one quarter tubular plates, T and L plates, spoon plates, dynamic compression plates, and cobra arthrodesis plates. In larger bones, such as the femur, so-called broad plates, with offset holes to minimize stress concentration, are used. The many different types and designs of plates can be grouped functionally into four categories: *neutralization plates, compression plates, buttress plates,* and *bridge plates.* In recent years there has been a proliferation of anatomically contoured specialty plates, particularly for periarticular fractures.

Neutralization plates are used in conjunction with interfragmentary screw fixation and neutralize torsional, bending, and shear forces. These are used commonly in fractures with butterfly or wedge-type fragments after interfragmentary screw fixation of the wedge portion of the fracture (Fig. 1.31). Stability of the plate is significantly improved by the interfragmentary screw. Common fractures fixed with neutralization plates are type B wedge fractures of the humerus, radius, ulna, and fibula. The technique for neutralization plate fixation essentially is the same as for compression plate fixation, except that compression is not applied through the screw holes.

Compression plates negate torsional, bending, and shear forces and create compression across the fracture site either through external tension devices or through specially designed self-compression holes in the dynamic compression plate design; these holes exert compression through translation of the plate as the screw engages it. Dynamic compression plates are used in type A shaft fractures, transverse or short oblique diaphyseal fractures, or type B fractures after interfragmentary fixation of the wedge fragment. Variations of the technique include inserting the interfragmentary screw outside the plate, applying compression through the plate with the two closest screws, and then filling in the remaining screws eccentrically from the fracture and middle of the plate. A semitubular plate also can be used as a compression plate, usually in the fixation of fibular fractures.

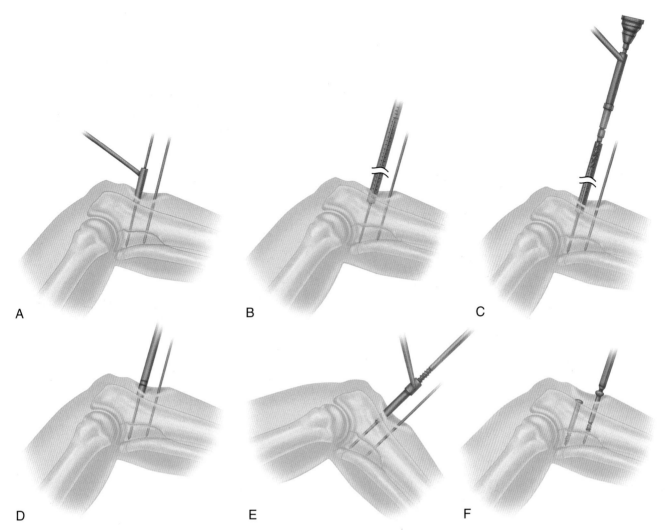

FIGURE **1.25** Insertion of small cannulated cancellous bone screws. **A,** After reduction of fragments, 1.25-mm threaded guide is inserted using small air drill and drill sleeve. Guidewire should cross fracture and penetrate far cortex. Guidewire position is confirmed with radiographs in three views, drill sleeve is removed, and second wire is inserted parallel to first wire. **B,** Guidewire insertion depth is determined by direct measuring device over wire; drilling depth is 5 mm less than reading on device to prevent penetration of far cortex. **C,** Cannulated drill bit is inserted into drill guide until coupling rests on guide. Drill is inserted into measuring device, knurled nut is loosened, drill guide is rotated until drill bit length corresponds to drilling depth, and nut is tightened. Drilling assembly is placed over guidewire, and drilling continues until coupling end contacts drill guide. **D,** Small cannulated countersink is placed over guidewire to create recess for screw head (a washer can be used if necessary). **E,** Near cortex is tapped using tapping assembly. **F,** Small cannulated bone screw of same length as depth drilled is inserted over guidewire. Guidewire is removed. Procedure is repeated for additional screws. (Redrawn after Müller ME, Allgöwer M, Schneider R, et al: *Manual of internal fixation: techniques recommended by the AO-ASIF group*, ed 3, Berlin, 1990, Springer-Verlag.)

The AO-ASIF low-contact dynamic compression plate system was designed to solve problems with biologic compatibility. The plate is contoured to improve circulation under the plate and to allow a narrow area of circumferential callus to regenerate at the fracture. The holes in the plate are uniformly positioned to optimize plate application about the fracture. Undercutting of the holes allows a greater angulatory capacity of the screw insertion angle up to 40 degrees. The compression feature of the screw holes also allows bidirectional compression through the holes. The plate is available in commercially pure titanium, as well as stainless steel.

Buttress plates negate compression and shear forces that frequently occur with metaphyseal-epiphyseal fractures, such as tibial plateau and tibial pilon fractures. They are frequently used in conjunction with interfragmentary screw fixation. They differ from other functional types of plates in that the plate is anchored to the main stable fragment but not necessarily to the fragment it is supporting. Correct contouring is mandatory, and the screws should be inserted so that they adhere to the shoulder of the screw hole closest to the fracture line to prevent axial deformation with loading.

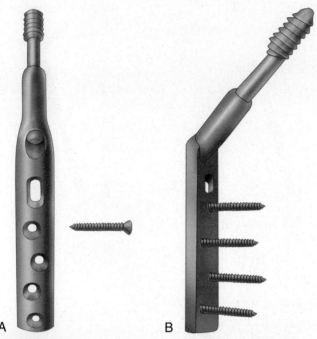

FIGURE 1.26 Examples of fixed and sliding hip screws and nails; sliding devices allow fracture site to collapse. (From Bechtold JE: Biomechanics of fracture fixation devices. In Gustilo RB, Kyle RF, Templeman DC, editors: *Fractures and dislocations*, St. Louis, 1993, Mosby.)

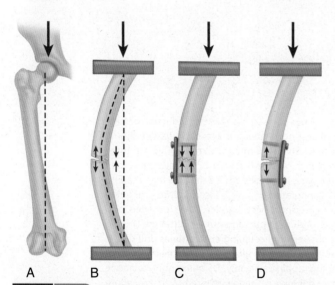

FIGURE 1.28 **A–D,** Principle of tension band plate. Because long bones are subject to eccentric loading, plate applied to outer (or convex) side counteracts tension forces and provides rigid internal fixation, whereas plate applied on inner (or concave) surface provides little fixation and would come under excessive bending stresses and soon show fatigue fracture. (Redrawn from Müller ME, Allgöwer M, Willenegger H: *Manual of internal fixation*, New York, 1970, Springer-Verlag.)

Bridge plates are used to span a comminuted unstable fracture or bone defect in which an anatomic reduction and rigid stability of the fracture cannot be restored by fracture reduction. This function is the most difficult for a plate to maintain. Biologic additions to this form of fixation frequently are required in the form of autogenous bone grafting. Indirect reduction techniques are

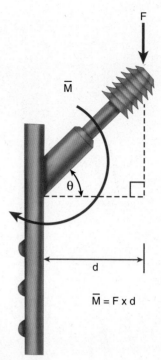

FIGURE 1.27 Influence of nail plate angle on bending moment: Larger angle results in smaller moment because of shorter distance *(d)*; conversely, smaller angle results in larger moment because of longer distance. (From Bechtold JE: Biomechanics of fracture fixation devices. In Gustilo RB, Kyle RF, Templeman DC, editors: *Fractures and dislocations*, St. Louis, 1993, Mosby.)

recommended to maximize the bone regeneration potential at the injury site.

After adequate bone regeneration has occurred, implant removal may be indicated because of patient preference or to restore skeletal strength. The risk of refracture after plate removal can be minimized by evaluating multiple radiographic views of the fracture. Restoration of the medullary canal and obliteration of all fracture lines suggest adequate healing, although refracture through screw holes still may occur. The AO-ASIF published general guidelines for implant removal that may be helpful (Table 1.10).

■ LOCKING PLATES

Locked plates are a hybrid of plate technology and percutaneous bridge plating using locked screws as a fixed-angle device. They have been shown to allow much greater load bearing than regular plates. The Less Invasive Stabilization System (LISS) (Synthes, Inc., West Chester, PA) uses unicortical locking screws to allow more elastic deformation than conventional plating systems. Locked plates also can be used in a hybrid fashion with locked and unlocked screws and are mechanically similar to pure locked constructs. Locked plates work best in osteoporotic bone where pull-out of the plate is problematic. They also provide adequate load-bearing strength to avoid medial and lateral plating in the distal femur, proximal tibia, and tibial plateau (see Fig. 1.31).

INTRAMEDULLARY NAIL FIXATION

Since the middle of the 1950s intramedullary nail techniques for fracture fixation have gained universal acceptance. Closed interlocking nail fixation is the procedure of choice for femoral

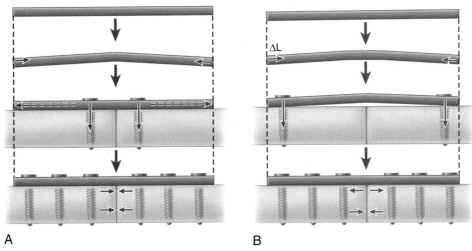

FIGURE 1.29 **A,** When prebent plate is used, inner screws are applied first, then outer screws. **B,** If outer screws are applied first, near cortex opens because plate is too long in relation to bone spanned between outer screw holes. (Redrawn after Müller ME, Allgöwer M, Schneider R, et al: *Manual of internal fixation: techniques recommended by the AO-ASIF group,* ed 3, Berlin, 1990, Springer-Verlag.)

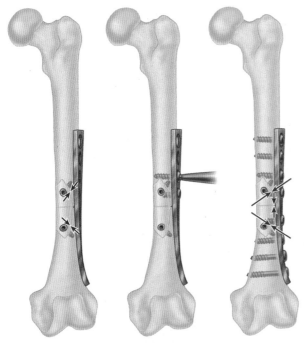

FIGURE 1.30 Plates can have more than one function. This plate is acting not only as protection plate but also as compression plate. For compression plate to serve as neutralization plate, plate must be contoured exactly, and screws must be inserted from fracture toward ends of plate. (Redrawn after Müller ME, Allgöwer M, Schneider R, et al: *Manual of internal fixation: techniques recommended by the AO-ASIF group,* ed 3, Berlin, 1990, Springer-Verlag.)

shaft fractures, especially in polytrauma patients, in most trauma centers in North America. This treatment method has been the subject of controversy since its introduction because of concerns of damage to the medullary circulation, possibilities of fat embolism, and complications from misapplication of the technique because of a lack of understanding of the biomechanical principles of intramedullary nail fixation. One by one these concerns have been answered by scientific

investigation to the point that intramedullary nailing has become the standard treatment for many fractures.

Satisfactory stabilization of a fracture by intramedullary fixation is possible under the following circumstances:

1. Unlocked nails can be considered when a noncomminuted fracture occurs through the narrowest part of the medullary canal; not only are side-to-side or shearing forces eliminated, but rotational forces also are well controlled. If the medullary canal is much larger in one fragment than in the other, poor control of rotational forces frequently results; in these situations, interlocking techniques are required. Generally, the interlocking screws should be positioned at least 2 cm from the fracture to provide sufficient stability to allow functional activity postoperatively. Axially unstable fractures are best treated with static or double-locked nails.

2. The curvature of the bone must be considered in selecting the type of nail and determining the degree of reaming necessary. Biomechanically, unlocked nails attain stability by a curvature mismatch between the bone and the nail, inducing a longitudinal interference fit. If curvature mismatch is large, more reaming will be required. The entry portal is critical for all nails and should be in the region that will minimize insertional forces. In the femur this is at the piriformis fossa in line with the medullary canal for straight nails, or in the medial greater trochanter for nails with a slightly lateral proximal bend. For the tibia and humerus, the offset between the entry portal and the alignment of the canal introduces strong forces on the posterior and medial cortices, respectively. Starting the nail at the level of the fibular head minimizes forces of insertion in the tibia.

3. Sufficient diameter and continuity of the medullary canal are prerequisites for intramedullary nail techniques. Excessive reaming should be avoided because it significantly weakens the bone and increases the risk of thermal necrosis. We recommend reaming until cortical "chatter" is encountered, known as "ream to fit." Never insert a nail larger than the diameter of the canal. In general, we use a nail 0.5 mm or 1.0 mm smaller than the largest reamer used.

4. Locked intramedullary nailing techniques should allow nailing of fractures to within 2 to 4 cm of the joint. These

techniques require the use of blocking screws or "poller" screws (Fig. 1.32). Newer nail designs with obliquely oriented distal locking screws and screws that can be locked into the nail to create a fixed-angle construct can increase stability in these metaphyseal fractures.

TABLE 1.10

Timing of Metal Removal

BONE FRACTURE	TIME AFTER IMPLANTATION (MO)
Malleolar fractures	8-12
Tibial pilon	12-18
Tibial shaft	
Plate	12-18
Intramedullary nail	18-24
Tibial head	12-18
Patella, tension band	8-12
Femoral condyles	12-24
Femoral shaft	
Single plate	24-36
Double plates	From mo 18, in two steps (interval, 6 mo)
Intramedullary nail	24-36
Peritrochanteric and femoral neck fractures	12-18
Pelvis (only in case of complaints)	From mo 10
Upper extremity (optional)	12-18

These data essentially relate to recent fractures with uncomplicated healing processes and do not apply to osteosyntheses in pseudarthroses, to major fragments, or after infections, which must be considered on an individual basis.

A perfect intramedullary nail has not yet been designed. The varying contours of bones make such a nail impossible, but improvement in the design of intramedullary nails continues. Special nails may be designed for each bone, for each kind of fracture, or for fractures in different regions of the same bone. An intramedullary nail should meet the following requirements:

1. It should be strong enough and provide sufficient stability to maintain alignment and position, including prevention of rotation; it should include interlocking transfixing screws as necessary.
2. It should be constructed so that contact-compression forces can impact the fracture surfaces, a desirable physiologic stimulus to union.
3. It should be placed so that it is accessible for easy removal; attachments are provided to facilitate removal.

Before selecting this technique, the surgeon should realize that complications are as possible with intramedullary fixation as with any other internal fixation. It is not a technique to be used casually. We recommend the following considerations:

1. Adequate preoperative planning is required to ensure that the fracture can be adequately stabilized within the working zone of the nail.
2. The patient should be able to tolerate a major surgical procedure. Special consideration should be given to patients with severe pulmonary injury because the added fat emboli from the procedure may intensify pulmonary problems.
3. Nails of suitable length and diameter must be available and identified before surgery.
4. Suitable instruments, trained assistants, and optimal hospital conditions are necessary for successful insertion of intramedullary nails.
5. A metal nail is not a substitute for union and will bend or break if subjected to undue strain during convalescence (Fig. 1.33).

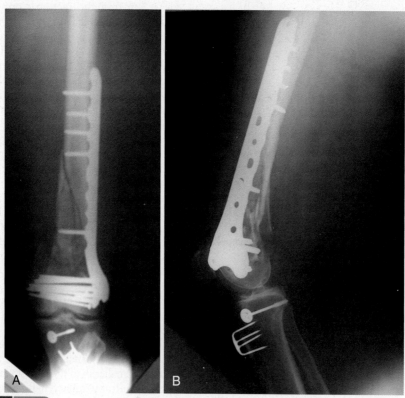

FIGURE 1.31 A and B, Fixation of comminuted distal femoral fracture with a locking plate.

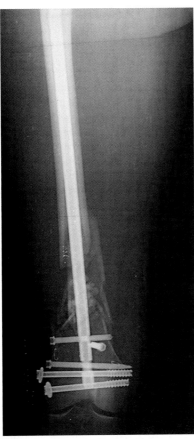

FIGURE 1.32 Blocking or poller screws can increase stability of intramedullary nail used for proximal or distal fracture, especially with small-diameter nail.

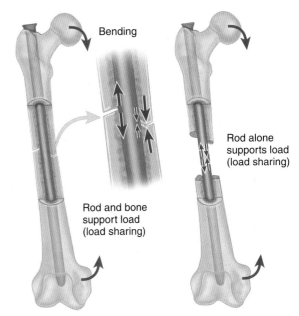

FIGURE 1.33 Load sharing in bending between intramedullary nail and bone; most of bending load is carried by nail, especially if there is segmental loss. (From Bechtold JE: Biomechanics of fracture fixation devices. In Gustilo RB, Kyle RF, Templeman DC, editors: *Fractures and dislocations*, St. Louis, 1993, Mosby.)

6. Closed nailing techniques should be used whenever possible. Higher union rates and fewer infections have been reported with the use of these techniques; however, the surgeon must be familiar with both open and closed techniques. As more experience is gained with closed techniques, fewer and fewer fractures will require open reduction. A limited open reduction, however, is preferable to accepting a poor closed reduction. This situation most frequently occurs in high-energy subtrochanteric femoral fractures in which traction will not adequately correct flexion and abduction.

■ TYPES OF INTRAMEDULLARY NAILS

Intramedullary nails, similar to plates, have anatomic and functional names. Centromedullary nails enter the bone in line with the medullary canal. They obtain contact with the bone through multiple points of longitudinal interference. They depend on restoration of bony contact and stability to avoid axial and rotational deformation of the fracture. Examples of centromedullary nails are the classic Küntscher cloverleaf and Sampson nails. Condylocephalic nails enter the bone in the condyles of the metaphysis and usually enter the opposite metaphyseal-epiphyseal area. They frequently are inserted in groups for added rotational stability. Examples of condylocephalic nails are Ender and Hackenthall pins. Cephalomedullary nails have a centromedullary portion but also permit fixation up into the femoral head. The Küntscher Y-nail and Zickel subtrochanteric nail are examples of this type.

Interlocking techniques further modified these classics by the addition of interlocking centromedullary and interlocking cephalomedullary nails. Interlocking nails allow a longer working length of the nail by the addition of interlocking screws to resist axial and rotational deformation of the fracture. Modney is credited with designing the first interlocking nail. Küntscher also designed an interlocking nail (the detensor nail), and this was modified by Klemm and Schellman and later by Kempf et al. and others. These pioneers developed the techniques and implants that formed the basis for several designs and techniques in use today. Cephalomedullary interlocking nails were designed to treat complex fractures extending into the proximal femur that were axially and rotationally unstable, such as complex subtrochanteric fractures, pathologic fractures, and ipsilateral hip and shaft fractures. These nails permit fixation with bolts, nails, and special lag screws, as exemplified by the Russell-Taylor reconstruction nail, the Williams Y-nail, and the Uniflex nail. Current intramedullary nails designed for femoral fixation reflect the area of insertion of the nail. Antegrade femoral nailing can be done through a piriformis or a trochanteric entry portal. Retrograde femoral nailing is done through an entry portal between the femoral condyles.

Interlocking fixation is defined as dynamic, static, and double locked. Dynamic fixation controls bending and rotational deformation but allows nearly full axial load transfer by bone. Dynamic fixation is used in axially stable fractures and some nonunions (Fig. 1.34A). Static fixation controls rotation, bending, and axial load and makes the implant a more load-bearing device with the potential for a reduced fatigue life. It is especially useful in comminuted, nonisthmal fractures of the femur and tibia. The double-locked mode controls bending, rotational forces, and some axial deformation, but because of the capability of axial translation of the screw within the nail, some shortening is possible (Fig. 1.34B). This mode of fixation is used in fractures of the humerus and occasionally in delayed unions and nonunions.

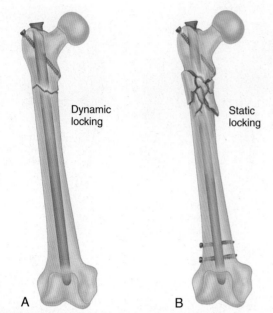

Dynamic
locking

Static
locking

A

B

FIGURE 1.34 Dynamic **(A)** and static **(B)** locking of intramedullary nail. (From Bechtold JE: Biomechanics of fracture fixation devices. In Gustilo RB, Kyle RF, Templeman DC, editors: *Fractures and dislocations*, St. Louis, 1993, Mosby.)

Dynamization of interlocking nails originally was described to avoid impairment of fracture healing because it was theorized that static interlocking would abort fracture repair. The technique involves conversion of the static mode to a dynamic mode by removing the screws from the longest fragment. Dynamization does potentially increase the fatigue life of the nail by decreasing its load bearing and also increases compression forces at the fracture site; however, if adequate cortical stability or bone regeneration has not occurred before dynamization, shortening results. Dynamization rarely is used today. Specific techniques of intramedullary nailing are discussed in the appropriate chapters.

■ REAMED VERSUS UNREAMED INTRAMEDULLARY NAILING

A continuing controversy in the management of long bone fractures in multiply injured patients is reaming of the canal for intramedullary nailing. Studies that support unreamed nailing emphasize the adverse physiologic effects of reaming, such as embolization of bone marrow fat to the lungs, and experimental evidence suggests that reaming adversely affects pulmonary function. This adverse effect is not clinically significant in most patients, however, and some authors have suggested that the development of pulmonary complications may be more closely related to the severity of an associated chest injury than to medullary reaming. Studies that support reamed nailing generally report no statistical difference in pulmonary complications between patients with reamed and unreamed nailings. Because of the multitude of factors contributing to the development of adult respiratory distress syndrome, a subset of patients in whom reaming may be harmful is difficult to define.

Another controversial area is whether reamed nailing of long bone fractures increases the frequency of infection. Currently available clinical data show no difference in infection rates after reamed and unreamed femoral nailing. Our experience with intramedullary nailing confirms this. Of 125 open femoral fractures treated with reamed (95 fractures) or unreamed (30 fractures) nailing, infection developed in 4% of all fractures, in 3.2%

of those with reamed nailing, and in 6.4% of those with unreamed nailing. Of 50 open tibial fractures treated with unreamed nailing, infection developed in four (8%); all four were type III injuries.

EXTERNAL FIXATION

External fixation is useful in trauma management, from damage control to definitive treatment. Although external fixation requires more careful clinical and radiographic monitoring than internal fixation, the general principles of application and management are relatively straightforward and its versatility allows its use in a wide variety of fractures. External fixation is not, however, appropriate for all fractures and should not be used when other forms of fixation, such as screws, plates, or nails, are more suitable.

■ ADVANTAGES

External fixation provides rigid fixation of the bones in cases in which other forms of immobilization, for one reason or another, are inappropriate. This is most common in severe, open types II and III fractures in which cast or traction methods would not permit access for management of the soft-tissue wounds and in which exposure and dissection to implant an internal fixation appliance would devitalize and contaminate larger areas and might significantly increase the risk of infection or loss of the limb itself.

1. Compression, neutralization, or fixed distraction of the fracture fragments is possible, as dictated by the fracture configuration. Uncomminuted transverse fractures can be optimally compressed, length can be maintained in comminuted fractures by pins in the major proximal and distal fragments (neutralization mode), or fixed distraction can be obtained in fractures with bone loss in one of paired bones, such as the radius or ulna, or in leg-lengthening procedures.

2. Direct surveillance of the limb and wound status is possible, including wound healing, neurovascular status, viability of skin flaps, and tense muscle compartments. Associated treatment (e.g., dressing changes, skin grafting, bone grafting, and irrigation) is possible without disturbing the fracture alignment or fixation. Rigid external fixation allows aggressive and simultaneous treatment of bone and soft tissues.

3. Immediate motion of the proximal and distal joints is allowed. This aids in reduction of edema and nutrition of articular surfaces and retards capsular fibrosis, joint stiffening, muscle atrophy, and osteoporosis.

4. The extremity is elevated without pressure on the posterior soft tissues. The pins and frames can be suspended by ropes from overhead frames on the bed, aiding edema resolution and relieving pressure on the posterior soft-tissue part.

5. Early patient mobilization is allowed. With rigid fixation the limb can be moved and positioned without fear of loss of fracture position. In stable, uncomminuted fractures early ambulation is usually possible; this may not be the case if these fractures are treated by traction or casting. Use of external fixation also allows mobilization of some patients with pelvic fractures.

6. The external fixation can be applied with the patient under local anesthesia, if necessary. If a patient's general medical condition is such that use of a spinal or general anesthetic is contraindicated, the fixator can be inserted using local anesthesia, although this is not optimal.

7. Rigid fixation can be used in infected, acute fractures or nonunions. Rigid fixation of the bone fragments in infected fractures or in infected established nonunions is a critical factor in controlling and obliterating the infection. This is rarely possible with casting or traction methods,

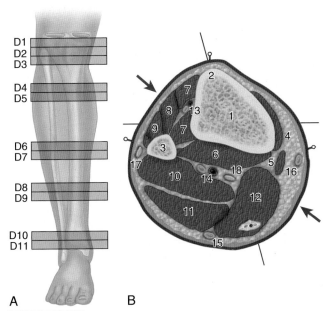

FIGURE 1.35 **A,** Eleven cross sections of leg, arranged into five groups corresponding to areas most commonly used for external fixation: D1 to D3, proximal epiphysis and metaphysis; D4 and D5, proximal diaphysis; D6 and D7, middle diaphysis; D8 and D9, distal diaphysis; D10 and D11, distal metaphysis and epiphysis. **B,** Cross-sectional anatomy of leg: 1, tibia; 2, tibial tuberosity; 3, fibular neck; 4, tibial collateral ligament of knee, semitendinosus, and gracilis; 5, sartorius; 6, popliteus; 7, anterior tibial; 8, extensor digitorum longus; 9, peroneus longus; 10, soleus; 11, lateral head of gastrocnemius; 12, medial head of gastrocnemius; 13, anterior tibial vessels (branches); 14, posterior tibial vessels; 15, short saphenous vein; 16, long saphenous vein; 17, common peroneal nerve; 18, tibial nerve. (From Faure C, Merloz PH: *Transfixation: atlas of anatomical sections for the external fixation of limbs*, Berlin, 1987, Springer-Verlag.)

and implantation of internal fixation devices is often ill advised. Modern external fixators in such instances can provide rigidity not afforded by other methods.

8. Rigid fixation of failed, infected arthroplasties can be obtained when joint reconstruction is not possible and arthrodesis is desired.

◼ DISADVANTAGES

1. Meticulous pin insertion technique and skin and pin track care are required to prevent pin track infection.
2. The pin and fixator frame can be mechanically difficult to assemble by the uninitiated surgeon.
3. The frame can be cumbersome, and the patient may reject it for aesthetic reasons.
4. Fracture through pin tracks may occur.
5. Refracture after frame removal may occur unless the limb is adequately protected until the underlying bone can again become accustomed to stress.
6. The equipment is expensive.
7. A noncompliant patient may disturb the appliance adjustments.
8. Joint stiffness may occur if the fracture requires that the fixator immobilize the adjacent joint. This is most common with fractures involving the proximal or distal limits of the bone, with the major fragment affording insufficient pin purchase and dictating a set of pins and frame above the joint.

9. External fixator components may interfere with the use of MRI. The induction of electric currents that can be produced and the possibility of heating of the external fixation device are two concerns; there are no reliable clinical data on either of these phenomena, however, and currently there is no industry standard for what is clinically "safe" in the use of MRI in patients with external fixator devices in place. Other concerns include the possibility of damage to the MRI machine and interference from external fixator components that make MRI scans invalid.

◼ COMPLICATIONS

Widespread use has brought about a series of unique complications. As with every other technique, however, adherence to basic principles and use of proper technique can keep complications to a minimum.

▌PIN TRACK INFECTION

Without proper technique for pin insertion and meticulous pin track care, pin track infection may be the most common complication, occurring in 30% of patients. Infection varies from minor inflammation remedied by local wound care; to superficial infection requiring antibiotics, local wound care, and occasional pin removal; to osteomyelitis requiring sequestrectomy. A comprehensive review of studies of pin care found one randomized, controlled study that showed no cleaning resulted in fewer infections than either saline solution cleansing or alcohol cleansing; another study found no difference between daily and weekly pin care. Because pin site irritation can lead to inflammation that results in infection, minimizing skin motion at the pin sites may be more important in preventing infection than the specific cleansing agent or schedule.

▌NEUROVASCULAR IMPALEMENT

The surgeon must be familiar with the cross-sectional anatomy of the limb and with the relatively safe zones and danger zones for pin insertion (Fig. 1.35). Several excellent manuals of cross-sectional anatomy are available and should be studied as part of the preoperative planning for external fixation. The radial nerve in the distal half of the arm and proximal half of the forearm, the dorsal sensory radial nerve just above the wrist, and the anterior tibial artery and deep peroneal nerve at the junction of the third and fourth quarters of the leg are the structures most often involved. Vessel penetration, thrombosis, late erosion, arteriovenous fistulas, and the formation of aneurysms also have been observed.

▌MUSCLE OR TENDON IMPALEMENT

Pins inserted through tendons or muscle bellies restrain the muscle from its normal excursion and can lead to tendon rupture or muscle fibrosis. Ankle stiffness is frequent if multiple transfixing pins are used in fractures of the tibia. Limbs must be placed in a position that avoids contractures before wires or pins are inserted impaling tendons and muscle.

▌DELAYED UNION

The rigid pins and frames can "unload" the fracture site, with cancellization and weakening of the cortex similar to that noted with internal rigid compression plate fixation if the fixator remains in place for several weeks or months. The callus produced is entirely endosteal, and delayed unions in 20% to 30% (up to 80%) of fractures have been reported in the literature with prolonged use of the rigid fixator.

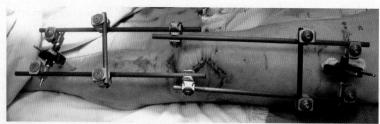

FIGURE 1.36 Spanning external fixation used for periarticular fracture fixation.

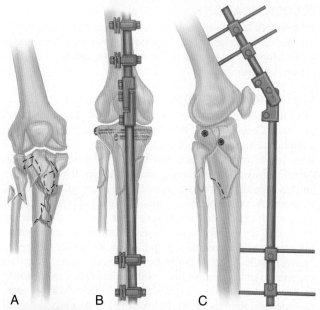

A B C

FIGURE 1.37 **A,** Comminuted proximal tibial plateau fracture extending into tibial diaphysis. **B** and **C,** Articular reconstruction and fixation with simple lag screw followed by spanning knee external fixation with moderate distraction provided by anterior unilateral frame to stabilize soft tissues by ligamentotaxis. (From Mast J, Jakob R, Ganz R: *Planning and reduction technique in fracture surgery*, Berlin, 1989, Springer-Verlag.)

COMPARTMENT SYNDROME

Increases in intracompartmental pressures of several millimeters of mercury in a tense muscle compartment may occur as the result of pins traversing the compartment, leading to a full-blown compartment syndrome.

REFRACTURE

Union resulting from the rigid fixation is largely endosteal, with little peripheral callus formation. The destressing of the cortical bone by the rigid fixation results in cancellization of the cortex; refracture is possible after fixator removal, unless the limb is adequately protected by the use of crutches, supplemental casts, or supports.

LIMITATION OF FUTURE ALTERNATIVES

Such methods as open reduction become difficult or impossible if pin tracks become infected.

INDICATIONS

Indications for external fixation are relatively specific and infrequent, but there are no absolute indications. Each case must be individualized. Routine use of the external fixator is not justified in patients in whom other conventional, time-tested methods, such as casting or open reduction and internal fixation, are applicable. Indications can be considered in three categories: (1) accepted, (2) possible, and (3) occasional.

ACCEPTED INDICATIONS

1. Severe types II and III open fractures
2. Fractures associated with severe burns
3. Fractures requiring subsequent cross-leg flaps, free vascularized grafts, or other reconstructive procedures
4. Certain fractures requiring distraction (e.g., fractures associated with significant bone loss or fractures in paired bones of an extremity in which maintenance of equal length of the paired bones is important)
5. Limb lengthening
6. Arthrodesis
7. Infected fractures or nonunions
8. Correction of malunions

POSSIBLE INDICATIONS

1. Certain pelvic fractures and dislocations
2. Open, infected pelvic nonunions
3. Reconstructive pelvic osteotomy (i.e., exstrophy of the bladder)
4. Fixation after radical tumor excision with autograft or allograft replacement
5. Femoral osteotomies in children (use of this method eliminates the necessity of subsequent removal of internal fixation appliances such as plates and screws)
6. Fractures associated with vascular or nerve repairs or reconstructions
7. Limb reimplantation

FIXATION OF MULTIPLE CLOSED FRACTURES

External fixation may be an alternative in polytrauma patients with fractures that could be managed singly by traction, casting, or open reduction and internal fixation, but that can be difficult to immobilize in combination. This technique of rapid reduction and fixation and spanning of periarticular fractures (Fig. 1.36) has been termed *damage control orthopaedics*.

SEVERELY COMMINUTED FRACTURES

External fixation can be used to supplement nonrigid internal fixation, for example, in comminuted fractures in which major fragments have been immobilized by Kirschner wires and screws but are not sufficiently rigid for definitive immobilization (Fig. 1.37).

LIGAMENTOTAXIS

The term *ligamentotaxis,* common in the European literature, suggests that certain intraarticular fractures can be treated by external fixation using traction by the fixator on the capsular and

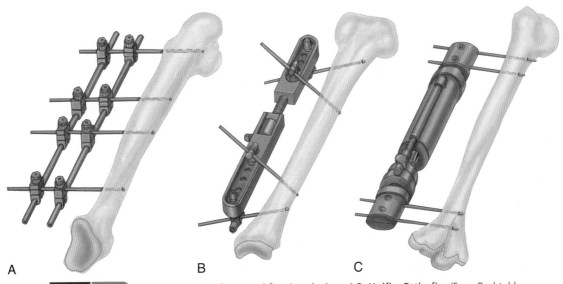

ligamentous structures around the joint (Fig. 1.37). This concept works well in comminuted intraarticular fractures of the distal radius, for which pins and plaster have commonly been employed.

FIXATION OF FRACTURES IN PATIENTS WITH HEAD INJURIES

Rigid external fixation can be used to immobilize fractures temporarily in patients with severe head injuries who are having severe elevations in intracranial pressure, seizures, or continual spasms, making traction, casting, or other forms of immobilization impractical. Unless rigidly fixed, the fracture can be compounded by seizures or frequent, severe muscle spasms. The external fixator can be removed and other forms of fracture management used when the head injury has improved.

FIXATION OF FRACTURES IN PATIENTS WHO REQUIRE FREQUENT TRANSPORTATION FOR DIAGNOSTIC TESTING, THERAPY, OR OTHER SURGICAL PROCEDURES

External fixation allows transportation without disturbing the fracture reduction in patients in whom traction does not allow transportation.

FIXATION OF FLOATING KNEE FRACTURES

External fixation of ipsilateral femoral and tibial fractures not suited for open reduction and internal fixation allows early knee function.

ASSESSMENT OF KNEE LIGAMENT STABILITY WITH FRACTURES OF THE UPPER TIBIA OR LOWER FEMUR IN PATIENTS IN WHOM INTEGRITY OF KNEE LIGAMENTS IS DIFFICULT TO ASSESS

The use of an external fixator to stabilize the adjacent fracture permits evaluation of the presence or absence of associated knee ligament disruption. When knee ligament repair or reconstruction is required with associated fractures, an external fixator can be used to immobilize the fracture and the ligament repair. Probably no more than 3 to 4 weeks of rigid

immobilization of the knee joint is required in such cases, after which time a hinged attachment can permit initiation of joint motion. Total immobilization of the joint for 6 to 8 weeks often results in some degree of joint ankylosis.

OCCASIONAL INDICATIONS

The use of external fixation in closed fractures, for which conventional methods have proved successful, must be questioned. Although the potential problems of pin track infections, delayed unions, and refractures can be reduced by careful attention to the basic principles, they do occur. The technique of external fixation is valuable in the treatment of fractures of long bones, but it should be reserved for patients in whom reduction and immobilization cannot be safely obtained by conventional techniques.

The general techniques for using external fixators are demanding, regardless of the specific fixator selected. Attention to detail is essential if maximal advantage of the device is to be gained and potentially serious complications are to be minimized. The initial treatment of the condition for which the external fixator is chosen must be considered first: irrigation, debridement, and reduction of the severe, open fracture; drainage, debridement, and sequestrectomy of the infected fracture or nonunion; or removal of the components and cement in the infected failed arthroplasty. Primary treatment in these and other conditions must be appropriately administered before fixator application.

■ DESIGN AND APPLICATION OF EXTERNAL FIXATORS

External fixators are composed of a bone anchorage system in the form of wires or pins, articulations, and longitudinal supports and are of two basic types: pin and ring. Pin fixators are subdivided into simple fixators, which provide independent application of single pins, and clamp fixators, which permit spatially constrained pin clusters (Fig. 1.38). Pin clamps often are connected to support members through "universal" articulations that permit adjustments after application. Pin fixators can be used in four basic configurations (Fig. 1.39). A unilateral frame with a support member and half-pins on

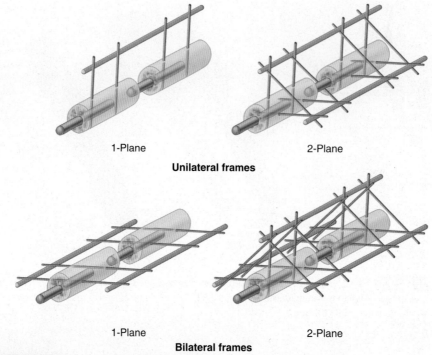

1-Plane

2-Plane

Unilateral frames

1-Plane

2-Plane

Bilateral frames

FIGURE 1.39 Four basic fixator configurations. (From Behrens F, Searls K: External fixation of the tibia: basic concepts and prospective evaluation, *J Bone Joint Surg* 68B:246, 1986.)

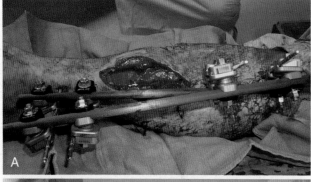

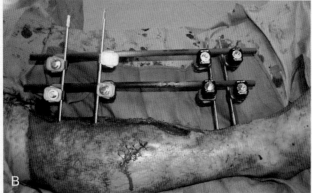

FIGURE 1.40 **A** and **B,** External fixation with unilateral frame.

one plane constitutes a unilateral one-plane configuration (Fig. 1.40). The addition of a second support member and a second plane of half-pins form a unilateral two-plane configuration. Transfixation pins connected to support members at either end are used to build the bilateral one-plane

configuration. The addition of a second plane of half-pins or possibly transfixation pins forms a bilateral two-plane configuration.

Ring fixators consist of complete or partial rings connected by rods or articulated members (Fig. 1.41). Rings are anchored to bone with half-pins or highly tensioned wires 1.5 to 2.0 mm in diameter. In addition to the fixation of acute fractures, elaborate hinged frames can be created to treat nonunions and malunions.

To prevent the problems of pin loosening, pin track infection, and possible neurovascular injury during pin insertion, the pinless external fixator was designed to be attached by clamps anchored in the cortex, rather than by pins that penetrate the medullary canal. Animal and cadaver studies showed this device to be strong enough for temporary fracture fixation, and it has been described as an ideal tool for emergency stabilization because the application technique is easy to learn, the device can be applied quickly (average of 20 minutes in their study), and it does not preclude the use of any further treatment methods (repeated debridements, soft-tissue coverage, and internal or external fixation of the fracture). Although this device is no longer commercially available in the United States, a 2015 report from China of 96 patients showed good results at an average follow-up of 2 years.

Hybrid external fixation techniques have been developed that combine wire fixation and half-pin fixation (Fig. 1.42). These devices have been used most frequently for fractures of the proximal or distal tibia with compromised soft tissue, diaphyseal extension, and minimal articular comminution. Several authors have reported good results with hybrid external fixation of proximal tibial fractures, but all emphasize that accurate reduction of articular surfaces, either open or percutaneous, is mandatory. Indications and techniques for hybrid external fixation are discussed in chapter 2.

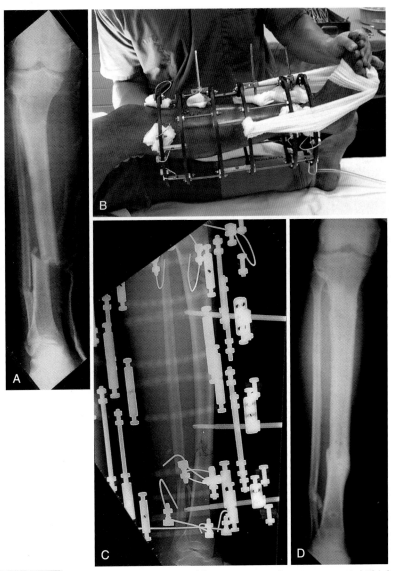

FIGURE 1.41   **A–D,** Ring fixator created for treatment of acute segmental tibial fracture.

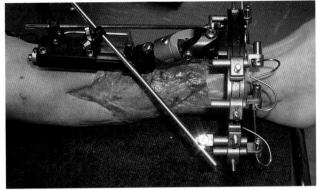

FIGURE 1.42   Hybrid external fixation of distal tibial and fibular fractures.

Combinations of internal and external fixation also have been reported to be effective for stabilization of severely comminuted fractures, with cited advantages of anatomic stable fixation, less soft-tissue dissection, and no large implants. Good results have been reported with limited internal fixation combined with external fixation in the treatment of complex tibial plateau fractures, distal tibial (pilon) fractures, and open tibial shaft fractures. One study, however, found no statistical differences in time to full weight bearing; time to union; or frequency of delayed union, osteomyelitis, malunion, infection, or pin loosening between open tibial fractures treated with external fixation alone and those treated with combined external fixation and lag screw fixation. Refractures and the need for bone grafting to obtain union were more than twice as frequent in the group with lag screw fixation. We have had good

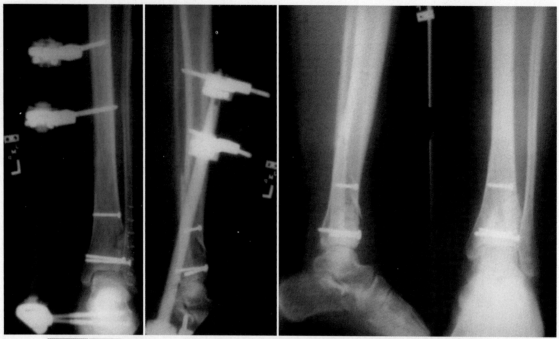

FIGURE 1.43   Screw fixation of articular fragment combined with external fixation.

results with screw fixation of articular fragments combined with external fixation (Fig. 1.43) but have not used this technique in diaphyseal fractures, which usually can be adequately stabilized with standard internal or external fixation methods.

A spectrum of fracture responses, from primary healing, to gap healing, to fusiform secondary callus, is seen with external fixation. Although initial stages of healing are improved by stability, later stages of healing, including the stimulation of callus indicative of secondary bone healing, may benefit from decreasing frame stability. Axial micromotion or dynamization may be especially beneficial. Most authors recommend at least partial early weight bearing after wound healing. Weight bearing must be gauged by increasing fracture stability. In segmental defects or comminuted fractures, weight bearing must be minimal so as not to exceed critical pressure at the pin-bone interface, which can cause resorption and loosening. In the late stages of fracture healing, several authors recommend gradual frame modification or "build down," in addition to axial dynamization, to continue stimulation of fracture healing.

GENERAL METHOD FOR HALF-PIN FIXATORS

The skin and other soft tissues must be handled with care. The skin should be sharply incised with short longitudinal incisions along safe zones. Bone is reached with gentle blunt dissection when the subcutaneous border of the tibia is not being used. Drill sheaths should be used during drilling, tapping (when indicated), and pin insertion. A new drill bit should be used with each procedure. Hand drilling or low-speed power drilling with pauses is preferred. Pins should be inserted by hand through sheaths. Thermal necrosis may be the initiating event in pin loosening and infection. Predrilling reduces bone temperature by approximately 50%. Pin sites should be cleaned daily with a washcloth and soap and water, usually in a shower, and covered by a light pressure dressing to minimize pin-skin motion.

GENERAL METHOD FOR CIRCULAR WIRE FIXATORS

In general, 1.5- and 1.8-mm wires need no incision or drill sheath. Larger, 2-mm wires can be inserted with a sheath and incision. Olive wires require a small incision through the skin only. Wires are used that have a special self-drilling tip so that no predrilling is required. A low-speed power drill with frequent pauses (or, preferably, an oscillating drill) or a hand drill should be used. After the safe angle for the transfixation wire at a given cross-sectional level is determined, the wire is stabbed through skin and muscle to bone. With a low-speed drill, the wire is drilled across both cortices of the bone. When the wire emerges from the far cortex, it is driven across the remaining soft tissues with a mallet. Care is taken to traverse soft tissue exactly as it lies without creating pressure or tension at the pin-skin interface. Wires are fixed to the external frame without bending to meet the frame, which occasionally may require small spacers. In general, large fracture fragments require two levels of fixation with two wires at each level. Short fragments can be fixed with one ring and a drop wire or with a wire offset from the main ring by a few centimeters. Stability is increased by increasing the angle between the wires at each level within anatomic constraints.

PIN INSERTION

TECHNIQUE 1.6

- Make a short longitudinal incision.
- Insert the drill sleeve and trocar into the pin clamp, and advance it to the cortex.
- Remove the trocar from the drill sleeve.

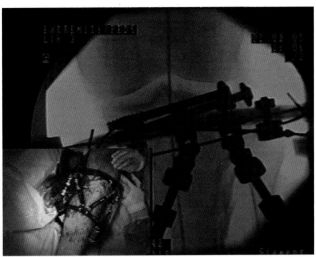

FIGURE 1.44 Application of spatial-frame external fixator with use of image intensification.

- Drill both cortices using the appropriate drill bit for the pin. Usually, 4-mm pins are used for the upper extremity and 5-mm or 6-mm pins are used for the femur and tibia.
- Use the depth gauge through the drill sleeve for depth measurement.
- Insert the appropriate pin though the sleeve and confirm bicortical purchase of the screws; this is easier with image intensification.
- Tighten the pin attachments; add additional pins and longitudinal supports as necessary for stability.
- Femoral fractures should be stabilized with at least six pins. Use at least three pins in a multiplane configuration to fix a short fragment at the hip or knee.

❚ ILIZAROV EXTERNAL FIXATOR

Ilizarov developed techniques to treat a variety of orthopaedic problems, including fractures, nonunions, and deformities, using an innovative modular circular external fixator with tensioned wires. Many changes in external fixation design and use have occurred in recent years, the most important of which is the shift toward half-pin frames and maintenance of the external fixator until union of unstable fractures. A trade-off exists between the need for initial rigidity to maintain fracture alignment and lessen the risk of infection in open fractures and the need for axial micromotion to stimulate fracture healing and prevent nonunion. Although it is only 25% as stiff axially as unilateral fixators, the Ilizarov external fixator is similar to pin fixators in its stiffness in bending and shear. Wire diameter and tension are the most important factors affecting frame stability. Other factors influencing frame stiffness include size, number, and location of the rings, divergence of the transfixing wires, use of olive wires, and distraction or compression loads at the fracture or nonunion. Intrinsic biomechanical factors unique to each patient include weight, cortical continuity, and integrity of the soft tissues.

The Ilizarov external fixator permits stabilization of high-energy fractures with minimal operative trauma to soft tissues, preserving critical blood supply (see Fig. 1.38). Early use of the limb, including weight bearing, is permitted and encouraged. The Ilizarov technique often eliminates the need for extensive soft-tissue procedures and bone grafting. Tensioned wire fixators are especially useful in treating chronic malunion and nonunion, with or without infection. Angulatory, translation, rotational, and length deformities can be corrected and union can be obtained in many of these difficult situations. Another application of the Ilizarov device is in salvage arthrodesis of the knee, ankle, and hindfoot.

The latest adaptation of the Ilizarov pin-to-ring concept is the spatial frame. This device uses a computer program to identify where the fracture is in space and, with mathematic calculations (also using a computer program), deformities can be corrected and fractures can be reduced without returning to the operating room. We also have used this device to reduce fractures acutely under image intensification (Fig. 1.44). Specific applications of external fixation to respective fractures are discussed further in the appropriate chapters (see chapters 2 and 4 to 6).

REHABILITATION

Rehabilitation of the patient and extremity should begin immediately, depending on the fracture and soft-tissue stability. We believe that adjacent joints should be mobilized as soon as possible; however, in open fractures, motion of musculotendinous units over fracture surfaces would irritate the soft tissues and may decrease resistance to infection. We usually incorporate immobilization of adjacent joints with splints, braces, or foot attachments to external fixation systems to prevent contracture. Physical therapy should include active and active-assisted exercises for joint mobilization as soon as soft-tissue healing permits. Neurologic deficits resulting in loss of active motion should be evaluated, and the appropriate joints should be splinted in functional positions to avoid contractures.

Weight bearing should be limited, depending on the stability of fixation, the type of fixation and its inherent fatigue life, and the systemic condition of the patient. Progression of weight bearing should be monitored radiographically according to evidence of stability and bone regeneration. We usually allow weight bearing as tolerated with most axially stable fractures treated with locked intramedullary nailing that do not have intraarticular extension. Weight bearing is protected in more unstable fractures until some fracture healing has occurred. With intraarticular fractures, weight bearing is not allowed for 3 months but early motion is encouraged. Range-of-motion and strengthening exercises should be monitored and directed by the physician and physical therapist; however, the patient should be instructed as to his or her responsibility for maximal functional return of the extremity. Vocational rehabilitation counseling should be initiated early to enable a productive return to society.

TREATMENT OF COMPLICATIONS FROM SURGICAL TREATMENT OF FRACTURES
INFECTION

Infections occur in 5% to 10% of open femoral and tibial fractures fixed with intramedullary nailing, and pin track infections occur in 0.5% to 42% treated with external fixation.

Orthopaedic surgical site infections have been reported to prolong total hospital stays by an average of 2 weeks, approximately double rehospitalization rates, and increase health care costs by more than 300%. In addition, patients with orthopaedic surgical site infections have substantially greater physical limitations and reductions in their health-related quality of life. Thus, it is important to prevent these infections when possible and to administer prompt and appropriate treatment when they occur.

A relatively recent concern has been the frequency of MRSA infections in trauma patients; the reported rate of MRSA infections (11%) in trauma patients is nearly double that reported in general orthopaedic patients (4% to 5.6%). One study found that MRSA carrier status at the time of admission, hip fracture, and advancing age (with an almost 2% increase in relative risk per year) were associated with higher rates of infection in orthopaedic trauma patients, whereas another large case-control study showed that vascular disease, chronic obstructive pulmonary disease, being admitted to an intensive care unit, having an open wound, and increased age were risk factors of the development of a deep infection with MRSA at the surgical site. Measurement of C-reactive protein levels has been reported to be valuable in the diagnosis of infection after internal fixation of fractures. In all patients studied, C-reactive protein levels increased after surgery, peaking on the second postoperative day, after which levels decreased. In those without infection, C-reactive protein levels continued to decrease but in those with infections a secondary elevation in C-reactive protein levels was noted beginning on the fourth day after surgery. A C-reactive protein value of greater than or equal to 96 mg/L on the fourth day after surgery was found to be predictive of infection.

These infections should be treated aggressively with repeat surgical debridements and appropriate antibiotic coverage (usually intravenous). When infection occurs in the presence of a skeletal fixation device (plate, nail, external fixator), there is a tradeoff between bony stability and foreign body response. Stability is necessary to eliminate the infection, but organisms may remain adherent to the orthopaedic implant, resulting in a persistent infection. If an implant is not needed to maintain bony stability, it should be removed. Implants needed for stability should be retained until bony stability occurs, or they should be replaced by another form of fixation (e.g., removing a plate and replacing it with an external fixator). A study of 121 patients who had early postoperative infections after internal fixation of fractures reported fracture union in 71% with operative debridement, retention of hardware, and culture-specific antibiotic treatment and suppression. Variables significantly associated with the success of obtaining osseous union were open fracture (58% success vs. 79% in closed fractures) and use of an intramedullary nail (46% vs. 77% with either plates or screws); other factors included tobacco use (66% vs. 76% in nontobacco users), *Pseudomonas* infection (44% vs. 73% with non-*Pseudomonas* infection), and MRSA infection (65% vs. 74% with non-MRSA infection).

If infections are not treated aggressively, surgical fixation becomes compromised. It is easier to treat a stable healed fracture with osteomyelitis than an unstable infected nonunion. For infections after intramedullary nailing of tibial fractures, most authors now recommend leaving the nail in place until fracture union, and then removing the nail and reaming the medullary canal. If sequestrectomy is required, exchange nailing usually is necessary.

Of 1520 femoral and tibial nailings performed at the Elvis Presley Regional Trauma Center between 1984 and 1993, 34 (2.2%) fractures became infected (17 femoral and 17 tibial). Debridement and irrigation with nail retention until fracture union, followed by nail removal and canal brushing or reaming at fracture union, led to 100% union and 100% eradication of infection in 17 infected femoral fractures. Infected tibial fractures had more complications. Two below-knee amputations were necessary because of soft-tissue problems. All remaining fractures united, whether converted to external fixators or treated with the nail left in situ; however, fractures treated with external fixation took twice as long to heal. When revision of fixation is needed to achieve fracture stability, exchange nailing may be preferable to external fixation to speed fracture union.

GAS GANGRENE

The term *gas gangrene* implies an infection with the *Clostridium* species of anaerobic bacteria, but many necrotizing soft-tissue infections are caused by mixed aerobic and anaerobic gram-negative and gram-positive bacteria. *Clostridium* can be cultured from approximately 30% of deep infections, but only a few progress to myonecrosis. *Clostridium* species, most commonly *C. perfringens, C. novyi*, and *C. septicum*, cause the most dramatic infections and are the most deadly, with mortality rates of 40% reported. More recent reports noted survival rates of greater than 90%, however.

C. perfringens, which causes approximately 90% of gas gangrene infections, contains four major toxins: alpha, beta, epsilon, and theta. The alpha toxin has been shown to be hemolytic, destroying platelets and polymorphonuclear leukocytes, and to cause widespread capillary damage. This toxin has been suggested to be important in infections that progress to gas gangrene.

Gas gangrene historically has been associated with war injuries. During World War I, gas gangrene occurred in 6% of open fractures and 1% of all open wounds; this frequency decreased to 0.7% during World War II, 0.2% during the Korean War, and 0.002% during the Vietnam War. Although gas gangrene usually is associated with open fractures or other severe soft-tissue trauma, it can occur after surgery or with no antecedent trauma.

Clostridial infections usually involve soft tissues and only rarely affect bone. They can cause a range of conditions, including simple contamination of a wound, localized infection of the skin and soft tissues without systemic symptoms, spreading cellulitis and fasciitis with systemic toxicity, and clostridial myonecrosis (gas gangrene). Localized infections usually spread slowly and cause little pain or edema, whereas spreading cellulitis and fasciitis progress rapidly; when suppuration, gas in the soft tissues, and toxemia are present, the condition usually is fatal within 48 hours.

Gas gangrene typically begins with the sudden appearance of pain in the region of the wound. In contrast to the pain with spreading cellulitis, the pain remains only in the infected regions and spreads only as the infection spreads; the infection can progress 10 cm per hour. The pulse rate may be elevated, but temperature generally is not, although fever, sweating, and anxiety or delirium may develop; profound shock and systemic toxemia can develop rapidly. The skin over the area usually is tense, white, and cooler than normal; it later progresses to dark red or purple. Muscle involvement is almost always more extensive than indicated by skin changes.

The diagnosis can be confirmed by local exploration of the wound and by radiographs, CT, or MRI; however, surgery should not be delayed in a patient in whom gas gangrene is highly suspected and whose symptoms are worsening. Prompt surgical removal of dead, damaged, and infected tissue (debridement) is necessary. Fasciotomy may be necessary for compartment syndrome. Amputation of an arm or leg may be indicated to control the spread of infection. Although penicillin G is effective against clostridial species, mixed infections are common and antibiotic treatment should include aminoglycosides, penicillinase-resistant penicillins, or vancomycin. For patients who are allergic to penicillin, alternative choices include clindamycin, a third-generation cephalosporin, metronidazole, and chloramphenicol. Tetanus prophylaxis should be ensured. Polyvalent antitoxin has not proved effective and is no longer used.

Hyperbaric oxygen therapy, as an adjunct to surgery and antibiotics, has had variable results in the treatment of gas gangrene. It generally is done with 100% oxygen at 3 atm of pressure for 1 to 2 hours every 8 to 12 hours, for a total of six to eight treatments. Proponents suggest that elevation of oxygen tension in the region of functioning capillaries in the infected wound halts alpha toxin production, and necrotic tissue can be debrided more conservatively, salvaging more viable tissue than would otherwise be possible. Several clinical studies have reported that lower morbidity and mortality rates were obtained with rapid initiation of hyperbaric oxygen therapy, whereas others have disputed the value of such a logistically difficult therapy.

The most important factors in the successful treatment of gas gangrene are early diagnosis and prompt treatment. To minimize morbidity and mortality, aggressive treatment, including surgical debridement and intravenous antibiotics, with or without hyperbaric oxygen therapy, must be instituted promptly.

TETANUS

Because of widespread vaccination programs, tetanus is a rare complication of open fractures in most developed countries. According to the Centers for Disease Control and Prevention (CDC), during 2001 through 2008 an average of 29 cases of tetanus were reported each year among the approximately one quarter billion individuals in the United States, for an annual incidence of 0.10 per million population. The overall mortality rate among the cases for which outcome was reported was 13%; the mortality rate in persons aged 65 or older was nearly three times higher. The CDC also reported tetanus vaccination coverage in only 57% of individuals between the ages of 18 and 64 and in only 44% of those 65 years of age and older.

When actively immunized with tetanus toxoid, patients require only a booster dose. Patients not immunized and patients with tetanus-prone wounds require human tetanus immune globulin, 250 U, for most wounds. The Subcommittee on Advanced Trauma Life Support of the American College of Surgeons identified several characteristics of tetanus-prone wounds: more than 6 hours old; stellate, avulsion, or abrasion configuration; depth of more than 1 cm; injury mechanism of missile, crush, burn, or frostbite; signs of infected, devitalized, denervated, or ischemic tissue; and contaminants (e.g., dirt, feces, soil, saliva). A tetanus toxoid active immunization series also should be started. Human tetanus immune globulin does not interfere with simultaneous active immunization with toxoid; however, separate syringes and separate sites of injection must be used for each. The protective level of antibodies provided by human tetanus immune globulin lasts longer than that provided by equine tetanus antitoxin, and by the time this level is decreasing, active immunization usually is effective. The second dose of tetanus toxoid should be given 4 weeks after the initial one, and a third dose should be given 6 to 12 months later. If manipulation of the wound or fracture is necessary at 1 to 2 months after injury, the dose of human tetanus immune globulin should be repeated.

Formerly, for patients who had been immunized with tetanus toxoid but had not received a booster dose during the previous 4 years, the administration of tetanus antitoxin was recommended for severe type III wounds. It is now known that the protection produced by active immunization lasts a long time and that a booster dose is effective in reactivating the immune mechanism for at least 6 and probably 10 years. An old open fracture that has healed and has been free of drainage for many months or years may still contain viable spores of *C. tetani*. Consequently, a reconstructive procedure such as bone grafting should not be done until the patient is actively immunized with tetanus toxoid.

According to the CDC 2011 report, 96% of those who sought care for their tetanus-prone wounds did not receive appropriate tetanus prophylaxis. Health care providers were encouraged to periodically assess their patients' tetanus vaccination status, especially those likely to be inadequately vaccinated or at increased risk for tetanus, such as individuals older than the age of 65, those with diabetes, and injection drug users.

SOFT-TISSUE COMPLICATIONS

Wound dehiscence may be a sign of occult or impending infection. The treatment is surgical debridement of all necrotic tissue. Plastic surgery consultation may be helpful. Many trauma patients are malnourished and have nutritional deficiencies during their hospitalization; this may result in impaired wound healing and infection. The treatment is nourishment through enteral or parenteral nutrition.

Fracture blisters or blebs may occur in high-energy trauma or in fractures adjacent to joints or areas of restricted skin mobility (Fig. 1.45). Fracture blisters generally are designated as bloody or clear. Bloody blisters are more likely to be infected, so surgery should be avoided in those areas. Clear blisters are less likely to be infected, and these areas may tolerate surgical intervention. If feasible, the blebs should be allowed to resolve, which may take 10 to 14 days and surgical treatment delayed, or the blebs can be treated aggressively.

Fracture blisters resemble second-degree burns histologically. We have used a burn treatment protocol for fracture

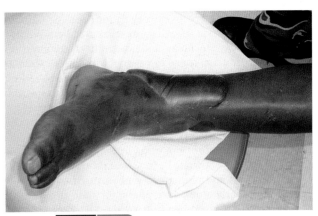

FIGURE 1.45 Blood blister.

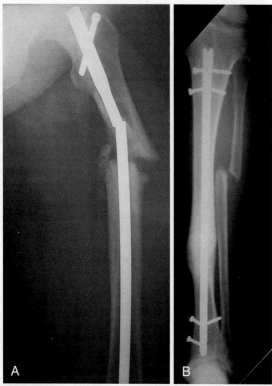

FIGURE 1.46 **A,** Broken femoral intramedullary nail resulted in nonunion that required bone grafting and plate fixation. **B,** Broken screws proximally and distally did not impede bony union.

blebs that calls for surgical excision using sterile technique and treatment of the wound base with Silvadene ointment dressings daily. With this protocol, we believe that stable epithelium usually is attained faster (within 5 to 10 days) and with less chance of superficial infection.

Swelling may not allow wound closure. We prefer to delay surgery until the skin can be wrinkled on examination, which usually indicates adequate pliability of the skin to support surgical intervention in that area.

THROMBOEMBOLIC COMPLICATIONS

Although fatal pulmonary emboli are rare in trauma patients, the occurrence of pulmonary emboli may complicate further the systemic demands on the patient. The difficulty is that no treatment for thromboembolic complications is without significant risk of morbidity or mortality, either from hemorrhagic complications secondary to anticoagulation or from migration or chronic venous stasis secondary to vena cava filters. Physical methods, such as stockings and intermittent compression, frequently are not applicable in patients with lower extremity fractures. Currently, we favor vena cava filters for polytrauma patients at high risk for pulmonary embolism, especially patients with spinal or pelvic and acetabular fractures.

Protocols for prophylaxis and treatment of deep vein thrombosis and pulmonary embolism currently are under evaluation. The combination of foot pumps and short-chain heparins has been shown to be the safest prophylaxis for deep vein thrombosis and pulmonary embolism. The use of foot pumps allows early prophylaxis after injury and after surgery, whereas the short-chain heparins are used later when bleeding is less likely.

BIOMECHANICAL CONSTRUCT COMPLICATIONS

All implants and external fixation systems eventually fail if bone regeneration does not occur in a timely fashion (Fig. 1.46). If possible, it is best to augment the fracture regeneration with autogenous bone grafts and weight-bearing methods as early as possible to maximize the fatigue life of the fracture fixation construct. Other treatment options for delayed unions and nonunions are described in the following chapters. Fracture management can be one of the most exciting and challenging problems that a physician faces. It requires an approach that is strategic and tactical.

Gill stated, "Study principles rather than methods. A mind that grasps principles will devise its own methods" (cited in Bick).

REFERENCES

GENERAL

Augat P, Faschingbauer M, Seide K, et al.: Biomechanical methods for the assessment of fracture repair, *Injury* 45(Suppl 2):S32, 2014.

Barcak EA, Beebe MJ: Bone morphogenetic protein. Is there still a role in orthopedic trauma in 2017? *Orthop Clin North Am* 48:301, 2017.

Bonyun M, Nauth A, Egol KA, et al.: Hot topics in biomechanically directed fracture fixation, *J Orthop Trauma* 28(Suppl 1):S32, 2014.

Bottlang M, Lorich DG, Dvorzhinskiy A, et al.: Biomechanics – hot topics part 1, *J Orthop Trauma* 32:S17, 2018.

Burns ER, Stevens JA, Lee R: The direct costs of fatal and non-fatal falls among older adults – United States, *J Safety Res* 58:99, 2016.

Centers for Disease Control and Prevention: *National vital statistics reports* 62:1, 2013, at www.cdc.gov/nchs/data_access/Vitalstatsonline.htm.

Davidson GH, Hamlat CA, Rivara FP, et al.: Long-term survival of adult trauma patients, *J Am Med Assoc* 305:1001, 2011.

Dietch ZC, Petroze RT, Thames M, et al.: The "high-risk" deep venous thrombosis screening protocol for trauma patients: is it practical? *J Trauma Acute Care Surg* 79:970, 2015.

Evans DC, Stawicki SP, Davido HT, et al.: Obesity in trauma patients: correlations of body mass index with outcomes, injury patterns, and complications, *Am Surg* 77:1003, 2011.

Foster BD, Kang HP, Buser Z, et al.: Effect of mental health conditions on complications, revision rates, and readmission rates following femoral shaft, tibial shaft, and pilon fracture, *J Orthop Trauma* 33:e210, 2019.

Garwe T, Cowan LD, Neas B, et al.: Survival benefit of transfer to tertiary trauma centers for major trauma patients initially presenting to nontertiary trauma centers, *Acad Emerg Med* 17:1223, 2010.

Giannoudis PV, Krettek C, Lowenberg DW, et al.: Fracture healing adjuncts – the world's perspective on what works, *J Orthop Trauma* 32:S43, 2018.

Gillespie WJ, Walenkamp GH: Antibiotic prophylaxis for surgery for proximal femoral and other closed long bone fractures, *Cochrane Database Syst Rev* (3):CD000244, 2010.

Gortler H, Rusyn J, Godbout C, et al.: Diabetes and healing outcomes in lower extremity fractures: a systematic review, *Injury Int J Care Injured* 48:177, 2018.

Hak DJ: The biology of fracture healing in osteoporosis and in the presence of anti-osteoporotic drugs, *Injury Int J Care Injured* 49:1461, 2018.

Hake ME, Young H, Hak DJ, et al.: Local antibiotic therapy strategies in orthopaedic trauma: practical tips and tricks and review of the literature, *Injury* 46:1447, 2015.

Hoff WS, Bonadies JA, Cachecho R, et al.: East Practice Management Guidelines Work Group: update to practice management guidelines for prophylactic antibiotic use in open fractures, *J Trauma* 70(3):751, 2011.

Inaba K, Siboni S, Resnick S, et al.: Tourniquet use for civilian extremity trauma, *J Trauma Acute Care Surg* 79:232, 2015.

Johansen K, Hansen Jr ST: MESS (mangled extremity severity score) 25 years on: time for a reboot? *J Trauma Acute Care Surg* 79:495, 2015.

Kates SL, Satpathy J, Petrisor BA, et al.: Outside the bone: what is happening systemically to influence fracture healing? *J Orthop Trauma* 32:S33, 2018.

Konda SR, Lack WD, Seymour RB, et al.: Mechanism of injury differentiates risk factors for mortality in geriatric trauma patients, *J Orthop Trauma* 29:331, 2015.

MacKenzie EJ, Weir S, Rivara FP, et al.: The value of trauma center care, *J Trauma* 69:1, 2010.

Masquelet A, Kanakaris NK, Obert L, et al.: Bone repair using the Masquelet technique, *J Bone Joint Surg Am* 101:1024, 2019.

Mitchell SL, Obremskey WT, Luly J, et al.: Inter-rater reliability of the modified radiographic union score for diaphyseal tibial fractures with bone defects, *J Orthop Trauma* 33:301, 2019.

Norris BL, Lang G, Russell TA, et al.: Absolute versus relative fracture fixation: impact on fracture healing, *J Orthop Trauma* 32:S12, 2018.

Patzakis MJ, Levin LS, Zalavras CG, et al.: Principles of open fracture management, *Instr Course Lect* 67:3, 2018.

Russell TA, Insley G: Bone substitute materials and minimally invasive surgery. A convergence of fracture treatment for compromised bone, *Orthop Clin N Am* 48:289, 2017.

Schluter PJ: The Trauma and Injury Severity Score (TRISS) revised, *Injury* 42:90, 2011.

Schottel PC, Warner SJ: Role of bone marrow aspirate in orthopedic trauma, *Orthop Clin N Am* 48:311, 2017.

Slobogean GP, O'Brien PJ, Brauer CA: Single-dose versus multiple-dose antibiotic prophylaxis for the surgical treatment of closed fractures, *Acta Orthop* 81:256, 2010.

Sterling JA, Guelcher SA: Biomaterial scaffolds for treating osteoporotic bone, *Curr Osteoporos Rep* 12:48, 2014.

Stevens NM, Tejwani N: Commonly missed injuries in the patient with polytrauma and the orthopaedist's role in the tertiary survey, *JBJS Reviews* 6(12):e2, 2018.

Vallier HA, Moore TA, Como JJ, et al.: Complications are reduced with a protocol to standardize timing of fixation based on response to resuscitation, *J Orthop Surg Res* 10:155, 2015.

Ward A, Iocono JA, Brown S, et al.: Non-accidental trauma injury patterns and outcomes: a single institutional experience, *Am Surg* 81:835, 2015.

Yacoub AR, Joaquim AF, Ghizoni E, et al.: Evaluation of the safety and reliability of the newly-proposed AO spine injury classification system, *J Spinal Cord Med*, 2015, [Epub ahead of print].

Yee MA, Hundal RS, Perdue AM, et al.: Autologous bone graft harvest using the reamer-irrigator-aspirator, *J Orthop Trauma* 32:S20, 2018.

POLYTRAUMA

Abdelfattah A, Core MD, Cannada LK, et al.: Geriatric high-energy polytrauma with orthopedic injuries: clinical predictors of mortality, *Geriatr Orthop Surg Rehabil* 5:173, 2014.

Gandhi RR, Overton TL, Haut ER, et al.: Optimal timing of femur fracture stabilization in polytrauma patients: a practice management guideline from the Eastern Association for the Surgery of Trauma, *J Trauma Acute Care Surg* 77:787, 2014.

Nahm NJ, Como JJ, Wilber JH, et al.: Early appropriate care: definitive stabilization of femoral fractures within 24 hours of injury is safe in most patients with multiple injuries, *J Trauma* 71:175, 2011.

Paffrath T, Lefering R, Flohé S, et al.: How to define severely injured patients? An Injury Severity Score (ISS) based approach alone is not sufficient, *Injury* 45(Suppl 3):S64, 2014.

Schreiber VM, Tarkin IS, Hildebrand F, et al.: The timing of definitive fixation for major fractures in polytrauma—a matched-pair comparison between a US and European level I centres: analysis of current fracture management practice in polytrauma, *Injury* 42:650, 2011.

SOFT-TISSUE INJURY

Bonilla-Yoon I, Masih S, Patel DB, et al.: The Morel-Lavallée lesion: pathophysiology, clinical presentation, imaging features, and treatment options, *Emerg Radiol* 21:35, 2014.

Investigators FLOW, Bhandari M, Jeray KJ, et al.: A trial of wound irrigation in the initial management of open fracture wounds, *N Engl J Med* 373:2629, 2015.

Nickerson TP, Zielinski MD, Jenkins DH, et al.: The Mayo Clinic experience with Morel-Lavallée lesions: establishment of a practice management guideline, *J Trauma Acute Care Surg* 76:493, 2014.

Sassoon A, Riehl J, Rich A, et al.: Muscle viability revisited: are we removing normal muscle? A critical evaluation of dogmatic debridement, *J Orthop Trauma*, 2015, [Epub ahead of print].

OPEN FRACTURES

Agel J, Rockwood T, Barber R, et al.: Potential predictive ability of the orthopaedic trauma association open fracture classification, *J Orthop Trauma* 28:300, 2014.

Berkes M, Obremskey WT, Scannell B, et al.: Maintenance of hardware after early postoperative infection following fracture internal fixation, *J Bone Joint Surg* 92A:923, 2010.

Chang Y, Bhandari M, Zhu KL, et al.: Antibiotic prophylaxis in the management of open fractures: a systematic survey of current practice and recommendations, *JBJS Reviews* 7(2), 2019.

Collinge CA, McWilliam-Ross K, Kelly KC, et al.: Substantial improvement in prophylactic antibiotic administration for open fracture patients: results of a performance improvement program, *J Orthop Trauma* 28(11):620, 2014.

Craig J, Fuchs T, Jenks M, et al.: Systematic review and meta-analysis of the additional benefit of local prophylactic antibiotic therapy for infection rates in open tibia fractures treated with intramedullary nailing, *Int Orthop* 38(5):1025, 2014.

Dirschl DR: Surgical irrigation of open fractures—a change in practice? *N Engl J Med* 373:2680, 2015.

Gardner MJ, Higgins TA, Harvin WH, et al.: What is important besides getting the bone to heal? Impact on tissue injury other than the fracture, *J Orthop Trauma* 32:S21, 2018.

Hao J, Cuellar DO, Herbert B, et al.: Does the OTA fracture classification predict the need for limb amputation? A retrospective observational cohort study on 512 patients, *J Orthop Trauma* 30(4):194, 2016.

Lack WD, Karunakar MA, Angerame MR, et al.: Type III open tibia fractures: immediate antibiotic prophylaxis minimizes infection, *J Orthop Trauma* 29:1, 2015.

Large TM, Douglas G, Erickson G, et al.: Effect of negative pressure wound therapy on the elution of antibiotics from polymethylmethacrylate beads in a porcine simulated open femur fracture model, *J Orthop Trauma* 26:506, 2012.

Lenarz CJ, Watson JT, Moed BR, et al.: Timing of wound closure in open fractures based on cultures obtained after debridement, *J Bone Joint Surg* 92A:1921, 2010.

Malhotra AK, Goldberg S, Graham J, et al.: Open extremity fractures: impact of delay in operative debridement and irrigation, *J Trauma Acute Care Surg* 76:1201, 2014.

Melvin JS, Dombroski DG, Torbert JT, et al.: Open tibial shaft fractures: I. Evaluation and initial wound management, *J Am Acad Orthop Surg* 18:10, 2010.

Obremskey W, Molina C, Collinge C, et al.: Current practice in the management of open fractures amount orthopaedic trauma surgeons. Part B: management of segmental long bone defects. A survey of Orthopaedic Trauma Association Members, *J Orthop Trauma* 28:e203, 2014.

Orthopaedic Trauma Association: Open Fracture Study Group: A new classification scheme for open fractures, *J Orthop Trauma* 24:457, 2010.

Pollak AN, Jones AL, Castillo RC, et al.: The relationship between time to surgical debridement and incidence of infection after open high-energy lower extremity trauma, *J Bone Joint Surg* 92A:7, 2010.

Poyanli O, Unay K, Akan K, et al.: No evidence of infection after retrograde nailing of supracondylar femur fracture in gunshot wounds, *J Trauma* 68:970, 2010.

Rehman S, Slemenda C, Kestner C, et al.: Management of gunshot pelvic fractures with bowel injury: is fracture debridement necessary? *J Trauma* 71:577, 2011.

Rodriguez L, Jung HS, Goulet JA, et al.: Evidence-based protocol for prophylactic antibiotics in open fractures: improved antibiotic stewardship with no increase in infection rates, *J Trauma Acute Care Surg* 77:400, 2014.

Rozell JC, Connolly KP, Mehta S: Timing of operative debridement in open fractures, *Orthop Clin N Am* 48:25, 2017.

Ryan SP, Pugliano V: Controversies in initial management of open fractures, *Scan J Surg* 103:132, 2014.

Sathiyakumar V, Thakore RV, Stinner DJ, et al.: Gunshot-induced fractures of the extremities: a review of antibiotic and debridement practices, *Curr Rev Musculoskelet Med* 8:276, 2015.

Sinha K, Chauhan VD, Maheshwari R, et al.: Vacuum assisted closure therapy versus standard wound therapy for open musculoskeletal injuries, *Adv Orthop* 2013:245940, 2013.

Srour M, Inaba K, Okoye O, et al.: Prospective evaluation of treatment of open fractures: effect of time to irrigation and debridement, *JAMA Surg* 150:332, 2015.

Truntzer J, Vopat B, Feldwtein M, et al.: Smoking cessation and bone healing: optimal cessation timing, *Eur J Orthop Surg Traumatol* 25:211, 2015.

Weber D, Dulai SK, Bergman J, et al.: Time to initial operative treatment following open fracture does not impact development of deep infection: a prospective cohort study of 736 subjects, *J Orthop Trauma* 28:613, 2014.

STIMULATION OF FRACTURE HEALING

Adie S, Harris IA, Naylor JM, et al.: Pulsed electromagnetic field stimulation for acute tibial shaft fractures: a multicenter, double-blind, randomized trial, *J Bone Joint Surg* 93A:1569, 2011.

Behrend C, Carmouche J, Millhouse PW, et al.: Allogeneic and autogenous bone grafts are affected by historical donor environmental exposure, *Clin Orthop Relat Res* 474:1405–1409, 2016.

Bhandari M, Schemitsch EH: Stimulation of fracture healing: osteobiologics, bone stimulations, and beyond, *J Orthop Trauma* 24(Suppl 1):S1, 2010.

Bhatt RA, Rozental TD: Bone graft substitutes, *Hand Clin* 28:457, 2012.

Dawson J, Kiner D, Gardner 2nd W, et al.: The reamer-irrigator-aspirator as a device for harvesting bone graft compared with iliac crest bone graft: union rates and complications, *J Orthop Trauma* 28:584, 2014.

Fleiter N, Walter G, Bösebeck H, et al.: Clinical use and safety of a novel gentamicin-releasing resorbable bone graft substitute in the treatment of osteomyelitis/osteitis, *Bone Joint Surg* 3:223, 2014.

Flierl MA, Smith WR, Mauffrey C, et al.: Outcomes and complication rates of different bone grafting modalities in long bone fracture nonunions: a retrospective cohort study in 182 patients, *J Orthop Surg Res* 8:33, 2013.

Garrison KR, Shemilt I, Donnell S, et al.: Bone morphogenetic protein (BMP) for fracture healing in adults, *Cochrane Database Syst Rev* 6:CD006950, 2010.

Geurts J, Chris Arts JJ, Walenkamp GH: Bone graft substitutes in active or suspected infection. Contra-indicated or not? *Injury* 42(Suppl 2):S82, 2011.

Goldstein C, Sprague S, Petrisor BA: Electrical stimulation for fracture healing: current evidence, *J Orthop Trauma* 24(Suppl 1):S62, 2010.

Goodman SB: Allograft alternatives: bone substitutes and beyond, *Orthopedics* 33:661, 2010.

Harmata AJ, Uppuganti S, Granke M, et al.: Compressive fatigue and fracture toughness behavior of injectable, settable bone cements, *J Mech Behav Biomed Mater* 51:345, 2015.

Kinaci A, Neuhaus V, Ring DC: Trends in bone graft use in the United States, *Orthopedics* 37:e783, 2014.

Kinney RC, Ziran BH, Hirshorn K, et al.: Demineralized bone matrix for fracture healing: fact or fiction? *J Orthop Trauma* 24(Suppl 1):S52, 2010.

Li X, Xu J, Filion TM, et al.: pHEMA-nHA encapsulation and delivery of vancomycin and rhBMP-2 enhances its role as a bone graft substitute, *Clin Orthop Relat Res* 471:2540, 2013.

Loeffler BJ, Kellam JF, Sims SH, et al.: Prospective observational study of donor-site morbidity following anterior iliac crest bone-grafting in orthopaedic trauma reconstruction patients, *J Bone Joint Surg Am* 94:1649, 2012.

Miller MA, Ivkovic A, Porter R, et al.: Autologous bone grafting on steroids: preliminary clinical results. A novel treatment for nonunions and segmental bone defects, *Int Orthop* 35:599, 2011.

Myeroff C, Archdeacon M: Autogenous bone graft: donor sites and techniques, *J Bone Joint Surg* 93:2227, 2011.

Nauth A, Miclau 3rd T, Li R, et al.: Gene therapy for fracture healing, *J Orthop Trauma* 24(Suppl 1):S17, 2010.

Roberts TT, Rosenbaum AJ: Bone grafts, bone substitutes and orthobiologics: the bridge between basic science and clinical advancements in fracture healing, *Organogenesis* 8:114, 2012.

Schlickewei CW, Laaff G, Andresen A, et al.: Bone augmentation using a new injectable bone graft substitute by combining calcium phosphate and bisphosphonate as composite – an animal model, *J Orthop Surg Res* 10:116, 2015.

Sloan A, Hussain I, Maqsood M, et al.: The effects of smoking on fracture healing, *Surgeon* 8:111, 2010.

Subramanian S, Mitchell A, Yu W, et al.: Salicylic acid-based polymers for guided bone regeneration using bone morphogenetic protein-2, *Tissue Eng Part A* 21:2013, 2015.

Tressler MA, Richards JE, Sofianos D, et al.: Bone morphogenetic protein-compared to autologous iliac crest bone graft in the treatment of long bone nonunion, *Orthopedics* 34:3877, 2011.

Tucci MA, Davis J, Beghuzzi HA: The effect of growth factor on osteoblast cell signaling, *Biomed Sci Instrum* 50:445, 2014.

Watanabe Y, Matsushita T, Bhandari M, et al.: Ultrasound for fracture healing: current evidence, *J Orthop Trauma* 24(Suppl 1):S56, 2010.

Xiao W, Fu H, Rahaman MN, et al.: Hollow hydroxyapatite microspheres: a novel bioactive and osteoconductive carrier for controlled release of bone morphogenetic protein-2 in bone regeneration, *Acta Biomater* 9:8374, 2013.

Zimmermann G, Moghaddam A: Allograft bone matrix versus synthetic bone graft substitutes, *Injury* 42(Suppl 2):S16, 2011.

Zingenberger S, Nich C, Valladares RD, et al.: Recommendations and considerations for the use of biologics in orthopedic surgery, *BioDrugs* 26:245, 2012.

INTERNAL FIXATION

Bassuener SR, Mullis BH, Harrison RK, et al.: Use of bioabsorbable pins in surgical fixation of comminuted periarticular fractures, *J Orthop Trauma* 26:607, 2012.

Bottlang M, Schemitsch CE, Nauth A, et al.: Biomechanical concepts for fracture fixation, *J Orthop Trauma* 29(Suppl 12):S28, 2015.

Brand S, Klotz J, Hassel T, et al.: Intraprosthetic fixation techniques in the treatment of periprosthetic fractures: a biomechanical study, *World J Orthop* 3:162, 2012.

Downey MW, Kosmopoulos V, Carpenter BB: Full threaded versus partially threaded screws: determining shear in cancellous bone fixation, *J Foot Ankle Surg* 54:1021, 2015.

Hak DJ, Toker S, Yi C, et al.: The influence of fracture fixation biomechanics on fracture healing, *Orthopedics* 33:752, 2010.

Makridis KG, Tosounidis T, Giannoudis PV: Management of infection after intramedullary nailing of long bone fractures: treatment protocols and outcomes, *Open Orthop J* 7:219, 2013.

Peck JB, Charpentier PM, Flanagan BP, et al.: Reducing fracture risk adjacent to a plate with an angulated locked end screw, *J Orthop Trauma* 29:e431, 2015.

Rose DM, Smith TO, Nielsen D, et al.: Expandable intramedullary nails in lower limb trauma: a systematic review of clinical and radiological outcomes, *Strategies Trauma Limb Reconstr* 8:1, 2013.

Scolaro JA, Routt ML: Intraosseous correction of misdirected cannulated screws and fracture malalignment using a bent tip 2.0 mm guidewire: technique and indications, *Arch Orthop Trauma Surg* 133:883, 2013.

EXTERNAL FIXATION

Andruszkow H, Pfeifer R, Horst K, et al.: External fixation in the elderly, *Injury* 46(Suppl 3):S7, 2015.

Bible JE, Mir HR: External fixation: principles and applications, *J Am Acad Orthop Surg* 23:683, 2015.

Eichinger JK, Herzog JP, Arrington ED: Analysis of the mechanical properties of locking plates with and without screw hole inserts, *Orthopedics* 34:19, 2011.

Flannery W, Balts J, McCarthy JJ, et al.: Are terminally threaded guide pins from cannulated screw systems dangerous? *Orthopedics* 34:e374, 2011.

Haller JM, Holt D, Rothberg DL, et al.: Does early versus delayed spanning external fixation impact complication rates for high-energy tibial plateau and plafond fractures? *Clin Orthop Relat Res* 474:1436–1444, 2016.

Harbacheuski R, Fragomen AT, Rozbruch SR: Does lengthening and then plating (LAP) shorten duration of external fixation? *Clin Orthop Relat Res* 470:1771, 2012.

Huang Z, Wang B, Chen F, et al.: Fast pinless external fixation for open tibial fractures: preliminary report of a prospective study, *Int J Clin Exp Med* 8(11):20805–20812, 2015.

Larsson S, Stadelmann VA, Arnoldi J, et al.: Injectable calcium phosphate cement for augmentation around cancellous bone screws. In vivo biomechanical studies, *J Biomech* 45:1156, 2012.

Lebel E, Blumberg N, Gill A, et al.: External fixator frames as interim damage control for limb injuries: experience in the 2010 Haiti earthquake, *J Trauma* 71:E128, 2011.

Logan C, Hess A, Kwon JY: Damage control orthopaedics: variability of construct design for external fixation of the lower extremity and implications on cost, *Injury* 46:1533, 2015.

Metcalfe D, Hickson CJ, McKee L, et al.: External versus internal fixation for bicondylar tibial plateau fractures: systematic review and meta-analysis, *J Orthop Traumatol* 16:275, 2014.

Oh JK, Hwang JH, Sahu D, et al.: Complication rate and pitfalls of temporary bridging external fixator in periarticular comminuted fractures, *Clin Orthop Surg* 3:62, 2011.

Qu H, Knabe C, Radin S, et al.: Percutaneous external fixator pins with bactericidal micron-thin sol-gel films for the prevention of pin tract infection, *Biomaterials* 62:95, 2015.

Shah CM, Babb PE, McAndrew CM, et al.: Definitive plates overlapping provisional external fixator pin sites: is the infection risk increased? *J Orthop Trauma* 28:518, 2014.

The complete list of references is available online at Expert Consult.com.

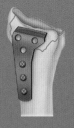

ANKLE	56	
Classification	56	
Isolated fractures of the medial and lateral malleoli	58	
Medial malleolar fracture	58	
Lateral malleolar fracture	59	
Bimalleolar fracture	59	
Syndesmotic injury	60	
Deltoid ligament tear and lateral malleolar fracture	64	
Irreducible fracture or fracture-dislocation	66	
Trimalleolar fracture	66	
Posterior tibial lip fracture	67	
Fracture of the anterior tibial margin at the ankle joint	68	
Ankle fractures in patients with diabetes	69	
Open ankle fractures	69	
Unstable ankle fracture-dislocation	69	
Tibial pilon fracture	70	
Open reduction and plate fixation	73	
Two-stage delayed open reduction and internal fixation	73	
Posterolateral approach to pilon fractures	76	
Combined internal and external fixation	77	

External fixation and fibular plating	78
Primary arthrodesis	82
FRACTURES OF THE TIBIAL SHAFT	**83**
Treatment	87
Cast bracing	87
Plate and screw fixation	87
Transfixation by screws	87
Intramedullary fixation	87
External fixation	95
Treatment of delayed union or nonunion	104
Fixation of the fibula for tibial fracture	104
Deformities of the foot and toes after tibial fracture	105
TIBIAL PLATEAU FRACTURE	**105**
Fracture classification	105
Fracture-dislocation classification	106
Evaluation	107
Treatment	109
Fracture of the lateral condyle	112
Ligament injury with condylar fracture	114
Arthroscopically assisted reduction and fixation of tibial plateau fractures	114
Fracture of the medial condyle	115
Comminuted proximal fractures	116

PATELLA	**117**
Treatment	118
Comminuted patellar fractures	123
DISTAL FEMUR	**124**
Plate and screw fixation	125
Dynamic condylar screw fixation	126
Intramedullary nailing	126
External fixation	128
Condylar fractures of the femur	128
Unicondylar fractures of the femur	128
Intercondylar fractures of the femur	130
Supracondylar fractures of the femur	134
SHAFT OF THE FEMUR	**134**
Traction and cast immobilization	134
External fixation	134
Fixation with plates and screws	135
Intramedullary fixation	136
Retrograde nailing of the femur	144
Errors and complications of intramedullary fixation	146
Intramedullary fixation in pathologic fractures	149
Fracture of the femoral shaft with dislocation of the hip	149

This chapter discusses the surgical management of common fractures in the lower extremity in adults. Basic techniques of fixation are discussed in chapter 1. The treatment of lower extremity fractures in children is discussed in other chapter.

Nonoperative treatment generally is restricted to stable, minimally displaced fractures or to fractures in patients with significant comorbidities that preclude surgery. Intramedullary nailing has become the treatment of choice for most femoral and tibial diaphyseal fractures, including select fractures with proximal and distal metaphyseal involvement; plating is most commonly indicated for periarticular fractures; and external fixation is most commonly indicated for periarticular fractures, fractures with severe soft-tissue injury, and temporary fixation before definitive fixation with another method. The indications, contraindications, and limitations of these techniques are discussed for each type of lower extremity fracture.

Operative management of fractures of the hip and pelvis is discussed in chapters 3 and 4. Fractures and dislocations of the foot are discussed in other chapter.

ANKLE

Injuries around the ankle joint cause destruction of not only the bony architecture but also often the ligamentous and soft-tissue components. Treatment of the soft-tissue and ligamentous components is discussed in other chapter. With fractures of the ankle, only slight variation from normal is compatible with good joint function. Radiographs after reduction should be studied with these requirements in mind: (1) the normal relationships of the ankle mortise must be restored, (2) the weight-bearing alignment of the ankle must be longitudinal axis of the leg, and (3) the contours of the articular surface must be satisfactorily reduced. The best results are obtained by anatomic joint restoration, and the method used to accomplish this may be either closed manipulation or open reduction and internal fixation (ORIF). For most fractures, the latter method most often ensures anatomic joint restoration and union.

CLASSIFICATION

Ankle fractures can be classified purely along anatomic lines as monomalleolar, bimalleolar, or trimalleolar. The

Lauge-Hansen Classification*

Supination-Adduction (SA)
Transverse avulsion-type fracture of the fibula below the level of the joint or tear of the lateral collateral ligaments
Vertical fracture of the medial malleolus

Supination-Eversion (External) Rotation (SER)
Disruption of the anterior tibiofibular ligament
Spiral oblique fracture of the distal fibula
Disruption of the posterior tibiofibular ligament or fracture of the posterior malleolus
Fracture of the medial malleolus or rupture of the deltoid ligament

Pronation-Abduction (PA)
Transverse fracture of the medial malleolus or rupture of the deltoid ligament
Rupture of the syndesmotic ligaments or avulsion fracture of their insertions
Short, horizontal, oblique fracture of the fibula above the level of the joint

Pronation-Eversion (External) Rotation (PER)
Transverse fracture of the medial malleolus or disruption of the deltoid ligament
Disruption of the anterior tibiofibular ligament
Short oblique fracture of the fibula above the level of the joint
Rupture of posterior tibiofibular ligament or avulsion fracture of the posterolateral tibia

Pronation-Dorsiflexion (PD)
Fracture of the medial malleolus
Fracture of the anterior margin of the tibia
Supramalleolar fracture of the fibula
Transverse fracture of the posterior tibial surface

* Classification into fracture type (A to C) and group (1-3).
From Geissler WB, Tsao AK, Hughes JL: Fractures and injuries of the ankle. In Rockwood CA Jr, Green DP, Bucholz RW, et al. editors: *Rockwood and Green's fractures in adults*, ed 4, Philadelphia, 1996, Lippincott-Raven.

Lauge-Hansen classification attempted to associate specific fracture patterns with the mechanism of injury and proposed a detailed classification, with each broad classification subdivided into four groups (Box 2.1). According to this classification, most fractures are supination-eversion, supination-adduction, pronation-abduction, and pronation-eversion injuries. In this classification system, the term *eversion* is a misnomer; it more correctly should be *external or lateral rotation*. The first word in the designation refers to the foot's position at the time of injury; the second word refers to the direction of the deforming force.

The most common mechanism is supination-eversion (supination-external rotation). The identifying feature is a spiral oblique fracture of the distal fibula and a rupture of the deltoid ligament or fracture of the medial malleolus. The supination-adduction type of injury is characterized by a transverse fracture of the distal fibula and a relatively vertical fracture of the medial malleolus. The pronation-abduction mechanism produces a transverse fracture of the medial malleolus and a short oblique fracture of the fibula

that appears relatively horizontal on the lateral radiograph. The pronation-eversion (pronation-external rotation) mechanism is characterized by a deltoid ligament tear or a fracture of the medial malleolus and a spiral oblique fracture of the fibula relatively high above the level of the ankle joint. Analysis of the fracture configuration, and hence the mechanism of forces producing the fracture, is especially important if closed reduction and immobilization are planned as definitive treatment. Generally, the mechanism of forces producing the fracture is reversed by the closed reduction manipulation; for example, if the fracture is produced by a supination, eversion, or external rotation mechanism, reduction is achieved by a pronation, inversion, or internal rotation manipulation.

Some authors caution against using the Lauge-Hansen classification alone to determine treatment and recommend that treatment be based on a clinical determination of stability. O'Leary and Ward described an abduction-external rotation mechanism that resulted in fracture of the medial malleolus and avulsion of the deltoid ligament, emphasizing the difficulty in determining the full extent of injury after high-velocity impact. This injury results from initial abduction and external rotation, followed by violent adduction that fractures the medial malleolus. Whitelaw et al. recommended evaluation of ankle joint stability by the anterior drawer and talar tilt tests after bony stabilization and surgical repair of any concomitant ligamentous disruption.

The Danis-Weber classification (Fig. 2.1) is based on the location and appearance of the fibular fracture. Type A fractures are caused by internal rotation and adduction that produce a transverse fracture of the lateral malleolus at or below the plafond, with or without an oblique fracture of the medial malleolus. Type B fractures are caused by external rotation resulting in an oblique fracture of the lateral malleolus, beginning on the anteromedial surface and extending proximally to the posterolateral aspect. The injury may include rupture or avulsion of the anteroinferior tibiofibular ligament, fracture of the medial malleolus, or rupture of the deltoid ligament. Approximately 80% to 90% of lateral malleolar fractures fall into the Danis-Weber type B category. Type C fractures are divided into abduction injuries with oblique fracture of the fibula proximal to the disrupted tibiofibular ligaments (C-1) and abduction-external rotation injuries with a more proximal fracture of the fibula and more extensive disruption of the interosseous membrane (C-2). Type C injuries may involve a medial malleolar fracture or a deltoid ligament rupture. Fracture of the posterior malleolus may accompany any of the three types. The AO classification divides the three Danis-Weber types further for associated medial injuries (Box 2.2). Malek et al. reported high interobserver and intraobserver reliability using the Danis-Weber classification system of 78% and 85%, respectively.

Authors have demonstrated that there is considerable interobserver variability between the classification systems for ankle fractures. In addition, although the Lauge-Hansen and Danis-Weber classifications have proved useful for understanding the mechanisms of injury and planning treatment, neither has been shown to have prognostic significance. Furthermore, the Lauge-Hansen classification scheme has demonstrated limitations in predicting associated soft-tissue injuries when evaluated with MRI.

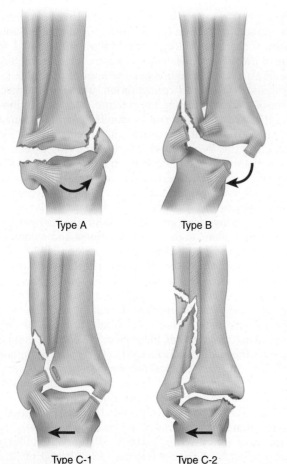

Type A　　　　Type B

Type C-1　　　　Type C-2

FIGURE 2.1 Danis-Weber classification of ankle fractures based on mechanism of injury and location and appearance of fibular fracture (see text). (Redrawn from Weber BG: *Die Verletzungen des oberen Sprunggelenkes*. In *Aktuelle Probleme in der Chirurgie*, Bern, 1966, Verlag Hans Huber.)

Fragments that are too small or comminuted for screw fixation can be stabilized with two Kirschner wires and a tension band (Fig. 2.2C). Alternatively, minifragment screws have become readily available and are an excellent option for stabilization of smaller fractures. Vertical fractures of the medial malleolus require horizontally directed screws or antiglide plating techniques (Fig. 2.2D and E). Dumigan et al. demonstrated that fixation of vertical medial malleolar fractures with neutralization plating is biomechanically advantageous.

Although stainless steel implants are used most commonly for medial malleolar fractures, the safety and efficacy of bioabsorbable implants have been investigated. The main theoretical advantage of these implants is that they reduce the incidence of late implant removal stemming from persistent prominence or tenderness around the screw heads. Although bioabsorbable implants have been used successfully, with no differences in outcomes noted between stainless steel and polyglycolide, drainage from sterile sinuses has been reported in 5% to 10% of patients, possibly related to the breakdown of polyglycolide. Also, in a series of 2528 patients, a 4.3% occurrence rate of clinically significant local inflammatory tissue reaction has been reported. Bioabsorbable implants are discussed in more detail in chapter 1.

Our preference is for metallic implants, typically screws or screw and plate combination, depending on the fracture morphology. Absorbable implants have a role in the treatment of associated articular fragments but are not a substitute for traditional internal fixation options.

ISOLATED FRACTURES OF THE MEDIAL AND LATERAL MALLEOLI
■ MEDIAL MALLEOLAR FRACTURE

Nondisplaced fractures of the medial malleolus usually can be treated with cast immobilization; however, in individuals with high functional demands, internal fixation may be appropriate to hasten healing and rehabilitation. Herscovici et al. obtained a high rate of union and functional outcome with conservative management of isolated medial malleolar fractures. Displaced fractures of the medial malleolus should be treated operatively because persistent displacement allows the talus to tilt into varus. Avulsion fractures involving only the tip of the medial malleolus are not as unstable as fractures involving the axilla of the mortise and do not require internal fixation, unless displacement is significant. Delayed internal fixation can be done if symptoms warrant. Fixation of the medial malleolus usually consists of two 4-mm cancellous lag screws oriented perpendicular to the fracture. Some authors have advocated fixation with bicortical 3.5-mm lag screws, rather than 4-mm cancellous screws, because biomechanical data suggest increased construct strength (Fig. 2.2A).

Smaller fragments can be fixed with one lag screw and one Kirschner wire to prevent rotation (Fig. 2.2B).

■ STRESS FRACTURE OF THE MEDIAL MALLEOLUS

Stress fractures of the medial malleolus usually present as localized pain, swelling, and tenderness over the medial ankle. Initially, they may not be apparent on radiographs but usually can be demonstrated on bone scan, CT, or MRI. Often stress fractures become apparent on follow-up radiographs. Shelbourne et al. recommended internal fixation for fractures

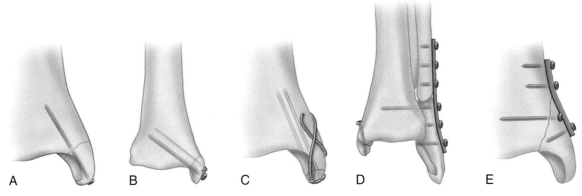

FIGURE 2.2 Fixation of medial malleolar fractures. **A,** Single lag screw through large fragment. **B,** Combination of 4-mm lag screw and Kirschner wire for small fragment. **C,** Tension band wiring for low transverse fracture. **D,** Vertical countersunk 4-mm lag screw for low transverse fracture. **E,** Plate fixation with horizontal screw fixation.

that are immediately apparent on radiographs and cast immobilization for those only apparent on bone scans. Stress fractures of the medial malleolus have a high risk of progression to complete fracture, delayed union, or nonunion. Often aggressive treatment, including surgery, is necessary.

■ LATERAL MALLEOLAR FRACTURE

Although fractures of the lateral malleolus without significant medial injury are common, the indications for open reduction of these fractures are still controversial. The maximal acceptable displacement of the fibula reported in the literature has ranged from 0 to 5 mm. In most patients, 2 to 3 mm of displacement is accepted, depending on their functional demands. Displacement of the talus has been shown to accompany displacement of the lateral malleolus in bimalleolar ankle fractures; therefore, anatomic reduction of the lateral malleolus is necessary in these injuries. Biomechanical studies have shown that isolated fractures of the lateral malleolus do not disturb joint kinematics or cause talar displacement with axial loading, and long-term clinical follow-up studies of closed treatment of supination-external rotation stage II fractures have demonstrated 94% to 98% good functional results, even with 3 mm of fibular displacement. Results after operative treatment are similar to those of closed treatment of supination-external rotation stage II injuries, regardless of whether anatomic reduction has been obtained. If the stability of a lateral malleolar fracture is uncertain, stress radiographs can be obtained to detect displacement of the talus indicative of medial injury. This can be done by a manual or gravity stress evaluation. Koval et al. evaluated whether a positive stress test predicts the need for operative fixation of lateral malleolar fractures. In their study, all patients with positive findings of stress radiographs of the ankles had an MRI to evaluate the integrity of the deltoid ligament complex. Only complete ruptures required operative stabilization. Patients with partial disruptions had successful nonoperative management with a minimum 1-year follow-up. Others have proposed ultrasonographic evaluation of the deltoid ligament to differentiate between a bimalleolar equivalent fracture and an isolated lateral malleolar injury. Others have proposed that preoperative radiographic and CT findings are effective in predicting syndesmotic injuries in supination-external rotation type ankle fractures. Choi et al. suggested that a fracture

height of more than 3 mm and medial joint space of more than 4.9 mm on CT, and fracture height of more than 7 mm and medial joint space of more than 4.0 mm on radiographs, is a good indicator of an unstable syndesmotic injury. However, the ideal preoperative diagnostic modality for assessing a medial-sided injury for decision-making regarding operative or nonoperative management remains unclear. We routinely obtain gravity or manual stress radiographs for appropriate injuries because of their simplicity.

BIMALLEOLAR FRACTURE

Bimalleolar ankle fractures disrupt the medial and lateral stabilizing structures of the ankle joint. Displacement reduces the tibiotalar contact area and alters joint kinematics. Closed reduction can often be accomplished but not maintained in anatomic position as swelling subsides. Nonunion has been reported in approximately 10% of bimalleolar fractures treated by closed methods, although these are not always symptomatic. Twenty percent of bimalleolar fractures involve intraarticular injuries to the talus and tibia; these injuries go untreated when closed methods are used. Randomized, prospective, and long-term follow-up studies of bimalleolar or bimalleolar-equivalent ankle fractures have shown superior results of operative over nonoperative treatment. A long-term follow-up study also showed superior results after operative treatment of supination-external rotation stage IV fractures. Tile and the AO group recommended ORIF of both malleoli for almost all bimalleolar fractures.

For most displaced bimalleolar fractures, we also recommend ORIF of both malleoli. Most Weber type B and type C lateral malleolar fractures are stabilized with plate and screw fixation. In some patients, lateral implants in the ankle may become symptomatic; however, in one study only half the patients had relief of pain after implant removal. Posterior plating of Weber type B fractures of the lateral malleolus using an antiglide technique has been advocated to avoid the possibility of intraarticular screws, decrease the incidence of palpable implants, and provide a stronger construct. In a prospective series of 32 patients, there were no nonunions, malunions, wound complications, loss of fixation, or intraarticular or palpable screws. Four patients had transient peroneal tendinitis, and in two patients the plates were removed because of symptoms caused by a poorly placed lag screw.

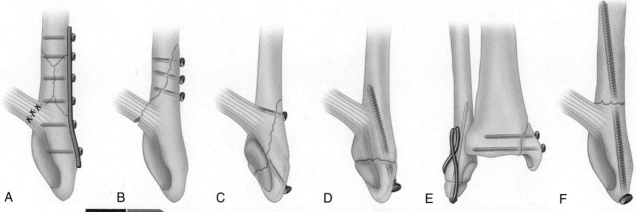

FIGURE 2.3   Fixation of lateral malleolar fractures. **A,** Standard fixation of fibular fracture with one third semitubular 3.5-mm plate and screws. **B,** Multiple 3.5-mm lag screws. **C,** Two lag screws for long oblique fracture. **D,** Single 3.5-mm malleolar screw for low transverse fracture. **E,** Tension band wiring; note 4-mm lag screw fixation of associated medial malleolar fracture. **F,** Fixation with 3.5-mm intramedullary screw.

Weber et al. documented peroneal tendon lesions precipitated by posterior antiglide plating of the lateral malleolus. In their series, 30% of patients demonstrated peroneal tendon injury at the time of implant removal. However, only 22% of these patients had symptoms preoperatively. The authors concluded that the tendon lesions correlated with distal plate placement and screw insertion through the most distal hole of the plate and therefore advocated either avoiding distal implant placement or removing the plate early.

Implant prominence also may be decreased in some lateral malleolar fractures by using a lag screw–only technique (Fig. 2.3). Several authors have reported successful treatment of lateral malleolar fractures with lag screw–only fixation, with no nonunions, loss of reduction, or soft-tissue complications. They cite less implant prominence and pain compared with patients who had plate fixation for similar injuries. Ideal candidates are patients younger than 50 years with a simple oblique lateral malleolar fracture and minimal comminution that allows the placement of two lag screws at least 1 cm apart.

Augmenting plate fixation with intramedullary Kirschner wires in osteopenic fibular fractures has been recommended in one study; 89% had minimal or no pain. In a biomechanical study, plates supplemented by Kirschner wires had an 81% greater resistance to bending than plates alone and twice the resistance to motion in torsional testing.

Operative treatment of periarticular fractures in general, ankle fractures in particular, probably is limited to two time periods: early and late. ORIF may be possible within the first 12 hours after injury but may not be possible again for 2 to 3 weeks because of excessive swelling, but this can be variable. Delayed closure and even skin grafting may be necessary when too much swelling exists at surgery. Equally good functional results have been found with immediate and delayed ORIF of Danis-Weber type B bimalleolar or bimalleolar equivalent ankle fractures, with no differences in complications, adequacy of reduction, range of motion, or operative time, although hospitalization was briefer and pain was diminished with immediate surgery in one study. Although delayed surgery may be technically more difficult, it is justified in patients with severe closed soft-tissue injury or fracture blisters. If open reduction of a fracture-dislocation is delayed, immediate closed reduction of the dislocation and splinting are mandatory to prevent skin necrosis.

SYNDESMOTIC INJURY

Injuries to the syndesmotic complex continue to be a center of controversy and continuing focus. Syndesmotic injuries are most commonly caused by pronation-external rotation, pronation-abduction and, infrequently, supination-external rotation mechanisms (Danis-Weber type C and type B injuries). These forces cause the talus to abduct or rotate externally in the mortise, leading to disruption of the syndesmotic ligaments.

Anatomic restoration of the distal tibiofibular syndesmosis is essential. If the fibular fracture is above the level of the distal tibiofibular joint, this joint is assumed to be disrupted and must be anatomically reduced. In the past, internal fixation of all syndesmotic injuries was considered mandatory, but a cadaver study showed that disruption of the syndesmosis did not cause ankle instability if no medial injury was involved. If a medial lesion was present, syndesmotic injuries extending more than 4.5 cm proximal to the ankle joint altered joint mechanics, but syndesmotic injuries extending less than 3 cm proximal to the ankle joint did not. Syndesmotic disruptions of 3.0 to 4.5 cm produced variable results. These findings suggested that syndesmotic fixation was unnecessary if the disruption extended less than 3 cm above the plafond or if the medial and the lateral injuries were stabilized by fixation of the medial malleolus or repair of the deltoid ligament.

A prospective study evaluating syndesmotic screw fixation of Weber type C ankle fractures in which the lateral malleolar fracture was located within 5 cm of the ankle joint found that syndesmotic screw fixation was not necessary if the fracture was anatomically reduced and was immobilized for 6 weeks postoperatively. This has not yet been extensively evaluated clinically, however. Others have more recently proposed an "anatomic" restoration of the syndesmosis, citing repair of the deltoid ligament and posteroinferior tibiofibular ligament to be equivalent to trans-syndesmotic fixation from a functional outcome perspective, but with improved syndesmotic reductions noted.

There is general agreement that syndesmotic fixation is indicated for (1) syndesmotic injuries associated with proximal fibular fractures for which fixation is not planned and that involve a medial injury that cannot be stabilized and (2) syndesmotic injuries extending more than 5 cm proximal to the plafond. Whether syndesmotic fixation should be used in lateral malleolar fractures located 3 to 5 cm from the ankle joint in which the medial injury (deltoid ligament) is not repaired remains controversial. If a high fibular fracture associated with a syndesmotic injury is not fixed, restoration of fibular length can be difficult to determine accurately. Furthermore, fixation of midshaft fibular fractures with associated syndesmotic injuries demonstrates improved biomechanical characteristics when compared with syndesmosis fixation alone.

The integrity of the syndesmosis can be evaluated intraoperatively by performing an external rotation stress test and Cotton test. Cotton described this test to determine incompetence of the ankle syndesmosis intraoperatively. Distraction is applied to the fibula with a bone hook to try to separate it from the tibia, to which an opposing force has been applied to prevent tibial motion. If no significant motion is noted between the distal tibia and fibula, the syndesmotic ligaments are intact. If more than 3 to 4 mm of lateral displacement occurs, syndesmotic fixation is necessary. Intraoperative radiographs should show a clear space of less than 5 mm between the medial wall of the fibula and the lateral wall of the posterior tibial malleolus. Persistent widening indicates an unreduced syndesmosis. A cadaver study showed that syndesmotic disruption, measured as posterior displacement of the fibula on an external rotation stress lateral radiograph, correlated more closely with anatomic diastasis than did displacement on stress mortise radiographs. Stark et al. recommended intraoperative external rotation stress evaluation for unstable Weber B fractures after identifying a 39% incidence of syndesmotic instability after lateral malleolar fixation.

Various methods have been used to fix the syndesmosis. Most commonly screws are inserted through the lateral malleolus and into the distal tibia. These screws not only hold the joint anatomically reduced but also stabilize the lateral buttress of the ankle mortise. If screw fixation is chosen, either one or two 3.5-mm or 4.5-mm cortical screws are necessary; both have been found to be equivalent biomechanically. Two syndesmotic screws have been found to provide more secure fixation than one screw, and the use of two screws has been suggested in large or noncompliant patients. The syndesmotic screw should be placed through both cortices of the fibula and either one or two cortices of the tibia. In a survey of members of the Orthopaedic Trauma Association and the American Orthopaedic Foot and Ankle Society, Bava et al. sought to identify the current state of syndesmotic injury management. Fifty-one percent used 3.5-mm cortical screws, 24% used 4.5-mm cortical screws, and 14% routinely used a suture fixation device. Forty-four percent used one screw, 44% used two screws, and the remainder was undecided. The most common construct was use of 3.5-mm screws engaging four cortices that were routinely removed at 3 months. Bioabsorbable screws also have been used for fixation of the syndesmosis and have shown comparable results to metallic implants. Suture bridge techniques have gained in popularity. The proposed benefit is decreased implant issues requiring secondary intervention and dynamic stabilization. Retrospective data have demonstrated some loss of syndesmotic reduction at short-term follow-up. Implant prominence and suture knot irritation can still occur. A recent meta-analysis demonstrated improved functional outcomes as well as lower rates of broken implants and syndesmotic malreduction with the use of suture button fixation when compared to traditional syndesmotic screws.

Whether and when syndesmotic screws need to be removed are controversial subjects. Recommendations in the literature range from routine removal of the screw before weight bearing is allowed (in 6 to 8 weeks) to removal after the fracture has healed only if symptoms develop. Advocates of screw removal contend that the syndesmotic fixation disrupts ankle mechanics by restricting the normal external rotation of the fibula that occurs with dorsiflexion. Removing the screw too early may allow recurrent diastasis of the syndesmosis, however. Syndesmosis displacement has been reported when the screw was removed before weight bearing was allowed, and screw breakage has been reported with weight bearing with the screw in place. If tricortical fixation is used, the screw usually loosens rather than breaks and may not disrupt normal ankle mechanics. If fixation through four cortices is used, both ends of the screw can be removed easily if breakage occurs. In general, late diastasis of the syndesmosis creates a much more difficult clinical problem than broken screws; it is advisable to leave the screw in place for at least 12 weeks. Furthermore, another study revealed that at 1-year follow-up there was no difference in clinical outcome of patients with intact or removed syndesmotic screws. In fact, the subset with broken screws had improved clinical outcomes; therefore, the authors recommended not removing intact or broken syndesmotic screws. We have transitioned toward not routinely removing syndesmotic fixation unless the ankle is symptomatic, primarily with stiffness limiting dorsiflexion. However, a recent small series has questioned the effect of syndesmotic screw removal, citing no significant improvements in dorsiflexion after implant removal.

The syndesmosis must be anatomically reduced and held with provisional Kirschner wires or a reduction clamp before the syndesmotic screws are inserted. Miller et al. noted a significant decrease in syndesmotic malreductions in a cohort of patients in whom the syndesmosis was directly viewed during reduction. We also advocate open reduction of the syndesmosis with direct viewing. The reduction can therefore be performed manually and maintained with a reduction clamp, in contrast to using the clamp to effect reduction, which can introduce rotational malreduction. The screw should be positioned 2 to 3 cm proximal to the tibial plafond, directed parallel to the joint surface, and angled 30 degrees anteriorly so that it is perpendicular to the tibiofibular joint. If the screw is placed too far proximally, it may deform the fibula and cause the mortise to widen. If the screw is not parallel to the joint, the fibula may shift proximally. If the screw is not perpendicular to the tibiofibular joint, the fibula may remain laterally displaced. The AO group recommended a fully threaded syndesmotic screw in a neutralization mode or position; however, others have suggested that a lag screw provides more secure fixation. Traditionally, it was recommended to maximally dorsiflex the ankle during syndesmotic fixation to prevent postoperative limitation of motion; however, there are data refuting this finding and noting that maximal dorsiflexion may induce an external rotation moment risking malreduction. A cadaver study found no loss of dorsiflexion when

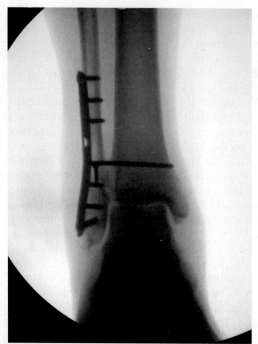

FIGURE 2.4 Fracture of fibula above level of syndesmosis, disruption of distal tibiofibular syndesmosis, and rupture of deltoid ligament. Deltoid ligament was repaired. Small fragment plate was applied to fibula, and syndesmosis was repositioned and held by transfixing screw through distal hole of fibular plate.

lag screws were used for fixation of the syndesmosis with the ankle in plantarflexion. Others have illustrated that postoperative radiographic measurements are unreliable markers of syndesmotic reduction, which is better assessed with CT.

If a small plate has been used to fix the fibular fracture, this transfixing screw can be one of the screws used to secure the plate to the lateral side of the fibula (Fig. 2.4). The reduced and fixed fibula must meet the three requirements for satisfactory function listed earlier in this section. Occasionally, the syndesmotic ligaments may avulse a small fragment of bone. If this is the case, syndesmotic stabilization can be accomplished by lag screw or minifragment fixation through this fragment.

Egol et al. evaluated outcomes after unstable ankle fractures with regard to the effects of syndesmotic fixation. They determined that at 1-year follow-up patients who underwent syndesmotic fixation had poorer outcomes than those who had malleolar fracture fixation alone.

FIXATION OF THE LATERAL MALLEOLUS

TECHNIQUE 2.1

- If the fractured fibula is part of a bimalleolar fracture pattern, we usually reduce and internally fix the lateral malleolar or fibular fracture before fixing the medial malleolar component. The exception to this is a comminuted

lateral malleolus as part of a bimalleolar or trimalleolar pattern. Occasionally, if comminution is severe, the lateral malleolus can be overreduced in the coronal plane, which inhibits anatomic reduction of the medial malleolar component of the injury. In this circumstance, it may be advisable to proceed with medial malleolar fixation initially.

- Expose the lateral malleolus and the distal fibular shaft through a lateral longitudinal incision. Protect the superficial peroneal nerve. Alternatively, a posterolateral incision can be used, and the plate can be inserted with a posterior antiglide technique. The advantage is the ability to achieve distal bicortical fixation in a posterior to anterior direction. An incision placed slightly posteriorly has the theoretical advantage of not being positioned directly over a laterally based implant; however, direct exposure of the syndesmosis (if needed) may be made increasingly difficult. Expose the fibula in extraperiosteal fashion.

- If the fracture is sufficiently oblique, if bone stock is good, and if there is no comminution, fix the fracture with one or two lag screws inserted from anterior to posterior to establish interfragmentary compression. Place the screws approximately 1 cm apart (Fig. 2.5). The length of the screws is important; the screws must engage the posterior cortex for secure fixation but must not protrude far enough posteriorly to encroach on the peroneal tendon sheaths.

- If the fracture is transverse, an intramedullary device can be used. Expose the tip of the lateral malleolus by splitting the fibers of the calcaneofibular ligament longitudinally.

- Insert a Rush rod, titanium elastic nail, interlocking fibular rod, or other intramedullary device across the fracture line into the medullary canal of the proximal fragment. If using an intramedullary device, do not tilt the lateral malleolus toward the talus. The insertion point for intramedullary fixation tends to be in line with the medullary canal of the fibula; because the intramedullary appliance is straight, the lateral malleolus may be inadvertently tilted toward the talus, resulting in narrowing of the ankle mortise and reduced motion. This mistake can be avoided by contouring the intramedullary rod.

- If the fracture is below the level of the plafond, if the distal fragment is small, and if the patient has good bone stock, use an intramedullary 3.5-mm malleolar screw for fixation. Rarely, a 4.5-mm lag screw can be used in large patients. Alternatively, orient the malleolar screw slightly obliquely to engage the medial cortex of the fibula proximal to the fracture.

- In patients with poor bone quality, place Kirschner wires obliquely from lateral to medial through the distal and proximal fibular fragments and secure them further with a tension band wire. Alternatively, precontoured periarticular locking constructs, which are now readily available, may afford increased stability.

- Anatomic reduction and maintenance of fibular length are necessary.

- If the fracture is above the level of the syndesmosis, use a small fragment, one third tubular plate for fixation after anatomic reduction has been obtained; a 3.5-mm dynamic compression plate can be used in larger individuals or for more proximal fractures. The plates can be used to supplement lag screw fixation or to span a comminuted segment. In general, place three cortical screws in the shaft of the fibula above the fracture and two or three screws distal to the fracture. Unicortical cancellous screws are placed below the level of the plafond. If the plate is placed posterolaterally, it acts as an antiglide plate. Several commercially available precontoured fixed angle distal fibular locking plates provide alternative fixation options distally, however, often at the expense of increased implant prominence.

■ Syndesmotic fixation, if necessary, can be done as described in the section on syndesmotic injuries.

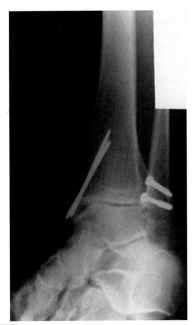

FIGURE 2.5 Bimalleolar ankle fracture with oblique fracture of lower fibula treated with interfragmentary screw fixation. Kirschner wires were used for internal fixation of medial malleolus. **SEE TECHNIQUE 2.1.**

FIXATION OF THE MEDIAL MALLEOLUS

TECHNIQUE 2.2

■ Make an anteromedial incision that begins approximately 2 cm proximal to the fracture line, extends distally and slightly posteriorly, and ends approximately 2 cm distal to the tip of the medial malleolus. We prefer this incision for two reasons: (1) the posterior tibial tendon and its sheath are less likely to be damaged, and (2) the surgeon is able to see the articular surfaces, especially the anteromedial aspect of the joint, which permits accurate alignment of the fracture and an opportunity to treat any associated impaction. However, this incision cannot be made extensile distally if associated foot injuries must be treated.

■ Handle the skin with care, reflecting the flap intact with its underlying subcutaneous tissue. The blood supply to the skin of this area is poor, and careful handling is necessary to prevent skin sloughing. Protect the greater saphenous vein and its accompanying nerve.

■ Usually the distal fragment of the medial malleolus is displaced distally and anteriorly and a small fold of periosteum commonly is interposed between the fracture surfaces. Remove this fold from the fracture site with a curet or periosteal elevator, exposing the small serrations of the fracture.

■ Debride small loose osseous or chondral fragments; large osteochondral fragments should be preserved and supported with a bone graft.

■ With a bone-holding clamp or pointed reduction tenaculum, bring the detached malleolus into the normal position, and, while holding it there, internally fix it with two 2-mm smooth Kirschner wires drilled across the fracture site as temporary fixation devices.

■ Check the fracture reduction with anteroposterior and lateral radiographs. If the reduction is satisfactory,

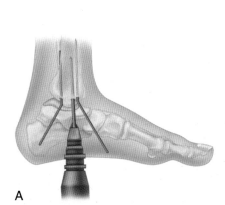

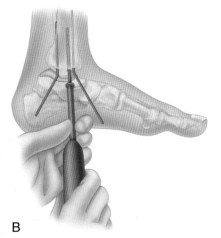

A   B

FIGURE 2.6 **A,** AO technique for internal fixation of medial malleolus. Hole (3.2 mm) is drilled while distal fragment is held reduced with two Kirschner wires bent to stay out of way. Length of hole is measured. **B,** Insertion of malleolar screw without tapping. Kirschner wires are removed after screw is tightened. If fragment tends to rotate, additional smaller screw or compression wiring can be added. **SEE TECHNIQUE 2.2.**

remove one of the Kirschner wires and insert a 4-mm lag screw; remove and replace the other Kirschner wire (Fig. 2.6). Alternatively, a drill with a 2.5- and a 3.5-mm bit can be used to create a path for the screws; a long pelvic drill bit will be necessary if bicortical lag screw fixation is chosen.

- Carefully inspect the interior of the joint, particularly at the superomedial corner, to ensure the screw has not crossed the articular surface, and to treat any associated anteromedial impaction if present.
- Use radiographs to verify the position of the screw and the fracture.
- If the medial malleolar fragment is very small or comminuted, fixation with a standard screw may be impossible; in these cases, use several Kirschner wires, minifragment screws, or tension band wiring for fixation. Large vertical fractures of the medial malleolus that involve proximal comminution often require a buttress plate to prevent loss of reduction; a small, one third tubular plate usually is sufficient. To avoid wound complications, extreme care must be taken when applying bulky implants to this area of poor skin coverage.

POSTOPERATIVE CARE The ankle is immobilized in a posterior plaster splint in neutral position and elevated. If the bone quality is good and the fixation is secure, the splint can be removed on the first postoperative visit and replaced with a removable splint or fracture boot. Range-of-motion exercises are begun. Weight bearing is restricted for 6 weeks, after which partial weight bearing can be started if the fracture is healing well and progressed accordingly.

If skin conditions, bone quality, comorbidities (e.g., diabetes), or other factors have prevented secure fixation, the fracture must be protected longer. The patient is placed in a short leg cast. The patient is not allowed to bear weight on the ankle until fracture healing is progressing well (8 to 12 weeks). A short leg walking boot is worn, and weight bearing is progressed.

DELTOID LIGAMENT TEAR AND LATERAL MALLEOLAR FRACTURE

A deltoid ligament tear accompanied by a fracture of the lateral malleolus is caused by the same mechanism that produces bimalleolar fractures, that is, supination with external rotation of the foot. Instead of the medial malleolus being fractured, however, the deltoid ligament is torn, allowing the talus to displace laterally (Fig. 2.7). Usually the anterior capsule of the ankle joint is also torn. The deltoid ligament, especially its deep branch, is important to the stability of the ankle because it prevents lateral displacement and external rotation of the talus. A deltoid ligament tear should be suspected if a fracture of the lateral malleolus is accompanied by tenderness, swelling, and hematoma on the medial side of the ankle. Historically, medial-sided ankle tenderness would lead the clinician to suspect a deltoid ligament disruption in the presence of a lateral malleolar fracture. However, it has been established that there

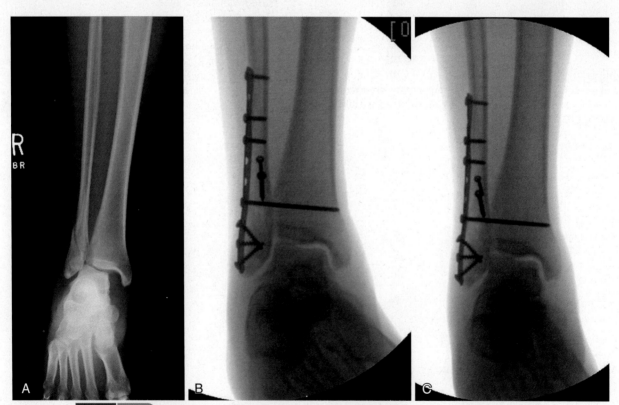

FIGURE 2.7 **A,** Lateral malleolar fracture with associated medial clear space widening and syndesmotic disruption. **B** and **C,** After surgical stabilization. Fibula is anatomically reduced and concentric tibiotalar reduction restored and maintained with a single quad-cortical syndesmotic screw.

is no statistically significant relationship between medial tenderness and deep deltoid ligament rupture. A routine anteroposterior radiograph may show no lateral displacement of the talus, but a radiograph made when the ankle is stressed into supination and external rotation shows displacement and tilting of the talus in the ankle mortise and a wide medial clear space (>4 mm). This radiograph should be obtained with the ankle in neutral position. With the ankle in plantarflexion, the narrowest portion of the talus is within the mortise, which may appear to be wide even without injury. Alternatively, a gravity external rotation stress radiograph can be obtained.

Closed treatment of these injuries is difficult because the talus tends to shift in the mortise. A 1-mm lateral shift of the talus can reduce the effective weight-bearing area of the talotibial articulation by 20% to 40%, and a 5-mm shift can reduce it by 80%. If closed treatment is chosen, the patient must be followed closely for displacement. Optimal treatment of this injury is controversial. Provided that the condition of the skin and the patient's age and general condition permit, ORIF of the fibula, with or without repair of the deltoid ligament, can be done. Nonoperative treatment also is feasible but requires careful radiographic monitoring to ensure maintenance of a congruent ankle mortise. If only the deltoid ligament tear is repaired, the talus is likely to become displaced laterally after surgery despite the use of a cast. If only the fibular fracture is repaired, the deltoid ligament may be caught between the medial malleolus and the talus, preventing accurate reduction, or the ligament may be relaxed after healing. One-year functional outcomes after nonoperative management are equivalent to ORIF of stress positive lateral malleolar fractures. However, complications may include residual medial clear space widening and lateral malleolar delayed union or nonunion.

Many surgeons advocate fixation of the fibula without routine exploration of the medial side, unless the reduction is blocked. We have found, however, that some fibers of the deltoid ligament can become trapped between the medial malleolus and the talus, even with a seemingly acceptable reduction, and this may lead to late displacement. Medial exploration requires little further surgical dissection; it allows the surgeon to ensure that the deltoid ligament has been cleared from the mortise, and it provides access for repair of the deltoid ligament if desired. We do not routinely repair the deltoid ligament and explore the medial side only in select cases, most often in injuries with a wide medial clear space and delayed presentation, because medial joint access may be required to restore a congruent tibiotalar joint.

Fractures of the lateral malleolus can be stabilized by several different methods, the most common being the use of a one third tubular plate and 3.5-mm cortical or locking screws. Long oblique fractures can be stabilized with lag screws alone. Fractures below the tibial plafond (Danis-Weber type A fracture) can be stabilized by a malleolar lag screw or with Kirschner wires and tension band fixation. We also have used oblique Kirschner wires placed from the distal fibular fragment into the tibia. Intramedullary devices can be used to stabilize transverse lateral malleolar fractures, but these rods do not prevent rotation. Interlocking intramedullary rods have been developed for the fixation of fibular fractures.

REPAIR OF THE DELTOID LIGAMENT AND INTERNAL FIXATION OF THE LATERAL MALLEOLUS

TECHNIQUE 2.3

- Make an anteromedial curved incision similar to, but slightly more distal than, the incision described for internal fixation of the medial malleolus (see Technique 2.2).
- Identify the deltoid ligament, which is composed of two parts: a fan-shaped superficial portion and a short, heavy, deep portion. The superficial portion is almost always torn across its middle or is avulsed from the medial malleolus; the fanned-out inferior attachment of this superficial portion makes an inferior tear less likely.
- Open the sheath of the posterior tibial tendon and displace the tendon to explore and repair the deep and more important portion of the deltoid ligament. This deep portion may be torn from the tip of the malleolus, avulsed from the side of the talus, or torn in the middle.
- If the deep portion has been avulsed from the medial aspect of the talus, place two No. 0 nonabsorbable sutures through the ligaments and pass these through holes drilled diagonally across the body and neck of the talus to exit in the sinus tarsi area. Leave these sutures untied until the fibular fracture has been anatomically reduced and internally fixed. Alternatively, suture anchors can be used.
- Make a lateral longitudinal incision and expose the lateral malleolus as described.
- Anatomically reduce and fix the fracture of the lateral malleolus as described previously (see Technique 2.1).
- When the lateral malleolar fracture has been rigidly fixed, snugly tie the sutures already placed in the deltoid ligament and passed through the talus.
- Close the lateral incision.
- Return to the medial side of the ankle, replace the posterior tibial tendon in its sheath, and close the sheath.
- Repair the superficial portion of the deltoid ligament with multiple interrupted, nonabsorbable sutures.
- If the entire deltoid ligament has been avulsed from the medial malleolus, drill two or three small holes in the malleolus and place interrupted sutures through them and the avulsed end of the ligament; alternatively, suture anchors can be used.
- Place the sutures in the ligament, but do not tie them before completing the fixation of the lateral malleolus because they may be torn loose during that procedure. If the lateral malleolus is fixed before these sutures are placed, repairing the ligament becomes much more difficult.

POSTOPERATIVE CARE The postoperative care is the same as that described after Technique 2.2.

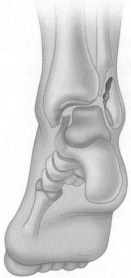

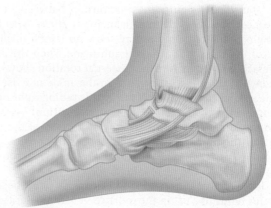

FIGURE 2.10 When deltoid ligament has been avulsed from its distal insertion, it may become reflected proximally and allow posterior tibial tendon to become interposed as shown. Spontaneous healing of ligament is impaired.

FIGURE 2.8 Deltoid ligament after being avulsed from medial malleolus may be caught between malleolus and talus.

talus and the intact medial malleolus. In this lesion, the deltoid ligament has been avulsed or torn and either the distal fibula has been fractured or the distal tibiofibular ligaments have been torn.

It may be impossible to reduce the gap by closed methods. The end of an avulsed deltoid ligament may be caught between the medial malleolus and the talus (Fig. 2.8). Less often, a deltoid ligament tear or an avulsion fracture of the tip of the medial malleolus may release the posterior tibial tendon and sometimes the tibial nerve and posterior tibial vessels and allow them to become trapped between the medial malleolus and the talus (Fig. 2.9). These obstructions must be removed surgically, and then the deltoid ligament tear or avulsion and any fracture of the lateral malleolus can be repaired (see Technique 2.1).

Occasionally, the posterior tibial tendon is interposed between the torn parts of the deltoid ligament and impairs healing (Fig. 2.10). In more severe fracture-dislocations, the posterior tibial tendon may be displaced far laterally between the distal tibia and fibula.

A lesion described by Bosworth (Fig. 2.11) may be the cause of failure to reduce a posterior fracture-dislocation of the ankle. The distal end of the proximal fragment of the fibula may be displaced posterior to the tibia and locked by the tibia's posterolateral ridge; the bone cannot be released by manipulation because of the pull of the intact interosseous membrane. The fibula is exposed, and a periosteal elevator is used to release the bone; considerable force may be necessary. The fibular fracture is fixed as described in Technique 2.1.

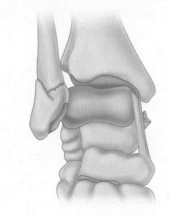

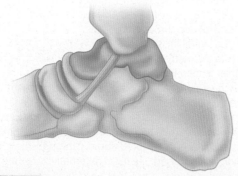

FIGURE 2.9 Trapping of posterior tibial tendon between medial malleolus and talus. Note widening of ankle mortise and avulsion fracture of medial malleolus.

IRREDUCIBLE FRACTURE OR FRACTURE-DISLOCATION

Anatomic reduction of fractures around the ankle is essential for acceptable functional results. One lesion that appears innocent but is nevertheless crippling if left untreated is the widened ankle mortise. Specifically, a widened ankle mortise is lateral displacement of the talus and the fibula that leaves an interval between the

TRIMALLEOLAR FRACTURE

Trimalleolar fractures require open reduction more often than any other type of ankle fracture. The results of treatment of trimalleolar fractures usually are not as good as the results obtained for bimalleolar fractures. Trimalleolar fractures usually are caused by an abduction or external rotation injury. In addition to fractures of the medial malleolus and fibula, the posterior lip of the articular surface of the tibia is fractured and displaced, allowing posterior and lateral displacement and external rotation with supination of the foot. The medial malleolus may remain intact, with a tear of the deltoid ligament occurring instead of a malleolar fracture.

The same principles and indications for open reduction as previously outlined for bimalleolar fractures apply to

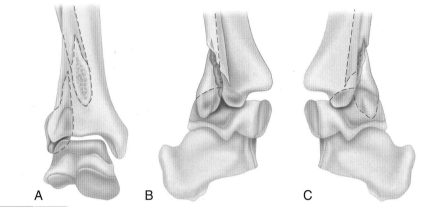

FIGURE 2.11 Bosworth fracture with entrapment of fibula behind tibia. **A,** Anteroposterior view. **B** and **C,** Lateral views.

trimalleolar fractures. Indications for open reduction of the posterior malleolus or posterior tibial fragment depend on its size, displacement, and, most important, its perceived contribution to stability of the injured ankle. A 50-degree external rotation view can be used for the most accurate assessment of the size and displacement of the posterior malleolar fragment. Historically, if the fragment of the posterior malleolus involves more than 25% to 30% of the weight-bearing surface, it should be anatomically reduced and held with internal fixation. Often, satisfactory reduction of the posterior tibial fragment, if small, occurs with anatomic and rigid fixation of the fibula because this fragment most often is posterolateral and attached to the fibula by the posterior tibiofibular ligament. Gardner et al. showed in a cadaver model that fixation of the posterior malleolus imparts syndesmotic stability to a greater extent than syndesmotic screws. If the posterior tibial fragment is small, a proximally displaced position may be of little consequence, but even the slightest posterior subluxation of the talus on the articular surface of the tibia is unacceptable. If there is a persistent step-off or gap of more than 2 to 3 mm or persistent posterior instability, open reduction is warranted. The posterior and proximal displacement of the tibial fragment creates an offset at the fracture. With the foot displaced posteriorly, this irregularity in the articular surface of the tibia is brought against the weight-bearing surface of the talus, and with motion and weight bearing severe traumatic arthritis develops. We routinely treat the posterior malleolus as part of the ankle injury complex because of its contribution to ankle stability. Very small fractures can be treated nonoperatively if ankle stability is proven, and frequently reduce well with anatomic fibular reconstruction. Our preference for larger displaced fragments is ORIF, and the decision for fixation should be made in the context of the extent of articular involvement and the expected contribution to restoring ankle stability.

POSTERIOR TIBIAL LIP FRACTURE
Fractures of the posterior lip of the tibia usually are associated with fractures of the medial and lateral malleoli, and the approach to the posterior malleolus may depend on what additional open reductions are required. Most often, an anteromedial incision is made to fix a fractured medial malleolus, and a posterolateral incision is used to fix the posterior lip of the tibia and the lateral malleolar fracture. If the posterior fragment is located more medially, a posteromedial approach can be used to treat the medial and posterior malleolar fractures. Alternatively, a separate posteromedial or posterolateral incision can be made adjacent to the Achilles tendon to allow indirect or direct reduction.

Preoperative CT scans are mandatory for evaluation of fracture morphology, including size, location, and any associated marginal impaction of the posterior malleolar fragment. The posterior lip fracture often reduces after reduction of the fibula. If this does not occur and internal fixation is necessary because of the size of the fragment or the presence of posterior instability, the posterior lip fracture should be reduced and internally fixed before reduction of either the medial or the lateral malleolus. The objective is to restore anatomically the articular surface of the distal tibia. Reduction and fixation of either malleolus reduce the distractibility of the tibial and talar joint surfaces, making exposure more difficult. Distraction of the tibiotalar joint can be increased by inserting a large Steinmann pin transversely through the calcaneus, to which a traction bow is applied. An assistant can distract the tibiotalar joint significantly using this technique if neither malleolus has been reattached. Alternatively, a large distractor may be of benefit. If the posterior malleolar fragment is small, a screw directed from posterior to anterior or a fully threaded screw placed by lag technique should be used because a partially threaded screw placed from anterior to posterior may leave screw threads crossing the fracture site. Preoperative planning, including CT scans, facilitates understanding of the orientation of the posterior malleolar segment and therefore aids in selection of an appropriate surgical approach and fixation. The frequent posterolateral position of this fragment often permits fixation through a posterolateral approach.

REDUCTION AND FIXATION OF POSTERIOR MALLEOLAR FRACTURE

TECHNIQUE 2.4

- Proper preoperative templating and review of imaging are necessary.

- The posterior malleolus can be exposed through a posteromedial incision by incising the posterior tibial tendon sheath adjacent to the posterior border of the tibia.
- Displace the medial malleolar fragment and dissect subperiosteally to gain access to the posterior malleolus. Although this approach permits direct access to a medially located posterior malleolus, fixation may be limited to screws.
- Insert two Kirschner wires 1 to 3 cm above the anterior tibial lip, directed from anterior to posterior, to engage the posterior fragment.
- When this temporary fixation has been achieved, make a hole from anterior to posterior with the appropriate size drill bit through both fragments; measure with a depth gauge; and insert a malleolar, small fragment screw, tightening the fragments together to produce interfragmentary compression (Fig. 2.12A-D).
- If a conventional screw is used, overdrill the anterior cortex so that a lag effect is achieved.
- Remove the Kirschner wires and anatomically reduce and internally fix the lateral and then the medial malleolus.
- If the posterior malleolar fragment is located more laterally, use a posterolateral incision. Make a 7.5-cm incision lateral to the Achilles tendon. Protect the sural nerve.
- Retract the Achilles tendon medially and the peroneal tendons laterally to expose the posterior malleolus.
- Establish the normal articular relationship between the talus and the tibia by anterior traction on the foot and by adduction and inversion.
- Correct the proximal displacement of the posterior lip of the tibia by placement of a joystick for manipulation and fix the fragment by inserting one or two lag screws from posterior to anterior into the tibial metaphysis, or alternatively place a posterior antiglide plate (see Fig. 2.12E), which is preferred because of its biomechanical advantage.
- After the posterior fracture has been fixed, repair the fractures of the medial and lateral malleoli as previously described (see Techniques 2.1 and 2.2).
- Carefully inspect the articular surface of the tibia through the anteromedial incision to confirm anatomic reduction of the articular surface.

POSTOPERATIVE CARE The postoperative care is the same as for internal fixation of bimalleolar fractures (see Techniques 2.1 and 2.2).

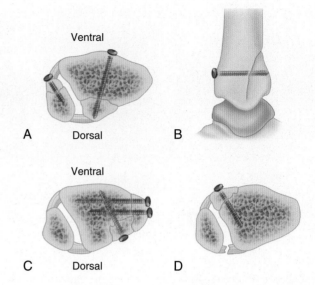

Ventral

A Dorsal B

Ventral

C Dorsal D

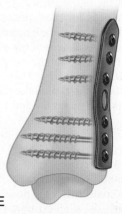

E

FIGURE 2.12 Fixation of posterior malleolar fracture. **A,** Anteroposterior 4-mm lag screw; lag screw also is used to fix avulsion fracture. **B,** Lateral view of 4-mm anteroposterior lag screw. **C,** Multiple lag screw fixation of comminuted fracture. **D,** Lag screw fixation of avulsion fracture of insertion of anterior tibiofibular ligament from distal tibia. **E,** Posterior plate fixation. (**A-D** from Johnson EE, Davlin LB: Open ankle fractures: the indications for immediate open reduction and internal fixation, *Clin Orthop Relat Res* 292:118, 1993.) **SEE TECHNIQUE 2.4.**

malleoli are treated as described previously. Surgery should be performed within the first 24 hours or delayed until the soft tissue is in good condition. CT is instrumental in preoperative templating to be prepared for treating segments of marginal impaction.

FRACTURE OF THE ANTERIOR TIBIAL MARGIN AT THE ANKLE JOINT

These fractures can be viewed as transitional fractures between traditional ankle fractures and pilon fractures, which typically are the result of axial loading. The treatment of fractures of the anterior margin of the tibia is about the same as that for the posterior margin, although in reverse. The fractures differ in one respect, however. Because fractures of the anterior margin usually are caused by a fall from a height that results in the foot and ankle being forcefully dorsiflexed, crushing of the articular surface of the tibia is likely to be more severe in these fractures. Perfect restoration of the articular surface of the tibia may be impossible. When necessary, associated fractures of the medial and lateral

REDUCTION AND FIXATION OF ANTERIOR TIBIAL MARGIN FRACTURES

TECHNIQUE 2.5

- Expose the fracture through an anterolateral incision 7.5 to 10 cm long, retract the extensor tendons medially, and continue the dissection until the entire anterior surface of the ankle joint has been exposed.

- Remove small, loose fragments of bone, preserving intact as much of the articular surface as possible.
- Reduce the anterior subluxation of the talus, appose the large anterior triangular fragment to the shaft of the tibia in its normal position, and transfix it with one or two screws or with threaded Kirschner wires if the fragments are small. If the fragment is comminuted, it may be necessary to apply a low-profile, small fragment buttress plate or span the ankle temporarily with an external fixator. Elevation of depressed articular segments can be supported with grafting.

POSTOPERATIVE CARE Postoperative care is the same as for internal fixation of bimalleolar fractures (see Technique 2.2).

ANKLE FRACTURES IN PATIENTS WITH DIABETES

Although malleolar fractures historically have been considered to be relatively benign injuries, operative treatment in patients with complicated diabetes mellitus is associated with significant complications. Significantly increased risk of unplanned readmission, unplanned reoperation, and mortality has been demonstrated. These patients often are older and may have peripheral vascular disease or peripheral neuropathy, which complicates their care. Complications have been reported to be as high as 43% compared with 15.5% in patients without diabetes. Complications may include deep and superficial infection, loss of fixation, malunion, wound necrosis, and amputation. Although diabetic patients treated nonoperatively have shown a high frequency of loss of reduction and malunion, they can be relatively minimally symptomatic. Nonoperative treatment is recommended for malleolar fractures in older diabetic patients with low functional demands. However, if surgical treatment of the ankle fracture is indicated, it should not be delayed or avoided simply because the patient is diabetic. Inadequate immobilization may lead to rapidly developing neuropathy. If the ankle fracture is nondisplaced or minimally displaced and has a stable configuration, closed management with prolonged casting is an acceptable alternative, but only with close supervision. If the fracture is displaced, and either considerable manipulation is necessary to reduce it or molding is required to maintain the reduction, an open approach with internal fixation is recommended. Regardless of the method of treatment, prolonged immobilization often is necessary to prevent the development of neuropathic complications.

In contrast, a study by Guo et al. compared patients with preoperatively neglected type 2 diabetes and a nondiabetic matched cohort and found no significant increase in postoperative infection after immediate operative stabilization of closed ankle fractures. Jones et al. demonstrated that operatively treated ankle fractures in diabetic patients without comorbidities had comparable complication rates to nondiabetic patients. The presence of diabetic comorbidities and, in particular, a history of Charcot arthropathy increased the likelihood of complications. In one large series, Costigan et al.

reported 84 patients who underwent ORIF for acute closed ankle fractures. Open fractures, insulin dependence, patient age, and fracture type affected outcome, and 83% of patients with absent pedal pulses and 92% of patients with preoperative neuropathy developed complications. Others have shown that operatively treated ankle fractures in diabetic patients are associated with higher rates of mortality and length of hospital stay, as well as total hospital charges. Ayoub reported the results of tibiotalar arthrodesis in 17 diabetic patients with unstable bimalleolar ankle fractures complicated by Charcot arthropathy. Results were better with surgery within 3 to 6 months of onset, with absence of dense peripheral neuropathy, and in patients with satisfactory extremity oxygenation. Amputation was required in 17.6% of patients.

We typically use standard fixation techniques in patients with controlled diabetes and unstable ankle fractures. However, in certain patients who are deemed at increased risk for fixation failure, the fixation strategy may be modified in the interest of obtaining rigid fixation. These include bicortical medial malleolar fixation, placement of multiple transfibular or transtibial syndesmotic position screws, adjuvant external fixation, and application of locking plate technology (Fig. 2.13).

OPEN ANKLE FRACTURES

Open ankle fractures caused by indirect injury are two to four times more likely to be open medially than laterally. Several studies have shown the advantages of primary internal fixation of open ankle fractures, including Gustilo type III wounds, compared with either closed immobilization with delayed fixation or immediate provisional fixation with Kirschner wires. We also prefer immediate internal fixation after surgical debridement. If the wound is severely contaminated, a temporary external fixator can be placed spanning the ankle and open reduction can be done when the wound is judged to be clean and swelling has decreased. Ngcelwane noted dirt and grass at the syndesmosis in some medial wounds, possibly sucked in by the vacuum created by dislocation of the ankle; he recommended a lateral incision for cross irrigation, especially for displaced Danis-Weber types B and C fractures with gas shadows. In addition to internal fixation, a temporary external fixator that spans the ankle joint can be used to make wound care easier. The fixator can be removed when soft-tissue healing is complete.

Although most patients (80%) can be expected to return to work after the fracture has healed, only approximately 18% return to their preinjury recreational level. The rate of deep infection in open ankle fractures is approximately 5%. We have found that open ankle fractures, especially fracture-dislocations, in diabetic patients, especially patients with neuropathy, are problematic and frequently become infected or have implant failure, sometimes resulting in amputation. Supplemental external fixation is advisable in these patients.

UNSTABLE ANKLE FRACTURE-DISLOCATION

Childress described a method that may be useful for unstable fracture-dislocations in the ankle when the usual treatment is inadvisable. This situation most often arises when an abrasion or superficial infection is present where an incision usually would be made for open reduction. Childress recommended this technique only as a last resort but found it useful several times. The ankle is stabilized by a pin inserted through the calcaneus into the medullary canal of the tibia. Our preferred

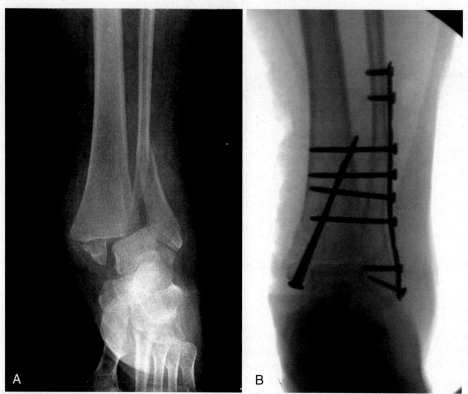

FIGURE 2.13 **A,** Elderly patient with osteoporosis, diabetes mellitus, and peripheral neuropathy who sustained an open comminuted bimalleolar ankle fracture-dislocation. **B,** After debridement, fracture is definitively treated with internal fixation. Because of patient's poor bone quality, multiple transfibular/transtibial screws were used to increase fixation purchase.

method of stabilization is application of a uniplanar external fixator with inclusion of the forefoot if warranted to prevent forefoot equinus posturing should a frame become necessary for definitive management. Use of a percutaneous tibiotalocalcaneal pin has been reserved for very rare instances in which existing implants preclude external fixation placement and stability is necessary for soft-tissue protection. We have modified the procedure so that the pin is directed to exit the anterior distal tibial metaphysis to facilitate later extraction should the implant fail. This pin can be directed from the calcaneal tuberosity, posterior to the talus, to enter the distal tibia, therefore remaining extra articular. We have used this technique to supplement more standard fixation when the patient is at risk for equinus contracture of the ankle or for stabilization of an injury before debridements.

STABILIZATION OF UNSTABLE ANKLE FRACTURE-DISLOCATION

TECHNIQUE 2.6

(CHILDRESS)
- Tape a Kirschner wire longitudinally on the medial side of the ankle exactly in the midline.

- Reduce the fracture-dislocation and obtain anteroposterior and lateral radiographs of the ankle.
- Using the Kirschner wire as seen in the radiograph as a guide, insert a 2.8-mm, smooth Steinmann pin in the midline on the sole 2.5 cm posterior to the calcaneocuboid joint and aim it toward the center of the tibia.
- Advance the pin about 10 cm into the distal tibia and check the position of it and the fragments by radiographs. Leave 1.3 cm of the pin protruding through the sole and pad it well.
- Apply a long leg cast that does not incorporate the end of the pin.

POSTOPERATIVE CARE The cast is removed at 4 to 6 weeks, and a short cast is applied. The pin is removed at 4 to 8 weeks, depending on the stage of healing and the original stability of the fracture. Weight bearing is not allowed until the pin has been removed, and then only as healing progresses.

TIBIAL PILON FRACTURE

Tibial pilon fractures encompass a spectrum of skeletal injury ranging from fractures caused by low-energy rotational forces to those precipitated by high-energy axial compression forces usually resulting from motor vehicle accidents or falls from a height. Rotational variants typically have a more favorable prognosis, whereas high-energy fractures frequently are

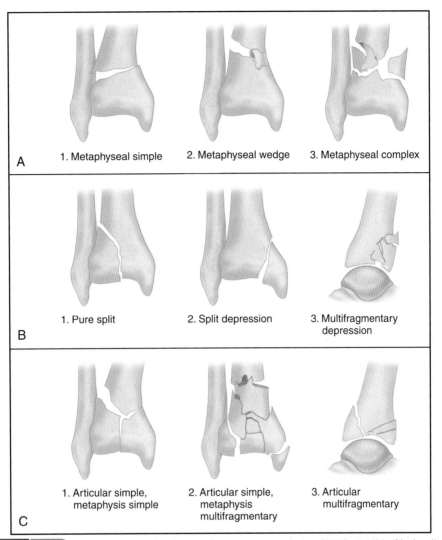

A
1. Metaphyseal simple   2. Metaphyseal wedge   3. Metaphyseal complex

B
1. Pure split   2. Split depression   3. Multifragmentary depression

C
1. Articular simple, metaphysis simple   2. Articular simple, metaphysis multifragmentary   3. Articular multifragmentary

FIGURE 2.14 Classification of Orthopaedic Trauma Association (OTA). **A,** Tibia/fibula, distal extraarticular. **B,** Tibia/fibula, distal, partial articular. **C,** Tibia/fibula complete articular. (From Orthopaedic Trauma Association Committee for Coding and Classification: Fracture and dislocation compendium, *J Orthop Trauma* 10(Suppl 1):1, 1996.)

associated with open wounds or severe, closed, soft-tissue trauma. The fracture may have significant metaphyseal or articular comminution or diaphyseal extension. Classification of these fractures is important in determining their prognosis and choosing the optimal treatment. The fibula is fractured in 85% of these patients, and the degree of talar injury varies.

Rotational fracture of the ankle can be viewed as a continuum, progressing from single malleolar fractures to bimalleolar fractures to fractures involving the distal tibial articular surface. Lauge-Hansen described a pronation-dorsiflexion injury that produces an oblique medial malleolar fracture, a large anterior lip fracture, a supraarticular fibular fracture, and a posterior tibial fracture. Giachino and Hammond described a fracture caused by a combination of external rotation, dorsiflexion, and abduction that consisted of an oblique fracture of the medial malleolus and an anterolateral tibial plafond fracture. These fractures generally have little comminution, no significant metaphyseal involvement, and minimal soft-tissue injury. They can be treated similarly to other ankle fractures with internal fixation of the fibula and lag screw

fixation of the distal tibial articular surface through limited surgical approaches.

Classification systems have been devised to describe more accurately the wide range of distal tibial articular fractures. The AO/OTA classification system provides a comprehensive description of distal tibial fractures. Type A fractures are extraarticular distal tibial fractures, which are subdivided into groups A1, A2, and A3, based on the amount of metaphyseal comminution. Type B fractures are partial articular fractures in which a portion of the articular surface remains in continuity with the shaft; these are subdivided into groups B1, B2, and B3, based on the amount of articular impaction and comminution. Type C fractures are complete metaphyseal fractures with articular involvement; these are subdivided into groups C1, C2, and C3, based on the extent of metaphyseal and articular comminution (Fig. 2.14).

Another commonly used system is that proposed by Rüedi and Allgöwer, which divides plafond fractures into three categories. Type I fractures are nondisplaced cleavage fractures that involve the joint surface; type II fractures have cleavage-type fracture lines with displacement of the articular surface but minimal comminution; type III fractures are associated with metaphyseal and articular comminution.

Studies have shown these classification systems to have only moderate interobserver reliability; nevertheless, they have proved to have some prognostic value. Treatment of fractures with little displacement or comminution (Rüedi and Allgöwer type I and type II spiral fractures) has yielded much better functional results with far fewer complications than treatment of the more severe fracture patterns (Rüedi and Allgöwer type III, AO types B3 and C3).

Intraarticular fractures of the distal tibia have been treated by a variety of methods, including plaster immobilization, traction, lag screw fixation, ORIF with plates, and external fixation with or without limited internal fixation. A variety of external fixators have been used: traditional half-pin fixators spanning the ankle, articulated half-pin fixators that allow ankle motion, half-pin fixators that do not span the ankle, and hybrid fixators that combine tensioned wires with half-pins in the tibial diaphysis and do not span the ankle joint. Hybrid frames may be composed of rings proximally and distally (Ilizarov, Monticell-Spinelli).

As a result of disappointing results after acute definitive management, staged protocols have been advocated consisting of temporary external fixation spanning the ankle joint, followed by ORIF with plates and screws after the condition of the soft tissues has improved, usually 2 to 3 weeks after injury. Percutaneous or minimally invasive plating techniques have been developed. Primary arthrodesis has been performed in selected severe fractures with extensive articular comminution and talar injury. In these patients, functional results are likely to be poor with attempts at anatomic restoration, which may not be feasible. There is some overlap in the indications for these differing methods of treatment. The surgeon's preference and experience should play a role in preoperative decision making.

Several variables must be considered when devising a treatment strategy. One must understand the mechanism of injury because this can reflect on the amount of associated soft-tissue damage. The fracture type should be determined according to the amount and location of displacement, comminution, impaction, and diaphyseal involvement. Fracture extension into the tibial diaphysis and ipsilateral fractures of the foot or tibia may influence the choice of treatment. Some authors have advocated early limited fixation of the fracture extensions into the diaphyseal region for certain fractures to facilitate later staged reconstruction. Radiographs of the contralateral ankle may be beneficial as a template for articular reconstruction.

In addition to plain radiographs, CT scans are extremely useful for determining accurately the direction of fracture lines, the size and displacement of articular fragments, and the extent of articular comminution and impaction. CT scans also are useful in planning surgical incisions and trajectory for screw or fine wire fixation. Traction can be applied using a calcaneal traction pin and Bohler frame or a uniplanar spanning external fixator. Radiographs in traction show the extent to which the articular surface can be reduced by ligamentotaxis. As a result, typically the CT scan should be obtained after the application of an external fixator. Unless a form of external fixation may be considered as definitive treatment, an acutely chosen preoperative CT scan can assist in planning

placement of limited internal fixation. Any impacted segments need to be reduced by open or limited open methods. Anatomic reduction may be impossible in some severely comminuted fractures.

The severity of soft-tissue injury should be clearly defined. Open injuries can be classified according to the Gustilo system. Although less obvious than open wounds, closed soft-tissue injuries can be quite severe and can adversely affect the functional outcome, especially if unrecognized.

The extremity should be examined carefully for signs of vascular injury, swelling, fracture blisters, soft-tissue crushing, closed degloving, and compartment syndrome. Blood-filled fracture blisters indicate more extensive cutaneous damage than blisters filled with clear fluid. The Tscherne classification system can be used to describe closed soft-tissue injury. Patient characteristics, such as smoking, alcoholism, peripheral vascular disease, and diabetes, should also be considered.

The ultimate goals of tibial pilon fracture management are restoring an anatomic articular surface, restoring mechanical alignment, maintaining joint stability, achieving fracture union, and regaining functional and pain-free weight bearing and motion, while avoiding complications. Ideal results are not attainable in some patients because of the severity of articular comminution and soft-tissue injury or comorbidities. Poor prognostic indicators are articular comminution (AO C3 and Rüedi-Allgöwer type III fracture), talar injury, severe soft-tissue injury, poor reduction of the articular surface, unstable fixation, and postoperative wound infection.

Many investigators have reported poorer results in the more severe fracture patterns. Anatomic reduction has a better prognosis than a fair or poor reduction but does not guarantee a good result. Some degree of arthrosis has been shown to develop in anatomic reductions; however, in fair or poor reductions (>2 mm of displacement), more severe arthrosis can be expected. In a series of 37 AO type B3 and C3 fractures treated with external fixation and delayed internal fixation of the articular surface, Dickson, Montgomery, and Field identified a subset of patients with "ground-glass" comminution, which was defined as more than three pieces of articular surface less than 2 mm in size seen on CT scan. Posttraumatic arthritis developed in 10 (38%) of the 26 ankles with ground-glass comminution and in none of the ankles without it. Overall, 17% of anatomically reduced fractures (5 of 29) developed arthritis, whereas five of seven nonanatomically reduced fractures developed arthritis.

In recent years, there has been a greater emphasis on functional outcome. Although there is no disagreement that anatomic reduction is desirable, the impact of anatomic reduction on overall outcome is less clear. An analysis of the effect of severity of injury and fracture reduction on clinical outcome found no correlation with clinical ankle score. In addition, no correlation has been found between radiographic arthrosis and clinical results. Williams et al. found that although radiographic arthrosis was related to injury severity and quality of reduction, there was no significant relationship between these variables and the 36-Item Short Form Health Survey (SF-36) score, clinical ankle score, or return to work. Functional outcome was more closely related to socioeconomic factors. Patients with a higher level of education were more likely to return to work and had higher ankle scores. The predictors of clinical outcome seem to be multifactorial and are not fully understood.

Other studies have found pilon fractures to have a negative long-term effect on general health as measured by the SF-36. Stiffness, swelling, persistent pain, and the use of an ambulatory aid were some of the reasons. Forty-three percent of previously employed patients were no longer employed, and of this subgroup, 68% attributed their inability to work to the pilon fracture. Poorer results were correlated with having two or more comorbidities and treatment with external fixation. Fractures treated with external fixation had more impairment of range of motion and worse pain scores than fractures treated with ORIF. External fixation tended to be used in more severe injuries (AO type C).

Factors to consider in the formulation of a treatment plan include the fracture pattern, soft-tissue injury, patient comorbidities, fixation resources, and surgical experience. The degree of articular comminution, talar damage, and soft-tissue injury is dictated by the injury; however, the surgeon does have some influence over other prognostic factors. The goal should be to obtain the best possible articular reduction and axial alignment while respecting the soft tissues. If the articular surface does not reduce by ligamentotaxis, some form of open reduction usually is indicated after the soft tissues have recovered. Fracture union can be enhanced by bone grafting areas of impaction, bone loss, or extensive metaphyseal comminution. The frequency of wound healing problems and infection can be decreased by recognizing open and closed soft-tissue injury and not operating through compromised soft tissue. In some cases, the surgeon must achieve a balance between the goals of anatomic reduction and prevention of wound complications. Anatomic reduction often is more difficult to achieve after a delay of 2 to 3 weeks; however, surgical incisions through swollen, contused soft tissues can lead to disastrous results, which may require free tissue transfer or even amputation.

Nondisplaced fractures, such as AO types A1, B1, and C1, have been treated successfully with operative and nonoperative methods. These are the only fracture types in which cast immobilization alone may be suitable. If casting is chosen, the patient should be observed closely for displacement, and weight bearing should be restricted for at least 8 to 12 weeks if the joint is nonarthritic. Calcaneal traction alone often is helpful in temporarily stabilizing severe fractures associated with soft-tissue swelling, but it seldom is used for definitive treatment. External fixation accomplishes the same goal of fracture reduction through ligamentotaxis and allows the patient to be mobilized. Limited fixation with 3.5- or 4.0-mm screws, inserted after either percutaneous or limited open reduction, combined with external fixation or minimally invasive plating techniques may be adequate treatment for AO types B1, B2, and stable C1 fractures.

■ OPEN REDUCTION AND PLATE FIXATION

For displaced fractures, operative treatment has been found to be superior to nonoperative treatment. Rüedi and Allgöwer popularized the technique of ORIF with plates and screws for tibial pilon fractures in the 1960s. This technique follows the AO principles of anatomic reduction, rigid stabilization, and early motion. The fibula is reduced first and stabilized with a plate. Then the articular surface of the tibia is reduced and provisionally fixed with Kirschner wires through an anteromedial incision. Metaphyseal defects are filled with bone graft, and the fracture is stabilized with a medial buttress plate. Rüedi and Allgöwer reported 70 good or excellent results in 75 fractures treated with this method. Only three fractures were open, and almost half were low-energy, sport-related injuries.

In the 1980s to the mid-1990s, series involving larger percentages of open and high-energy injuries reported far fewer successful results and a high incidence of complications with this technique, especially in Rüedi and Allgöwer type III (AO type C3) fractures. When complications occur, they can be devastating. Free tissue transfer often is necessary to salvage the extremity, and the final result in some cases is amputation. Satisfactory results in Rüedi and Allgöwer types I and II fractures have been reported to be between 60% and 82% and 37% and 40% in type III fractures treated with ORIF, respectively. Infection rates after type III fractures have been reported to be 12.5% to 37%.

Plate and screw fixation has been associated with more frequent wound breakdown and infection than in similar fractures treated with external fixation. Watson et al. reported more excellent and good results at 5-year follow-up with external fixation (81%) than with open plating (75%) in 94 pilon fractures. They based their treatment choices on the severity of the soft-tissue injury: Tscherne grade 0 and grade I were treated with plating, and grade II and grade III and open fractures were treated with external fixation.

■ TWO-STAGE DELAYED OPEN REDUCTION AND INTERNAL FIXATION

The high incidence of wound complications after ORIF of pilon fractures reported in the 1980s and in the early to mid-1990s is attributable to operating through a poor soft-tissue envelope. In an effort to improve overall results, protocols for staged ORIF were developed, and these have decreased the frequency of wound complications and infections associated with plating of pilon fractures. Initially, the fibula is plated and an external fixator is placed, spanning the ankle. Preoperatively, the proposed incision for tibial reduction is planned and the fibular incision is placed so that the skin bridge between the two incisions is at least 7 cm, although smaller soft-tissue bridges have been shown to be tolerable. If the soft tissue overlying the fibula is compromised, fibular plating should be delayed. External fixation pins should be placed well away from planned incisions and out of the zone of injury and potential plate fixation.

Watson et al. described a two-pin "traveling traction" type of external fixator that is useful in this situation. An AO delta frame spanning the ankle or a medial half-pin fixator consisting of one half-pin in the talus, one half-pin in the calcaneus, and two half-pins in the tibial shaft have been recommended; however, the use of a talar pin may compromise certain surgical approaches. Tibial pilon open reduction is done after the soft tissues have improved and swelling has decreased (usually between 10 and 21 days). Skin wrinkling and healing of fracture blisters are clinical indicators of improved soft-tissue condition. Careful soft-tissue handling and low-profile plates are recommended. When the soft-tissue swelling has significantly diminished, anatomic reduction and internal fixation can be done with fewer wound complications than with early ORIF.

Several authors have recommended staged protocols for treatment of complex pilon fractures with severe soft-tissue injuries. Patterson and Cole described immediate fibular fixation and placement of a medial spanning external fixator, followed at an average 24 days later by removal of the fixator and ORIF. Of 22 type C3 pilon fractures, 21 healed within an average of 4.2 months with no infections or soft-tissue complications. These authors cited as advantages of this protocol (1) better soft-tissue management, because the first stage aims to obtain anatomic fibular realignment and restore anatomic length of the distal tibia with little disruption of the soft tissues, and (2) the ability to obtain anatomic realignment of the articular surface under direct vision in the second stage. Disadvantages include the need for a large soft-tissue dissection initially and the difficulty of reduction techniques and maneuvers in a fracture 3 weeks or more after injury. Patterson and Cole also cautioned against creating large soft-tissue dissections and bone stripping.

Blauth et al. compared three different treatment methods in 51 patients with predominantly AO type C pilon fractures. They found no significant difference among the methods in regard to soft-tissue infection. There was no statistical correlation between arthritis and soft-tissue injury or treatment group. There was a trend toward better range of motion, less pain, more frequent return to previous occupation, and increased ability to return to leisure activities in the staged treatment group; however, it was not statistically significant. Based on these results, the authors stated a preference for the staged procedure in patients with severe soft-tissue compromise that involved limited screw fixation of the articular surface through stab incisions and spanning external fixation followed by a less invasive plating technique after soft-tissue healing.

Most pilon injuries are treated in staged fashion owing to the reported decrease in associated complications. However, investigation continues to further our understanding of these difficult fractures in an effort to minimize soft-tissue complications and maximize treatment results. Graves et al. revealed that the larger soft-tissue envelope associated with obesity resulted in a trend toward increased wound complications. White et al. evaluated 95 OTA 43.C-type tibial pilon fractures, 88% of which were managed within 48 hours of injury, and found results comparable to those previously reported for other treatment modalities. The lateral approach has been advocated for treating certain fracture patterns in a staged fashion, as have combined posteromedial and posterolateral approaches. Boraiah et al. reported outcomes of open pilon fractures treated with ORIF in a staged fashion. Despite a 3% and 5% deep and superficial infection rate, respectively, functional outcome scoring for most patients was poor. Harris et al. determined that patients sustaining a type C3 fracture developed more complications, required secondary interventions, and had worse functional scoring at a mean follow-up of 98 months.

PLATING TECHNIQUE

Open anatomic reduction and rigid fixation with plate and screw devices can be used effectively to treat tibial pilon fractures if strict attention is paid to fracture reduction and soft-tissue management. This technique is suitable for low-energy fractures with large displaced fragments, little comminution, and no diaphyseal extension (Fig. 2.15). An extremity with minimal swelling and a good soft-tissue envelope is of paramount importance if complications are to be prevented. Skin wrinkling is a good indication that edema has subsided. Soft-tissue handling must be meticulous, and strict "no-touch" techniques have been advocated. The most prudent course is temporization with placement of an external fixator until the soft tissues can be definitively treated. Formal open plating techniques should be used cautiously in open fractures and Rüedi and Allgöwer type III fractures (AO type C3) because of the high reported incidences of poor results and complications.

MINIMALLY INVASIVE PLATING

In an effort to decrease the wound complications associated with traditional open plating techniques, less invasive methods of plating have been developed. The fracture is primarily reduced by ligamentotaxis, and further reduction and plating are performed through limited incisions. Open medial plating has been found to disrupt the blood supply of the distal tibia to a greater extent than percutaneous plating, which might predispose to delayed union or nonunion.

Borens et al. reported their results in 17 patients treated with minimally invasive plating of selected tibial pilon fractures with a low-profile medial plate. All fractures healed. Results were rated as excellent in eight patients (47%), fair in seven patients (41%), and poor in two patients (12%). The authors concluded that this technique was effective and reduced soft-tissue complications associated with open plating of pilon fractures. They advocated the use of this technique in a staged protocol.

Minimally invasive plating techniques have been further enhanced with the widespread development of precontoured locking-plate technology, particularly those with outriggers to target proximal fixation. We do not routinely perform open reduction of the fibular component during the initial setting and prefer to maintain length through application of an external fixator alone, particularly if the fibular fracture is highly comminuted. Alternatively, a small anterolateral surgical approach can be used for articular reduction and then fixation can be done in submuscular fashion and proximal fixation percutaneously positioned. This can be done with a medially based large distractor for facilitation of reduction. The anterolateral approach is described in other chapter. Care must be taken to ensure adequate soft-tissue bridging if a separate incision is necessary to treat the fibula. When the anterolateral approach is used, a separate incision occasionally is needed to place a percutaneous small medial plate if the fracture pattern demands.

Understanding the typical morphology of tibial pilon fractures is paramount to devising an appropriate reduction strategy, whether the fibula is fixed acutely or not. Mapping of tibial pilon fractures has revealed characteristic fracture fragments that can be identified in most fractures. These consist of anterolateral, medial, and posterolateral fragments, with a central component that may be significantly comminuted. As with many ankle fractures, reduction of the fibular component can improve the reduction of the posterior fragment. These fragments must be recognized whether a formal open or a limited technique is used. With open approaches, the reduction sequence (after fixation of the fibula in many cases) begins posteriorly and then progresses medially, followed by central reduction, and finally the anterolateral fragment.

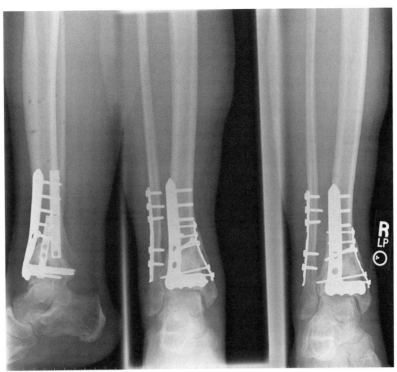

FIGURE 2.15   Plate and screw fixation of distal tibial and fibular fractures.

STAGED MINIMALLY INVASIVE OPEN REDUCTION AND INTERNAL FIXATION

TECHNIQUE 2.7

Stage 1
- Place the patient supine on a radiolucent operating table and place a tourniquet.
- For ORIF, make a standard posterolateral incision.
- Reduce the fracture, and fix the fibula with a one third tubular plate.
- Close the wound with 3-0 nylon.
- Place a triangular external fixator spanning the ankle joint.
- Place two pins proximally in the anteromedial aspect of the tibia and place one threaded pin through the calcaneus.
- Using ligamentotaxis and the reestablished lateral column, the pilon fracture is temporarily reduced and secured (Fig. 2.16).

Stage 2
- Definitive reconstruction can be done as soon as healing of the soft tissues permits, typically as judged by the return of skin wrinkling.
- Place the patient supine on a radiolucent table with a tourniquet. If preoperative planning has shown that percutaneous plating is impossible, reduce articular surfaces through a limited anterior arthrotomy, chosen by the location of primary fracture lines, which can also allow bone grafting or application of a small anterior plate or both.
- If percutaneous plating is possible, estimate the length of the plate based on preoperative films. Place the plate on the skin while checking the position with fluoroscopy.

- Contour the plate to fit on the anteromedial aspect of the distal tibia. After bending and twisting the plate using plate benders, check the anticipated position using fluoroscopy.
- Make one anteromedial incision at the proximal end of the anticipated plate position and one at the distal end.
- Make a tunnel connecting these two incisions in an extraperiosteal fashion by advancing a clamp from distal to proximal or from proximal to distal.
- Tie a strong suture (e.g., Ethibond No. 5) through the first hole in the plate. Use the Kelly clamp to help pull the plate through the subcutaneous tunnel under radiographic control. Through small stab incisions, fix the plate with 3.5-mm cortical low-profile screws. Locking screws may be used if a bridge plate construct is deemed necessary.
- If necessary, place a cortical screw through the midportion of the plate. Because the plate is flexible, good bone-plate contact can be achieved (Fig. 2.17).
- When final radiographic control shows adequate reduction and fixation, remove the external fixator.
- Deflate the tourniquet and obtain hemostasis. Close the wound over drains in standard layered fashion.
- Place a bulky cotton dressing with a posterior plaster splint to maintain the ankle in neutral position.

POSTOPERATIVE CARE Postoperatively, the limb is immobilized with the use of a splint. Closed suction drains are typically removed on postoperative day 1 or 2. Depending on the rigidity of fixation, splint immobilization is discontinued as wound healing permits. Passive and active range-of-motion exercises are then initiated. Sutures are removed between 2 and 3 weeks postoperatively. Full weight bearing is not permitted until full bony healing is confirmed radiographically, usually by 12 weeks.

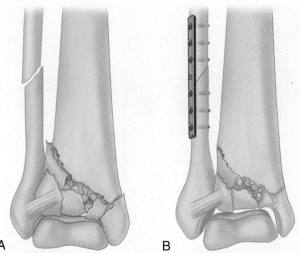

FIGURE 2.16 **A,** Comminuted pilon fracture with fibular fracture. **B,** Fibular length is restored and secured with six-hole plate as first step in reconstruction of pilon fracture. (From deSouza LJ: Fractures and dislocations about the ankle. In Gustilo RB, Kyle RF, Templeman DC, editors: *Fractures and dislocations*, St. Louis, 1993, Mosby.) **SEE TECHNIQUE 2.7.**

If minimally invasive techniques are not deemed appropriate for the fracture pattern, open techniques should be used. Similar to the technique above, once the soft-tissue envelope is appropriate after staged external fixation, the surgeon can embark on definitive fixation. The selected surgical approach should take into account the primary fracture lines or "lines of access" to effect the reduction with the most direct access to minimize soft-tissue undermining. This may consist of multiple smaller surgical incisions. Multiple surgical approaches have been described for definitive fixation, the most common being anterolateral and anteromedial.

■ POSTEROLATERAL APPROACH TO PILON FRACTURES

Alternatives to the traditional anteromedial approach for ORIF of pilon fractures have been advocated in an attempt to reduce the incidence of soft-tissue complications. The interval is between the peroneal tendons and the flexor hallucis longus. A thicker soft-tissue envelope overlying the plate (flexor hallucis longus muscle) was thought to potentially decrease problems with wound healing and deep infection. A disadvantage of this approach is poor exposure of the ankle joint, which limits its utility in fractures with anterior comminution. Some authors suggest the posterolateral approach should be considered as an alternative surgical approach in fractures that can be effectively reduced posteriorly.

Bhattacharyya examined the complications associated with the use of the posterolateral approach for pilon fractures in 19 patients. Complications occurred in nine of the 19 patients. Six patients (31%) had wound problems (three superficial infections, three deep infections). Four patients (21%) had nonunions (two aseptic, two infected), three patients required ankle arthrodesis, and one patient had a 3-mm step-off. The authors concluded that the posterolateral approach did not reduce the incidence of wound complications compared with

other approaches. They recommended this surgical approach only for pilon fractures in which the articular displacement and comminution are predominantly located posteriorly or when an anterior approach is not recommended because of the condition of the soft tissues.

The posterolateral approach is rarely indicated as the sole approach for management of pilon injuries. Instead, it can be a component of an overall strategy to treat these injuries. Some have advocated its use early in the treatment of the fibula and posterior fragment. Definitive ORIF of the plafond from a staged anterior-based approach has the benefit of a stable posterior column to serve as the base for reconstruction.

POSTEROLATERAL APPROACH TO PILON FRACTURES

TECHNIQUE 2.8

- With the patient under general anesthesia, remove the temporary external fixator that was previously placed. Administer antibiotics preoperatively.
- Place the patient prone and exsanguinate the extremity and inflate the tourniquet.
- Make a posterolateral incision into the distal tibia between the peroneal tendons and flexor hallucis longus, adjacent to the Achilles tendon. The approach can be carried proximally if needed.
- Identify and protect the sural nerve.
- Apply a femoral distractor if necessary to gain length or view the joint. Apply the distractor through new pins in the tibia to the calcaneus (Fig. 2.18).
- If necessary, plate the fibula through the same incision and fix with a 3.5-mm one third tubular plate.
- Obtain articular reduction by direct manipulation of the fracture fragments through the fracture sites under direct exposure. Confirm reduction with fluoroscopy.
- Fix the articular fragments with 3.5-mm lag screws or 4.0-mm cancellous screws.
- For the metaphyseal component of the injury, apply an appropriate plate for the injury type. C-type injuries typically require a 3.5-mm plate. B-type injuries can be treated with lower-profile implants placed in an antiglide fashion.
- For large bone defects caused by comminution, consider using iliac crest bone grafting or appropriate bone graft substitutes.
- Perform wound closure in standard layered fashion and consider insertion of a subfascial closed suction drain.

POSTOPERATIVE CARE The leg is splinted and elevated for 48 hours. We routinely place a closed suction drain postoperatively for posterolateral approaches. Early ankle motion is encouraged with physical therapy once the wound permits and sutures have been removed. Weight bearing begins at 12 weeks when radiographs permit.

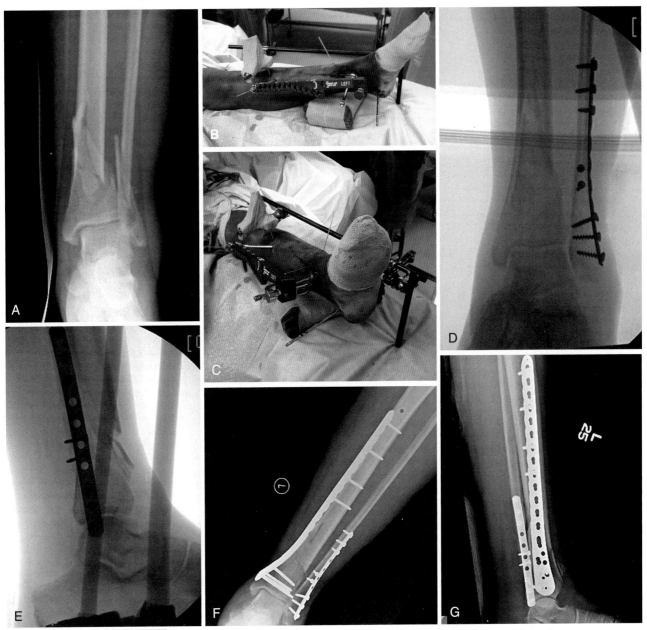

FIGURE 2.17 **A,** Closed, comminuted fracture involving tibial pilon and fibula. **B** and **C,** Application of uniplanar external fixation and fibular ORIF facilitates indirect reduction of distal tibial comminution. **D-G,** After healing of soft tissues, patient returned for definitive fixation with limited open reduction and minimally invasive plate osteosynthesis. **SEE TECHNIQUE 2.7.**

◼ COMBINED INTERNAL AND EXTERNAL FIXATION

In response to reports of unacceptable results with plating of high-energy tibial pilon fractures with traditional techniques, external fixation combined with limited internal fixation of the fibula and articular surface of the tibia has been advocated as an alternative approach. Reports of external fixation combined with limited internal fixation for tibial pilon fractures have shown a decreased incidence of infection compared with similar fractures treated with plate and screw devices. However, a 20% incidence of pin complications and wound healing problems over the fibular incision were noted in one study.

In a long-term follow-up study (5 to 12 years) by Marsh et al., of 35 pilon fractures treated with monolateral spanning external fixation, reduction was rated as good in 14, fair in 15, and poor in 6. Osteoarthrosis was grade 0 in 3, grade 1 in 6, grade 2 in 20, and grade 3 in 6. Arthrosis was correlated with severity of injury and quality of reduction but did not correlate with clinical result (15 excellent, 10 good, and 7 poor). Fifteen patients rated their outcome as excellent, 10 as good, 7 as fair, and 1 as poor. Most patients (27 of 31) were unable to run.

Another study by Dickson et al. of 37 high-energy tibial pilon fractures (AO B3 and C3) treated by spanning external fixation and a second-stage open reduction of the articular surface at 10 to 21 days reported 81% good and excellent

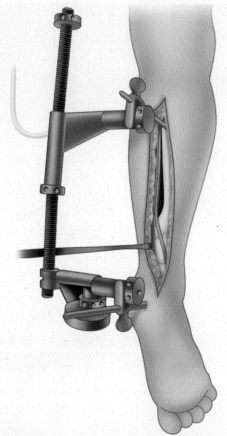

FIGURE 2.18   Posterior approach. Femoral distractor has been applied, and sural nerve is dissected free. **SEE TECHNIQUE 2.8.**

results. Complications included infection in 8%, loss of reduction in 11%, secondary arthrosis in 8%, and one (3%) amputation in a diabetic patient with a failed arthrodesis.

Studies have shown good to excellent results with the use of hybrid external fixation in 67% to 69% of intraarticular or Rüedi-Allgöwer type II fractures and 75% to 97% good results. Complications have been reported in 23% to 66% of patients and include deep and superficial infections and malunion.

■ EXTERNAL FIXATION AND FIBULAR PLATING

Although an integral part of the AO principles for ORIF of tibial pilon fractures, the role of fibular plating is controversial when external fixation is used as the definitive treatment. Potential advantages of fibular plating include increasing mechanical stability, assisting in reduction of the anterolateral articular fragment, and restoring the length and alignment of the tibia. Potential disadvantages include increased operative time, possible wound complications, and potential malreduction resulting in inability to accurately reduce the plafond. In addition, fibular plating restricts the ability of the fixator to be dynamized and may lead to delayed union or varus malunion if metaphyseal defects are not bone grafted. Fibular reduction may be difficult in some fractures, and malreduction impairs the ability to reduce the tibia.

In a study by Williams et al. of patients treated with fibular plating, complications included fibular wound infections (23%), fibular nonunions (9%), and angular malalignment (4.5%). Complications in patients without fibular plating

included angular malunions (19%) and tibial wound infection (3%). An increased frequency of delayed union or varus malunion in the fractures with fibular plating was not found; however, the authors concluded that plating of the fibula in tibial pilon fractures treated with external fixation spanning the ankle is associated with significant complications and that good results can be obtained without fibular fixation. Limitations of the study included the small number of patients.

Watson et al. analyzed 39 tibial pilon fractures that were treated with a variety of external fixation devices and were considered treatment failures. They found that 64% of the failures consisted of malunion or nonunion of the diaphyseal-metaphyseal junction in fractures with plated or intact fibulas and unrecognized bone loss or comminution of the tibia that was never bone grafted. The authors contended that this complication may be avoided by early recognition and bone grafting of tibial bone loss or comminution before frame dynamization. Alternatively, bone grafting potentially can be avoided by not plating the fibula and by using a screw or wire to maintain fibular reduction at the ankle mortise. There currently is no definitive evidence to support or condemn fibular fixation in tibial pilon fractures treated with external fixation. The risks and benefits of fibular fixation must be weighed for each individual fracture. We do not routinely stabilize the fibular fracture at the time of initial external fixator application, particularly if the definitive management will be with external fixation. However, we do in select patients treat the fibular fracture early if a posterolateral approach is used to treat a posterior plafond fragment and then return in a staged fashion once the soft-tissue envelope allows for fixation of the remaining components of the injury.

Although external fixation techniques have been shown to reduce the incidence of wound complications and deep infection compared with open reduction and plating, malunions and pin site infections remain problematic. Comparative series have shown that articular reduction was better in the open reduction group than in the external fixation group, although external fixation was used more commonly for more severe fractures.

■ SPANNING EXTERNAL FIXATION

Traditional half-pin external fixation that spans the ankle joint has the advantages of requiring less soft-tissue dissection and of leaving no large implants in a subcutaneous position, which theoretically should lead to fewer wound complications and infections, especially in open fractures or fractures with severe closed soft-tissue injury. Limited open reduction may be necessary, however, if the fracture does not reduce by ligamentotaxis. External fixation can be used to stabilize almost any fracture of the distal tibia, regardless of comminution, and is especially useful in fractures with diaphyseal extension. Half-pin external fixators are relatively easy to apply, and most surgeons are familiar with this technique. Potential disadvantages include pin track infection and pin loosening, which are common with any type of external fixator; loss of reduction, which can occur if the fixation is removed before the fracture heals; and ankle stiffness, which may occur because half-pin fixators span the ankle and subtalar joints. At least one half-pin usually is inserted into the calcaneus, which makes this technique more difficult if an ipsilateral calcaneal fracture is involved. Half-pins in the hindfoot loosen with time, and bone grafting may be needed in comminuted fractures to promote fracture union before fixator removal.

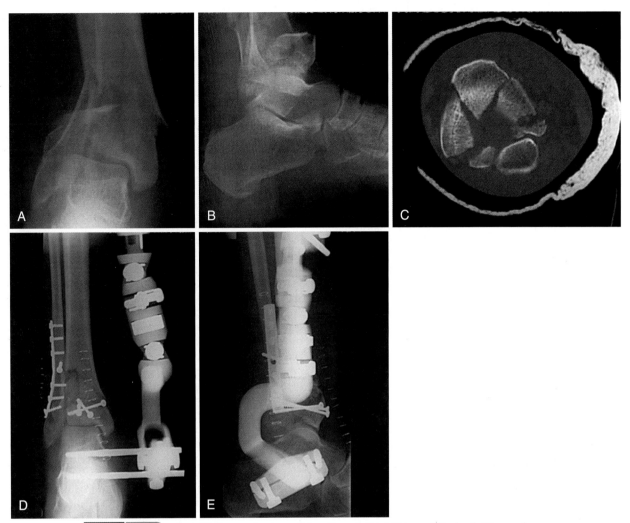

FIGURE 2.19 **A** and **B,** Severe fracture-dislocation of distal tibia and fibula. **C,** CT scan shows fracture pattern. **D** and **E,** After fixation with plate and screws in fibula, lag screws in tibia, and articulated fixator to maintain reduction.

The articulated half-pin fixator, with a hinge to allow ankle motion, was developed to prevent immobilization of the tibiotalar joint. The axis of the hinge is aligned as closely as possible to the true axis of the ankle, and the articulated hinge can be loosened to allow ankle motion. It has not been proved, however, that the articulating feature improves overall functional results.

Marsh et al. compared 19 patients with pilon fractures treated in a spanning external fixator without ankle motion with 22 patients treated with an articulated spanning external fixator and early ankle range of motion (within 2 weeks of surgery). Patients were placed in a short leg cast or walking boot for 4 to 6 weeks after fixator removal. The authors found no significant differences between the groups in range of motion, pain, or functional scores. The authors cautioned that follow-up was short and that numbers may have been too small to detect differences.

Half-pins are placed in the calcaneus and talus and connected to half-pins in the diaphysis. The fracture is reduced by distraction and ligamentotaxis. The fibula can be plated if the overlying soft tissues have not been damaged. The articular surface is reduced further percutaneously, under fluoroscopic guidance, or through limited incisions made directly over fracture lines. The articular reduction is fixed with 3.5- or 4.0-mm screws (Fig. 2.19). Bone grafting of metaphyseal defects is necessary in 25% to 60% of fractures; it can be done acutely if soft-tissue coverage is good, or it can be delayed 4 to 6 weeks until the soft tissues have healed.

SPANNING EXTERNAL FIXATION OF TIBIAL PILON FRACTURE

TECHNIQUE 2.9

(BONAR AND MARSH)

- Fix a hinged, articulated fixator to two screws distally, one in the calcaneus and one in the talus, and to two screws proximally in the tibia. Insert all screws after predrilling. To protect the soft tissues, perform all drilling and screw insertion through sleeves.

- Place the calcaneal and talar screws as indicated in Fig. 2.20A to straddle the neurovascular bundle.
- Using fluoroscopy, place the talar screw first without using the fixator template. Locate the starting point of the talar screw on the distal medial neck of the talus (see Fig. 2.20A); place the screw parallel to the dome of the talus, as seen fluoroscopically on an anteroposterior view of the ankle (Fig. 2.20B), and roughly perpendicular to the long axis of the foot (Fig. 2.20C). The placement and direction of this screw are important because they align the template used to insert the rest of the screws.
- Ensure bicortical purchase by making sure that two threads penetrate the lateral neck of the talus on an anteroposterior fluoroscopic view.
- Place the calcaneal and tibial screws through the template based on the talar screw. The calcaneal screw can be placed high or low in the tuberosity of the calcaneus by rotating the articulated hinge. The high position allows more postoperative dorsiflexion and is recommended.
- Confirm bicortical purchase of the calcaneal screw on an axial fluoroscopic view of the hindfoot. The center of the hinge of the articulated fixator should be near the middle of the talus.
- After the screws have been placed, remove the template, apply the fixator, and lock the proximal ball joint. Use a compression distraction apparatus to distract the ankle joint and evaluate the reduction fluoroscopically.
- Based on preoperative planning and the intraoperative appearance after distraction, make limited incisions to aid in exact reduction of the articular surface and obtain fixation with small fragment screws. Choose incision locations that coincide directly with the major fracture lines to provide a view of the articular surface, using the fracture as a window. Large tenaculum reduction forceps may help reduce the major fragments.
- Use screw fixation for the articular fragments only; do not attempt to obtain screw fixation across the metaphyseal fracture. Tibial plates are not used. Use cannulated screws for percutaneous insertion and keep periosteal stripping to a minimum.
- Apply bone graft to the metaphyseal defect through the same incision or through a separate incision if needed.

POSTOPERATIVE CARE The limb is kept elevated until soft-tissue healing allows mobilization. Most patients are kept non–weight bearing and are not allowed to bear more than 20 kg of weight during the first 6 weeks. The external fixator is dynamized (the locking nut is released to allow sliding of the telescoping body) at 4 to 12 weeks, at which time weight bearing is increased. The fixator is removed when healing of the fracture is evident on radiographs and the patient can walk without pain when the fixator body is removed. Ankle joint motion is begun when soft-tissue conditions permit, usually at 1 to 2 weeks. An Orthoplast (Johnson & Johnson, New Brunswick, NJ) splint is worn to maintain the ankle in neutral except during range-of-motion exercises.

▌HYBRID EXTERNAL FIXATION

Hybrid external fixators consist of tensioned wires in the epiphyseal fragment of the tibia connected to half-pins placed in the diaphysis. Similar to half-pin fixators, these devices provide greater preservation of the soft tissues and greater ease in spanning diaphyseal fracture lines than do plating devices. The tensioned wires, which can be used in a manner similar to lag screws, can aid in the reduction and fixation of articular fragments. Confining the fixation to above the ankle joint has potential advantages and disadvantages. The tibiotalar and subtalar joints are not immobilized, which theoretically should diminish stiffness in these areas.

The surgeon must be familiar with the biomechanics of these fixators to ensure a stable construct. In a biomechanical study, Yang et al. found that a bar-ring hybrid fixator consisting of a unilateral fixator body connected to a ring/wire assembly was too flexible. The addition of diagonally placed struts significantly improved the stability of this construct. A two-ring hybrid fixator seemed to have the best mechanical performance. In fractures with extreme articular comminution, the wires may not provide adequate fixation, however. Fixation wires may need to be placed intracapsularly for adequate fixation, and although septic arthritis caused by pin track infection is a potential complication, this has not been a problem in the ankle as it has been in the knee. Neurologic, vascular, or tendinous impalement can occur if safe corridors for wire placement are not recognized. Fractures associated with tibiotalar instability also are not adequately stabilized with this method. Many surgeons do not have experience with tensioned wire techniques. Hybrid fixators are most appropriate for AO type A, type C1, and type C2 fractures.

Early ligamentotaxis reduction is important to close large fracture gaps and to reduce fracture hemorrhage and tension on the tenuous soft-tissue envelope. A delay of more than a few days may make it impossible to disimpact the metaphyseal fragments and makes realignment of any shaft extension and comminution difficult; it also makes indirect reduction difficult and may require a larger or more extensile incision. Calcaneal traction can be applied immediately after evaluation in the emergency department or, for open fractures, in the operating room during emergency irrigation and debridement. Watson et al. described the use of a "traveling traction" device consisting of a 6-mm, centrally threaded Steinmann pin through the calcaneal tuberosity and a similar pin through the proximal tibia at the level of the fibular head. A simple quadrilateral external fixator frame is constructed by applying medial and lateral radiolucent external fixation bars, and manual distraction is done to obtain a ligamentotaxis reduction. A CT scan of the extremity in traction allows formulation of an operative plan. If ligamentotaxis has obtained a relative reduction, percutaneous olive wires can be used, with or without cannulated screws. If the joint is not reduced, a limited open approach is indicated.

Based on review of more than 150 CT scans of these injuries, Watson developed a four-quadrant approach to wire insertion (Fig. 2.21). Incisions are made to correspond with the anatomically "safe" corridors for transfixation wire placement to stabilize the metaphyseal fragments. The only region inaccessible to tension wire fixation is a fracture line that is exactly transverse in the coronal plane. Because of anatomic restraints, olive wires cannot be placed from directly anterior to posterior, and fracture lines in this orientation are best stabilized with small cannulated screws.

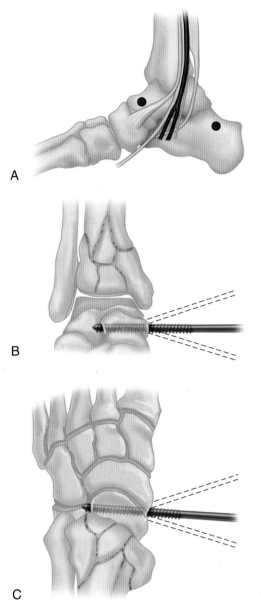

A

B

C

FIGURE 2.20 **A,** Placement of calcaneal and talar screws to avoid neurovascular bundle and subtalar joint. **B,** Talar screw is parallel to talar dome on anteroposterior view (*dashed lines* indicate inaccurate screw placement). **C,** Screw is perpendicular to long axis of foot, and two threads should protrude through far cortex of talus. **SEE TECHNIQUE 2.9.**

DEFINITIVE RING EXTERNAL FIXATION OF TIBIAL PILON FRACTURES

TECHNIQUE 2.10

(WATSON)

- Place the patient on a radiolucent table on a beanbag patient-positioning device. Bolster the beanbag to elevate the entire lower extremity and to allow placement of a circular fixator without its impinging on the table. Maintain

calcaneal traction through a table extension with a sterile traction bow. If a two-pin external fixator is in place, use it to maintain traction.
- Stabilize the fibula first. If the condition of the soft tissues allows, use a limited open reduction technique to apply a four-hole or six-hole plate. If the soft tissues along the lateral aspect of the fibula are compromised, use percutaneous tenaculum forceps to pull the fibula out to length and pin it temporarily to the lateral tibia with a percutaneous Kirschner wire, which later is replaced with a tensioned olive wire.
- The external fixation frame usually consists of three or four rings. Begin the frame with a distally based ring located at the level of the ankle joint. Locate the second ring just proximal to any shaft extension. If there is a wide zone of diaphyseal-metaphyseal extension, an additional middle ring is necessary. Connect the proximal two or three rings above the fracture by long, threaded rods. Leave the distal ring free.
- Open the proximal ring construct in a "clamshell" fashion and place it over the tibial shaft. Place a transverse reference wire parallel to the knee joint and level with the fibular head, and attach the proximal ring to this wire. Obtain appropriate soft-tissue clearance and position the proximal ring on the limb to ensure that it is parallel to the knee joint and collinear with the intact proximal shaft of the tibia.
- Place a Schanz pin into the proximal tibial shaft and attach it to the most proximal ring. At this point, the proximal ring construct is firmly attached to the tibia above the fracture. Place additional transfixation wires or Schanz pins on the additional proximal rings to obtain two levels of fixation on each ring of the intact proximal shaft. Do not yet place olive wires through any area of comminution.
- Articular fixation is performed next. If ligamentotaxis was successful, stabilize the fracture by placing percutaneous olive wires across the major fragments in accordance with the preoperative CT data (Fig. 2.22A). This approach differs from techniques in which a standardized pattern of transfixation wire placement is used; in this technique, the transfixation wires are placed where the fracture patterns dictate. For coronal plane fractures, use cannulated screws to facilitate fixation of the wires.
- If ligamentotaxis was unsuccessful, an open approach is indicated.
- Based on the CT data, select an appropriate corridor and make a 4- to 6-cm incision, avoiding undermining any large cutaneous flaps. If the placement of the incision has been selected carefully, it should lead directly to the major fracture line.
- Minimal periosteal stripping is necessary, and the fracture line is opened like a book to reveal the joint. The impacted articular fragments also are visible because the joint is distracted.
- Use a small elevator to disimpact the articular surface and reduce it under direct vision.
- Use Kirschner wires to hold the fragments temporarily and apply any bone graft necessary to maintain the segment in position and fill any cancellous defects. Reduce the metaphyseal fragments and hold them with temporary Kirschner wire fixation. Use screws for de-

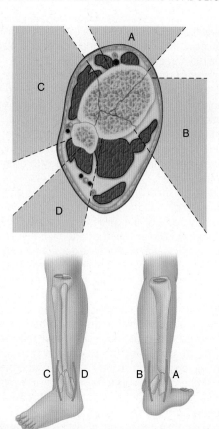

FIGURE 2.21 Fracture patterns found on CT scans of pilon fracture: anterolateral, posterolateral, anteromedial, or postero-medial fragments with central impaction or compression. Based on anatomically safe corridors, wires can be passed obliquely through safe zones *A* and *D* or *B* and *C*; wires cannot be passed safely directly from anterior to posterior. Safe zones *A, B, C,* and *D* correspond to incisions. (Redrawn from Watson JT: Tibial pilon fractures, *Tech Orthop* 11:150, 1996.)

finitive articular fixation of any coronal fracture lines. Alternatively, for most fracture lines, place olive wires percutaneously or directly through the incision to fix the fragments.

- At least three or four olive wires are necessary to obtain adequate fixation of the articular surfaces. If the distal tibial-fibular joint has been disrupted, use an olive wire to reduce the diastasis by passing the wire from the fibula across the tibia. If the fibula has not been plated, ensure that it is pulled out to its full length and that appropriate rotation is maintained before placing the tibia-fibula transfixation wire. Place the final wire, a transverse reference wire, just anterior to the fibula. Pass the wire only through the tibia to ensure that it is parallel to the joint, approximately 1 cm proximal to the ankle joint. Then "clamshell" the distal ring and place it around the wires, positioning the ring on the reference wire (Fig. 2.22B). This ensures that the knee and ankle joints are parallel when the distal and proximal rings have been connected.
- Attach the remainder of the wires to the free ring. Because the wires may not lie directly in apposition to the ring, build up to the ring by using various posts of different heights (Fig. 2.22C).

- Tension the opposing olive wires symmetrically using two-wire tensioners. Perform this tensioning under fluoroscopic control to prevent asymmetric compression of the fracture lines.
- Attach the distal ring to the proximal rings with threaded rods with conical washers, allowing some variability in reducing and maintaining the overall mechanical axis.
- Use the ring at the level of proximal shaft extension to reduce proximal shaft comminution. Use olive or smooth wires to manipulate and maintain shaft alignment and to reduce any large fracture lines in this area. Attach these wires to the mid-distal ring and tension them under fluoroscopy so that the reduction can be observed.
- For AO type C injuries with extensive joint involvement and large areas of metaphyseal comminution, it is helpful to preconstruct a four-ring frame with an attached foot frame to maintain distraction at the ankle joint. The distraction construct can be as simple as a calcaneal pin or wire attached to a distal calcaneal ring or as extensive as a full foot frame attached to the distal tibial ring.
- Use a distraction frame similar to that described earlier and attach the proximal tibial rings first, providing appropriate soft-tissue clearance.
- Attach the foot frame or calcaneal pin and perform distraction ligamentotaxis across the ankle joint by adjusting the threaded rods.
- If ligamentotaxis reduction is inadequate, do an open procedure as described previously.
- When reduction is satisfactory, position the distal tibial ring at the level of the fracture; pass the fixation wires across the fracture fragments, attach them to the ring, and tension them as described earlier. The only difference in this technique is that the distal tibial ring is already attached to the frame and it is not necessary to "clamshell" the ring to place it around the wires.

POSTOPERATIVE CARE In fractures with significant periarticular comminution or fragments with minimal soft-tissue attachment, Watson recommended maintaining distraction across the ankle for 6 weeks. When tentative healing has occurred at the joint line, the foot frame or calcaneal pin is removed in an outpatient procedure. Physical therapy is begun to increase range of motion and general strength. Total non–weight bearing is maintained in patients with severely comminuted (AO type C3) fractures. In fractures with shaft extension, tentative weight bearing is begun when early callus and some signs of healing are seen on radiographs, usually at 8 to 10 weeks. Progressive weight bearing is begun, and by 12 to 14 weeks the patient usually is ambulatory with the aid of one crutch or a cane.

■ PRIMARY ARTHRODESIS

Primary arthrodesis has been suggested as a method of treating severely comminuted tibial pilon fractures. Several investigators have noted, however, that severe skeletal injury and

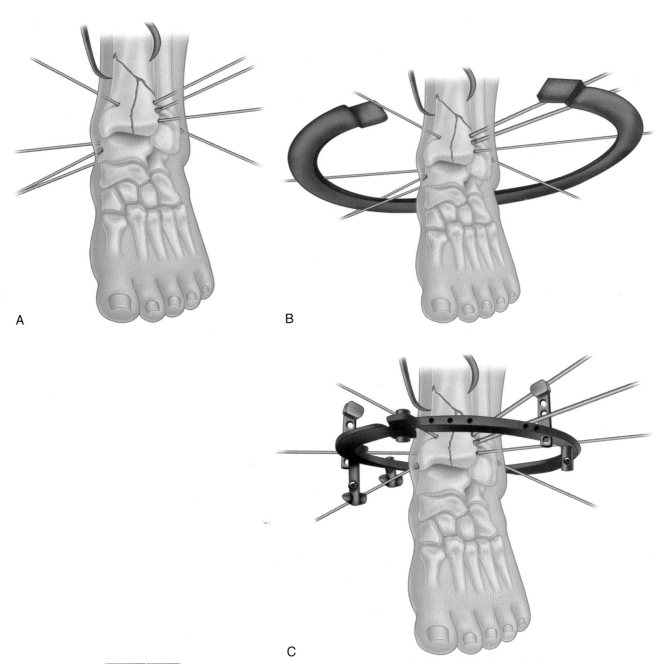

A

B

C

FIGURE 2.22   **A,** Fracture lines are reduced and compressed with multiple olive wires, based on preoperative CT data. **B,** Distal ring is "clam-shelled" and placed parallel to ankle joint. **C,** Posts of various heights are used to attach wires to ring. (From Watson JT: Tibial pilon fractures, *Tech Orthop* 11:150, 1996.) **SEE TECHNIQUE 2.10.**

nonanatomic reduction do not preclude a satisfactory clinical result. We recommend stabilization of these fractures with an external fixator to maintain alignment and allow bony consolidation. Arthrodesis can be done later if the patient is sufficiently symptomatic. Primary arthrodesis may be considered for severe open injuries with extensive loss of cartilage from the tibial and talar articular surfaces (Fig. 2.23). The wound is debrided, and the remaining cartilage is removed from the talus and tibia. An external fixator can be used to stabilize the fracture. Bone grafting may be necessary when the soft tissues have healed.

FRACTURES OF THE TIBIAL SHAFT

Fractures of the shaft of the tibia cannot be treated by following a simple set of rules. Because of its location, the tibia is exposed to frequent injury; it is the most commonly fractured long bone. Because one third of the tibial surface is subcutaneous throughout most of its length, open fractures are more common in the tibia than in any other major long bone. The blood supply to the tibia is more precarious than that of bones enclosed by heavy muscles. High-energy tibial fractures may be associated with compartment syndrome or neural or vascular injury. The presence of hinge joints at the knee and the

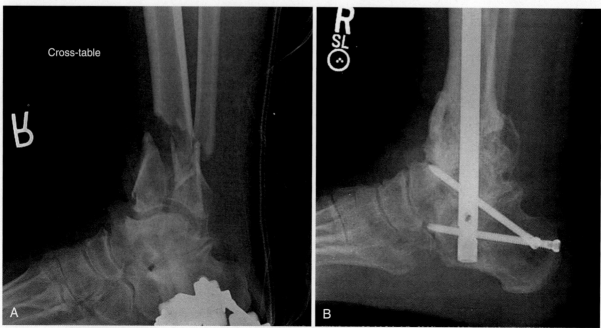

FIGURE 2.23 **A,** Comminuted fracture of tibial pilon after a fall from height. Patient had previous talar fracture resulting in posttraumatic arthritis of tibiotalar and subtalar articulations. **B,** Definitive management with primary tibiotalocalcaneal arthrodesis with retrograde intramedullary implant secondary to preexisting arthrosis.

ankle allows no adjustment for rotary deformity after fracture, and special care is necessary during reduction to correct such deformity. Delayed union, nonunion, and infection are relatively common complications of tibial shaft fractures.

Evaluation of tibial fractures should include a detailed history and physical examination. The limb is inspected for open wounds and soft-tissue crush or contusion, and a thorough neurovascular examination is performed. A pulse deficit or neurologic deficit may be a sign of compartment syndrome or vascular injury, which must be identified and treated immediately. The ipsilateral femur, knee, ankle, and foot also must be examined. When the examination is completed, the limb is realigned gently and splinted. Appropriate tetanus and antibiotic prophylaxes are administered. Plain anteroposterior and lateral radiographs that include the knee and ankle are obtained. Oblique radiographic views at 45 degrees sometimes are required to detect a nondisplaced spiral fracture. Radiographs of the contralateral tibia sometimes are necessary to evaluate length in fractures with severe comminution or bone loss.

The indications for operative and nonoperative treatment of tibial shaft fractures continue to be refined. Although commonly advocated in the past, nonoperative treatment now is generally reserved for closed, stable, isolated, minimally displaced fractures caused by low-energy trauma and some stable low-velocity gunshot fractures. Operative treatment is indicated for most tibial fractures caused by high-energy trauma. These fractures usually are unstable, comminuted, and associated with varying degrees of soft-tissue trauma. Operative treatment allows early motion, provides soft-tissue access, and avoids complications associated with immobilization. The goals of treatment are to obtain a healed, well-aligned fracture; pain-free weight bearing; and functional range of motion of the knee and ankle joints. The optimal treatment method should assist in meeting these goals while minimizing complications, especially infection. These goals may not be attainable in severely injured limbs.

Sarmiento, Nicoll, and others found that closed treatment with casting or functional bracing is an effective method of treatment for many tibial shaft fractures that avoids the potential complications of surgical intervention. For closed treatment to succeed, the cast or brace must maintain acceptable fracture alignment and the fracture pattern must allow early weight bearing to prevent delayed union or nonunion. Repeated attempts at manipulation should be avoided. If the fracture cannot be well aligned, an alternative method of treatment should be chosen. Axial or rotational malalignment and shortening cause cosmetic deformities and alter the loading characteristics in adjacent joints, which may hasten the development of posttraumatic arthritis.

The amount of malalignment and shortening considered acceptable also is controversial. Distal tibial malalignment may be more poorly tolerated than more proximal malalignment. The recommendations in the literature vary widely: 4 to 10 degrees of varus-valgus malalignment, 5 to 20 degrees of anteroposterior malalignment, 5 to 20 degrees of rotatory malalignment, and 10 to 20 mm of shortening. In general, we strive to achieve less than 5 degrees of varus-valgus angulation, less than 10 degrees of anteroposterior angulation, less than 10 degrees of rotation, and less than 15 mm of shortening. Maintaining fracture alignment is difficult in certain fracture types, and if repeated attempts at realignment have been unsuccessful, operative fixation is indicated.

The important factors in prognosis are (1) the amount of initial displacement, (2) the degree of comminution, (3) whether infection has developed, and (4) the severity of the soft-tissue injury excluding infection. Torsional fractures with or without simple comminution have been found to have a better prognosis than high-energy patterns, such as short oblique or transverse fractures, with or without comminution. Torsional fractures tend to create a longitudinal tear of the periosteum and may not disrupt endosteal vessels, whereas transverse fractures usually tear the periosteum circumferentially and completely disrupt the endosteal circulation. Reduction is difficult in displaced spiral fractures of the distal third of the tibia.

Hoaglund and States classified fractures of the tibia as being caused by either high-energy or low-energy trauma and found this classification useful in prognosis. Fractures in the high-energy group resulted from accidents such as motor vehicle collisions and crush injuries. This group included more than half the total fractures and 90% of the open fractures; fractures in this group healed in an average of 6 months. Fractures in the low-energy group resulted from accidents such as falls on ice and while skiing; these healed in an average of about 4 months. These researchers found that the level of fracture was not significant in the prognosis but that the amount of bony contact was. Fractures in which contact between the fragments after reduction was 50% to 90% of normal healed significantly faster than fractures in which contact was less.

Displacement of more than 50% of the width of the tibia at the fracture site has been noted to be a significant cause of delayed union or nonunion. Fractures with more than 50% comminution are considered unstable and usually are associated with high-energy trauma and significant open or closed soft-tissue injury. The presence or absence of a fibular fracture does not influence the prognosis, although inhibited fracture healing of closed tibial fractures associated with intact fibulas treated with cast immobilization has been reported.

Patient characteristics also can influence the success of closed treatment of tibial shaft fractures. Alignment can be difficult to maintain with casts or braces in patients with edematous or obese extremities. Loss of reduction may occur in noncompliant patients with closed treatment, whereas delayed union and nonunion are common in patients in whom weight bearing must be restricted for a prolonged time. An individual's functional demands also must be considered when planning treatment.

In comparative studies of intramedullary nailing and casting for the treatment of isolated closed tibial shaft fractures, intramedullary nailing has been found to achieve higher union rates and better functional scores. Although these studies show the superiority of intramedullary nailing over casting for closed unstable tibial shaft fractures, further comparative studies are necessary to confirm these results and establish more rigid treatment guidelines.

Nicoll, an advocate of closed treatment, listed the following indications for internal fixation: (1) open fracture requiring complicated plastic surgery, (2) associated fracture of the femur and other major injuries, (3) paraplegia with sensory loss, (4) segmental fracture with displaced central fragments, and (5) gaps resulting from missing bone fragments. Internal fixation has been recommended for unstable, comminuted, or segmental fractures; bilateral tibial fractures; and ipsilateral femoral fractures. Operative treatment also currently is favored for open fractures, fractures with severe closed soft-tissue injury, fractures associated with compartment syndrome, fractures involving vascular injury, and fractures in patients with multiple trauma.

Fractures in which closed treatment is inappropriate can be treated with plate and screw fixation, intramedullary fixation (interlocking intramedullary nails), and external fixation. Locked intramedullary nailing currently is the preferred treatment for most tibial shaft fractures requiring operative fixation. Plating is used primarily for fractures at or proximal to the metaphyseal-diaphyseal junction. External fixation is useful for fractures with periarticular extension and for severe open fractures. In severely mangled extremities, amputation should be considered.

For open high-energy tibial fractures, results of treatment have improved significantly because of important contributions made by large trauma services. Several factors are important for a good outcome in these fractures. Aggressive and repeated debridements of all devitalized tissue, including large fragments of bone, are essential. Because vascular soft tissue and bone are essential for resisting infection and providing a bed for reconstruction, Gustilo and others stressed the importance of leaving the wound open and repeating debridement every 24 to 48 hours until closure at 5 to 7 days by delayed primary closure, skin grafting, or skin flaps. Our protocol is repeat debridement and irrigation at 48 to 72 hours if there is evidence of continuing demarcation of the zone of injury. All Gustilo type III fractures routinely have repeat debridement. Antibiotics should be used routinely with open fractures. Aminoglycosides are added to cephalosporins for type III open fractures, and penicillin is included for fractures with severe contamination. Soft-tissue coverage by 5 to 7 days should be obtained by delayed closure, skin grafting, or flap coverage.

Although there is no dispute that soft-tissue management is the most important factor in determining the outcome of open tibial fractures, the optimal method of fixation is debated. Sufficient stability of the fracture fragments and soft tissues usually can be obtained only by locked intramedullary nails or external fixation. Plate fixation has been associated with an unacceptably high incidence of infection. For Gustilo type I, type II, and type IIIA open fractures, most orthopaedic traumatologists prefer intramedullary nailing.

Studies comparing unreamed nailing with external fixation have shown that tibial fractures treated with unreamed nailing required fewer additional operations and achieved better functional outcomes with fewer superficial infections than fractures treated with external fixation. Comparisons of reamed with unreamed nailing (two studies with 132 patients) have shown a reduced risk of reoperation with a reamed technique.

Type IIIB open tibial fractures have been associated with a relatively high incidence of infection when treated with external fixation and with unreamed nailing. There are, however, specific open fractures for which acute intramedullary nailing is almost certainly not the best treatment option. Open fractures secondary to war injuries; fractures with severe contamination, especially involving the medullary canal; and type IIIC open tibial fractures, especially those in which limb salvage is questionable, all are potentially better treated with external fixation.

The time to debridement for open tibial fractures has not been found to be predictive of infection; however, fracture severity has. Negative-pressure wound therapy is being used more frequently for open wound management, although similar infection and nonunion rates with negative-pressure wound therapy compared with historical controls have been reported.

We prefer intramedullary nailing for most open tibial fractures. Our protocol (Fig. 2.24) includes planning of postoperative management to decrease the frequency of delayed union and implant failure. With this protocol, union was obtained in 48 (96%) of 50 open tibial fractures. Additional procedures to promote union were done in 18 patients at an average of 4 months after injury.

Mangled extremities are severe open fractures often associated with vascular injury or nerve disruption. Surgeons treating these injuries face the difficult decision of whether to attempt limb salvage or perform early amputation. Salvage often is technically possible but may result in disastrous medical, social, psychologic, and financial consequences for the patient.

Complete anatomic disruption of the tibial nerve in adults and crush injuries with a warm ischemia time of more than 6 hours have been suggested as absolute indications for primary amputation; suggested relative indications include serious associated polytrauma, severe ipsilateral foot trauma, and a projected long course to full recovery. Other factors are the patient's age, occupation, and medical condition; the mechanism of injury; fracture comminution; bone loss; the extent and location of neurologic and vascular injury; and the severity and duration of shock. Various authors have attempted to formulate scores predicting the likelihood of

salvage or amputation, but none has proved entirely accurate. In a long-term study of functional results and quality of life in patients with severe open tibial fractures treated with either salvage or amputation, recovery time and long-term disability were reduced with early below-knee amputation, while another study reported a high rate of preservation of a functional weight-bearing limb in patients with type IIIB open tibial fractures treated with aggressive wound management and early soft-tissue coverage.

In an effort to resolve questions about the indications for limb salvage or amputation in a mangled extremity, the Lower Extremity Assessment Project (LEAP) study group was formed. In a multicenter, prospective, longitudinal study, the investigators identified risk factors that predisposed patients to poor outcomes in the salvage and amputee groups. Poor prognostic indicators were attributable to low educational level, income below poverty level, nonwhite racial background, lack of insurance, poor social support network, smoking, and pending legal action. Patients with salvaged limbs without risk factors for poor outcomes had results equivalent to the results of amputees at 2 and 7 years but required more surgical procedures and more rehospitalizations. Patients with tibial nerve injury and insensate feet had substantial impairment at 12 and 24 months; however, outcomes were no different in patients with amputated or salvaged limbs. The LEAP study group also found that muscle injury, absence of sensation, arterial injury, and vein injury

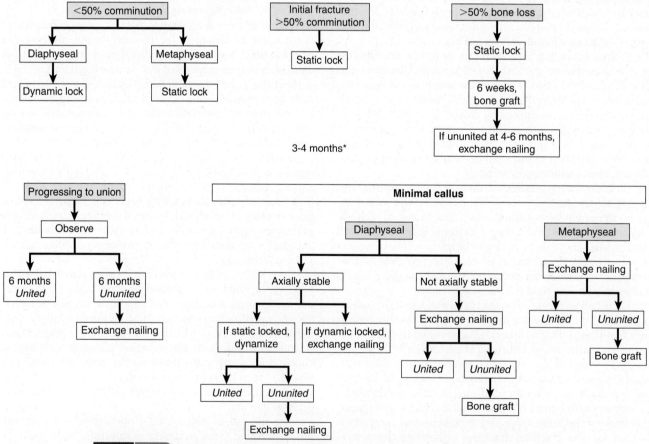

FIGURE 2.24 Protocol for initial unreamed nailing and postoperative treatment of open tibial fractures. *Bone graft may be indicated at 6 weeks in type IIIB open fractures. (From Whittle AP: Clinical results of unreamed nailing of tibial and femoral fractures, *Tech Orthop* 11:67, 1996.)

were factors that had the greatest impact on the surgeon's decision to amputate or salvage the extremity. However, the group of patients with insensate limbs recovered intact sensation in 67%, questioning insensibility as an absolute indication for amputation.

TREATMENT
■ CAST BRACING

The use of a short cast or functional brace for treatment of a tibial shaft fracture resulted in a 97% union rate in a study by Sarmiento et al. The incidence of nonunion ranged from 0% to 13%. Sarmiento narrowed his indications for bracing to closed fractures and low-energy open fractures. Other studies all resulted in recommendations for some type of closed treatment.

Although good functional results without deformity have been reported in more than 95% of patients, the immobilization required with closed treatment may adversely affect ankle motion. Ankle stiffness has been reported in 20% to 30% of patients who had closed treatment. Angular deformity of more than 5 degrees occurs in 10% to 55% of fractures treated with a cast or brace, and shortening of at least 12 to 14 mm occurs in 5% to 27% of patients. Sarmiento's series of carefully selected fractures had the best results, whereas series with more unstable fractures reported poorer results. Loss of reduction requiring operative treatment has been reported in 2.4% to 9.3% of patients in several larger series. Anatomic reduction and rigid immobilization are highly advantageous to the healing of a fracture, but not at the risk of infection and delayed union. The closed, early weight-bearing method of treatment often concedes minor complications in favor of a predictably high union rate and no major complications. It is a method applicable to many types of tibial shaft fractures, but it requires a good deal of patience and time from the physician and a cooperative patient. We prefer casting for minimally displaced, stable, low-energy tibial fractures.

■ PLATE AND SCREW FIXATION

Plate fixation has been recommended for treatment of tibial fractures that are unsuitable for nonoperative management historically. Open reduction and plating provide stable fixation, allow early motion of the knee and ankle, and maintain length and alignment. The greatest disadvantage of plating is that it requires soft-tissue stripping, which can lead to wound complications and infection. Before the 1960s, plating of open and closed tibial fractures often was complicated by delayed union, nonunion, implant failure, soft-tissue sloughing, and infection, especially if performed within the first week after injury.

The AO group subsequently developed compression plating techniques and implants that remain in use today. Good functional results were reported in 98% of closed fractures with a 6% complication rate, and 90% good results in open fractures; these had, however, a 30% complication rate. A significant increase in complications was noted in progressively higher-energy fractures that were treated by ORIF, and complications increased from 9.5% for torsional fractures to 48.3% for comminuted fractures. Likewise, increased infection rates from 2.1% for torsional fractures to 10.3% for comminuted fractures were noted. Also, nonunion was twice as common and infection five times more likely when open fractures were treated with plating.

Other investigators also have reported increased complications when plating open tibial fractures (infections 1.9% in closed fractures and 7.1% in open fractures; implant failure 0.6% in closed fractures and 10.3% in open fractures). Most authors now recommend plating for tibial shaft fractures associated with displaced intraarticular fractures of the knee and ankle. Refinements in plating and indirect reduction should be used when plating extended shaft fractures, and soft-tissue handling should be meticulous.

In an effort to decrease the frequency of delayed union, non-union, and infection after tibial shaft fractures, "percutaneous" plating was developed to obtain stable fixation while preserving the fracture environment. This technique involves plating of any associated fibular fracture, prebending a 3.5-mm dynamic compression plate to match the tibial anatomy, and placing the plate and screws through small incisions. Current indications for percutaneous plating are (1) a tibial shaft fracture with periarticular metaphyseal comminution that precludes locked intramedullary nailing and (2) a tibial fracture that cannot be treated with intramedullary fixation because of a preexisting implant, such as a tibial base plate from a total knee arthroplasty. Percutaneous plating is technically challenging, and malalignment is more frequent than with other methods of fixation.

■ TRANSFIXATION BY SCREWS

Lag screws can be used for fixation of long oblique (more than three shaft diameters) or spiral fractures that extend into the metaphysis, although these fractures more commonly are treated using other methods. These evenly placed lag screws are oriented perpendicular to the fracture and are placed away from narrow fracture ends. This technique may be useful to supplement external fixation in open fractures by stabilizing large butterfly fragments to one of the principal fragments. Furthermore, we have found this technique useful for open fractures with short periarticular segments that are difficult to control with external fixation alone before definitive fixation (Fig. 2.25).

■ INTRAMEDULLARY FIXATION

Locked intramedullary nailing currently is considered the treatment of choice for most type I, type II, and type IIIA open and closed tibial shaft fractures (Fig. 2.26) and is especially useful for segmental and bilateral tibial fractures. Busse et al. polled orthopaedic trauma surgeons with regard to management of tibial fractures. Eighty percent preferred operative treatment for closed fractures. Intramedullary nailing preserves the soft-tissue sleeve around the fracture site and allows early motion of the adjacent joints. The ability to lock the nails proximally and distally provides control of length, alignment, and rotation in unstable fractures and permits stabilization of fractures located below the tibial tubercle or 3 to 4 cm proximal to the ankle joint. Nailing is not recommended in patients with open physes, anatomic deformity, or burns or wounds over the entry portal.

Küntscher developed his V-shaped and cloverleaf nails in the 1930s, but it was not until nearly 50 years later that rigid intramedullary nailing became a widely accepted treatment for tibial shaft fractures, with 98% good results in closed fractures and in 97.5% of open fractures treated with unreamed straight Küntscher nails. Herzog modified the straight Küntscher nail to accommodate the eccentric proximal portal. Some authors proposed reaming of the medullary canal

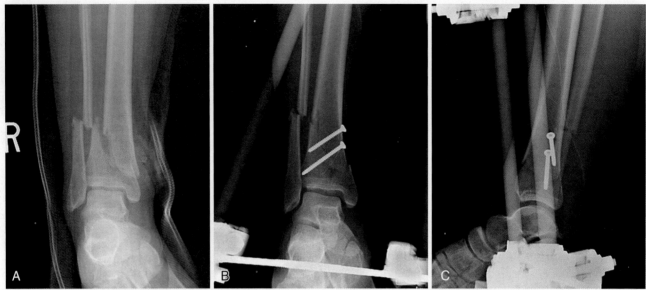

FIGURE 2.25 **A,** Patient with medially open extraarticular distal tibia and fibular fractures. **B** and **C,** At time of uniplanar external fixation application, coronal plane stability was difficult to control and resulted in continued soft-tissue endangerment from displaced underlying tibial metaphyseal spike. Anatomic reduction of tibia and interfragmentary lag screw fixation as temporizing measure to provide stability as adjunct to external fixator.

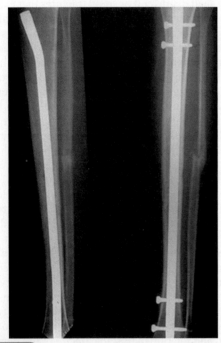

FIGURE 2.26 Open tibial fracture stabilized with intramedullary nail.

to improve the fit of the nail and to increase its rotational control and strength. Biomechanical data suggest substantial improvement in fracture site mobility when increasing to a larger diameter implant.

In the 1970s, Grosse and Kempf and Klemm and Schellmann developed nails with interlocking screws, which expanded the indications for nailing to include more proximal, distal, and unstable fractures. Reports of interlocking nails inserted with reaming showed good results (97% union

rate; 2.2% complication rate), especially in closed fractures, but some authors have cautioned against their use in the dynamic or simple unlocked mode, noting that most complications in their series occurred with dynamic locked nails; they also did not recommend routine dynamization.

REAMED VERSUS UNREAMED NAILING

Studies published in the 1970s and 1980s reported unacceptably high infection rates (13.6% to 33%) in small series of open tibial fractures treated with reamed nailing. These reports led to the conclusion that medullary reaming is contraindicated in open tibial fractures, especially Gustilo type II and type III. Studies of open tibial fractures treated with unreamed Ender pins and Lottes nails during the same time period reported infection rates of 6% to 7%. Animal experiments showed that insertion of reamed nails disturbs cortical blood flow to a greater extent than insertion of unreamed nails, possibly increasing susceptibility to infection. These factors led to the development of interlocking intramedullary nails suitable for unreamed insertion.

In our series of 50 unreamed tibial nailings of three type I, 13 type II, and 34 type III (11 type IIIA and six type IIIB) open fractures, there were four infections, all in type III fractures. Two infections occurred in type IIIB fractures after failure of initial rotational or free flaps. One infection in a type IIIA open fracture developed at 10 months, immediately after bone grafting of a bone defect. All infections resolved with no chronic osteomyelitis. This series and subsequent studies reported union in 96% to 100% of fractures, infection in 2% to 13%, nail failure in 0% to 6%, screw failure in 6% to 41%, and secondary surgery to achieve union in 35% to 48%.

Implant failure most often is associated with smaller (8 mm) nails, axially unstable fractures, metaphyseal fractures, delayed union or nonunion, open fracture, and severe comminution. Nail failure may require additional surgery. In one study, failure occurred most often at the transverse proximal locking screw when a single screw was used. Fractures in the distal third of the tibia had the highest frequency of nail breakage.

Problems with delayed union and implant failure with the smaller implants used in unreamed nailing have led some investigators to return to the use of reamed nailing in open tibial fractures. Using perioperative antibiotics and modern techniques of wound closure, infection rates have been reported to be 1.8% of type I, 3.8% of type II, and 9.5% of type III open tibial fractures (5.15% in type IIIA and 12.5% in type IIIB) treated with reamed nailing. These results are similar to the results obtained with unreamed locked tibial nails.

A randomized, prospective study comparing reamed with unreamed locked nailing of open tibial fractures found no statistically significant difference in the results of treatment of open tibial fractures with reamed nailing and with unreamed nailing except for the higher incidence of screw failure in the unreamed nailings.

Other investigators still caution against reamed nailing in open tibial fractures, especially high-grade open fractures, reporting a 21% occurrence of deep infection in type I and type II fractures treated with reamed nailing. The severity of soft-tissue injury and adequacy of debridement and soft-tissue coverage are more important in the prevention of infection than is the type of implant used. Currently, most orthopaedic traumatologists in North America accept the use of reamed nails in type I and type II open fractures; however, the use of reamed nailing in type III open fractures is controversial.

The successful use of unreamed nailing in patients with open tibial fractures has led some investigators to recommend this technique for closed fractures as well. Potential advantages of unreamed nailing over the reamed technique include shorter operative time, less blood loss, and less disruption of the endosteal blood supply in patients with severe closed soft-tissue injuries. No significant differences have been found in outcomes and complications between reamed and unreamed nailing of closed tibial shaft fractures. However, a trend toward improved union has been noted with reamed nailing. In one study, significantly more screws failed in unreamed than reamed nails. These and other studies seem to indicate that fracture and soft-tissue characteristics are more important in determining fracture outcome than the choice of treatment, and reamed nailing is recommended for most closed unstable tibial shaft fractures.

A meta-analysis showed a decreased nonunion rate with reamed intramedullary nailings for closed injuries. Furthermore, the results of the Study to Prospectively Evaluate Reamed Intramedullary Nails in Patients with Tibial Fractures (SPRINT) illustrate a possible benefit to reaming when compared with unreamed devices. In addition, it also found that delaying reoperation until at least 6 months may decrease the need for secondary interventions for fractures of the tibia. Lefaivre et al. evaluated long-term (median 14 years) functional outcomes after intramedullary tibial nailing. They found outcome measures comparable to the normal population, but with some insignificant sequelae still present.

INTRAMEDULLARY NAILING OF FRACTURES OF THE PROXIMAL THIRD OF THE TIBIAL SHAFT
The enthusiasm for locked nailing of tibial shaft fractures has led some surgeons to expand the indications to include

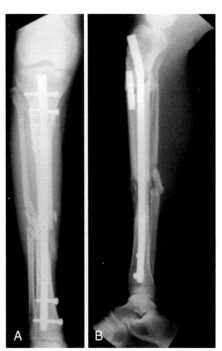

FIGURE 2.27 **A** and **B,** Proximal tibial fracture treated with intramedullary nailing and lateral plate.

more proximal and distal fractures. Malalignment is a common problem in proximal-third fractures treated with locked nails because of the large discrepancy in size between the tibial nail and the wide tibial metaphysis. Valgus angulation and anterior displacement of the proximal fragment are the most common deformities. Valgus deformity can be caused by a portal that starts too far medially and is directed laterally. A medial parapatellar incision and impingement from the patella may cause a portal to be directed in this manner.

A biomechanical study found that medial to lateral screws in one plane can allow the nail to slide on the screws. Apex anterior angulation or anterior displacement can be caused by a portal that starts too distally or is directed too posteriorly. A proximal bend that is at or below the fracture site can cause anterior translation of the proximal fragment when the nail wedges against the cortex. Locking the nail proximally with the knee flexed causes extension of the proximal fragment owing to the pull of the patellar tendon. Refinements in technique, including more precise placement of the entry portal and the use of some form of supplemental fixation such as blocking screws, unicortical plates (Fig. 2.27), and two-pin medial external fixation, have greatly reduced the frequency of this complication.

Some proximal-third tibial fractures can best be treated by other methods. Bono et al. developed an algorithm that is helpful in treatment decision-making (Fig. 2.28). Tornetta et al. described a technique of nailing with the knee in a semiextended position with a medial parapatellar arthrotomy to mitigate against extension deformity of the proximal fragment. The technique was later revised to include a smaller superomedial incision, which is facilitated by newly available instrumentation permitting this application in a more percutaneous manner. Investigations are ongoing with regard to this technique's effect on the patellofemoral articulation. A 22% trochlear articular damage rate has been reported

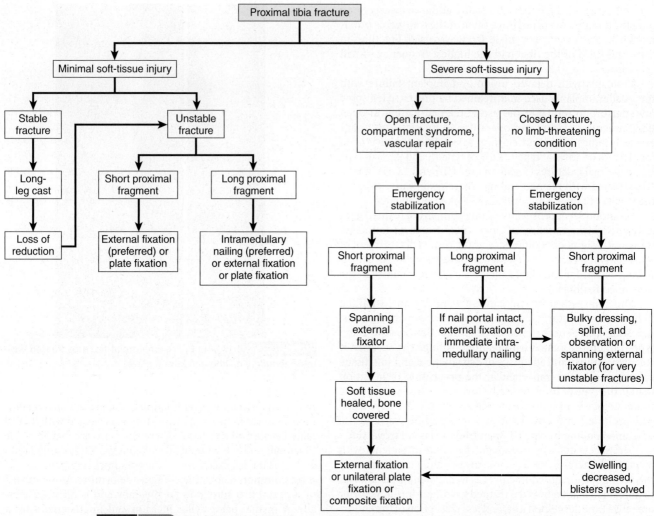

FIGURE 2.28   Treatment algorithm for proximal tibial fractures with minimal or severe soft-tissue injury. (From Bono CM, Levine RG, Rao JP, Behrens FF: Nonarticular proximal tibia fractures: treatment options and decision making, *J Am Acad Orthop Surg* 9:176, 2001.)

in one study after the semiextended nailing; however, these patients were early in the series and results were attributed to errors in technique. In a recent cadaver investigation, patellofemoral contact pressures were examined and found to be higher in the suprapatellar portal compared with traditional approaches. The authors thought the pressure exerted was below that necessary for cartilage damage and therefore concluded that the surgical approach is viable. Further investigation is necessary to determine the long-term functional implications for the patellofemoral joint. Data continue to emerge regarding this technique. Sanders et al. recently reported a series of 55 patients who underwent tibial nailing through a semiextended approach with a suprapatellar portal. Radiographic and clinical follow-up were performed at a minimum of 12 months postoperatively including follow-up arthroscopy and MRI. The authors concluded that this technique results in no significant differences in pain, disability, or knee range of motion after 12 months of follow-up when compared to infrapatellar nailing. A recent meta-analysis found no superiority of the semi-extended technique compared to the intra-patellar technique with regard to functional and knee pain outcomes.

Currently, we use this technique for most difficult proximal third fractures. The technique has several advantages beyond reduction of proximal tibial fractures. It likely lessens the need for supplementary reduction aids, such as blocking screws, and the intraoperative radiographs are significantly easier to obtain.

INTRAMEDULLARY NAILING OF FRACTURES OF THE DISTAL TIBIAL SHAFT

Intramedullary nailing of more distal fractures is possible, but the ability to maintain a mechanically stable reduction becomes more difficult the farther the fracture extends distally. Two distinct fracture patterns have been identified. Direct bending forces produce simple transverse and oblique tibial fractures with same-level fibular fractures and no intraarticular extension, but soft-tissue injury is more severe. Torsional forces cause spiral fractures, usually with different-level fibular fracture and frequent intraarticular involvement of either the medial or the posterior malleolus. One must also be cognizant of the potential for distal fracture extension to the tibial plafond or associated ankle pathology. Stuermer and Stuermer identified that in the presence of certain injury markers, namely, pronation-eversion mechanisms, spiral fractures, proximal fibular fractures, or an intact fibula, associated ankle injuries were diagnosed in 20.1% of patients. We typically recommend a CT scan for distal fractures with radiographic evidence or concern about distal intraarticular extension.

Two distal locking screws are required to prevent recurvatum deformity from rotation around a single distal locking screw. Cancellous lag screws can be used to stabilize medial and posterior malleolar fractures. Open reduction is done if there is intraarticular displacement. The fibula is plated if necessary for the stability of the ankle joint or if it is severely displaced. Distal fibular fixation can be useful in very distal fractures to facilitate alignment of the tibia.

Although not advocated by Robinson et al., some investigators believe that plating same-level fibular fractures helps prevent malalignment in distal tibial fractures treated with intramedullary nailing. We analyzed the influence of fibular fractures on maintaining alignment in 40 distal-fourth tibial fractures treated with locked intramedullary nailing. The five tibial fractures with intact fibulas and four fractures with fibular fixation all healed in anatomic alignment. All 11 unfixed fibular fractures located at levels different from the tibial fracture were in anatomic alignment, whereas 12 (60%) of 20 unfixed fibular fractures occurring at the same level as the tibial fracture were malaligned. This study suggests that internal fixation of some fibular fractures improves stability in distal-fourth tibial fractures treated with intramedullary nailing. For transverse fractures of the fibula, we prefer a medullary device if fixation is deemed necessary.

Overall union rates of 96% have been reported after reamed nailing of distal tibial fractures. A biomechanical study determined that the fixation strength achieved in fractures 4 cm from the tibiotalar joint with a shortened nail (1 cm removed) was comparable with that of standard intramedullary nailing of fractures 5 cm from the joint. They cautioned, however, in neither construct was fixation strong enough to resist moderate compression-bending loads and that patients with distal tibial fractures treated with intramedullary nailing must follow weight-bearing restrictions until significant fracture healing occurs to prevent coronal plane malalignment. It is clear that intramedullary nail fixation of distal tibial fractures is challenging. Newer implant designs with tighter distal screw clusters have facilitated treatment of these injuries without need for implant modification.

Vallier et al. investigated the factors influencing outcomes after distal tibial shaft fractures in 104 patients. Functional testing identified residual dysfunction when compared with the uninjured population. Mild pain was noted but was not typically limiting. No patients reported unemployment as a result of their fracture. The same investigators reported a prospective comparison of plate with intramedullary nail fixation for distal tibial fractures. In their series, intramedullary nailing was associated with more malalignment.

ANTERIOR KNEE PAIN AFTER INTRAMEDULLARY NAILING

Anterior knee pain is the most commonly reported complication after intramedullary nailing of the tibia. Historically, 56% of patients have some degree of chronic knee pain and have difficulty kneeling. The cause of this knee pain is still unclear.

Suggested contributing factors include younger, more active patients, nail prominence above the proximal tibial cortex, meniscal tear, unrecognized articular injury, increased contact pressure in the patellofemoral articulation, damage to the infrapatellar nerve, and surgically induced scar formation.

Some authors have suggested that a transpatellar approach is associated with more frequent anterior knee pain than is a medial paratendinous approach, although others disagree. Investigations have shown no difference in anterior knee pain whether a transtendinous or paratendinous surgical approach was used. Anterior knee pain improves with time, yet quadriceps weakness and lower functional knee scores correlated with knee pain in the long term. In an effort to circumvent this issue, semiextended nailing techniques have been advocated, but have yet to demonstrate clear benefit with regard to anterior knee pain.

INTRAMEDULLARY INTERLOCKING NAILS

Currently, a variety of interlocking tibial nails are available. Most can be inserted using a reamed or unreamed technique. There are differences in nail composition (stainless steel, titanium) and location of the proximal bend. Some nails have medially to laterally directed locking screws, and others have additional proximal oblique screw holes and anteroposterior distal screw holes. Nails with more distally placed distal locking screws improve the ability to treat very distal tibial fractures. The surgeon should be familiar with the strengths and limitations of the various nailing systems to choose the appropriate implant for a specific fracture. All unstable fractures should be locked with two screws distally and two proximally to maintain length and prevent rotation. We routinely statically lock most fractures. A proximal drill guide allows accurate nail insertion and placement of the proximal screws, whereas distal fixation is typically performed free-hand.

PREOPERATIVE PLANNING

Preoperative radiographs of the uninjured tibia can be used to establish the proper nail diameter, the expected amount of reaming, and the final nail length for severely comminuted fractures. (Radiographic templates are available for preoperative planning.) The nail length should permit the proximal end to be countersunk with the distal end centered in the distal epiphysis. Diaphyseal fractures must be slightly distracted with traction before closed antegrade medullary nailing.

Further impaction occasionally occurs when severely comminuted fractures are later dynamized. This risk should be considered during the selection of nail length to prevent later nail migration into the ankle or nail protrusion out of the proximal tibia.

Measurement is especially important for very tall or very short patients who may require a nail either longer or shorter than is commonly kept in inventory. Colen and Prieskorn found that the most accurate method for determining correct nail length of four methods tested (full-length scanograms, "spotograms," acrylic template overlays, and tibial tubercle–medial malleolar distance [TMD]) was the TMD. The TMD is determined by measuring the length between the highest (most prominent) points on the medial malleolus and the tibial tubercle. Eleven of 14 nails selected by scanograms were incorrect, 6 of 14 selected by spotograms were incorrect, and 14 of 14 selected by templates were too small. TMD correctly selected 10 of 14 nail lengths. The authors suggested that the TMD is an easy, inexpensive, and accurate method of preoperative determination of correct nail length. The diameter of the nail is assessed by measuring the tibia at its narrowest point, which is best appreciated on lateral radiographs.

The decision to insert the nail with or without reaming should be made preoperatively. "Reamed" and "unreamed" refer to technique, rather than implants. Unreamed nail insertion usually requires nails with diameters ranging from 8 to 10 mm, depending on canal diameter, and cannot be used in patients with medullary canals narrower than 8 mm. Reaming allows insertion of stronger implants with larger diameters. We recommend reamed nail insertion for fractures, open or closed, with minor soft-tissue injury and only consider the unreamed nail technique for fractures with more extensive soft-tissue injury.

Nailing can be done using either a fracture table or a standard radiolucent operating table. A fracture table may be preferable if a skilled assistant is unavailable or if the fracture is not nailed acutely. Disadvantages of a fracture table include the longer time required for patient positioning, increased risk of nerve injury from traction or pressure on the posterior thigh from the crossbar, and the possibility of elevation of compartment pressures with prolonged traction. Multiple injuries are more easily treated on a standard operating table. Other advantages of the standard operating table include lower risk of iatrogenic nerve injury and greater flexibility in manipulating the fracture site and changing position of the extremity as needed. Without skeletal traction, however, fracture reduction is more difficult to maintain, and an assistant is needed to help stabilize the limb. We prefer a standard radiolucent table with the limb positioned over a bolster.

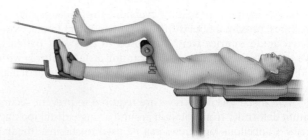

FIGURE 2.29   Patient is positioned supine, and traction is applied through calcaneal traction pin or special foot holder. **SEE TECHNIQUE 2.11.**

INTRAMEDULLARY NAILING OF TIBIAL SHAFT FRACTURES

TECHNIQUE 2.11

Fracture Table

- If a fracture table is used, place a calcaneal traction pin before positioning. Place the patient supine with the hip flexed 45 degrees and the knee flexed 90 degrees (Fig. 2.29).
- Place a well-padded crossbar proximal to the popliteal fossa to support the thigh in the flexed position. Adequate padding should reduce the risk of compression neuropathy.
- Attach the calcaneal pin to the traction apparatus on the fracture table, apply traction, and reduce the fracture under fluoroscopic guidance.
- To decrease the risk of traction injury to neurologic structures, release the traction after the ability to reduce the fracture has been confirmed.
- Prepare and drape the limb, allowing full exposure of the knee to above the patella and enough access to the distal tibia for locking screw placement. Reapply traction after the entry portal is made.

Standard Operating Table

- If a standard operating table is used, place the patient supine with the thigh supported in a flexed position over a padded bolster.
- A skilled assistant is needed to assist with fracture reduction and help support the limb during the procedure.
- A femoral distractor or two-pin external fixator can be used to help maintain reduction. Place a Schanz pin 1 cm distal to the knee joint and place a second pin 1 cm proximal to the ankle joint. The proximal pin must be placed in the posterior portion of the tibial condyle to avoid the path of the nail.

Measurement of Rotation

- Before nailing, measure rotation by the method described by Clementz. Measure the amount of tibial torsion in the uninjured extremity with the knee fully extended and a C-arm image intensifier placed in the lateral position with the beam parallel to the floor.
- Rotate the leg until a perfect lateral view of the distal femur is obtained with the condyles superimposed exactly. Hold the knee and foot in this position while the C-arm is brought into the anteroposterior position with the beam perpendicular to the floor to image the ankle.
- Rotate the C-arm until a tangential image of the inner surface of the medial malleolus is seen. This is the reference line at the ankle.
- Tilt the beam cranially 5 degrees to obtain a better image of the ankle. Center the structures to be imaged in the radiographic field.
- The amount of tibial torsion is equal to the difference between the reference line at the ankle and a line perpendicular to the floor. If the tangential view of the medial malleolus is obtained with the C-arm rotated laterally 10 degrees from perpendicular, tibial torsion is 10 degrees.
- Alternatively, obtain rotational alignment by aligning the iliac crest, patella, and second ray of the foot.
- Close attention to operative technique can greatly decrease the risk of complications after tibial nailing.

Nail Placement

- Begin the entry portal by making a 3-cm incision along the medial border of the patellar tendon, extending from the tibial tubercle in a proximal direction. It may be necessary to extend the incision farther proximally through skin and subcutaneous tissue only to protect the soft tissues around the knee during reaming and nail insertion.
- Insert a threaded tip guidewire through the metaphysis anteriorly to gain access to the medullary canal (Fig. 2.30). With the appropriate soft-tissue sleeve, advance

the guidewire into the correct starting portal as noted on multiplanar imaging. This typically is located along the medial slope of the lateral tibial eminence on the anteroposterior view and just anterior to the articular margin on lateral imaging.

- Confirm the proper position on anteroposterior and lateral fluoroscopic views before guidewire insertion. Obtain a true anteroposterior view of the tibia when assessing the placement of the guidewire. If the limb is externally rotated, the portal may be placed too medially and violate the tibial plateau and injure the intermeniscal ligament. A portal placed too distally may damage the insertion of the patellar tendon or cause the nail to enter the tibia at too steep of an angle, which may cause the tibia to split or cause the nail to penetrate the posterior cortex. Check the process of insertion on lateral fluoroscopic views. The safe zone for tibial nail placement is just medial to the lateral tibial spine on the anteroposterior view and immediately adjacent and anterior to the articular surface on the lateral view.
- Direct the guidewire to a position nearly parallel to the shaft as it is inserted more deeply to prevent violation of the posterior cortex. Once appropriate provisional guidewire trajectory is achieved, create the entry portal with the cannulated entry reamer with matching soft-tissue protection sleeve. Alternatively, the starting portal can be created with a cannulated curved awl.
- Insert a ball-tipped guidewire through the entry portal into the tibial canal and pass it across the fracture site into the tibia under fluoroscopic guidance (Fig. 2.31). The guide rod should be centered and slightly lateral within the distal fragment on anteroposterior and central lateral views and advanced to within 1.0 to 0.5 cm of the ankle joint.
- If a reamed technique is chosen, ream the canal in 0.5-mm increments, starting with a reamer smaller than the measured diameter of the tibial canal (Fig. 2.32). Ream with the knee in flexion to avoid excessive reaming of the anterior cortex. Hold the fracture reduced during reaming to decrease the risk of iatrogenic comminution. Prevent the guide rod from being partially withdrawn during reaming. We prefer "minimal" reaming, with no more than 2 mm of reaming after cortical contact ("chatter") is first initiated. Newer larger diameter end-cutting reamers simplify the medullary preparation. It is advised to ream with the tourniquet deflated because its use may lead to thermal necrosis of bone and soft tissue.
- Choose a nail diameter that is 1.0 to 1.5 mm smaller than the last reamer used. Ream the entry site large enough to accept the proximal diameter of the chosen nail.
- Do not undersize the nail because a loose-fitting nail would be less stable and the smaller implants are not as strong and may be more prone to implant failure. In general, the largest implant suitable for a given patient should be used.
- When reaming is completed, determine the length of the nail by using the system-specific depth gauge to accurately determine the necessary implant length. Alternatively, place the tip of a guidewire of the same length at the most distal edge of the entry portal. Subtract the length of the overlapped portions of the guide rods from the full length of the guide rod to determine the length of the

nail, making sure the fracture is held out to length during this measurement. Comminuted fractures may require preoperative radiographic measurement of the contralateral tibia to assess length properly.

- Attach the insertion device and proximal locking screw guide to the nail. Direct the apex of the proximal bend in the nail posteriorly. Some nail systems use oblique proximal locking screws, which are directed anteromedial to posterolateral and anterolateral to posteromedial. Insert the nail with the knee in flexion (except in some proximal third fractures) to avoid impingement on the patella. Evaluate rotational alignment by aligning the iliac crest, patella, and second ray of the foot. This is imperative for not only fracture alignment but also the rotation of the implant in relation to the limb. This ensures that the interlocking holes remain in their intended orientation and that the sagittal bend of the nail does not induce deformity. Tremendous force should not be necessary to insert the nail. Moderate manual pressure with a gentle back-and-forth twisting motion usually is sufficient for nail insertion. If a mallet is used, the nail should advance with each blow. If the nail does not advance, withdraw the nail and perform further reaming or insert a smaller diameter nail. It is important to keep the fracture well aligned during nail insertion to prevent iatrogenic comminution and malalignment.
- When the nail has passed well into the distal fragment, remove the guidewire to avoid incarceration; and during final seating of the nail, release traction to allow impaction of the fracture. Do not shorten fractures excessively with segmental comminution. When the nail is fully inserted, the proximal end should lie 0.5 to 1.0 cm below the cortical opening of the entry portal. This position is best seen on a lateral fluoroscopic view. If the nail protrudes too far proximally, knee pain and difficulty with kneeling may result. Excessive countersinking also should be avoided because it makes nail removal more difficult. The distal tip of the nail should lie 0.5 to 2.0 cm from the subchondral bone of the ankle joint. Distal fractures require nail insertion near the more distal end of this range. If compression of the fracture is planned, the nail should be appropriately countersunk to prevent prominence once the fracture is compressed.
- Insert proximal locking screws using the jig attached to the nail insertion device. Place the drill sleeve through a small incision down to bone. Measure the length of the screw from calibrations on the drill bit. The number of interlocking screws is dependent on fracture characteristics. Tighten all connections between the insertion device, drill guide, and nail before screw insertion.
- Perform distal locking by using a freehand technique after "perfect circles" are obtained by fluoroscopy. In the lateral position, adjust the fluoroscopic beam until it is directed straight through the distal screw holes and the holes appear perfectly round.
- Place a drill bit through a small incision overlying the hole and center the tip in the hole. Taking care not to move the location of the tip, bring the drill bit in line with the fluoroscopic beam and drill through the near (medial) cortex. Detach the drill from the bit and check the position of the drill bit with fluoroscopy to ensure that it is passing through the screw hole. When proper position is confirmed, drive the drill bit through the far (lateral) cortex.

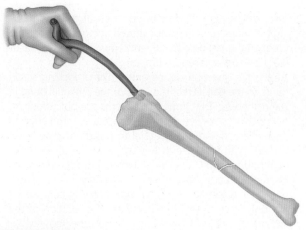

FIGURE 2.30 Opening of medullary canal with curved awl. **SEE TECHNIQUE 2.11.**

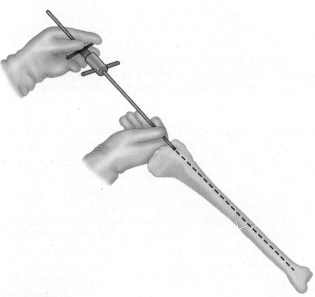

FIGURE 2.31 Reduction of fracture with guide rod. **SEE TECHNIQUE 2.11.**

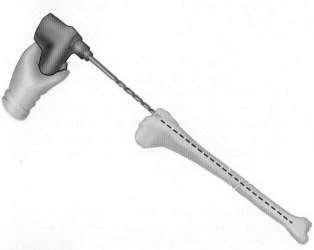

FIGURE 2.32 Reaming of tibia in 0.5-mm increments, using cannulated reamers over guide rod. **SEE TECHNIQUE 2.11.**

- Measure the screw length using drill sleeves and calibrated bits or check the anteroposterior view on the fluoroscopy screen, using the known diameter of the nail as a reference for length, or a system-specific depth gauge.
- After screw insertion, obtain a lateral image to ensure the screws have been inserted through the screw holes. Two distal locking screws are used in most fractures.
- Some nail systems have the option of placing an anteroposterior distal locking screw. "Perfect circles" are obtained in the anteroposterior fluoroscopic view. Do not injure the anterior tibial tendon or extensor hallucis longus or nearby neurovascular structures. Meticulous attention to technique can minimize complications from anteroposterior distal interlocking. Careful soft-tissue protection and retraction both during drilling and screw insertion are critical to prevent soft-tissue injury or tethering as the screw head engages anterior tibial cortex. A drill sleeve can be valuable for protection of the associated soft tissues during this portion of the procedure.
- Before interlocking, inspect the fracture site for possible distraction. If the fracture is distracted, place the distal locking screws first. Some intramedullary implants now have the capability to provide axial compression, for properly selected fracture patterns, during the process of interlocking.
- After distal locking is complete, impact the fracture by carefully driving the nail backward while watching the fracture site under fluoroscopy. Keep the knee flexed until the nail insertion instruments are removed to avoid damage to the soft tissues around the patella.
- Most nails are statically locked. Minimally comminuted transverse diaphyseal fractures can be dynamically locked; however, comminuted or metaphyseal fractures should be statically locked. If there is any question about stability, perform static locking. Because the nail may not prevent malalignment of unstable fractures before it is locked, it is crucial to maintain accurate reduction until proximal and distal locking is complete.
- Modifications in technique have decreased the incidence of malalignment in proximal-third fractures. The reduction can be manipulated more freely if nailing is not done on a fracture table.
- To prevent valgus, start the entry portal in line with the lateral intercondylar eminence and center it on the medullary canal on the anteroposterior fluoroscopic image. An incision lateral to the patellar tendon can be used.
- To prevent anterior angulation and displacement, move the portal more proximally and posteriorly and direct it more vertically in a line more parallel with the anterior tibial cortex. Interlocking the nail proximally with the knee extended relaxes the pull of the patellar tendon and prevents anterior angulation. Many nail systems require removal of the insertion jig, however, to extend the knee to avoid impingement on soft tissues.
- Tornetta et al. recommended nailing proximal-third tibial fractures in a semiextended position (15 degrees of flexion) using two thirds of a medial parapatellar arthrotomy to retract the patella laterally. This technique prevents the patella from causing the portal to be angled from medial to lateral and allows proximal interlocking to be performed with the knee extended. Using a nail with a more proximally located bend decreases the risk of ante-

rior displacement of the proximal fragment. A nail with proximal locking screws oriented obliquely at 90 degrees to each other provides more resistance to varus-valgus angulation than one-plane, medial-to-lateral screws. Semiextended nailing through a suprapatellar portal also has been described and is gaining in popularity. In this technique, a midline incision is created approximately two fingerbreadths proximal to the superior pole of the patella. The quadriceps mechanism is divided sharply in line with its fibers. It is critical to use suprapatellar specific instrumentation to provide protection to the patellofemoral joint. The cannula and trocar are inserted atraumatically in a retropatellar fashion, allowing the femoral trochlea to act as a guide to positioning the instrumentation in line with the medullary canal. The guide pin placement, medullary reaming, and nail insertion can then proceed as previously described.

- In contrast to diaphyseal fractures, the nail does not "automatically" reduce the fracture because it is inserted through the wide tibial metaphysis. Accurate fracture reduction before nail insertion helps to decrease the risk of malalignment. Reduction can be accomplished by using an AO distractor medially or by limited open reduction and application of a unicortical plate as described by Benirschke et al. This technique can be particularly useful in open fractures.
- Malalignment also can be prevented by using blocking screws as described by Krettek et al. Overcorrect the deformity and insert blocking screws anteriorly to posteriorly on the concave side of the deformity. The screws effectively reduce the diameter of the metaphysis and physically block the nail by creating an artificial "cortex," thus preventing angulation by increasing stability. Use of blocking screws to prevent malalignment in distal metaphyseal fractures also can be valuable (Fig. 2.33).

POSTOPERATIVE CARE The patient initially is placed in a removable splint or orthosis and early range-of-motion exercises are begun. Noncompliant patients or patients with unstable fracture fixation are placed in a patellar tendon-bearing brace or orthosis until enough healing occurs to ensure stability. Unrestricted weight bearing is permitted in axial stable patterns (i.e., transverse diaphyseal). Weight bearing is restricted until early callus occurs (4 to 6 weeks) and then is progressed as tolerated in fractures without axial stability and those at the proximal or distal metadiaphyseal junction. Nail removal is not routinely necessary but may be needed to relieve pain in patients with prominent implants. Nail removal usually is delayed until at least 12 to 18 months after injury, when all fracture lines are obliterated and there is full cortical remodeling. Conversely, removal of interlocking screws for symptomatic implants is not uncommon and can be done once sufficient healing and fracture stability are achieved.

■ EXTERNAL FIXATION

External fixation is a useful and versatile tool in the treatment of tibial fractures, both as a temporizing and definitive treatment. Three distinct types of fixators are

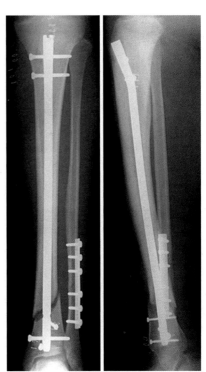

FIGURE 2.33   Malalignment after intramedullary nailing can be prevented by use of blocking screws in addition to standard locking screws. **SEE TECHNIQUE 2.11.**

commonly used: half-pin fixators, wire and ring fixators, and hybrid fixators that combine half-pins and tensioned wires. Although commonly used in the past, transfixion pins currently are used mainly in the calcaneus or as part of a two-pin "traveling traction" fixator. These devices can be used to stabilize almost any fracture, whether open or closed, throughout the length of the tibia. External fixation provides stable fixation, preserves soft tissues and bone vascularity, leaves wounds accessible, and causes little blood loss. Frame designs provide uniplanar or multiplanar fixation and can be modified to allow axial compression with weight bearing, which stimulates fracture union. External fixators that use tensioned wires for fixation extend the indications for external fixation to include periarticular fractures (Fig. 2.34). Pin site infection, malunion, joint stiffness, patient acceptance, and delayed union remain the greatest problems, however, associated with external fixation.

External fixation as definitive management usually is indicated for severe open fractures (type IIIB and type C), especially fractures with gross contamination of the tibial canal or if the adequacy of the initial debridement (shotgun wound, crush injuries) is a concern. External fixation also can be used in the delayed management of fractures with bone loss, either by providing stabilization for autogenous bone grafting or by creating regenerated bone with circular wire fixators. External fixators also are preferable in patients with very small medullary canals, fractures associated with burns or wounds over the tibial nail entry portal, open fractures receiving delayed treatment (>24 hours), severely contaminated fractures, fractures with vascular injury in which

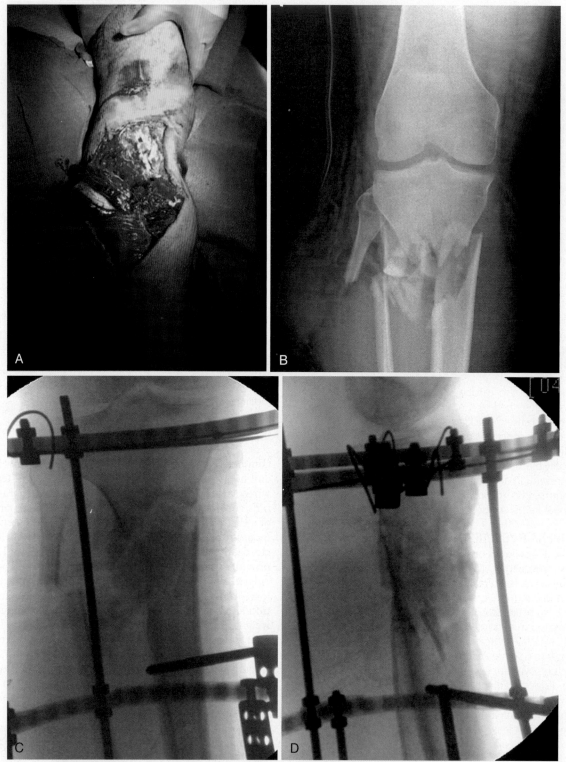

FIGURE 2.34 **A** and **B,** Clinical photograph and initial radiograph of pedestrian struck by vehicle at high speed. Presented with Gustilo 3B open proximal fibular and tibial fractures. Note large bone defect. **C** and **D,** Fracture managed with multiplanar ring external fixator secondary to overlying soft-tissue injury requiring skin grafting. Osseous defect managed with bulk autogenous bone grafting and acute compression/shortening of fracture in wire frame after removal of large antibiotic spacer.

salvage may be questionable, war injuries, and in some patients with multiple-system trauma in whom blood loss must be kept to a minimum.

External fixation may be indicated for patients with unstable closed fractures, fractures complicated by compartment syndrome, diaphyseal fractures with periarticular extension, segmental fractures with a periarticular component, and head injury or impaired sensation.

Initial healing of a fracture, especially a comminuted open fracture, depends on the blood supply from surrounding soft tissues. Fracture and soft-tissue stability must be maintained to allow continued capillary ingrowth into the injured areas. If external fixation is used for open tibial fractures, temporary fixation of the foot to eliminate ankle and soft-tissue motion at the fracture site should be considered. If fixation of the foot is not important for fracture stability, it is removed when the soft tissues have healed, and ankle motion is encouraged.

The amount of stiffness that provides the most favorable environment for fracture healing in an external fixator is unknown. More rigid frames are preferred initially during the phase of soft-tissue healing and usually have fewer pin site problems. Fractures with more inherent instability require stiffer frames than more stable fracture patterns. There is evidence that gradually destabilizing the frame to permit more weight bearing by the bone stimulates fracture healing. Destabilization usually includes converting the frame from a static to a dynamic construct by loosening the pin-to-bar clamps on one side of the fracture. Axial compression is allowed while maintaining angular and rotational alignment. Frames also can be made less rigid by increasing the distance between the bar and the bone and removing the outer bar in a double-bar frame. The fracture should be stable enough to resist excessive shortening or angulation before fracture destabilization.

Although external fixation long has been proposed for provisional soft-tissue care, a growing number of reports advocate it for definitive fracture care, especially for high-energy fractures with significant diastasis or dissociation of the tibia and fibula and little intrinsic stability. These reports cite high complication rates, especially of malunion, with conversion of high-energy fractures from external fixation to casts. External fixators now usually are retained until fracture union. External fixation also provides stability for fractures that require subsequent bone grafting. Although open fractures with bone loss clearly require bone grafting or bone transport with ring fixators, open fractures with periosteal stripping (type IIIB) also frequently require autogenous bone grafting for union. These especially difficult fractures have led some authors to recommend early bone grafting in all such injuries.

To avoid intrinsic problems of delayed union, nonunion, pin loosening, and pin track infection, conversion to internal fixation after soft tissues and all pin sites have healed (8 to 12 weeks) has been suggested as the ideal time for such conversion, while others have cautioned against early removal of the fixator in high-energy fractures with disruption of the interosseous membrane, comminution, or bone loss. In a prospective evaluation of 78 patients, Bråten et al. demonstrated that time to union and full weight bearing were similar between intramedullary nails and external fixation. However, the cohort receiving a nail achieved unprotected weight bearing sooner. External fixation resulted in more reoperations, whereas 64% of the patients with intramedullary nails had anterior knee pain at 1 year. Others have evaluated the factors that influence fracture healing with external fixation and found significant disparities of healing associated with lack of supplemental fixation techniques and pin track infections.

HALF-PIN FIXATORS

Numerous brands of external fixators are available. The fixator chosen should provide adequate stability, permit progressive weight bearing, and allow dynamization and destabilization as the fracture heals. Fixator systems that accommodate pin placement in more than one plane and have the ability to include the foot are most useful. Lighter weight, lower cost, and less interference with visualization of the bone on radiographs also are desirable attributes if they do not compromise the stability and versatility of the system. Single-unit fixators with large universal joints readily permit adjustments to fracture reduction after the frame is applied. These fixators tend to be less stable because they do not allow wide pin spacing, and it is more difficult to add a second plane of fixation. Modular fixators allow greater freedom in placement but are more difficult to adjust when the frame is completed. Pin removal and replacement may be necessary to improve reduction. Newer pin clamp designs with ball joint or pivoting mechanisms increase the adjustability of these constructs to some extent.

PREOPERATIVE PLANNING

The initial frame should be rigid enough to minimize motion at the fracture site. Stability can be increased in several ways, as follows: increasing pin diameter, increasing the distance between the pins, increasing the number of pins, increasing the number of stabilizing bars, decreasing the distance from the bar to the limb, and adding a second plane of fixation. Tibial fixators use pins ranging from 4.5 to 6.0 mm in diameter. The pin should be less than one third the diameter of the bone to prevent fracture. Uncomminuted fractures require a minimum of two pins for each major fragment (including large segmental fragments). A uniplanar construct usually provides sufficient stability for many tibial fractures. The addition of a third pin to a fragment significantly increases rigidity, especially if it is in another plane. A fourth pin in a single fragment provides minimal additional stability and usually is unnecessary. Comminuted fractures may benefit from three pins per major fragment, and two-plane fixation is preferred. Two-plane fixation can be achieved by connecting pins in different planes to a single bar. Alternatively, the pins placed in a second plane can be attached to a second bar, and the bars can be connected with bar-to-bar clamps. Rigidity can be increased in a uniplanar construct by connecting the pins to the two bars stacked on top of each other.

Widely spaced pins in each fragment provide stability in the plane of fixation and in the plane perpendicular to it. Short fragments do not allow wide pin spread, however. Two pins placed in the same plane in a short fragment provide stability in the plane of the pins but are less stable in the plane perpendicular to the pins. Adding a pin in a different plane enhances stability. Because the major bending moments in the tibia occur in the sagittal plane, fixation in this plane is more stable. Tibial fractures associated with unstable ipsilateral ankle injuries or with severe soft-tissue wounds of the distal leg require extension of the fixation into the foot to facilitate soft-tissue healing.

EXTERNAL FIXATION FOR TIBIAL SHAFT FRACTURES

At our institution, this technique is most applicable for provisional stabilization of open tibial fractures or in the setting of multiple trauma for fractures that will typically be managed definitively by other means.

TECHNIQUE 2.12

- Before fixator application, review cross-sectional anatomy to confirm the "safe zones" for pin placement and to minimize the risk of neurologic, vascular, or tendinous injury.
- Place pins through either the anterior or the anteromedial cortex along the subcutaneous border of the tibia to avoid soft-tissue tethering. Direct the pins perpendicular to the long axis of the bone and parallel to the joint surfaces and insert them through small longitudinal incisions.
- Bluntly dissect soft tissues to bone.
- Place a drill sleeve against the bone and predrill the pin hole with an appropriate-size bit. Predrilling lowers the risk of thermal necrosis and pin loosening.
- Insert a pin with the correct thread length through the sleeve by power drill and into the bone. Bicortical purchase is necessary to prevent loosening. Threads should not protrude through the skin at the insertion site because this can cause pin site irritation. Some pins have conical rather than cylindrical threaded portions to create a radial preload with tightening. These pins cannot be backed out after insertion without causing loosening. Do not insert them too deeply.
- Some systems have different thread designs for cortical and cancellous bone, which use different drill bits. The following is a technique for the application of a generic modular fixator.
- Pins should be nearly perpendicular to the long axis of the tibia and parallel to the knee and ankle joints. If the length of the segments allow, place the most proximal and distal pins at the metaphyseal-diaphyseal junction, where the bone is thicker and better pin purchase is obtained than in the cancellous bone of the metaphysis. Proximally, place the pin at least 15 mm from the joint to avoid penetration of the joint capsule and avoid the pes tendons and patellar tendon.
- Place the inner pin in each fragment at least 1 cm from the fracture site, avoiding undisplaced areas of comminution. The fracture site could become secondarily infected from a pin site infection if the pin is too close. If the length of the segment allows, place inner pins 2 to 3 cm from the fracture site. Keep in mind that wide pin spread enhances stability.
- Apply multiple pin-to-bar connections and connect the bars positioned.

- Perform reduction. If the injury is open, the traumatic wound provides an excellent opportunity to effect reduction under direct vision or with provisional clamps.
- Securely tighten all connections. Assess fracture reduction with fluoroscopy and adjust as needed.
- Additional bars can increase construct stability.
- If stability warrants, expand the external fixation to include the foot. To include the foot, insert 4-mm or 3-mm pins through the subcutaneous border of either the first or the fifth metatarsal respectively or, if necessary, place larger half-pins or transfixation pins in the posterior tuberosity of the calcaneus. Avoid equinus, inversion, and eversion of the foot.
- Connect the foot pins to the tibial frame using either specialized pin clamps or additional bars and bar-to-bar clamps.
- Combining external fixation with lag screw fixation of the diaphysis is discouraged.

POSTOPERATIVE CARE Pin site care is started after the initial postoperative dressing has been removed. Pin sites are cleaned daily using a diluted hydrogen peroxide solution or antibacterial soap and water. Pin sites are inspected to ensure that the pins are tight. A removable splint is used to prevent equinus, with definitive fixation performed later.

COMPLICATIONS

When the soft-tissue techniques previously described are used and the safe zones of the tibia are observed, especially with half-pin fixation in the subcutaneous tibial border, immediate complications are rare. Vascular injury more often is the result of late erosion of a vessel than of direct injury; however, direct injury is possible, especially with transfixation pins in bilateral uniplanar frames. Persistent bleeding at the time of surgery or late spontaneous bleeding must be investigated to rule out direct injury, late erosion, or pseudoaneurysm of a major vessel. We have seen persistent bleeding around the pins from small periosteal arteries in children.

Pin track irritation is common and requires daily pin site care with soap and water cleansing and gentle pressure dressings. Oral antibiotics may be required for secondary cellulitis.

Removal of the external fixator and application of a cast before union in high-energy tibial fractures may result in malunion or nonunion. Intramedullary nailing after external fixation, especially with a history of a pin track infection, results in a high rate of infection, although a low rate of malunion or nonunion. In our experience, with an average delay in nailing of 7 weeks after fixator removal, intramedullary nailing of delayed union or nonunion of the tibia has been extremely successful. Gustilo recommended delaying any reconstructive surgery for severe open tibial fractures, including bone grafting and delayed nailing, until all wounds are reepithelialized.

ILIZAROV EXTERNAL FIXATION DEVICE

The tensioned wire external fixator has proved valuable in the acute and subacute care of tibial fractures. It has been used more frequently for difficult fractures, especially metaphyseal fractures with significant shaft extension. Difficult nonunions with bone loss, deformity, or infection also have been managed effectively with this type of fixation (Fig. 2.35). Preoperative planning and frame construction, early mobilization of the patient, daily cleansing of skin and frame, and close follow-up minimize complications.

Our experience with the Ilizarov external fixator has been primarily with tibial fractures. Stabilization of short periarticular fragments is possible with this appliance. Four 1.8-mm diameter wires used to stabilize a bicondylar tibial plateau fracture provide the effective cross section of fixation of 7.2 mm. Four wires also provide eight cortical interfaces and, because of the multiplanar orientation, virtually eliminate any late displacement of fragments. Because the wires are highly tensioned and supported circumferentially, a trampoline of fixation is provided (Fig. 2.36). Spanning the knee or ankle for 4 to 6 weeks occasionally is necessary, especially after elevation of a joint surface and bone grafting.

The Taylor spatial frame (Smith & Nephew, Memphis, TN) is a unique ring-and-wire fixator consisting of two rings connected by six oblique struts (Fig. 2.37). Its application is similar to that of the Ilizarov except that FastFx struts are used, and reduction is performed manually under image intensification until the best possible reduction is obtained in the anteroposterior and lateral planes. The struts are then locked in place. Additional rings can be added as necessary, and the foot can be incorporated. With the aid of a computer software-generated prescription, the struts can be adjusted as a procedure in the outpatient setting to effect anatomic reduction at the fracture site. Radiographic parameters are entered into a computer. Length, rotation, translation, and coronal and sagittal alignment all can be corrected by changing the lengths of the six struts as dictated by the computer program. We have used this fixator primarily to correct malunions, but it can be useful in treating acute fractures as well.

Open fractures with extensive bone loss are another indication for the Ilizarov method. The unstable fracture, soft-tissue defect, and bone loss all are managed successfully with one device and method. The first step in the management of complex fractures is to determine if the limb is salvageable, however. Occasionally, these injuries are managed best by early amputation, especially in the presence of major arterial or nerve injury. A dysvascular, insensate terminal limb does not function better than a prosthetic limb. The number of operations, the length of treatment, and the psychologic factors associated with salvage of a severely injured limb must be considered. Other relative indications for the Ilizarov fixator in acute trauma are open fractures, unstable closed fractures, and compartment syndrome.

Up to 100% union rates have been reported after this technique. We examined 40 unstable tibial fractures treated with the Ilizarov external fixator, 37.5% of which were open fractures; 12 of the 15 open fractures were Gustilo grade III fractures. Nineteen fractures were bicondylar tibial plateau fractures with extensive shaft extension. Four autogenous bone grafts were required for open fractures with bone loss. One fracture failed to unite and required

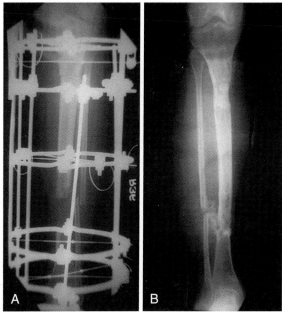

FIGURE 2.35 **A,** Infection after open tibial fracture was treated with bone resection and Ilizarov bone transplant, with bone graft at docking site. **B,** After removal of fixator.

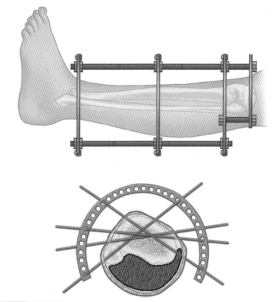

FIGURE 2.36 Ilizarov external fixation provides trampoline effect because of highly tensioned wires that are supported circumferentially.

reapplication of a frame, after which union was obtained. The average active range of motion of the knee after fracture healing was 110 degrees.

Time to union probably is related to the quality of reduction and restoration of normal alignment. We prefer accurate apposition and alignment at the initial application of a simpler trauma frame rather than the use of articulated frames and subsequent reduction. Our preference for tibial fractures for which definitive external fixation has been selected is multiplanar ring external fixation as opposed to a modular half-pin fixator.

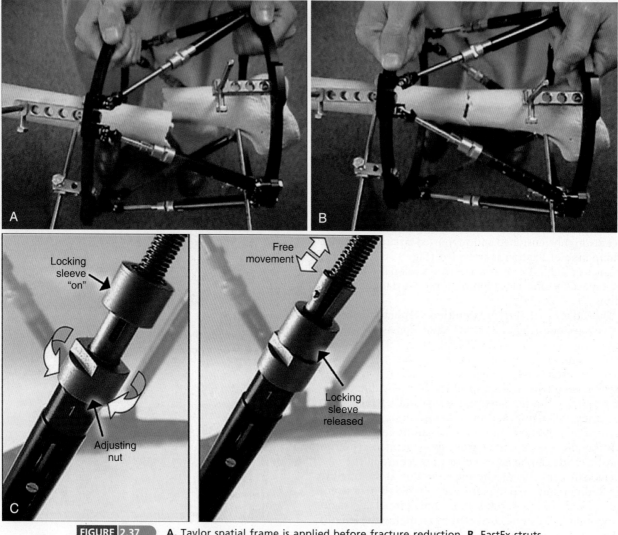

FIGURE 2.37 **A,** Taylor spatial frame is applied before fracture reduction. **B,** FastFx struts allow reduction under direct vision or C-arm control. If reduction is satisfactory, no adjustments are necessary; if not, gradual adjustments can be made using the deformity correction computer program. **C,** FastFx struts have dual actions. With the locking sleeve released, strut lengths can be changed to effect fracture reduction. (Courtesy Smith & Nephew, Memphis, TN.)

ILIZAROV METHOD IN OPEN FRACTURES

In open fractures with bone loss, the Ilizarov external fixator should be strongly considered as the primary treatment. Conventional treatment consists of debridement and delayed coverage with a rotation or free flap, followed by autogenous bone grafting. The tensioned wire fixator allows serial debridement of all necrotic tissue. If bone is not exposed, a split-thickness skin graft can be placed onto the remaining muscle. Later, a corticotomy is performed with transport of bone into the gap. The tendency of soft tissue is to move with the transported bone and the normal tendency of split-thickness grafts to contract and fill the soft-tissue and bony defects, eliminating the need for more difficult rotation or free flaps. If an insignificant length of vascular exposed bone is present after debridement, further shortening of fragment ends should be considered to avoid the necessity of flap coverage. Then a simple skin graft can be used as just described. Alternatively, the Taylor Spatial Frame can be used. It permits soft-tissue closure followed by gradual correction of osseous alignment for injuries that would otherwise require more involved soft-tissue coverage procedures.

If a significant amount of vascular bone remains uncovered after debridement, a free flap or rotation flap should be used (Fig. 2.38A). At flap coverage, a corticotomy is made and a fragment is prepared for transport into the bony defect (Fig. 2.38B and C). Ilizarov recommended a metaphyseal corticotomy for bone transport.

RECONSTRUCTIVE PROCEDURES

Reconstructive soft-tissue procedures are possible with circular tensioned wire fixators. Typical fracture frames are composed of four threaded rods linking four complete rings. Temporary removal of one rod allows 180-degree access to the leg for bone grafting of delayed unions or for free flap grafts. Removal of the anterolateral rod allows access to a dorsalis pedis donor, and removal of the posteromedial rod allows access to the posterior tibial artery.

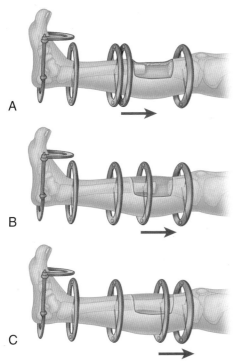

FIGURE 2.38 **A,** Free flap or rotation flap. **B** and **C,** Corticotomy and preparation of fragment for transport into bony defect.

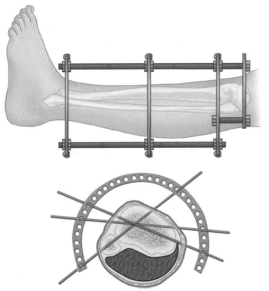

FIGURE 2.39 Open section ring used for most proximal ring in tibial mounting and attached to complete ring.

PREOPERATIVE PLANNING

Preparation is essential to success with the Ilizarov fixator. We modify the standard Ilizarov method by assembling the frames preoperatively, which greatly reduces intraoperative time. Radiographs are used to determine correct ring positions, and ring size is determined by the uninjured extremity. Two fingerbreadths of clearance are necessary for tibial mountings (Fig. 2.39). Rings that are too large do not support the transfixing wires adequately, and osteogenesis is impaired. Because of the anatomic constraints of safe wire placement, 90-degree divergence generally is unobtainable. A

second level of fixation in each segment improves frame stiffness to anteroposterior bending and torsion. Two rings are used on large fragments, and a ring and drop post are used for smaller fragments.

The midfemur is the most proximal level to accommodate a complete ring comfortably. Fixation to the proximal femur usually is accomplished with hybrid frames and half-pins. The entire lower extremity can be treated with a simple cylindrical frame from midfemur to the ankle. The thigh dictates ring size, usually one or two sizes larger than that normally used for the tibia. The frame should be situated parallel to the tibia on anteroposterior and lateral views. The femur is centered at the level of the patella and inclined in anatomic valgus with respect to the frame. An open section ring can be used as the distal femoral ring to allow full flexion at the knee (Fig. 2.40). This ring can be attached to a complete ring with heavyweight sockets to make it more resistant to deformity when tensioned wires are applied to the open section ring. Likewise, the most proximal ring in a tibial mounting can be an open section ring attached to a complete ring, allowing maximal flexion and providing two levels of fixation (see Fig. 2.39).

In open tibial fractures, the foot can be included in the frame to prevent soft-tissue motion at the fracture. Pilon fractures also may require foot fixation for fracture stability. The foot frame is removed after the soft tissues have healed, unless it is required for fracture stability. If the peroneal nerve or anterior or lateral compartment is injured, at least temporary incorporation of the foot should be considered to prevent contracture. The foot may be included in a tibial lengthening or bone transport to prevent equinus. A stable foot mounting consists of two half-rings joined by plates threaded on one end (Fig. 2.41). These special plates prevent distortion of the foot frame when wires are tensioned. Half-rings of the same size used for the tibial frame usually are used for the foot frame.

Swelling and dependent edema create late changes in extremity dimensions and must be anticipated. More clearance is needed posteriorly for the lower extremity, and the thigh requires more room for swelling than the leg.

ILIZAROV EXTERNAL FIXATION FOR TIBIAL SHAFT FRACTURES

TECHNIQUE 2.13

- Place the patient on a radiolucent table extension, using the external fixator for traction and subsequent reduction. Longitudinal traction reduces most fractures to within 10 to 15 degrees of anatomic alignment. In our experience, the addition of hinges to the trauma frame has been unnecessary. Excessive or prolonged traction should be avoided to prevent neurologic or vascular injury.
- After preparing and draping the extremity, disconnect the ring connection bolts on one side of the preassembled frame and open the frame.

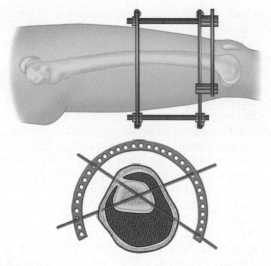

FIGURE 2.40   Open section distal femoral ring.

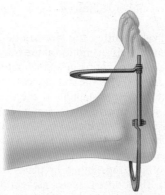

FIGURE 2.41   Stable foot mounting consisting of two half-rings joined by plates.

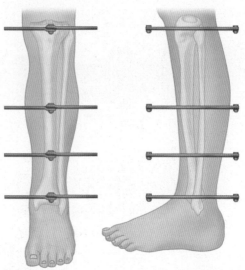

FIGURE 2.42   Frame reassembled around tibia and aligned parallel to crest of tibia in anteroposterior plane. **SEE TECHNIQUE 2.13.**

- Place the frame around the extremity, reassemble it with adequate soft-tissue clearance, and align it with coupling bolts parallel to the crest of the tibia in the anteroposterior and lateral planes (Fig. 2.42).
- If used to treat the fracture shown in Fig. 2.43A, hold the frame in this position with proximal and distal transverse reference wires placed parallel to the knee and ankle (Fig. 2.43B). As the wires are secured to the frame (Fig. 2.43C) and tension is applied, further correction of the fracture in the coronal plane is achieved (Fig. 2.43D).
- Alternatively, suspend the frame with ordinary suction tubing placed around the extremity and secured to the frame with towel clips. Tilt eccentrically the proximal and distal rings until they are parallel to the knee and ankle joints. After secure fixation with at least two wires to the proximal and distal rings, bring these two rings parallel to their counterparts in the center of the frame for further fracture reduction.
- Use arched olive wires for final fracture reduction (Fig. 2.43E). For final coronal plane correction of the residual displacement (Fig. 2.43F), place an olive wire in a transverse fashion (if safe) (Fig. 2.43G) and apply tension, without securing it tightly to the frame, to pull the fragment toward the tensioner. Use image intensification to ensure adequate reduction.

- After adequate correction is obtained in this plane, secure the wire to the frame on the olive side. If further correction is needed in the sagittal plane, connect this olive wire in an arched fashion (Fig. 2.43H) and tension the wire to obtain final correction (Fig. 2.43I and J). Eliminate any residual distraction (Fig. 2.44).
- In rare cases, two olive wires inserted from opposite sides perpendicular to the fracture plane can effect reduction and apply compression to the fracture (Fig. 2.45). This pattern of wire placement may not always be safe, however. These fractures should be fixed with one or more lag screws followed by external fixator placement (Fig. 2.46). Preoperative axial CT scans help determine the appropriate method of fixation. Interfragmentary screws or wires in the diaphyseal region usually should be avoided because they negate the axial flexibility of the Ilizarov external fixator, which ideally promotes secondary fracture healing.
- Handle skin and other soft tissues with care. In general, 1.5-mm and 1.8-mm wires need no incision or drill sheath. If desired, use a sheath and incision for insertion of the larger 2-mm wires. Glove paper can facilitate grasping the wire close to the insertion site for increased control.
- Use a small skin incision for olive wires. Predrilling is not required for wire insertion. Use a low-speed power drill with frequent pauses or a hand drill to drill the wires through bone.
- After determining the safe angle for the transfixation wires at a given level, stab the wire through the skin and muscle to bone. (Several references for safe transfixation using cross-sectional anatomy are available.)
- Use a low-speed drill to insert the wire across both cortices of the bone. When the wire emerges from the far cortex, tap it through the remaining soft tissues to reduce the risk of neurovascular injury. Avoid undue pressure or tension on the pin-skin interface.
- Attach the wires to the rings without bending them to meet the frame; this may require small spacers to build the connecting bolts off the frame.

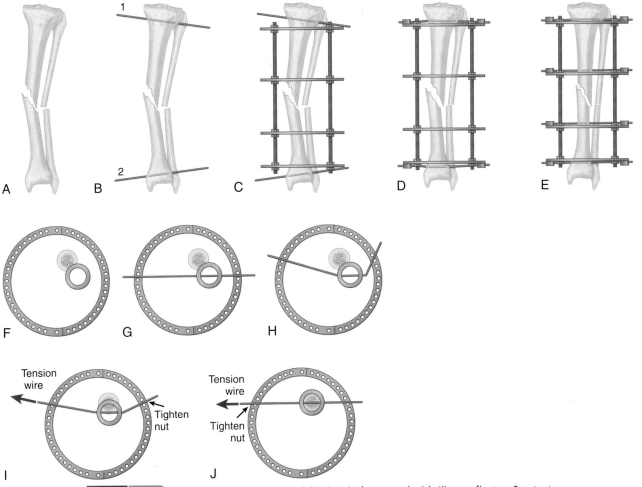

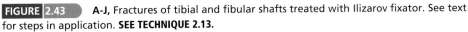

FIGURE 2.43 **A-J,** Fractures of tibial and fibular shafts treated with Ilizarov fixator. See text for steps in application. **SEE TECHNIQUE 2.13.**

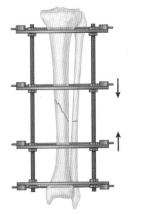

FIGURE 2.44 Residual distraction eliminated. **SEE TECHNIQUE 2.13.**

▌ COMPLICATIONS

With careful determination of safe zones by level of fixation, acute neurovascular injury with transfixation wires is rare. In the immediate postoperative period, an unusually painful wire should be suspected of passing through a larger nerve and should be removed. Late neurovascular injury is exceedingly rare, unless bone transport or relative motion of fragments exists, and usually occurs during a reconstructive procedure rather than during simple fracture immobilization. Flexion contractures of the knee and ankle occur less frequently with fracture treatment than with lengthening and can be prevented by active exercises and weight bearing in the frame. Pin irritation is common, although serious pin track infection is unusual. Wire-skin interfaces should be cleaned daily with soap and water. After wounds have healed, showers are encouraged and swimming in chlorinated pools is allowed with a clear water rinse afterward. Gentle pressure dressings prevent pin and skin motion. A loose wire must be suspected at the first signs of pain and inflammation. Suspect wires should be retensioned. Generalized cellulitis should be managed by assessment of all pin sites and administration of oral antibiotics until it resolves. Pin track infection that fails to respond to these measures should be treated by wire exchange.

Patients with head injuries may have excessive dependent edema because they rarely are moved enough to change the dependency or to help lymphatic pumping. If skin impinges on the frame toward the end of treatment (Fig. 2.47A), thin cardboard can be slotted to accommodate any wires and slipped between the skin and the frame to prevent pressure necrosis (Fig. 2.47B). If skin impinges on the frame early in the treatment, the frame must be modified. When problems

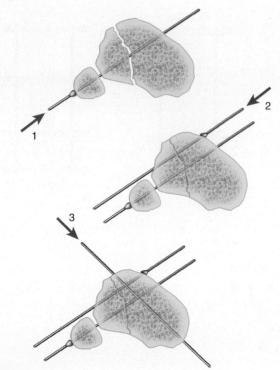

FIGURE 2.45 Insertion of two olive wires from opposite sides perpendicular to fracture plane. **SEE TECHNIQUE 2.13.**

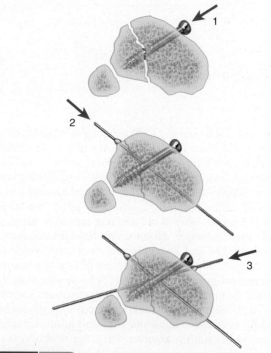

FIGURE 2.46 Fixation with one or more lag screws and application of external fixator. **SEE TECHNIQUE 2.13.**

exist at short-arc segments of several rings, the frame may be shifted toward the impingement by reattaching all wire fixation bolts in new holes away from the impingement. If the skin impinges on a single ring, that ring can be modified by introducing two short plates between the ends of the half-rings to create an ellipse with its major axis toward the impingement.

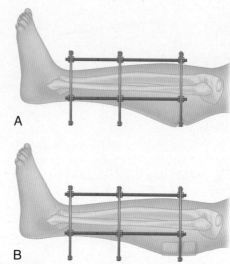

FIGURE 2.47 **A,** Impingement of skin on frame. **B,** Thin cardboard used to prevent pressure necrosis.

Alternatively, a saw can be used to remove a segment of a ring if sufficient stability remains. Major problems with circumferential impingement at several levels can be solved by constructing a larger frame around the first frame. The rings of this larger frame are positioned at exactly the same levels. Curled wire ends are straightened, and the wires are attached to the outer frame at both ends. Finally, wire fixation bolts on the smaller frame are loosened and the smaller frame is disassembled. Cannulated wire fixation bolts from the smaller frame may be taped against the new frame. This modification can be made without loosening wires or losing reduction.

■ TREATMENT OF DELAYED UNION OR NONUNION

Delayed union after unreamed nailing can be treated by nail exchange or by removal of the nail and insertion of a larger nail using a reamed technique. This technique is indicated for delayed unions in fractures with small (8 mm) or loose implants, axially unstable fractures, and perimetaphyseal fractures. The technique is unsuccessful in fractures with bone loss of more than one third to one half of the cortical circumference and may precipitate infection in type IIIB open fractures. Percutaneous bone grafting, the time-tested method for delayed union and nonunion of the tibia, is used most frequently for type IIIB open fractures and fractures with significant bone loss and after other methods have failed. Other methods for treatment of delayed union are external bone stimulation and historically dynamization of the nail to allow axial impaction of the fracture and to stimulate healing, provided that the fibula has not healed. Loss of reduction has been reported to occur in 16% of proximal and distal fractures after dynamization.

■ FIXATION OF THE FIBULA FOR TIBIAL FRACTURE

Internal fixation of the fibula is unnecessary in treating fibular shaft fractures but may be useful in stabilizing other structures. Fixation of a fibular fracture by a plate and screws or by an intramedullary nail inserted through the lateral malleolus partially stabilizes comminuted fractures of the distal tibial shaft or metaphysis when damage of the soft tissues or contamination of the wound makes internal fixation of the tibia inadvisable. Furthermore, internal fixation of the fibula may be considered as an adjuvant in very distal tibial fractures treated with intramedullary fixation to prevent valgus deformity.

DEFORMITIES OF THE FOOT AND TOES AFTER TIBIAL FRACTURE

A checkrein deformity of the great toe can occur after fracture of the distal third of the tibia. The flexor hallucis longus muscle adheres to callus at the fracture, with its tendon forming a bowstring between this point and the site of insertion of the tendon into the great toe. When the ankle is dorsiflexed, the great toe is sharply flexed, but when the ankle is plantarflexed, the interphalangeal joint extends completely. The pressure of the plantar surface of the great toe against the sole of the shoe on dorsiflexion of the ankle produces a painful callus. If it is impossible to free the muscle in the distal third of the leg after the fracture has united, the tendon is lengthened in the foot.

Clawfoot or cavus deformity has been reported after fractures of the tibial shaft and are believed to be the result of fibrous contracture of the muscles of the deep compartment from muscle trauma and ischemia in the deep posterior compartment of the leg. This deformity may be misinterpreted as an inward malrotation of the tibial fracture.

TIBIAL PLATEAU FRACTURE

Proximal tibial articular fractures caused by high-energy mechanisms may be associated with neurologic and vascular injury, compartment syndrome, deep vein thrombosis, contusion, crush injury to the soft tissues, or open wounds. Tscherne and Lobenhoffer emphasized the importance of distinguishing between the "pure" plateau fracture pattern and the fracture-dislocation pattern. In their review of 190 proximal tibial articular fractures, 67% of meniscal injuries occurred in plateau fracture patterns, whereas 96% of cruciate injuries and 85% of medial collateral ligament injuries occurred in fracture-dislocation patterns. Peroneal nerve injury was twice as common in fracture-dislocation patterns. These authors also introduced the term *complex knee trauma* to describe injuries associated with significant damage to two or more of the following compartments: the soft-tissue envelope of the knee, the ligamentous stabilizers, and the bony structures of the distal femur and proximal tibia. Complex fractures involving the femoral and tibial articular surfaces had a 25% incidence of vascular injury and 25% incidence of compartment syndrome. In 19 complex fractures with severe soft-tissue injury, vascular injury occurred in 31%, compartment syndrome in 31%, and peroneal nerve injury in 23%. Accurate determination of fracture pattern and soft-tissue injury is necessary when developing a treatment plan.

Proximal tibial articular fractures can be caused by motor vehicle accidents or bumper strike injuries; however, sports injuries, falls, and other less violent trauma frequently produce them, especially in elderly patients with osteopenia. The frequency of the type of fracture produced has been shown to be related to the frequency of collateral ligament injury to the type and mechanism of forces applied to the knee (Fig. 2.48). Considering the "pure" fracture patterns, ligamentous injuries occur more frequently in minimally displaced, local compression, and split compression fractures, and it is wise to obtain stress radiographs of the knee to evaluate these structures.

The classification of intraarticular proximal tibial fractures originally proposed by Hohl and later modified by Moore and Hohl is commonly used to describe tibial plateau fractures (Fig. 2.49). The classification distinguishes between five primary fracture patterns and five fracture-dislocation patterns, with fracture-dislocations occurring one seventh as frequently as fractures. Tibial plateau fracture patterns according to Hohl and Moore include type 1, minimally displaced; type 2, local compression; type 3, split compression; type 4, total condyle; and type 5, bicondylar. (Fracture-dislocation patterns are described in a later section.) Hohl observed that this classification may be an intermediate step in the evolution of a classification that separates the myriad ligamentous and soft-tissue injuries that, along with the bony injury, determine outcome. Our involvement with a level I trauma center has shown several fractures that defy conventional classification and treatment methods. These extremely high-energy fractures, frequently open, usually include bicondylar comminution and extensive shaft comminution with dissociation of the metaphysis and the diaphysis, as in Schatzker type VI. The Schatzker classification closely corresponds to the fracture patterns of Hohl and Moore with the addition of type VI, metaphyseal-diaphyseal dissociation. Schatzker, McBroom, and Bruce, in a review of 94 tibial condylar fractures, proposed the following classification and treatment methods when the fracture is significantly displaced or when significant joint instability is present.

FRACTURE CLASSIFICATION

Fracture patterns as classified by Schatzker:

Type I—pure cleavage (Fig. 2.50A). A typical wedge-shaped uncomminuted fragment is split off and displaced laterally and downward. This fracture is common in younger patients without osteoporotic bone. If displaced, it can be fixed with two transverse screws, or the addition of a low-profile condylar plate.

Type II—cleavage combined with depression (Fig. 2.50B). A lateral wedge is split off, but in addition the articular surface is depressed down into the metaphysis. This tends to occur in older individuals, and, if the depression is more than 5 to 8 mm or instability is present, most should be treated by open reduction, elevation of the depressed plateau "en masse." Then bone grafting of the metaphysis, fixation of the fracture with screws, and buttress plating of the lateral cortex are performed.

Type III—pure central depression (Fig. 2.50C). The articular surface is driven into the plateau. The lateral cortex is intact. These tend to occur in osteoporotic bone. If the depression is severe, or if instability can be shown on stress, the articular fragments should be elevated and bone grafted and the reduced articular injury is supported with subchondral rafting fixation, with or without plate augmentation.

Type IV—fractures of medial condyle (Fig. 2.50D). These may be split off as a single wedge or may be comminuted and depressed. The tibial spines often are involved. These fractures tend to angulate into varus and should be treated by open reduction and fixation with a medial buttress plate and screws.

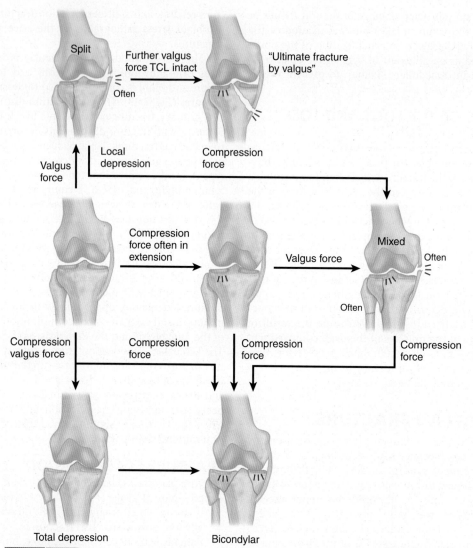

FIGURE 2.48 Relationship of force to tibial condylar fractures. Tibial collateral ligament injuries commonly occur in split and mixed fractures of lateral plateau. In mixed fractures, fibula is often fractured. In total depression fractures, proximal fibular fracture or proximal tibiofibular diastasis occurs.

Type V—bicondylar fractures (Fig. 2.50E). Both tibial plateaus are split off. The distinguishing feature is that the metaphysis and diaphysis retain continuity. Both condyles can be fixed with buttress plates and cancellous screws, to avoid stabilizing condyles with large bulky implants. The less involved condyle can be stabilized with a small antiglide plate placed at the apex of the fracture with minimal soft-tissue dissection, our preferred method.

Type VI—plateau fracture with dissociation of metaphysis and diaphysis (Fig. 2.50F). A transverse or oblique fracture of the proximal tibia is present in addition to a fracture of one or both tibial condyles and articular surfaces. The dissociation of the diaphysis and metaphysis makes this fracture unsuitable for treatment in traction, and most should be treated with buttress plates and screws, one on either side if both condyles are fractured. Pin and wire fixators also have been advocated for fixation of these difficult fractures.

FRACTURE-DISLOCATION CLASSIFICATION

The fracture-dislocation patterns classified by Hohl and Moore (Fig. 2.51), in addition to occurring with a higher incidence of associated ligamentous injuries, occur with more frequent meniscal injuries, and a much higher incidence of neurovascular injury, increasing from 2% for type I to 50% for type V, with an overall average of 15%, approximately that of classic dislocation of the knee.

Type I—coronal split fracture. These fractures account for 37% of tibial plateau fracture-dislocations. The fracture involves the medial side, is apparent on the lateral view, and has a fracture line running at 45 degrees to the medial plateau in an oblique coronal-transverse plane. The fracture may extend to the lateral side, and avulsion fractures of the fibular styloid, insertion of the cruciates, and Gerdy's tubercle are common. Half of these fracture-dislocations are stable on stress views, and although they conceivably could be managed in a cast in extension or traction with limited range of motion, we frequently

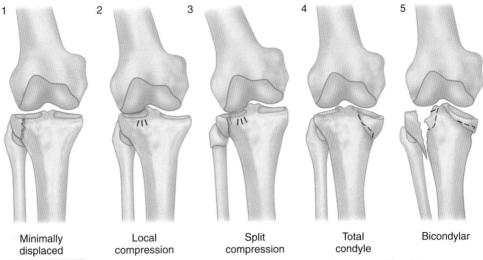

FIGURE 2.49 Classification of tibial plateau fractures as described by Hohl and Moore: type 1, minimally displaced; type 2, local compression; type 3, split compression; type 4, total condyle; and type 5, bicondylar.

use closed reduction and percutaneous screw fixation to improve reduction and allow early range of motion in a cast brace; protected weight bearing is continued for 8 to 10 weeks. If open reduction is required, the fragment usually reduces in extension and can be fixed with interfragmentary screws. Associated ligamentous injuries can be repaired along with the invariable capsular disruption.

Type II—entire condyle fracture. This fracture-dislocation may involve the medial or lateral plateau and is distinguished from the type IV fracture by a fracture line extending into the opposite compartment beneath the intercondylar eminence (Fig. 2.52). The opposite collateral ligament is involved in half of fractures, resulting in fracture or dislocation of the proximal fibula. This type constitutes 25% of all fracture-dislocations, and 12% result in neurovascular injuries. Stress testing is necessary to determine occult ligament injury. Stable fractures can be managed by cast bracing, frequent follow-up, and delayed weight bearing. Unstable or poorly reduced fractures can be fixed with interfragmentary screws after closed or open reduction and repair of any ligament injury, cast bracing, and delayed weight bearing.

Type III—rim avulsion fracture. Constituting 16% of fracture-dislocations, this type involves almost exclusively the lateral plateau, with avulsion fragments of the capsular attachment, Gerdy's tubercle, or the plateau. Disruption of either or both cruciate ligaments is common. Although meniscal injury is rare, neurovascular injuries occur in 30% of fractures and nearly all type III fractures are unstable. A lateral approach allows screw fixation of the articular rim and repair of avulsed iliotibial band and collateral ligaments. Cruciate ligament repair or augmentation may be necessary.

Type IV—rim compression fracture. This injury accounts for 12% of all fracture-dislocations. It is almost always unstable. The opposite collateral ligament complex and usually (75% of patients) the cruciate ligaments are avulsed or torn, allowing the tibia to sublux to the extent that the femoral condyle compresses a portion of the anterior, posterior, or "middle" articular rim. Stable injuries can

be treated by casting until the ligaments heal. If surgery is necessary, a parapatellar approach allows debridement of small fragments, elevation and stabilization of larger fragments, and repair of cruciate and opposite collateral ligaments. Postoperative mobilization is largely dictated by the nature of the ligamentous injury and repair.

Type V—four-part fracture. Constituting 10% of all fracture-dislocations, this injury is nearly always unstable. Neurovascular injury occurs in 50% of fractures; the popliteal artery and the peroneal nerve are injured in more than one third. Both collateral ligament complexes are disrupted with the bicondylar fracture, and the stabilization provided by the cruciates is lost because the intercondylar eminence is a separate fragment. Although a bicondylar approach has been recommended, others have been more cautious, recommending plating of the more comminuted plateau and lag screw fixation of the more intact condyle. Realizing the high incidence of infection and dehiscence with bicondylar plating and the extensive exposure necessary, a method of lateral plateau plating with temporary medial external fixation was described by Mast. We have used limited open reduction techniques combined with multiplanar external fixation. As with Schatzker type V bicondylar fractures, extreme care must be taken with soft tissues. Motion is not allowed until the skin has healed. Weight bearing is delayed according to the method of fixation; with Ilizarov fixation, early weight bearing is allowed to tolerance.

EVALUATION

A thorough history should be obtained, including determination of the mechanism of injury and the patient's overall medical status, age, and functional and economic demands. A detailed physical examination is necessary to detect concomitant ligamentous injuries, neurovascular injuries, compartment syndrome, additional fractures, and other injuries. Compartmental pressures should be measured with an accurate method if clinical suspicion of compartment syndrome exists in patients unable to provide a reliable clinical examination. Ankle-brachial indices should be obtained, and

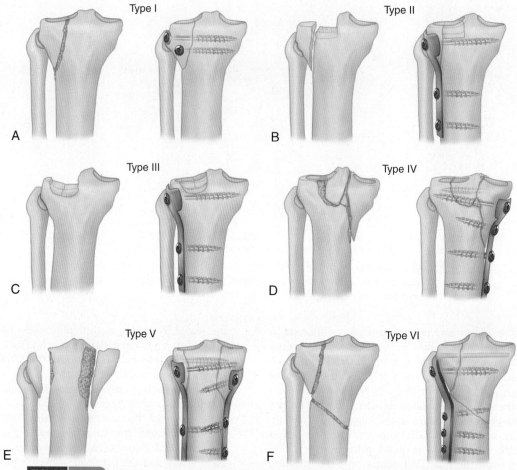

Type I   Type II   Type III   Type IV   Type V   Type VI

A   B   C   D   E   F

FIGURE 2.50   **A,** Type I, pure cleavage fracture. **B,** Type II, cleavage combined with depression. Reduction requires elevation of fragments with bone grafting of resultant hole in metaphysis. Lateral wedge is lagged on lateral cortex, protected with buttress plate. **C,** Type III, pure central depression. There is no lateral wedge. Depression also can be anterior or posterior or involve whole plateau. After elevation of depression and bone grafting, lateral cortex is best protected with buttress plate. **D,** Type IV. Medial condyle is split off as wedge (type A) as illustrated, or it can be crumbled and depressed (type B), which is characteristic of older patients with osteoporosis (not illustrated). **E,** Type V. Note continuity of metaphysis and diaphysis. In internal fixation, both sides must be protected with buttress plates. **F,** Type VI. Essence of this fracture is fracture line that dissociates metaphysis from diaphysis. Fracture pattern of condyles varies, and all types can occur. If both condyles are involved, proximal tibia should be buttressed on both sides.

further vascular studies should be obtained in patients with suspected vascular injury. Patients with obvious vascular injuries should be taken promptly to the operating room for vascular exploration and revascularization. Provisional stabilization with external fixation may be required.

Anteroposterior, lateral, and oblique radiographs and CT scans are necessary to evaluate these fractures. Assessment of the degree and the size of depressed articular fragments may be possible only with CT. Often the classification of the fracture made from standard radiographs is changed to another type after the CT scans are evaluated. The upper tibial articular surface normally is inclined posteriorly 10 to 15 degrees, and an anteroposterior radiograph with the beam angled caudally 10 to 15 degrees provides better views of the tibial plateaus. Stress radiographs for collateral ligament injury have been mentioned previously. Analysis of MRI findings in 29 tibial plateau fractures found tibial collateral injuries

in 55%, lateral meniscal tears in 45%, fibular collateral ligament injuries in 34%, anterior cruciate ligament injuries in 41%, posterior cruciate ligament injuries in 28%, and medial meniscal tears in 21%. Mustonen et al. demonstrated a 42% incidence of abnormal meniscal findings on MRI in patients who sustained tibial plateau fractures, and 88% of patients with meniscal tears had unstable injuries. The exact role of MRI in evaluating patients with tibial plateau fractures is still evolving. MRI is probably most appropriate in the evaluation of fracture-dislocation patterns when there is a high suspicion for injury to the associated soft-tissue stabilizers. Radiographic predictors for fractures with an increased incidence of compartment syndrome include tibial widening and femoral displacement.

Ruffolo et al. reported complication rates after ORIF of bicondylar injuries treated through dual incisions. Nonunion and deep infection occurred commonly after staged ORIF of

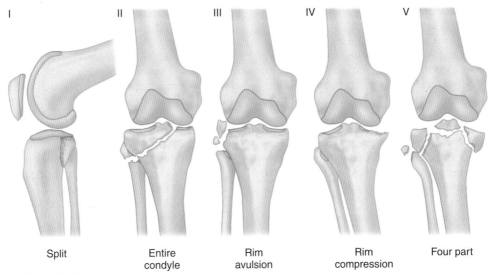

I	II	III	IV	V
Split	Entire condyle	Rim avulsion	Rim compression	Four part

FIGURE 2.51 Hohl and Moore classification of proximal tibial fracture-dislocations. (Redrawn from Hohl M, Moore TM: Articular fractures of the proximal tibia. In Evarts CM, editor: *Surgery of the musculoskeletal system*, ed 2, New York, 1990, Churchill Livingstone.)

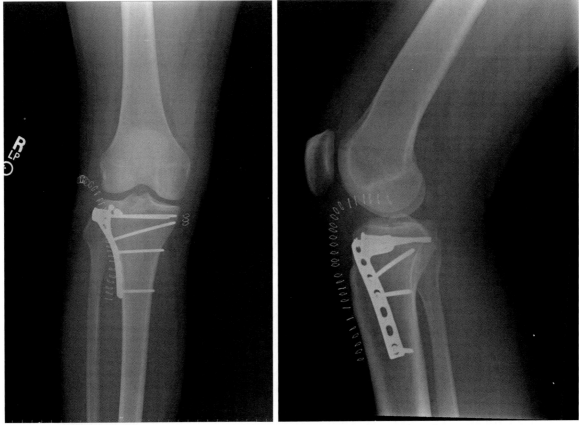

FIGURE 2.52 Type II fracture-dislocation of tibial plateau fixed with plate and screws.

high-energy tibial plateau fractures. Open fractures and open fasciotomy wounds at the time of internal fixation are associated with higher infection rates, 43.8% and 50.0%, respectively. Ahearn et al. noted poor patient-reported outcome measures after complex bicondylar tibial plateau fractures and similar clinical and radiographic outcomes with internal fixation and Taylor Spatial Frame.

Whatever the injury, the damage to the joint usually is more extensive than the radiographs indicate. The bony attachments of one or both cruciate ligaments may be avulsed and lie as free fragments in the joint. Comminuted fragments of the articular surface often lie at angles to their normal plane and may be upside down. The meniscus often is torn at its periphery, and a part or all of it may lie between the comminuted fragments.

TREATMENT

Goals of treatment of proximal tibial articular fractures include restoration of articular congruity, axial alignment, joint stability, and functional motion. If operative treatment is chosen, fixation must be stable enough to allow early motion and the technique should minimize wound complications. Surgical treatment is usually recommended for fractures associated with instability, ligamentous injury, and significant articular displacement; open fractures; and fractures associated with compartment syndrome. Ligamentous instability must be distinguished from osseous instability. After the articular surfaces of a joint have been fractured, joint function usually is proportionate to the accuracy of reduction. For displaced fractures, most authors point out that the most significant factor influencing long-term results, and hence treatment approach, is the degree of displacement and depression.

The degree of acceptable articular displacement is controversial. Some authors recommend surgical reduction for an articular stepoff of more than 2 mm, whereas others advocate surgical reduction for 5 mm or more of joint depression or displacement of more than 5 degrees axial alignment. Still others have reported similar clinical results with operative and nonoperative treatment of fractures with 8 mm of depression. Most authors agree that if depression or displacement exceeds 10 mm, surgery to elevate and restore the joint surface is indicated. If the depression is less than 5 mm in stable fractures, nonoperative treatment consisting of early motion in a hinged knee brace and delayed weight bearing usually is satisfactory. If the depression is 5 to 8 mm, the decision for nonoperative or operative treatment depends to a great degree on the patient's age, activity demands on the knee, and coronal plane stability. If a patient is elderly and sedentary, nonoperative treatment usually is suitable. If a patient is young or active, attempts at surgical reconstruction of the joint surface are justified.

Long-term follow-up studies have shown that posttraumatic arthritis is associated with residual instability or axial malalignment and not the degree of articular depression. Instability is another indication for operative treatment. Instability may result from ligamentous disruption, osseous depression of the articular surface, or translational displacement of a fracture fragment. Ligament injuries occur in 10% to 33% of tibial plateau fractures. The major indication for surgery is not the measure of depression of the fragment or articular surface but the presence of varus or valgus instability of 10 degrees or more with the knee flexed less than 20 degrees.

Treatment methods proposed for fractures of the tibial condyles include extensile exposure with arthrotomy and reconstruction of the joint surface with plate and screw fixation (Fig. 2.53), arthroscopy or limited arthrotomy and percutaneous screw fixation or external fixation with pin or wire fixators, and nonoperative management with a cast brace for selected patients. Newer plating techniques are capable of fixation with less iatrogenic soft-tissue elevation and use minimally invasive approaches. If more than one incision is used, a large soft-tissue bridge is left between them. No method can be used routinely for all fractures, and each patient must be evaluated individually. Extensive surgery on a severely comminuted fracture may result in less than optimal internal fixation and a need for postoperative immobilization, often resulting in the joint being neither stable nor freely movable.

In undisplaced fractures, after the integrity of the collateral ligaments is established, treatment should consist of a few days of splinting followed by early active knee motion. Weight bearing should be delayed until fracture healing is evident, generally at 8 to 10 weeks. Eighty-nine percent good results have been reported in fractures treated with closed reduction and cast bracing with little correlation between the late radiographic appearance and the functional result. Reduction and alignment were lost most often in medial condylar and bicondylar fractures.

Sarmiento et al. found that often the condition of the fibula, whether fractured or intact, determines the angular behavior of these fractures under weight-bearing and functional conditions. Isolated fractures of the lateral condyle with an intact fibula did not collapse further because of the support of the fibula. Conversely, fractures of the lateral condyle with associated fibular fractures had a tendency to collapse into valgus because of the loss of fibular support. Fractures of both condyles did not collapse further or angulate when the proximal fibula was fractured and displaced. If the fibula was intact, however, the medial condyle usually collapsed, creating a varus deformity.

Lateral split fractures can be reduced open or percutaneously using traction and reduction forceps under arthroscopic or fluoroscopic control. If the displaced rim of the condyle cannot be reduced into a supporting position under the femoral condyle using closed manipulation, open reduction is required. Arthroscopic evaluation of all Schatzker type I fractures that are treated operatively has been recommended to ensure that the lateral meniscus is not trapped within the fracture site. Many lateral split fractures can be stabilized adequately by percutaneously placed large cancellous screws. If the lateral condylar fracture is associated with a fibular head fracture, a lateral buttress plate provides additional stability.

Depressed articular segments cannot be reduced by ligamentotaxis alone and require elevation through a cortical window, bone grafting, and fixation with either subchondral screws or a buttress plate. Patil et al. reported biomechanical data suggesting that four 3.5-mm screws were superior to two 6.5-mm screws in axial compression. Traditionally, the reduction has been observed through an arthrotomy and submeniscal incision; however, investigators have successfully used fluoroscopic or arthroscopically assisted reduction, bone graft or bone graft substitute, and percutaneous screw fixation to treat tibial plateau fractures with articular depression (Schatzker type II and type III). Displaced fractures of the medial condyle (Schatzker type IV) often are quite unstable and generally are best treated with open reduction and fixation with a medial buttress plate, which is biomechanically the most sound.

The treatment of severe or "complex" tibial plateau fractures can be quite difficult. Severe or complex tibial plateau fractures include bicondylar fractures (Schatzker type V), tibial plateau fractures with metaphyseal-diaphyseal discontinuity (Schatzker type VI), and fractures with open wounds, severe closed soft-tissue abrasions, contusions or crush injuries (Tscherne type II or III), compartment syndrome, or vascular injury. Closed methods of treatment with traction or cast bracing usually are unsuccessful in maintaining articular reduction and axial alignment. Traditional methods of open reduction and plating require extensive exposure, which may

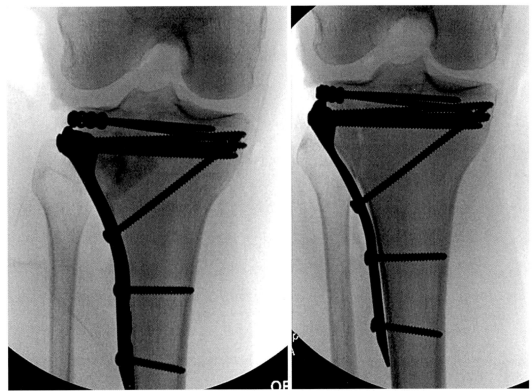

FIGURE 2.53   Lateral split depression tibial plateau fractures can be managed with anatomic reduction of articular injury and subchondral rafting screws to support articular elevation. Lateral condyle supported with buttress plate construct. With lateral peripheral rim comminution, subchondral rafter screws can be coupled with plate to act as washer.

compromise soft tissue further and devascularize bone fragments, leading to infection.

Attempts have been made to reduce the incidence of complications in these fractures by using less extensile exposures and indirect reduction techniques and by supplementing lateral buttress plate fixation with a small antiglide plate rather than a second bulky medial buttress plate. Mills and Nork suggested that dual plating could be achieved with minimal soft-tissue dissection by using a more anterior skin incision and limiting subperiosteal dissection to fracture margins and to the area of anticipated plate application. The use of small-fragment (3.5-mm screws) AO/ASIF T-plates has been reported for fixation of tibial plateau fractures. Anatomic or nearly anatomic reductions were obtained in 86.7% without infections or soft-tissue complications. The smaller diameter and increased malleability of the small fragment T-plate is thought to have provided better buttressing of the osteochondral fragments than the larger precontoured AO/ASIF T-plates and L-plates (6.5-mm screws).

Others have obtained good results without infection in grade II and grade III open complex (Schatzker types V and VI) tibial plateau fractures treated by experienced surgeons with a standard protocol of thorough debridement, immediate rigid internal fixation, and delayed closure at 5 days. Temporarily spanning the knee with an external fixator has been recommended in patients with severe soft-tissue injury. Internal fixation can be done after swelling has decreased, much akin to the current strategies for management of pilon injuries.

External fixation using either half-pin fixators or ring-and-wire fixators also has been advocated as definitive fixation for complex tibial plateau fractures. Cannulated screws can be used as accessory fixation of the articular surface. An external fixator placed below the knee can maintain articular reduction and axial alignment and allow early motion (Fig. 2.54). Minimal soft-tissue dissection is required for application of an external fixator, which theoretically should reduce wound complications.

Not all fractures reduce with ligamentotaxis alone, and a limited open reduction sometimes is necessary with bone grafting. One potential disadvantage of external fixation is the risk of pin site infection. Pin site infections usually are minor and can be treated with oral antibiotics. Septic arthritis has been reported to develop, however, as a result of infection around periarticular pins and wires. Anatomic studies have shown that pins or wires placed within 14 mm of the knee joint may be intracapsular. To prevent septic arthritis, intracapsular placement of pins and wires should be avoided.

Clinical studies have shown that ring-and-wire fixation is an acceptable method of treatment for complex tibial plateau fractures (87% to 88% good or excellent results with 6.5% to 12% superficial infections). A four-wire construct has been shown to provide stability comparable to that obtained with dual plating.

We frequently use ring-and-wire fixation for the treatment of complex tibial plateau fractures (Fig. 2.55). In 57 patients with Schatzker type VI tibial plateau fractures treated with Ilizarov fixation, four fractures became infected

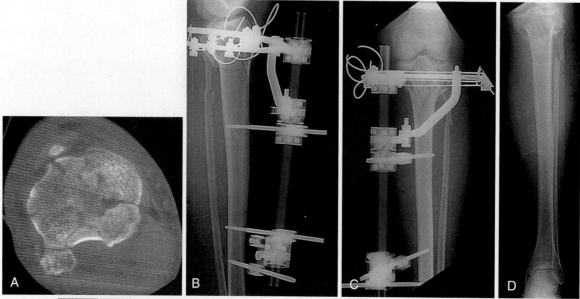

FIGURE 2.54   **A,** CT scan of open fracture of tibial plateau. **B** and **C,** Fixation with hybrid external fixator. **D,** After fixator removal.

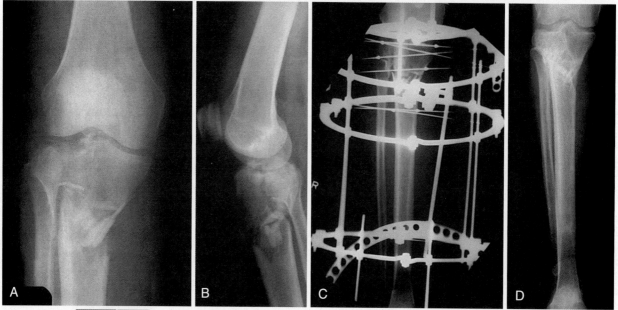

FIGURE 2.55   **A** and **B,** Fracture of tibial plateau. **C,** Stabilization with Ilizarov circular external fixator. **D,** After fixator removal.

(7%), including two with septic arthritis. Twenty-two fractures (38%) were open. In 45 fractures (84%) with acceptable reductions, knee range of motion averaged 115 degrees. In nine patients (16%) with poor reductions, knee motion averaged 79 degrees.

Monolateral half-pin external fixation placed below the knee is another technique that has been used to treat complex tibial plateau fractures. Accessory cancellous screws are used to maintain the articular reduction. This is technically easier for surgeons unfamiliar with ring-and-wire fixation techniques; however, half-pins may not achieve as secure fixation as small tensioned wires in comminuted metaphyseal bone.

Occasionally, a tibial plateau fracture is so comminuted or the soft-tissue injury so severe that accurate reduction and stable fixation are impossible in the acute setting. In this situation, the knee can be spanned by a half-pin external fixator as temporary or definitive fixation. This technique allows the patient to be mobilized while maintaining axial alignment of the limb. Immobilization of the knee for 6 weeks does not seem to affect adversely the ultimate knee range of motion.

■ FRACTURE OF THE LATERAL CONDYLE

An understanding of the mechanism producing fractures of the lateral tibial condyle is necessary for intelligent treatment. This fracture usually is produced by a valgus strain on the knee, with the ligaments and muscles on the medial side resisting separation of the tibial and femoral condyles. The lateral femoral condyle is driven downward into the weight-bearing surface of the lateral tibial condyle, depressing the central portion of the articular surface into the cancellous metaphysis well below its normal level. In addition, the lateral margin of the articular surface of the tibia bursts laterally and one or more fractures extend longitudinally down into the metaphysis of the tibia, producing a lateral fragment. This fragment usually is fairly large and, when seen from the lateral side, often is triangular, with the base of the triangle proximal. Usually the fragment is held at joint level by the intact fibula. Less often, the lateral condyle fractures the fibula at its neck and may be displaced as one large fragment with only slight central depression and comminution.

Open treatment of tibial plateau fractures is made easier by the use of the AO large distractor. For lateral plateau fractures, one bicortical pin is inserted just anterior to the lateral femoral epicondyle, parallel to the joint. The second pin is inserted into the lateral tibial cortex, distal to the site of proposed fixation, in the midcoronal plane, perpendicular to the tibia. As the distractor is lengthened, much of the reduction is attained by ligamentotaxis. The use of this device also permits improved intraarticular visualization for reduction. Because the femoral pin is located near the center of rotation of the femoral condyle, the fracture is minimally disturbed by flexion and extension of the knee in attempts to locate the fracture lines and fix the plateau.

OPEN REDUCTION AND FIXATION OF A LATERAL TIBIAL PLATEAU FRACTURE

TECHNIQUE 2.14

- The procedure typically is done under tourniquet control.
- For fractures of the lateral condyle, make a straight or slightly curvilinear anterolateral incision, starting 3 to 5 cm above the joint line proximally and extending distally below the inferior margin of the fracture site from just anterior to the lateral femoral epicondyle to Gerdy's tubercle. This incision provides good exposure while avoiding skin complications.
- Make the fascial incision in line with the skin incision. Do not undermine soft-tissue flaps more than necessary. Reflect the iliotibial band from its insertion on Gerdy's tubercle both anteriorly and posteriorly. Gain intraarticular exposure by incising the coronary or inframeniscotibial ligament by submeniscal arthrotomy and retract the meniscus superiorly after placement of nonabsorbable meniscocapsular tagging sutures.
- Inspect and debride or repair any meniscal tears to preserve as much of the meniscus as possible.
- To expose the longitudinal fracture of the lateral condyle, elevate the origin of the extensor muscles from the anterolateral aspect of the condyle in an extraperiosteal

fashion. Reflect the muscle origin laterally until the fracture line is exposed.
- Retract the lateral fragment to gain access to the central part of the tibial condyle. This lateral fragment often hinges open like a book, exposing the depressed articular surface and cancellous bone of the central depression.
- Alternatively, make a cortical window below the area of depression to allow reduction of this fragment. This approach generally requires less soft-tissue dissection than hinging open the lateral condylar fragment.
- Insert a periosteal elevator or osteotome well beneath the depressed articular fragments, and by slow and meticulous pressure elevate the articular fragments and compressed cancellous bone in one large mass (Fig. 2.56). Take as much cancellous bone as possible. This produces a large cavity in the metaphysis that must be filled with bone graft or substitute. Unless this is done, redisplacement and settling can occur. Various types of grafts have been proposed, from transverse cortical supports to full-thickness iliac grafts. We prefer injectable bone substitutes or allograft for metaphyseal subchondral defect management after elevation of depressed articular segments. Recent data support the use of structural allograft to reduce the risk of articular subsidence with satisfactory clinical outcomes.
- The standard lateral approach gives only a limited view of the posterolateral plateau and provides no access to the posterior wall of the lateral tibial plateau. Certain fractures located in the posterolateral plateau require a more extensile approach. In this situation, the fascial incision follows the insertion of the extensor muscles and continues over the subcapital fibula. The entire layer is stripped distally as required. Expose the peroneal nerve and cut the fibular neck with an oscillating saw. This allows retraction of the upper segment to the back or rotation of the fibular head upward, exposing the posterolateral plateau and the lateral and posterior flare of the proximal tibia.
- If displacement of the peripheral rim is slight and central depression of the condyle is the main deformity, remove an anterior cortical window with its proximal edge distal to the articular surface.
- Insert a curved bone tamp through the cortical window or fracture line into the cancellous subchondral bone, and elevate to the normal level the depressed fragments of the articular surface as seen through the submeniscal arthrotomy. As the fragments are elevated and reduced, temporarily fix them with multiple small Kirschner wires. Stabilize with subchondral raft screw fixation. The Kirschner wires can be advanced through the soft-tissue envelope medially and then extracted from the medial side until flush with the lateral cortex.
- Apply a buttress plate to the anterolateral proximal tibia. Precontoured periarticular plates designed for tibial plateau fractures are readily available, typically in either a 3.5- or 4.5-mm dimension. Depending on the fit of the implant, one may choose to place separate raft screws before affixing the plate to ensure subchondral support of newly elevated articular segments. Typically, for simple lateral condylar fractures alone, nonlocking 3.5-mm implants are sufficient.
- Augment the defect with cancellous bone or bone graft substitute.

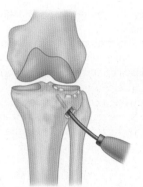

FIGURE 2.56 Periosteal elevator or similar instrument is introduced below level of depressed tibial plateau fragment. With careful and gentle upward pressure, articular fragments are elevated. **SEE TECHNIQUE 2.14.**

- The meniscocapsular tagging sutures can then be incorporated in the repair, either through the plate or the iliotibial band.

POSTOPERATIVE CARE The knee is placed into a removable knee immobilizer. At 1 to 2 days postoperatively, physical therapy is initiated with quadriceps exercises and gentle active-assisted exercises are begun, or a passive motion machine can be used. Crutch walking is begun, but no weight bearing is permitted for 10 to 12 weeks.

■ LIGAMENT INJURY WITH CONDYLAR FRACTURE

Collateral and cruciate ligament injuries occurring with tibial condylar fractures are much more common than previously realized and, if untreated, may be responsible for instability and a poor late result, despite a well-healed condylar fracture. An increased incidence of posttraumatic arthritis has been found after tibial plateau fractures with concomitant ligamentous injury. Ligamentous injuries have been reported in 4% to 33% of tibial plateau fractures and 60% of fracture-dislocations. The medial collateral ligament is most commonly injured, usually with undisplaced or local depression fractures of the lateral tibial condyle. Stress radiographs are helpful in making this diagnosis. A prospective study of 30 tibial plateau fractures with operative repair, found a 56% incidence of additional soft-tissue injury; 20% of fractures were associated with meniscal tears, 20% had medial collateral ligament injury, 10% had anterior cruciate ligament injury, 3% had lateral collateral ligament injury, and 3% had peroneal nerve injury. Medial collateral ligament injury occurred most often with Schatzker type II fractures, whereas meniscal injury occurred most often with Schatzker type IV fractures.

Preoperative and postoperative stress examination of the knee is recommended to detect ligamentous injury. Residual laxity after anatomic reduction of the tibial plateau indicates ligamentous injury. If the intercondylar eminences of the tibia are fractured and displaced, these should be replaced and secured at the time of open reduction of the condyle. Fixation can be done with sutures passed through

bony tunnels or with a small fragment screw if the eminence fragment is large enough. Midsubstance tears of the anterior cruciate ligament should be reconstructed later if significant laxity remains after fracture healing. Acute midsubstance tears of the medial collateral ligament usually heal satisfactorily with nonoperative treatment. Because the increased surgical exposure necessary to repair the ligament and postoperative immobilization that is required can lead to increased knee stiffness, acute repair of the medial collateral ligament is infrequently indicated. Collateral ligament injuries should be protected with a hinged knee brace. If the medial collateral ligament is repaired, a separate medial incision is required as described for the repair of the medial collateral ligament. Although early motion after fixation of tibial condylar fractures is desirable, motion may be delayed if repair of an acute collateral ligament injury also is involved.

■ ARTHROSCOPICALLY ASSISTED REDUCTION AND FIXATION OF TIBIAL PLATEAU FRACTURES

Arthroscopic techniques require minimal soft-tissue dissection, afford excellent exposure of the articular surface, and can be used to diagnose and treat concomitant meniscal injury.

Buchko and Johnson described an arthroscopic technique in which the affected extremity is placed in a thigh holder, a tourniquet is inflated, and an anterolateral arthroscopic portal is placed approximately 2 cm above the joint line to enable the surgeon to look downward on the tibial plateau. A complete diagnostic assessment is performed. A low-pressure arthroscopic pump can be used but is not mandatory, although it improves exposure and facilitates joint lavage. If the pump is used for extracapsular fractures, the metaphyseal portion of the fracture site should be exposed to prevent extravasation of irrigation fluid into the soft tissues. This incision can be used later to create a bony window for reduction and bone grafting. Schatzker type III fractures usually are intraarticular, and extravasation is less of a concern. The joint should be thoroughly lavaged to evacuate the hemarthrosis and remove loose bony and chondral fragments. When the diagnostic evaluation has been completed, the reduction can be performed with the pump off or as a dry arthroscopic technique. If the lateral meniscus is entrapped in the fracture site, it can be lifted out with a hook. Meniscal tears usually can be repaired and should be treated accordingly.

Depressed fragments can be elevated through a small cortical window. The depressed fragment can be localized by using an anterior cruciate ligament tibial guide to place a Kirschner wire into the displaced fragment. The fragment can be elevated using a cannulated impactor. The reduction can be evaluated accurately through the arthroscope, and the resulting defect can be filled with autogenous bone graft or appropriate bone graft substitute. Fixation is achieved with percutaneously placed 3.5-mm cortical screws. Because buttress plating may be necessary in patients with osteoporotic bone, arthroscopically assisted reduction is less suitable for this patient population. Small clinical series using arthroscopically assisted reduction and fixation techniques in predominantly Schatzker type I, type II, and type III tibial plateau fractures have shown good or excellent results in 80% to 100% of patients.

■ FRACTURE OF THE MEDIAL CONDYLE

If open reduction, elevation, and internal fixation of the medial tibial condyle are required, a technique similar to that previously described for the lateral tibial condyle is done. The fracture can be approached through a straight anterior, anteromedial, or posteromedial incision. For split compression and total depression fractures of the medial tibial condyle, in addition to elevating the depressed fragment and packing bone beneath it, a medial buttressing plate should be applied. This can be bent to an accurate contour to fit the tibial metaphysis and the tibial condyle, and the fracture can be secured with cancellous or cortical locking screws in the proximal portion of the plate and standard cortical screws in the distal portion (Fig. 2.57). More complex fractures of the medial plateau may require a more extensile exposure. Alternatively, for isolated medial injuries with joint impaction, an anterior parapatellar approach can be used to permit visualization of the articular reduction.

POSTEROMEDIAL EXPOSURE

TECHNIQUE 2.15

- Critically evaluate the preoperative imaging and the patient's soft-tissue envelope to ensure satisfactory edema resolution before proceeding.

- The location of the distal extent of the medial condyle on CT aids in determining the ideal location for the surgical incision.
- The goal of internal fixation application should be a stable buttress construct. To achieve this goal, internal fixation should be positioned over the apex of the fracture distally.
- Most medial and posteromedial condyle fractures can be fixed through a posteromedial surgical approach, otherwise a posterior approach should be considered.
- Mark the proposed skin incision with surgical indelible ink just posterior and parallel to the posteromedial tibial border.
- Divide the skin and subcutaneous tissues sharply and mobilize the inferior border or the pes anserinus tendons, and then use the interval created with the medial head of the gastrocnemius.
- At times, mobilization of the superior border of the pes anserinus tendons may be necessary for fracture fixation. Alternatively, if a more extensile exposure is necessary, the pes anserinus tendons can be released and subsequently repaired.
- Perform reduction and internal fixation using a 3.5-mm small fragment plate centered over the apex of the distal fracture extension. This approach can be used in conjunction with lateral condylar fixation through an anterolateral approach to treat bicondylar injuries.
- The incision can be placed farther anteriorly if the fracture pattern dictates. Although infrequently necessary, extensile medial approaches have been advocated through anterior midline incisions for medial condyle fractures of the proximal tibia.

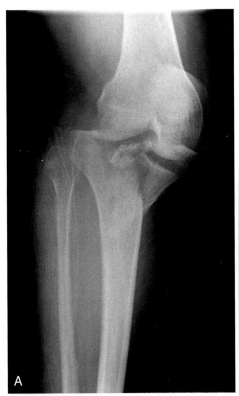
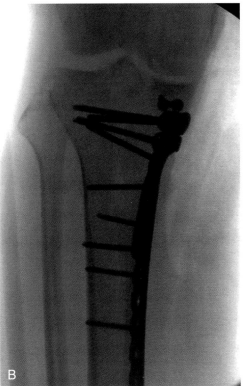

FIGURE 2.57 **A,** Medial tibial plateau fracture-dislocation injury. **B,** Reduction and stabilization of displaced medial tibial condyle through posteromedial approach allowing buttress plate fixation.

■ COMMINUTED PROXIMAL FRACTURES

In the past, anatomic reduction through extensive exposures and rigid fixation with multiple large fragment plates have been advocated for the treatment of bicondylar tibial plateau fractures. The unacceptable incidence of wound and infectious complications often associated with these techniques has led to the development of alternative treatment strategies. Currently accepted techniques include indirect reduction, less extensive surgical exposures, buttress plate fixation of the most comminuted condyle, and fixation of the less involved condyle with smaller implants, such as cannulated screws, and antiglide plates. Ring-and-wire fixators with or without limited open reduction are also being used to treat these difficult fractures. Preoperative CT scans are essential in planning a strategy for treatment. ORIF is delayed for 7 to 10 days (sometimes longer) until edema and soft-tissue injury have subsided. If surgery is delayed, temporary uniplanar external fixation spanning the knee is a valuable technique for both skeletal and soft-tissue stabilization until definitive fixation can occur.

OPEN REDUCTION AND INTERNAL FIXATION OF BICONDYLAR INJURIES

The surgical approach to complex tibial plateau fractures must be individualized on the basis of particular fracture configuration. The following is a general approach applicable to many of these fractures.

TECHNIQUE 2.16

- Place the patient supine on the fluoroscopic table.
- Based on imaging studies, as well as careful preoperative planning, mark the proposed surgical incisions, both medially and laterally, which aids in confirming that a sufficient soft-tissue bridge will be present to minimize the potential for soft-tissue complications.
- Typically, the posteromedial approach is performed as described earlier. This permits reduction and stabilization of the medial condylar segment of the injury, thus effectively converting the injury to a unicondylar fracture. Small fragment plates (3.5-mm; one third tubular, reconstruction, or T-plates) are commonly used. Fortunately, medial condylar impaction is rare. Medial condylar fixation can be applied as a true antiglide buttress plate, without proximal screw fixation, particularly when comminution is absent. When apical comminution is present, proximal fixation may be necessary to maintain reduction. We have found temporary unicortical locking screws to be of benefit. This technique prevents longer screws from interfering with the lateral reduction. Once the lateral reduction and fixation are complete, these unicortical screws can be exchanged for longer implants if necessary.
- Expose the lateral condylar component as described earlier, through an anterolateral approach, with meticulous soft-tissue handling as also described earlier. Correct articular comminution or depression and any meniscal pathologic process and stabilize the fracture provisionally. Large periarticular clamps often are used to effect compression be-tween the medial and lateral condyles. Subchondral rafting screws can then be positioned. The ability to use these screws is somewhat dependent on the "fit" of the lateral plate, given the variable proximal tibial anatomy. If the plate seems to fit more distally, then proceed with placement of subchondral rafting interfragmentary lag screws independent of the plate. Otherwise, the proximal-most screws of the plate can serve this function.
- Perform definitive anterolateral fixation with a precontoured proximal tibial plate, whose proximal fixation allows capture of the medial condylar segment.
- Any residual cancellous void from elevation of articular depression can then be treated as previously described. (see Technique 2.14)

POSTOPERATIVE CARE Active and active-assisted exercises, including controlled passive motion, are instituted. Weight bearing is not permitted for 10 to 12 weeks postoperatively. Any associated soft-tissue issues may delay initiation of aggressive motion, as do certain fracture patterns such as those involving the tibial tubercle.

CIRCULAR EXTERNAL FIXATION

TECHNIQUE 2.17

(WATSON)

- Position the patient on a fracture table or radiolucent operating table.
- Apply calcaneal or distal tibial pin traction. Ensure that sufficient clearance exists around the limb for placement of appropriately sized circular rings. Fixator rings should allow 1.5 cm of clearance over the anterior crest of the tibia and 3 to 4 cm of clearance around the posterior calf.
- When the patient is positioned, apply traction and obtain reduction using ligamentotaxis.
- Achieve further closed manipulation by using large reduction forceps.
- If any articular depression is not reduced by ligamentotaxis alone, use a limited approach through a CT-directed incision to ensure minimal soft-tissue dissection and reduction of the articular surface (Fig. 2.58A).
- Perform bone grafting.
- After reduction of the condyles, use olive wires (1.8-mm Kirschner wires with a 4-mm bead located eccentrically on the wire) to achieve interfragmentary compression of the condylar surface (Fig. 2.58B). Place counteropposed olive wires through the fragments, coming from opposite sides of the major condylar fracture lines to maintain condylar reduction. Cannulated screws can be substituted for olive wires if fragments are not extensively comminuted. Use fluoroscopy for placement and direction of the periarticular olive wires and for tensioning of the wires. Three or four olive wires usually are required for stabilization of the condylar and metaphyseal fragments.

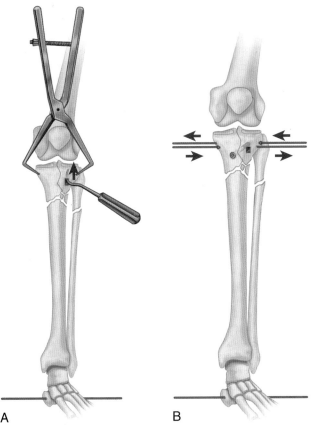

FIGURE 2.58 **A,** Elevation of depressed plateau. **B,** Placement of opposing olive wires and cannulated screw after bone grafting. **SEE TECHNIQUE 2.17.**

- Open the frame by removing the anterior connecting bolts of each ring and place the frame over the leg.
- Reattach the anterior connecting bolts.
- Temporarily place the proximal ring below the level of condylar involvement. After condylar reduction, it is slid proximally on the threaded rods to the level of the fibular head, and eventually all the proximal wires are attached to this fixation ring. Position the middle ring just distal to any shaft fracture component and place the distal ring at the level of the ankle joint. If extensive shaft comminution is present, apply an additional ring to the midportion of the shaft to complete a four-ring frame. Attach the proximal ring to the proximal wires, taking care that the proximal ring is parallel to the joint. Pass a distal transfixion wire at the level of the distal tibia and parallel to the ankle joint. When this wire is attached and tensioned to the distal ring, ensure appropriate alignment of the mechanical axis by forcing the proximal and distal rings to become parallel to each other; the joints also are parallel.
- It also is possible to use the fibular head as a buttress plate. By placing an olive wire through the fibular head obliquely into the lateral condyle and tensioning this olive wire, the fibular head is compressed onto the lateral condyle.

POSTOPERATIVE CARE Weight bearing is delayed for 10 to 12 weeks to allow all intraarticular fracture lines and bone grafts to consolidate, and progressive weight

PATELLA

Fractures of the patella constitute almost 1% of all skeletal injuries, resulting from either direct or indirect trauma. The anterior subcutaneous location of the patella makes it vulnerable to direct trauma, such as the knee striking the dashboard of a motor vehicle or from a fall on the anterior knee. These injuries often are comminuted or displaced and may include chondral injury to the distal femur or patella. Fractures caused by indirect mechanisms result from a violent contraction of the quadriceps with the knee flexed. These fractures usually are transverse and may be associated with tears of the medial and lateral retinacular expansions. Most patellar fractures are caused by a combination of direct and indirect forces. The most significant effects of fracture of the patella are loss of continuity of the extensor mechanism of the knee and potential incongruity of the patellofemoral articulation.

Fractures of the patella can be classified as undisplaced or displaced and subclassified further according to fracture configuration (Fig. 2.59). Transverse fractures usually involve the central third of the patella but can involve the proximal (apical) or distal (basal) poles. A variable amount of comminution of the poles may be present. Most fractures in reported series are transverse. Vertical fractures usually involve the middle and lateral thirds of the patella. If only the medial or lateral edge of the patella is affected, the fracture is called marginal. Vertical fractures are seen best on axial radiographs of the patella; displacement and retinacular disruption rarely occur in vertical fractures. Another common fracture pattern is the comminuted or stellate patellar fracture, which is associated with a variable amount of displacement.

Patellar fractures generally are associated with a hemarthrosis and localized tenderness. In fractures that are displaced or have concomitant retinacular tears, a palpable defect may be present. Inability of the patient to extend the affected knee actively usually indicates a disruption of the extensor mechanism and a torn retinaculum, which require surgical treatment. Occasionally, if active knee extension is limited by pain, the hemarthrosis can be aspirated under sterile conditions and followed by intraarticular injection of local anesthetic. In patients without significant impairment of the extensor mechanism, active knee extension should be restored. An open wound in the vicinity of a patellar fracture may be a sign of an open fracture, which requires urgent surgical treatment. If uncertainty exists as to whether the open wound communicates with the joint, the saline load test can be used. This test may not be 100% reliable in open fractures with very small traumatic arthrotomies.

Patellar fractures should be radiographically evaluated with anteroposterior, lateral, and axial (Merchant) views. Transverse fractures usually are best seen on a lateral view, whereas vertical fractures, osteochondral fractures, and articular incongruity are best evaluated on axial views. A comparison view of the opposite knee sometimes is necessary to differentiate an acute fracture from a bipartite patella, which

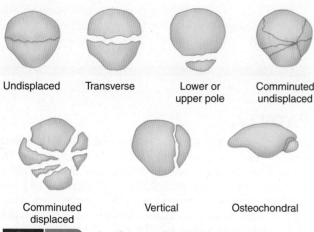

Undisplaced   Transverse   Lower or
upper pole   Comminuted
undisplaced

Comminuted
displaced   Vertical   Osteochondral

FIGURE 2.59 Classification of patellar fractures. (Redrawn from Wiss DA, Watson JT, Johnson EE: Fractures of the knee. In Rockwood CA Jr, Green DP, Bucholz RW, et al. editors: *Rockwood and Green's fractures in adults*, ed 4, Philadelphia, 1996, Lippincott-Raven.)

is a failure of fusion of the superolateral portion of the patella and which usually is bilateral.

TREATMENT

The initial treatment of acute patellar fractures should consist of splinting the extremity in extension and applying ice to the knee. To prevent soft-tissue damage, the ice should not be applied directly to the skin. Closed fractures with minimal displacement, minimal articular incongruity, and an intact extensor retinaculum can be successfully treated nonoperatively. Nonoperative treatment consists of immobilizing the knee in extension in a cylinder cast or orthosis from ankle to groin for 4 to 6 weeks, with weight bearing allowed as tolerated. Boström considered 3 to 4 mm of fragment separation and 2 to 3 mm of articular incongruity to be acceptable for nonoperative treatment; if either separation or articular incongruity is greater, operative treatment is indicated. In his long-term follow-up study, fractures treated nonoperatively had the best overall results.

Fractures associated with retinacular tears, open fractures, and fractures with more than 2 to 3 mm of displacement or incongruity are best treated operatively. The goal is restoration of articular congruity and repair of the extensor mechanism with fixation secure enough to allow early motion. When the skin is normal, the operation should be done as soon as is practical. Delay retards convalescence and to some extent unfavorably affects the result. If contusion or laceration of the skin is present, it usually is best to perform the indicated operation immediately on admission to the hospital or very soon thereafter. When lacerations or abrasions become superficially infected, surgery must be delayed 7 to 10 days until the danger of contaminating the operative wound is minimal.

Opinions differ as to the optimal treatment of patellar fractures. Accepted methods include a variety of wiring techniques, screw fixation, partial patellectomy, and total patellectomy. Open fractures of the patella are a surgical urgency and should be treated with immediate debridement and irrigation. Early soft-tissue coverage (within 5 days) should reduce the incidence of infection. The same surgical techniques used to treat closed patellar fractures can be used successfully for open fractures. Two series reported 77% good or excellent results after operative treatment of open patellar fractures. In open fractures, soft-tissue stripping should be kept to the minimum necessary to stabilize the fracture adequately. Torchia and Lewellen discouraged the use of cerclage wires in open fractures because of the potential adverse effects on vascularity.

Wiring techniques are used most often for transverse fractures. They also can be used in comminuted fractures if the fragments are large enough to lag together with screws, converting it to a transverse fracture. Many different wiring techniques have been described, including cerclage wiring, alone or in combination; tension band wiring, alone or modified with longitudinal Kirschner wires or screws; Magnusson wiring; and Lotke longitudinal anterior band wiring (Fig. 2.60).

In experimental studies, the most secure fixation was obtained with modified tension band wiring. This is especially useful in osteopenic and comminuted fractures. Anchoring the fixation wiring directly in bone rather than threading it through the soft tissue around the patella has been recommended if early motion is to be initiated. Also, a second tension band wire through tendon has been shown to provide improved fixation.

Two screws alone provide adequate fixation in fractures with good bone stock; however, displacement of fragments is slightly greater with screws alone without tension band wiring. A cadaver study found that specimens fixed with the tension band through cannulated screws failed at the highest load.

Good-to-excellent results have been described after fixation of displaced transverse patellar fractures with figure-of-eight wiring through parallel cannulated compression screws. Suggested advantages of this technique included a low-profile construct that caused less implant irritation of local soft-tissue structures, the possibility of early restricted motion, and its use as a salvage method after failure of traditional tension band wiring. We currently prefer a tension band modified with Kirschner wires or screws for transverse fractures with large fragments. If comminution is present, a cerclage wire can be added. The results of tension band wiring techniques generally are good (81%), but 2 mm of displacement has been reported in 22% of fractures treated with tension band fixation and early motion. Noncompliance and technical errors have been cited as reasons for displacement. Braided polyester and braided cable have been used and seem to provide fixation similar to stainless steel wire.

Arthroscopically assisted percutaneous screw fixation also has been described for fixation of displaced transverse patellar fractures with good results. If the amount of comminution and the articular damage preclude salvage of the entire patella, partial or total patellectomy may be indicated. Although Brooke proposed in 1937 that the patella is not a functional organ, later studies refuted this claim. Haxton studied patients with and without patellae and showed that the power of extension of the knee increases as the joint extends; that is, the power of extension is greater with the knee at 30 degrees of flexion than at 60, 90, or 120 degrees. Kaufer compared intact and patellectomized cadaver knees and found that 15% to 30% more quadriceps force was required to fully extend patellectomized knees than intact knees. The effect of patellectomy was eliminated by elevation of the tibial tubercle 1.5 cm. Because extension is the

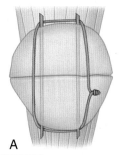 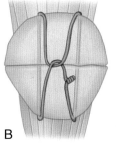 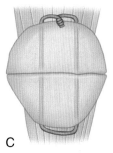

A   B   C

FIGURE 2.60 Types of patellar fixation. **A,** Modified tension band. **B,** Lotke longitudinal anterior band (LAB) wiring. **C,** Magnusson wiring. **SEE TECHNIQUE 2.20.**

most important function of the knee, it must be concluded that patellectomy definitely impairs the efficiency of the quadriceps mechanism. This may not be enough to interfere with ordinary activities, and we have not found tibial tubercle elevation after patellectomy to be necessary. Two separate series with long-term follow-up reported reduction in quadriceps strength of 33% and 44%, respectively, after patellectomy. Comparison of anterior tension band fixation with patellectomy found 80% excellent results after osteosynthesis compared with 50% excellent results after patellectomy.

In an effort to maintain the length of the patella and allow earlier motion, techniques have been developed to preserve rather than excise the inferior pole of the patella in comminuted fractures. Yang and Byun reported good functional results and no implant failure, infections, delayed unions, or nonunions in 25 patients treated with a separate vertical wiring technique for comminuted fractures of the inferior pole of the patella. The vertical wire technique also proved to be stronger than a partial patellectomy and pull-out sutures in biomechanical testing on cadavers. Matejcic et al. described the use of a basket plate for fixation of comminuted inferior pole patellar fractures. In 51 patients, results were excellent in 30, good in 16, and satisfactory in five. There were no poor results.

Because of the objections to patellectomy, we try to save all of the patella or at least the proximal or distal third if practical. If the distal or proximal pole of the patella is comminuted, the small fragments are removed but the largest fragment is preserved. When comminution is extensive and reconstruction of the articular surface is impossible, complete patellectomy is performed. Despite the frequent occurrence of quadriceps weakness and atrophy, good or excellent results are noted after patellectomy in 78% of patients at long-term follow-up. A recent comparison of ORIF with partial patellectomy for patellar fractures found persistent functional impairment and equal range of motion, functional scores, and complication rates between the two modalities.

When partial patellectomy is chosen, as much of the patella as possible should be salvaged. Larger pieces can be secured together with interfragmentary screws to increase the size of the patellar remnant. The comminuted fragments are removed, and the extensor mechanism is reattached to the patella through drill holes. The size of the patellar fragment worth salvaging is controversial. Measurement of patellofemoral contact areas and patellofemoral pressures in cadaver knees before and after partial patellectomy found marked alterations in patellofemoral contact area in specimens after 60% patellectomy with a contact area less than 50% of controls. Saltzman et al. found that the area of the salvaged

fragment averaged 11.8 cm^2 and that only one specimen was less than 4.1 cm^2. At an average 8-year follow-up, 78% of patients had good or excellent results, range of motion averaged 94% of normal, and average strength was 85% of normal. Patellofemoral arthritis developed in 53%. The size of the retained fragment did not correlate with the result.

The proper site of insertion of the patellar tendon into the patellar remnant after partial patellectomy also has been controversial. Reinserting the patellar tendon anteriorly on the patella has been shown to cause excessive tilting of the lower pole of the patella toward the femoral articular surface and lead to patellofemoral arthritis, and reattachment of the patellar tendon near the articular edge of the patella has been recommended. However, posterior attachment of the patellar tendon near the articular surface was found to cause tilting of the proximal pole of the patella toward the femoral articular surface and that anterior reattachment of the patellar tendon restored a more normal pattern of patellofemoral contact. In a cadaver model, the forces required to extend the knee were significantly higher when the patellar tendon was reattached near the articular surface, but forces were increased when the tendon was reattached to the anterior cortex.

Whatever site of reattachment is chosen, intraoperative radiographs should be evaluated carefully to ensure that the extensor mechanism is not excessively shortened and that the remaining patella is not tilted. Comparison of the results of simple patellectomy with the results of patellectomy with advancement of the vastus medialis obliquus at a minimum 3-year follow-up determined that results were significantly better in patients with vastus medialis obliquus advancement.

Open reduction and external fixation using superior and inferior pins placed transversely, adjacent to the proximal and distal poles, and connected externally to compressive clamps has been used successfully to treat transverse and comminuted fractures. Others have advocated application of circular external fixation under arthroscopic control and plating techniques. Recent series have advocated the use of mini-fragment augmentation to tension band fixation and locked mesh-plate fixation for comminuted fractures of the patella.

Lazaro et al. reported a series of 36 patients. They demonstrated 37% removal of implants, patella baja in 57%, and anterior knee pain in 80% during activities of daily living. Improvement was noted over the first 6 months; however, functional impairments persisted at 1-year follow-up, noting deficits in strength, power, and endurance. Bonnaig et al. reported 73 patients with functional outcome data at 1 year, noting that functional impairment persisted at 1-year minimum follow-up, and ORIF scored similarly to partial patellectomy for range of motion, functional scores, and complications. Lazaro et al. reported outcomes after operative fixation of complete articular patellar fractures. Functional impairment was noted with a decrease in extensor mechanism strength, power, and endurance. In this series, 37% underwent removal of symptomatic implants, and 80% had anterior knee pain during activities of daily living. LeBrun et al. also noted persistent symptoms at a mean of 6.5-year follow-up. Removal of symptomatic implants occurred in 52%.

COMMON APPROACH AND TECHNIQUE FOR PATELLAR FRACTURES

TECHNIQUE 2.18

- Make a longitudinal midline incision, our preference. Alternatively, a transverse curved incision can be made approximately 12.5 cm long with the apex of the curve on the distal fragment, which gives enough exposure for reduction of the fracture and repair of the ruptured extensor expansion and synovium. If an area of skin is severely contused, attempt to avoid it or elect to excise a small area because skin closure produces no significant difficulty.
- Reflect the skin and subcutaneous tissue proximally and distally to expose the entire anterior surface of the patella and the quadriceps and patellar tendons. If the fracture fragments are significantly separated, tears in the extensor expansion are presumed, and these must be carefully explored medially and laterally.
- Remove all small, detached fragments of bone and inspect the interior of the joint and especially the patellofemoral groove for an osteochondral fracture.
- Thoroughly irrigate the interior of the joint to remove blood clots and small particles of bone.
- Anatomically reduce the fracture fragments using large towel clips or appropriate bone-holding forceps and fix the fragments internally by the method preferred by the surgeon. Inspect the articular surface after fixation to ensure that the reduction is anatomic.
- Carefully repair with interrupted sutures the synovium, ruptured capsule, and extensor mechanism from their outer ends toward the midline of the joint.

CIRCUMFERENTIAL WIRE LOOP FIXATION

Circumferential wire loop fixation was formerly the most popular technique. With the loop threaded through the soft tissues around the patella, rigid fixation is not achieved, so a delay of 3 to 4 weeks in starting knee motion is necessary if this technique is used. It has largely been replaced by more rigid fixation techniques to permit early motion of the joint, although it can be used in conjunction with other techniques for fixation of comminuted fractures. We frequently use a variation of this technique for augmentation of a repair with nonabsorbable suture.

TECHNIQUE 2.19

(MARTIN)
- Begin threading a No. 18 stainless steel wire at the superolateral border of the patella, passing it transversely immediately next to the superior pole of the patella through the quadriceps tendon.
- Pass the wire through the tissue using a large Gallie needle, or thread it through a large Intracath needle inserted with the sharp point exiting at the site where the next suture is desired.
- Fit the No. 18 wire into the sharp end of the Intracath needle, and as the needle is withdrawn, pass the No. 18 wire along its path within the needle. This usually is easier than using the large Gallie needle because of the stiffness of the No. 18 wire.
- Pass the medial end of the wire in a similar manner along the medial border of both fragments midway between the anterior and posterior surfaces.
- Pass the medial end of the wire transversely through the patellar tendon from the medial to the lateral side around the distal border of the patella and then proximally along the lateral side of the patella to the superolateral border. The wire must be placed close to the patella, especially above and below; if it is inserted through the tendons away from the fragments, fixation is insecure because the wire cuts through the soft tissues when under tension and allows separation of the fragments. Centering the wire midway between the anterior and posterior surfaces keeps the fracture line from opening anteriorly or posteriorly as the circumferential wire is tightened.
- Approximate the fragments and hold them in position with a towel clip or bone-holding forceps; draw both ends of the wire until they are tight and twist them together.
- Confirm the position of the fragments, especially the relationship of the articular surfaces, by radiographs of the knee in the anteroposterior and the lateral planes and by direct inspection and palpation before the capsular tears are repaired.
- Cut off the redundant wire and depress the twisted ends into the quadriceps tendon.
- Repair the capsular tears with interrupted suture.
- A pretwisted wire that is tightened by twists at two points opposite each other supplies more even pressure and fixation across the fracture site. Placing the first twist in the wire before beginning its insertion allows for this extra site for tightening.

POSTOPERATIVE CARE A posterior splint from groin to ankle provides sufficient immobilization during the early postoperative period. The patient is encouraged to perform quadriceps-setting exercises and within a few days should be lifting the leg off the bed. At 10 to 14 days, the sutures are removed and a cylinder cast or knee immobilizer is applied with the knee in extension. The patient is allowed to be ambulatory, using crutches when active muscular control of the leg has been obtained. As muscle power returns, the crutches are discarded, usually at 6 to 8 weeks. After fracture union, the wire can be removed; if not, it eventually may break, become painful, and be difficult to remove. The twisted ends usually can be located through a small stab incision; the wire is cut near the ends and is withdrawn with little difficulty. We have used heavy synthetic sutures instead of wire, and some data suggest comparable performance with potentially less soft-tissue irritation compared to traditional wire.

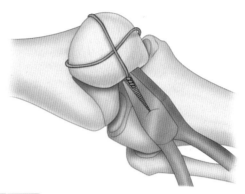

FIGURE 2.61 Schauwecker technique of tension band wiring of patella. **SEE TECHNIQUE 2.20.**

TENSION BAND WIRING FIXATION

The AO group has used and recommended a tension band wiring principle for fixation of fractures of the patella. By proper placement of the wires, the distracting or shear forces tending to separate the fragments are converted into compressive forces across the fracture site (see Fig. 2.60), resulting in earlier union and allowing immediate motion and exercise of the knee. Generally, two sets of wire are used. One is passed transversely through the insertion of the quadriceps tendon immediately adjacent to the bone of the superior pole and then passed anteriorly over the superficial surface of the patella and in a similar way through the insertion of the patellar tendon. This wire is tightened until the fracture is slightly overcorrected or opened on the articular surface. The second wire is passed through transverse holes drilled in the superior and inferior poles of the anterior patellar surface and tightened.

The capsular tears are repaired in the usual manner. The knee is immobilized in flexion, and early active flexion produces compressive forces to keep the edges of the articular surface of the patella compressed together. Early active flexion exercises are essential for the tension band principle to work. Schauwecker described a similar technique in which the wire is crossed in a figure-of-eight over the anterior surface of the patella (Fig. 2.61). Supplemental lag screws or Kirschner wires can be used to increase fixation in comminuted fractures (Fig. 2.62). Our preference is to use cannulated screws with a figure-of-eight tension band wire for those fractures that can be anatomically reduced.

TECHNIQUE 2.20

- Approach the patellar fracture in the usual fashion.
- Carefully clean the fracture surfaces of blood clot and small fragments.
- Explore the extent of the retinacular tears and inspect the trochlear groove of the femur for damage.
- Thoroughly lavage the joint.

- If the major proximal and distal fragments are large, reduce them accurately, with special attention to restoring a smooth articular surface.
- With the fracture reduced and held firmly with clamps, drill two 2-mm Kirschner wires from inferior to superior through each fragment. Place these wires about 5 mm deep to the anterior surface of the patella along lines dividing the patella into medial, central, and lateral thirds. Insert the wires as parallel as possible. In some cases, it is easier to insert the wires through the fracture site into the proximal fragment in a retrograde manner before reduction. This is made easier by tilting the fracture anteriorly about 90 degrees.
- Withdraw the wires until they are flush with the fracture site, accurately reduce the fracture and hold it with clamps, and drive the wires through the distal fragment. Leave the ends of the wires long, protruding beyond the patella and quadriceps tendon attachments to the inferior and superior fragments.
- Pass a strand of 18-gauge wire transversely through the quadriceps tendon attachment, as close to the bone as possible, deep to the protruding Kirschner wires, over the anterior surface of the reduced patella, transversely through the patellar tendon attachment on the inferior fragment and deep to the protruding Kirschner wires, and back over the anterior patellar surface; tighten it at the upper end. Alternatively, place the wire in a figure-of-eight fashion.
- Check the reduction by palpating the undersurface of the patella with the knee extended. If necessary, make a small longitudinal incision in the retinaculum to allow insertion of the finger.
- Bend the upper ends of the two Kirschner wires acutely anteriorly and cut them short.
- When they are cut, rotate the Kirschner wires 180 degrees; with an impactor, embed the bent ends into the superior margin of the patella posterior to the wire loops. Cut the protruding ends of the Kirschner wires short inferiorly.
- Repair the retinacular tears with multiple interrupted sutures.
- Alternatively, 4.0-mm partially threaded cannulated screws can be used instead of Kirschner wires (Fig. 2.63). Minifragment lag screws also can be placed horizontally to join comminuted fracture fragments, converting a comminuted fracture to a transverse fracture pattern. A

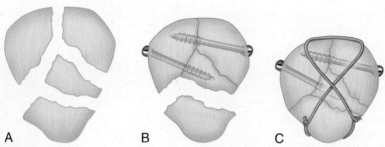

FIGURE 2.62 **A-C,** Schauwecker method of compression wiring of patella using supplemental screws for comminuted fracture **(C)**. Comminuted fragments **(A)** are transformed with screws into bifragmental fracture **(B)**. **SEE TECHNIQUE 2.20.**

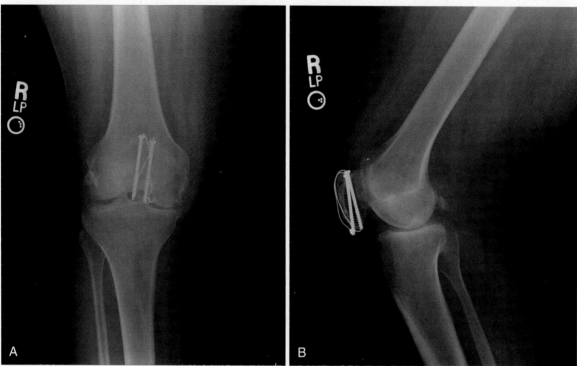

FIGURE 2.63 **A** and **B,** Displaced transverse fracture of patella fixed with tension band wires using two anterior wire loops and two longitudinally directed screws. **SEE TECHNIQUE 2.20.**

modified anterior tension band technique can be used. If the anterior cortex is split from the articular surface in the coronal plane, the fragment often can be secured with the anterior tension band wire. If this is unsuccessful, the fragment can be excised. As with all patellar repairs, a gravity flexion test is performed intraoperatively to determine stability, and range of motion can be initiated early in the postoperative course.

POSTOPERATIVE CARE The limb is placed in extension in a posterior plaster splint or removable knee brace. The patient is allowed to ambulate while bearing weight as tolerated on the first postoperative day. Isometric and stiff-leg exercises are encouraged, beginning on the first postoperative day. The extent of active motion permitted in the immediate postoperative period is determined intraoperatively based on the fracture repair stability. Active range-of-motion exercises can be performed when the wound has healed, at 2 to 3 weeks. Progressive resistance exercises can be begun and

the brace discontinued at 6 to 8 weeks if healing is evident on radiograph. Unrestricted activity can be resumed when full quadriceps strength has returned, at 18 to 24 weeks. In patients with less stable fixation or extensive retinacular tears, active motion should be delayed until fracture healing has occurred. Initiating range-of-motion exercises by the sixth postoperative week is desirable but not always possible. A controlled motion knee brace can be used, allowing full extension and flexion to the degree permitted by the fixation as determined intraoperatively.

If fixation is lost and the fragments separate 3 to 4 mm, or 2 to 3 mm of articular incongruity is present, revision surgery may be required. If the reduction improves with the knee in full extension, the patient can be treated by 6 weeks of splinting or casting with the knee in full extension. If the reduction does not improve, revision fixation or partial patellectomy should be considered. The implant can be removed after healing of the fracture if it causes symptoms.

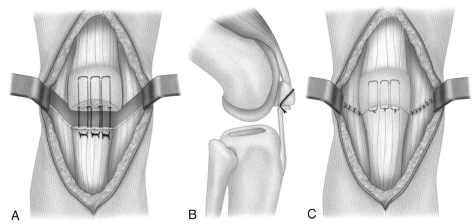

FIGURE 2.64 Partial patellectomy (see text). **A,** Retained fragment is approximated to tendon with large, nonabsorbable sutures. **B,** Drill holes are oriented to reattach tendon close to articular surface. **C,** Quadriceps expansions are completely repaired. **SEE TECHNIQUE 2.21.**

COMMINUTED PATELLAR FRACTURES

Often, only the distal pole of the patella is fragmented, leaving a substantial and relatively normal proximal fragment. This fragment is an important part of the extensor mechanism and should be preserved. The details of suture of the patellar tendon to the fragment should be observed carefully to prevent a tilt of the fragment, which can cause erosion of the trochlear groove.

PARTIAL PATELLECTOMY

TECHNIQUE 2.21

- Expose the fracture as previously described. If at least one third of the proximal third of the patella is intact, preserve it.
- Clear the joint of loose fragments of bone and cartilage. Trim away the edges of the capsule and tendon. Excise the comminuted fragments. Small flecks of bone can be left within the patellar tendon to make anchorage easier.
- Trim the articular edge of the proximal fragment and smooth it with a rasp.
- Beginning on the fracture surface of the proximal fragment just anterior to the articular cartilage, use a 2-mm Kirschner wire or 2.5-mm drill bit to drill three parallel holes in a proximal direction (one hole in the center and one each in the medial and lateral thirds). Alternatively, we routinely use a Beathe pin to create the bone tunnels and pass the suture simultaneously.
- Weave two heavy nonabsorbable sutures through the patellar tendon, one through the medial and one through the lateral half of the tendon (Fig. 2.64). Use a suture passer to pass the free proximal ends of the sutures through the holes in the patella. Place one suture end each through the medial and lateral holes and two through the central hole.

- With the knee slightly hyperextended, tie the sutures securely over the superior pole of the patella. The patellar tendon should evaginate and lie against the raw fractured surface of the patellar remnant near the articular surface. This prevents tilting of the fragment and contact of the raw surface with the femur.
- Occasionally, the proximal pole of the patella is comminuted, leaving a single distal fragment consisting of half or more of the bone. This fragment, provided that it contains a smooth articular surface, also should be preserved by applying the principles outlined in the technique just described. Much of the lower pole at its inferior limits is uncovered by articular cartilage.

PARTIAL PATELLECTOMY USING FIGURE-OF-EIGHT LOAD-SHARING WIRE OR CABLE

Because of the powerful forces generated by the quadriceps mechanism, protection of the repair often is necessary. This can be accomplished by a figure-of-eight, load-sharing wire or cable, as described by Perry et al. The cable protects the patellar tendon repair by transmitting tensile loads directly from the quadriceps tendon or proximal pole of the patella to the tibial tubercle. This technique also can be used to protect tenuous internal fixation of patellar fractures, and it allows more aggressive rehabilitation. We frequently augment an extensor mechanism repair with a nonabsorbable suture in this fashion, thus facilitating earlier range of motion.

TECHNIQUE 2.22

(PERRY ET AL.)
- After internal fixation or partial patellectomy with extensor mechanism repair has been done, drill a 2-mm

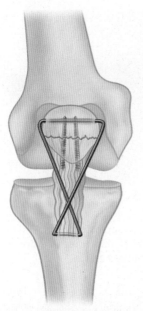

FIGURE 2.65   After reduction and internal fixation of patellar fracture, two cables are inserted through transverse holes drilled in tibial tubercle and proximal pole of patella; they are crossed anteriorly to patellar ligament to form figure-of-eight and are crimped to each other. **SEE TECHNIQUE 2.22.**

hole transversely across the proximal pole of the patella and drill a second hole transversely across the tibial tubercle.

- Hyperextend the knee to relax the patellar tendon.
- Pass a heavy braided suture or a 16-gauge stainless steel wire through each of the two drill holes (Fig. 2.65). Alternatively, pass the wire or cable through the quadriceps insertion adjacent to the patella proximally, rather than through the proximal pole of the patella.
- Cross the sutures or wires anterior to the patellar tendon and tighten and crimp them to each other to form a figure of eight. As the wires are tightened, the patella tracks distally; the patellar tendon should be completely lax during this step. Avoid patella baja.
- Gently flex the knee to 90 degrees to confirm that displacement of the fracture does not occur. It is important to cross the wires anteriorly over the patellar tendon; otherwise, flexion of the knee causes the wire to displace posteriorly, which prevents it from sharing the load across the fracture site. The wire can be removed as an outpatient procedure in about 3 months or after healing of the fracture has occurred.

TOTAL PATELLECTOMY

In fractures in which comminution is so severe that no sizable fragments are salvageable, a total patellectomy may be indicated.

TECHNIQUE 2.23

- Excise all the fragments, preserving as much of the patellar and quadriceps tendons as possible.
- Clear the joint of bone chips and debris by thorough irrigation.
- Place a heavy, nonabsorbable suture with a grasping technique through the margins of the patellar and quadriceps tendons and through the medial and lateral capsular expansions in a purse-string manner.
- Pull the suture taut and evaginate the tendon ends completely outside the joint. When the suture has been tightened until it makes a circle about 2 mm in diameter, tie it securely.
- Although small, this rosette of tendon may give the appearance of a small patella. Use supplemental interrupted sutures to repair the capsular rupture and to appose the quadriceps and patellar tendon ends further. The purse-string suture shortens the quadriceps mechanism and helps prevent extensor lag, which is common after patellectomy.
- A quadriceps tie-down technique can be used if insufficient tendon is available to suture the quadriceps and patellar tendons primarily. One such technique is an inverted V-plasty of the quadriceps tendon.

DISTAL FEMUR

Supracondylar and intercondylar fractures of the distal femur historically have been difficult to treat. These fractures often are unstable and comminuted and tend to have a bimodal distribution, occurring in elderly or younger multiple-injured patients. Because of the proximity of these fractures to the knee joint, regaining full knee motion and function may be difficult. The incidences of malunion, nonunion, and infection are relatively high in many reported series. In older patients, treatment may be complicated by previous joint arthroplasty.

The classification of distal femoral fractures described by Müller et al. and expanded in the AO/OTA classification is useful in determining treatment and prognosis. It is based on the location and pattern of the fracture and considers all fractures within the transepicondylar width of the knee (Fig. 2.66). Type A fractures involve the distal shaft only with varying degrees of comminution. Type B fractures are condylar fractures; type B1 is a sagittal split of the lateral condyle, type B2 is a sagittal split of the medial condyle, and type B3 is a coronal plane fracture. Type C fractures are T-condylar and Y-condylar fractures; type C1 fractures have no comminution, type C2 fractures have a comminuted shaft fracture with two principal articular fragments, and type C3 fractures have intraarticular comminution.

In the 1960s, nonoperative treatment methods, such as traction and cast bracing, produced better results than operative treatment because of the lack of adequate internal fixation devices. With the development of improved internal fixation devices by the AO group, treatment recommendations began to change and operative treatment produced better results than nonoperative treatment, especially for intercondylar and extraarticular fractures.

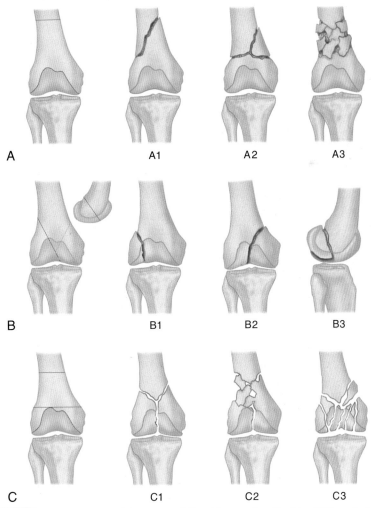

FIGURE 2.66 Classification of fractures of distal femur described by Müller et al. (Redrawn from Müller ME, Nazarian J, Koch P, Schatzker J: *The comprehensive classification of fractures of long bones*, Berlin, 1990, Springer-Verlag.)

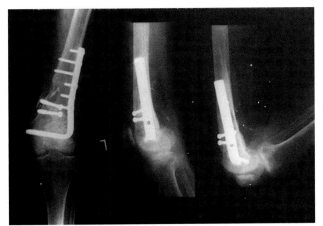

FIGURE 2.67 Patient with displaced comminuted supracondylar fracture of femur internally fixed with AO supracondylar blade plate and multiple screws.

Advances in implant technology, technical execution of surgical fixation, rehabilitation, and surgeon understanding have largely contributed to the shift toward operative intervention for these injuries. Operative treatment is recommended for all fractures of the distal femur in the appropriate patient, with the exception of simple, nondisplaced fractures. Early mobilization of the knee is important in obtaining a good result.

PLATE AND SCREW FIXATION

The blade plate designed by the AO group in Switzerland was one of the first plate-and-screw devices to gain wide acceptance for treatment of fractures of the distal femur. Although it provides stable fixation of most fractures (Fig. 2.67), the technique is technically demanding; early problems included infection and inadequate fixation in osteoporotic bone and refracture after plate removal.

As experience with AO plating techniques increased and the use of perioperative antibiotics became routine, the results reported with these devices improved. In 1989, Siliski, Mahring, and Hofer reported good or excellent results in 81% of fractures, with infection occurring in 7.7%, unintentional shortening in 7.6%, and malalignment in 5.8%. Results were better in type C1 fractures (92% good or excellent results) than in type C2 and type C3 fractures (77% good or excellent results).

More biologic techniques of plating have been advocated using indirect reduction techniques, minimal soft-tissue stripping, and gentle retraction. Femoral distractors or

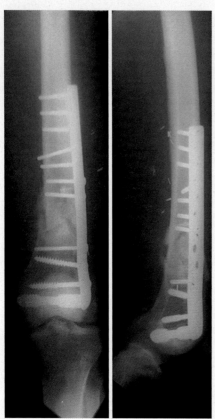

FIGURE 2.68 Fixation of medial condylar fracture with dynamic condylar screw.

external fixators are used to regain length and alignment of the fracture, and metaphyseal comminution is left in situ with no attempt made to reduce comminuted fragments anatomically. Because the soft tissues are left relatively undisturbed, bone grafting is less often necessary (see **Video 2.1**).

DYNAMIC CONDYLAR SCREW FIXATION

A less technically demanding alternative to the blade plate is the dynamic condylar screw (Fig. 2.68). The blade plate requires accurate insertion in three planes simultaneously, whereas the dynamic condylar screw allows freedom in the flexion-extension plane. A minimum of 4 cm of uncomminuted bone in the femoral condyles above the intercondylar notch is necessary for successful fixation. The main disadvantage of the dynamic condylar screw is that insertion of the condylar lag screw requires removal of a large amount of bone, which makes revision surgery, should it be necessary, more difficult. Reported results of distal femoral fractures treated with the dynamic condylar screw were similar to results obtained with blade plates with 87% excellent or satisfactory results. Nonunion occurred in 0% to 5.7%, infection in 0% to 5.3%, and malunion in 5.3% to 11%. Bone grafting was used in about one third of the fractures. In one study, all poor results occurred in elderly, osteopenic patients with comminuted intraarticular fractures. This technique may be unsuitable for patients with osteoporosis.

Blade plates and condylar screws are unsuitable for use in fractures with less than 3 to 4 cm of intact femoral condylar bone and in fractures with a large amount of articular comminution. For these fractures, the condylar buttress plate is the most commonly used implant. The multiple holes in the distal end of the plate allow multiple screws to be directed into comminuted fragments. Fractures with a comminuted medial buttress, segmental bone loss, or very low transcondylar fractures may angulate into varus because of movement at the screw-plate interface. Devices developed to lock the screws into the plate increase the stability of the construct to prevent varus deformation. Some authors have used methyl methacrylate to improve screw purchase in osteopenic bone. Traditionally, if medial instability is present after application of a lateral buttress plate, the addition of a medial plate is recommended. An inverted large fragment T-plate inserted through a separate medial subvastus incision, double plating with bone grafting, and a locked dual plating technique all have been recommended. Bolhofner et al. advocated percutaneous plating. They treated 57 supracondylar femoral fractures with open reduction and plating using indirect methods, and all fractures healed. Using the Schatzker scoring method, they reported good results in 84% but admitted that surgical skill was a factor. We agree that this is a good technique for bridging a highly comminuted fracture.

Condylar plates with screws that are locked to the plate have been used (Fig. 2.69). These plates provide stability similar to the dynamic condylar screw and mitigate the varus angulation that can occur with a medial femoral defect. This fixation may eliminate the need for a medial femoral plate.

The less invasive stabilization system (LISS) plate, which uses locked screws and percutaneous fixation, was developed to circumvent the problems with previous fixation methods. The biomechanical properties of this fixation device have been compared with the properties of the dynamic condylar screw and condylar buttress plate. The LISS allowed higher elastic deformation than the other systems, placing it between rigid fixation and intramedullary nailing. Our experience with this method has been satisfactory, but our implant preference is locking condylar plating systems. Locking implants with polyaxial capability also are available, which provide utility for certain fractures, particularly periprosthetic injuries.

INTRAMEDULLARY NAILING

Intramedullary nailing has received increased attention for the treatment of distal femoral fractures. These devices obtain more "biologic" fixation than plates because they are load-sharing, rather than load-sparing, implants. They offer greater soft-tissue preservation, and bone grafting is required less often. The major disadvantage of nail fixation is that it provides less rigid stabilization of distal femoral fractures than plate fixation in biomechanical testing. Implant failure has been reported in 15% of distal-third femoral fractures treated with antegrade interlocking nailing using slotted designs. The frequency of implant failure increases if the fracture is within 5 cm of the most proximal screw hole. It has been suggested that implant failure can be prevented by driving the nail to subchondral bone, delaying full weight bearing, and increasing the wall thickness of the nail. By using these principles, intramedullary nailing has been used successfully to treat fractures of the distal femur.

When antegrade interlocked intramedullary nailing is done with the patient in the lateral decubitus position, the weight of the leg can cause valgus angulation. When the patient is supine, however, the pull of the gastrocnemius muscles cause posterior angulation. Smooth Steinmann pins in the distal femur, medial and lateral to the patella, can be used to manipulate the fragment and maintain proper alignment. A traction pin also can be placed anteriorly in the distal femur

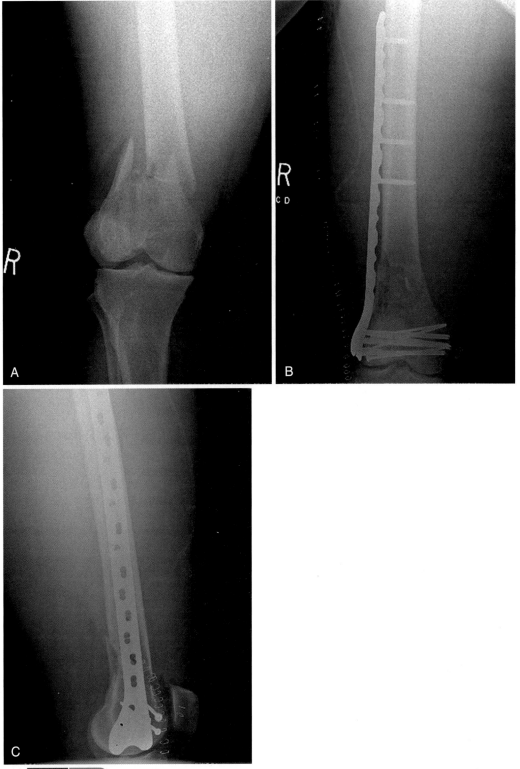

FIGURE 2.69 **A,** Comminuted fracture of distal femur with intraarticular extension. **B** and **C,** Open reduction and internal fixation through lateral parapatellar arthrotomy to view anatomic reduction of articular component, and submuscular plate is then positioned percutaneously.

to prevent posterior angulation when the supine position is used. Overall, excellent or good results have been reported in 95% after antegrade nailing.

We evaluated the results of 57 supracondylar and intercondylar fractures of the femur treated with antegrade interlocking nailing at our institution. These included eight AO type A2, 13 type A3, eight type C1, 25 type C2, and three type C3 fractures; 44% of the fractures were open. All fractures united, and 3.5% required bone graft. Malunion occurred in 7% of fractures, and two type IIIB open fractures (3.5%) became infected. One nail

(1.7%) failed but did not require reoperation. Range of motion averaged 115 degrees. Poor results occurred in all three AO type C3 fractures, one caused by infection and two by malreduction of unrecognized coronal fracture lines.

If nailing is considered for treatment of an intercondylar femoral fracture, preoperative radiographs and CT scans must be scrutinized carefully for the presence of coronal fracture lines. AO type C3 fractures generally are best treated with plating techniques, whereas retrograde nailing probably is preferable for distal femoral fractures with extensive shaft extension. Anteroposterior medial and lateral blocking screws can increase the primary stability of these fractures.

Retrograde femoral nails inserted through the intercondylar notch have become a popular method of treating supracondylar fractures. Similar to antegrade nails, these nails have the theoretical advantages of being load-sharing devices, requiring little soft-tissue dissection and infrequently needing bone grafting. Retrograde nailing of distal femoral fractures is preferable to antegrade nailing in the vast majority of situations involving the distal femur. Retrograde nailing is technically easier than antegrade nailing in obese patients. Distal femoral fractures below hip implants or above total knee implants with an open notch design also can be treated effectively with retrograde nailing. Retrograde nailing also can be used to stabilize distal femoral fractures associated with ipsilateral hip fractures, allowing the hip fracture to be stabilized with a separate device.

In mechanical testing comparing antegrade nailing with retrograde nailing in femoral shaft fractures with and without bony contact, no difference was found in the nails when used for stable fracture configurations, but in unstable fracture configurations, the nail size (larger), not the method of insertion, determined stability.

Reports of retrograde supracondylar nailing have shown acceptable results (90% to 100% union; knee range of motion 100 to 116 degrees). Reported complications have included infection in 0% to 4%; malunion in 0% to 8%; implant failure in 4% to 10%; nail fracture in 0% to 8%; and nail impingement on the patella in 0% to 12%, which can be avoided by properly countersinking the nail. Flexible intramedullary implants, such as the Zickel supracondylar device, Ender rods, and Rush rods, also have been used with some success to treat distal femoral fractures; however, since the development of more rigid plate and screw devices and interlocking intramedullary nails, the indications for their use are limited. Newer implant designs with minimally invasive insertion techniques have antiquated the use of flexible devices.

Successful use of retrograde intramedullary nail fixation as an adjuvant to distal femoral plating has been reported, particularly in elderly patients.

EXTERNAL FIXATION

External fixation can be used as either temporary or definitive fixation in severe open distal femoral fractures, especially fractures associated with vascular injury. If the fracture has significant comminution with shortening, consideration should be given to application of an external fixator. Because of the potential for pin track infection and knee stiffness, this technique should be reserved for the most severe open fractures. We use this technique to provide local traction while allowing mobility for patients with multiple trauma. This technique also allows better CT evaluation of the distal femoral fracture. Early conversion from a spanning external fixator to an intramedullary nail is safe in patients with multiple injuries.

If a patient is placed in a spanning external fixator and is not medically ready for intramedullary nailing or plating, a period of skeletal traction can be instituted during a pin site holiday in preparation for definitive fixation if the initial fixator has been in place longer than 14 days or the pin sites are of concern.

CONDYLAR FRACTURES OF THE FEMUR
■ UNICONDYLAR FRACTURES OF THE FEMUR

Unicondylar fractures (AO type B) occur less frequently than supracondylar or intercondylar femoral fractures. Concomitant injuries to the ipsilateral extremity are present in about one third of patients. Careful radiographic evaluation, including anteroposterior, lateral, and tunnel views, is necessary to diagnose accurately associated injuries to the knee and coronal fractures of the posterior condyle (AO type B3 or Hoffa fractures). A CT scan is necessary to describe the fracture more accurately. Nondisplaced fractures can be treated nonoperatively but must be followed closely for loss of reduction. Displaced unicondylar fractures require surgical fixation to prevent the complications of axial malalignment, posttraumatic arthritis, knee stiffness, and instability frequently reported after nonoperative treatment. Some minimally displaced fractures can be treated with percutaneous reduction and fixation, but open reduction usually is necessary to obtain an anatomic articular reconstruction. Cancellous lag screws or a small-fragment buttress plate provide sufficient fixation to allow movement after a few days. In patients with osteoporotic bone, a buttress plate may be necessary to prevent cephalad migration of the condyle.

FRACTURE FIXATION OF THE MEDIAL CONDYLE

If only one condyle is fractured, the operation is relatively simple, and because the shaft is not involved, internal fixation usually is secure enough to allow movement early in the postoperative course. Often condylar fractures can be reduced with traction on a fracture table or flat-topped radiolucent table and provisionally maintained with various periarticular clamps. The fracture can then be secured with a percutaneous lag screw, a conical, headless compression screw, or placement of a buttress plate. However, we recommend open reduction to ensure anatomic articular reconstruction.

TECHNIQUE 2.24

- On the anteromedial aspect of the knee, begin a longitudinal incision 10 cm proximal to the joint line and extend it distally to below the level of the joint. Incise the capsule and synovium at the joint level in line with the skin incision, and extend the incision proximally along the lateral edge of the vastus medialis muscle at its junction with the quadriceps tendon. Extend this incision proximally enough to expose the medial femoral condyle, the patellofemoral groove, and the intercondylar area.
- Insert a Steinmann pin into the large fragment so that it can be used as a lever during reduction.

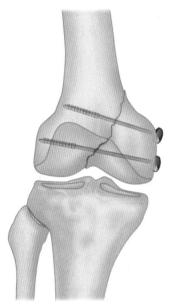

FIGURE 2.70 Fracture of medial condyle fixed with 6.5-mm cancellous screws. **SEE TECHNIQUE 2.24.**

- Clear the joint of all debris, thoroughly irrigate and reduce the fracture under direct vision using the pin as a lever. A periarticular reduction clamp can be inserted percutaneously on the lateral femoral condyle to effect interfragmentary compression after articular reduction.
- Multiple Kirschner wires can be inserted across the fracture fragments into the intact lateral femoral condyle for provisional fixation.
- Place two cancellous screws perpendicular to the fracture site to fix the medial femoral condylar fragment to the intact lateral femoral condyle (Fig. 2.70). The size of the implant depends on the fragment size but can range from 3.5- to 6.5-mm screws. If the bone is osteoporotic, a washer under the head of the screw prevents the head from sinking through the cortex.
- Remove the multiple Kirschner wires used for temporary fixation, and confirm the reduction with radiographs made in two planes. Ensure that the ends of the pins or cancellous screws penetrate the lateral femoral cortex because osteoporotic bone within the condyle does not afford good purchase. The lag screw effect of the cancellous screws should produce good fixation and interfragmentary compression.
- In some patients with osteoporotic bone, fixation with screws alone may be inadequate; therefore, a buttress plate is contoured to fit the medial condyle.
- An alternative is the use of small fragment fixation, in which interfragmentary compression can be achieved with 3.5-mm interfragmentary screws and further stabilized with the addition of a small-fragment buttress plate, which is our preference in most cases.
- Whichever internal fixation construct is selected, the key principle remains anatomic articular reduction.

POSTOPERATIVE CARE The patient is placed in a removable long-leg splint or a bulky soft dressing with light compression wrap and knee immobilizer. Continuous passive motion can be initiated immediately after surgery if desired. Gentle active and active-assisted exercises are begun when swelling subsides. Ambulation with a walker or crutches is started on postoperative day 2 or 3, allowing only non–weight bearing. Range-of-motion exercises and quadriceps and hamstring exercises are increased gradually. If the fracture is healing satisfactorily, partial weight bearing can be allowed at 8 to 10 weeks. By 12 to 14 weeks, the patient usually has gradually progressed to full weight bearing. The residual disability after isolated fractures of the medial femoral condyle usually is minor, and good range of motion can be regained when reduction and fixation are satisfactory and joint motion is begun early.

FRACTURE FIXATION OF THE POSTERIOR PART OF THE MEDIAL CONDYLE

If the posterior part of the medial femoral condyle is sheared off, ORIF with lag screws is recommended. Although this fracture looks harmless on the radiographs, it may produce a marked disability. Initially undisplaced fractures frequently displace if treated conservatively. As seen on the lateral view, the loose fragment consists of approximately the posterior half of the condyle. The fragment has minimal soft-tissue attachments and may be devoid of blood supply. Almost its entire surface is covered with articular cartilage. The amount of displacement may be minimal. If the fragment is not reduced properly, roughening of the articular surface and osteonecrosis occur. Ordinarily, the fragment should not be removed because it is an important part of the articular surface when the knee is flexed at 90 degrees. Treatment consists of fixation of the fracture in proper position.

TECHNIQUE 2.25

- Adequate exposure can require anteromedial and posteromedial incisions. Anatomic reduction of the articular surface is of paramount importance.
- Replace the posterior portion of the medial femoral condyle using a posteromedial Henderson incision and fix it temporarily with multiple Kirschner wires.
- Depending on the size of the fragment, insert two 3.5-mm or 4.5-mm appropriately countersunk interfragmentary lag screws from the anterior to posterior. We also have used cannulated differential thread headless compression screw fixation. Place the screws medial to the patellofemoral articulation, if possible, and direct them perpendicular to the fracture site.
- Countersink all screws that are placed through the articular surface. Inspect to see that the screw does not penetrate the articular surface posteriorly.
- Remove the transfixing Kirschner wires. Occasionally, a portion of the medial head of the gastrocnemius may require reflection for adequate exposure.
- After the screws have been inserted, check the reduction and position of the screw by radiographs and close the wound.

POSTOPERATIVE CARE Postoperative care is the same as that recommended after fixation of the medial femoral condyle (see Technique 2.24).

■ INTERCONDYLAR FRACTURES OF THE FEMUR

ORIF of comminuted intercondylar and supracondylar fractures of the femur demands experience and surgical skill. A complete set of instruments and familiarity with their use are required for this method of fixation. Strict adherence to basic principles and technique is required to prevent unsatisfactory results. ORIF of these difficult fractures is justified only if (1) the joint surfaces can be restored anatomically, (2) fixation is sufficiently rigid that external immobilization is not required, (3) rigidity of fixation is sufficient to allow early and active motion of the knee joint, and (4) the skin and soft tissues are satisfactory for a major operation.

Historically, insertion of a 95-degree condylar blade plate is technically difficult and unforgiving. The broad surface area of the plate provides excellent fixation and resistance to bending and torsional forces. If the blade is inserted correctly into the condyles, anatomic alignment of the femur can be obtained by fixing the plate to the shaft of the femur. If the blade is inserted incorrectly, malalignment occurs. Difficulty in application and design advancements have largely eliminated the use of blade plates and dynamic condylar screws as first-line fixation devices. Evolution of fracture fixation devices for the distal femur has led to most extramedullary implants being condylar plates with the capability for locking screws, at times polyaxial, and typically with some form of targeting instrumentation that has allowed for considerably less soft-tissue dissection. Refer to earlier editions of this text for detailed techniques on distal femoral blade plate or dynamic condylar screw implant insertion.

Fracture morphology will dictate the required surgical approach for appropriate reduction and fracture stabilization. The need for significant proximal extensile exposure is rare, particularly with modern targeting instrumentation. Supracondylar fractures or simple intercondylar fractures often can be treated through direct lateral surgical approaches distally. Those with more extensive articular involvement necessitate direct exposure to ensure anatomic reduction. This is most frequently accomplished through an anterior approach with lateral parapatellar arthrotomy. In fracture-specific cases, a small accessory medial incision may be required for fracture manipulation or screw placement. Most frequently, we use the distal aspect of the approach described next (swashbuckler approach) or a more lateral parapatellar approach for those in need of anatomic reduction of comminuted articular injuries. The most distal extent of the approach is necessary for direct articular reduction and implant insertion. Care should be taken to avoid dissection or manipulation of the metaphyseal region in an effort to retain the fracture biology and lessen the chance for healing difficulties.

To provide better exposure of the distal articular surface of the femur, Starr, Jones, and Reinert used a modified anterior approach they called the "swashbuckler approach." Cited advantages to this approach, in addition to improved exposure, are sparing of the quadriceps muscle bellies and a surgical scar that does not interfere with subsequent total knee arthroplasty.

SWASHBUCKLER APPROACH TO THE DISTAL FEMUR

TECHNIQUE 2.26

(STARR ET AL.)

- Place the patient supine, preferably on a radiolucent table.
- Use a sterile tourniquet only if necessary to avoid medial retraction of the quadriceps.
- Place a roll or triangle under the knee. Make a midline incision from above the fracture laterally to across the patella (Fig. 2.71A).
- Extend the incision directly down to the fascia of the quadriceps. Incise the quadriceps fascia in line with the skin incision. Sharply dissect the quadriceps fascia off the vastus lateralis muscle laterally to its inclusion with the iliotibial band.
- Retract the iliotibial band and fascia laterally, continuing the dissection down to the linea aspera.
- Incise the lateral parapatellar retinaculum, separating it from the vastus lateralis (Fig. 2.71B).
- Make a lateral parapatellar arthrotomy to expose the femoral condyles.
- Place a retractor under the vastus lateralis and medialis, exposing the distal femur and displacing the patella medially (Fig. 2.71C).
- Ligate the perforating vessels and elevate the vastus lateralis, exposing the entire distal femur.
- Proceed with the internal fixation as needed.
- Close the wound by suturing the fascia back in place.

■ LOCKING CONDYLAR PLATE FIXATION

Locking condylar plate fixation is indicated for intraarticular and extraarticular condylar fractures, bridging of highly comminuted distal femoral fractures, and treatment of distal femoral malunions. Current implants offer the stability of fixed angle devices with the ability to be placed in a biologically appropriate manner and therefore are our current choice for most AO/OTA Type A and C fractures requiring plate osteosynthesis.

Authors have attempted to identify factors contributing to nonunion and failures in these difficult fractures. Obesity, open fractures, infection, and stainless steel implants have been identified as risk factors for development of nonunion. Ricci et al. evaluated risk factors for reoperation. In their series, 19% required reoperation to achieve union. Diabetes and open fracture were independent risk factors for deep infection and delayed union. Factors associated with implant failure included open fractures, smoking, increased body mass index, and shorter plate length. Barei et al. evaluated their series of open distal femoral fracture. They concluded that despite metaphyseal bone loss, locking plates obviate the need for routine bone grafting of some open distal femoral fractures. Fractures demonstrating posterior cortical contact were strongly correlated with primary union. Because of the inconsistent callus these injuries exhibit through comminuted metaphyseal regions, alterations of the fixation strategy

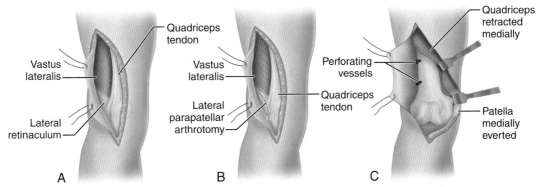

FIGURE 2.71 Swashbuckler technique. **A,** Fascia overlying quadriceps is incised longitudinally and lifted laterally off underlying muscle. **B,** Farther laterally, fascia over quadriceps becomes confluent with iliotibial band. Lateral parapatellar arthrotomy is performed. Proximally, arthrotomy incision is made between vastus lateralis muscle and lateral retinaculum of knee. **C,** Proximal release of vastus lateralis fibers from lateral intermuscular septum allows further mobilization of quadriceps. Perforating vessels can be controlled with cautery. **SEE TECHNIQUE 2.26.**

have been proposed. Dynamic locking or far cortical locking, as a method to increase micromotion on the lateral cortex to increase the callus response, has been advocated.

SUBMUSCULAR MINIMALLY INVASIVE LOCKING CONDYLAR PLATE APPLICATION

TECHNIQUE 2.27

- Position the patient supine on a radiolucent table. Place a well-padded bump under the ipsilateral hip to maintain the femur in neutral rotation. Prepare and drape the limb in normal fashion. Position the limb on a sterile bump or triangular bolster. Contralateral rotation films can be helpful to gauge rotation reduction and for intraoperative referencing.
- Expose the distal femur as previously described (see Technique 2.26). Typically, only the distal extent of the approach is necessary with lateral parapatellar arthrotomy for articular reduction. Alternatively, a direct lateral approach may be used in extraarticular fractures or those with simple articular components (Fig. 2.72).
- Reduce the condylar fragments with Kirschner wires and reduction forceps.
- Place the condylar plate guide on the lateral cortex to determine the proper position for the placement of interfragmentary lag screws to maintain the condylar reduction without interfering with the plate.
- Using anatomic landmarks and C-arm imaging, place the plate in a submuscular fashion on the reconstructed condyles with or without attempting to reduce the proximal fragments, and insert a 2.5-mm guidewire through the wire guide central hole parallel to the femorotibial joint line. Obtain an image to confirm placement parallel to the joint line. For this portion of the procedure, wire placement is critical because it "sets" the distal position

of the plate in the coronal plane. Nonparallel positioning of this initial reference wire can inadvertently induce a varus or valgus coronal plane malalignment. Beware of anatomic variances, such as a hypoplastic lateral condyle, which can make reconstruction and implant positioning quite difficult. Close scrutiny of contralateral knee films can facilitate identification of anatomic nuances when preoperative templating is performed.

- On the lateral fluoroscopic plane, confirm that the distal positioning of the plate parallels the posterior cortex of the distal femur to ensure appropriate coronal plane flexion and extension. Once appropriate positioning is noted, place additional guidewires through the locking guides to secure the plate on the distal segment.
- Longitudinal traction can be applied and the targeting instrumentation used to permit placement of a provisional guidewire in the most proximal hole of the plate chosen. It is critical that the length and rotational reduction be noted before this step. Additionally, in particularly comminuted fractures of the distal femoral metaphysis, a single proximal wire may not provide sufficient length maintenance alone.
- Once the length and rotational alignment are "set," place a small bolster under the metaphyseal portion of the fracture to determine flexion and extension.
- Many periarticular plates do not fit every patient's anatomy, and consequently there can be variable offset of the plate from the femoral shaft. As a result, failure to recognize this can induce varus or valgus malalignment when threaded reduction instrumentation or nonlocking cortical screws are used to seat the plate on bone. When offset is identified, the plate should be applied as an "internal-external fixator," with locking screw fixation to maintain anatomic coronal plane reduction. The reduction is more important than plate to bone contact.
- Locking screws can be inserted in any order, but we usually prefer to insert the central screw first, followed by the surrounding screws in the distal segment. Proximal fixation is achieved with placement of 4.5-mm cortical screws or 5.0-mm locking cortical screws through the targeting instrumentation. A minimum of eight cortices should be used proximally.

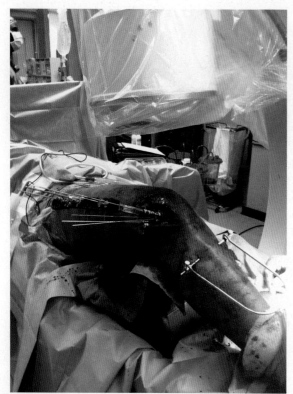

FIGURE 2.72   Minimally invasive plate insertion for fixation of supracondylar *or* intercondylar distal femoral fractures using specially designed outriggers for targeting proximal fixation. This permits accurate fixation while minimizing further biologic insult to comminuted metaphyseal zones. Note proximal tibial traction pin and bow used for greater control of axial length and rotational alignment. **SEE TECHNIQUE 2.27.**

- Take care when placing proximal fixation into the shaft. Consider filling the most proximal hole in the construct with a unicortical locking screw or a bicortical nonlocking screw to minimize stress riser formation.
- Ideally, long plate constructs with well-spaced fixation is sought. Locking screw fixation in close proximity to metaphyseal comminution can result in a very rigid construct that may contribute to inconsistent callus formation and should be avoided if possible.
- Securely tighten all screws again before wound closure.
- Perform fascial and skin closure in the standard fashion.

POSTOPERATIVE CARE Early passive motion with some active motion is begun as tolerated. Focus also is placed on passive extension exercises to minimize contracture formation. Weight bearing is avoided for 10 to 12 weeks. Active and passive range of motion should be encouraged during this time.

LESS INVASIVE STABILIZATION SYSTEM

The technique for use of the LISS system is in many respects very similar to application of the locking condylar plate in a minimally invasive fashion (Fig. 2.73). One can refer to the previous technique. However, several key differences should be mentioned. The LISS system is constructed of titanium and, therefore, its modulus of elasticity is different than many available locking condylar plating systems and permits more flexibility. Whereas

the design of many locking condylar plates allows for plate reduction techniques, the LISS relies on the reduction being achieved before implant positioning. Furthermore, it truly is an "internal-external fixator," and therefore fixation with locking screws near and far from the fracture provides the greatest stability. This is better tolerated with the LISS as compared with locking condylar plates because of the increased flexibility in LISS. In addition, the screw fixation is solely unicortical.

DOUBLE PLATE FIXATION

Very low distal femoral fractures with extensive articular and metaphyseal comminution may not be stabilized adequately by lateral plating alone. Application of an additional medial plate may be necessary. A separate medial incision is preferred to reduce the amount of soft-tissue stripping required for plate application.

TECHNIQUE 2.28

(CHAPMAN AND HENLEY)

- After lateral fixation, assess whether the fracture stabilization is sufficient to permit early functional range of motion. If not, proceed with application of medial fixation through a separate longitudinal medial approach.
- Alternatively, very distal fractures may require an accessory medial approach for reduction purposes in addition to lateral intervention and before definitive fixation.
- Make an anteromedial incision from the anterior margin of the pes anserinus, following the adductor canal (Fig. 2.74A). The deep dissection follows the subvastus (Southern) approach. Incise the fascial envelope surrounding the vastus medialis along the posterior margin of the muscle.
- Use blunt dissection to elevate the muscle off the periosteum and the intermuscular septum from the adductor tubercle to the intact proximal femoral shaft.
- Distally, sharply incise the 2- to 3-cm wide tendinous insertion of the vastus medialis into the medial capsule.
- Expose the joint through a medial parapatellar arthrotomy. This approach does not require formal dissection of the superficial femoral artery because the artery is retracted posteriorly with the sartorius muscle.
- Protect the descending genicular artery and saphenous nerve by bluntly dissecting the posterior margin of the vastus medialis and retracting the artery and nerve anteriorly. Leave the superficial and deep fibers of the medial collateral ligament attached to the femoral condyle.
- If a posterior medial condylar fragment is present, make an additional arthrotomy just posterior to the medial collateral ligament to allow access to this portion of the articular surface. Flexion of the knee and posterior retraction of the sartorius and adductor longus make this easier.
- Inspect the medial compartment, including the meniscus, and remove any loose fragments from the joint.
- Continue posterior exposure until the intact medial femoral shaft is visible, minimizing soft-tissue stripping during dissection and retraction.
- Reduce and provisionally stabilize each of the femoral condyles as described for application of a locking condy-

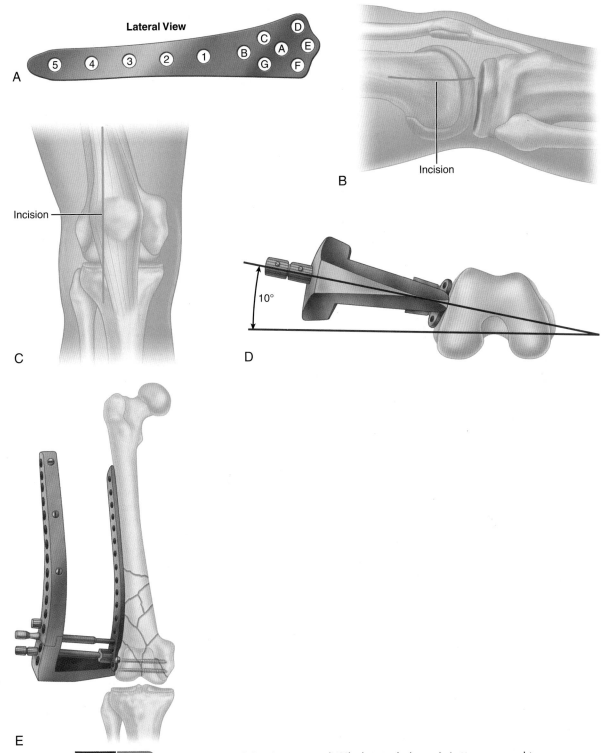

FIGURE 2.73 Less invasive stabilization system (LISS) plate technique. **A,** Letters are used to identify distal plate holes; numbers are used to identify diaphyseal plate holes. **B,** Lateral incision. **C,** In complex intraarticular fracture, lateral parapatellar approach is necessary. **D,** Insertion guide has tendency to tilt toward floor. When positioned properly on lateral condyle, insertion guide is internally rotated approximately 10 degrees to femoral shaft. Plate position is adjusted if necessary. **E,** Kirschner wire inserted through stabilization bolt. (Redrawn from *Less Invasive Stabilization Technique (LISS): technique guide*, Paoli, PA, 2001, Synthes.)

lar plate and reduce and fix the medial and lateral femoral condyles to each other, incorporating any intercalary fragments.

- Use Kirschner wires, pointed reduction tenaculums, or large periarticular clamps for temporary stabilization.
- Reduce the reconstructed distal articular block and provisionally fix it to the femoral shaft. Position a lateral plate and temporarily fix it to the distal femur.
- When reduction is satisfactory, secure it with two to four proximal and distal screws inserted with image intensification guidance.
- Bend the medial buttress plate to match exactly the contour of the medial femur. We prefer small-fragment fixation, typically.
- Place the transverse portion of the plate distally so that the screw holes allow placement of screws into the anterior and posterior portions of the femoral condyles. The anterior screw should permit bicondylar-transcondylar fixation (Fig. 2.74B).
- For the proximal end of the medial plate, use at least four cortices of fixation (Fig. 2.75).
- After screws are placed, consider filling bone defects with autologous cancellous grafts in closed injuries. Otherwise, antibiotic cement spacers may be advisable in open injuries and in preparation for future grafting. Repair the arthrotomy and close the medial approach in routine fashion.

POSTOPERATIVE CARE Postoperative care is the same as after that for locking condylar plate fixation, with initiating motion based on stability of fracture repair.

■ SUPRACONDYLAR FRACTURES OF THE FEMUR

Most supracondylar fractures of the femur can be treated with interlocking intramedullary nailing or plate-and-screw devices. Even those with simple intraarticular fracture components often can be treated with intramedullary nail fixation. Distal screw configurations vary and are often the determinants in whether a supracondylar femoral fracture can be adequately stabilized with an intramedullary device. In patients who are poor operative risks, nonoperative treatment with acute skeletal traction followed by cast bracing is an option. Historically, flexible intramedullary implants with supplemental bracing have been used in some low-demand elderly patients; however, current minimally invasive nailing and plating techniques have the advantages of minimizing surgical trauma and providing stable fixation, which typically requires no adjuvant bracing. Refer to techniques for retrograde intramedullary nail fixation and minimally invasive locking condylar plate insertion.

SHAFT OF THE FEMUR

Fractures of the shaft of the femur are among the most common fractures encountered in orthopaedic practice. Because the femur is the largest bone of the body and one of the principal load-bearing bones in the lower extremity, fractures can cause prolonged morbidity and extensive disability unless treatment is appropriate. Fractures of the femoral shaft often are the result of high-energy trauma and may be associated with multiple system injuries. Several techniques are now available for their treatment, and the orthopaedic surgeon must be aware of the advantages, disadvantages, and limitations of each to select the proper treatment for each patient. The type and location of the fracture, the degree of comminution, the age of the patient, the patient's social and economic demands, and other factors may influence the method of treatment. Possible treatment methods for fractures of the femoral shaft include the following:

- Closed reduction and spica cast immobilization
- Skeletal traction
- Femoral cast bracing
- External fixation
- Internal fixation
- Intramedullary nailing with open or closed technique
- Antegrade interlocking intramedullary nailing with or without reaming
- Retrograde interlocking intramedullary nailing
- Plate fixation

Locked intramedullary nailing is currently considered to be the treatment of choice for most femoral shaft fractures. Regardless of the treatment method chosen, the following principles are agreed on: (1) restoration of alignment, rotation, and length, (2) preservation of the blood supply to aid union and prevent infection, and (3) rehabilitation of the extremity and the patient.

TRACTION AND CAST IMMOBILIZATION

Skeletal traction methods most often are a preliminary phase to other definitive methods of femoral shaft fracture management, for instance, before plating or closed intramedullary nailing. Rarely are balanced skeletal or roller traction methods used as definitive treatment in adults. These are mentioned for historical reasons only. The length of confinement to bed, with its potential for complications, and the economic consequences of several weeks or months in the hospital make this an impractical method when used alone.

EXTERNAL FIXATION

Although we recommend immediate debridement, irrigation, and interlocking intramedullary nailing for most open femoral shaft fractures, half-pin fixators have proved effective, especially for massively contaminated fractures and fractures requiring rapid stabilization for vascular repair. Infections have occurred in some of our patients after nailing of fractures previously treated with external fixation, as has been reported by other authors. After wound coverage, early conversion (2 weeks) of external fixation to intramedullary fixation may decrease the incidence of infection. Temporary rapid external fixation of femoral fractures can be used in unstable, severely injured polytraumatized patients, especially if further blood loss is a major concern. External fixation can be maintained until union, but this is rare. Most commonly, a uniplanar external fixator is applied anteriorly or anterolaterally in polytraumatized patients or in patients with massive contaminated wounds as a means of temporary skeletal stabilization for later definitive management. For diaphyseal fractures, the knee joint rarely is immobilized; however, more distal fractures of the supracondylar or intercondylar variety most frequently require fixation to the tibia.

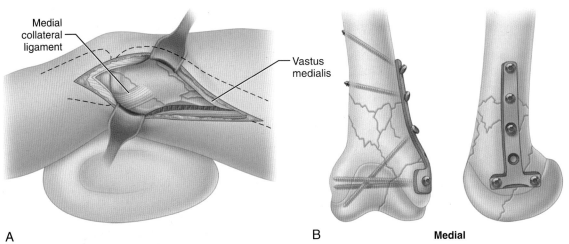

FIGURE 2.74 Double plating of distal femoral fracture. **A,** Subvastus (Southern) approach (see text). **B,** Application of large fragment T-plate. **SEE TECHNIQUE 2.28.**

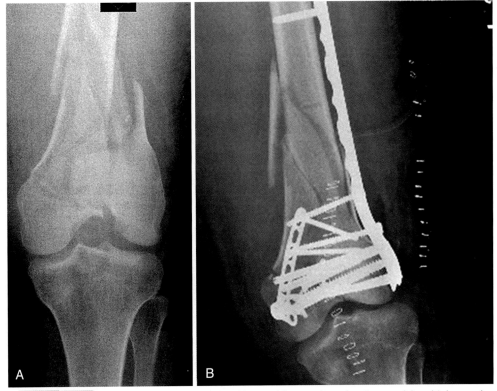

FIGURE 2.75 **A,** Highly comminuted distal femoral fracture in pedestrian struck by a high-speed vehicle. Note very low fracture involvement of medial femoral condyle. Lateral-based constructs would not typically provide adequate fixation into this fragment. **B,** Small fragment fixation of medial femoral condyle through subvastus approach, as adjuvant to more typical lateral-based fixation construct. **SEE TECHNIQUE 2.28.**

FIXATION WITH PLATES AND SCREWS

Since the 1960s, the AO surgeons in Switzerland have used either intramedullary fixation or compression plate fixation for almost all femoral shaft fractures. Their methods have many proponents. The most accurate reduction of comminuted fractures of the femoral shaft can be obtained with interfragmentary compression and plate and screw fixation. This treatment allows early motion and good function, but the risk of infection (2% to 5%), failure of fixation (6% to 10%), and delayed union (up to 19%) have been reported at unacceptable levels. However, if rigid internal fixation with interfragmentary compression is achieved successfully, complications are few.

Several reports have recommended the routine application of a bone graft medially in all comminuted fractures fixed with AO plates, or if rigid fixation is not obtained. Plating of femoral shaft fractures requires experience and judgment. Misuse of this method produces more poor results than any other.

Excellent results have been obtained with plating of comminuted shaft fractures without medial bone grafting when indirect reduction of intermediate fragments, preservation of soft-tissue attachments to bone especially medially, and final compression have been obtained. Femoral plating in patients with blunt polytrauma has been recommended, especially patients with ipsilateral femoral neck and shaft fractures, arterial injuries, or unstable spinal injuries. The technique involves indirect reduction, posterolateral plate application, and medial bone graft. Plating does not require the fracture table or fluoroscopic image intensifier that is necessary for closed femoral nailing. Plating preserves the endosteal blood supply; however, the cortex underlying the plate is devitalized. Low-contact dynamic compression plates with scalloped recesses permit less iatrogenic insult to the periosteal blood supply (Fig. 2.76).

Seligson et al. reviewed the results of femoral plating in 15 patients with multiple trauma. They noted a reduced postoperative morbidity from adult respiratory distress syndrome after plating as compared to that reported after intramedullary nailing. Complications of fracture healing were significantly greater (30%) after plating, however, than after intramedullary nailing (12%).

If plate and screw fixation is indicated, we prefer the 4.5-mm dynamic compression plate. In general, the broad plate should be used with approximately eight cortices (four holes) of screw purchase on either side of a transverse fracture. If plates and screws are used for internal fixation of femoral shaft fractures, weight bearing and unprotected ambulation usually are not possible as soon as after intramedullary nailing.

A lateral approach is used for fractures of the femoral shaft when plates and screws are used for fixation. It is essential that the plate be sufficiently long so that at least four screws are proximal and distal to the limits of the fracture. Cancellous screws at the distal end of the femur improve purchase, especially if the bone is osteoporotic. Plates can be removed 2 to 3 years after injury, provided that union is complete; however, plate removal is not routinely necessary. Cortical bone beneath a rigid AO plate remodels more like cancellous bone. For the cortex to return to its normal strength and structure, stress has to be gradually reapplied after removal of the plate. When two plates at 90 degrees to each other have been used, both plates should not be removed at the same time because the bone is doubly weak, and thus refracture is likely. The second plate can be removed 6 months after the first. The bone should be protected from excessive stress for at least 6 weeks after plate removal.

INTRAMEDULLARY FIXATION

Internal fixation of fractures of the femoral shaft became popular after World War II, when open intramedullary nailing was introduced. In a young adult patient with an uncomminuted fracture through the narrowest portion of the medullary canal, an intramedullary nail, barring complications, provides the ultimate treatment for femoral shaft fractures. Successful intramedullary nailing results in a short hospital stay, a rapid return of motion in all joints, prompt return to walking, and a relatively short total disability time. With current implant designs, fractures in the proximal or distal thirds of the shaft or fractures with severe comminution are also suitable for this form of internal fixation.

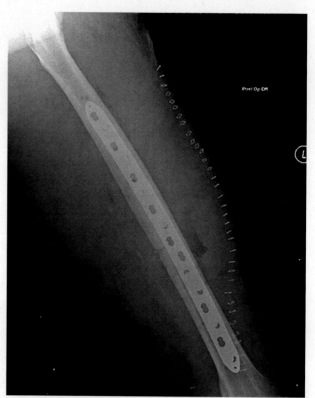

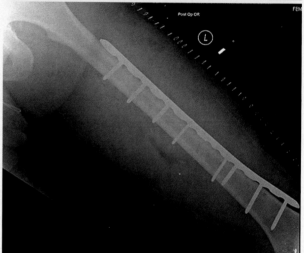

FIGURE 2.76 Polytraumatized patient with extensive pulmonary injuries and femoral diaphyseal fracture treated with ORIF using large fragment compression plating.

Although Küntscher introduced closed intramedullary nailing in the 1940s, it did not gain popularity in North America until the 1970s. With improvements in technique and especially the availability of image intensifiers, closed nailings have replaced the open technique. Historical improvements in design have expanded the indications for nailing of proximal and distal fractures. A variety of intramedullary devices are available; the most commonly used today are interlocking intramedullary nails, through which transverse or oblique transfixing screws can be inserted to control the major proximal and distal fragments, providing length and rotational stability. The nail can be inserted in either an antegrade or retrograde fashion.

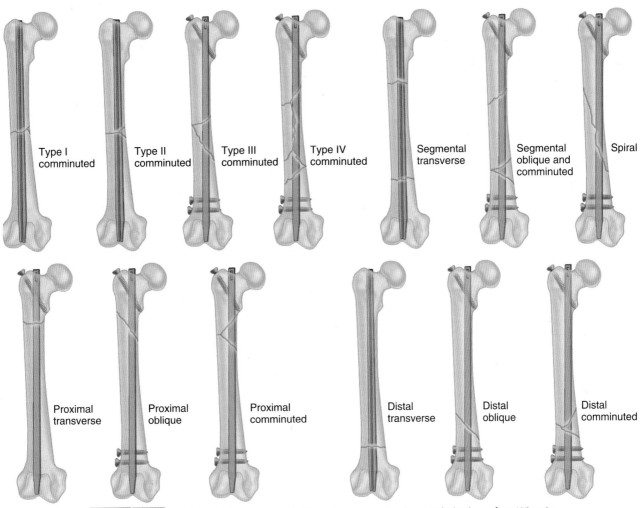

FIGURE 2.77 Winquist-Hansen classification of comminution (see text). (Redrawn from Winquist RA, Hansen RT, Clawson DK: Closed intramedullary nailing of femoral fractures: a report of five hundred and twenty cases, *J Bone Joint Surg* 66A:529, 1984.)

Historically, plating of femoral fractures has had higher rates of infection and nonunion than closed intramedullary nailing. Because there was some concern that interlocking nails might promote healing difficulties, the Winquist-Hansen classification of comminution (Fig. 2.77) was routinely used to determine whether static locking was necessary. Winquist and Hansen classified fractures into the following categories: (1) type I fracture, a comminuted fracture in which a small piece of bone has broken off, not affecting fracture stability; (2) type II fracture, in which at least 50% contact of the abutting cortices remains to prevent shortening and help control rotation, and in which sufficient proximal and distal cortical contact of the nail is possible to prevent translation and shortening; (3) type III comminuted fracture, which has less than 50% cortical contact or in which purchase of the nail would be poor in either the proximal or the distal fragment, allowing rotation, translation, and shortening; and (4) type IV comminuted fracture, in which the circumferential buttress of bone has been lost and no fixed contact exists between the major proximal and distal fragments to prevent shortening.

The optimal time for intramedullary nailing of closed and open fractures has been an area of controversy, particularly in the presence of multisystem trauma; however, current data support early (within 24 hours) nailing for most femoral fractures. Authors have demonstrated significant decreases in patient morbidity with stabilization of femoral fractures within 24 hours compared with delayed fixation after 48 hours, especially in patients with multiple injuries. Another series suggested that delayed femoral fixation beyond 12 hours in polytrauma patients can result in mortality reduction of approximately 50%. Pape et al. suggested that immediate reamed femoral nailing may precipitate adult respiratory distress syndrome in patients with blunt thoracic trauma. In follow-up clinical studies, patients were subclassified to assess the risk for complications after reamed femoral nailing. Those identified as "borderline" patients, or those with multiple injuries who were at risk for complications after early reamed intramedullary femoral nailing, were found to have a higher incidence of pulmonary complications with early definitive intervention. The authors advocated that in the presence of multiple injuries, the preoperative condition should be considered when deciding on treatment modalities for femoral shaft fractures to minimize complications.

Other studies have not confirmed the findings of Pape et al. Controversy remains regarding the impact of reamed intramedullary nail fixation of femoral fractures in patients with multisystem trauma. The current consensus seems to be that immediate fixation of femoral fractures with reamed intramedullary nailing does not increase the risk of clinically significant pulmonary complications in most patients. However, those who are identified as being "borderline" or at very high risk for complications may be best served with an approach using "damage control orthopaedics" to provide necessary stabilization while minimizing early surgical insult. At our institution, most femoral shaft fractures that can be treated with intramedullary nail fixation are treated with early total care. Patients identified to be at risk, primarily based on concomitant multisystem injuries and physiologic parameters, are temporized with either external fixation or skeletal traction, both of which have been demonstrated to be efficient as early measures.

Winquist and others have shown that elevation in intramedullary pressures and thermal damage caused by reaming can be decreased by using sharp reamers with deep cutting flutes and narrow shafts and by using minimal force during reamer insertion. In addition to causing marrow embolization, reaming also damages the endosteum and decreases the torsion strength of the femoral fragments.

Because of the possible effects of medullary reaming, unreamed nailing has received increased attention. Interlocked intramedullary nailing without reaming requires smaller implants capable of not only sustaining the loads of weight bearing but also withstanding the prolonged healing time generally required for severe open fractures. Russell-Taylor Delta nails (Smith and Nephew, Memphis, TN) have functioned well in this situation. Our first 100 Delta femoral nailings of acute fractures included all grades and 35 open fractures. In a population that formerly would have been treated with nails averaging 13.5 mm in diameter, 62 10-mm nails and 38 11-mm nails were used. No infections developed in the 100 fractures. One screw broke in a patient with a delayed union, and thus renailing was required before union. One other delayed union also required renailing before union.

Studies have found similar results between reamed and unreamed nailing with no differences in operative time, transfusion requirements, or pulmonary complications. Although there was no overall difference in time to union, delayed unions have been reported more often after unreamed than reamed nailing. When distal fractures were analyzed separately, fractures with reamed nailing were found to heal more quickly. No advantage to unreamed nail insertion has been demonstrated. In contrast to the tibia, the femur is surrounded by vascular soft tissue and infection of femoral fractures is less of a concern.

Although the incidence of infection with open nailing of closed fractures is nearly 10% in some series, the incidence in closed nailing of closed fractures generally is less than 1%. The incidence of infection after closed reamed nailing of open femoral fractures is 2% to 5%. In the past, delayed nailing was recommended to prevent infection; however, more recent reports indicate that immediate nailing of open femoral fractures does not significantly increase the risk of infection.

In our early use of locked intramedullary nails for segmentally comminuted fractures, we attempted to delay definitive intramedullary fixation for 2 to 3 weeks until soft tissues had theoretically stabilized and the granulation tissue around the fracture would serve as a better recipient bed for reaming. In our first 100 fractures treated with the Russell-Taylor

nail (1985-1986), including 23 open fractures of all grades, we were forced to intervene earlier, however, to prevent further deterioration of patients with multiple injuries, and the average delay to nailing of open fractures was only 8.4 days. Two of the three infections after nailing of open femoral fractures in our series occurred in patients with persistent initial wounds (20 and 24 days after injury) who had delayed reamed nailing. In our first 125 open femoral fractures treated with the Russell-Taylor nail, with immediate or delayed fixation, with or without reaming, the overall infection rate was 4%.

Currently, we strive to operatively treat all open fractures within 8 hours of injury. Open femoral fractures are treated with initiating immediate intravenous antibiotic coverage depending on the wound type, followed by urgent debridement and irrigation. The femur is stabilized with a statically locked reamed intramedullary nail. The isthmus diameter is approximated radiographically as part of preoperative templating. The traumatic wound is closed, if surgically clean, over closed suction drains in lower-grade open injuries. Massive open wounds or those that are grossly contaminated are left open or covered with vacuum-assisted wound closure dressings. Repeat debridements are performed every 24 to 48 hours, depending on the characteristics of the wound environment, until delayed primary closure can be safely obtained. Otherwise, we aim to obtain wound closure by 2 to 7 days using skin grafting or, rarely, flap coverage.

We also have found locked intramedullary nailing to be a safe and effective treatment for femoral fractures with vascular injury. Although repair of the popliteal artery can withstand 18 kg of traction, we prefer to fix the femoral fracture at the time of vascular repair if possible because little additional surgical exposure is required for closed nailing. Early fixation allows the benefits of early mobilization. We also have found that intramedullary nailing is easier to perform early because usually less traction is required and the fragments are easier to reduce. In a review of femoral fractures with vascular injuries treated at our institution between 1986 and 1994, 17 fractures treated with either immediate or delayed intramedullary nailing all were successfully salvaged. Gunshot wounds caused most injuries, and only one fracture was nailed before vascular repair. A patient with a femoral fracture and suspected vascular injury ideally should be taken to the operating room for arteriography after sufficient imaging to accurately assess the fracture morphology for preoperative planning purposes, and, of course, to identify any other limb or life-threatening injuries. Time is critical in these injuries. Close coordination with the general trauma and vascular surgical services is a prerequisite, and rapid external fixation can be applied to provide a stable skeletal environment for vascular repair. Alternatively, a temporary vascular shunt can be placed while skeletal fixation is performed, which thus permits vascular repair without the potential impedance that an external fixator may impose. In our experience, an anterolateral external fixator orientation is preferred because it does not interfere with medial access and does not place pin tracks in line with any potential lateral approach or interlocking incisions.

Retrograde intramedullary nailing has been advocated for patients with morbid obesity, ipsilateral femoral neck and shaft fractures, ipsilateral femoral and tibial fractures (floating knee injuries), pregnancy, and multiple trauma. Current techniques recommend using a portal in the intercondylar notch. Retrograde and antegrade femoral nailing in femoral shaft fractures have been compared. Healing, delayed union, and malunion were nearly identical in both groups. Patients in the antegrade group reported more hip pain (9%) at follow-up, and patients in the retrograde group reported more knee pain (36%). Retrograde nailing also is a viable option for open femoral fractures. The incidence of associated knee sepsis was 1.1% in a series by O'Toole et al.

Closed nailing of acute femoral fractures using either a femoral distractor or manual traction without a fracture table has been advocated. We continue to use a fracture table routinely. The newer fracture tables allow total body imaging without moving the patient, decreasing the risk to the patient and minimizing setup time.

We recommend early static locked nailing, with reaming, of open and closed femoral fractures as soon as possible. Relative contraindications to nailing include the presence of previously inserted fixation device, preexisting deformity, massive contaminated open wounds, or borderline patient parameters. Absolute but correctable contraindications to femoral nailing are hypovolemia, hypothermia, and coagulopathy.

Most femoral shaft fractures at our institution are treated with the patient supine on a fracture table. Lateral positioning typically is reserved for proximal subtrochanteric fractures for which lateral positioning is much more conducive to fracture reduction as opposed to the supine position. Distal interlocking is performed using a freehand "perfect circle" technique. This technique can be performed rapidly; we routinely use two locking screws distally, primarily in comminuted fractures that require not only rotational but also length stability. Although some studies have found no difference when one or two screws were used for locking, we believe that weight bearing can potentially begin earlier when two distal locking screws are used rather than one.

We do not routinely perform dynamization for those fractures that demonstrate healing difficulties. For delayed union at 6 to 8 months in Winquist-Hansen grade 3 or grade 4 comminuted fractures, we prefer bone grafting in situ or closed reamed exchange nailing. Small and moderate bone defects usually fill in spontaneously.

▌PREOPERATIVE PLANNING

After deciding that the fracture is suitable for intramedullary nailing, careful planning before surgery is necessary. There is no correlation between the length of the bone and size or contour of its canal. Young athletes with strong bones usually have a small medullary canal at the isthmus where the thick cortices encroach on the canal. In contrast, elderly patients usually have large canals; even a 15-mm nail may not be large enough. In an average patient, the smallest diameter of the canal is in the distal part of the proximal third of the shaft. The canal gradually enlarges proximally and distally. Fractures through an expanded part of the canal are less securely fixed by a standard intramedullary nail than fractures through the narrowest part.

The proper length of the nail should be determined preoperatively; this is best done by radiography to ensure the appropriate array of sizes are available intraoperatively. Even with this information, the proper diameter of the nail is best determined at the time of surgery because of inherent measurement errors that may be present in electronic imaging software if no calibration tool is used. Regardless of its diameter, the canal in an adult should be prepared to 1.0 to 1.5 mm greater in diameter than the anticipated nail diameter.

Insertion instrumentation for closed nailing procedures is commonplace, with the general concepts being standard. Different manufacturers may have a variety of features permitting, for example, variable interlocking options. Therefore, familiarity with the available implant systems translates directly into the surgeon's understanding of their utility in special or unexpected circumstances intraoperatively. Ensuring the availability and presence of the implants and instrumentation is one of the most important preoperative planning steps for a successful procedure.

One must also consider the advantages and disadvantages of the use of a fracture table in treating these injuries. Fracture tables can be time-consuming to set up, continuous traction generated by a fracture table can lead to postoperative nerve palsies, and fracture tables pose difficulties for other surgeons who may need to operate on associated injuries. Their primary indications for this technique were an ipsilateral acetabular or vertical shear pelvic fracture, associated unstable spinal injuries, and bilateral extremity injuries. McFerran and Johnson initially excluded obese or very muscular patients, very small or skeletally immature patients, and patients with ipsilateral neck and shaft fractures; however, as they gained experience, only patients with ipsilateral neck and shaft fractures and fractures more than 24 hours old were excluded.

McFerran and Johnson recommended preoperative scanograms of the uninvolved femur in the emergency department to evaluate length. Because of their success in performing femoral nailings with a femoral distractor, their technique evolved to femoral nailing without a fracture table using manual traction only. This technique saves the time that is necessary to place the femoral distractor. A skilled assistant is necessary to perform this technique. Reduction of uncomminuted fractures can be difficult. Reduction of comminuted fractures is easier, but it is more difficult to judge length and rotation.

There has been debate as to the ideal entry portal for antegrade closed femoral nailing. Stannard et al. reported their prospective randomized comparison of piriformis fossa and greater trochanteric starting portals. There was no difference in hip function at 1-year follow-up. Intraoperative parameters favored a trochanteric entry portal, primarily because of less operative and fluoroscopy time. A recent meta-analysis did not identify functional superiority when comparing trochanteric and piriformis entry points or antegrade and retrograde starting portals.

In our institution, most acute fractures are treated with the use of a fracture table for antegrade intramedullary nailing procedures through a trochanteric entry portal. Lateral piriformis entry tends to be reserved for select subtrochanteric femoral fractures where trochanteric entry can potentiate deformity of the proximal segment. We have not found the added time of patient positioning or table setup to be excessive and have found the ease of imaging to outweigh the disadvantages of the table.

ANTEGRADE FEMORAL NAILING

TECHNIQUE 2.29

Patient Positioning and Preparation
- Based on preoperative templating and surgical plan, decide on a radiolucent flat-topped or fracture table and patient position. We prefer the use of a fracture table.

- We have used the lateral and supine positions extensively, and each has its relative indications (Fig. 2.78). The supine position is more universal. It provides easier access for the anesthesiologist, especially in severely injured patients. The circulating and scrub nurses and the radiographic technicians also are more comfortable with the patient in this position. It is most useful for bilateral femoral fractures, fractures of the distal third of the femur, and femoral fractures with contralateral acetabular fractures. Gaining the correct entry portal to the proximal femur usually is only somewhat more difficult with the patient supine, primarily in obese patients.
- If the patient is supine, adduct the trunk and affected extremity. Flex the affected hip 15 to 30 degrees.
- Apply traction through a skeletal pin or to the foot with a well-padded traction boot. A well-padded perineal post is positioned, and the uninjured extremity is placed in a well-padded traction boot. The legs are positioned in a scissor configuration.
- Estimate correct rotational alignment with respect to the normal anteversion of the hip as determined with the image intensifier. This can be accomplished by taking fluoroscopic views of the uninjured knee and hip at the same rotation of the image intensifier and saving these for later reference. Therefore, comparable anteroposterior fluoroscopic views of the injured limb, both knee and hip, can then allow for rotational correction based on the profile of the lesser trochanter. Similarly, the angle difference between a radiographic true lateral of the knee and hip will represent hip anteversion.
- Rotate the foot and distal fragment of the femur to match the proximal fragment by observing the image C-arm. By taking successive views with the C-arm, it is possible to obtain a lateral view of the proximal femur in which the femoral neck and shaft are parallel but offset about 1 cm. The angle of the C-arm necessary to obtain this "true lateral" usually can be read directly off the C-arm. Taking into account the normal femoral anteversion of 15 to 20 degrees, it is possible to determine exactly the angle at which to place the foot. For example, if the femoral neck and shaft were superimposed when the C-arm was angled 40 degrees from the horizontal, assuming a femoral anteversion of 20 degrees, it would be necessary to externally rotate the foot 20 degrees to match proximal and distal fragments.
- If the patient is in the lateral decubitus position with the perineal post, ensure that most of the trunk weight is on the trochanteric rest of the unaffected hip.
- Place the fractured side in 15 to 30 degrees of hip flexion. The normal side is in neutral to slight hip extension. Use the image intensifier to view the entire femur in the anteroposterior and lateral projections from the knee to the hip.
- Prepare the patient in the standard manner. Drape the buttocks and lateral thigh to the popliteal crease. Cover the image intensifier arm with a sterile isolation drape.

Preparation of Femur
- Make a short oblique skin incision starting 2 to 3 cm from the proximal tip of the greater trochanter and continue it proximally and medially. A longer incision may be necessary in obese patients.
- Incise the fascia of the gluteus maximus in line with its fibers.
- Identify the subfascial plane of the gluteus maximus and palpate the piriformis fossa or trochanteric portal.
- Advance the threaded tip guidewire to the approximate level of the piriformis fossa. If a trochanteric antegrade technique is used, the entry point is along the medial slope of the greater trochanter (Fig. 2.79).
- Image the trochanteric region to adjust the position of the guidewire such that the trajectory will permit placement into the center of the medullary canal distally.
- Check the pin position with anteroposterior and lateral imaging. If the pin is not central in the femoral canal, but appropriate on one image plane, then the soft-tissue guide with multiple-pin "honeycomb" insert may be used. This device permits fine tuning of the starting guidewire to the proper position by the addition of a second pin.
- When the pin is properly placed, advance it to below the lesser trochanter.

Proximal Entry Portal Preparation
- Remove the honeycomb insert, leaving the guidewire and the entry portal tool in the wound. If the insert was not needed, place the soft-tissue sleeve before creating the entry portal to protect the abductor muscular insertion.
- Place the entry reamer assembly, consisting of a 14-mm channel reamer, entry reamer connector, and entry reamer (Fig. 2.80), into the entry portal tool and over the guidewire.
- Ream the assembly into the femur until it bottoms out on the entry portal tool.
- Check the position of the reamer during the insertion with anteroposterior and lateral imaging.
- Remove the entry reamer and guidewire, leaving the entry portal tube and the channel reamer in place.
- Alternatively, the channel reamer may not be used. The cannulated entry reamer may be positioned over the starting guidewire. For simple diaphyseal fractures the channel reamer generally is not necessary. The device's advantages become clearly evident with more proximal fractures as a means of externally controlling the characteristic deformity often seen in subtrochanteric fracture patterns.

Reduction and Guidewire Insertion
- Place the reduction tool consisting of the reducer and a T-handle into the channel reamer and connector in the femur (Fig. 2.81).
- Advance the reduction tool to the fracture site. Use the tool to manipulate the proximal fragment and engage the distal fragment with the tool's tip. Alternatively, if the intramedullary reduction tool is not used, percutaneous unicortical reduction "joysticks" can be employed for facilitating reduction or external reduction devices also are available.
- When the distal fragment is reached and engaged, advance the 3.0-mm ball-tipped guidewire across the fracture. Use the vice-grip device to advance the guidewire (see Fig. 2.81).
- Confirm the reduction and position of the guidewire with anteroposterior and lateral images at multiple lev-

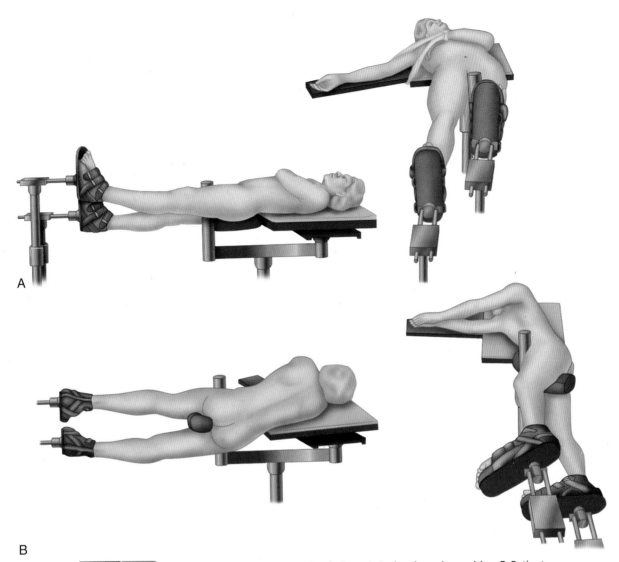

A

B

FIGURE 2.78 Russell-Taylor interlocking nail technique. **A,** Patient in supine position. **B,** Patient in lateral decubitus position. **SEE TECHNIQUE 2.29.**

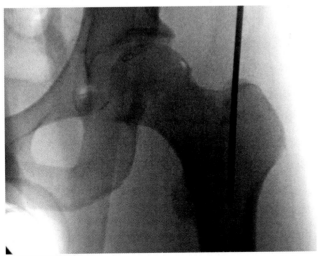

FIGURE 2.79 Trochanteric starting portal for antegrade intramedullary nailing procedures of femur. **SEE TECHNIQUE 2.29.**

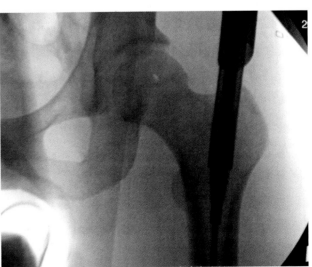

FIGURE 2.80 Insertion of the channel reamer into proximal femoral metaphysis for creating a starting portal for antegrade nailing. **SEE TECHNIQUE 2.29.**

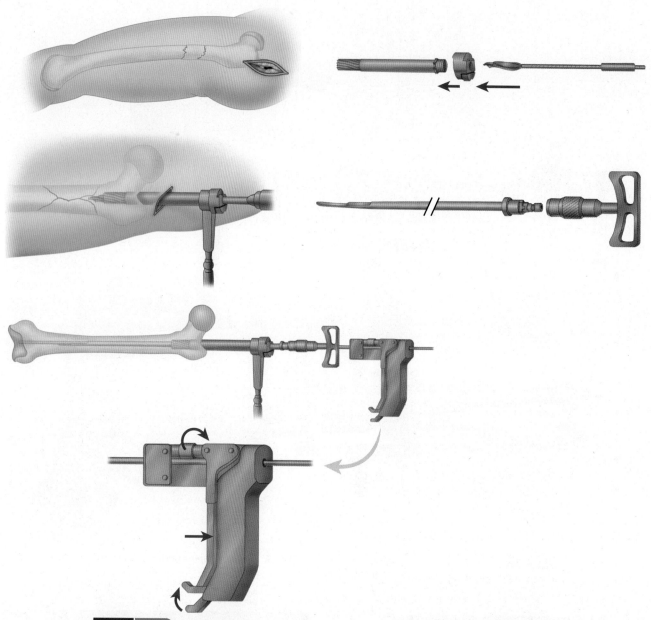

FIGURE 2.81   Antegrade femoral nailing. When reducer is in medullary canal and has captured distal fragment, ball-tipped guide rod is inserted through it with use of gripper into distal femur in region of old epiphyseal scar. (Redrawn from Femoral antegrade nailing: technique manual, Memphis, TN, 2001, Smith & Nephew Richards.) **SEE TECHNIQUE 2.29.**

els. The goal should be concentric central placement of the wire distally to the level of the epiphyseal scar (Fig. 2.82).
- Remove the reduction tool with the T-handle if used.

Canal Preparation
- Remove the reducer and ream the canal sequentially at 0.5-mm intervals until there is moderate "chatter" or until the reaming exceeds the selected nail diameter by 1.0 to 1.5 mm. The channel reamer must be removed for reamers larger than 12.5 mm (Fig. 2.83). An obturator is used to prevent inadvertent removal of the ball-tipped wire from the proper position within the distal segment of the femur. This must be done during withdrawal of the reamer with each pass. If the wire is withdrawn, re-

position and confirm the location on fluoroscopy before further reaming.
- Confirm the proper nail length by positioning the guide-wire at the point of desired distal position, usually between the superior pole of the patella and the level of the distal epiphyseal scar on the anteroposterior image.
- The proper nail length can be determined by either of several methods.
- Using the guidewire method, with the distal end of the rod between the proximal pole of the patella and the distal femoral epiphyseal scar, overlap a second guide rod on the portion of the reduction guide rod extending proximally from the femoral entry portal. The difference in length of the two guidewires is the desired length of the nail.

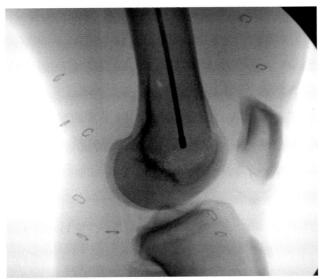

FIGURE 2.82 Intramedullary bead-tipped guidewire inserted concentrically to distal femur at level of distal femoral physeal scar or midportion of patella. **SEE TECHNIQUE 2.29.**

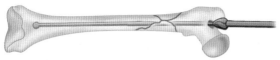

FIGURE 2.83 Reaming of femoral canal over 3.2-mm guide rod. **SEE TECHNIQUE 2.29.**

- Alternatively, most nail systems now supply cannulated depth gauges designed to be placed over the 3.0-mm wire, permitting length determination. This is the preferred method.
- Insert the ruler over the guidewire and place it at the level of the femoral insertion.
- Check this with the anteroposterior image. Read the measurement off the measurement device.

Nail Insertion
- Attach the drill guide assembly to the selected nail.
- Remove the entry portal tube and channel reamer, leaving the guidewire in place.
- Place the nail into the femur and advance it manually. The nail may require gentle impaction to fully seat.
- If there is significant resistance, remove the nail and ream the canal 0.5 mm larger.
- Seat the nail completely as confirmed on multiplanar image intensification.

Interlocking of Nail
- For proximal and distal interlocking, use the 5-mm locking screws. Depending on the chosen implant's configuration, proximal and distal locking options may vary. Standard static locking with this implant is from the greater trochanter directed obliquely to the lesser trochanter.
- Place the gold drill sleeve into the proximal guide and dimple the skin.

- Make a stab wound at that point and spread the tissue to the bone.
- Insert the gold drill sleeve with the silver inner liner and use the long pilot drill to go to the inner cortex but not through it.
- Measure the length on the calibrated drill bit at the silver guide top. Then penetrate the far cortex. Remove the drill and silver sleeve.
- Insert the screw of the proper length and advance it manually until seated.
- Check the position with an anteroposterior image.
- Evaluate that satisfactory length and rotational alignment has been restored before proceeding with distal interlocking.

Freehand Technique for Distal Targeting
- Place the image intensifier in the lateral position and scan the distal femoral metaphysis. A true lateral image should be sought. This is confirmed with visualization of the distal interlocking screw holes appearing as perfect, clear circles. If the holes appear oblong or to have double density, then the proper image has not been obtained. Note that this represents a true lateral image of the nail and not necessarily the distal femur.
- When the holes are completely circular, center a ring forceps or the tip of a scalpel over the chosen interlocking hole on the lateral side of the leg. Make a longitudinal stab incision through the skin, subcutaneous tissue, and iliotibial band centered over the interlocking hole in the nail.
- Place a trocar-tip drill bit over the screw hole, angled approximately 45 degrees to permit viewing under fluoroscopy (Fig. 2.84). Make appropriate adjustments until the tip is centered over the desired hole; each adjustment should be accompanied by a fluoroscopic image until the proper position is obtained.
- Bring the drill parallel and in line with the fluoroscopic beam. Take care to maintain constant pressure to avoid movement of the drill tip.
- Penetrate the lateral cortex. Remove the drill bit from the driver and confirm on the lateral image the drill bit placed within the interlocking hole. If it is not, make appropriate adjustments in alignment. Then reattach the driver and penetrate the medial cortex.
- Calibrated drill bits are used for this portion of the procedure and it greatly increases the ease of determining screw length. Alternatively, a standard depth gauge can be used. Place the appropriate length interlocking bolt by hand, confirming satisfactory purchase.
- Repeat if additional distal interlocking screws are desired.
- Anteroposterior and lateral imaging should confirm appropriate screw position and length.
- Irrigate and close the wounds in a standard layered fashion.

Final Evaluation
- Before leaving the operative suite, several key elements must be evaluated.
- First, if the nail has been locked in standard fashion, evaluate the femoral neck with multiplanar fluoroscopic imaging to ensure that no occult femoral neck fracture is identified. Dynamic stress fluoroscopy has been shown to

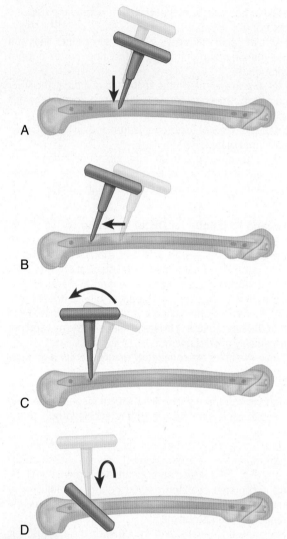

FIGURE 2.84 Freehand technique. **A,** Awl is placed over proximal screw hole with its handle angled 45 degrees. **B-D,** Awl is adjusted under image intensification until point is centered in screw hole and then is swung perpendicular to axis of bone **(C)** and driven to lateral side of rod **(D). SEE TECHNIQUE 2.29.**

be superior to static imaging for identifying occult fractures intraoperatively.

- Next, confirm the length and rotational reductions and compare with the uninjured limb to ensure symmetry. This can prove to be challenging with significantly comminuted fractures and is best performed with a combination of methods. Comparison to the contralateral uninjured femur has been questioned from an accuracy standpoint, given inherent side-to-side differences in individuals. The fracture rotation also can be estimated based on the inherent anteversion of the cephalomedullary nail intraoperatively. Length can be assessed with measurement of the contralateral uninjured femur radiographically, clinical assessment, or use of postoperative CT scanogram scout imaging.
- Evaluate the thigh compartments, and if clinical concern exists, then obtain objective compartment measurements.

- Examine the ligaments of the ipsilateral knee.
- A postoperative anteroposterior pelvis radiograph with both hips internally rotated provides the optimal profile view of the femoral neck as a further check for occult femoral neck fractures and should be obtained and reviewed before anesthesia is discontinued.

POSTOPERATIVE CARE Weight bearing depends on the stability of the fracture fixation. Weight bearing to tolerance is allowed immediately regardless of the nail size if satisfactory cortical contact is achieved. In the rare circumstance that an adolescent nail is used in an adult, protected weight bearing should be initiated until early radiographic healing is noted. Touch-down or partial weight bearing is allowed in comminuted injuries. Hip and knee range of motion are encouraged. Quadriceps-setting and straight-leg raising exercises are begun before hospital discharge. Hip abduction exercises are begun after wound healing. Weight bearing is progressed as callus formation occurs. Ambulatory aids such as crutches or a walker are used for the first 6 weeks. Hip and knee range-of-motion and strengthening exercises are recommended during this time. Unassisted ambulation is permitted as strength recovery and radiographic healing progress.

■ RETROGRADE NAILING OF THE FEMUR

Retrograde femoral nailing may be beneficial in the following clinical situations: (1) obese patients, in whom it is difficult to obtain an antegrade entry portal; (2) patients with ipsilateral femoral neck and shaft fractures, to allow the use of separate fixation devices for the shaft and neck fractures; (3) patients with floating knee injuries, to allow fixation of the femoral and tibial fractures through the same anterior longitudinal incision; (4) multiply-injured trauma patients, to decrease operative time by not using a fracture table, which allows multiple injuries to be treated by preparing and draping simultaneously; and (5) pregnant patients, such that intraoperative fluoroscopy is minimized around the pelvis. An intercondylar portal is favored for insertion. It is important to remember that retrograde nailing is more reliable in controlling distal shaft fractures, whereas antegrade nailing provides better control of proximal shaft fractures. Satisfactory results were reported by Moed and Watson and Herscovici and Whiteman in early trials of this technique and have been reported in more recent series. Supracondylar fractures have lower union rates (80% to 84%) with this technique than femoral shaft fractures (85% to 100%). Retrograde nailing of the femur is not without frequent complications, however, including knee pain (13% to 60%) and secondary surgery (12% to 35%). The infection rate is acceptable (0% to 14%). Varus-valgus malunion, common with the initial extraarticular entry site (12% to 29%), is less common with the current intercondylar entry site.

Nonetheless, retrograde intramedullary nail stabilization provides significant benefits in certain clinical circumstances and has an acceptable risk profile compared with antegrade procedures.

RETROGRADE FEMORAL NAILING

TECHNIQUE 2.30

- Place the patient on a radiolucent flattop operating room table. A small bolster can be positioned under the ipsilateral hip to prevent external rotation of the proximal femur. Surgical preparation and draping must include the hip girdle and lower flank.
- Position the leg over a sterile bump or triangle. Tibial traction may be used and affixed to the traction bow holder. Alternatively, a tibial traction pin and traction bow can be used as a "handle" for more exacting control of the distal segment when manual traction is used.
- Make an incision through the lateral parapatellar, medial parapatellar, or transpatellar tendon based on surgeon preference. The retropatellar fat pad must be incised and an arthrotomy performed. Insert a guidewire into the intercondylar notch. Position the pin directed centrally into the medullary canal on anteroposterior imaging. Confirm its position and trajectory on lateral imaging; the pin placement should be in line with the medullary canal at the anterior extent of Blumensaat's line (Fig. 2.85).
- Advance the guidewire into the distal femoral metaphysis. Place the soft-tissue protection sleeve over the guidewire for protection of the articular surfaces and patellar tendon.
- Similar to the antegrade technique, a multiple-pin "honeycomb" insert can aid in perfecting the guidepin placement. If this is used, remove the honeycomb insert and place the cannulated entry reamer over the initial guidewire.
- Advance into the femur until the reamer is within the distal femur, taking special care to maintain the soft-tissue protection sleeve in place to avoid iatrogenic intraarticular injury. (Do not use the channel reamer and entry reamer connector for this procedure.)
- Take care to ensure appropriate trajectory of the pin in the distal segment, particularly with fractures involving the distal femoral metaphysis. Otherwise, coronal and sagittal plane malalignments can result secondary to nail-canal mismatch. Blocking screws may be indicated to maintain alignment.
- Remove the reamer and guidewire and insert a 3-mm bead-tipped guidewire into the distal fragment.
- Reduce the fracture and advance the guidewire into the proximal segment to the level of the lesser trochanter. A cannulated reduction tool or external devices, such as a large distractor, can be used for reduction maneuvers in combination with axial traction. Small bumps or bolsters can be placed along the posterior surface of the thigh as determined by fluoroscopy to aid in sagittal plane reduction.
- Prepare the medullary canal by introducing cannulated reamers over the guidewire to a diameter 1.0 to 1.5 mm larger than the nail to be used.
- Recheck the position of the guidewire to confirm its position at the lesser trochanter.
- Apply traction to the leg to ensure proper length. Measure for the appropriate length of the nail with a ruler

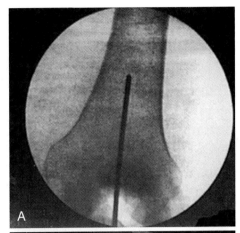

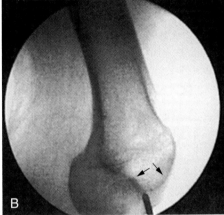

FIGURE 2.85 Retrograde femoral nailing (see text). **A,** Anteroposterior view of guide pin being passed 10 cm into medullary canal through intercondylar notch. **B,** On lateral view, medullary canal tapers distally *(arrows)* to form V; guide pin is placed at apex of canal. (From Herscovici D, Whiteman KW: Retrograde nailing of the femur using an intercondylar approach, *Clin Orthop Relat Res* 332:98, 1996.) **SEE TECHNIQUE 2.30.**

placed over the guidewire. Check to ensure the ruler is countersunk. This is most easily performed on the lateral image plane.
- Remove the entry portal tool and insert the nail attached to the targeting guide, seating it to the level of the lesser trochanter (Fig. 2.86).
- Maintain traction on the leg to avoid shortening.
- Check the lateral image to ensure the nail is properly inset.
- When the nail is at the proper level, remove the guidewire.
- Proceed with distal locking of the nail using the guide.
- Insert the drill sleeve and trocar through the targeting guide and dimple the skin.
- Make a stab wound at the site and enlarge the hole with blunt dissection to bone.
- Reinsert the drill guide to bone. Advance the drill until the far cortex is encountered and read the measurement off the drill bit calibrations for length approximation. Complete the penetration of the cortex.
- Insert the screw by hand until fully seated.
- Check the length and position of the screws with anteroposterior and lateral imaging.

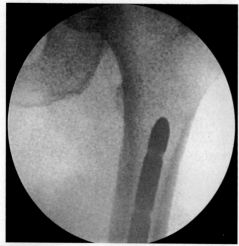

FIGURE 2.86 Nail is seated at level of distal trochanter. (From Herscovici D, Whiteman KW: Retrograde nailing of the femur using an intercondylar approach, *Clin Orthop Relat Res* 332:98, 1996.) **SEE TECHNIQUE 2.30.**

- Repeat this procedure until the desired number of interlocking screws have been positioned.
- Recheck the alignment and length of the femur using a Bovie cord from the anterior superior iliac crest, middle of the femoral head, middle of the knee, and middle of the tibial plafond. Check the lateral reduction.
- When the final reduction and length are acceptable, move to the proximal locking hole, which should be placed in the anteroposterior plane at the level of the lesser trochanter to avoid nerve and vessel injury. Identify the hole by the perfect circle technique.
- Using the image intensifier, localize the interlocking holes proximally because this will assist in placement of the incision. Make a longitudinal skin incision, sharply dividing the subcutaneous tissue and deep fascia, and bluntly dissect to bone. Avoid damage to the branches of the femoral nerve.
- Drill into the femur when the position is acceptable by the perfect circle technique.
- Use the same technique to determine the screw length as described previously.
- Place the interlocking screw using the captured screwdriver.
- Recheck the alignment and reduction with multiple anteroposterior and lateral views.
- Image the hip in full fluoroscopic mode with internal and external rotation and push-pull to check for an occult femoral neck fracture.
- Close the wounds in a standard layered fashion and apply a dressing.
- Perform the same series of checks as described for antegrade nail procedures.

POSTOPERATIVE CARE Postoperative rehabilitation depends on the stability of fixation, and the fracture pattern and must be individualized for each patient. All patients are initially placed in a knee immobilizer. Patients with stable fixation can be started on a continuous passive motion program in the first 24 to 48 hours after surgery. Frac-

tures with less secure fixation may require hinged bracing. Initial weight bearing depends on fracture stability after fixation. Patients with intercondylar fractures or supracondylar fractures require protected weight bearing until radiographic progression permits advancement of weight bearing (usually between 10 and 12 weeks).

■ ERRORS AND COMPLICATIONS OF INTRAMEDULLARY FIXATION

Given the correct indications for intramedullary nailing, the necessary equipment and assistance, and adequate training, the following are the most common difficulties in interlocking nailing. Although locked femoral nailing generally is considered to yield good functional results, many patients report symptoms related to their fracture and fixation more than 1 year after injury, including pain related to changes in weather, limping, difficulty with walking, climbing, or standing, and trochanteric pain or thigh pain. A significant decrease in hip abductor strength also has been noted. The presence of heterotopic ossification, femoral shortening, or proximal nail prominence has not been shown to correlate with this loss of abductor strength. It has been hypothesized that postoperative abductor weakness is caused by injury to the gluteus medius and minimus muscles or to the superior gluteal nerve during portal creation or by inadequate postoperative rehabilitation. Retracting the gluteus medius and minimus anteriorly when exposing the nail insertion site has been suggested to prevent injury to these muscles and their nerve supply. Patients should be counseled about their expected postoperative recovery.

▌ PATIENT POSITIONING AND TRACTION

Femoral nailing with the patient supine on a fracture table is our preferred method when an antegrade approach is used. In this technique, the hip is adducted to improve access to the piriformis fossa or trochanteric entry portal and intraoperative traction is used. Hip adduction has been found to increase pressure on the pudendal nerve, resulting in pudendal nerve palsy. Traction should be minimized to avoid this complication. Use of a well-padded perineal post and minimizing operative and traction time have been recommended.

We recommend the following technique modifications to limit intraoperative hip adduction and traction when using a fracture table. The patient is placed on the fracture table, and traction is applied with the hip in neutral position to confirm the ability to reduce the fracture. Traction is released during preparation and draping of the extremity and during creation of the entry portal. The hip is adducted to gain access to the nail insertion site but is brought back to neutral position when the entry portal has been created. Traction is reapplied for fracture reduction.

We have identified two patterns of injury in which excessive traction may be required for fracture reduction, leading to a higher incidence of pudendal and peroneal nerve palsies: segmental femoral fractures and floating knee injuries (which necessitate antegrade femoral nailing). Because of the soft-tissue stripping that often occurs with segmental femoral fractures, the segmental fragment may not reduce with the application of even large amounts of traction. In these rare cases, we prefer a limited open reduction or percutaneous joystick manipulation to the use of excessive traction. For floating knee injuries, we prefer to nail the femur first, applying traction through a pin inserted in either the distal femur or the proximal tibia, flexing the knee, and supporting the tibial fracture with a splint to reduce tension on the peroneal nerve.

Early nailings are technically easier than delayed nailings. Less traction force is required, and fragment reduction is easier. If nailing is delayed more than 12 hours, the femur should be stabilized with traction, which can facilitate length maintenance in anticipation of definitive fixation.

Compartment syndrome and peroneal nerve palsy as a result of elevation in a calf-supporting, well-leg holder have been described. We recommend placing the unoperated leg, regardless of injury, in the extended supine position on the fracture table.

ERRORS IN NAIL INSERTION

We recommend the supine position for many reasons. True lateral views of the hip and proximal femur are easily obtained, and it is imperative that the starting portal be directly in line with the center of the shaft on both views. This usually is in the piriformis fossa close to the medial wall of the greater trochanter, sometimes slightly within the greater trochanter. Determining the correct starting portal is worth extra time and effort. An eccentric portal can cause comminution and loss of fixation.

If difficulty exists in passage of the reamer guidewire, several techniques can be used. A cannulated intramedullary reduction tool can be invaluable in effecting a difficult reduction in a closed manner. If one is not available, the proximal segment can be reamed to accommodate a small intramedullary nail that can then be placed in lieu of a reduction tool to accomplish the same goal. The proximal fragment usually must be extended and, depending on the level of the fracture with respect to the perineal post, either adducted or abducted. The containment of the guidewire must be confirmed on orthogonal views. If a guidewire is inadvertently partially withdrawn with the reamer, its position should be immediately evaluated fluoroscopically. The passage of the nail across the fracture must be seen on orthogonal views to prevent impingement on the cortex.

Complications of reaming are eliminated by the unreamed technique. Closed section nails can be driven over the initial guidewire. Short distal fragments should be supported as the nail is being driven to prevent extension at the fracture. The guidewire must enter the distal fragment well centered and must stay centered to the intercondylar notch for very short distal fragments to prevent varus or valgus malalignment. All fractures should be locked statically (proximal and distal screws), and blocking screws may be indicated to provide an artificial "cortex" for containment of nails when metaphyseal canal-nail mismatch exists.

A nail that is larger than the medullary canal may become firmly incarcerated and resist all efforts to drive it farther or to extract it. To remove the nail, a small incision is made laterally at the level of incarceration, two 5- to 6-mm holes are drilled in the lateral cortex 3 to 4 cm apart, and they are connected with an osteotome or sagittal saw. The nail can then be withdrawn. If the starting portal is correct, a smaller nail should be used or the constricting

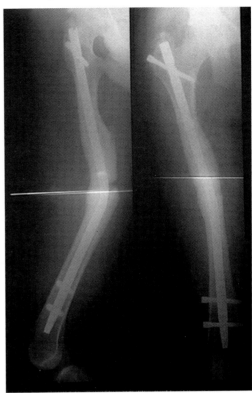

FIGURE 2.87 Bending of femoral intramedullary nail after repeated secondary trauma.

section of the canal should be reamed to a larger diameter. Careful preoperative templating and canal preparation should virtually eliminate the complication of nail incarceration.

BENT OR BROKEN NAILS

The femoral nails in common use today have a smooth, bullet-shaped leading tip to make insertion easier and are slightly bowed anteriorly. This preformed anterior bow should be directed anteriorly when the nail is inserted. Improper selection (inserting a "right" nail in a left femur) results in improper alignment of the proximal interlocking screw hole.

A bent nail usually indicates an injudicious act on the part of the patient or a nail that was too small (Fig. 2.87). A bent nail is not an indication for manipulation; it only succeeds in further weakening the nail. Instead, the bent nail should be removed and a new one should be inserted. When bending of the nail has occurred, it is wishful thinking to expect that union will occur before further bending or breaking of the nail, a far more complicated situation. Just before a bent nail is extracted, the leg should be manipulated into as nearly normal alignment as possible. A broken nail almost always can be extracted through the buttock incision, using an assortment of extraction hooks to engage the distal tip and deliver both halves. If a hook is unsuccessful, the proximal half is removed by its normal driver extractor. Next, a ball-tip guidewire is placed through the distal half of the nail and jammed into position with other guidewires. The initial guidewire is withdrawn with the distal segment of nail.

EXTRACTION OF AN UNBROKEN ANTEGRADE FEMORAL NAIL

TECHNIQUE 2.31

- Place the patient in the straight lateral position using a beanbag or other positioning device on a radiolucent operating table.
- Prepare the entire leg, lateral buttock, and torso to the ribs. Drape the leg to allow full hip and knee motion for positioning.
- Flex the hip to almost 90 degrees.
- Remove the proximal and distal locking screws in the standard fashion.
- Lay a guidewire on the thigh and obtain a fluoroscopic image of the proximal hip. Adjust the wire to coincide with the femoral nail on the lateral view. Draw a line along the wire, extending it onto the buttock. Externally rotate the thigh and, using fluoroscopic imaging, mark a line in a similar fashion to determine the anteroposterior nail position. The intersection of the two lines indicates the site of the incision for placement of the extractor. The incision may be different than what was used initially to insert the device, particularly if it was originally placed with the patient supine.
- If heterotopic bone is to be removed, the incision will need to be made larger.
- Insert a guidewire along the scissors until it touches the nail.
- Adjust the guide pin until it advances into the nail.
- Obtain anteroposterior and lateral images of the hip to confirm placement of the guidewire into the nail.
- Insert the cone-shaped femoral extractor on the extraction bar into the wound over the guide pin. Screw the extractor into the nail. If there is overgrown bone, use a soft-tissue protection sleeve and place a cannulated entry reamer over the guidewire to remove the osseous cap before insertion of the nail extractor. The first pass may not engage the nail fully, but it removes much of the interposed soft tissue.
- Reinsert the extractor over the guide pin or wire and tighten it onto the nail with force sufficient to require the use of the wrenches.
- Use the slotted mallet to hammer the nail out. Irrigate and close the wound in the standard fashion.

EXTRACTION OF A BROKEN FEMORAL ANTEGRADE NAIL

TECHNIQUE 2.32

- Position the patient as described previously.
- Remove all locking screws.
- Approach the proximal femur as described previously with the long 3.2-mm guide pin.

- Insert the pin into the nail.
- Remove the heterotopic bone with curets or a reamer.
- Remove the guide pin, and insert a hooked guidewire and advance it to the tip of the broken nail.
- Wedge the hooked guidewire with multiple smaller guidewires. This should align the broken ends to make the broken nail more like one piece and avoid catching the sides of the femur. Manipulation of the femur may be necessary if deformity is present to allow for "linear" removal.
- Grasp the multiple guidewires with locking (vice-grip) pliers attached to a universal sliding extractor.
- Carefully extract the nail with gentle mallet blows. If unsuccessful, an open approach may be necessary.

▌INFECTIONS

A deep infection after either open or closed intramedullary fixation is a serious complication. The literature reports infection rates of 1.5% to 10% after open reduction and intramedullary fixation; after closed reduction and nailing, most authors report less than a 1% deep infection rate. This in and of itself is justification for mastering the closed nailing technique.

If a deep infection occurs after intramedullary nailing, the involved site (usually the fracture site) should be surgically opened and widely drained. All devitalized tissue, small bone fragments, granulation tissue, and hematoma should be removed, and the surgical site may require multiple debridements, depending on the virulence of the organism. The intramedullary nail can be left in place, however, if it is providing fixation because removal of the nail usually results in an infected nonunion. At times, infections that are difficult to control may require early deep implant removal and temporary antibiotic cement nail insertion before definitive fixation in an effort to eradicate the infection. Cultures should be obtained, and appropriate antibiotics should be begun. We usually give the patient intravenous antibiotics for 6 weeks after this surgery. The patient is then given an oral suppressive antibiotic, often until union if the implant is retained. The patient's progress is monitored by repeated measuring of erythrocyte sedimentation rate and C-reactive protein.

The infection usually remains localized to the fracture site, and although drainage may continue indefinitely and a medullary sequestrum may form, the nail should be left in place if possible. Involucrum and callus form despite infection if the fixation remains fairly rigid. The nail should not be removed until the healing is strong enough to support the fracture. At this time, a sequestrectomy is performed and the nail is removed. Rarely, infection extends from one end of the medullary canal to the other and may follow the nailing of an open fracture of the femur. This complication is serious and usually results in drainage for a long time, with exacerbations and remissions. The nail is left in place despite the infection until the fracture unites, provided that fixation is reasonably firm.

If the fracture is infected and the nail is broken or providing little stability, it can be removed at the time of the open drainage procedure and a larger nail can be inserted or an external fixator applied. With either choice, the fragments

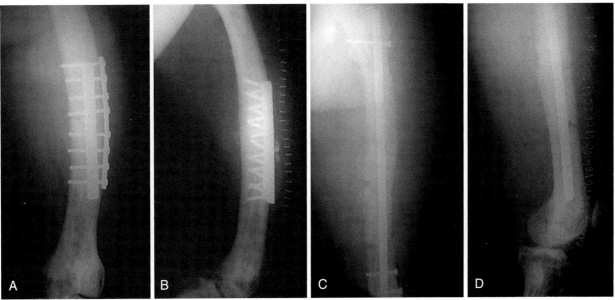

FIGURE 2.88 **A** and **B,** Femoral fracture in patient with Paget disease was fixed with double plates. **C** and **D,** Fracture occurred below plates; plates were removed, and femur was stabilized with intramedullary nail.

must be immobilized; the wound may be left open, and an appropriate antibiotic regimen is begun.

In our experience, infection occurs after closed nailing of closed fractures in about 0.5% of patients. Of the femoral fractures we treat, 25% are open and infection occurs after closed nailing of open fractures in 2% to 3% of patients. To date, in more than 2500 femoral nailings, all infections were controlled with debridement and antibiotics during fracture healing. After healing of the fracture, the nails were removed and the medullary canals underwent debridement and irrigation. No evidence of infection returned after nail removal.

INTRAMEDULLARY FIXATION IN PATHOLOGIC FRACTURES

For pathologic fractures resulting from metastatic tumors, intramedullary fixation is usually rigid enough to allow the patient to be up and about in relative comfort for the remaining months of life. If the metastatic deposit is discovered before fracture, closed prophylactic intramedullary nailing is justified if a pathologic fracture is impending. If a fracture occurs through a large metastatic tumor, a large intramedullary nail supplemented by methyl methacrylate may afford good fixation. Union may even occur. The theoretical disadvantage that the passage of an intramedullary nail through the tumor may dislodge tumor cells and accelerate metastatic spread does not justify condemnation of the method. In these fractures, because the bone is often severely osteoporotic, fixation usually is more secure after intramedullary nailing than after the application of plates and screws. Local radiation therapy can be given after nailing without ill effect.

Grundy reported 63 fractures of the femur in patients with Paget disease. The most common site of fracture was the subtrochanteric area, with the upper shaft the next most common (Fig. 2.88). He recommended treatment of shaft fractures with traction followed by cast immobilization. In subtrochanteric fractures, he suggested using a short intramedullary nail,

pointing out that there is usually bowing and that a long nail would become incarcerated or would cut out because of the deformity. The short nail fixation did allow the fractures to heal and prevented the progressive varus deformity that tends to result with nonoperative treatment of subtrochanteric fractures in Paget disease.

Metastatic lesions frequently are in the subtrochanteric region and may be multicentric. They are slow to heal because of bone loss, tumor extension, and radiation therapy. Therefore intramedullary implants are well suited for treatment of pathologic processes because they allow immediate weight bearing. Furthermore, modern cephalomedullary nails provide rigid fixation of the entire femur from the femoral neck to the intercondylar notch, and rotation and length are maintained by the proximal and distal locking screws. In a multicenter prospective study, 25 metastatic femoral lesions in 22 patients were treated with the Russell-Taylor reconstruction nail. Pathologic fractures had occurred in 15 femurs, and 10 had impending pathologic fractures. Twenty-four of the 25 lesions produced incapacitating pain, and pain relief was evident immediately after surgery in all. At an average 1-year follow-up, fixation had not been lost in any patient, and of the 22 patients, 16 were still alive.

FRACTURE OF THE FEMORAL SHAFT WITH DISLOCATION OF THE HIP

It was previously believed that the same mechanism that produces a fracture of the neck of the femur with a fracture of the shaft also may produce a dislocated hip. In a cadaver study, the combination of dislocation of the hip and fracture of the shaft could be produced only by two separate forces. The hip is dislocated by a force applied in line with the shaft while the knee and hip are flexed 90 degrees and the hip is adducted; the femoral shaft is fractured by another force applied to the lateral aspect of the thigh. The fact that in this injury the shaft fracture usually is transverse supports these

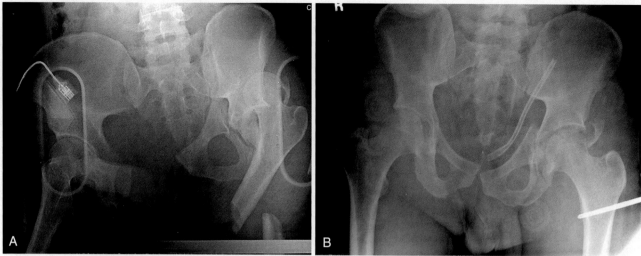

FIGURE 2.89 **A,** Polytraumatized patient with left femoral diaphyseal fracture and associated femoroacetabular dislocation. Also note concomitant complex pelvic ring and left-sided acetabular injury. **B,** Proximal femur was reduced using percutaneous positioned Schanz pin at time of patient's exploratory laparotomy. Pin was then incorporated into uniplanar external fixator for temporary stabilization of femoral fracture secondary to patient's overall condition on presentation.

findings. Adduction of the proximal fragment as seen in the radiographs of the femur is strong evidence that the hip is dislocated; in most fractures of the femoral shaft without dislocation of the hip, the proximal fragment is abducted. This illustrates and supports the importance of a thorough systematic radiographic evaluation in the setting of high-energy trauma to include at a minimum orthogonal imaging of joints adjacent to the anatomic area of primary injury.

In this combined injury, the dislocation of the hip is an emergency and must be reduced promptly to prevent osteonecrosis of the femoral head (Fig. 2.89). We prefer to treat the femoral shaft fracture definitively, in the same setting, if the patient's condition permits early total care. Rarely will the femoracetabular dislocation reduce closed, and percutaneous instruments are necessary for a successful reduction.

REFERENCES

ANKLE (PILON FRACTURES)

Alexandropoulos C, Tsourvakas S, Papchristos J, et al.: Ankle fracture classification: an evaluation of three classification systems: Lauge-Hansen, A.O. and Broos-Bisschop, *Acta Orthop Belg* 76:521, 2010.

Amorosa LF, Brown GD, Greisberg J: A surgical approach to posterior pilon fractures, *J Orthop Trauma* 24:188, 2010.

Bava E, Charlton T, Thorderson D: Ankle fracture syndesmosis fixation and management: the current practice of orthopaedic surgeons, *Am J Orthop* 39:242, 2010.

Boraiah S, Kemp TJ, Erwteman A, et al.: Outcome following open reduction and internal fixation of open pilon fractures, *J Bone Joint Surg* 92A:346, 2010.

Briceno J, Wusu T, Kaiser P, et al.: Effect of syndesmotic implant removal on dorsiflexion, *Foot Ankle Int* 40:499, 2019.

Cannada LK: The no-touch approach for operative treatment of pilon fractures to minimize soft tissue complications, *Orthopedics* 33:734, 2010.

Choi Y, Kwon SS, Chung CY, et al.: Preoperative radiographic and CT findings predicting syndesmotic injuries in supination-external rotation-type ankle fractures, *J Bone Joint Surg* 96A:1161, 2014.

Egol KA, Pahk B, Walsh M, et al.: Outcome after unstable ankle fracture: effect of syndesmotic stabilization, *J Orthop Trauma* 24:7, 2010.

Gougoulia N, Knanna A, Sakellariou A, Maffulli N: Supination-external rotation ankle fractures: stability a key issue, *Clin Orthop Relat Res* 468:243, 2010.

Grassi A, Samuelsson K, D'Hooghe P, et al.: Dynamic stabilization of syndesmosis injuries reduces complications and reoperations as compared with screw fixation: a meta-analysis of randomized controlled trials, *Am J Sports Med* 48:1000, 2020.

Graves ML, Porter SE, Fagan BC, et al.: Is obesity protective against wound healing complications in pilon surgery? Soft tissue envelope and pilon fractures in the obese, *Orthopedics* 11:33, 2010.

Ketz J, Sanders R: Staged posterior tibial plating for the treatment of Orthopaedic Trauma Association 43C2 and 43C3 tibial pilon fractures, *J Orthop Trauma* 26:341, 2012.

Little MM, Berkes MB, Schottel PC, et al.: Anatomic fixation of the supination external rotation type IV equivalent ankle fractures, *J Orthop Trauma* 29:250, 2015.

Liu JW, Ahn J, Raspovic KM, et al.: Increased rates of readmission, reoperation, and mortality following open reduction and internal fixation of ankle fractures are associated with diabetes mellitus, *J Foot Ankle Surg* 58:470, 2019.

Peterson KS, Chapman WD, Hyer CF, Berlet GC: Maintenance of reduction with suture button fixation devices for ankle syndesmotic repair, *Foot Ankle Int* 36:679, 2015.

Pollard JD, Deyhim A, Rigby RB, et al.: Comparison of pullout strength between 3.5 mm fully threaded bicortical screws and 4.0 mm partially threaded, cancellous screws in the fixation of medial malleolar fractures, *J Foot Ankle Surg* 49:248, 2010.

Raeder BW, Figved W, Madsen JE, et al.: Better outcome for suture button compared with single syndesmotic screw for syndesmosis injury: five-year results of a randomized controlled trial, *Bone Joint Lett J* 102-B:212, 2020.

Sanders DW, Tieszer C, Corbett B: Operative versus nonoperative treatment of unstable lateral malleolar fractures: a randomized multicenter trial, *J Orthop Trauma* 26:129, 2012.

Shimozono Y, Hurley ET, Myerson CL, et al.: Suture button versus syndesmotic screw for syndesmosis injuries: a meta-analysis of randomized controlled trials, *Am J Sports Med* 47:2764, 2019.

Tantigate D, Ho G, Kirschenbaum J, et al.: Functional outcomes after fracture-dislocation of the ankle, *Foot Ankle Spec* 13:18, 2020.

Wake J, Martin JD: Syndesmosis injury from diagnosis to repair: physical examination, diagnosis, and arthroscopic-assisted reduction, *J Am Acad Orthop Surg*, 2020, [Epub ahead of print].

Wawrose RA, Grossman LS, Tagliaferro M, et al.: Temporizing external fixation vs splinting following ankle fracture dislocation, *Foot Ankle Int* 41:177, 2020.

White TO, Guy P, Cooke CJ, et al.: The results of early primary open reduction and internal fixation for treatment of OTA 43.C-type tibial pilon fractures: a cohort study, *J Orthop Trauma* 24:757, 2010.

TIBIAL SHAFT

Cain ME, Hendrickx LAM, Bleeker NJ, et al.: Prevalence of rotational malalignment after intramedullary nailing of tibial shaft fractures: can we reliably use the contralateral uninjured side as the reference standard? *J Bone Joint Surg Am* 102:582, 2020.

Chan DS, Serrano-Riera R, Griffing R, et al.: Suprapatellar versus infrapatellar tibial nail insertion: a prospective randomized control pilot study, *J Orthop Trauma* 30:130, 2016.

Connelly CL, Bucknall V, Jenkins PJ, et al: Outcome at 12 to 22 years of 1502 tibial shaft fractures, *Bone Joint J* 96B:1370, 2014.

Foote CJ, Guyatt GH, Vignesh KN, et al.: Which surgical treatment for open tibial shaft fractures results in the fewest reoperations? A network meta-analysis, *Clin Orthop Relat Res* 473:2179, 2015.

Frihagen F, Madsen JE, Sundfeldt M, et al.: Taylor Spatial Frame™ or reamed intramedullary nailing for closed fractures of the tibial shaft. A randomized controlled trial, *J Orthop Trauma*, 2020, [Epub ahead of print.].

Hendrickx LAM, Virgin J, van den Bekerom MPJ, et al.: Complications and subsequent surgery after intra-medullary nailing for tibial shaft fractures: review of 8110 patients, *Injury*, 2020, [Epub ahead of print.].

Ibrahim I, Johnson A, Rodriguez EK: Improved outcomes with semi-extended nailing of tibial fractures? a systematic review, *J Orthop Trauma* 33:155, 2019.

Lack WD, Starman JS, Seymour R, et al.: Any cortical bridging predicts healing of tibial shaft fractures, *J Bone Joint Surg* 96:1066, 2014.

Lam SW, Teraa M, Leenen LP, van der Heijden GJ: Systematic review shows lowered risk of non-union after reamed nailing in patients with closed tibial shaft fractures, *Injury* 41:671, 2010.

Vallier HA, Cureton BA, Patterson BM: Randomised, prospective comparison of plate versus intramedullary nail fixation for distal tibia shaft fractures, *J Orthop Trauma* 25:736, 2011.

Zamorano DP, Robicheaux GW, Law J, Mercer J: *Semiextended nailing: is the patellofemoral joint safe? Paper #58*, presented at the annual meeting of the Orthopaedic Trauma Association, 2010.

TIBIAL CONDYLE AND TIBIAL PLATEAU

Ahearn N, Oppy A, Halliday R, et al.: The outcome following fixation of bicondylar tibial plateau fractures, *Bone Joint Lett J* 96B(95):6–62, 2014.

Berkes MB, Little MT, Schottel PC, et al.: Outcomes of Schatzker II tibial plateau fracture open reduction internal fixation using structural bone allograft, *J Orthop Trauma* 28:97–102, 2014.

Colman M, Wright A, Gruen G, et al.: Prolonged operative time increases infection rate in tibial plateau fractures, *Injury* 44:249, 2013.

Evangelopoulos D, Chalikias S, Michalos M, et al.: Medium-term results after surgical treatment of high-energy tibial plateau fractures, *J Knee Surg* 33:394, 2020.

Haller JM, Holt DC, McFadden ML, et al.: Arthrofibrosis of the knee following a fracture of the tibial plateau, *Bone Joint Lett J* 97B:109, 2015.

Haller JM, McFadden M, Kubiak EN, Higgins TF: Inflammatory cytokine response following acute tibial plateau fracture, *J Bone Joint Surg* 97A:478, 2015.

Hap DXF, Kwek EBK: Functional outcomes after surgical treatment of tibial plateau fractures, *J Clin Orthop Trauma* 11(Suppl 1):S11, 2020.

Hong G, Huang X, Lv T, et al.: An analysis on the effect of the three-incision combined approach for complex fracture of tibial plateau involving the posterolateral tibial plateau, *J Orthop Surg Res* 15:43, 2020.

Ruffolo MR, Gettys FK, Montijo HE, et al.: Complications of high energy bicondylar tibial plateau fractures treated with dual plating through 2 incisions, *J Orthop Trauma* 29:85, 2015.

Sanders R, DiPasquale TG, Jordan CJ, et al.: Semiextended intramedullary nailing of the tibia using a suprapatellar approach: radiographic results and clinical outcomes at a minimum of 12 months follow-up, *J Orthop Trauma* 28:245, 2014.

Stewart CC, O'Hara NN, Mascarenhas D, et al.: Predictors of symptomatic implant removal after open reduction and internal fixation of tibial plateau fractures: a retrospective case-control study, *Orthopedics* 43:161, 2020.

Zeng ZM, Luo CF, Putnis S, Zeng BF: Biomechanical analysis of posteromedial tibial plateau split fracture fixation, *Knee* 18:51, 2011.

Ziran BH, Becher SJ: Radiographic predictors of compartment syndrome in tibial plateau fractures, *J Orthop Trauma* 27:612, 2013.

PATELLA

Bonnaig NS, Casstevens C, Archdeacon MT, et al.: Fix it or discard it? A retrospective analysis of functional outcomes after surgically treated patella fractures comparing ORIF with partial patellectomy, *J Orthop Trauma* 29:80, 2015.

Busel G, Barrick B, Auston D, et al.: Patella fractures treated with cannulated lag screws and Fiberwire® have a high union rate and low rate of implant removal, *Injury* 51:473, 2020.

Camarda L, La Gutta A, Butera M, et al.: FiberWire tension band for patellar fractures, *J Orthop Traumatol* 17:75, 2016.

Cho JW, Kent WT, Cho WT, et al.: Miniplate augmented tension-band wiring for comminuted patella fractures, *J Orthop Trauma* 33:e143, 2019.

Lazaro LE, Wellman DS, Sauro G, et al.: Outcomes after operative fixation of complete articular patellar fractures: assessment of functional impairment, *J Bone Joint Surg* 95A(e96):1–8, 2013.

LeBrun CT, Langford JR, Sagi HC: Functional outcomes after operatively treated patella fractures, *J Orthop Trauma* 26:422, 2012.

Lorich DG, Fabricant PD, Sauro G, et al.: Superior outcomes after operative fixation of patella fractures using a novel plating technique: a prospective cohort study, *J Orthop Trauma* 31:241, 2017.

Sillander M, Koueiter DM, Gandhi S, et al.: Outcomes following low-profile mesh plate osteosynthesis of patella fractures, *J Knee Surg* 31:919, 2018.

Taylor BC, Mehta S, Castaneda J, et al.: Plating of patella fractures: techniques and outcomes, *J Orthop Trauma* 28:e231, 2014.

Wagner FC, Neumann MV, Wolf S, et al.: Biomechanical comparison of a 3.5 mm anterior locking plate to cannulated screws with anterior tension band wiring in comminuted patellar fractures, *Injury*, 2020, [Epub ahead of print.].

FEMUR

Adams Jr JD, Tanner SL, Jeray KJ: Far cortical locking screws in distal femur fractures, *Orthopedics* 38:e153, 2015.

Avilucea FR, Joyce D, Mir HR: Dynamic stress fluoroscopy for evaluation of the femoral neck after intramedullary nails: improved sensitivity for identifying occult fractures, *J Orthop Trauma* 33:88, 2019.

Barei DP, Beingessner DM: Open distal femur fractures treated with lateral locked implants: union, secondary bone grafting, and predictive parameters, *Orthopedics* 35:e843, 2012.

Becher S, Ziran B: Retrograde intramedullary nailing of open femoral shaft fractures: a retrospective case series, *J Trauma Acute Care Surg* 72:696, 2012.

Bottlang M, Fitzpatrick DC, Sheerin D, et al.: Dynamic fixation of distal femur fractures using far cortical locking screws: a prospective observational study, *J Orthop Trauma* 28:181, 2014.

Brewster J, Grenier G, Taylor BC, et al.: Long-term comparison of retrograde and antegrade femoral nailing, *Orthopedics* 20:1, 2020.

Croom WP, Lorenzana DJ, Auran RL, et al.: Is contralateral templating reliable for establishing rotational alignment during intramedullary stabilization of femoral shaft fractures? A study of individual bilateral differences in femoral version, *J Orthop Trauma* 32:61, 2018.

Even JL, Richards JE, Crosby CG, et al.: Preoperative skeletal versus cutaneous traction for femoral shaft fractures treated within 24 hours, *J Orthop Trauma* 26:e177, 2012.

Gheraibeh P, Vaidya R, Hudson I, et al.: Minimizing leg length discrepancy after intramedullary nailing of comminuted femoral shaft fractures: a quality improvement initiative using the scout computed tomography scanogram, *J Orthop Trauma* 32:256, 2018.

Harvin WH, Oladeji LO, Della GJ, et al.: Working length and proximal screw constructs in plate osteosynthesis of distal femur fractures, *Injury* 48:2597, 2017.

Hussain N, Hussai FN, Sermer C, et al.: Antegrade versus retrograde nailing techniques and trochanteric versus piriformis intramedullary nailing entry points for femoral shaft fractures: a systematic review and meta-analysis, *Can J Surg* 60:19, 2017.

Karahan G, Yamak K, Kocoglu T, et al.: The effect of implant choice on varus angulation and clinical results in the management of subtrochanteric fractures, *J Orthop* 20:46, 2020.

Linn MS, McAndrew CM, Prusaczyk B, et al.: Dynamic locked plating of distal femur fractures, *J Orthop Trauma* 29:447, 2015.

Liporace FA, Yoon RS: Nail plate combination technique for native and periprosthetic distal femur fractures, *J Orthop Trauma* 33:e64, 2019.

O'Toole RV, Riche K, Cannada LK, et al.: Analysis of postoperative knee sepsis after retrograde nail insertion of open femoral shaft fractures, *J Orthop Trauma* 24:677, 2010.

Patterson JT, Ishii K, Tornetta 3rd P, et al.: Open reduction is associated with greater hazard of early reoperation after internal fixation of displaced femoral neck fractures in adults 18-65 years, *J Orthop Trauma* 34:294, 2020.

Ricci WM, Streubel PN, Morshed S, et al.: Risk factors for failure of locked plate fixation of distal femur fractures: an analysis of 335 cases, *J Orthop Trauma* 28:83, 2014.

Ries Z, Hansen K, Bottlang M, et al.: Healing results of periprosthetic distal femurs fractures treated with far cortical locking technology: a preliminary retrospective study, *Iowa Orthop J* 33:7–11, 2013.

Rodriquez EK, Boulton C, Weaver MJ, et al.: Predictive factors of distal femoral fracture nonunion after lateral locked plating: a retrospective multicenter case-control study of 283 fractures, *Injury* 45:554, 2014.

Rogers NB, Hartline BE, Achor TS, et al.: Improving the diagnosis of ipsilateral femoral neck and shaft fractures: a new imaging protocol, *J Bone Joint Surg Am* 102:309, 2020.

Scannell BP, Waldrop NE, Sasser HC, et al.: Skeletal traction versus external fixation in the initial temporization of femoral shaft fractures in severely injured patients, *J Trauma* 68:633, 2010.

Stannard JP, Bankston L, Futch LA, et al.: Functional outcome following intramedullary nailing of the femur: a prospective randomized comparison of piriformis fossa and greater trochanteric entry portals, *J Bone Joint Surg* 93A:1385, 2011.

Steinberg EL, Elis J, Steinberg Y, et al.: A double-plating approach to distal femur fracture: a clinical study, *Injury* 48:2260, 2017.

Vaidya R, Dimoyski R, Cizmic Z, et al.: Use of inherent anteversion of an intramedullary nail to avoid malrotation in comminuted femur fractures: a prospective case- control study, *J Orthop Trauma* 32:623, 2018.

The complete list of references is available online at ExpertConsult.com.

CHAPTER 3

FRACTURES AND DISLOCATIONS OF THE HIP

John C. Weinlein

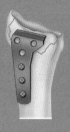

FEMORAL NECK FRACTURES	153	Classification	168	Intramedullary nailing	179	
		Treatment	168	Plate fixation	182	
Classification	153	Treatment with screw–side plate devices	169	**HIP DISLOCATIONS AND FEMORAL HEAD FRACTURES**	187	
Diagnosis	154					
Treatment	154	Treatment with intramedullary nails	173	Reduction maneuvers for posterior hip dislocation	187	
Operative treatment	155					
Outcomes and complications	161	Plate fixation compared with intramedullary nail fixation	174	Reduction maneuver for anterior hip dislocation	192	
Failure of fixation	161					
Nonunion and osteonecrosis	161	**SUBTROCHANTERIC FEMORAL FRACTURES**	179	**FRACTURES OF THE IPSILATERAL FEMORAL NECK AND SHAFT**	196	
Arthroplasty	164	Classification	179			
Basicervical femoral neck fractures	167	Treatment	179			
INTERTROCHANTERIC FEMORAL FRACTURES	168					

As the number of hip fractures continues to increase in the United States (with an estimated 458,000 to 1,037,000 hip fractures per year by 2050 in patients 45 years old or older), orthopaedic surgeons will be called on to help deal with this impending public health crisis. Although most hip fractures occur in the geriatric population, more and more young patients are surviving motor vehicle accidents and presenting with high-energy injuries about the hip. Hip fractures in these two populations can be very different, and an understanding of these differences will help determine the appropriate treatment to minimize morbidity and mortality and restore the patient to his or her preinjury functional status.

FEMORAL NECK FRACTURES

Fractures of the neck of the femur occur predominantly in the elderly, typically resulting from low-energy falls, and may be associated with osteoporosis. Fractures of the femoral neck in the young are a very different injury and are treated in very different ways. Femoral neck fractures in young patients typically are the result of a high-energy mechanism, and associated injuries are common. Most fractures of the femoral neck are intracapsular and may compromise the tenuous blood supply to the femoral head (Fig. 3.1). This blood supply must also be understood for approaches to the proximal femur as well as implant placement. While the superior retinacular artery has been well described as being the main provider of perfusion to the femoral head, the inferior retinacular artery has more recently been shown to also provide significant perfusion and the anatomic course has been demonstrated to be consistent.

CLASSIFICATION

Femoral neck fractures can be classified by the location of the fracture line (subcapital, transcervical, or basicervical [Fig. 3.2]), the Garden classification, or Pauwels classification. The Garden classification (Fig. 3.3) is the most commonly used classification system and is based on the degree of displacement:

Stage I: incomplete fracture line (valgus impacted)
Stage II: complete fracture line; nondisplaced
Stage III: complete fracture line; partially displaced
Stage IV: complete fracture line; completely displaced

Stages III and IV can be differentiated radiographically by carefully scrutinizing the trabecular patterns of the femoral head and acetabulum. Stage III femoral neck fractures maintain contact between the femoral neck and femoral head, and the trabecular patterns between the head and acetabulum are no longer aligned. Stage IV fractures do not maintain contact between the femoral neck and femoral head, and the trabecular patterns between the head and acetabulum have realigned. Interobserver reliability between stages is low; however, most surgeons are able to differentiate between nondisplaced femoral neck fractures (stages I and II) and displaced femoral neck fractures (stages III and IV). A shortcoming of the Garden classification is that angulation and displacement in the sagittal plane are not considered.

The Pauwels classification (Fig. 3.4) was initially described in 1935 in the German literature and was thought to describe the major forces present at the fracture site. The classification has been misquoted in the literature over the years, causing some confusion, but the basic premise remains: increasing verticality of the femoral neck fracture line is associated with increased presence of shear at the fracture site. The classification is based on the angle the fracture line makes in reference to the horizontal. The fracture line in a Pauwels type I fracture is between 0 and 30 degrees in reference to the horizontal, type II is between 30 and 50 degrees, and type III is more than 50 degrees (Fig. 3.5). More recently, Collinge et al. reported significant comminution in 96% of femoral neck fractures with high Pauwels angles. The Pauwels classification is relevant because optimal treatment may vary with the Pauwels angle.

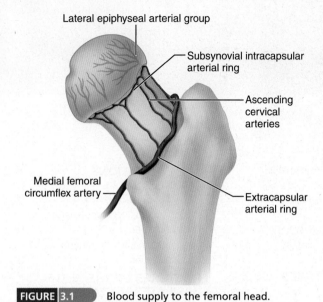

FIGURE 3.1 Blood supply to the femoral head.

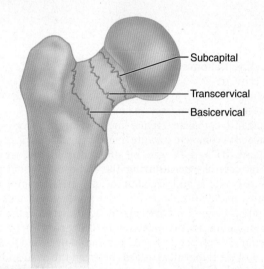

FIGURE 3.2 Classification of femoral neck fractures by location: subcapital, transcervical, basicervical.

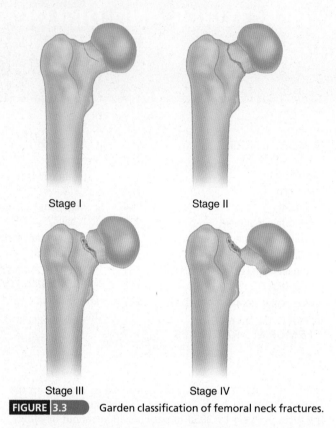

FIGURE 3.3 Garden classification of femoral neck fractures.

DIAGNOSIS

The diagnosis of a femoral neck fracture is based on history, physical examination, and radiographs. Most patients with femoral neck fractures give a history of a traumatic event, with the exception of patients who have stress fractures of the femoral neck. Also, many young patients with high-energy femoral neck fractures have associated injuries, including head injuries, and may not be able to give a history. The index of suspicion for a femoral neck fracture must be extremely high because the consequences of a missed femoral neck fracture can be disastrous. The physical examination typically reveals an extremity that is shortened and externally rotated. Standard anteroposterior pelvic and cross-table lateral views of the hip are necessary, and a traction internal rotation view often is helpful. The cross-table lateral view, while often difficult to obtain, is probably essential in enabling prediction of failure with fixation in Garden I and II femoral neck fractures. The entire femur should be imaged. MRI has become the imaging study of choice to evaluate occult femoral neck fractures. CT scans to evaluate femoral neck fractures, often available as part of the trauma work up (CT scan of the chest, abdomen, and pelvis), can yield useful information including degree of comminution.

TREATMENT

A satisfactory reduction is paramount in minimizing the complications associated with treatment of femoral neck fractures, including nonunion and osteonecrosis. "Radiographic" or "visual" reduction continues to be debated; however. studies that have associated reduction quality with outcomes are generally based on radiographs. A closed reduction can be attempted in every patient for whom internal fixation is planned. The Whitman technique involves applying traction to the abducted, extended, externally rotated hip with subsequent internal rotation. Reduction attempts should not be forceful and should not be repeated more than two or three times. Once reduction has been attempted, the angulation and alignment must be critically evaluated. The Garden alignment index (Fig. 3.6) can be used to evaluate femoral neck angulation and alignment. The trabecular alignment pattern (Fig. 3.7) is evaluated with both anteroposterior and lateral radiographs or fluoroscopy. On the anteroposterior image, the angle between the medial shaft and the central axis of the medial compressive trabeculae should measure between 160 and 180 degrees. An angle of less than 160 degrees indicates varus, whereas an angle of more than 180 degrees indicates excessive valgus. On the lateral image, angulation should be approximately 180 degrees and deviation of more than 20 degrees indicates excessive anteversion or retroversion. Interestingly, Liporace et al. reported a high percentage of retroversion of the femoral neck (approximately 20% of Caucasians in their series), and this relatively high frequency of retroversion

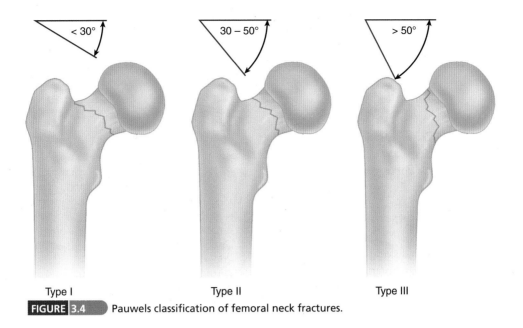

Type I Type II Type III

FIGURE 3.4 Pauwels classification of femoral neck fractures.

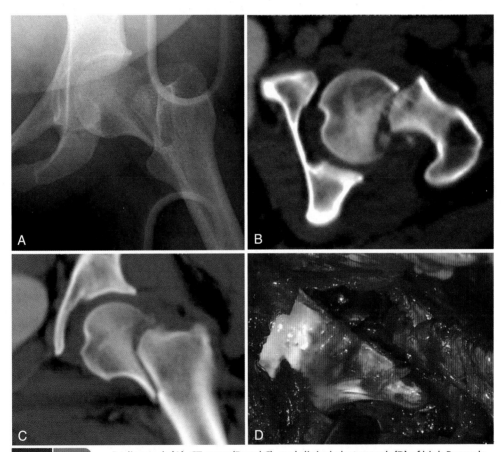

FIGURE 3.5 Radiograph **(A)**, CT scans **(B and C)**, and clinical photograph **(D)** of high Pauwels angle femoral neck fracture.

must be considered in the care of not just femoral neck fractures but other fractures of the proximal femur and femoral shaft. Lowell et al. described the radiographic or fluoroscopic appearance of an anatomically reduced femoral neck as "shallow-S– or reverse-S–shaped curves" (Fig. 3.8); these "curves" may be more useful than the Garden alignment index for intraoperative evaluation of alignment. We find

using the fluoroscopic appearance of the contralateral uninjured hip useful intraoperatively as a reference for these "curves" as well as varus/valgus angulation.

■ OPERATIVE TREATMENT

Most femoral neck fractures require operative treatment. Possible exceptions include stress fractures on the compression side of the femoral neck and femoral neck fractures in patients who are nonambulatory and comfortable or are too infirm for operative treatment.

▌ IMPLANT CHOICE

The choice of implant and operation is largely dependent on the patient's physiologic age. Patients with displaced femoral neck fractures who are physiologically older are best treated with arthroplasty. Younger patients are treated with internal fixation. With hemiarthroplasty, controversy exists to some degree over the use of cemented or cementless stems, as well as unipolar or bipolar prostheses. Data from several studies indicate that many community ambulators may be better treated with THA than with hemiarthroplasty. A major concern with THA for femoral neck fracture is dislocation, which has led to an increased interest in using an anterior or anterolateral approach when THA is done for treatment of a femoral neck fracture.

FIXATION OF FEMORAL NECK FRACTURE WITH CANNULATED SCREWS

TECHNIQUE 3.1

- Place the patient supine on a fracture table. Attempt closed reduction with the Whitman or other reduction technique. We typically scissor the lower extremities (unaffected hip extended relative to the injured side), but a well-leg holder also can be used.

- Fluoroscopically assess the quality of the reduction. If reduction is satisfactory, proceed with fixation.
- We typically use three partially threaded screws (6.5, 7.0, or 7.3 mm) in an inverted triangle configuration (Fig. 3.9A and B).
- Use fluoroscopy in both planes to localize placement of the inferocentral wire. Make a skin incision extending 2 to 3 cm proximally. Split the fascia in line with the skin incision, and use a Cobb elevator to gently split the fibers of the vastus lateralis muscle longitudinally.
- Place the inferocentral wire in perfect position on both views. Placing a guidewire along the anterior femoral neck can be helpful in determining appropriate anteversion. Make sure not to begin below the lesser trochanter and to continue proximally along the calcar. We use smooth or drill-tipped guidewires to optimize tactile feel and minimize cortical extrusion.
- Once the first guide pin is in place, use a parallel guide to place the posterosuperior and then anterosuperior pins to obtain posterior and anterior cortical support in the femoral neck. The posterosuperior guidewire should not be above the equator on the anteroposterior view. The anterosuperior guidewire should be above the equator on the anteroposterior view. Advance the guide pins just short of the articular surface. Be very careful not to violate the articular surface.
- To determine appropriate screw length, measure the length of the guide pin and subtract 5 mm. Self-drilling, self-tapping screws generally are used, but sometimes predrilling of the outer cortex is necessary in patients with dense bone. Washers are used where space permits.
- A fourth screw (diamond configuration) may be used in patients with significant posterior comminution (Fig. 3.9C). Use extreme care if a fourth screw is used because of the possibility of being extraosseous if the screw is placed posteriorly.

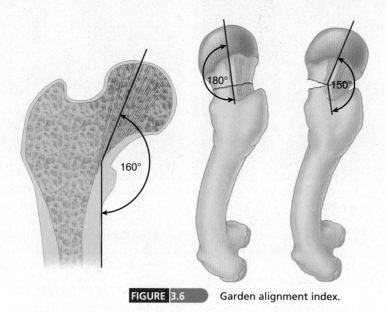

FIGURE 3.6 Garden alignment index.

Guide pins should be placed with the goal of obtaining femoral neck cortical support for screws. The femoral neck is not circular; it is more of an anterior-leaning ellipse. Zhang et al. warned of a cortical perforation risk of almost 20% in a two-dimensional 6.5-mm screw placement simulation (Fig. 3.10). The risk of perforation was 6.7% posterosuperiorly and 10.7% anteroinferiorly, and the authors illustrated "risk zones" for screw placement. Concerns about cortical perforation have also been noted, specifically in regard to the posterosuperior screw placement in an inverted triangle configuration.

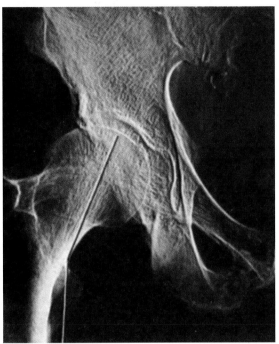

FIGURE 3.7 Anteroposterior radiograph shows angle between medial trabecular stream in femoral head and medial cortex of femoral shaft. (From Garden RS: Reduction and fixation of subcapital fractures of the femur, *Orthop Clin North Am* 5:683, 1974.)

They reported a 70% screw extrusion rate (Fig. 3.11) for posterosuperior screw (6.5 mm) placement using fluoroscopy in a cadaver model.

Care must be taken in the starting of guide pins on the lateral cortex because inaccurate passage of the pins (multiple attempts or attempts below the level of the lesser trochanter) has been associated with subtrochanteric femoral fractures. In a biomechanical model, screw configuration was shown to influence the occurrence of subtrochanteric femoral fracture. Femoral neck fractures fixed with an apex-distal configuration exhibited a greater load to failure (before subtrochanteric femoral fracture) than those fixed with an apex-proximal configuration. The concern of subtrochanteric femoral fracture, as well as the increased possibility of nonunion, was reported in a recent clinical study as well. Although a randomized trial suggested no difference between long (32 mm) and short (16 mm) threaded screws for femoral neck fractures, we attempt to maximize thread length proximal to the fracture line, but not crossing the fracture line, when compressing femoral neck fractures. Interestingly, Liu et al. suggested a redesign of screw thread length (26 mm) to accomplish this goal. Washers are used whenever possible because their use has been suggested to reduce the risk of failure, likely because of increased compressive forces generated when they are used.

Cannulated screw fixation can be done only after satisfactory reduction has been obtained. If satisfactory closed reduction cannot be obtained, open reduction, or arthroplasty in an elderly patient, is indicated. An inadequate closed reduction must not be accepted. An open reduction can be done through either a Watson Jones-approach or a modified Smith-Petersen approach. Subcapital or transcervical femoral neck fractures can be better seen and more easily reduced through a modified Smith-Petersen approach; however, this approach does require a second incision for placement of fixation. A recent cadaver study supports increased anatomic exposure with the modified

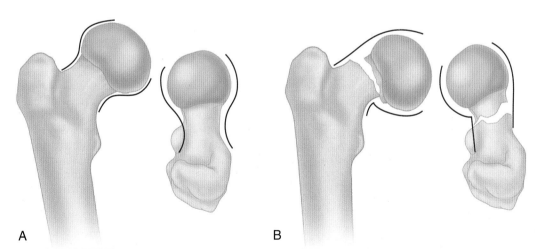

A B

FIGURE 3.8 **A,** Concave outline of femoral neck meets convex outline of femoral head in "S" or reversed-"S" curve superiorly, inferiorly, anteriorly, and posteriorly. **B,** Failure of restoration of these "S" signs is indicative of nonanatomic alignment. (Redrawn from Lowell JD: Results and complications of femoral neck fractures, *Clin Orthop Relat Res* 152:162, 1980.)

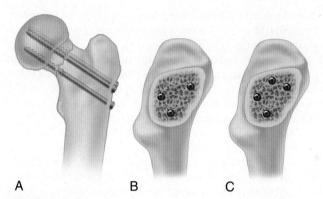

A   B   C

FIGURE 3.9   For fixation of femoral neck fractures, three partially threaded screws can be inserted in an inverted triangle configuration (**A and B**). Four screws can be placed in a diamond configuration when significant comminution is present (**C**). **SEE TECHNIQUE 3.1.**

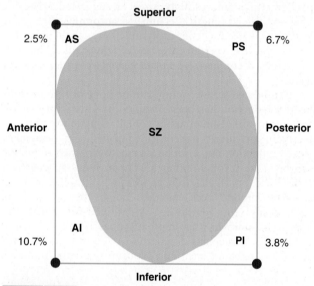

FIGURE 3.10   SZ indicates the safe zone. (From Zhang YQ, Chang SM, Huang YG, et al: The femoral neck safe zone: a radiographic simulation study to prevent cortical perforation with multiple screw insertion, *J Orthop Trauma* 29:e178, 2014.)

Smith-Petersen approach (with or without a rectus tenotomy) versus the Watson-Jones approach.

OPEN REDUCTION AND INTERNAL FIXATION

TECHNIQUE 3.2

(MODIFIED SMITH-PETERSEN)
- Position the patient supine on a flat-topped or fracture table. A fracture table makes lateral fluoroscopy easier.
- Make a longitudinal incision beginning at the anterior superior iliac spine and extending approximately 10 cm distally toward the lateral aspect of the patella.

- Incise the fascia of the tensor fascia latae and develop the interval between the tensor fascia latae and the sartorius muscle. Cauterize ascending branches of the lateral femoral circumflex artery as they are encountered.
- Identify and tag the direct head of the rectus femoris and then release it off the anterior inferior iliac spine if desired. Repair it at the conclusion of the procedure either directly (if stump has been left) or with a suture anchor.
- Reflect the indirect head of the rectus femoris muscle from the capsule, along with the iliocapsularis muscle if present.
- Perform a capsulotomy in the shape of a T, inverted-T, Z, or H. We most often use a T-shaped capsulotomy; however, a Z-shaped capsulotomy also is reasonable. The vascular anatomy of the proximal femur must be considered, and portions of the capsulotomy must be carefully extended (e.g., if a capsulotomy in the shape of an inverted T or H is made, posterior extension of the transverse limb at the base of the femoral neck should be avoided to prevent injury to the blood supply to the femoral head). Hohmann retractors can be placed within the capsule and used for gentle retraction, always being cognizant of femoral head perfusion.
- Place a 5.0-mm Schanz pin in the proximal femoral diaphysis to control the distal segment and place a T-handle on the Schanz pin to aid in manipulation.
- Insert two 2.0-mm threaded Kirschner wires into the head segment and use them as joysticks to reduce the fracture. We also have used a reduction clamp (Farabeuf) to gain compression across the fracture of the femoral neck, as described by Molnar and Routt (Fig. 3.12).
- Once satisfactory reduction is confirmed both visually and radiographically, insert cannulated screws (see Technique 3.1), screw–side plate (SSP) device with derotational screw, or proximal femoral plate.

POSTOPERATIVE CARE   Patients with high-energy femoral neck fractures are kept at touch-down (weight of leg) weight bearing for 10 to 12 weeks. Older patients are allowed protected weight bearing with a walker if their balance and other medical comorbidities allow. Patients who cannot safely ambulate are encouraged to mobilize to a chair to minimize pulmonary complications.

Controversy exists about the best method of fixation for displaced subcapital and transcervical femoral neck fractures, and there are strong advocates of both cannulated screws (Fig. 3.13) and compression hip screws. The recent FAITH (Fixation using Alternative Implants for the Treatment of Hip Fractures) randomized controlled trial showed no difference in reoperation rates between cancellous screws and SSP in the treatment of low-energy femoral neck fractures in patients older than 50 years. Subgroup analysis did suggest a potential advantage of SSP devices in displaced fractures, basicervical fractures, and in smokers, although there was a higher rate of osteonecrosis in patients treated with SSP devices (9% vs. 5%). Based on study protocol, none of the patients treated with SSP devices had supplemental fixation such as a derotational screw. Biomechanical studies suggest that a compression hip screw coupled with a derotational screw (Fig. 3.14) is

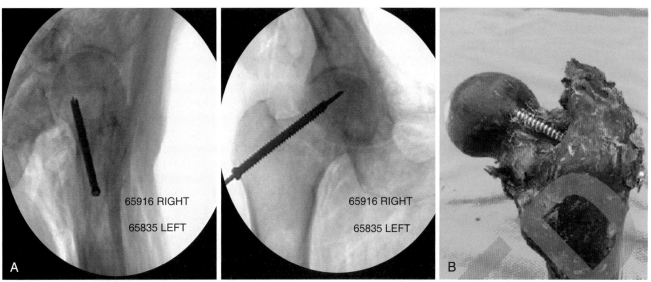

FIGURE 3.11   **A,** Anteroposterior and lateral fluoroscopic images showing contained screw. **B,** Stripped cadaver specimen with posterior-cranial screw breach with thread extrusion. (From Hoffmann JC, Kellam J, Kumaravel M, et al: Is the cranial and posterior screw of the "inverted triangle" configuration for femoral neck fractures safe? *J Orthop Trauma* 33:331, 2019.)

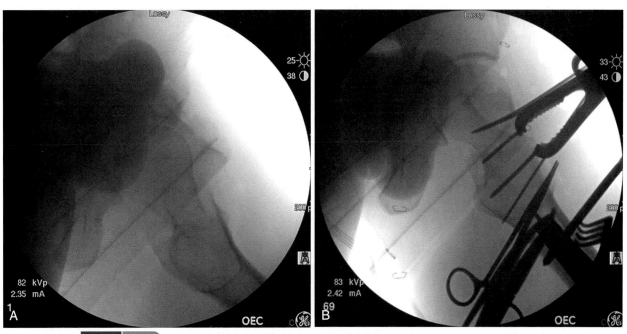

FIGURE 3.12   Reduction (Farabeuf) clamp can be used to gain compression across femoral neck fracture. **A,** Displaced fracture. **B,** Reduced fracture. **SEE TECHNIQUE 3.2.**

stronger than three cannulated screws in the treatment of unstable basicervical femoral neck fractures. A retrospective clinical study comparing fixation devices for Pauwels type III femoral neck fractures found no definitive evidence indicating the optimal fixation device. There was a higher nonunion rate with cannulated screws than with fixed angle devices (dynamic hip screw, cephalomedullary nail, dynamic condylar screw); however, this difference was not statistically significant. Biomechanical data suggest that a proximal femoral locking plate may be superior to both cannulated screws and a compression hip screw in

a Pauwels type III femoral neck model, but clinical studies have not been encouraging. Berkes et al. reported a high incidence of catastrophic failure with proximal femoral locking plates. A different design of plate has shown improved results compared with cannulated screws; this design allows some controlled shortening. We typically reserve use of proximal femoral locking plates for fractures with significant femoral neck comminution (Figs. 3.15 and 3.16). The Targon dynamic proximal femoral locking plate (Aesculap AG, Tuttlingen, Germany) (Fig. 3.17A), which has been used in Europe for more than a decade with generally favorable results, is currently not available in United States. The Conquest dynamic proximal femoral locking plate (Smith & Nephew, Memphis, TN) (Fig. 3.17B) is a similar option; however, clinical data currently are lacking.

Other options include a trochanteric lag screw and medial buttress plating. A trochanteric lag screw for high Pauwels angle femoral neck fractures is supported by biomechanical data; however, a recent clinical series specifically using this technique did not have favorable results.

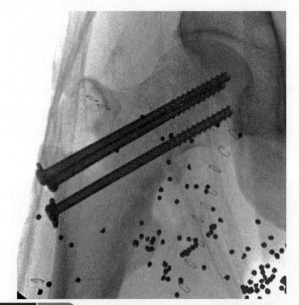

FIGURE 3.13 Cannulated screw fixation of displaced femoral neck fracture after open reduction.

The technique for placement of a compression hip screw is described in the section on intertrochanteric femoral fractures (see Technique 3.4). Care must be taken with placement of a large diameter lag screw in patients with nonosteoporotic bone, and consideration should be given to routinely using a tap as well as placing a derotational screw.

Femoral neck shortening (Fig. 3.18) appears to be common after fixation of femoral neck fractures. Shortening of more than 1 cm was reported to occur after 42% of Garden I fractures and 63% of Garden II fractures fixed with cannulated screws. The importance of femoral neck length in influencing functional outcome has been emphasized in several reports. Femoral neck shortening was associated with pain and decreased mobility in a study of over 500 patients with femoral neck fractures treated with the Targon dynamic femoral locking plate. The mean age of patients in this study was 76.1 years. Zlowodzki et al. retrospectively evaluated the effect of femoral neck shortening on functional outcome in 70 patients with healed femoral neck fractures, 64% of which were nondisplaced intracapsular fractures. All patients were treated with screw fixation, and 69 of 70 had acceptable reductions according to the Garden alignment index. Interestingly, 46 (66%) of the 70 patients healed with shortening of more than 5 mm and 27 (39%) had more than 5 degrees of varus. The primary outcome measure, the SF-36 physical functioning score, correlated with the degree of femoral neck shortening, suggesting that femoral neck shortening negatively impacts functional outcome. Similarly, Slobogean et al. reported decreased functional outcomes (Harris Hip Score, Timed Up and Go, SF-36 Physical Component Summary) in patients younger than 55 years of age (mean, 43.7 years) who had shortening of 10 mm or more after treatment of a femoral neck fracture with multiple cancellous screws.

Boraiah et al. reported treatment of 54 intracapsular femoral neck fractures with anatomic reduction, intraoperative

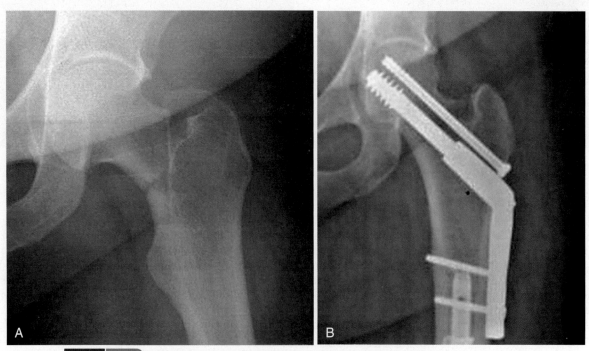

FIGURE 3.14 Displaced femoral neck fracture **(A)**, in this case ipsilateral to femoral shaft fracture, fixed with compression hip screw and derotational screw **(B)**.

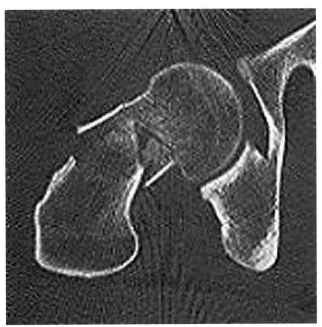

FIGURE 3.15 Axial CT scan of femoral neck fracture with significant posterior femoral neck comminution.

compression, and length-stable implants. Various open reduction techniques were used depending on fracture pattern and physiologic age. Intraoperative compression was achieved before placement of a dynamic hip screw (or dynamic helical hip screw) and fully threaded screws. The overall union rate was 94%, with an average shortening of the femoral neck of 1.7 mm. The average 36-Item Short Form Health Survey (SF-36) physical functioning score was 42, and the Harris Hip Score was 87. The Bodily Pain subscore of the SF-36 correlated with the "abductor lever arm" (distance from the center of the femoral head to a tangential line along the greater trochanter). Patients with greater differences in the abductor lever arm between the fractured and unaffected sides had lower Bodily Pain subscores. Weil et al. reported a small series demonstrating minimal shortening after the treatment of femoral neck fractures with fully threaded screws; 23 of 24 fractures were classified as Garden I or II. There was no statistically significant difference in complication or reoperation rates when compared to a historical control treated with partially threaded screws. Larger series supporting this technique currently are lacking in the literature, and at least one study reported high complication rates.

Only slight changes in technique are necessary to stabilize femoral neck fractures at length. Obviously, the reduction is paramount. Using length-stable implants in fractures that are not well reduced may result in nonunion. Potentially, the goals of union and maintenance of femoral neck length can both be achieved. Closed reduction of displaced fractures can be attempted, followed by open reduction through either a Smith-Petersen or Watson-Jones approach if closed reduction fails to obtain an anatomic reduction. In older patients and fractures with less displacement, more limited open reductions can be done if needed with the use of ball-spike pushers, Cobb elevators, and Kirschner wires to obtain anatomic reductions. After reduction has been obtained, partially threaded cannulated screws can be placed for

compression across the fracture site. Once adequate compression is achieved, the cannulated screws are replaced one by one with fully threaded screws with washers. If a compression hip screw is to be used, such as for a high Pauwels angle femoral neck fracture, a guide pin is placed perpendicular to the fracture line, and a partially threaded cannulated screw is inserted, followed by the SSP device. The partially threaded screw is then changed to a fully threaded screw (Fig. 3.19). Two fully threaded screws also can be used if patient's femoral neck anatomy will allow. As previously noted, large series demonstrating the effectiveness of these techniques are lacking in the literature.

Femoral neck shortening also may lead to prominent implant placement. Implant removal was the most frequent reoperation (24%) reported in 796 young patients after treatment of femoral neck fractures. Zielinski et al. reported a similar rate of reoperation for implant removal (23%), but implant removal generally had a positive impact on patients' quality of life. Surgeons and patients should be aware of the possibility of femoral neck fracture after implant removal.

OUTCOMES AND COMPLICATIONS
■ FAILURE OF FIXATION
Internal fixation may fail because of many factors, including inadequate reduction, poor implant selection or position, nonunion, osteonecrosis, and infection. Determining the cause of fixation failure is extremely important in planning revision surgery. In young patients, early recognition of inadequate reduction or poor implant selection or position can be treated with revision open reduction and internal fixation (Fig. 3.20) and femoral neck nonunions or malunions can be treated with valgus intertrochanteric osteotomy. Femoral neck nonunion, malunion, and osteonecrosis in elderly patients can be treated with THA. Infection after the treatment of femoral neck fractures can be quite problematic. The goal is to suppress the infection with debridement and culture-specific antibiotics, maintaining the hardware until union at which time it is removed. Hardware failure with infection requires hardware removal and possibly resection arthroplasty. Occasionally, total hip arthroplasty can be done after implant failure with infection but only in a staged fashion and after infection has been eradicated.

■ NONUNION AND OSTEONECROSIS
Nonunion (Fig. 3.21) and osteonecrosis (Fig. 3.22) are two major problems that lead to revision surgery after treatment of intracapsular femoral neck fractures. In a meta-analysis of 18 studies involving younger patients (ages 15 to 50 years) with femoral neck fractures, the overall incidence of osteonecrosis was 23% and the incidence of nonunion was 9%. The 564 patients in these studies included those with both displaced and nondisplaced intracapsular femoral neck fractures. In a series of 73 femoral neck fractures in patients between the ages of 15 and 50 years treated at a single institution, Haidukewych et al. found an overall frequency of osteonecrosis of 23% and nonunion of 8%. Osteonecrosis developed in 27% of displaced fractures and 14% of nondisplaced fractures. Thirteen patients (18%) had conversion to arthroplasty; 11 of these arthroplasties were done purely for osteonecrosis. Initial fracture displacement and the quality of radiographic reduction were found to affect results. In another series including 62 Pauwels type III femoral neck fractures, osteonecrosis developed in

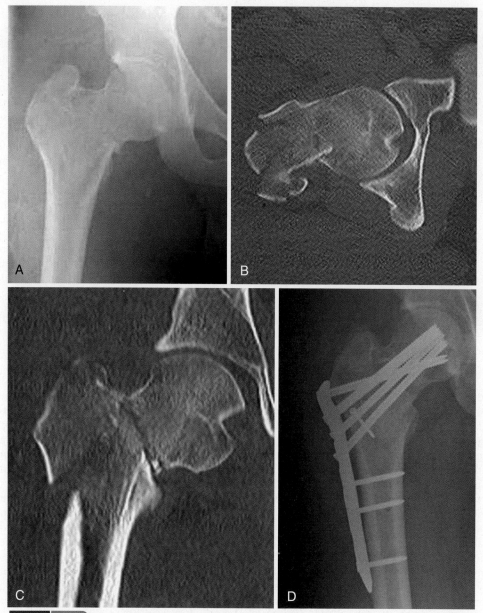

FIGURE 3.16 Preoperative radiograph **(A)** and axial **(B)** and coronal **(C)** CT scans of a femoral neck fracture with posterior femoral neck comminution with extension into the greater trochanter. **D,** United fracture after fixation.

11% and nonunion in 16%. The average age of patients in this series was 42 years (range 19 to 64 years). The higher non-union rate in this study is likely a result of the difficulty of treating higher Pauwels angle femoral neck fractures.

Osteonecrosis continues to be a problem after femoral neck fractures, even nondisplaced fractures. In fact, higher intracapsular pressures have been demonstrated with non-displaced femoral neck fractures than with displaced frac-tures. Routine capsulotomy is controversial. Capsulotomy probably is most effective in Garden types I and II frac-tures in which the capsule may not be torn or completely torn and tamponade may be a major cause in the develop-ment of osteonecrosis. We usually perform capsulotomies in young patients with nondisplaced femoral neck frac-tures and only occasionally do so in the geriatric popula-tion. Although there is no conclusive study proving that

capsulotomy decreases the frequency of osteonecrosis, it can be done quickly and safely and may reduce the risk of osteonecrosis.

FLUOROSCOPICALLY GUIDED CAPSULOTOMY OF THE HIP

TECHNIQUE 3.3

- After fixation of the femoral neck fracture, prepare a no. 10 scalpel blade by placing an approximately 2-cm strip of Ioban around the blade/handle junction to decrease the

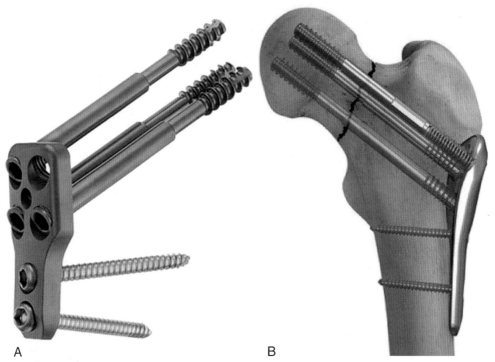

FIGURE 3.17 Dynamic locking constructs for proximal femoral fractures. **A,** Targon FN (Aesculap B. Braun Medical Inc, Tuttlingen, Germany). **B,** CONQUEST FN (Smith & Nephew, Memphis, TN).

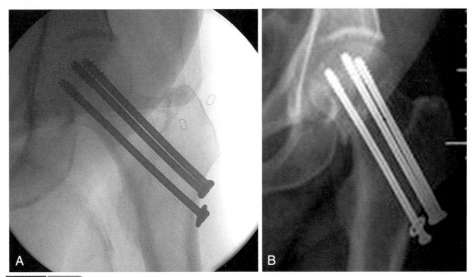

FIGURE 3.18 Significant femoral neck shortening after treatment of minimally displaced femoral neck fracture with partially threaded cannulated screws. **A,** Intraoperative fluoroscopic anteroposterior view. **B,** Anteroposterior radiograph revealing significant femoral neck shortening.

likelihood of dissociation of the blade from handle within the body.

- Through the lateral incision made for fixation with cannulated screws, compression hip screw, or proximal femoral locking plate, using tactile feel and fluoroscopic guidance, advance the scalpel along the anterior femoral neck with the blade directed inferiorly.
- Once the femoral head is encountered, rotate the blade 90 degrees and withdraw the scalpel with a posterior directed force to complete the capsulotomy.

Christal et al. showed in a cadaver series that fluoroscopically guided capsulotomy is safe and effective at decreasing intracapsular pressure. Dissections of the cadavers after capsulotomy found that the average distances from the femoral artery and lateral most branch of the femoral nerve were 40.3 and 19.5 mm, respectively. The minimal distances in individual cadavers were 36 mm from the femoral artery and 15 mm from the lateral most branch of the femoral nerve. Intracapsular pressure was substantially decreased after capsulotomy.

A meta-analysis of 106 reports of displaced femoral neck fractures in older patients (65 years or older) reported overall

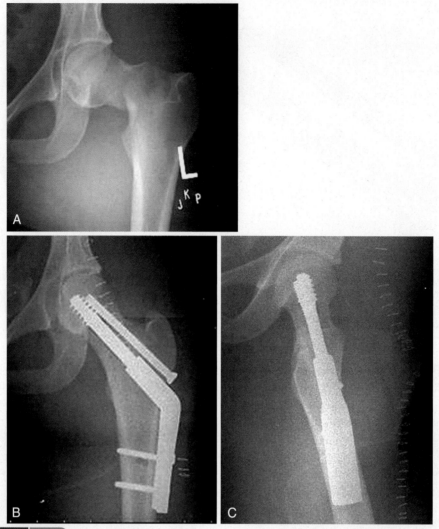

FIGURE 3.19 In an attempt to minimize femoral neck shortening, partially threaded screw used for compression is changed to fully threaded screw. **A,** Radiograph at time of injury. **B** and **C,** After operative reduction and fixation.

rates of osteonecrosis and nonunion of 16% and 33%, respectively. The rate of reoperation within 2 years ranged from 20% to 36% after internal fixation, which was higher than after hemiarthroplasty. Interestingly, a recent randomized controlled trial revealed a 20% major reoperation rate for *nondisplaced* femoral neck fractures treated with screws in patients 70 years of age or older. Although there was no difference in Harris Hip Scores between those treated with screws and those with hemiarthroplasty, patients with hemiarthroplasty were more mobile and had a lower rate of major reoperations.

ARTHROPLASTY

The decision to proceed with fixation or arthroplasty depends on fracture characteristics and physiologic patient age. Displaced femoral neck fractures in physiologic younger patients (<65 years of age) generally should be treated with anatomic reduction and stable internal fixation. Displaced femoral neck fractures in most older patients should be treated with arthroplasty. The role of arthroplasty for geriatric patients with nondisplaced femoral neck fractures deserves further exploration. A high-quality meta-analysis that included nine

randomized trials showed that arthroplasty substantially reduced the risk of revision surgery compared with internal fixation in the treatment of displaced femoral neck fractures in patients 65 years of age or older. Arthroplasty, however, was associated with greater blood loss, longer operative time, and more frequent infections. Hudson et al. found a higher rate of reoperation after internal fixation than after hemiarthroplasty in patients older than 80 years but did not find a difference in reoperation rates in patients between 65 and 80 years of age. In a randomized trial, Rogmark et al. compared internal fixation and arthroplasty for treatment of displaced femoral neck fractures in ambulatory patients aged 70 years or older. Failure, defined as early fracture displacement, nonunion, osteonecrosis with collapse, or infection, occurred in 43% of patients treated with internal fixation and in 6% of those treated with arthroplasty at 2 years. A follow-up study of the same cohort of patients at 10 years revealed that these results were stable over time: at no point in time did patients with successful internal fixation display better outcomes in regard to hip pain or mobility than did patients with successful arthroplasty. The American Academy of Orthopaedic

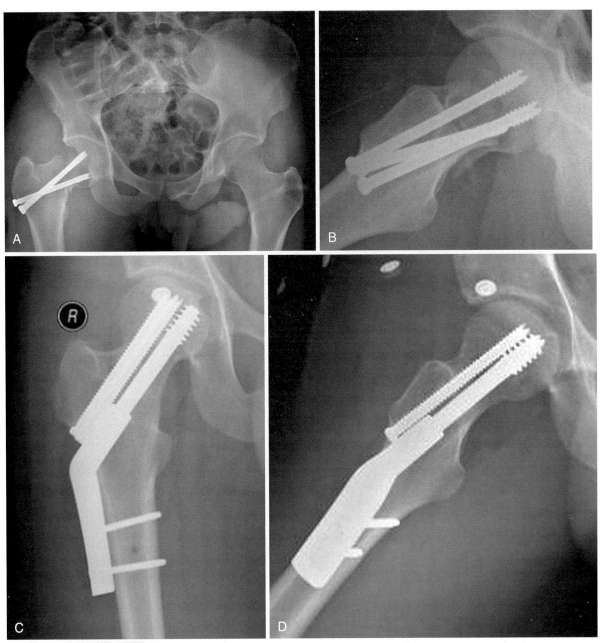

FIGURE 3.20   Malreduction of femoral neck fracture resulting in varus **(A)** and apex posterior **(B)** deformity. **C** and **D,** After revision open reduction and internal fixation.

Surgeons Clinical Practice Guideline for Management of Hip Fractures in the Elderly (2014) states "Strong evidence supports arthroplasty for patients with unstable (displaced) femoral neck fractures" (Table 3.1).

Once the decision has been made to proceed with arthroplasty, several controversial issues still need to be considered: type of arthroplasty (hemiarthroplasty or total hip arthroplasty [THA]), unipolar or bipolar (if hemiarthroplasty has been chosen), cemented or uncemented femoral stem, and surgical approach. Total hip arthroplasty is superior to hemiarthroplasty (Fig. 3.23) for displaced femoral neck fractures in active, physiologically older patients without significant comorbidities. Many studies have identified several potential benefits of THA over hemiarthroplasty, including superior functional outcome scores, decreased pain, improved ambulation, and

lower reoperation rates. A disadvantage of THA appears to be a slightly higher dislocation rate. A change in approach (direct anterior) may alleviate some of the dislocation concerns with THA. In community ambulators with a longer than 5-year life expectancy, THA generally is a better option than hemiarthroplasty. Those with a short life expectancy, significant medical comorbidities, or cognitive impairment are better served with hemiarthroplasty. If hemiarthroplasty is chosen, unipolar or bipolar heads appear to yield similar results. Moderate evidence appears to favor cemented over noncemented stems.

Interestingly, only 21% of respondents to a recent survey reported that the 2014 Clinical Practice Guidelines (CPG) led to changes in their practice. The two changes most frequently cited were increased use of THA and cemented stems. Not surprisingly, arthroplasty-trained surgeons were more likely

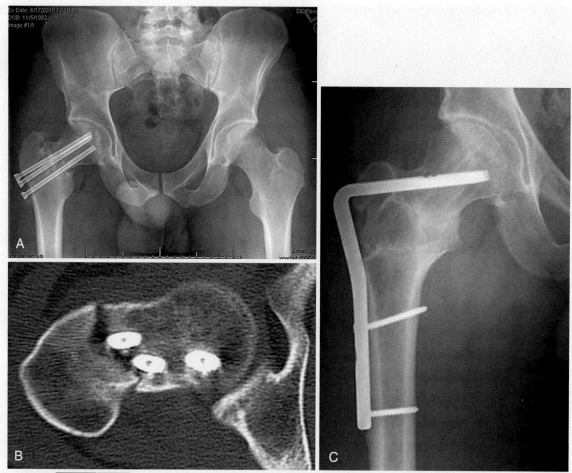

FIGURE 3.21 Nonunion of femoral neck fracture. Anteroposterior radiograph **(A)** and CT scan **(B)**. **C,** Union after fixation with blade plate. (Courtesy David Templeton MD, Minneapolis, MN.)

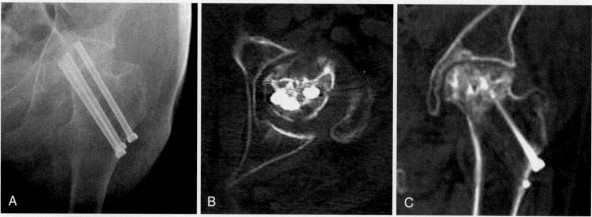

FIGURE 3.22 Osteonecrosis after treatment of femoral neck fracture: **(A)** anteroposterior radiograph, **(B)** axial CT scan, and **(C)** coronal CT scan.

than trauma-trained surgeons to use THA in the two femoral neck fracture examples contained in the survey.

Although the CPG highlight recommendations for geriatric fracture care, financial data suggest that arthroplasty rather than fixation should be considered for patients younger than 65 years. THA was found to be a cost-effective option for displaced femoral neck fractures in patients older than 54 years. The age at which THA was cost-effective decreased with increasing comorbidities. THA was cost-effective for patients older than 47 years with mild comorbidity (Charlson Comorbidity Index [CCI] 1 or 2) and for patients older than 44 years with multiple comorbidities (CCI ≥ 3). Complications are more frequent after THA for failed internal fixation than after THA for acute femoral neck fracture.

TABLE 3.1

American Academy of Orthopaedic Surgeons Clinical Practice Guideline for Management of Hip Fractures in the Elderly

FRACTURE/TREATMENT CONSIDERATION	RECOMMENDATION/COMMENT	STRENGTH OF RECOMMENDATION
Stable (nondisplaced) femoral neck fracture	Operative fixation	Moderate
Unstable (displaced) femoral neck fracture	Arthroplasty	Strong
Unipolar vs. bipolar	Similar outcomes in unstable (displaced) femoral neck fractures	Moderate
Hemi vs. total hip arthroplasty	Total hip arthroplasty more beneficial in properly selected patients with unstable (displaced) femoral neck fractures	Moderate
Cemented femoral stems	Cemented femoral stems preferred in arthroplasty for femoral neck fracture	Moderate
Surgical approach	Higher dislocation rates with posterior approach for arthroplasty in treatment of displaced femoral neck fractures	Moderate
Stable intertrochanteric fractures	Sliding hip screw or cephalomedullary device	Moderate
Subtrochanteric or reverse obliquity fractures	Cephalomedullary device	Strong

Moderate recommendation—evidence from two or more "moderate" strength studies with consistent findings, or evidence from a single "high" quality study for recommending for or against the intervention.
Strong recommendation—evidence from two or more "high" quality studies with consistent findings for recommending for or against the intervention.
Modified from https://www.aaos.org/CustomTemplates/Content.aspx?id=6395.

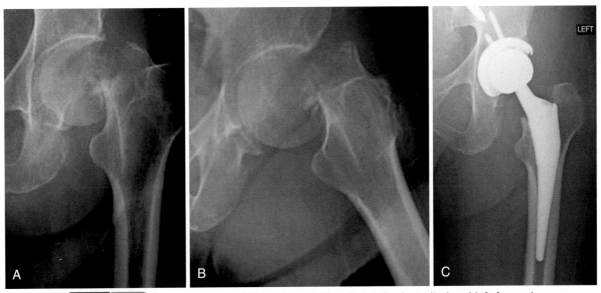

FIGURE 3.23 Anteroposterior **(A)** and lateral **(B)** radiographs show displaced left femoral neck fracture. **C,** After total hip arthroplasty.

BASICERVICAL FEMORAL NECK FRACTURES

Basicervical femoral neck fractures are extracapsular femoral neck fractures, and much controversy exists regarding their treatment. These fractures are rare, with some estimates as low as 1.6% of all hip fractures. They are often misclassified as well, sometimes being grouped with transcervical femoral neck fractures and other times with intertrochanteric femoral fractures. Su et al. showed that basicervical femoral neck fractures are more unstable than intertrochanteric femoral fractures. Both biomechanical and clinical studies have concluded that these fractures are not ideally treated with cannulated screws. Watson et al. reported failure in six of 11 patients with basicervical neck fractures treated with intramedullary nailing. Five of the six failures were associated with screw cut-out despite all six having a tip-apex distance less than 22 mm (mean, 17.4 mm). None of these patients had a derotational screw placed. Another study suggested better outcomes with intramedullary nailing than with a screw and side-plate device (SSP) for basicervical femoral neck fractures. Authors of a recent biomechanical study were unable to determine the optimal implant for basicervical femoral neck fractures. Different modes of failure were noted between intramedullary nails and SSP devices with a derotational screw. While all of the SSP failures involved screw cut-out, only one of 18 intramedullary nails failed with screw cut-out. Seventeen failed either rotationally or with medial trochanteric wall migration. The failure mode in this biomechanical study is obviously different from the failure mode outlined by Watson et al. Hopefully, future studies will evaluate intramedullary nails with an additional screw, either independent or part of the proximal interlocking mechanism. There also may be a role for arthroplasty in physiologically older patients with a basicervical femoral neck fracture.

INTERTROCHANTERIC FEMORAL FRACTURES
CLASSIFICATION

Many classifications of pertrochanteric and intertrochanteric femoral fractures have been proposed over the years. Boyd and Griffin initially described four types of pertrochanteric femoral fractures in 1949 (Fig. 3.24):

Type 1: Fractures that extend along the intertrochanteric line

Type 2: Comminuted fractures with the main fracture line along the intertrochanteric line but with multiple secondary fracture lines (may include coronal fracture line seen on lateral view)

Type 3: Fractures that extend to or are distal to the lesser trochanter

Type 4: Fractures of the trochanteric region and proximal shaft with fractures in at least two planes

Probably the most useful classification of intertrochanteric femoral fractures is the AO/OTA classification (Fig. 3.25):

31A1: Fractures are not comminuted (single fracture line extending medially).

31A2: Fractures have increasing comminution (separate lesser trochanteric fragment).

31A3: Fractures include reverse obliquity, transverse, or subtrochanteric extension patterns.

Each group contains subgroups to further describe the characteristics of each fracture. The AO/OTA classification has been very useful in evaluating the results of treatment of intertrochanteric femoral fractures and allowing comparisons among reports in the literature.

TREATMENT

Nonoperative treatment of intertrochanteric femoral fractures is rare but may still have a role in nonambulatory patients in whom adequate pain control can be achieved without surgery.

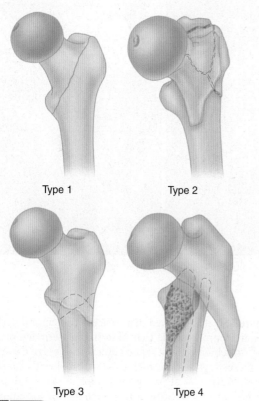

FIGURE 3.24 Boyd and Griffin classification of trochanteric fractures.

Type 1   Type 2

Type 3   Type 4

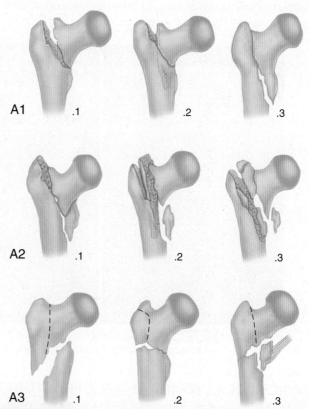

A1 .1 .2 .3

A2 .1 .2 .3

A3 .1 .2 .3

FIGURE 3.25 AO classification of trochanteric fractures. Group A1, simple two-part fracture; group A2, fracture extends over two or more levels of medial cortex; group A3, fracture extends through lateral cortex of femur distal to vastus ridge. (Redrawn from Müller ME, Nazarian S, Koch P, et al: *The comprehensive classification of fractures of long bones,* Berlin, 1990, Springer-Verlag.)

Internal fixation is appropriate for most intertrochanteric femoral fractures. Optimal fixation is based on the stability of the fracture. The mainstay of treatment of intertrochanteric femoral fractures is fixation with a SSP device (Fig. 3.26) or intramedullary device (Fig. 3.27).

■ TREATMENT WITH SCREW–SIDE PLATE DEVICES

Compression or dynamic hip screws are a good option for the treatment of stable intertrochanteric femoral fractures (AO/OTA 31A1 and many 31A2 fractures), particularly in patients with lower preinjury functional status. The implant cost is less with SSP than with intramedullary nails, and the technique of placement of a SSP is familiar to most experienced orthopaedic surgeons; however, orthopaedic surgeons who have completed their training more recently may not be as familiar with the procedure.

SCREW–SIDE PLATE FIXATION OF INTERTROCHANTERIC FEMORAL FRACTURES

TECHNIQUE 3.4

- Place the patient on a fracture table with a perineal post.
- Either place the foot of the contralateral lower extremity in a boot and scissor the leg (unaffected hip extended relative to the injured side) (Fig. 3.28) or use a well-leg holder.
- Place the affected extremity into a boot after the reduction maneuver has been carried out. Reduction of the affected extremity usually is done with traction and internal rotation. The typical sagittal plane deformity, posterior sag, may require correction with an anterior applied force to the posterior distal fragment before completing the reduction with traction and internal rotation.
- We typically place the affected extremity in 20 to 30 degrees of hip flexion.
- Position the fluoroscopy unit on the contralateral side or between the patient's legs depending on the position of the uninjured leg. Adequate fluoroscopy must be attainable before proceeding.
- Obtain fluoroscopy views in the sagittal and coronal planes. Make any necessary adjustments by increasing or decreasing traction or altering abduction/adduction and internal/external rotation. Carefully scrutinize the fluoroscopic images to avoid the most common malalignments: varus deformity, posterior sag, and excessive internal rotation. Be aware that excessive internal rotation is common, particularly when the greater trochanter is not attached to the distal segment.
- The fracture mechanism (low-energy and high-energy) should have already been noted, because standard reduction maneuvers are not likely to be successful with high-energy intertrochanteric femoral fractures (Fig. 3.29) and limited open reduction or more formal open reduction through a Watson-Jones approach will likely be required.

EXPOSURE

- Begin the incision at the vastus ridge and carry it distally. Continue dissection through the iliotibial band and split the fascia of the vastus lateralis longitudinally.
- Elevate the vastus lateralis anteriorly off the lateral intermuscular septum while coagulating branches of the profunda femoris artery as they are encountered.
- Complete the exposure by sharply incising the origin of the vastus lateralis to allow retraction and subsequent plate placement.

STABILIZATION

- Insert a guide pin through the angled guide into the center-center position within the femoral head (Fig. 3.30A). A guide pin can be placed anteriorly along the femoral neck to approximate the anteversion. Insert the guide pin to approximately 5 mm from the articular surface and measure (Fig. 3.30B).
- Set a triple reamer 5 mm less than the above measurement and ream (Fig. 3.30C). Be sure not to advance the guide pin into the pelvis when reaming. A tap may need to be used in patients with good bone quality (Fig. 3.30D).
- Select a lag screw that is the same length as the measurement from the triple reamer. If significant shortening is expected or desired, choose a lag screw that is 5 mm shorter than the measurement from the triple reamer. Ensure that the lag screw is sufficiently covered by not placing a lag screw any shorter than 5 mm less than the measurement from the triple reamer.
- Using the insertion wrench, insert the lag screw with the plate to the appropriate depth (Fig. 3.30E). Realize that 180 degrees of rotation of the lag screw results in 1.5 mm of lag screw advancement. When advancement is completed, the handle of the insertion wrench must be perpendicular to the axis of the femur and not the axis of the floor.
- Advance the side plate onto the lateral aspect of the femur. Use a tamp to fully seat the plate onto the lag screw (Fig. 3.30F). Unscrew the lag screw retaining rod and remove the insertion wrench and then the guide pin.
- Secure the plate to bone with a screw or a plate clamp (Fig. 3.30G). Place two to three bicortical screws in total into the shaft, typically through a two-hole to four-hole plate (Fig. 3.30H). If a screw is used to reduce the plate to the bone, the initial screw may need to be changed because of excessive length.
- Release traction and insert a compression screw if desired (Fig. 3.30I); alternatively, apply manual compression. Obtain fluoroscopic images to evaluate reduction and hardware placement.

POSTOPERATIVE CARE Patients with intertrochanteric femoral fractures treated with a compression hip screw are allowed to bear weight as tolerated in most circumstances because this device is used in more stable fracture patterns.

Proper placement of the lag screw is important in reducing the incidence of implant failure (cut-out). The tip-apex distance (Fig. 3.31) is calculated from the sum of the distances

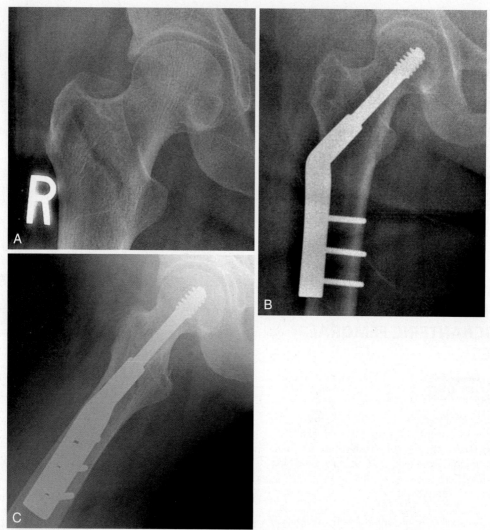

FIGURE 3.26 Fixation of intertrochanteric fracture with compression hip screw. **A,** Preoperative anteroposterior radiograph. **B** and **C,** After fixation.

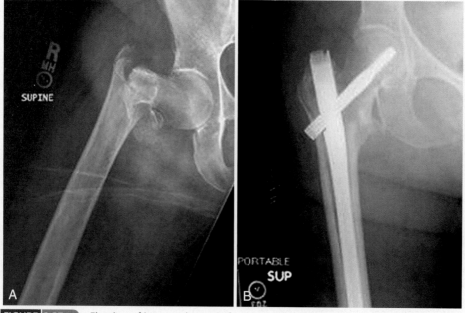

FIGURE 3.27 Fixation of intertrochanteric fracture with Gamma nail. **A,** Preoperative radiograph. **B,** After fixation.

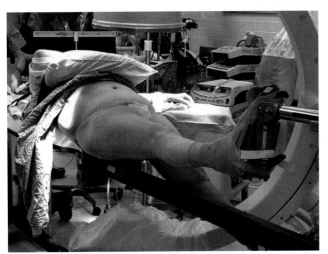

FIGURE 3.28 "Scissor" position for compression hip screw fixation of intertrochanteric femoral fracture. **SEE TECHNIQUE 3.4.**

between the tip of the lag screw to the apex of the femoral head on both the anteroposterior and lateral views. As the tip-apex distance increases above 25 mm, the risk of failure increases exponentially (Fig. 3.32). This recommendation for tip-apex distance may not apply when a helical blade is used in place of a lag screw; medial helical blade migration has been reported with tip-apex distances of less than 20 mm.

Integrity of the lateral wall of the trochanter is another consideration when treating intertrochanteric femoral fractures with a compression hip screw device. In a series of intertrochanteric femoral fractures treated with compression hip screws, 22% of patients with a fractured lateral wall (A3 fractures or iatrogenic fractures in A1 and A2 fractures) required a second operation within 6 months; 74% of the lateral wall fractures occurred intraoperatively (A1 and A2 fractures). Interestingly, only 3% of patients with A1.1, A1.2, A1.3, and A2.1 fractures had intraoperative fractures of the lateral wall, whereas 31% of patients with A2.2 and A2.3 fractures had such fractures. In another study evaluating factors associated

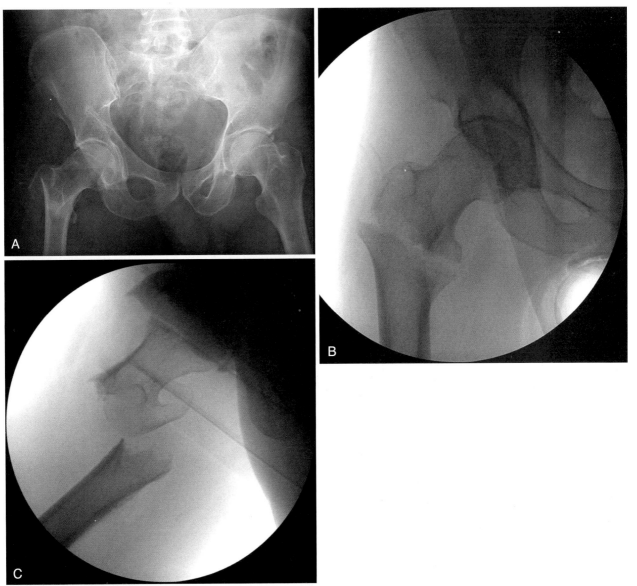

FIGURE 3.29 High-energy intertrochanteric fracture. **A,** Preoperative radiograph. **B** and **C,** Intraoperative fluoroscopic views. **SEE TECHNIQUE 3.4.**

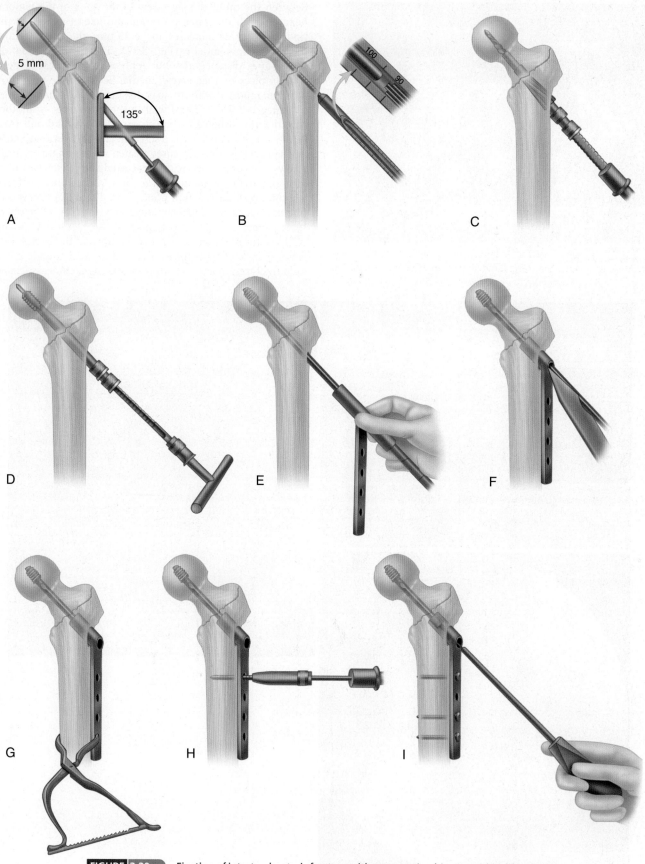

FIGURE 3.30 Fixation of intertrochanteric fracture with compression hip screw. (Modified from Baumgaertner MR: *Compression hip screw plates: technique manual,* Memphis, 2000, Smith & Nephew.)
SEE TECHNIQUE 3.4.

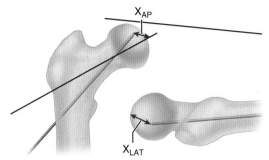

FIGURE 3.31 Calculation of tip-apex distance (TAD). Distances from tip of implant to apex of femoral head on anteroposterior *(left)* and lateral *(right)* views are summed ($X_{AP} + X_{Lat}$). TAD of less than 25 mm should be achieved. (Redrawn from Powell J, Dirschl DR: Fractures of the proximal femur. In Baumgaertner MR, Tornetta P, editors: *OKU Trauma 3, Rosemont, American Academy of Orthopaedic Surgeons,* 2005; and Lindskog DM, Baumgaertner MR: Unstable intertrochanteric hip fractures in the elderly, *J Am Acad Orthop Surg* 12:179, 2004.)

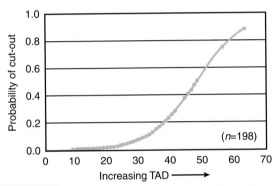

FIGURE 3.32 Tip-apex distance (TAD) graph. (Redrawn from Baumgaertner MR, Curtin SL, Lindskog DM, Keggi JM: The value of the tip-apex distance in predicting failure of fixation of peritrochanteric fractures of the hip, *J Bone Joint Surg* 77A:1058, 1995.)

with failure in the treatment of stable (31A1) intertrochanteric femoral fractures with compression hip screws, Kim et al. identified iatrogenic lateral wall comminution as the most significant predictor of excessive displacement and suggested using a trochanteric stabilizing plate (Fig. 3.33) or proceeding with a different fixation device (intramedullary nail) if iatrogenic comminution is identified intraoperatively. These studies suggest caution in using a compression hip screw for fractures more complex than A2.1 and that the lateral wall must be carefully evaluated when a compression hip screw is considered for more stable fracture patterns. More recently, Pradeep et al. suggested using lateral wall thickness to predict lateral wall fracture. Lateral wall thickness was defined as the distance between a point 3 cm caudal to the innominate tubercle of the greater trochanter extending 135 degrees to the fracture line. Lateral wall thickness of less than 21 mm predicted lateral wall fracture with 95% sensitivity and 88.2% specificity. Interestingly, lateral wall fracture also appears to be a risk factor for cut-out with intramedullary nail treatment (Fig. 3.34).

Another device purported to decrease the risk of lateral wall fracture is the Gottfried plate (percutaneous compression plate), which is fixed with two screws placed percutaneously into the femoral neck and head. The two screws provide intraoperative compression but also allow dynamic compression as the patient ambulates. The first published results of this plate included 97 intertrochanteric femoral fractures (21 A1, 18 A2.1, and 58 A2.2 fractures) in which few complications were reported. Two randomized trials have compared the percutaneous compression plate with the compression hip screw; both reported decreased intraoperative blood loss, and one reported decreased operative time as well. At 6 weeks, patients treated with the percutaneous compression plate had significantly less pain and could bear significantly more weight on the injured extremity than those treated with a compression screw device. They also had less pain with activity at all time points, but this difference was significant only at 3 months. Other potential benefits of the percutaneous compression plate include a lower risk of lateral wall fracture and improved rotational stability. Carvajal-Pedrosa et al. reported satisfactory results in almost 300 31A2 fractures treated with the percutaneous compression plates. We have no experience with this technique.

■ TREATMENT WITH INTRAMEDULLARY NAILS

Unstable intertrochanteric femoral fractures (A3 and probably many A2 fractures) are best treated with an intramedullary implant. For some time, second-generation cephalomedullary devices such as the Gamma nail have been used with success. The theoretical benefits of intramedullary nails over SSP devices include improved biomechanics (shortened lever arm), decreased blood loss, smaller incisions, and decreased femoral neck shortening. The largest meta-analysis comparing intramedullary nails with side-plate devices from the Cochrane database concluded that side plates are superior to intramedullary nails in the treatment of intertrochanteric femoral fractures. This meta-analysis, however, included older versions of cephalomedullary nails, which had problems with fracture at the distal tip of the nail. Although this complication does still occur, it is much less frequent with newer nail designs.

INTRAMEDULLARY NAILING OF INTERTROCHANTERIC FEMORAL FRACTURES

TECHNIQUE 3.5

PATIENT POSITIONING

■ Patient positioning is similar to that described in Technique 3.4. We generally prefer to place the patient supine, but the lateral position may be beneficial with certain fracture patterns and with morbidly obese patients.

■ Place the patient on a fracture table with a perineal post.

■ Place the contralateral lower extremity in a boot and scissor the leg (hip extended relative to contralateral side).

- Place the affected extremity into a boot after the reduction maneuver has been carried out (see Technique 3.4). We typically place the affected extremity in 20 to 30 degrees of hip flexion.
- Adduct the patient's torso and secure the ipsilateral arm over the patient's chest.
- Position the fluoroscopy unit on the contralateral side. Adequate fluoroscopy must be attainable before proceeding.
- Obtain fluoroscopy views in the sagittal and coronal planes. Make any necessary adjustments by increasing or decreasing traction or altering abduction/adduction and internal/external rotation. Carefully scrutinize the fluoroscopic images to avoid the most common malalignments: varus deformity, posterior sag, and excessive internal rotation. Be aware that excessive internal rotation is common, particularly when the greater trochanter is not attached to the distal segment.

ENTRY PORTAL

- For fixation of intertrochanteric femoral fractures, as well as many other fractures of the femur, we use a modified medial trochanteric portal (Fig. 3.35). The modified medial trochanteric portal is located on the medial aspect of the greater trochanter along the trochanteric ridge on the anteroposterior view and in line with the femoral shaft on the lateral view. A cadaver study found no damage to the gluteus medius tendon with this portal, which may be associated with less abductor weakness than the standard trochanteric portal.
- Make an approximately 3-cm incision, beginning 3 cm proximal to the tip of the greater trochanter and extending proximally (this incision may need to be extended depending on the body habitus of the patient).
- Incise the aponeurosis of the gluteus maximus.
- Localize a guide pin on the medial aspect of the greater trochanter (modified medial trochanteric portal). Insert the guide pin 2 to 3 cm distally into the proximal fragment. At this point use fluoroscopy to assess the guide pin placement in both planes. Make any corrections of the guide pin with a two-pin technique and a honeycomb type guide. We believe that the use of a two-pin technique saves significant fluoroscopic time in the operating room.
- Use the proximal reamer to ream over the guide pin to a depth just below the level of the lesser trochanter. Correct any malreduction before reaming.
- Place the ball-tip guide pin down the shaft of the femur to the physeal scar and measure the guide pin to determine the appropriate length of the intramedullary nail.
- We typically use a 10-mm diameter nail for intertrochanteric femoral fractures. We believe there is no significant benefit to placing a larger diameter nail in most situations and that placing a larger nail may increase the risk of anterior cortical perforation.
- Ream to a diameter 1.5 mm larger than the diameter of the intramedullary nail. Pay careful attention to the anterior bow of the femur and, if necessary, ream 2 mm larger than the nail diameter.
- After selecting the appropriate nail angle, length, and diameter, assemble the nail and drill guide. We generally choose a 130-degree nail because nails with less than the native neck-shaft angle (NSA) have been associated with

varus malreductions (contralateral fluoroscopic evaluation allows estimation of NSA). Ciufu et al. identified neck-shaft malreduction as a predictor of nail cut-out.
- Insert the nail with the guide facing anteriorly to use the bow of the nail to make insertion easier. Rotate the guide laterally after the nail has been inserted approximately halfway down the intramedullary canal. During nail placement, evaluate its placement with lateral fluoroscopically to avoid anterior cortical perforation.
- Insert the nail to a depth that allows center-center positioning in the femoral head with the lag screw. Remove the ball-tipped guide pin.
- Evaluate version of the nail on the lateral fluoroscopic view; version is correct when the nail, guide, and femoral neck and head are all aligned.
- Make a small incision laterally through the skin and fascia and place the appropriate drill sleeve into the lateral aspect of the femur.
- Advance a guide pin to within 5 mm of subchondral bone. Confirm appropriate center-center position in the femoral head.
- Measure for the length of the lag screw.
- Ream for lag screw.
- Use a tap if the patient does not have osteoporotic bone.
- Insert the lag screw. If compression is desired with a Gamma nail, turn the thumbwheel of the Gamma lag screw driver clockwise against the lag screw guide sleeve. The lag screw guide sleeve must be unlocked (knob of target device must be turned counterclockwise). Place the set screw.
- See specific technique guide if an intramedullary nail with a helical blade is selected.
- Place distal interlocking screws as desired.

POSTOPERATIVE CARE Patients with intertrochanteric femoral fractures treated with an intramedullary device are allowed to bear weight as tolerated in most circumstances; however, this device may be used in more unstable fracture patterns and occasionally weight-bearing status needs to be modified based on these fracture patterns.

SHORT OR LONG NAILS FOR INTERTROCHANTERIC FEMORAL FRACTURES

Both short and long nails are options for 31A1 and most 31A2 intertrochanteric femoral fractures. Two recent systematic reviews revealed slightly longer operative times (13 to 19 minutes), increased blood loss (37 to 39 mL), and increased transfusion rates with long intramedullary nails. Neither study demonstrated a statistically significant difference in periimplant femoral fracture rate, with both studies having overall fracture rates of less than 2%. However, implant-specific periimplant fracture rates may exist and should be considered when such data are available. Fractures do appear to increase with time and generally are associated with nails that are not interlocked distally.

PLATE FIXATION COMPARED WITH INTRAMEDULLARY NAIL FIXATION

The decision to use a compression hip screw or an intramedullary nail is multifactorial and is based on surgeon training and preference, cost, and patient and fracture

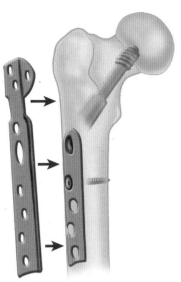

FIGURE 3.33 Trochanteric stabilizing plate can be used as adjunct to compression hip screw and side plate fixation. (Redrawn from Synthes [USA]: Trochanter stabilization plate for DHS: technique guide, Paoli, 2000, Synthes.)

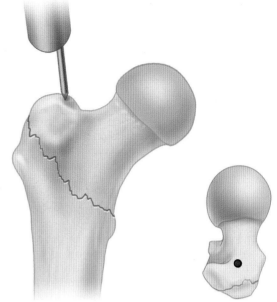

FIGURE 3.35 Modified medial trochanteric portal. **SEE TECHNIQUE 3.5.**

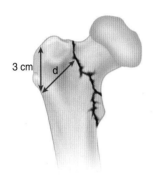

3 cm   d

FIGURE 3.34 Diagram showing lateral wall thickness (*d*) defined as the distance in millimeters from a reference point 3 cm below innominate tubercle of the greater trochanter, angled 135 degrees upwards to the fracture line of the distal fragment on an anteroposterior radiograph. (Redrawn from Pradeep AR, KiranKumar A, Dheenadhayalan J, et al: Intraoperative lateral fractures during dynamic hip screw fixation for intertrochanteric fractures. Incidence, causative factors and clinical outcome, *Injury* 49:334, 2018.)

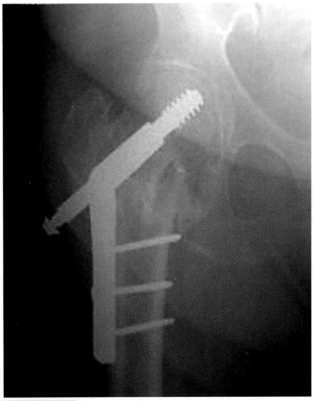

FIGURE 3.36 Significant shortening (malunion) after treatment of intertrochanteric fracture with compression hip screw.

characteristics. Proponents of intramedullary nail fixation argue that less shortening occurs with an intramedullary nail than with a compression hip screw (Fig. 3.36). Minimal shortening (mean 5.9 mm) was found at union in a series of intertrochanteric femoral fractures considered "stable" and treated with a compression hip screw; similar shortening (5.3 mm) was found in "unstable" fractures treated with intramedullary nailing. The purpose of the study was not to compare shortening in stable and unstable fractures treated with different devices, but to show that experienced surgeons can identify stable intertrochanteric femoral fractures and that these stable intertrochanteric femoral fractures can be treated with a compression hip screw with minimal shortening. In femoral neck fractures, a correlation has been identified between femoral neck length (shortening)

and decreased functional outcome, and the same correlation may exist with intertrochanteric femoral fractures. Although more shortening does occur with the use of compression hip screws, the amount of shortening that is functionally relevant has not been well defined. Shortening does appear to affect gait, as Gausden et al. demonstrated with gait analysis; a correlation was found between shortening after intertrochanteric femoral fractures and decreased cadence, increased double support time, decreased step length, and increased single support asymmetry.

There is some evidence in the literature that the functional outcomes in patients with certain fracture types may be influenced by the choice of implant. In a randomized trial by Utrilla et al., there was no overall difference in functional outcomes in patients 65 years of age or older with an intertrochanteric femoral fracture treated with either a Gamma nail or a compression hip screw; however, when patients with unstable fracture patterns were analyzed, those with an intramedullary nail had better walking ability at 12 months than those treated with a compression hip screw. Pajarinen et al. compared outcomes of proximal femoral nailing with compression hip screw fixation in the treatment of AO/OTA 31A fractures. At 4 months after surgery a much larger percentage of patients (76%) treated with intramedullary nail fixation had returned to their preinjury walking ability than patients treated with compression hip screws (54%). The mean shortening of the femoral neck also was much less in patients treated with intramedullary nail fixation (1.3 mm) than in those with compression hip screws (6.1 mm).

A randomized controlled trial by Parker demonstrated improved mobility at 8 weeks, 3 months, and 6 months after surgery with intramedullary nailing compared to placement of a SSP device. No other clinically significant differences were found between groups. The 400 patients in this study were then combined with an additional 600 patients from a separate randomized controlled trial with the goal of analyzing the three different OTA/AO fracture subdivisions (A1, A2, A3). There were no differences in peri-implant

fracture (0.8% in both groups) or any other fracture-related complications. The author reported a "consistent finding of superior regaining of mobility for those treated with the intramedullary nail with A1 and A2 fractures." One year after treatment of 538 A2 and A3 fractures, Bretherton et al. noted greater medialization in those treated with SSP than in those with intramedullary nailing. Patients with more than 50% medialization had worse pain and mobility scores at 1 year.

A unique intramedullary device (InterTAN, Smith & Nephew, Memphis, TN) (Fig. 3.37) uses two integrated proximal interlocking screws that allow linear intraoperative compression. The nail's geometry and integrated proximal interlocking at least theoretically improve rotational stability in the proximal segment. The first series of patients treated with this nail, reported by Ruecker et al., included 100 patients (32 AO/OTA A1-1 fractures, 54 A2.1-3 fractures, and 14 reverse obliquity fractures), with 48 patients available for follow-up at 1 year. No malunions or nonunions occurred, 73% of fractures had no postoperative shortening, 27% had shortening of less than 5 mm, and 58% of patients had returned to their pre-fracture functional status at 1-year follow-up. Although there were no femoral fractures reported in this study, fracture distal to the tip of the nail has been reported by others, primarily with the use of short nails. Theoretical benefits of this device are promising, and we have used it for unstable intertrochanteric femoral fractures with good results. Matre et al. reported a large randomized trial comparing the InterTAN nail (Smith & Nephew, Memphis, TN) with the sliding hip screw. Unfortunately, the patient group was very heterogeneous and 42% of fractures were stable OTA-AO 31A1 fractures. Only 20% of fractures were unstable OTA-AO 31A3 fractures. A

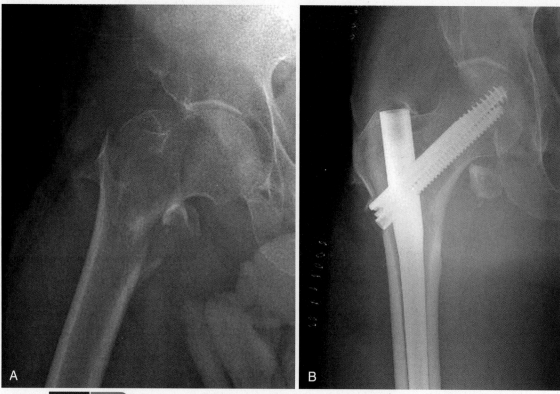

FIGURE 3.37 InterTAN device uses two integrated proximal interlocking screws that allow linear compression intraoperatively. **A,** Preoperative radiograph. **B,** After fixation.

trochanteric buttress plate was used for all A3 fractures and "considered" for A1 and A2 fractures with osteoporotic bone. Outcomes were similar between the two groups with a small, questionably clinically significant, benefit in pain with early mobilization in patients treated with the InterTAN. According to the authors, the addition of the trochanteric buttress plate did not prevent excessive medialization, which was associated with postoperative pain.

In a randomized controlled trial, Sanders et al. compared the InterTAN to SSP for fixation of 249 A1 and A2 fractures and found no difference in primary outcomes (Functional Independence Measure [FIM] and Timed Up and Go [TUG] test). They did find significantly less shortening in those treated with InterTAN fixation. Subgroup analysis demonstrated that patients who could mobilize independently before injury and had an unstable fracture (31A-2) had less shortening and improved FIM and TUG scores after treatment with the InterTAN compared to SSP. Biomechanical studies support integrated two-screw proximal locking. Clinically, there may be a benefit to integrated two-screw proximal locking for intramedullary nails in the treatment of intertrochanteric femoral fractures; however, large, high-quality, comparative studies are still lacking.

INTRAMEDULLARY NAILING OF INTERTROCHANTERIC FEMORAL FRACTURES WITH INTEGRATED PROXIMAL INTERLOCKING SCREWS (INTERTAN)

TECHNIQUE 3.6

- Patient positioning, reduction, and establishment of the entry portal are as described for intramedullary nailing of intertrochanteric femoral fractures (see Technique 3.5).
- Once the guide pin has been localized under fluoroscopy, introduce the 12.5-mm entry reamer/16-mm channel reamer combination through the soft-tissue guide (entry portal tube) over the guide pin. Insert the channel reamer to the level of the lesser trochanter (positive stop on the entry portal tube) (Fig. 3.38A). We usually use a long InterTAN and remove the entry reamer and guide pin at this time, leaving the channel reamer in place.
- Introduce the ball-tipped guide pin or the reducer and then the guide pin and advance it to the level of the physeal scar.
- Measure for the length of the intramedullary nail.
- If necessary, ream sequentially to a diameter 1.5 mm larger than the nail to be used (Fig. 3.38B). We typically use a 10-mm diameter nail for intertrochanteric femoral fractures and ream sequentially to 11.5 mm.
- Assemble the nail and advance it into the femur. As with all antegrade femoral nails inserted through a trochanteric or modified medial trochanteric portal, place the nail with the guide facing anteriorly to use the bow of the nail

to make insertion easier (Fig. 3.38C). Rotate the guide laterally after the nail has been inserted approximately halfway down the intramedullary canal. Monitor insertion of the nail with lateral fluoroscopy to avoid anterior cortical perforation.
- Before seating the nail completely, evaluate anteversion with lateral fluoroscopy and rotate the nail to make sure that the wire within the insertion handle transects the nail and femoral head/neck.
- Confirm appropriate nail depth with the alignment arm and fluoroscopy in the anteroposterior plane.
- Remove the ball-tipped guide pin.
- Make a small incision laterally through the skin and fascia and place the appropriate drill sleeve on the lateral aspect of the femur (Fig. 3.38D).
- Place two integrated proximal interlocking screws. Use the 4.0-mm drill to create a pilot hole for the 3.2-mm guide pin and place the guide pin in the center-center position within the femoral head to within 5 mm of subchondral bone (Fig. 3.38E). Measure for the length of the lag screw, subtracting 5 to 10 mm from the length of the pin depending on the amount of compression desired.
- Use the 7.0-mm compression screw starter drill and then the 7.0-mm compression screw drill inferior to the guide pin to drill for the derotational bar and subsequent compression screw (Fig. 3.38F), and place the derotation bar.
- Use the 10.5-mm drill to drill over the 3.2-mm guide pin (Fig. 3.38G) and insert the appropriate-length lag screw (Fig. 3.38H).
- Remove the derotation bar and insert the integrated compression screw (Fig. 3.38I). Relax traction before completely compressing the fracture.
- Remove the drill guide handle and engage the set screw proximally if desired.
- Insert a distal screw or screws for dynamic or static locking if desired.

POSTOPERATIVE CARE Patients with intertrochanteric femoral fractures treated with an InterTAN device are allowed to bear weight as tolerated in most circumstances; however, this device may be used in more unstable fracture patterns, and occasionally weight bearing needs to be modified based on the fracture patterns.

Regardless of implant selected, malrotation appears to be frequent with intertrochanteric femoral fractures. Ramanoudjame et al. found malrotation of more than 15 degrees in 16 (40%) of 40 fractures on postoperative CT scans; 14 of these were excessively internally rotated. Studies have shown that neutral rotation or internal rotation is most often necessary for appropriate reduction; however, external rotation may be necessary if the greater trochanter is not part of the distal segment. Although some malrotation, particularly in younger patients with femoral shaft fractures, may be fairly well compensated, similar compensation may not occur in geriatric patients. Interestingly, retroversion of the proximal femur has been found to be fairly common in the general population, present in up to 21% of Caucasian males; retroversion of more than 10 degrees was found in approximately 6% of African Americans. The method

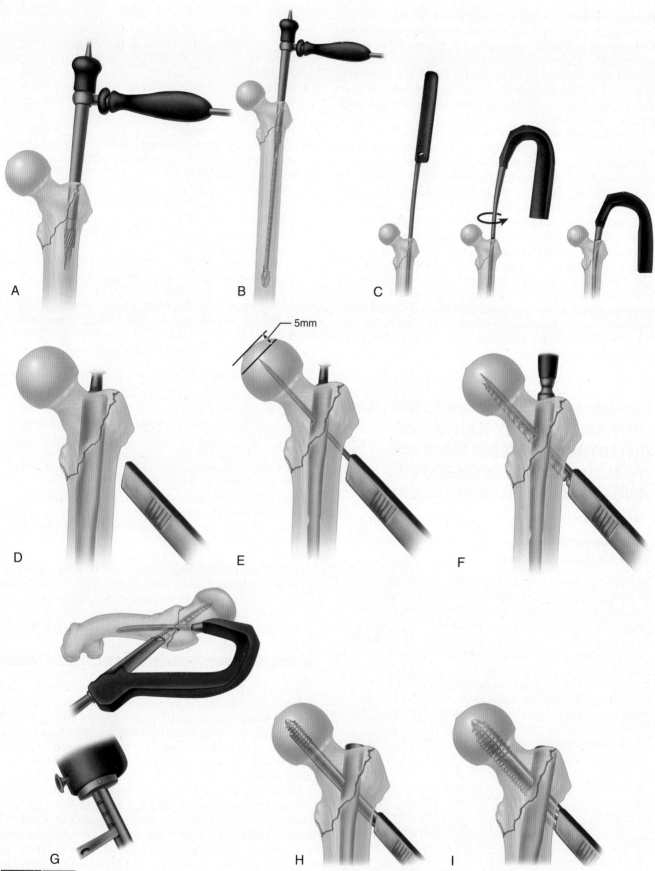

FIGURE 3.38   Fixation of intertrochanteric fracture with InterTAN. **A,** Insertion of entry reamer/channel reamer to level of lesser trochanter. **B,** Sequential reaming through channel reamer. **C,** Placement of nail beginning with guide facing anteriorly. **D,** Insertion of drill sleeve through small incision. **E,** Placement of guide pin in center-center position in femoral head. **F,** Drilling for derotational bar and subsequent compression screw. **G,** Drilling for lag screw with derotational bar in place. **H,** Insertion of lag screw. **I,** Insertion of integrated compression screw.   (Modified from Ruecker AH, Russell TA, Sanders RW, Tornetta P: *TRIGEN InterTAN: surgical technique*, Memphis, 2006, Smith & Nephew.) **SEE TECHNIQUE 3.6.**

of calculating the version of the uninjured side initially described by Tornetta for femoral shaft fractures also can be used for intertrochanteric femoral fractures. The version of the contralateral, uninjured side is calculated by obtaining a true lateral image of the hip and knee. The difference between the values at the hip and knee is the version. This value can then be used as a template for the injured side. The only real drawback to this method is time, adding approximately 15 minutes to the procedure. This method therefore may not be ideal for the sickest of patients for whom operating room time should be minimized.

SUBTROCHANTERIC FEMORAL FRACTURES

Fractures occurring in the area between the lesser trochanter and the isthmus of the femoral canal are considered subtrochanteric fractures. These fractures also have been described as those occurring within the first 5 cm distal to the lesser trochanter. Initially described by Boyd and Griffin as a variant of peritrochanteric femoral fractures with a high incidence of unsatisfactory results, treatment of these fractures continues to be a challenge.

CLASSIFICATION

Many classifications have been described since that of Boyd and Griffin in 1949, but none has been proven to be superior to any other. The Russell-Taylor classification (Fig. 3.39) considers the integrity of the lesser trochanter and extension of fracture lines into the piriformis fossa.

Type I: Fractures do not extend into the piriformis fossa.
    IA: Lesser trochanter is intact.
    IB: Lesser trochanter is not intact.
Type II: Fractures extend into the piriformis fossa.
    IIA: Lesser trochanter is intact.
    IIB: Lesser trochanter is not intact.

This classification is descriptive and still guides treatment, albeit to a lesser degree than it once may have because of advances in intramedullary nailing implants and techniques. Reverse obliquity fractures often are considered Russell-Taylor IB subtrochanteric femoral fractures based on their behavior.

TREATMENT

The mainstay of treatment for subtrochanteric femoral fractures is intramedullary nailing. Evidence exists that intramedullary implants are superior to extramedullary implants in the treatment of most fractures in this difficult region. Certainly, there are circumstances in which blade plates and proximal femoral locking plates are useful, and we occasionally use both of these devices.

■ INTRAMEDULLARY NAILING

Understanding the deforming forces (Fig. 3.40) is extremely important in avoiding the typical malalignments and malunions associated with subtrochanteric femoral fractures. The proximal fragment is affected by the pull of the abductors, external rotators, and iliopsoas. The distal fragment is affected by the pull of the adductors. The results of these muscle insertions include abduction, external rotation, and flexion of the proximal fragment and medialization of the distal fragment. More proximal subtrochanteric femoral fractures are influenced to a much greater degree by these deforming forces than subtrochanteric femoral fractures that occur farther from the lesser trochanter. The overall pull of the quadriceps and hamstrings results in shortening of the extremity. The integrity of the lesser trochanter also affects deforming forces, and subtrochanteric femoral fractures that involve the lesser trochanter may not be affected by the iliopsoas and therefore experience less flexion and external rotation.

The choice of positioning also can be influenced by the characteristics of the fracture. Intramedullary nailing of subtrochanteric femoral fractures can be done with the patient in a supine or lateral position. We prefer the supine position with a modified medial trochanteric portal for most subtrochanteric femoral fractures, and we reserve the lateral position for obese patients. A lateral starting point will result in varus malalignment with resultant increased nonunion risk. We typically use a fracture table, but a free-hand technique also can be effective if an adequate number of assistants are available. We typically use a nailing system that allows standard proximal interlocking as well as locking in reconstruction mode (two cephalomedullary screws). Russell-Taylor IB, IIA, and IIB fractures are proximally locked in reconstruction mode. Russell-Taylor IA fractures can be locked in standard or reconstruction mode (Fig. 3.41); however, for IA fractures closer to the lesser trochanter we tend to proximally interlock the nail in reconstruction mode. Patients without adequate bone stock in the femoral head may be treated with a Gamma nail type device or InterTAN. These nails also may be more appropriate for subtrochanteric femoral fractures in geriatric patients because they more closely match the radius of curvature of the femur.

We also advocate "trajectory control" (Fig. 3.42) in the treatment of subtrochanteric femoral fractures. Trajectory control involves precise establishment of the proximal nail portal under fluoroscopic guidance (Fig. 3.42A), obtaining anterior and lateral cortical support, and reaming through a channel (Channel Reamer, Smith & Nephew, Memphis, TN) (Fig. 3.42B), which we believe results in less eccentric reaming and less malalignment. A retrospective study revealed much less malalignment after the concept of "trajectory control" was implemented and a channel reamer was used routinely in the treatment of subtrochanteric femoral fractures.

INTRAMEDULLARY NAILING IN RECONSTRUCTION MODE

TECHNIQUE 3.7

- Place the patient supine (or lateral) on a fracture table, with the injured extremity in traction through a skeletal traction pin or boot and the hip flexed 30 to 40 degrees (Fig. 3.43A).
- Use fluoroscopy to determine appropriate version. This determination can be made by the Tornetta method described earlier. Alternatively, if the fracture does not involve the lesser trochanter (distal to the lesser trochanter), the profile of the lesser trochanter relative to the knee can

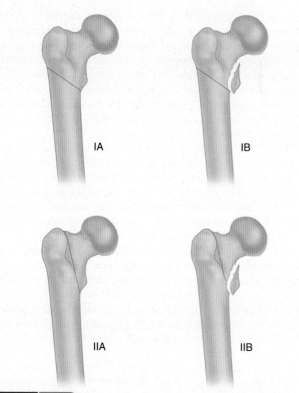

FIGURE 3.39 Russell-Taylor classification of subtrochanteric femoral fractures.

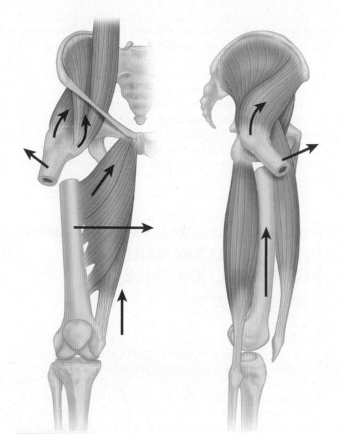

FIGURE 3.40 Deforming forces acting on subtrochanteric femoral fracture.

be compared with the contralateral side. This method has been shown to be fairly sensitive in detecting rotational abnormalities. A side-to-side difference of 20% in the size of the lesser trochanter correlates to approximately 15 degrees of rotational difference.

- After making an incision (Fig. 3.43B), place a guide pin on the proximal femur in a position to proceed with a modified medial trochanteric portal (or piriformis fossa portal) and insert the guide pin (Fig. 3.43C). If localization of the guide pin is difficult because of abduction, flexion, and external rotation of the proximal fragment, enlarge the proposed lateral incision for placement of reconstruction screws and introduce a large bone-holding forceps to correct the proximal segment deformity and simplify guide pin placement.

- If a piriformis nail is used, the guide pin must be "cheated" approximately 5 mm anteriorly on the lateral view to allow placement of the two cephalomedullary screws.

- Correct the typical deformities of the proximal segment and hold them corrected before reaming the proximal segment. Correct any residual abduction and flexion with a combination of ball spike pusher and elevator (Fig. 3.44). Alternatively, place a clamp through the same incision that will be used for insertion of the cephalomedullary screws. If instability persists after clamp removal, a cerclage wire can be used to hold the deformities corrected (Fig. 3.45).

- Use the combination entry reamer/channel reamer (Fig. 3.43D) to ream the proximal femur (Fig. 3.43E), avoiding eccentric reaming.

- Use the reduction tool (Fig. 3.43F) to aid with fracture reduction.

- Insert the ball-tipped guide rod across fracture (Fig. 3.43H).

- Measure for length of the intramedullary nail (Fig. 3.43I).

- Ream the femoral shaft sequentially through the channel reamer (Fig. 3.43J).

- Place the appropriate-size intramedullary nail and, in most patients, lock it proximally in reconstruction mode (Fig. 3.43K).

- Drill a hole for the most distal of the cephalomedullary screws first, just above the calcar. Leave the drill bit in place while drilling for the second screw and also leave this drill bit in place. Place the distal screw first and then the more proximal screw, placing both screws in the center of the femoral head on the lateral view.

- Lock the nail distally with a free-hand technique (see Technique 2.29).

- Check rotation for any external or internal rotational malalignments. Move the hip through a range of motion at 90 degrees of flexion and compare this range of motion to the contralateral side. A significant side-to-side difference can be corrected by removing the distal interlocking screws, correcting the rotation, and then relocking the nail.

See also Video 3.1.

POSTOPERATIVE CARE Patients with subtrochanteric femoral fractures treated with an intramedullary device typically are allowed touch-down weight bearing for the first 6 weeks and advanced based on healing as shown on follow-up radiographs.

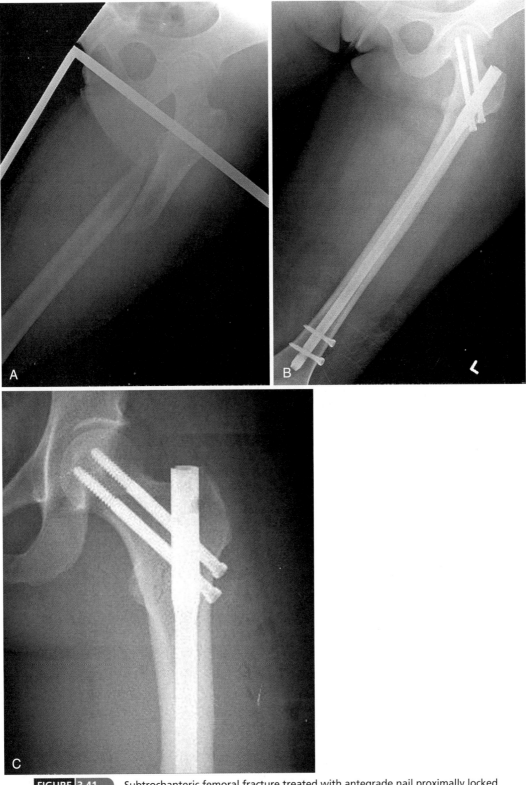

FIGURE 3.41 Subtrochanteric femoral fracture treated with antegrade nail proximally locked in reconstruction mode. **A,** Preoperative radiograph. **B** and **C,** After fixation with intramedullary nail.

A common error in nailing of subtrochanteric femoral fractures is a lateral starting portal, which will lead to varus malalignment (Fig. 3.46). Proponents of piriformis entry nails argue that there is less likelihood of a lateral starting portal with a piriformis entry nail and theoretically less varus malalignment. Clear evidence does not exist that nailing of subtrochanteric femoral fractures with a piriformis entry nail results in less varus malalignment than does the use of a modified medial trochanteric portal. If a suboptimal portal is made, it can be corrected by placing a small plate within

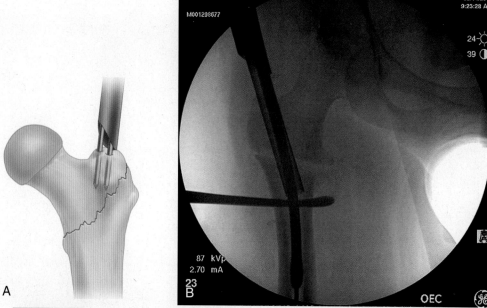

FIGURE 3.42 "Trajectory control" (see text). Establishment of precise entry portal **(A)** and protection of portal by reaming through channel **(B)**. (Modified from Ruecker AH, Russell TA, Sanders RW, Tornetta P: *TRIGEN InterTAN: surgical technique*, Memphis, 2006, Smith & Nephew.)

the reamed lateral track and re-reaming a more medial portal (Fig. 3.47) or by using the original portal and adding an anterior-to-posterior blocking screw to correct the malaligned lateral to medial trajectory (Fig. 3.48).

■ PLATE FIXATION

Although most RT-IIA and RT-IIB fractures can be treated with intramedullary nailing, the procedure can be more technically difficult. Fractures that compromise the entry portal often are reconstructed with a cannulated screw or small plate before intramedullary nailing. A very small percentage of subtrochanteric femoral fractures with proximal extension that compromises the integrity of the starting portal are best treated with a proximal femoral locking plate (Fig. 3.49). Some clinical reports have questioned the effectiveness of one manufacturer's proximal femoral locking plate because of frequent early failures; however, biomechanical data comparing proximal femoral locking plates to blade plates are promising. Placement of a proximal femoral locking plate may be technically easier than placement of a blade plate. A proximal femoral locking plate can be placed with either a percutaneous or open technique based on fracture characteristics. A blade plate can be placed using direct or indirect reduction techniques; however, percutaneous placement is not an option. A blade plate can be very useful in revision situations.

FIXATION OF SUBTROCHANTERIC FEMORAL FRACTURE WITH A PROXIMAL FEMORAL LOCKING PLATE

TECHNIQUE 3.8

- Position the patient supine on a fracture table as described in Technique 3.7.
- If the lesser trochanter on the affected side is intact, obtain a fluoroscopic anteroposterior view of the contralateral hip with the patella facing directly anteriorly toward the ceiling (this position can be confirmed with a true anteroposterior view of the knee). Save this image to the fluoroscopy machine to allow later referencing of the contour of the lesser trochanter (Fig. 3.50).
- Make a lateral approach to the proximal femur.
- Split the fascia lata in line with the skin incision. Split the fascia of the vastus lateralis and elevate the muscle off the intermuscular septum. Release the origin of the vastus lateralis from the trochanteric ridge.
- Based on preoperative imaging, choose bridge plating or direct reduction with interfragmentary fixation and neutralization plating. We typically use a bridge plating technique and rely on preoperative templating of the contralateral side for assessing length.
- Once appropriate alignment has been achieved, introduce the plate through the proximal wound to the level that allows placement of a guide pin just proximal to calcar (Fig. 3.51A). We generally use a long plate that allows placement of four or five well-spaced screws (low screw density).
- Pin the plate in place proximally and distally with provisional pins (Fig. 3.51B). A cortical screw can be placed to reduce the plate to bone as necessary.
- Place the locking screw just above the calcar (Fig. 3.51C) and then place a cortical screw distal to the fracture into the shaft and reduce the shaft to the plate, paying particular attention to the fracture alignment.

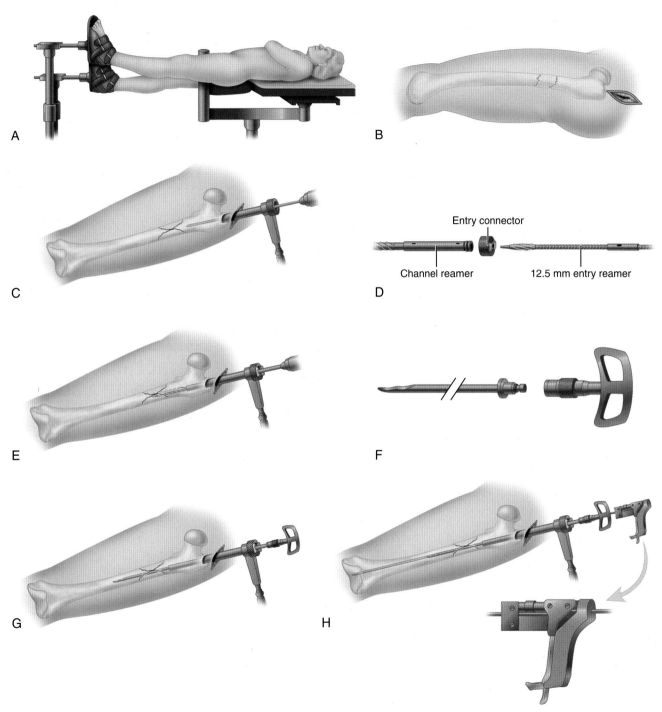

Entry connector

Channel reamer   12.5 mm entry reamer

FIGURE 3.43   Fixation of subtrochanteric fracture with antegrade intramedullary nail locked in reconstruction mode. **A,** Patient placed supine (or lateral) on fracture table. **B,** Small incision beginning approximately 3 cm proximal to greater trochanter and extended proximally. **C,** Establishment of precise entry portal (medial trochanteric portal or piriformis fossa portal, depending on nail selected). **D,** Introduction of combination entry reamer/channel reamer and **(E)** proximal reaming. **F,** Reduction tool used to reduce fracture **(G). H,** Insertion of ball-tipped guide rod across fracture.

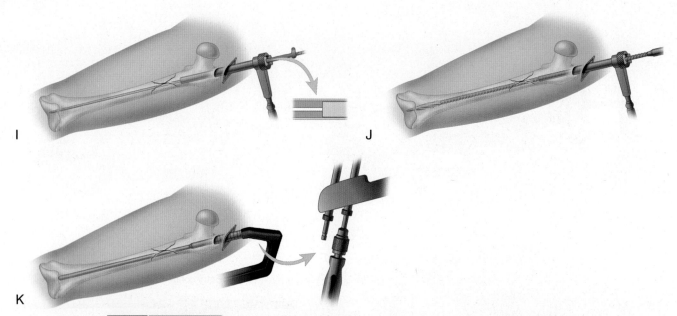

FIGURE 3.43, Cont'd   **I,** Measurement for length of nail. **J,** Reaming of femoral shaft sequentially through the channel reamer. **K,** Placement of intramedullary nail and locking proximally in reconstruction mode. **SEE TECHNIQUE 3.7.**

- Because of concerns about creating a significant stress riser at the end of the plate, we tend to avoid a bicortical locking screw and prefer either a bicortical nonlocking screw or a unicortical locking screw. If a bicortical nonlocking screw is to be used, it should be placed before placement of any locking screws in the shaft. Also, if a bicortical nonlocking screw and outrigger are used together, the outrigger should be set at least one hole shorter than the length of the plate.
- Fill the plate proximally with as many locking screws as possible based on the individual patient's anatomy. If an initial proximal cortical screw was placed, change it to a locking screw.
- At this point, evaluate rotation. If the lesser trochanter is intact, rotate the foot to face the patella directly anteriorly. Compare the contour of the lesser trochanter to the other side using the fluoroscopic image obtained at the beginning of the procedure. Careful evaluation of rotation is important because the typically externally rotated proximal segment may have been internally rotated at least to a degree with reduction of the fracture and plate placement.
- Place two or three additional screws in the shaft to complete the final construct (Fig. 3.51D). The decision to use locking or nonlocking shaft screws is influenced by the patient's bone quality.
- After all screws are placed, close the incision in standard fashion.
- Clinically evaluate length and rotation before the patient is awakened from anesthesia.

POSTOPERATIVE CARE Touch-down weight bearing is allowed for the first 6 weeks and is advanced based on evidence of healing on follow-up radiographs.

FIXATION OF SUBTROCHANTERIC FEMORAL FRACTURE WITH A BLADE PLATE

TECHNIQUE 3.9

- Preoperative planning for the placement of a blade plate is extremely important. Even with computerized radiographs, we use printed radiographs if available to create an accurate template.
- Position the patient supine on a fracture table as described in Technique 3.7. Make a similar lateral exposure as used for placement of proximal femoral locking plate (Technique 3.8), but extend incision significantly farther distally, making the incision as long as the anticipated plate length.
- Insert a Kirschner wire into the lateral aspect of the proximal femur at a 95-degree angle relative to the shaft and based on preoperative templating. Evaluate the position of the Kirschner wire and anteversion of the hip in both planes on a lateral fluoroscopic view. Some systems have guides available that simplify preparation for chisel seating.
- Use a 3.2-mm drill bit to prepare an entrance for the chisel just distal to the Kirschner wire into the lateral cortex.
- Advance the chisel into the lateral aspect of the femur and into the femoral neck using the Kirschner wire as a guide. Make sure the chisel is continually oriented to the alignment of the proximal fragment with disregard for the orientation of the distal fragment.

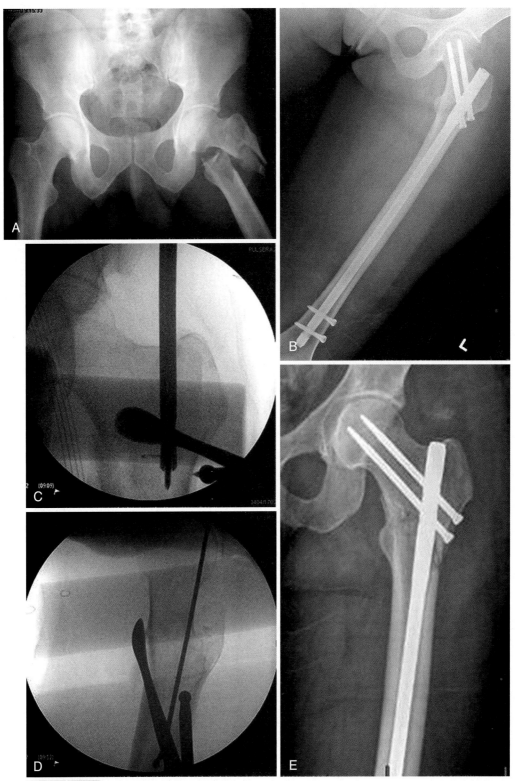

FIGURE 3.44   Use of elevator and ball spike pusher for correction of residual deformity of proximal segment. **A,** Preoperative deformity. **B,** Intraoperative lateral fluoroscopic image without reduction aids. Intraoperative anteroposterior **(C)** and lateral **(D)** fluoroscopic images showing elevator and ball spike pusher used to correct sagittal and coronal plane deformities. **E,** After reduction.   (Courtesy Richard Kyle, MD, Minneapolis, MN.) **SEE TECHNIQUE 3.7.**

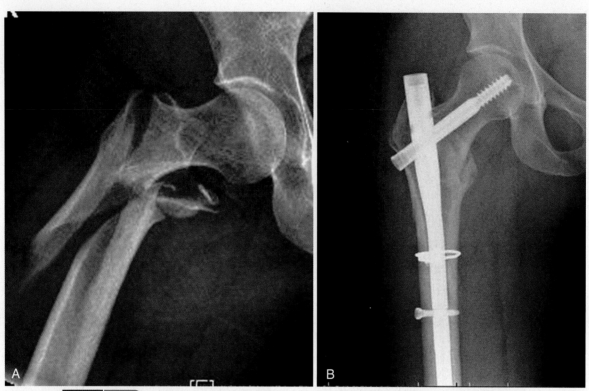

FIGURE 3.45   Use of cerclage wire to hold correction of proximal segment deformity. Preoperative **(A)** and postoperative **(B)** radiographs. (Courtesy William Albers, MD, Memphis, TN.) **SEE TECHNIQUE 3.7.**

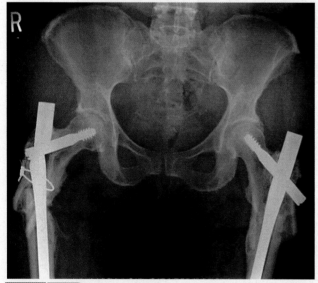

FIGURE 3.46   Varus malalignment with implant failure resulting from lateral starting point.

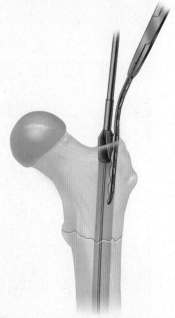

FIGURE 3.47   To correct suboptimal portal, a small plate can be placed in reamed lateral track and more medial portal established. (Redrawn from Gardner MJ, Henley HB: *Harborview illustrated tips and tricks in fracture surgery,* Philadelphia, 2010, Lippincott Williams and Wilkins.)

- Withdraw the chisel every 10 to 15 mm to avoid incarcerating the seating chisel. Advance the chisel to the appropriate depth determined from preoperative templating.
- Introduce the blade plate.
- Once fully seated, use the plate to reduce the fracture. Bone-holding forceps can be used to provisionally reduce the plate to the bone distally while screws are inserted.

Insert an eccentrically placed screw first. If compression provided by this screw is insufficient, an articulating tensioner can be used.

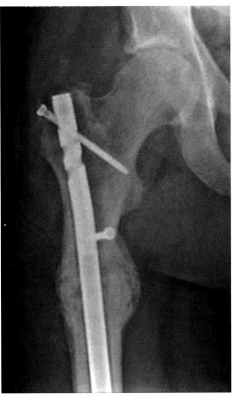

■ Evaluate rotation as described with fixation with a proximal femoral locking plate (see Technique 3.8). Any rotational abnormality can be corrected by removing the distal screws, correcting the rotational abnormality, and reinserting the screws.

POSTOPERATIVE CARE Postoperative care is the same as for that after fixation with a proximal femoral locking plate (see Technique 3.8).

HIP DISLOCATIONS AND FEMORAL HEAD FRACTURES

Hip dislocations and femoral head fractures typically are the result of a high-energy mechanism. The most common mechanism of injury is a motor vehicle accident. In addition to the hip dislocation or hip dislocation with associated femoral head fracture, associated ipsilateral knee pathology is quite common. One study noted an 89% incidence of ipsilateral knee pathology on MRI evaluation. A high index of suspicion is necessary to avoid missing knee injuries and injuries to other areas of the body. Associated systemic injuries have been documented in 40% to 75% of patients. Sciatic nerve injuries also are common with posterior hip dislocations and have been documented in 10% to 15% of patients.

The clinical presentation of the injured limb can give important information regarding the likely type and direction of hip dislocation. Most hip dislocations are posterior, and the position of the injured extremity is shortened, internally rotated, and adducted. Anterior dislocations are much more rare (<10%) and present as a shortened and externally rotated limb. A rare type of fracture-dislocation includes a pure hip dislocation with a femoral head fracture, and this injury pattern presents uniquely as slight hip and knee flexion and neutral hip rotation (Fig. 3.52). Mehta and Routt described this injury pattern and warned about the consequences of attempted closed reduction.

The evaluation of a patient with suspected hip dislocation should be expedited, beginning with an immediate anteroposterior pelvic radiograph before any attempt at reduction. The size of the femoral head and the projection of the lesser trochanter compared with the contralateral side yield important information about the direction of the dislocation. With a posterior dislocation, the femoral head typically appears smaller and the lesser trochanter may not be seen because of internal rotation of the extremity (Fig. 3.53). With an anterior dislocation, the femoral head typically appears larger and the lesser trochanter may be seen in its entirety because of external rotation of the extremity. Loss of concentricity of the femoral head with the acetabulum also is seen with dislocation.

A pure hip dislocation should be reduced as soon as possible to minimize the risk of osteonecrosis. There has been some discussion as to the location (emergency department or operating room) where reductions should take place; this decision should be based on the resources of individual hospitals. The risk of osteonecrosis clearly increases with increasing time to reduction of the dislocation. Osteonecrosis may complicate 1% to 22% of posterior hip dislocations. Multiple attempts at closed reduction should be avoided to minimize the risk of iatrogenic damage to the femoral head. Repeat plain films and a CT scan of the pelvis should be obtained after closed reduction. Intraarticular fragments from either the posterior wall or femoral head that result in an incongruous reduction are an indication for surgical treatment. Patients with incongruous hip joints secondary to intraarticular fragments (Fig. 3.54) after closed reduction are placed in distal femoral skeletal traction. The size and location of intraarticular fragments are evaluated on CT scan (Fig. 3.55). Patients are then treated on an emergent or urgent basis depending on the size of the fragment and the patient's condition.

REDUCTION MANEUVERS FOR POSTERIOR HIP DISLOCATION

Many closed reduction maneuvers have been described, including the Rochester Method (Fig. 3.56), the East Baltimore lift, and the Allis, Bigelow, and Stimson maneuvers. The Rochester Method is effective and convenient for the surgeon but can be used only when the patient does not have a contralateral lower extremity injury. The surgeon performing the reduction maneuver stands on the side of the patient's affected extremity. The patient's hips and knees are flexed to 90 degrees bilaterally. An assistant supports the contralateral hip and maintains knee flexion

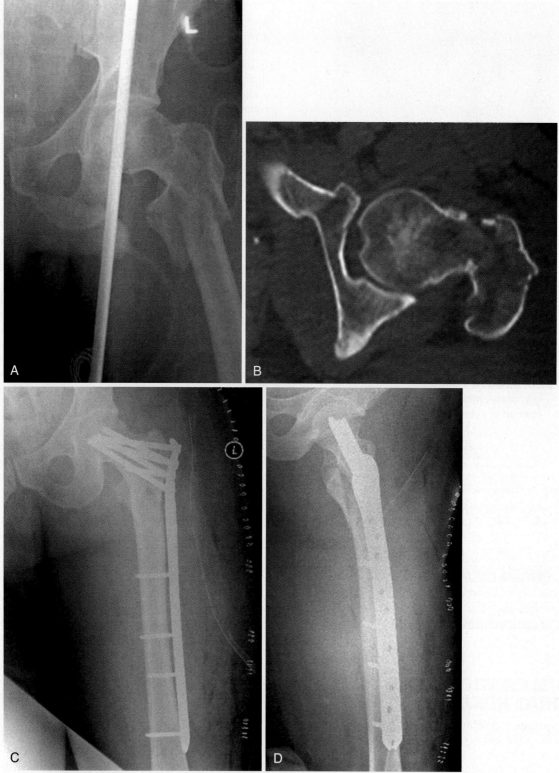

FIGURE 3.49   Proximal femoral locking plate fixation of subtrochanteric femoral fracture with proximal extension. **A,** Preoperative radiograph. **B,** Preoperative axial CT scan shows extension proximally into piriformis fossa. **C** and **D,** After fixation with locking plate.

by holding the foot/ankle. The surgeon's more cephalad arm is passed beneath the patient's proximal calf and placed on the contralateral patella, while the more caudal arm is used to control the patient's ipsilateral ankle and

rotate the extremity as needed. A second assistant stabilizes the pelvis if needed. The surgeon internally rotates the extremity before using the contralateral patella as a fulcrum to apply an anterior-directed force to reduce the

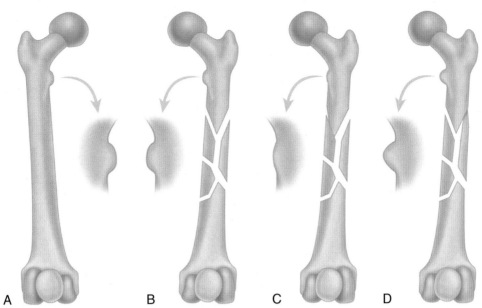

FIGURE 3.50 Rotation can be assessed by comparison of contour of affected lesser trochanter to that of contralateral hip. **A,** The contour of the lesser trochanter from the contralateral uninjured side with the patella oriented anteriorly. **B,** The contour of the lesser trochanter from the injured side should match the uninjured side after correct rotation has been restored. **C,** The contour of the lesser trochanter is diminished as the proximal fragment is internally rotated relative to the distal fragment. This indicates an overall external rotation deformity of the extremity. **D,** The contour of the lesser trochanter is enlarged as the proximal fragment is externally rotated relative to the distal fragment. This indicates an overall internal rotation deformity of the extremity. (Redrawn from Krettek C: Fractures of the distal femur. In Browner BD, Jupiter JB, Levine AM, et al, editors: *Skeletal trauma*, 4th ed. Philadelphia, 2009, Elsevier.) **SEE TECHNIQUE 3.8.**

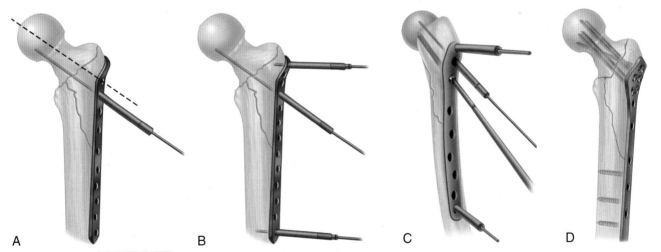

FIGURE 3.51 Fixation of subtrochanteric fracture with proximal femoral locking plate (see text). **A,** Plate is introduced through proximal wound and advanced distally to the level that allows placement of guide pin just proximal to calcar and in the center of the femoral head on the lateral view. **B,** Plate is pinned in place proximally and distally once placement has been optimized. **C,** Locking screw is placed just proximal to calcar. **D,** Final construct after placement of proximal and distal screws. (Modified from Peri-Loc locked plating system: surgical technique, Memphis, Smith & Nephew, 2011.) **SEE TECHNIQUE 3.8.**

dislocation. As the hip is reduced the surgeon externally rotates the extremity.

The East Baltimore lift (Fig. 3.57) is also convenient and effective. This maneuver does require some additional effort from an assistant but can be used in patients with contralateral lower extremity injuries. The surgeon performing the reduction maneuver stands on the side of the patient's affected extremity. The patient's ipsilateral hip and

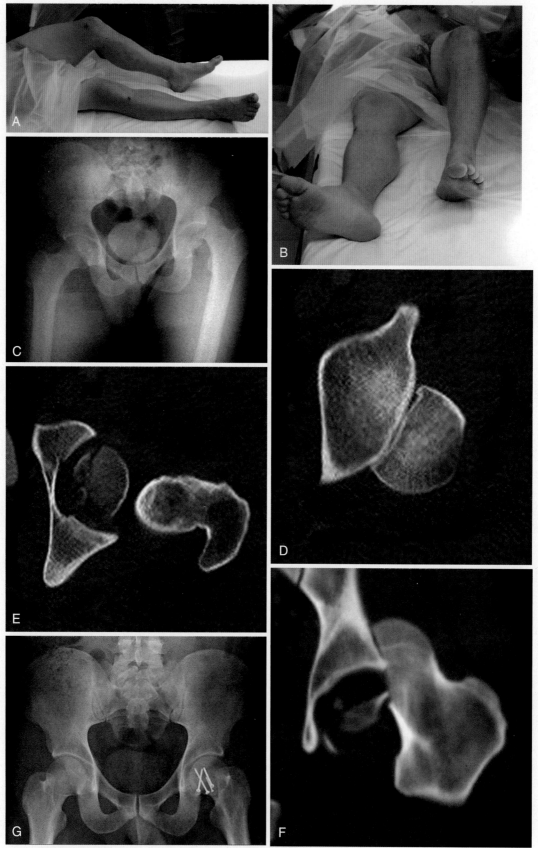

FIGURE 3.52   Pure hip dislocation with concomitant femoral head fracture. **A** and **B**, Characteristic extremity posture. **C**, Preoperative radiograph. Preoperative axial (**D** and **E**) and coronal (**F**) CT scans. **G**, Anteroposterior pelvic radiograph shows union.

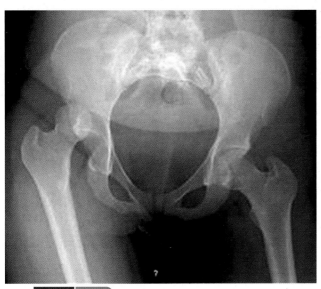

FIGURE 3.53 Posterior hip dislocation.

knee are flexed to 90 degrees. The surgeon's more cephalad arm is passed beneath the patient's proximal calf and placed on an assistant's shoulder. The assistant reciprocates by placing his or her hand on the surgeon's shoulder for stability. The surgeon's more caudal arm is used to control the patient's ankle and rotate the extremity if necessary. A second assistant stabilizes the pelvis as needed. The surgeon internally rotates the extremity, and the surgeon and first assistant then stand (extending at the hips and knees), resulting in an anterior-directed force to reduce the dislocation. As the hip is reduced the surgeon externally rotates the extremity.

The Allis maneuver (Fig. 3.58) can be done with one less assistant than the East Baltimore lift. The patient is positioned supine, an assistant stabilizes the pelvis, and the surgeon applies traction in the direction opposite the deformity. While traction is being applied, the hip is flexed to 90 degrees and the extremity is internally and externally rotated as necessary to achieve reduction.

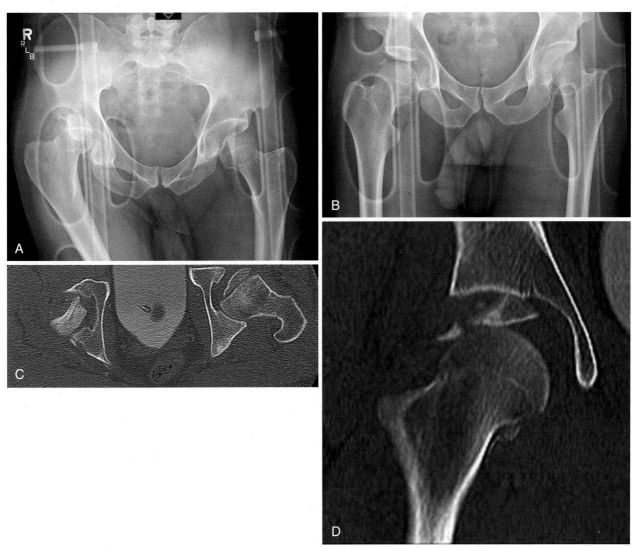

FIGURE 3.54 Incongruous joint after closed reduction as a result of intraarticular fragments. **A,** Pre-reduction radiograph. **B,** Radiograph after reduction. Axial **(C)** and coronal **(D)** CT scans after reduction.

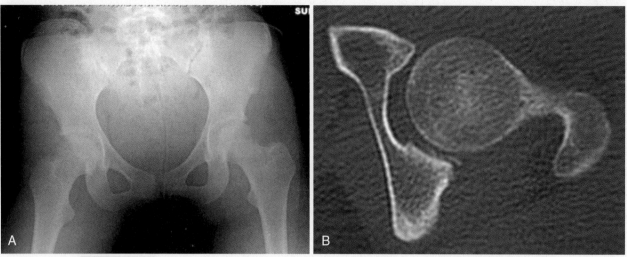

FIGURE **3.55** Subtle incongruity on a plain radiograph **(A)** can be further evaluated on CT scan **(B)**.

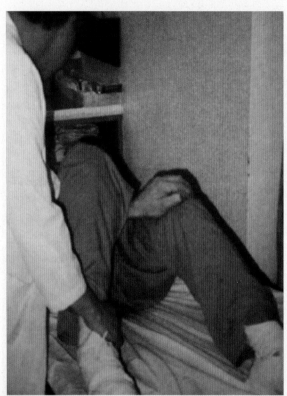

FIGURE **3.56** Rochester maneuver for reduction of posterior hip dislocation. (Redrawn from Stefanich RJ: Closed reduction of posterior hip dislocation: the Rochester method, *Am J Orthop (Belle Mead NJ)* 28:64, 1999.)

The Bigelow maneuver (Fig. 3.59) requires the same number of individuals as the Allis maneuver. The patient is again positioned supine, and an assistant stabilizes the pelvis. The surgeon places one arm beneath the patient's proximal calf and grasps the ankle with his or her other arm. The surgeon applies traction in the direction opposite the deformity and then flexes the hip to 90 degrees.

Traction is maintained at 90 degrees of flexion, keeping the extremity adducted and internally rotated. The femoral head is then levered into the acetabulum with a combination of abduction, external rotation, and extension of the hip.

The Stimson maneuver (Fig. 3.60) is not very practical because the patient must be placed prone with the affected extremity off the end of the table.

If reduction cannot be obtained by closed methods with adequate sedation, an immediate CT scan is ordered to determine the presence of any block to reduction. One additional closed reduction attempt can be made in the operating room with the patient under general anesthesia, proceeding with open reduction if necessary.

REDUCTION MANEUVER FOR ANTERIOR HIP DISLOCATION

Anterior hip dislocations typically can be reduced with longitudinal traction, laterally directed force on the thigh, and often internal rotation to complete the reduction. If closed reduction fails, the Smith-Petersen approach is used for open reduction.

OPEN REDUCTION OF POSTERIOR HIP DISLOCATION THROUGH A POSTERIOR APPROACH

TECHNIQUE 3.10

- Place the patient in the lateral position with the hip extended and the knee flexed to relieve tension on the sciatic nerve. Consider the use of traction if there is an intraarticular fragment.
- Make a standard Kocher-Langenbeck approach to the hip.

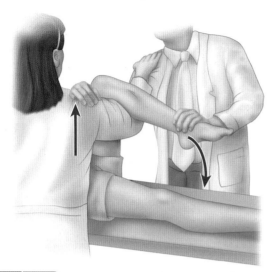

FIGURE 3.57 East Baltimore lift for reduction of posterior hip dislocation.

- Identify the sciatic nerve, which can be difficult because of the altered anatomy. Attempt to locate the nerve on the posterior aspect of the quadratus femoris muscle.
- To avoid further potential insult to the blood supply of the femoral head, do not release the quadratus femoris from the femur; release the piriformis and obturator tendons at least 15 mm from their respective insertions, and make any necessary capsulotomy extension off the acetabular rim.
- Remove any impediments to reduction in the acetabulum, including osteochondral fragments or labrum.
- Guide the femoral head back into the acetabulum while protecting the sciatic nerve.

POSTOPERATIVE CARE After reduction of pure hip dislocations, weight bearing is allowed as tolerated on crutches, with progression as pain allows. Patients with posterior hip dislocations are instructed in posterior hip precautions and follow these for at least 6 weeks. Patients are followed closely for the first 2 years because, if osteonecrosis is going to develop, it likely will present within this time frame.

Associated posterior wall fractures are common with posterior hip dislocations; their treatment is described in chapter 4. Femoral head fractures occur in association with 5% to 15% of hip dislocations. The most frequently used classification system of femoral head fractures is the Pipkin classification (Fig. 3.61):

Type I: Femoral head fracture caudal to fovea

Type II: Femoral head fracture cephalad to fovea

Type III: Femoral head fracture (Pipkin I or II) with femoral neck fracture

Type IV: Femoral head fracture (Pipkin I, II, or III) with acetabular fracture

Similar to pure hip dislocations, reduction of a hip dislocation with an associated femoral head fracture (Pipkin types I and II) should be performed as soon as possible and after considering features consistent with an irreducible fracture-dislocation. After reduction, CT should be used to assess the size, location, and reduction of the femoral head fragment. Most would argue that large Pipkin type I femoral head fragments, especially with fragment displacement, should be rigidly fixed. With larger femoral head fragments, the likelihood of instability increases. More controversy exists over smaller femoral head fragments. Some recommend acute excision, whereas others believe the fragment can be treated nonoperatively. Assessment of reduction with CT is essential. Any Pipkin type II fracture that is not anatomically reduced should be treated surgically. Reduction and fixation can be accomplished through an anterior (Smith-Petersen) or posterior (Kocher-Langenbeck) approach or a posterior approach with surgical dislocation. We typically use a Smith-Petersen approach or surgical dislocation for Pipkin type I and II femoral head fractures, and the fractures usually are fixed with countersunk 2.7-mm or 3.5-mm cortical screws or headless compression screws.

Pipkin type III fractures are rare, and data to guide management of these injuries are lacking. In young patients, we

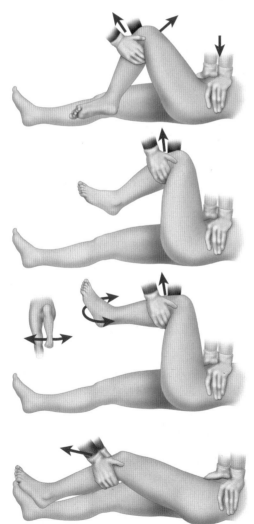

FIGURE 3.58 Allis reduction maneuver for posterior hip dislocation.

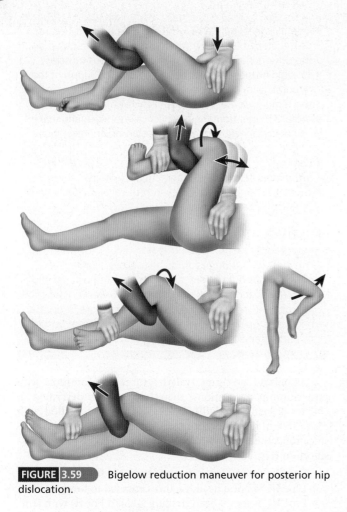

FIGURE 3.59 Bigelow reduction maneuver for posterior hip dislocation.

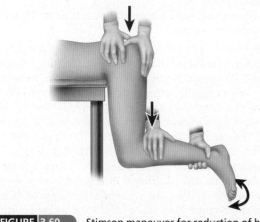

FIGURE 3.60 Stimson maneuver for reduction of hip dislocation.

usually proceed with open reduction and internal fixation. Older patients are treated with arthroplasty.

Pipkin type IV fractures most commonly consist of a femoral head fracture with a posterior wall acetabular fracture. This combination may be best treated with surgical dislocation (Fig. 3.62). Treatment generally is dictated by the acetabular fracture. A multicenter study evaluating the complications associated with surgical hip dislocation concluded that the procedure is safe with a low incidence of

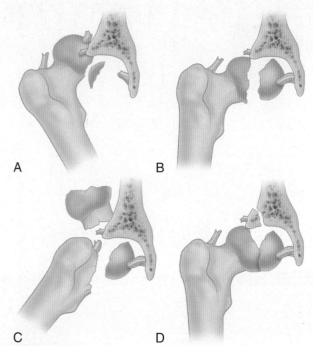

FIGURE 3.61 Pipkin classification of posterior dislocation of hip with femoral head fracture. **A,** Type I: femoral head fracture caudal to fovea capitis. **B,** Type II: femoral head fracture cephalad to fovea capitis. **C,** Type III: type I or II fracture with associated femoral neck fracture. **D,** Type IV: type I, II, or III fracture with associated acetabular fracture.

complications. Of 334 hips treated with surgical hip dislocation for various hip pathologic processes, none developed osteonecrosis. The rate of trochanteric nonunion was 1.8%. Although the number of hips in this series is large, only one patient had surgical dislocation for trauma. Osteonecrosis also has not been reported as a complication in a series in which this approach was used for treatment of femoral head fractures or for joint debridement and treatment of acetabular fractures. The technique for surgical dislocation of the hip (Ganz) is described in other chapter. Surgical dislocation allows excellent visualization for open reduction and internal fixation of large femoral head fragments or debridement or excision of small femoral head fragments.

Hip dislocations with associated femoral head fractures are managed with touch-down weight bearing for 12 weeks. An exception to this management is a patient with femoral head excision, who is allowed to bear weight as tolerated on crutches. Patients also are instructed on hip precautions and are told to follow these for at least the first 6 weeks after surgery.

Closed reduction of a posterior hip dislocation can be complicated by the presence of an ipsilateral femoral neck or femoral shaft fracture. An anteroposterior view of the pelvis must be obtained and reviewed before any reduction attempt because attempts at closed reduction of a posterior hip dislocation with an associated femoral neck fracture may result in displacement or further displacement of the femoral neck fracture and further injury to the vessels supplying the femoral head. Physiologically older patients with this injury should be treated with arthroplasty. Younger patients should be treated with open reduction of the femoral neck

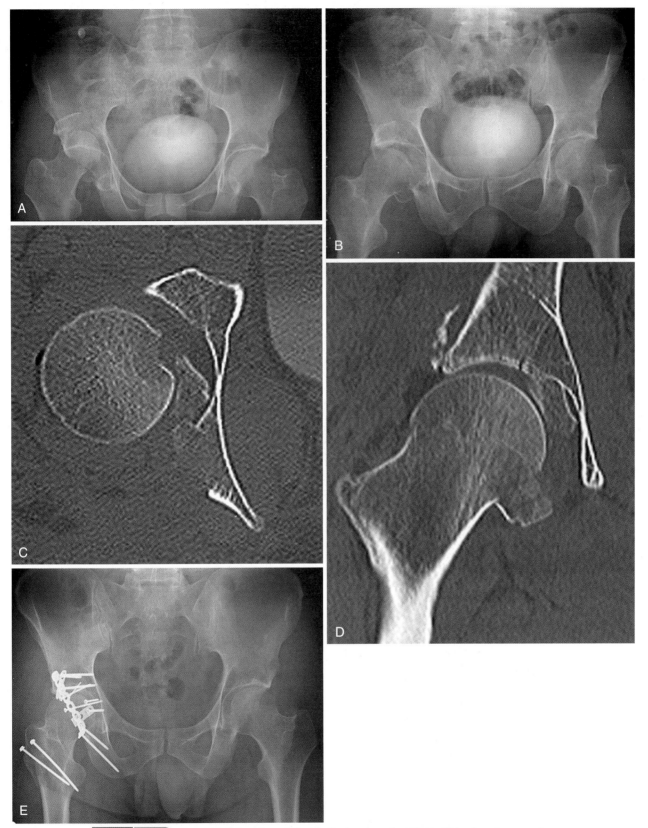

FIGURE 3.62 Surgical dislocation of the hip for treatment of Pipkin IV fracture (open reduction and internal fixation of posterior wall acetabular fracture and debridement of infrafoveal femoral head fracture). **A,** Injury pelvic radiograph. **B,** After reduction. Axial **(C)** and coronal **(D)** CT scans after reduction. **E,** Postoperative pelvic radiograph.

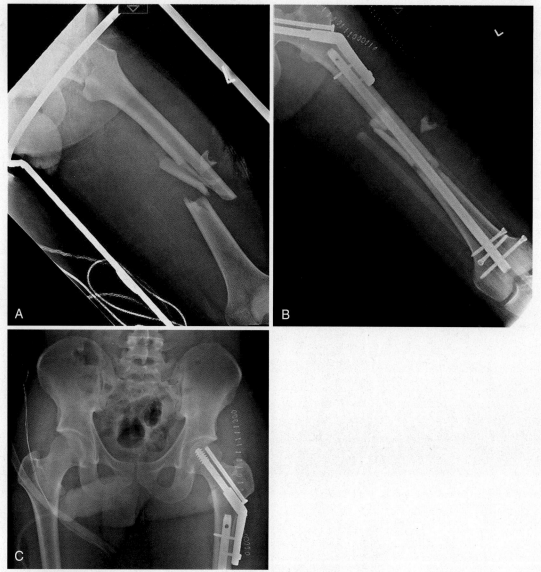

FIGURE 3.63 Fixation of ipsilateral femoral neck and shaft fractures. **A,** Preoperative radiograph. **B** and **C,** Postoperative radiographs.

fracture if displaced and then with reduction of the hip dislocation. We do not attempt closed reduction of dislocated hips with associated femoral neck fractures unless the neck fracture is nondisplaced and can be stabilized (provisionally or definitively) before any reduction attempt. Dislocated hips with femoral shaft fractures are treated differently, and an attempt at closed reduction should be made. If difficulty is encountered, the patient is taken to the operating room and a Schanz pin in the proximal aspect of the femoral shaft is used to aid reduction.

FRACTURES OF THE IPSILATERAL FEMORAL NECK AND SHAFT

Ipsilateral femoral neck fractures occur in association with femoral shaft fractures between 1% and 9% of the time. Timing of the diagnosis of the femoral neck fracture has a dramatic impact on outcomes, and late diagnosis of concomitant femoral

neck fractures can have disastrous complications. Radiographs must be carefully scrutinized to avoid missing an associated femoral neck fracture. The evaluation of femoral fractures includes anteroposterior and lateral views of the femur, as well as an anteroposterior view of the pelvis and lateral view of the affected hip. Because a high-quality lateral image of the affected hip can be difficult to obtain in a patient with a femoral fracture, a pelvic CT scan is obtained on every patient who has a femoral fracture caused by blunt trauma. The pelvic CT scan should be 2-mm cuts and include coronal and sagittal reconstructed images in addition to the standard axial images.

If the femoral neck fracture is diagnosed preoperatively, its treatment is the priority, followed by treatment of the femoral shaft. If the femoral neck is displaced, open reduction generally is performed through a Smith-Petersen or Watson-Jones approach, and stabilization is obtained with either cannulated screws or a compression hip screw (Fig. 3.63). If the femoral neck is nondisplaced, it also can be stabilized with either cannulated screws or a compression hip screw. As

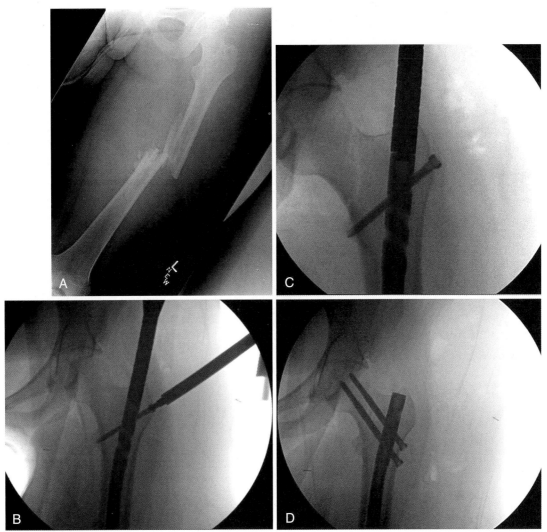

FIGURE 3.64 Ipsilateral femoral neck fracture discovered intraoperatively after placement of intramedullary nail. **A,** Preoperative radiograph. **B,** Intraoperative fluoroscopic view after placement of intramedullary nail. **C,** Intraoperative fluoroscopic view after range of motion of hip under live fluoroscopy. **D,** Intraoperative fluoroscopic view after removal of standard proximal interlocking screw and placement of reconstruction screws.

previously noted in the section on femoral neck fractures, reduction and fixation are done with the patient on a fracture table to allow the highest quality lateral imaging. A nondisplaced femoral neck fracture with an associated femoral shaft fracture can be treated with a single device (antegrade reconstruction nail), but this is technically difficult and the potential complications are greater. If using an antegrade nail, we generally place a cannulated screw across the femoral neck fracture before intramedullary nailing.

To avoid missing associated femoral neck fractures, live fluoroscopic images are obtained after placement of an intramedullary nail. Stress examination of the femoral neck also has been advocated by some authors. A standard anteroposterior view of the pelvis with the lower extremities in internal rotation and a lateral view of the hip are obtained in the operating room with the patient under anesthesia. Even with this protocol it is possible to miss a femoral neck fracture, and repeat imaging of the hip is indicated if the patient has any complaints of hip pain.

If a femoral neck fracture is diagnosed after placement of an intramedullary nail (Fig. 3.64), treatment is based on the amount of displacement and the nail system that has been used. If the femoral neck fracture has not been diagnosed until this point, the fracture is likely nondisplaced or minimally displaced. If the fracture is nondisplaced and the nail system has a reconstruction option, the standard proximal interlocking screw can be removed and two cephalomedullary screws placed. Occasionally, the nail position must be adjusted cranial or caudal to allow placement of the two cephalomedullary screws. If this adjustment is necessary, two guide pins are placed across the femoral neck to avoid displacement of the fracture. If the nailing system does not allow a reconstruction option, cannulated screws can be placed around the intramedullary nail.

Ostrum et al. reported 92 proximal femoral fractures (68 of which were femoral neck fractures) with associated ipsilateral femoral shaft fractures. Only 15 of the femoral neck fractures were transcervical or subcapital, and overall only 39%

of the 92 proximal femoral fractures were displaced. All fractures were treated with either a sliding hip screw or cannulated screws. Nonunion occurred in two (3%) of 68 femoral neck fractures, and 8 (8%) of 92 femoral shaft fractures developed delayed unions or nonunions that required secondary intervention. No differences were detected between the two fixation devices.

Patients with ipsilateral femoral neck and shaft fractures are allowed only touch-down weight bearing for the first 10 to 12 weeks after surgery.

REFERENCES

GENERAL

American Academy of Orthopaedic Surgeons: Management of hip fractures in the elderly: evidence-based clinical practice guideline, September 5, 2014. Available at: https://www.aaos.org/CustomTemplates/Content.aspx?id=6395&ssopc=1. Accessed May 14, 2019.

Berry SD, Kiel DP, Colón-Emeric C: Hip fractures in older adults in 2019, *J Am Med Assoc*, 2019 May 10, [Epub ahead of print].

Bretherton CP, Paraker MJ: Early surgery for patients with a fracture of the hip decreases 30-day mortality, *Bone Joint Lett J* 97B:104, 2015.

Brox WT, Roberts KC, Taksali S, et al.: The American Academy of Orthopaedic Surgeons evidence-based guideline on management of hip fractures in the elderly, *J Bone Joint Surg* 97A:1196, 2015.

Cha YH, Ha YC, Park HJ, et al.: Relationship of chronic obstructive pulmonary disease severity with early and late mortality in elderly patients with hip fracture, *Injury*, 2019 May 22, [Epub ahead of print].

Harrison T, Robinson P, Cook A, Parker MJ: Factors affecting the incidence of deep wound infection after hip fracture surgery, *J Bone Joint Surg* 94B:237, 2012.

Kanis JA, Odén A, McCloskey EV, et al.: A systematic review of hip fracture incidence and probability of fracture worldwide, *Osteoporos Int* 23:2239, 2012.

Kim SM, Moon YW, Lim SJ, et al.: Prediction of survival, second fracture, and functional recovery following the first hip fracture surgery in elderly patients, *Bone* 50:1343, 2012.

Larsson G, Strömberg RU, Rogmark C, Nilsdotter A: Prehospital fast track care for patients with hip fracture: impact on time to surgery, hospital stay, post-operative complications and mortality: a randomised controlled trial, *Injury* 47:881, 2016.

Mariconda M, Costa GG, Cerbasi S, et al.: Fractures predicting mobility and change in activities of daily living after hip fracture: a 1-year prospective cohort study, *J Orthop Trauma* 30:71, 2016.

Modi K, Erdefelt A, Mellner C, et al.: "Obesity paradox" hold true for patients with hip fracture: a registry-based cohort study, *J Bone Joint Surg Am* 101:888, 2019.

Modig K, Erdefelt A, Mellner C, et al.: "Obesity paradox" holds true for patients with hip fracture: a registry-based cohort study, *J Bone Joint Surg Am* 101:888, 2019.

Mundi S, Pindiprolu B, Simunovic N, Bhandari M: Similar mortality rates in hip fracture patients over the past 31 years, *Acta Orthop* 85:54, 2014.

Palm H, Krasheninnikoff M, Holck K, et al.: A new algorithm for hip fracture surgery, *Acta Orthop* 83:26, 2012.

Patel JN, Klein DS, Sreekumar S, et al.: Outcomes in multidisciplinary team-based approach in geriatric hip fracture care: a systematic review, *J Am Acad Orthop Surg*, 2019 May 30, [Epub ahead of print].

Peeters CM, Visser E, Van de Ree CL, et al.: Quality of life after hip fracture in the elderly: a systematic literature review, *Injury* 47:1369, 2016.

Pollock FH, Bethea A, Samanta D, et al.: Readmission within 30 days of discharge after hip fracture care, *Orthopedics* 38:e7, 2015.

Roberts KC, Brox WT, Jevsevar DS, Sevarino K: Management of hip fractures in the elderly, *J Am Acad Orthop Surg* 23:131, 2015.

Sanzone AG: Current challenges in pain management in hip fracture patients, *J Orthop Trauma* 30(Suppl 1):S1, 2016.

Stirton JB, Maier JC, Nandi S: Total hip arthroplasty for the management of hip fracture: a review of the literature, *J Orthop* 16:141, 2019.

FRACTURES OF THE FEMORAL NECK

Archibeck MJ, Carothers JT, Tripuraneni KR, White Jr RE: Total hip arthroplasty after failed internal fixation of proximal femoral fractures, *J Arthroplasty* 28:168, 2013.

Avilucia FR, Joyce D, Mir HR: Dynamic stress fluoroscopy for evaluation of the femoral neck after intramedullary nails: improved sensitivity for identifying occult fractures, *J Orthop Trauma* 33:88, 2019.

Berkes MB, Little MT, Lazaro LE, et al.: Catastrophic failure after open reduction internal fixation of femoral neck fractures with a novel locking plate implant, *J Orthop Trauma* 26:e170, 2012.

Boraiah S, Paul O, Hammond S, et al.: Predictable healing of femoral neck fractures treated with intraoperative compression and length-stable implants, *J Trauma* 69:142, 2010.

Christal AA, Taitsman LA, Dunbar Jr RP, et al.: Fluoroscopically guided hip capsulotomy: effective or not? A cadaveric study, *J Orthop Trauma* 25:214, 2011.

Ciufu DJ, Zaruta DA, Lipof JS, et al.: Risk factors associated with cephalomedullary nail cut-out in the treatment of trochanteric hip fracture, *J Orthop Trauma* 31(11):583, 2017.

Collinge CA, Mir H, Reddix R: Fracture morphology of high shear angle "vertical" femoral neck fractures in young adult patients, *J Orthop Trauma* 28:270, 2014.

Cronin PK, Freccero DM, Kain MS, et al.: Garden 1 and 2 femoral neck fractures collapse more than expected after closed reduction and percutaneous pinning, *J Orthop Trauma* 33:116, 2019.

Davidovitch RI, Jordan CJ, Egol KA, Vrahas MS: Challenges in the treatment of femoral neck fractures in the nonelderly adult, *J Trauma* 68:236, 2010.

Deangelis JP, Ademi A, Staff I, Lewis CG: Cemented versus uncemented hemiarthroplasty for displaced femoral neck fractures: a prospective randomized trial with early follow-up, *J Orthop Trauma* 26:135, 2012.

DeHaan AM, Groat T, Priddy M, et al.: Salvage hip arthroplasty after failed fixation of proximal femur fractures, *J Arthroplasty* 28:855, 2013.

Dolatowski FC, Frihagen F, Bartels S, et al.: Screw fixation versus hemiarthroplasty for nondisplaced femoral neck fractures in elderly patients: a multicenter randomized controlled trial, *J Bone Joint Surg Am* 101:136, 2019.

Duckworth AD, Bennet SJ, Aderinto J, Keating JF: Fixation of intracapsular fractures of the femoral neck in young patients: risk factors for failure, *J Bone Joint Surg* 93B:811, 2011.

Gjertsen JE, Vinje T, Engesaeter LB, et al.: Internal screw fixation compared with bipolar hemiarthroplasty for treatment of displaced femoral neck fractures in elderly patients, *J Bone Joint Surg* 92A:619, 2010.

Griffin J, Anthony TL, Murphy DK, et al.: What is the impact of age on reoperation rates for femoral neck fractures treated with internal fixation and hemiarthroplasty? A comparison of hip fracture outcomes in the very elderly population, *J Orthop* 13:33, 2016.

Grosso MG, Danoff JR, Padgett DE, et al.: The cemented unipolar prosthesis for the management of displaced femoral neck fractures in the dependent osteopenic elderly, *J Arthroplasty* 31:1040, 2016.

Hopley C, Stengel D, Ekkernkamp A, Wich M: Primary total hip arthroplasty versus hemiarthroplasty for displaced intracapsular hip fractures in older patients: a systematic review, *BMJ* 340:c2332, 2010.

Hoffmann JC, Kellam J, Kumaravel M, et al.: Is the cranial and posterior screw of the "inverted triangle" configuration for femoral neck fractures safe? *J Orthop Trauma* 33:331, 2019.

Inngul C, Blomfeldt R, Ponzer S, Enocson A: Cemented versus uncemented arthroplasty in patients with a displaced fracture of the femoral neck: a randomised controlled trial, *Bone Joint Lett J* 97B:1475, 2015.

Jiang J, Yang CH, Lin Q, et al.: Does arthroplasty provide better outcomes than internal fixation and mid- and long-term follow-up? A meta-analysis, *Clin Orthop Relat Res* 473:2672, 2015.

Johansson T: Internal fixation compared with total hip replacement for displaced femoral neck fractures: a minimum fifteen-year follow-up study of a previously reported randomized trial, *J Bone Joint Surg* 96A:e46, 2014.

Kain MS, Marcantonio AJ, Iorio R: Revision surgery occurs frequently after percutaneous fixation of stable femoral neck fractures in elderly patients, *Clin Orthop Relat Res* 472:4010, 2014.

Kim KH, Han KY, Kim KW, Lee JH, Chung MK: Local postoperative complications after surgery for intertrochanteric fractures using cephalomedullary nails, *Hip Pelvis* 30(3):168, 2018.

Langslet E, Frihagen F, Opland V, et al.: Cemented versus uncemented hemiarthroplasty for displaced femoral neck fractures: 5-year followup of a randomized trial, *Clin Orthop Relat Res* 472:1291, 2014.

Leonardsson O, Rolfson O, Hommel A, et al.: Patient-reported outcome after displaced femoral neck fracture: a national survey of 4467 patients, *J Bone Joint Surg* 95A:1693, 2013.

Leonardsson O, Sernbo I, Carlsson A, et al.: Long-term follow-up of replacement compared with internal fixation for displaced femoral neck fractures: results at ten years in a randomised study of 450 patients, *J Bone Joint Surg* 92B:406, 2010.

Lewis DP, Waever D, Thorninger R, et al.: Hemiarthroplasty vs total hip arthroplasty for the management of displaced neck of the femur fractures: a systematic review and meta-analysis, *J Arthroplasty*, 2019 Apr 6, [Epub ahead of print].

Liao L, Zhao JM, Su W, et al.: A meta-analysis of total hip arthroplasty and hemiarthroplasty outcomes for displaced femoral neck fractures, *Arch Orthop Trauma Surg* 132:1021, 2012.

Liodakis E, Antoniou J, Zuko DJ, et al.: Major complications and transfusion rates after hemiarthroplasty and total hip arthroplasty for femoral neck fractures, *J Arthroplasty* 31:2008, 2016.

Liu C, Von Keudell A, McTague M, et al.: Ideal length of thread forms for screws used in screw fixation of nondisplaced femoral neck fractures, *Injury* 50:727, 2019.

Lorich DG, Lazaro LE, Boraiah S: Femoral neck fractures: open reduction internal fixation. In Wiss D, editor: *Master techniques in orthopaedic surgery: fractures*, ed 3, Philadelphia, 2012, Wolters Kluwer.

Mahmoud SS, Pearse EO, Smith TO, Hing CB: Outcomes of total hip arthroplasty, as a salvage procedure, following failed internal fixation of intracapsular fractures of the femoral neck: a systematic review and meta-analysis, *Bone Joint Lett J* 98B:452, 2016.

Miller BJ, Callaghan JJ, Cram P, et al.: Changing trends in the treatment of femoral neck fractures: a review of the American Board of Orthopaedic Surgery database, *J Bone Joint Surg* 96A:e149, 2014.

Murphy DK, Randell T, Brennan KL, et al.: Treatment and displacement affect the reoperation rate for femoral neck fracture, *Clin Orthop Relat Res* 471:2691, 2013.

OHara NN, Slobogean GP, Stockton DJ, et al.: The socioeconomic impact of a femoral neck fractures on patients aged 18-50: a population-based study, *Injury*, 2019 May 29, [Epub ahead of print].

Pala E, Trono M, Bitoni A, Lucidi G: Hip hemiarthroplasty for femur neck fractures: minimally invasive direct anterior approach versus postero-lateral approach, *Eur J Orthop Surg Traumatol* 26:423, 2016.

Porter SE, Russell GV, Sledge JC, et al.: A novel way to prevent lost scalpel blades during percutaneous placement of iliosacral screws, *J Orthop Trauma* 24:194, 2010.

Rogmark C, Leonardsson O: Hip arthroplasty for the treatment of displaced fractures of the femoral neck in elderly patients, *Bone Joint Lett J* 90B:291, 2016.

Rudelli S, Viriato SP, Meireles TL, Frederico TN: Treatment of displaced neck fractures of the femur with total hip arthroplasty, *J Arthroplasty* 27:246, 2012.

Samuel AM, Russo GS, Lucasiewicz AM, et al.: Surgical treatment of femoral neck fractures after 24 hours in patients between the ages of 18 and 49 is associated with poor inpatient outcomes: an analysis of 1361 patients in the National Trauma Data Bank, *J Orthop Trauma* 30:89, 2016.

Sassoon A, D'Apuzzo M, Sems S, et al.: Total hip arthroplasty for femoral neck fracture: comparing in-hospital mortality, complications, and disposition to an elective patient population, *J Arthroplasty* 28:1659, 2013.

Slobogean GP, Sprague SA, Scott T, Bhandari M: Complications following young femoral neck fractures, *Injury* 46(3):484, 2015.

Souder CD, Brennan ML, Brennan KL, et al.: The rate of contralateral proximal femoral fracture following closed reduction and percutaneous pinning compared with arthroplasty for the treatment of femoral neck fractures, *J Bone Joint Surg* 94A:418, 2012.

Stockton DJ, Dua K, O'Brien PJ, et al.: Failure patterns of femoral neck fracture fixation in young patients, *Orthopedics*, 2019 March 26, [Epub ahead of print].

Støen RØ, Lofthus CM, Nordsletten L, et al.: Randomized trial of hemiarthroplasty versus internal fixation for femoral neck fractures: no differences at 6 years, *Clin Orthop Relat Res* 472:360, 2014.

Thürig G, Schmitt JW, Slankamenac K, Werner CM: Safety of total hip arthroplasty for femoral neck fractures using the direct anterior approach: a retrospective observational study in 86 elderly patients, *Patient Saf Surg* 10:12, 2016.

Travis EC, Tan RS, Funaki P, et al.: Clinical outcomes of total hip arthroplasty for fractured neck of femur in patients over 75 years, *J Arthroplasty* 30:230, 2015.

von Roth P, Abdel MP, Harmsen WS, Berry DJ: Cemented bipolar hemiarthroplasty provides definitive treatment for femoral neck fractures at 20 years and beyond, *Clin Orthop Relat Res* 473:3595, 2015.

Weil YA, Khoury A, Zualter I, et al.: Femoral neck shortening and varus collapse after navigated fixation of intracapsular femoral neck fractures. *J Orthop Trauma* 26(1):19, 2012.

Wendt MC, Cass JR, Trousdale RR: Incidence of radiographic cam-type impingement in young patients (<50) after femoral neck fracture treated with reduction and internal fixation, *HSS J* 9:113, 2013.

Yang Z, Liu H, Xie X, et al.: Total hip arthroplasty for failed internal fixation after femoral neck fracture versus that for acute displaced femoral neck fracture: a comparative study, *J Arthroplasty* 30:1378, 2015.

Yu L, Wang Y, Chen J: Total hip arthroplasty versus hemiarthroplasty for displaced femoral neck fractures: meta-analysis of randomized trials, *Clin Orthop Relat Res* 470:2235, 2012.

Zhang YQ, Chang SM, Huang YG, et al.: The femoral neck safe zone: a radiographic simulation study to prevent cortical perforation with multiple screw insertion, *J Orthop Trauma* 29:e178, 2015.

Zielinski SM, Keijers NL, Praet SFE, et al.: Femoral neck shortening after internal fixation of a femoral neck fracture, *Orthopedics* 36(7):e849, 2013.

Zi-Sheng A, You-Shui G, Zhi-Zhen J, et al.: Hemiarthroplasty vs primary total hip arthroplasty for displaced fracture of the femoral neck in the elderly: a meta-analysis, *J Arthroplasty* 27:583, 2012.

INTERTROCHANTERIC FRACTURES

Aktselis I, Kokoroghiannis C, Fragkomichalos E, et al.: Prospective randomised controlled trial of an intramedullary nail versus a sliding hip screw for intertrochanteric fractures of the femur, *Int Orthop* 38:155, 2014.

Barton TM, Gleeson R, Topliss C, et al.: A comparison of the long Gamma nail with the sliding hip screw for the treatment of AO/OTA 31-A2 fractures of the proximal part of the femur: a prospective randomized trial, *J Bone Joint Surg* 92A:792, 2010.

Bohl DD, Basques BA, Golinvaux NS, et al.: Extramedullary compared with intramedullary implants for intertrochanteric hip fractures: thirty-day outcomes of 4432 procedures from the ACS NSQIP database, *J Bone Joint Surg* 96A:1871, 2014.

Boone C, Carlberg KN, Koueiter DM, et al.: Short versus long intramedullary nails for treatment of intertrochanteric femur fractures (OTA 31-A1 and A2), *J Orthop Trauma* 28:e96, 2014.

Bretherton CP, Parker MJ: Femoral medialization, fixation failures, and functional outcome in trochanteric hip fractures treated with either a sliding hip screw or an intramedullary nail from within a randomized trial, *J Orthop Trauma* 30:642, 2016.

Carvajal-Pedtosa C, Gómez-Sánchez RC, Hernández-Cortés P: Comparison of outcomes of intertrochanteric fracture fixation using percutaneous compression plate between stable and unstable fractures in the elderly, *J Orthop Trauma* 30:e201, 2016.

Ciufo DJ, Zaruta DA, Lipof JS, et al.: Risk factors associated with cephalomedullary nail cutout in the treatment of trochanteric hip fractures, *J Orthop Trauma* 31:583, 2017.

Dunn J, Kusnezov N, Bader J, et al.: Long versus short cephalomedullary nail for trochanteric femur fractures (OTA 31-A1, A2, and A3): a systematic review, *J Orthop Traumatol* 17:361, 2016.

Egol KA, Marcano AJ, Lewis L, et al.: Can the use of an evidence-based algorithm for the treatment of intertrochanteric fractures of the hip maintain quality at a reduced cost? *Bone Joint Lett J* 96B:1192, 2014.

Erez O, Dougherty PJ: Early complications associated with cephalomedullary nail for intertrochanteric hip fractures, *J Trauma Acute Care Surg* 72:E101, 2012.

Forte ML, Virnig BA, Eberly LE, et al.: Provider factors associated with intramedullary nail use for intertrochanteric hip fractures, *J Bone Joint Surg* 92A:1105, 2010.

Gausden EB, Sin DM, Levack AE, et al.: Gait analysis after intertrochanteric hip fracture: does shortening result in gait impairment? *J Orthop Trauma* 32:554, 2018.

Gavaskar AS, Tummala NC, Srinivasan P, et al.: Helical blade of the integrated lag screws: a matched pair analysis of 100 patients with unstable trochanteric fractures, *J Orthop Trauma* 32:274, 2018.

Guerra MT, Pasqualin S, Souza MP, Lenz R: Functional recovery of elderly patients with surgically-treated intertrochanteric fractures: preliminary results of a randomised trial comparing the dynamic hip screw and proximal femoral nail techniques, *Injury* 45(Suppl 5):S26, 2014.

Hoffmann S, Paetzold R, Stephan D, et al.: Biomechanical evaluation of interlocking lag screw design in intramedullary nailing of unstable pertrochanteric fractures, *J Orthop Trauma* 27:483, 2013.

Hong JY, Suh SW, Park JH, et al.: Comparison of soft-tissue serum markers in stable intertrochanteric fracture: dynamic hip screw versus proximal femoral nail—a preliminary study, *Injury* 42:204, 2011.

Horwitz DS, Tawari A, Suk M: Nail length in the management of intertrochanteric fracture of the femur, *J Am Acad Orthop Surg* 24:e50, 2016.

Huang Y, Zhang C, Luo Y: A comparative biomechanical study of proximal femoral nail (InterTAN) and proximal femoral nail antirotation for intertrochanteric fractures, *Int Orthop* 37:2465, 2013.

Hulet DA, Whale CS, Beebe MJ, et al.: Short versus long cephalomedullary nails for fixation of stable versus unstable intertrochanteric femur fractures at a Level 1 trauma center, *Orthopedics* 42:e202, 2019.

Kazemian GH, Manafi AR, Najafi F, Najafi MA: Treatment of intertrochanteric fractures in elderly high risk patients: dynamic hip screw vs. external fixation, *Injury* 45:568, 2014.

Kim Y, Dheep K, Lee J, et al.: Hook leverage technique for reduction of intertrochanteric fracture, *Injury* 45:1006, 2014.

Kleweno C, Morgan J, Redshaw J, et al.: Short versus long cephalomedullary nails for the treatment of intertrochanteric hip fractures in patients older than 65 years, *J Orthop Trauma* 28:391, 2014.

Gavaskar AS, Tummala NC, Srinivasan P, et al.: Helical blade of the integrated lag screws: a matched pair analysis of 100 patients with unstable trochanteric fractures, *J Orthop Trauma* 32:274, 2018.

Langford J, Pillai G, Ugliailoro AD, Yang E: Perioperative lateral trochanteric wall fractures: sliding hip screw versus percutaneous compression plate for intertrochanteric hip fractures, *J Orthop Trauma* 25:191, 2011.

Ma KL, Wang X, Luan FJ, et al.: Proximal femoral nails antirotation, Gamma nails, and dynamic hip screws for fixation of intertrochanteric fractures of the femur: a meta-analysis, *Orthop Traumatol Surg Res* 100:859, 2014.

Matre K, Havelin LI, Gjertsen JE, et al.: Intramedullary nails result in more reoperations than sliding hip screws in two-part intertrochanteric fractures, *Clin Orthop Relat Res* 471:1379, 2013.

McCormack R, Panagiotopolous K, Buckely R, et al.: A multicenter, prospective, randomised comparison of the sliding hip screw with the Medoff sliding screw and side plate for unstable intertrochanteric hip fractures, *Injury* 44:1904, 2013.

Nherera L, Trueman P, Horner A, et al.: Comparison of a twin interlocking derotation and compression screw cephalomedullary nail (InterTAN) with a single screw derotation cephalomedullary nail (proximal femoral nail antirotation): a systematic review and meta-analysis for intertrochanteric fractures, *J Orthop Res* 13:46, 2018.

Nherera L, Trueman P, Horner A, et al.: Comparing the costs and outcomes of an integrated twin compression screw (ITCS) nail with standard of care using a single lag screw or a single helical blade cephalomedullary

nail in patients with intertrochanteric hip fractures, *J Orthop Surg Res* 30:217, 2018.

Parker MJ: Sliding hip screw versus intramedullary nail for trochanteric hip fractures: a randomised trial of 1000 patients with presentation of results related to fracture stability, *Injury* 48:2762, 2017.

Parker MJ, Bowers TR, Pryor GA: Sliding hip screw versus the Targon PF nail in the treatment of trochanteric fractures of the hip: a randomised trial of 600 fractures, *J Bone Joint Surg* 94B:391, 2012.

Parker MJ, Cawley S: Sliding hip screw *versus* the Targon PFT nail for trochanteric hip fractures: a randomised trial of 400 patients, *Bone Joint Lett J* 99-B:1210, 2017.

Pradeep AR, KiranKumar A, Dheenadhayalan J, et al.: Intraoperative lateral wall fractures during Dynamic Hip Screw fixation for intertrochanteric fractures-Incidence, causative factors and clinical outcome, *Injury* 49:334, 2018.

Ramanoudjame M, Guillon P, Dauzac C, et al.: CT evaluation of torsional malalignment after intertrochanteric fracture fixation, *Orthop Traumatol Surg Res* 96:844, 2010.

Reindl R, Harvey EJ, Berry GK, et al.: Intramedullary versus extramedullary fixation for unstable intertrochanteric fractures: a prospective randomized controlled trial, *J Bone Joint Surg* 97A:1905, 2015.

Santoni BG, Diaz MA, Stoops TK, et al.: Biomechanical investigation of an integrated 2-screw cephalomedullary nail versus a sliding hip screw in unstable intertrochanteric fractures, *J Orthop Trauma* 33:82, 2019.

Schmidt-Rohlfing B, Heussen N, Knobe M, et al.: Reoperation rate after internal fixation of intertrochanteric femur fractures with the percutaneous compression plate: what are the risk factors? *J Orthop Trauma* 27:312, 2013.

Sanders D, Bryant D, Tieszer C, et al.: A Multicenter Randomized Control Trial Comparing a Novel Intramedullary Device (InterTAN) Versus Conventional Treatment (Sliding Hip Screw) of Geriatric Hip Fractures, *J Orthop Trauma* 31(1):1, 2017.

Serrano R, Blair JA, Watson DT, et al.: Cephalomedullary nail fixation of intertrochanteric femur fractures: are two proximal screws better than one? *J Orthop Traum* 31:577, 2017.

Shen J, Luo F, Sun D, et al.: Mid-term results after treatment of intertrochanteric femoral fractures with percutaneous compression plate (PCCP), *Injury* 46:347, 2015.

Swart E, Makhni EC, Macaulay W, et al.: Cost-effectiveness analysis of fixation options for intertrochanteric hip fractures, *J Bone Joint Surg* 96A:1612, 2014.

Vaughn J, Cohen E, Vopat BG, et al.: Complications of short versus long cephalomedullary nail for intertrochanteric femur fractures, minimum 1 year follow-up, *Eur J Orthop Surg Traumatol* 25:665, 2015.

Yang E, Qureshi S, Trokhan S, Joseph D: Gotfried percutaneous compression plating compared with sliding hip screw fixation of intertrochanteric hip fractures: a prospective randomized study, *J Bone Joint Surg* 93A:942, 2011.

Yoon PW, Kwon JE, Yoo JJ, et al.: Femoral neck fracture after removal of the compression hip screw from healed intertrochanteric fractures, *J Orthop Trauma* 27:696, 2013.

Zhang Y, Zhang S, Wang S, et al.: Long and short intramedullary nails for fixation of intertrochanteric femur fractures (OTA 31-A1, A2, and A3): a systematic review and meta-analysis, *Orthop Traumatol Surg Res* 103:685, 2017.

SUBTROCHANTERIC FRACTURES

Beingessner DM, Scolaro JA, Orec RJ, et al.: Open reduction and intramedullary stabilization of subtrochanteric femur fractures: a retrospective study of 56 cases, *Injury* 44:1910, 2013.

Codesido P, Mejia A, Riego J, et al.: Subtrochanteric fractures in elderly people treated with intramedullary fixation: quality of life and complications following open reduction and cerclage wiring versus closed reduction, *Arch Orthop Trauma Surg* 137:1077, 2017.

Forward DP, Doro CJ, O'Toole RV, et al.: A biomechanical comparison of a locking plate, a nail, and a 95° angled blade plate for fixation of subtrochanteric femoral fractures, *J Orthop Trauma* 26:334, 2012.

Gardner MJ, Henley HB: *Harborview illustrated tips and tricks in fracture surgery*, Philadelphia, 2010, Lippincott Williams and Wilkins.

Georgiannos D, Lampridis V, Bosbinas I: Subtrochanteric femoral fractures treated with long Gamma nail: a historical control case study versus long trochanteric Gamma nail, *Orthop Traumatol Surg Res* 101:675, 2015.

Grisell M, Moed BR, Bledsoe JG: A biomechanical comparison of trochanteric nail proximal screw configurations in a subtrochanteric fracture model, *J Orthop Trauma* 24:359, 2010.

Hak DJ, Wu H, Dou C, et al.: Challenges in subtrochanteric femur fracture management, *Orthopedics* 38:498, 2015.

Hoskins W, Bingham R, Joseph S, et al.: Subtrochanteric fracture: the effect of cerclage wire on fracture reduction and outcome, *Injury* 46:1992, 2015.

Imerci A, Canbek U, Karatosun V, et al.: Nailing or plating for subtrochanteric femoral fractures: a non-randomized comparative study, *Eur J Orthop Surg Traumatol* 25:889, 2015.

Joglekar SB, Lindvall EM, Martirosian A: Contemporary management of subtrochanteric fractures, *Orthop Clin North Am* 46:21, 2015.

Kim KK, Won Y, Smith DH, et al.: Clinical results of complex subtrochanteric femoral fractures with long cephalomedullary hip nail, *Hip Pelvis* 29:113, 2017.

Krappinger D, Wolf B, Dammerer D, et al.: Risk factors for nonunion after intramedullary nailing of subtrochanteric femoral fractures, *Arch Orthop Trauma Surg*, 2019 Feb 7, [Epub ahead of print].

Mingo-Robinet J, Torres-Torres M, Moreno-Barrero M, et al.: Minimally invasive clamp-assisted reduction and cephalomedullary nailing without cerclage cables for subtrochanteric femur fractures in the elderly: surgical technique and results, *Injury* 46:1036, 2015.

Persiani P, Noia G, de Cristo C, et al.: A study of 44 patients with subtrochanteric fractures treated using long nail and cerclage cables, *Musculoskelet Surg* 99:225, 2015.

Riehl JT, Koval KJ, Langford JR, et al.: Intramedullary nailing of subtrochanteric fractures—does malreduction matter?, *Bull Hosp Jt Dis* 72:159, 2013, 2014.

Saini P, Kumar R, Shekhawat V, et al.: Biological fixation of comminuted subtrochanteric fractures with proximal femur locking compression plate, *Injury* 44:226, 2013.

Shin WC, Moon NH, Jang JH, et al.: Technical note and surgical outcomes of percutaneous cable fixation in subtrochanteric fracture: a review of 51 consecutive cases over 4 years in two institutions, *Injury* 50:409, 2019.

Streubel PN, Wong AHW, Ricci WM, Gardner MJ: Is there a standard trochanteric entry site for nailing of subtrochanteric femur fractures? *J Orthop Trauma* 25:202, 2011.

Thomás J, Teixidor J, Batalla L, et al.: Subtrochanteric fractures: treatment with cerclage wire and long intramedullary nail, *J Orthop Trauma* 27:e157, 2013.

Wang J, Ma JX, Jia HB, et al.: Biomechanical evaluation of four methods for internal fixation of comminuted subtrochanteric fractures, *Medicine (Baltimore)* 95:e3382, 2016.

Yeh WL, Su CY, Chang CW, et al.: Surgical outcomes of atypical subtrochanteric and femoral fracture related to bisphosphonates use in osteoporotic patients with or without teriparatide treatment, *BMC Musculoskelet Disord* 18:527, 2017.

Yoon RS, Donegan DJ, Liporace FA: Reducing subtrochanteric femur fractures: tips and tricks, do's and don'ts, *J Orthop Trauma* 29(Suppl 4):S28, 2015.

FRACTURE, DISLOCATION, AND FRACTURE-DISLOCATION OF THE HIP

Anakwenze OA, Kancheria V, Major NM, Lee GC: Isolated sciatic nerve entrapment by ectopic bone after femoral head fracture-dislocation, *Am J Orthop (Belle Mead NJ)* 42:275, 2013.

Berkes MB, Cross MB, Shindle MK, et al.: Traumatic posterior hip instability and femoroacetabular impingement in athletes, *Am J Orthop (Belle Mead NJ)* 41:166, 2012.

Berry SD, Kiel DP, Colón-Emeric C: Hip fractures in older adults in 2019, *J Am Med Assoc*, 2019 May 10, [Epub ahead of print].

de Joode SGCJ, Kalmet PHS, Fiddelers AAA, et al.: Long-term functional outcome after a low-energy hip fracture in elderly patients, *J Orthop Traumatol* 20:20, 2019.

Foulk DM, Mullis BH: Hip dislocation: evaluation and management, *J Am Acad Orthop Surg* 18:199, 2010.

Groff H, Kheir MM, George J, et al.: Causes of in-hospital mortality after hip fractures in the elderly, *Hip Int*, 2019 Mar 25, [Epub ahead of print].

Keel MJB, Bastian JD, Büchler L, Siebenrock KA: Surgical dislocation of the hip for a locked traumatic posterior dislocation with associated femoral neck and acetabular fractures, *J Bone Joint Surg* 92B:442, 2010.

Kokubo Y, Uchilda K, Takeno K, et al.: Dislocated intra-articular femoral head fracture associated with fracture-dislocation of the hip and acetabulum: report of 12 cases and technical notes on surgical intervention, *Eur J Orthop Surg Traumatol* 23:557, 2013.

Lin D, Lian K, Chen Z, et al.: Emergent surgical reduction and fixation for Pipkin type 1 femoral fractures, *Orthopedics* 36:778, 2013.

Masse A, Aparto A, Alluto C, et al.: Surgical hip dislocation is a reliable approach for treatment of femoral head fractures, *Clin Orthop Relat Res* 473:3744, 2015.

Mostafa MF, El-Adl W, El-Sayed MA: Operative treatment of displaced Pipkin type I and II femoral head fractures, *Arch Orthop Trauma Surg* 134:637, 2014.

Sink EL, Beaulé PE, Sucato D, et al.: Multicenter study of complications following surgical dislocation of the hip, *J Bone Joint Surg* 93A:1132, 2011.

Steppacher SD, Albers CD, Siebenrock KA, et al.: Femoroacetabular impingement predisposes to traumatic posterior hip dislocation, *Clin Orthop Relat Res* 471:1937, 2013.

Tannast M, Pleus F, Bonel H, et al.: Magnetic resonance imaging in traumatic posterior hip dislocation, *J Orthop Trauma* 24:723, 2010.

Wikerøy AK, Clarke-Jenssen J, Ovre SA, et al.: The natural history of bone bruise and bone remodeling in the traumatised hip: a prospective 2-year follow-up study of bone bruise changes and DEXA measurements in 13 patients with conservatively treated traumatic hip dislocations and/or fractures, *Injury* 43:1672, 2012.

Wylie JD, Abtahi AM, Beckmann JT, et al.: Arthroscopic and imaging findings after traumatic hip dislocation in patients younger than 25 years of age, *J Hip Preserv Surg* 2:303, 2015.

Zlotorowicz M, Caubak J, Caban A, et al.: The blood supply to the femoral head after posterior fracture/dislocation of the hip, assessed by CT angiography, *Bone Joint Lett J* 95B:1453, 2013.

The complete list of references is available online at expertconsult.inkling.com.

CHAPTER 4

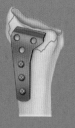

FRACTURES OF THE ACETABULUM AND PELVIS

Michael J. Beebe

ACETABULAR FRACTURES	202	Choice of surgical approach	216	Radiographic evaluation	237
Anatomy	202	Specific fracture patterns	218	Classification	238
Radiographic evaluation	204	Postoperative care	227	Treatment	244
Classification	207	Outcome and complications	228	Initial management	244
Treatment	208	Acute total hip arthroplasty as		Indications for nonoperative and	
Initial treatment	209	treatment of acetabular fracture	231	operative treatment	246
Indications for nonoperative		Complications of acute total hip		Timing of surgery	250
treatment	210	arthroplasty for acetabular		Choice of treatment	250
Secondary congruence in displaced		fracture	235	Internal fixation of the anterior	
both-column fractures	212	Total hip arthroplasty for		pelvis	257
Indications for operative		posttraumatic arthritis	235	Posterior approach and	
treatment	215	**PELVIC FRACTURES**	235	internal fixation	260
Timing of surgery	216	Anatomy	237	Outcomes	266

ACETABULAR FRACTURES

The management of acetabular fractures is one of the most, if not the most, complex aspect of orthopaedic trauma. It involves a definite learning curve, probably best documented in a report by Matta and Merritt of the first 121 acetabular fractures treated operatively by Matta. Grouping the surgical reductions chronologically in groups of 20 clearly showed that experience improved the ability to avoid unsatisfactory reductions and to perform anatomic reductions (Fig. 4.1). Kebaish, Roy, and Rennie demonstrated this same concept by comparing the reductions obtained by experienced pelvic trauma surgeons with those obtained by less experienced surgeons, who had a much lower rate of anatomic reduction (Fig. 4.2).

ANATOMY

The acetabulum is an incomplete hemispherical socket with an inverted horseshoe-shaped articular surface surrounding the medial nonarticular cotyloid fossa. The acetabulum can best be described as a partial ball and socket joint composed of six components: (1) anterior, or iliopubic, column, (2) posterior, or ilioischial, column, (3) anterior wall, (4) posterior wall, (5) acetabular dome/roof, and (6) medial wall or quadrilateral plate.

The two columns of bone, described by Letournel and Judet as an inverted Y, support and transmit load to the remainder of the pelvis (Fig. 4.3). The anterior column is composed of the anterior half of the iliac crest, the iliac spines, the anterior half of the acetabulum, and the pubis. The posterior column is the ischium, the ischial spine, the posterior half of the acetabulum, and the dense bone forming the sciatic notch. The shorter posterior column ends at its intersection with the anterior column at the top of the sciatic notch. Classification of these fractures used the column concept, and its understanding is central to the discussion of fracture patterns, operative approaches, and internal fixation.

The articular surface of the acetabulum is divided into the remaining four parts. The posterior wall is larger than the anterior wall and more often presents as a separate fragment because of the flexed position of the hip during the occurrence of many acetabular fractures. The iliopectineal eminence is the prominence in the anterior column that lies directly over the femoral head and represents the inferior half of the anterior wall. This area can be especially difficult to access and provide stable fixation when represented as a separate fragment. The dome, or roof, of the acetabulum is the weight-bearing portion of the articular surface that supports the femoral head when in an upright bipedal position (Fig. 4.4). While it is a confluence of the anterior and posterior walls, the ability to provide anatomic restoration must be considered when choosing an approach. Further, it must be recognized that when the dome occurs as a separate fragment or impacted articular segment, it is important to optimize reduction, fixation, and thus, patient outcomes. Anatomic restoration of the dome with concentric reduction of the femoral head beneath this dome is the goal of both operative and nonoperative treatment.

The quadrilateral surface is the flat plate of bone forming the lateral border of the true pelvic cavity and lying adjacent to the medial wall of the acetabulum (Fig. 4.5). The quadrilateral surface may be comminuted and incompetent, especially in acetabular fractures in the elderly, and the thin nature of this bone may limit the types of fixation that can be used in this region.

The neurovascular structures passing through the pelvis are at risk during the original injury and subsequent treatment, and the various surgical approaches are designed around these structures. The sciatic nerve exiting the greater sciatic notch inferior to the piriformis muscle frequently is injured with posterior fracture-dislocations of the hip and fractures with posterior displacement (Fig. 4.6). The functioning of both the tibial and common peroneal components of the sciatic nerve must be carefully documented in the emergency department and after subsequent interventions (including reduction of a hip dislocation and changes in traction). The sciatic nerve has frequent variation in its relationship to the piriformis muscle as

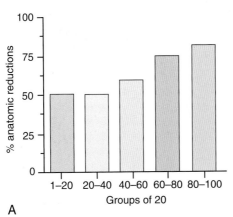

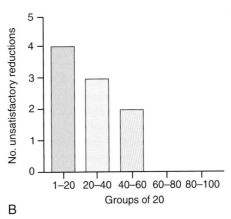

FIGURE 4.1 **A,** Percentage of anatomic reductions per group of 20 for first 100 cases. **B,** Number of unsatisfactory reductions of displaced acetabular fractures per group of 20 for Matta's first 100 surgical cases. (From Matta JM, Merritt PO: Displaced acetabular fractures, *Clin Orthop Relat Res* 230:83, 1988.)

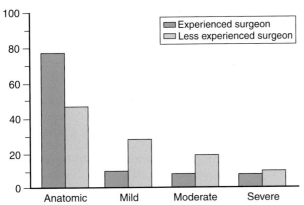

FIGURE 4.2 Quality of reduction of acetabular fractures obtained by experienced pelvic trauma surgeons compared with surgeons with less experience. Mild incongruency is defined as up to 4 mm of fracture displacement; moderate incongruency, as 4 to 10 mm; and severe incongruency, as more than 10 mm. (From Kebaish AS, Roy A, Rennie W: Displaced acetabular fractures: long-term follow-up, *J Trauma* 31:1539, 1991.)

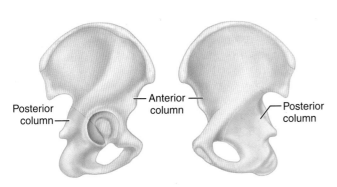

FIGURE 4.3 Two-column concept of Letournel and Judet used in classification of acetabular fractures (see text).

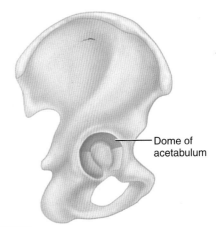

FIGURE 4.4 Superior dome of acetabulum.

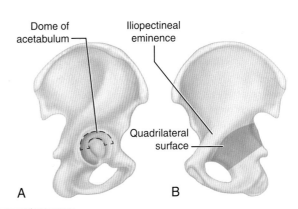

FIGURE 4.5 **A,** Iliopectineal eminence overlies dome of acetabulum. **B,** Quadrilateral surface lies adjacent to medial wall of acetabulum.

it exits the sciatic notch, with common separation of tibial and peroneal branches at this level.

The superior gluteal artery and nerve exit the greater sciatic notch at its most superior aspect and can be tethered to the bone at this level by variable fascial attachments. Fractures that enter the superior portion of the greater sciatic notch can be associated with significant hemorrhage, possibly requiring angiography with embolization of the superior gluteal artery (Fig. 4.7). Selective and nonselective angiography may play a role in operative indications and approaches and should be as selective as possible to limit these risks.

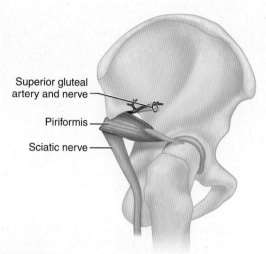

FIGURE 4.6   Piriformis divides greater sciatic notch and is key to this region. Sciatic nerve is shown leaving pelvis below this muscle; superior gluteal artery, vein, and nerve are above it.

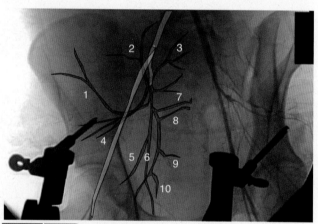

FIGURE 4.7   Diagram depicting the pelvic arterial system, overlaid on a pelvic angiogram. The common iliac artery is shown in aqua; the external artery, in yellow; the internal iliac artery, in green; the posterior branch of the internal iliac artery, in red; and the anterior branch of the internal iliac artery, in blue. Smaller vessels include the superior gluteal artery (1), iliolumbar artery (2), lateral sacral artery (3), inferior gluteal artery (4), umbilical artery (5), obturator artery (6), internal pudendal artery (7), medial rectal artery (8), uterine artery or ductus deferens (9), and superior vesical artery (10). (From Viadya R, Waldron J, Scott A, et al: Angiography and embolization in the management of bleeding pelvic fractures, *J Am Acad Orthop Surg* 26:e68, 2018.)

Knowledge of the intrapelvic relationships of the lumbosacral trunk, common and external iliac vessels, and inferior epigastric vessels as well as of the obturator artery and nerve becomes crucial as retractors, reduction forceps, drills, and screws are placed through anterior approaches. One particularly noteworthy anatomic relationship is the anastomosis between obturator and external iliac systems, which occurs in more than 80% of patients (Fig. 4.8). Failure to ligate this vascular connection during the ilioinguinal or Stoppa approach can lead to significant hemorrhage that is difficult to control as the vessels retract into the pelvis.

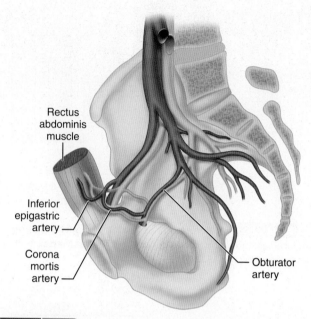

FIGURE 4.8   Schematic drawing showing arterial and venous anastomosis between external iliac and obturator systems.

RADIOGRAPHIC EVALUATION

The acetabulum is evaluated radiographically with an anteroposterior pelvic view as well as with the 45-degree oblique views of the pelvis described by Judet and Letournel, commonly called Judet views. In the iliac oblique view, the radiographic beam is roughly perpendicular to the iliac wing. In the obturator oblique view, the radiographic beam is roughly perpendicular to the obturator foramen. Inclusion of the opposite hip in the radiographic field on the anteroposterior and Judet views is essential for evaluation of symmetric contours that may have slight individual variations and to determine the width of the normal articular cartilage in each view.

Six radiographic landmarks were defined by Judet and Letournel and should be appreciated on all plain films. The iliopubic line, or arcuate line, represents the medial cortex of the anterior column, while the ilioischial line signifies the medial cortex of the posterior column. The radiographic graphic U, more commonly referred to as the teardrop, represents the most inferior and anterior aspect of the acetabular fossa laterally and the anterior aspect of the quadrilateral plate medially. The sourcil represents the acetabular roof and extends to the lateral aspect of the teardrop superiorly. The anterior and posterior lips represent the most lateral aspect of the anterior and posterior walls, respectively.

The radiographic landmarks seen on each view are depicted in Figures 4.9 and 4.10. Fractures that traverse the anterior column disrupt the iliopectineal line, whereas fractures that traverse the posterior column disrupt the ilioischial line. Each fracture pattern in the classification of Letournel and Judet has typical radiographic characteristics with respect to the disruption or intactness of the radiographic landmarks, as shown for a posterior column fracture in Figure 4.11. Evaluation of the various fracture patterns from the standard radiographs requires an understanding of the three-dimensional implications of the status of each of the radiographic landmarks, as well as a three-dimensional grasp of pelvic bony anatomy and the possible variations of fracture

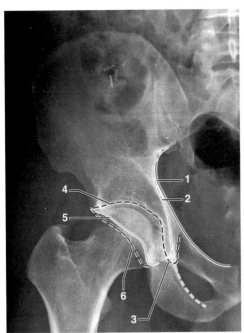

FIGURE 4.9 Landmarks of standard anteroposterior radiograph of hip. 1, Iliopectineal line beginning at greater sciatic notch of ilium and extending down to pubic tubercle. 2, Ilioischial line formed by posterior four fifths of quadrilateral surface of ilium. 3, Radiographic teardrop composed laterally of most inferior and anterior portion of acetabulum and medially of anterior flat part of quadrilateral surface of iliac bone. 4, Roof of acetabulum. 5, Edge of anterior lip of acetabulum. 6, Edge of posterior lip of acetabulum.

lines within a given fracture pattern. In the operating room, the three standard views can be obtained with fluoroscopy. The restoration of the radiographic landmarks is a guide to the adequacy of fracture reduction. Borrelli et al. described the use of Judet view radiographs generated from computed tomography (CT) data that they found to be as good as or better than conventional radiographs in identifying fracture characteristics and classification; however, it should be noted that classically described radiographic findings such as the "spur sign" may not be as readily apparent when the patient is not tilted, as in traditional Judet views.

The anatomic dome is a three-dimensional structure composed of subchondral bone and its overlying cartilage that articulates with the weight-bearing portion of the femoral head. Multiple studies have concluded that the single most important factor affecting long-term outcome in both operatively and nonoperatively treated acetabular fractures is maintenance of a concentric reduction of the femoral head beneath an intact or anatomically reconstructed dome. The dome, or roof, can be seen on the anteroposterior and Judet views of the pelvis, but the subchondral bone shown on each of these views is only 2 to 3 mm wide and represents only that small portion of the actual articular weight-bearing surface that is tangential to the x-ray beam. Matta et al. developed a system for roughly quantifying the acetabular dome after fracture, which they called the "roof arc" measurements. These measurements involve determination of how much of the roof remains intact on each of the three standard radiographic views: anteroposterior, obturator oblique, and iliac oblique. The medial roof arc is measured on the anteroposterior view

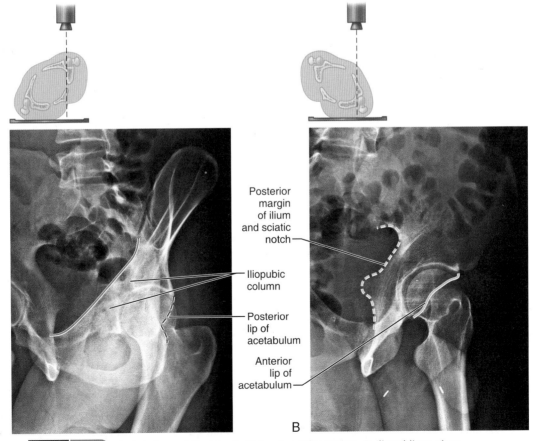

Posterior margin of ilium and sciatic notch

Iliopubic column

Posterior lip of acetabulum

Anterior lip of acetabulum

A

B

FIGURE 4.10 Judet views of the hip. **A,** Obturator oblique view. **B,** Iliac oblique view.

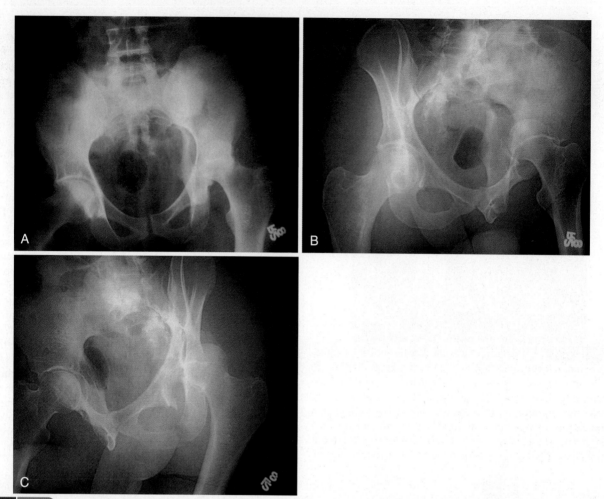

FIGURE 4.11   Fracture of posterior column of acetabulum. **A,** Anteroposterior view shows intact iliopectineal line, with disrupted ilioischial line. **B,** Iliac oblique (Judet) view shows disrupted posterior column and intact anterior wall. **C,** Obturator oblique (Judet) view shows intact anterior column in profile.

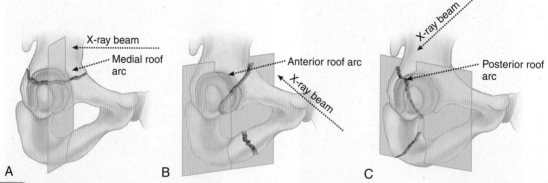

FIGURE 4.12   "Roof arc" measurement, as described by Matta et al. **A,** Medial roof arc is measured on anteroposterior view. **B,** Anterior roof arc is measured on 45-degree angle obturator oblique view. **C,** Posterior roof arc is measured on 45-degree angle iliac oblique view.

by drawing a vertical line through the roof of the acetabulum to its geometric center. A second line is then drawn through the point where the fracture line intersects the roof of the acetabulum and again to the geometric center of the acetabulum. The angle thus formed represents the medial roof arc (Fig. 4.12A). The anterior and posterior roof arcs are similarly determined on the obturator oblique and iliac oblique views, respectively (Fig. 4.12B and C). Although these are rough calculations, they are useful in the assessment of fractures of the posterior or anterior column, transverse fractures,

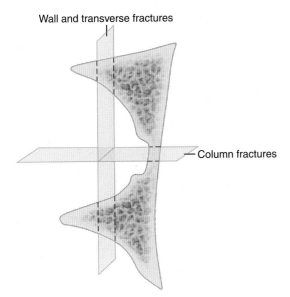

Wall and transverse fractures

Column fractures

FIGURE 4.13 Orientation of fracture lines through acetabulum as seen on CT scan.

T-type fractures, and associated anterior column and posterior hemitransverse fractures; they have limited usefulness for evaluation of both-column fractures and fractures involving the posterior wall. According to Matta et al., if any of the roof arc measurements in a displaced fracture are less than 45 degrees, operative treatment should be considered.

CT is invaluable in the diagnosis and planning of treatment for acetabular fractures, as even fellowship-trained orthopaedic trauma surgeons can more reliably classify fractures on CT as compared to multiplanar radiographs. Axial cuts should be taken with thin (3-mm or less) intervals and corresponding slice thicknesses. The entire pelvis generally is included to avoid missing a portion of the fracture, and comparison to the opposite hip is performed routinely. The surgeon should learn to move from image to image, following the fracture lines and envisioning the obliquities and displacements of the fracture lines shown. A plastic pelvic model is helpful in learning this technique and later for drawing more complex fractures directly on the model. In general, the transverse fracture lines and fractures of the anterior and posterior walls are in the sagittal plane, paralleling the quadrilateral surface when they are viewed on axial CT images (Figs. 4.13 and 4.14). Anterior and posterior column fractures usually extend through the quadrilateral surface and into the obturator foramen with a more coronal orientation; variant fracture types, however, may not follow these generalities.

Some authors have suggested that axial CT images overestimate the extent of comminution of acetabular fractures; however, only existing fracture lines are shown on the images. For example, in transverse fractures, moving proximally on successive cuts, small fragments of the anterior and posterior walls enlarge to coalesce through the roof, becoming the axial cross section of the ilium. What may appear to be separate anterior and posterior wall fracture fragments on more inferior cuts is the distal extent of a single proximal fragment. An oblique fracture line divides the acetabulum, so the more inferior CT cuts appear to have three fragments when there are only two. By studying the individual fragments on multiple successive cuts, the entire fracture can

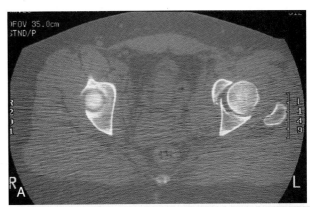

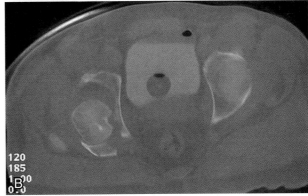

FIGURE 4.14 **A,** Anterior column fracture with typical fracture orientation. **B,** Posterior wall fracture.

be appreciated, giving a true mental three-dimensional picture. High-resolution coronal and sagittal reconstructions of the fracture are helpful in the preoperative evaluation of complex fractures by delineating fractures that lie directly in the plane of a given axial CT image. Even CT scans can give the same information about the acetabular dome as the roof arc measurements on the anteroposterior and oblique radiographs. Axial CT scans showing the superior 10 mm of the acetabular roof to be intact have been shown to correspond to radiographic roof arc measurements of 45 degrees. Fracture of the cotyloid fossa does not appear to jeopardize stability of the femoral head under the dome if the fossa extends to within 10 mm of the apex of the roof and the articular surface is intact.

Three-dimensional CT reconstructions (Fig. 4.15) of a fracture have been described for several decades, but are readily fabricated with modern CT software and can be projected in many different views with subtraction of the femoral head that show unique features of the various fracture patterns. These images can be extremely helpful with complicated fractures, especially in the educational setting. While 3-D imaging is a useful tool, it is essential to take time to understand both plain film radiographs and single-plane CT imaging of these fractures.

CLASSIFICATION

The classification of acetabular fractures described by Letournel and Judet (Fig. 4.16) is the commonly used classification system. In this system, acetabular fractures are divided into two basic groups: *simple fracture types* and the more complex *associated fracture types* (Box 4.1).

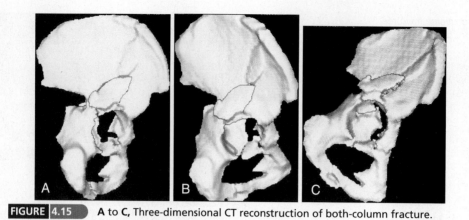

FIGURE 4.15 **A** to **C**, Three-dimensional CT reconstruction of both-column fracture.

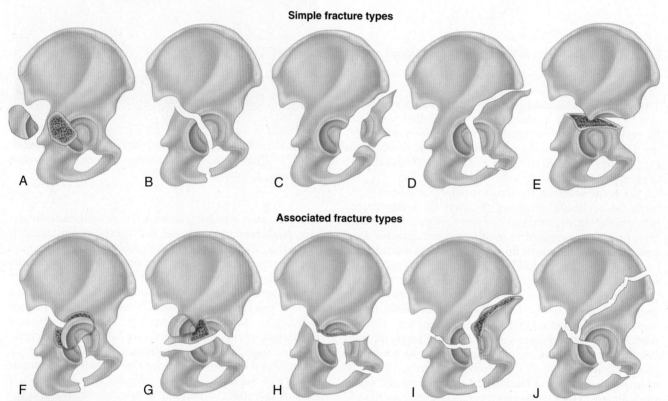

FIGURE 4.16 Letournel and Judet classification of acetabular fractures. **A**, Posterior wall fracture. **B**, Posterior column fracture. **C**, Anterior wall fracture. **D**, Anterior column fracture. **E**, Transverse fracture. **F**, Posterior column and posterior wall fracture. **G**, Transverse and posterior wall fracture. **H**, T-shaped fracture. **I**, Anterior column and posterior hemitransverse fracture. **J**, Complete both-column fracture.

Although several of the associated fracture types involve both columns of the acetabulum, the designation *associated both-column fracture* in this classification denotes that none of the articular fracture fragments of the acetabulum maintain bony continuity with the axial skeleton: a fracture line divides the ilium, so the sacroiliac joint is not connected to any articular segment. The spur sign, shown on the obturator oblique view, is pathognomonic of a both-column fracture. It represents the remaining portion of the ilium still attached to the sacrum and is seen projected lateral to the medially displaced acetabulum (Fig. 4.17).

TREATMENT

With longer follow-up of operatively treated acetabular fractures it has become clear that fractures with even small residual incongruencies of the critical portion of the acetabulum lead to long-term arthritis more often than do similar fractures with more anatomic reductions. Based on this information, the indications for open reduction and internal fixation (ORIF) of acetabular fractures have become more inclusive in the young patient; however, the indications in the geriatric patient are still being actively investigated.

BOX 4.1

Letournel and Judet Classification of Acetabular Fractures

Simple (Elementary) Patterns
- Anterior wall fracture
- Anterior column fracture
- Posterior wall fracture
- Posterior column fracture
- Transverse fracture

Complex (Associated) Patterns
- Posterior column and posterior wall fractures
- Transverse and posterior wall fractures
- T-shaped fracture
- Anterior column and posterior hemitransverse fractures
- Associated both-column fractures

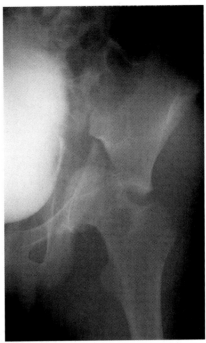

FIGURE 4.18 Transverse acetabular fracture with true central fracture-dislocation; intrapelvic femoral head can become locked between superior and inferior fracture fragments.

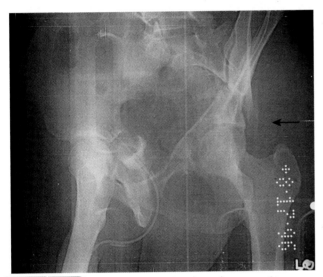

FIGURE 4.17 Spur sign in both-column fracture of acetabulum.

INITIAL TREATMENT

Acetabular fractures generally are caused by high-energy trauma, and associated injuries are frequent. Management of the entire patient should follow accepted Advanced Trauma Life Support (ATLS) protocol, with orthopaedic treatment of the acetabular fracture appropriately integrated into the treatment plan. In general, operative treatment of an acetabular fracture is not considered an orthopaedic emergency/urgency (requiring operative intervention within 1 to 24 hours), except when it is part of open fracture management, or is performed for a fracture associated with an irreducible dislocation of the hip. In the latter case, urgent open reduction of the hip dislocation followed by treatment of the associated fracture should be performed as expediently as possible to decrease the risk of complications of osteonecrosis and ongoing cartilaginous damage to the femoral head.

Closed reduction of hip dislocations should be performed with full relaxation through sedation in the emergency department or with general anesthesia. Reduction should be confirmed with either radiography or fluoroscopy. Not all patients with acetabular fractures require skeletal traction. When the hip is stable with the legs in an abduction pillow and a congruent reduction is achieved, we prefer to send the patient to CT prior to placing traction. We then evaluate if the femoral head articular cartilage will tend to undergo further damage from displaced intraarticular fractures through edge loading, such as a displaced transverse fracture, or due to retained intraarticular fragments. If either of these conditions exist, the hip remains unstable, or the reduction is noncongruent because of soft-tissue interposition, the patient is placed in skeletal traction, while they are resuscitated before surgical intervention. We prefer the use of distal femoral traction pins to facilitate knee flexion during subsequent surgery, if a prone traction position is required. We generally start with a weight equal to 10% of the patient's body weight, up to a maximum of 20 to 25 lb.

Historically, *central fracture-dislocation* of the hip was used to describe any acetabular fracture with medial subluxation of the femoral head. Although this terminology has been replaced with more descriptive fracture classification systems, a true central fracture-dislocation with the femoral head completely dislocated medially into the pelvis is an unusual injury that requires urgent treatment (Fig. 4.18). The femoral head can be locked between the fracture fragments, making reduction extremely difficult or impossible through closed means. Closed reduction with general anesthesia and fluoroscopic assistance should be attempted. After reduction, the femoral head is extremely unstable and will easily displace back into the pelvis if skeletal traction is not maintained.

If closed reduction of a hip dislocation associated with an acetabular fracture is unsuccessful, the immediate treatment

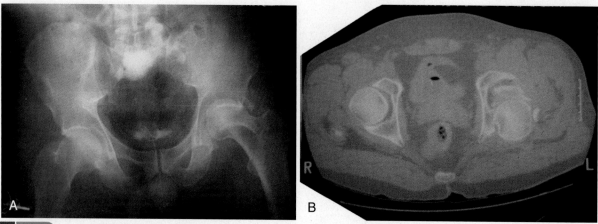

FIGURE 4.19 Anteroposterior pelvic radiograph **(A)** and CT scan **(B)** of irreducible hip dislocation with posterior wall acetabular fracture. Posterior wall fragment is incarcerated, blocking reduction.

TABLE 4.1

Relationship of Classification Systems for Pelvic Ring Fractures

	BUCHOLZ	TILE	OTA/AO	YOUNG-BURGESS	LETOURNEL	DENIS
Stable Pelvic Ring	I	A1, B2	61A, 61B2	Anterior-posterior compression I Lateral compression I Combined mechanical injury*	*	*
Partial Instability	II	B1	61B2	Anterior-posterior compression II Lateral compression II Combined mechanical injury* Lateral compression III	*	*
Complete Instability	III	C	61C	Anterior-posterior compression III Lateral compression III Vertical shear Combined mechanical injury*	*	*

*Can be associated with all types of instability.
OTA/AO, Orthopaedic Trauma Association/Arbeitsgemeinschaft für Osteosynthesefragen.
From Olson SA, Burgess A: Classification and initial management of patients with unstable pelvic ring injuries, *Instr Course Lect* 54:383, 2005.

of the hip depends on the experience of the surgeon. A rapid CT scan of the pelvis will demonstrate the acetabular fracture pattern, and may demonstrate the obstruction to reduction of the hip dislocation, which will allow formulation of an operative plan for ORIF (Fig. 4.19). If the block to reduction is as simple as an intraarticular fragment and the patient is too unstable for formal ORIF, Marecek and Routt described a percutaneous fluoroscopic technique for displacing intraarticular fragments blocking concentric hip reduction after closed reduction, allowing further planning and resuscitation of the patient. If an experienced acetabular surgeon is not readily available, transfer to a facility capable of managing such injuries should be done swiftly, as outcome after these injuries is time-dependent.

▣ INDICATIONS FOR NONOPERATIVE TREATMENT
▮ NONDISPLACED AND MINIMALLY DISPLACED FRACTURES

Fractures that traverse the weight-bearing dome, but are displaced less than 2 mm, may be appropriate for treatment with non–weight bearing for 6 to 12 weeks, depending on

the fracture characteristics (Table 4.1). Radiographs should be obtained immediately after the patient is first mobilized and frequently thereafter to ensure that no displacement has occurred. Occasionally this requires a repeat CT scan to assess maintenance of reduction.

▮ FRACTURES WITH SIGNIFICANT DISPLACEMENT BUT IN WHICH THE REGION OF THE JOINT INVOLVED IS JUDGED TO BE UNIMPORTANT PROGNOSTICALLY

This determination is made with the roof arc measurements at 45 degrees for each roof arc: medial, anterior, and posterior (Fig. 4.20). Vrahas, Widding, and Thomas questioned whether the 45-degree value is the most appropriate for each roof arc. In a study of cadaver hips, they proposed acceptable roof arc measurements as 25 degrees for the anterior roof arc, 45 degrees for the medial roof arc, and 70 degrees for the posterior roof arc. As a rough guide, they recommended ORIF of displaced fractures exiting the posterior column above the upper border of the ischial spine, as well as of fractures exiting the anterior column through the iliac wing.

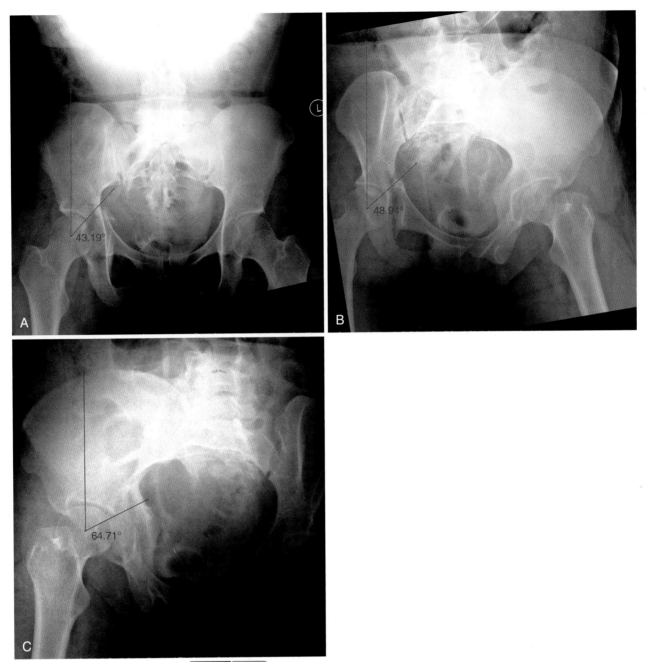

FIGURE 4.20 Matta roof-arc measurements. See text.

Displaced fractures through the weight-bearing dome in a young patient with more than 2 mm of displacement should be treated operatively. These fractures tend to displace, leading to inferior results. In the modern era, virtually no fractures are treated definitively by traction to maintain a reduction involving the acetabular dome.

Fractures with a posterior wall component, especially when associated with posterior fracture-dislocations of the hip, require separate consideration and are evaluated after closed reduction. Larger posterior wall fragments lead to posterior hip instability and require fixation. Three well-described methods, that of Calkins (Fig. 4.21), Keith (Fig. 4.22), and Moed (Fig. 4.23), have been used for determination of wall size in comparison to the normal acetabulum. Critical wall size resulting in instability is determined by the method

of measurement, with Calkins, Keith, and Moed hypothesizing that walls larger than 40%, 65.7%, and 50%, respectively, based on their measurements, were going to be unstable. They also theorized that fragments smaller than 20%, 44.8%, and 20% based on measurements by the methods of Calkins, Keith, and Moed, respectively, would be stable. However, only 2 years later Moed et al. published another study warning against the use of CT findings as the sole predictor of stability. Their follow-up found that inappropriate nonoperative treatment (i.e., nonoperative management of an unstable hip) would have occurred in 6% (11/180) of patients and inappropriate operative treatment (i.e., operative fixation of a stable hip) would have occurred in 16% (28/180) of patients. This finding was further reinforced by Firoozabadi et al. when they showed that 23% of fractures smaller than 20% of the wall

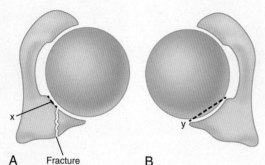

FIGURE 4.21 Straight-line measurement of posterior wall as described by Calkins et al. for calculation of "approximate acetabular fracture index" (ApAFI). **A,** Straight line medial-lateral measurement is made of remaining intact articular posterior wall acetabular segment at level of greatest amount of fracture involvement (X). **B,** Length of posterior acetabular arc is determined from uninjured, contralateral hip at same level (Y). X divided by Y multiplied provides the index percentage. (Redrawn from Moed BR, Ajibade DA, Israel H: Computed tomography as a predictor of hip stability status in posterior wall fractures of the acetabulum, *J Orthop Trauma* 23:7, 2009.)

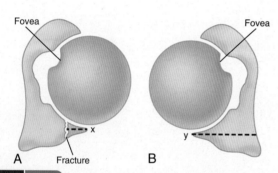

FIGURE 4.22 Method of Keith et al. **A,** Approximate medial-lateral dimension (depth) of fractured segment (X) is determined at level of fovea. **B,** Percentage of fragment size is calculated from ratio of measured depth of fractured segment to intact matched contralateral acetabular depth measured to medial extent of quadrilateral plate (Y) at comparable level of fovea. (Redrawn from Moed BR, Ajibade DA, Israel H: Computed tomography as a predictor of hip stability status in posterior wall fractures of the acetabulum, *J Orthop Trauma* 23:7, 2009.)

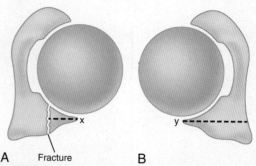

FIGURE 4.23 Method of Moed. **A,** Approximate medial-lateral dimension (depth) of fractured segment (X) is determined at level of greatest size of posterior wall fracture fragment. **B,** Percentage of depth size is calculated from ratio of measured depth of fractured segment to intact matched contralateral acetabular depth measured to medial extent of quadrilateral plate (Y) at level comparable to that used for measurement of fracture fragment. (Redrawn from Moed BR, Ajibade DA, Israel H: Computed tomography as a predictor of hip stability status in posterior wall fractures of the acetabulum, *J Orthop Trauma* 23:7, 2009.)

were unstable. These fractures did tend to extend more cranially (5.0 mm from the dome compared to 9.5 mm from the dome); however, this was not found to be a reliable predictive factor in determining stability. While these measurements can aid the surgeon, an examination under anesthesia (EUA) remains the gold standard for predicting posterior instability after acetabular fracture involving less than 50% of the wall, with operative management without EUA indicated for those involving more than 50%.

Tornetta described EUA of the acetabulum after utilizing fluoroscopic stress views of 41 hips with acetabular fractures for which ORIF was not indicated based on roof arcs of 45 degrees, a subchondral CT arc of 10 mm, displacement of less than 50% of the posterior wall, and congruence on the anterior-posterior and Judet views of the hip. He either sedated or

anesthetized patients and stressed their fractures in the direction of the deforming force for each fracture pattern while fluoroscopically viewing the fractures on all three standard radiographic views. He found that three of these hips subluxated on stress views without frank instability noted clinically, and these fractures underwent ORIF. These hips would have passed the traditional clinical test of stability by flexing the hip to 90 degrees. The same preference for dynamic fluoroscopic stress testing has been stated by other authors when comparing CT criteria for stability in posterior wall fractures to fluoroscopic EUA.

We have adopted this technique of performing stress views under fluoroscopy when patients are considered for nonoperative treatment of smaller posterior wall fractures. We view the pelvis in the obturator oblique view, flexing the hip to 90 degrees, providing adduction and internal rotation. A static fluoroscopic image is then obtained. While posteriorly directed pressure is applied through the knee with enough force to rock the pelvis (50 to 100 lb), a spot fluoroscopic view is obtained and scrutinized to assess subluxation (Fig. 4.24).

Stable hips are treated like a pure dislocation of the hip. We still prescribe posterior hip precautions for the first 6 weeks, with touch-down weight bearing on crutches for 2 weeks, followed by progressive weight bearing, then full return to activity at 6 weeks. Following this assessment and treatment technique, Grimshaw and Moed reported the radiographic outcome of 15 nonoperatively treated patients with small posterior wall fractures that were stable with EUA. At a minimum of 2 years after injury, none of the patients showed incongruence or joint space narrowing.

SECONDARY CONGRUENCE IN DISPLACED BOTH-COLUMN FRACTURES

An associated both-column (ABC) fracture, by definition, has all its fragments free to move independent of the remaining ilium attached to the axial skeleton. Occasionally, comminuted both-column fracture fragments assume a position of

and occasionally exceptional results. The concept applies only to specific both-column fractures where all the articular fragments are free to conform around the displaced femoral head and cannot be applied to other fracture types.

While biomechanical analysis of secondary congruence displays increased mean pressures (122%) and peak pressures (280%), the clinical relevance of this is still not fully delineated, as nearly 70% (11/16) of patients treated nonoperatively by Letournel had excellent results at 4.3 years of average follow-up. At our institution, patients with ABC acetabular fractures with secondary congruence, who are of an age and activity level that make total hip arthroplasty a reasonable alternative if posttraumatic arthritis were to develop, are treated with nonoperative management. Patients who are not candidates for a total hip arthroplasty as a salvage option are treated with operative intervention, if they meet all other criteria.

MEDICAL CONTRAINDICATIONS TO SURGERY

In patients with multiple trauma, medical contraindications from multisystem injury are common, even in previously healthy patients. Although early fracture fixation and mobilization are basic tenets of polytrauma treatment protocols, complex fractures may require long operative procedures with significant blood loss. On occasion, the severity of the medical condition mandates that operative intervention be delayed. If deemed needed, the articular cartilage of the hip should be protected during these delays by placing the patient in skeletal traction. On occasion, severe head trauma with a tenuous, evolving spectrum of injury may preclude a surgical procedure; however, a head injury in itself is not necessarily a contraindication to surgery. The eventual neurologic outcome frequently cannot be reliably assessed in the immediate postinjury period, when acetabular ORIF can most reliably be performed.

Percutaneous fluoroscopic screw fixation has been recommended for suitable fractures in severely injured patients, in patients with significant medical comorbidities, and by some authors for patients over the age of 60. In our practice, although not a substitute for formal ORIF, it serves as an excellent alternative in select patients (Fig. 4.26). Gary et al. reported the use of percutaneous screw fixation in acetabular fractures in patients 60 years of age and older assessed 6.8 years after the index surgery. At final follow-up, approximately 30% had been converted to total hip arthroplasty. They found that in the patients who retained their native hips, their short musculoskeletal functional assessment was similar to two series of formal ORIF in this age group, and that the Harris Hip Scores in those patients converted to total hip replacement were similar to those reported for acute total hip replacement for acetabular fracture. In medically compromised patients in whom a full open approach may not be possible, percutaneous management may offer improved pain control, earlier mobilization, and prevention of skin breakdown, deep venous thrombosis (DVT), and other medical complications.

LOCAL SOFT-TISSUE PROBLEMS, SUCH AS INFECTION, WOUNDS, AND SOFT-TISSUE LESIONS FROM BLUNT TRAUMA

An open wound in the anticipated surgical field is a relative contraindication, as is systemic infection. More ominous in

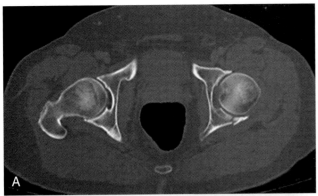

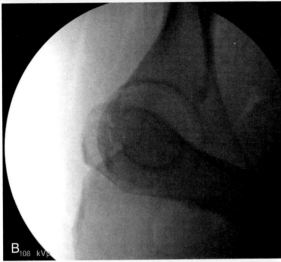

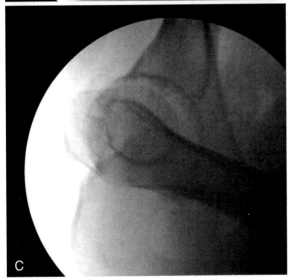

FIGURE 4.24 **A,** CT of minimally displaced left posterior wall. **B,** Obturator oblique view obtained fluoroscopically with no stress applied shows concentric reduction. **C,** Same view with posterior stress applied demonstrates hip subluxation. Open reduction and internal fixation were performed.

articular "secondary congruence" around the femoral head, even though the femoral head is displaced medially and there may be gaps between the fracture fragments (Fig. 4.25). The concept of secondary congruence was described by Letournel, and closed treatment of these fractures has yielded reasonable

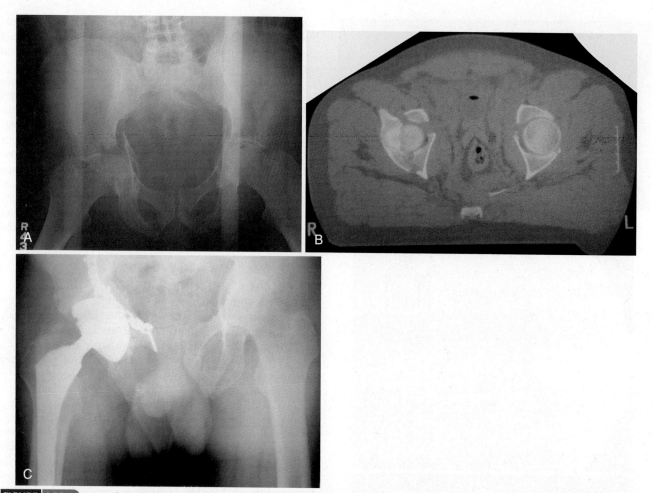

FIGURE 4.25 **A** and **B,** Right hip displays comminuted both-column acetabular fracture with secondary congruence. Left hip has T-shaped fracture with medial dome impaction. **C,** Three years after open reduction and internal fixation of right T-type fracture, patient developed posttraumatic arthritis that required total hip arthroplasty, while left hip with both-column fracture with secondary congruence treated nonoperatively remained minimally symptomatic.

fractures around the acetabulum is the Morel-Lavallée lesion, a localized area of subcutaneous fat necrosis over the lateral aspect of the hip caused by the same trauma that caused the acetabular fracture (see chapter 1). Judet and Letournel found that in their series approximately 8% of patients who sustained a blow to the greater trochanter had a clinically significant Morel-Lavallée lesion. The size and extent of this lesion are variable, with as many as 46% of "closed" injuries being culture-positive at initial debridement, and operating through it has been associated with a higher rate of postoperative infection, with as high as 12% infection rates being reported with repeated postoperative wound debridement, packing, and healing by secondary intention. However, Tseng and Tornetta described an alternative method of percutaneous decompression and debridement with delayed ORIF until at least 24 hours after drains were removed, which was performed when output was less than 30 mL per day. While they reported no infections in any patient treated percutaneously, of the two fractures that were fixed through a Kocher-Langenbeck approach, one required a surgical exploration of the wound because of persistent drainage (see Technique 53.1). Alternatively, some fractures can be treated through anterior approaches, thus

avoiding the affected area. The presence of a significant Morel-Lavallée lesion should be suspected in any patient with hypermobility of the skin or a fluid wave in the subcutaneous tissue. The CT scan, if available, should be scrutinized for a fluid collection in the subcutaneous tissues.

The presence of a suprapubic catheter was previously considered a contraindication to acetabular ORIF by the ilioinguinal and anterior intrapelvic (AIP) approaches. Bacterial colonization of the catheter had been anecdotally reported to increase the rate of infection; however, a recent series using the National Trauma Data Bank (NTDB) showed no increase in infectious complications in patients undergoing pelvic or acetabular surgery who had a suprapubic catheter. As a large database study, these findings are certainly promising but not always representative of findings in smaller controlled groups; thus, when possible, through primary repair of the bladder rupture and Foley catheter drainage, we still attempt to avoid suprapubic catheter placement.

ELDERLY PATIENTS WITH OSTEOPOROTIC BONE

Traditionally, there was a concern for loss of reduction due to inadequate fixation in osteoporotic bone; however, a small

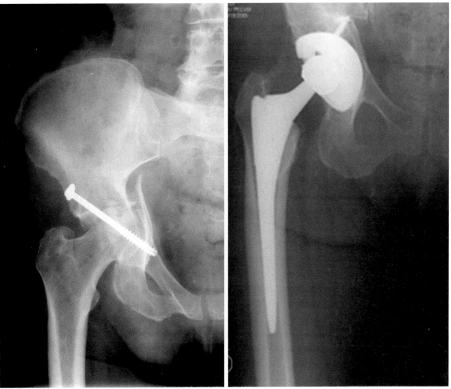

FIGURE 4.26   Total hip arthroplasty after percutaneous fixation of acetabular fracture in elderly patient.

series by Helfet et al. questioned this this concern, as only one patient in 18 lost reduction during the healing period. Carroll et al. found that in 84 patients over the age of 55 years who had initial ORIF for their acetabular fractures, nearly 31% (26/84) required conversion to total hip arthroplasty within 5 years of their initial surgery. Similarly, a study from a level 1 trauma center found that 28% of patients over the age of 60 years required a total hip arthroplasty within 2.5 years of their injury. Superior medial impaction of the dome, or the "gull sign," particularly correlated with a poor outcome (Fig. 4.27).

Ryan et al. reported a series of patients ages 60 years or older who had acetabular fractures that met traditional operative criteria. Although this was a small series of only 27 patients, they found that only 15% (4/27) required conversion to total hip arthroplasty and the remaining 85% had WOMAC and SF-8 scores consistent with those of patients with a normal hip.

In our practice, elderly patients with fracture morphology consistent with poor outcomes (e.g., large areas of impaction or "gull sign") are routinely treated with ORIF and acute total hip arthroplasty. Comminuted and impacted fractures in high-comorbidity elderly patients often are treated with early mobilization and nonoperative management, with a discussion that delayed surgery may be required if the patient develops symptomatic arthritis. The benefit of nonoperative management in these patients is that many will do well without any surgery and those who do require surgery will have a more predictable delayed total hip arthroplasty that requires less time, less blood loss, and a lower rate of transfusion than patients who have had ORIF.

■ INDICATIONS FOR OPERATIVE TREATMENT
▌FRACTURE CHARACTERISTICS

Operative indications for acetabular fractures traditionally include (1) 2 mm or more of displacement in the dome of the acetabulum as defined by any roof arc measurements of less than 45 degrees on any of the three Judet views or 10 mm on CT cuts, (2) subluxation of the femoral head noted on any of the three standard radiographic views or CT, (3) posterior wall fractures involving more than 40% of the joint, and (4) dynamic instability of the hip allowing subluxation in posterior wall fractures involving less than 40% of the joint.

▌INCARCERATED FRAGMENTS IN THE ACETABULUM AFTER CLOSED REDUCTION OF A HIP DISLOCATION

Small avulsed fragments of the ligamentum teres that stay sequestered in the cotyloid fossa and do not affect the congruency of the hip probably do not require excision. Fragments noted on CT to be lodged between the articular surfaces of the femoral head and the acetabulum warrant excision, as do fragments in the cotyloid fossa large enough to cause subluxation of the joint. Fluoroscopic and arthroscopic techniques of fragment removal have been described, although most often this is performed through an open approach, up to and including need for surgical dislocation.

▌PREVENTION OF NONUNION AND RETENTION OF SUFFICIENT BONE STOCK FOR LATER RECONSTRUCTIVE SURGERY

This last indication for ORIF should be applied only in cases of extreme deformity because total hip arthroplasty after failed ORIF of an acetabular fracture may be more difficult than hip arthroplasty after nonoperative management. Scarring from

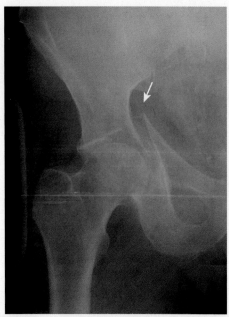

FIGURE 4.27 "Gull sign" on this transverse fracture indicates impaction of medial portion of weight-bearing dome.

previous surgeries, implants, and heterotopic bone can complicate such secondary reconstruction. Percutaneous fixation may be considered in patients who are at high risk of conversion to total hip arthroplasty but have displacement that is concerning for nonunion of the columns required for standard cup placement. We use this technique to mobilize these patients, using limited column fixation to prevent gross displacement of the fracture. After fracture healing, conversion to total hip arthroplasty can be done if the patient's symptoms warrant (see Fig. 4.27). This topic is covered in more detail later (see Total Hip Arthroplasty as Treatment of Acetabular Fracture).

■ TIMING OF SURGERY

Acetabular fractures associated with irreducible hip dislocation, open fracture, vascular compromise, or worsening neurologic deficit require urgent surgical intervention. Conversely, in most circumstances, acetabular fracture surgery should be done only after the patient is medically optimized and the surgeon has studied the fracture in detail with adequate preoperative planning and assembly of an experienced surgical team. There is a general belief that delaying surgery for 2 to 3 days may result in less bleeding at the time of surgery. This belief has been called in question by Dailey and Archdeacon, who studied patients with posterior wall fractures treated through the Kocher-Langenbeck approach, and associated both-column and anterior column/posterior hemitransverse fractures treated through anterior intrapelvic approaches, with surgery either before 48 hours or after 48 hours postinjury. They found no difference in blood loss or operative times in the two groups. This has been further supported by subsequent studies from Parry et al. and Furey et al.

Ideally, ORIF of acetabular fractures should be performed within 5 to 7 days of injury, if not sooner. As time passes, anatomic reduction becomes more difficult as hematoma organization, soft-tissue contracture, and subsequent early callus

formation hinder the process of fracture reduction, especially if more limited exposures are utilized. Madhu et al. found a decreased ability to attain anatomic reductions in associated fracture patterns after 5 days and in elementary patterns after 15 days. After a delay of more than 3 weeks, an extensile exposure may be necessary to obtain operative reduction of fractures that could have otherwise been treated through more limited exposures.

■ CHOICE OF SURGICAL APPROACH

If surgical stabilization is indicated, detailed evaluation of the fracture configuration and classification is necessary to plan the operative approach. Some fracture patterns are routinely reduced through an ilioinguinal or AIP approach (also known as the modified Stoppa approach), whereas the posterior Kocher-Langenbeck approach is more appropriate for others.

Generally, transverse-posterior wall and T-shaped fractures with either posterior wall involvement or principally posterior displacement, and transverse fractures with predominantly posterior displacement, are treated through a Kocher-Langenbeck approach. Prone positioning of the patient may aid the reduction of some acetabular fractures treated through the Kocher-Langenbeck approach, such as fractures with a displaced transverse component, by not allowing the weight of the leg to displace the fracture medially. Digastric osteotomy of the trochanter, as described by Siebenrock, can aid exposure of transverse fractures or supraacetabular extension of fractures of the posterior column and wall. This osteotomy, when performed correctly, does not affect the vascularity of the femoral head, and has a high rate of union. This osteotomy also has been combined with surgical dislocation of the femoral head in the treatment of selected fractures and is especially useful for acetabular fractures associated with Pipkin fractures of the femoral head, which can be treated in conjunction with the acetabular fracture through a single approach. An anterior approach is generally used for anterior wall, anterior column, anterior-column posterior-hemitransverse, associated both-column fractures, or any combination of such. T-shaped or transverse fractures with predominately anterior displacement can also be treated with an anterior approach.

The AIP, or modified Stoppa, approach uses a Pfannenstiel skin incision with a vertical split in the rectus abdominis though the linea alba. The rectus on the involved side is elevated off the superior surface of the pubis and any anastomoses between the obturator vessels and the external iliac or inferior epigastric vessels (the corona mortis) are ligated to expose the internal surface of the anterior column and the quadrilateral surface. It can be used for many fractures previously treated through the ilioinguinal approach. The use of the AIP approach with the lateral window of the ilioinguinal approach has been promoted as a way of avoiding the dissection of the middle window of the ilioinguinal approach and thus exposure of the femoral vein, artery, nerve, and lymphatics. Addition of an osteotomy of the anterior superior iliac spine can significantly improve visualization of the anterior wall or psoas gutter, traditionally only accessible through the middle window of an ilioinguinal approach. It can also be used to improve visualization from the lateral window in patients with a large abdomen.

ANTERIOR INTRA-PELVIC APPROACH

TECHNIQUE 4.1

- Generally, a Pfannenstiel incision is used, approximately 2 cm above the pubic symphysis. As an alternative, a vertical midline skin incision may be used, starting 1 cm inferior to the symphysis, and ending 2 cm to 3 cm inferior to the umbilicus (Fig. 4.28A).
- Divide the subcutaneous tissues in line with the skin incision to expose the fascia overlying both rectus muscles of the abdomen and identify the decussation of fascial fibers at the midline.
- A 0.5 to 1 cm transverse incision in the fascia near midline can help identify the interval between the heads of the rectus muscle bellies prior to extension of the incision vertically. Once the interval is identified, incise the rectus fascia longitudinally along the linea alba and gently retract both bellies of the rectus abdominis muscle laterally (Fig. 4.28B).
- In the proximal part of the incision, take care not to incise the peritoneum. The entire approach should stay in the preperitoneal space. However, extension proximally will increase the muscular excursion and is necessary for optimal visualization.
- Loosely pack a wet sponge in the retropubic space to protect the urinary bladder and place a malleable retractor to protect the bladder (Fig. 4.28C).
- Release the rectus over and onto the anterior aspect of the pubic tubercle; again, increased release will increase later visualization.
- Sharply dissect the thick periosteum from the superior pubic bone to allow deeper blunt dissection. (Fig. 4.28D).
- Identify the upper border of the superior pubic ramus (pectin pubis) and carry the dissection laterally along the pelvic brim. Once past the pubic tubercle, place a sharp Hohmann retractor over the lateral aspect of the tubercle.
- Place a Deaver retractor laterally, with care to avoid injury to the iliac vessels. Dissecting carefully along the medial surface of the superior ramus, identify the corona mortis vessels and ligate (or clip) them as necessary (Fig. 4.28E).
- Continue subperiosteal dissection laterally, following the upper border of the superior pubic bone to the direction of the pelvic brim, exposing the beginning of the iliopectineal eminence.
- Dissect the beginning of the iliopectineal arch from the bone to allow elevation of the femoral vessels and nerve (Fig. 4.28F).
- Continue lateral dissection in a subperiosteal fashion, following the upper border of the pelvic brim. A sharp Hohmann or custom retractor may be placed over the acetabular rim near the ilio-pubic eminence. At this point, the entire internal surface of the superior pubic ramus has been exposed adequately for plate fixation.
- As the quadrilateral surface is reached, the obturator neurovascular bundle should be identified and may require mobilization. Use a custom pelvic floor retractor or malleable retractor placed into the lesser sciatic notch to protect the obturator neurovascular bundle and bladder.
- With a Cobb elevator, elevate the periosteum and obturator internus to expose the quadrilateral surface (Fig. 4.28G).
- After development of the subperiosteal dissection over the pelvic brim, a sharp Hohmann retractor can be impacted on the posterior top of the acetabulum into the ilium. Take great care not to injure the external iliac vein, which may be in proximity to the elevators, if not adequately retracted. (Fig. 4.28H).

Developed by Letournel in the 1960s, the traditional ilioinguinal approach consists of three windows through a single skin incision, extending from the iliac crest to the midline, above the symphysis. The lateral window extends lateral to the iliopsoas (iliopectineal fascia), the middle window is between the iliopsoas and the external iliac vessels, and the medial window is medial to the external iliac vessels. The originally described ilioinguinal approach involved a medial window developed lateral to the rectus muscle or through a tenotomy of the rectus tendon; however, most surgeons who use the ilioinguinal approach now combine the ilioinguinal and AIP approaches, working through a window between the rectus muscle bodies along the linea alba. Traditionally, most surgeons prefer to use skeletal traction on a radiolucent flat-top table for most fractures treated through an anterior approach. Use of a triangle under the hip helps to relax the iliopsoas and improve visualization through the lateral window.

More complicated fractures may require one of the extensile approaches, such as the extended iliofemoral approach described by Letournel and Judet, the triradiate approach of Mears and Rubash, or the T-approach described by Reinert et al. The use of extensile approaches have largely fallen out of favor in the last decade, mostly because of the morbidity of these extensive dissections, but they remain a viable option for certain fracture patterns. The historic indications include associated both-column fractures with posterior wall displacement or a segmental posterior column or transtectal T-shaped fractures with significant displacement of both columns, especially in a young patient. If an extensile exposure is used, confirmation of the patency of the superior gluteal artery with angiography has been recommended because this may be the only vascular pedicle supplying the abductor muscles. This recommendation was based primarily on clinical observation of patients with extensile exposures as well as concerns about the collateral circulation of the abductor muscle mass, and was further supported by cadaver studies. This recommendation is not universally accepted and was not supported by a canine study with ligation of the superior gluteal artery followed by various surgical approaches showing ischemia, yet no frank necrosis with extensile approaches. Caution is still recommended in considering the use of an extensile approach with a suspected superior gluteal artery injury.

To prevent complications of extensile exposures, limited exposures and indirect reduction techniques have been recommended, as have combined anterior and posterior approaches for some fractures. Our preference is to perform consecutive approaches separately, with an anterior approach and then a posterior one, or vice versa, depending on the fracture pattern, rather than performing such approaches simultaneously with the patient in a "floppy lateral" position. When

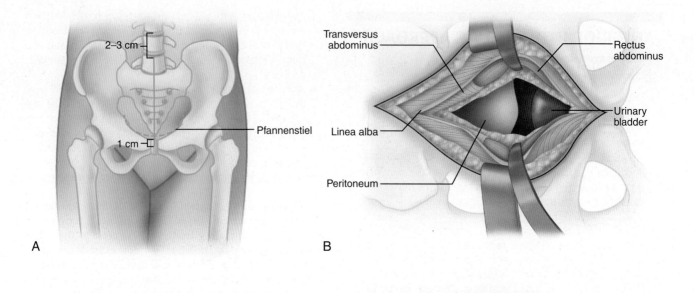

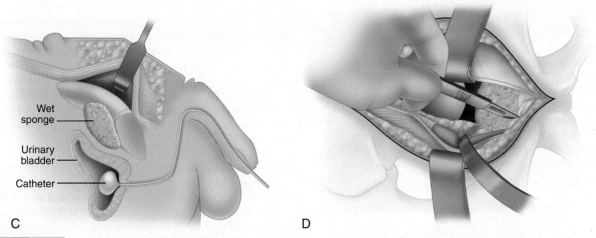

FIGURE **4.28** Stoppa approach for open reduction and internal fixation of acetabular fracture. **A,** Incision. **B,** Retraction of rectus abdominis muscle. **C,** Wet sponge packed into retropubic space to protect the urinary bladder. **D,** Dissection of periosteum from the superior pubic bone. (From AO Surgery Reference, www.aosurgery.org. Copyright by AO Spine International, Switzerland.)

Continued

performing sequential anterior and posterior approaches, care must be taken to avoid placing implants into the portion of the fracture that will be accessed by the opposite approach. While the "floppy lateral" position with simultaneous anterior and posterior exposures avoids this problem, visibility and access are compromised, especially from the anterior approach, because the patient is not truly supine.

■ SPECIFIC FRACTURE PATTERNS

Detailed surgical recommendations and techniques for acetabular fracture stabilization are too numerous to be included here, and the reader is referred to the traditional texts of Letournel and Judet, as well as the more recent publication by Tile, Helfet, Kellam, and Vrahas. Specialized pelvic equipment, implants, and facilities are required for optimal treatment of these fractures, including a radiolucent fracture table, a full array of screw sizes and lengths (up to 110 mm), and reconstruction plates that can be contoured in three dimensions as required by the convoluted configuration of the bony pelvis (Fig. 4.29). Pelvic clamps developed by the AO/ASIF group for reduction of fracture fragments are especially helpful. Custom clamps have also been developed

and are commercially available. Improved retractors, including custom radiolucent retractors, are also available and may improve visualization and reduce risk by decreasing the need for removal and replacement. Treatment strategies for specific fractures are shown in Figure 4.30.

▌POSTERIOR WALL FRACTURES

The most common acetabular fracture treated by the average orthopaedist is the posterior wall fracture. These fractures are, for the most part, treated through a Kocher-Langenbeck approach (see Technique 1.74) with the patient positioned either prone or in the lateral decubitus position on a fracture table or with the leg free. When positioning the patient, the sciatic nerve should be considered; flexion of the knee with slight extension of the hip can reduce tension throughout the case. If the fracture extends superiorly into the dome, the modified Gibson approach or a digastric trochanteric osteotomy can be done to allow additional exposure. The trochanteric fragment can be displaced anteriorly to expose the supraacetabular surface of the ilium. If a modification of the standard approach is planned, this also should be taken into

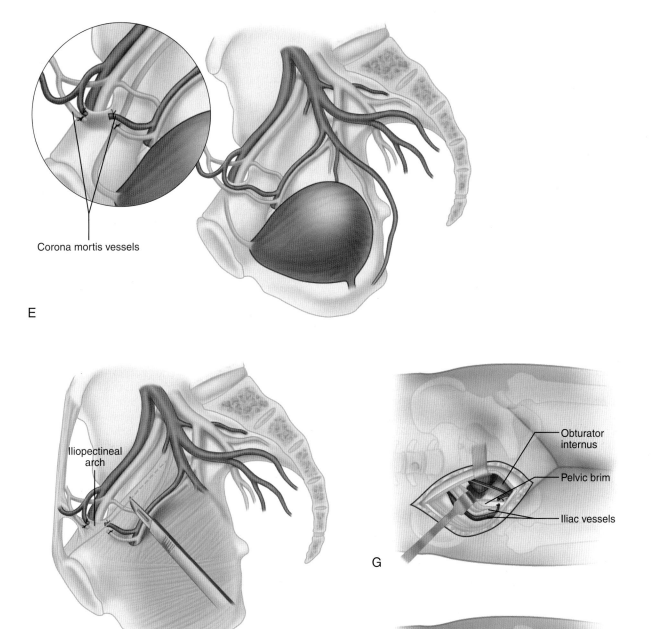

FIGURE 4.28, Cont'd   **E,** Identification of the corona mortis vessels. **F,** Dissection of the iliopectineal arch from the bone. **G,** Elevation of the periosteum and obturator internus to expose the quadrilateral surface. **H,** Placement of Hohmann retractors to expose acetabulum. (Redrawn from AO Foundation, Davos Platz, Switzerland.) **SEE TECHNIQUE 4.1.**

consideration. While the digastric osteotomy can be done with the patient prone, if there is any possibility of requiring a surgical dislocation, this can be done only with the patient in the lateral position. During the approach, care should be taken to avoid splitting the gluteus maximus past the first neurovascular branches, which can result in denervation and abductor weakness. The short external rotators must be released approximately 1 cm from their insertion to avoid injury to the deep branch of the medial femoral circumflex artery as it arises from the muscle body of the quadratus femoris and passes posterior to the obturator internus tendon immediately adjacent to its insertion on the femur.

The hip is distracted to clear any incarcerated fragments before reduction of the wall fragments. A close inspection is made for marginal impaction of articular fragments into the intact posterior column. Marginal impaction, which occurs in more than 22% of isolated wall fractures and should be scrutinized on the preoperative CT scan and intraoperatively, is elevated and bone grafted or fixed using a bone graft substitute. If necessary, the technique described by Giannoudis, Tzioupis, and Moed for two-level reconstruction of comminuted posterior wall fractures with marginal fragments secured by subchondral mini-fragment screws is used (Fig. 4.31). After reduction of the wall fragments, provisional fixation with Kirschner wires can be used while definitive fixation is performed with lag screws, when possible, and a contoured reconstruction plate placed from the ischium, over the retroacetabular surface onto the lateral ilium (Fig. 4.32). Intraarticular screw placement must be avoided. Intraoperative fluoroscopy in multiple views should be used to ensure that all screws are extraarticular. When necessary, the

C-arm position can be modified to allow further "over the top" range of motion to obtain the necessary views (Fig. 4.33).

The use of spring plates has been advocated to improve stability in comminuted fractures. These can be made from one third tubular plates by cutting or breaking the plate through the last screw hole and bending down the remaining end as tines, which are used to capture bone fragments that cannot be easily fixed with screws. Premade spring plates also are available, which are preferable because of their metallurgy, which uses spring steel. The spring plate is slightly overcontoured so that when the reconstruction plate is applied over the spring plate the captured fragments are held firmly in position. A Kirschner wire can be used to sound the edge of the bony acetabulum and ensure the tines of the plate are not overlying the femoral head. The tines should be placed over bone and not over the soft tissues of the labrum alone. This technique is useful in fractures with multiple fragments and fractures that extend close to the acetabular rim (Fig. 4.34).

Other less commonly used techniques for the fixation of posterior wall fractures include the use of locking reconstruction plates with unicortical locking screws in the posterior wall to allow positioning of the plate closer to the acetabular rim without penetrating the articular surface of the wall. Another reported technique is the use of cervical H-shaped plates to substitute for comminuted posterior wall cortical bone while supporting underlying articular fragments that have been reduced.

Although a posterior wall fracture is the easiest fracture pattern to reduce, the reported long-term results after this fracture have varied, with upwards of 20% of patients requiring conversion to total hip arthroplasty at some point and those

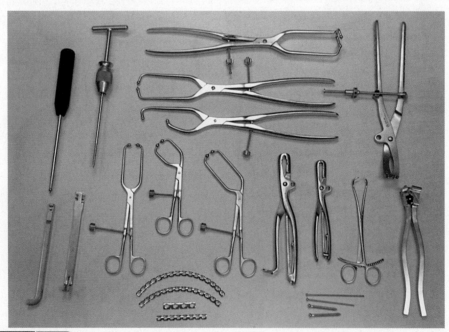

FIGURE 4.29   Specialized instruments and implants for treatment of acetabular fractures.

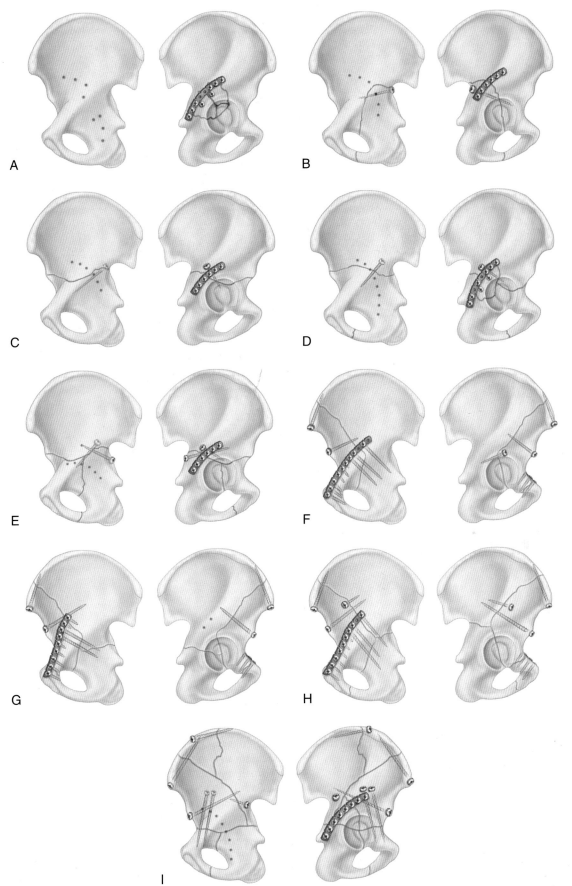

FIGURE 4.30 **A,** Multifragmented posterior wall fracture with intraarticular comminution. **B,** Posterior column fracture with lag screw reaching anterior column. **C,** Transverse fracture with lag screw reaching anterior column. **D,** Associated transverse and posterior wall fracture. **E,** Associated T-type acetabular fracture. Lag screws are inserted into both anterior and posterior columns. **F,** Anterior column fracture. Several lag screws are placed between inner and outer tables of innominate bone. **G,** Associated anterior column and posterior hemitransverse fracture. Screws inserted from pelvic brim must reach distal to fracture line and engage in posterior column. **H,** Both-column fracture operated on through ilioinguinal approach. Screws inserted from pelvic brim reach posterior column. **I,** Both-column fracture. Internal fixation is performed through extended iliofemoral approach. Two very long screws are inserted into anterior column and reach superior pubic ramus.

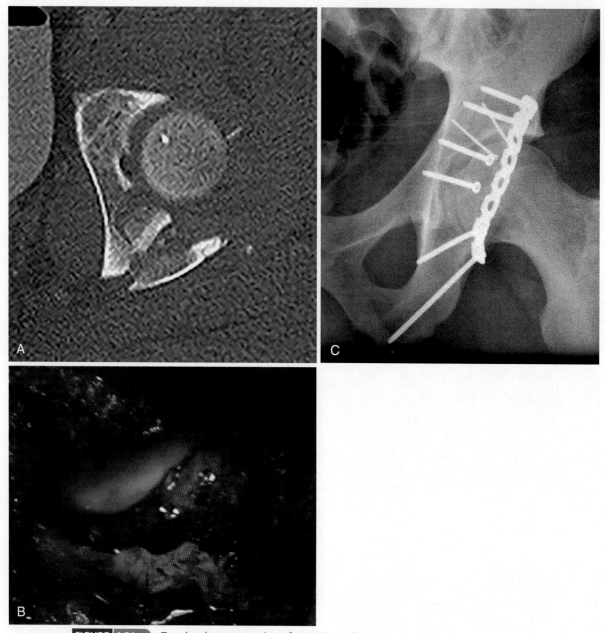

FIGURE 4.31   Two-level reconstruction of comminuted posterior wall fracture.

with more complex fracture characteristics having even higher rates of conversion. Osteonecrosis of the femoral head because of associated hip dislocation, marginal impaction, multiple fracture fragments, and osteochondral injuries of the femoral head all adversely affect the outcome of these fractures.

POSTERIOR COLUMN FRACTURES

Isolated posterior column fractures are relatively uncommon and, if significantly displaced, require ORIF (Fig. 4.35). The main indication is instability of the hip, and low column fractures with a posterior roof arc angle of 70 degrees or more can be treated nonoperatively. The utility of dynamic stress for evaluation of posterior column fractures has not been as well described as it has for posterior wall fractures. Traumatic injury to the sciatic nerve is relatively more common compared with other fracture patterns, as is entrapment of the superior gluteal

bundle due to the cranial extension of the fracture line into the greater sciatic notch. The Kocher-Langenbeck approach is used routinely. Rotational deformity in addition to displacement must be corrected by placement of a Schanz screw in the ischium to control rotation while the fracture is reduced with a small fragment Jungbluth reduction clamp. Typical fixation is with lag screws combined with a contoured reconstruction plate along the posterior column. A secondary plate, more peripheral, can assist with rotational control.

ANTERIOR WALL AND ANTERIOR COLUMN FRACTURES

Isolated anterior wall fractures are uncommon and sometimes associated with anterior hip dislocation. Fractures requiring surgery are best accessed through an ilioinguinal approach or a lateral window with an anterior superior iliac spine osteotomy.

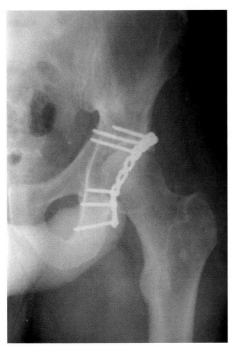

FIGURE 4.32 Posterior wall fracture fixed with contoured 3.5-mm pelvic reconstruction plate.

Anterior column fractures are approached similarly, with the addition of an AIP approach when necessary. Reduction is through correction of medialization and external rotation. This most often is done with a Farabeuf clamp and ball spike or an offset clamp. Fixation is with a contoured plate or LC-2 style screw along the pelvic brim (Fig. 4.36). The acetabulum here is thin, and screws generally should not be placed in this region. Anterior column fractures that exit higher through the iliac wing require fixation along the iliac crest, as well as either plate or screw fixation. Kazemi and Archdeacon have advocated percutaneous fixation of select minimally displaced anterior column fractures with immediate weight bearing. While they achieved excellent radiographic outcomes in 19 of 22 patients followed more than 1 year, our preference is to protect weight bearing in most patients. In elderly patients, for whom protected weight bearing may not be possible, placement of percutaneous fixation may prevent future displacement and allow earlier mobilization.

TRANSVERSE FRACTURES

These fractures, although classified as simple, present a spectrum of difficulty. Selection of the appropriate approach is crucial because fractures with primarily anterior displacement can be difficult to reduce through a posterior approach. Transtectal fractures, or fractures that occur through the dome above the cotyloid fossa, have the worst prognosis, and accurate reduction is essential. Juxtatectal fractures, those that occur at the junction of the cotyloid fossa with the articular surface, also usually require reduction, whereas infratectal fractures frequently can be treated nonoperatively if roof arc measurements are appropriate with no subluxation of the femoral head.

Reduction and fixation can be performed through either an anterior or a posterior approach. This should be based on the aspect of the fracture with the most displacement. Most isolated transverse acetabular fractures without an associated

pelvic ring injury have posterior displacement, as the fracture hinges on the intact symphysis. If a posterior approach is used, this should be done with the patient prone rather than in the lateral decubitus position, unless a surgical dislocation is planned. If the patient is placed in the lateral decubitus position, the weight of the leg tends to displace the ischiopubic fragment medially. Collinge, Archdeacon, and Sagi studied patients with transverse fractures treated either in the lateral or prone positions and found that using Matta's radiographic criteria for reduction, prone positioned patients had anatomic reductions in 61% (<2 mm of residual fracture displacement), whereas in lateral-positioned patients 42% were graded as anatomic.

Typically, we use a small Jungbluth clamp on the posterior column to reduce the fracture while rotation is controlled by a Schanz screw in the ischium. Alternately, a short-angled pelvic clamp can be placed through the greater sciatic notch to control the anterior reduction. This technique is especially pertinent with an associated wall fracture that extends medially over the entire outer table, limiting the ability to place a Jungbluth clamp. Care must be taken to not place pressure on the sciatic nerve with clamps placed through the sciatic notch. The reduction can be assessed directly by palpating the reduction of the quadrilateral surface through the greater sciatic notch. Anterior column fixation is usually achieved first, with a lag screw placed with fluoroscopic guidance. Care must be taken with placement of the anterior lag screw to prevent shearing of the fracture. Often a transverse lag screw will provide more optimal trajectory than a traditional anterior column screw down the ramus. Posterior fixation typically is with a contoured plate along the posterior column preceded by a lag screw if the fracture orientation is appropriate.

From the ilioinguinal approach, reduction is usually accomplished by using plate reduction along the anterior column to close the fracture gap; a large spiked reduction clamp placed on the quadrilateral surface and the lateral surface of the ilium in the region of the anterior inferior spine controls medial displacement and rotation of the caudal fragment. Typical fixation is a contoured plate along the pelvic brim with lag screws directed down the posterior column (Fig. 4.37). On occasion, combined approaches are necessary for more complex transverse fractures or those that are delayed in operative intervention.

POSTERIOR COLUMN FRACTURE WITH ASSOCIATED POSTERIOR WALL FRACTURE

A Kocher-Langenbeck approach is used, rarely with a trochanteric osteotomy. The column fracture is reduced first. This is, in general, performed as described above. Once any marginal impaction has been treated, the posterior column fracture line is reduced. The wall should then be reduced and pinned in place. A traditional wall plate can be placed with the clamps left in place, allowing the clamps to be removed before placement of the posterior column plate (Fig. 4.38).

TRANSVERSE FRACTURE WITH ASSOCIATED POSTERIOR WALL FRACTURE

This common fracture usually is treated through the Kocher-Langenbeck approach alone. However, in the case of a wall fracture extending medial to the inner table, it can be exceptionally difficult, using this approach, to obtain anatomic reduction of the transverse fracture line. In cases such as this, use of a dual approach with fixation of the transverse fracture from anterior and fixation of the wall from posterior should be considered.

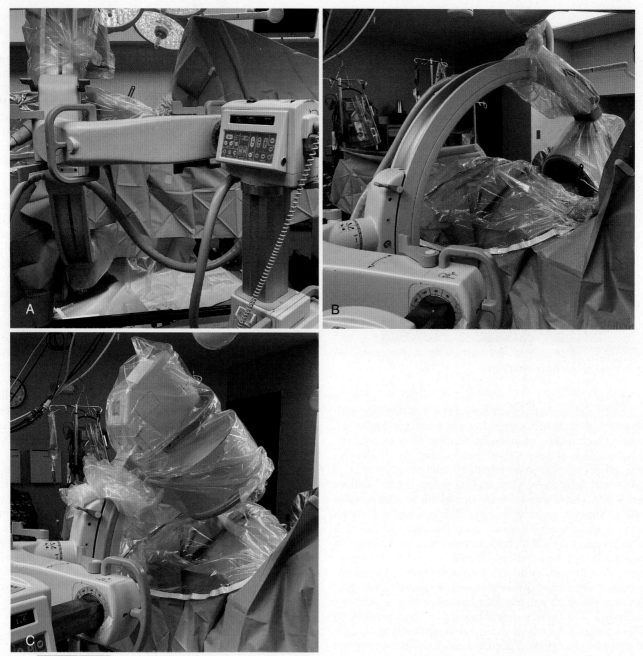

FIGURE 4.33 A-C, Positioning of C-arm to allow further "over-the-top" range of motion to obtain necessary views.

The intraarticular portion of the transverse fracture can be seen through the defect created by the retraction of the posterior wall fragment. Marginal impaction along the transverse fracture line should be considered. As above, the transverse fracture line often can be reduced with a Jungbluth clamp on the posterior column, relying on an intact symphyseal hinge. When this is not sufficient, care must be taken not to injure the sciatic nerve when a reduction clamp is being placed through the greater sciatic notch to reduce the transverse component of this fracture. Rotational control of the distal segment is accomplished by placing a Schanz pin in the ischium. Typically, the transverse component is fixed with lag screws into the anterior column and the posterior wall is plated, followed by placement of a second posterior column plate (Fig. 4.39).

T-SHAPED FRACTURES

T-shaped, or T-type, fractures span a range of severity, requiring different reduction and fixation methods. These fractures most often can be treated through a Kocher-Langenbeck approach with the patient prone, because the fracture line of the posterior column is more significantly displaced than that of the anterior column. The anterior column fracture line can be reduced through the sciatic notch after reduction of the posterior column portion, or reduced first with displacement of the posterior column, facilitating clamp placement. The anterior column is fixed with screws placed down the anterior column from a position above the acetabulum using fluoroscopic guidance; the posterior column portion can be fixed with a lag screw and a reconstruction plate.

However, these fractures occasionally necessitate an anterior approach when the anterior segment is more significantly displaced than that of the posterior component. Fixation is achieved through a contoured plate placed along the pelvic brim with lag screws extending into the posterior column.

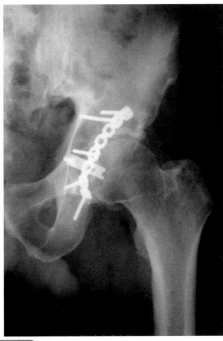

FIGURE 4.34 Posterior wall acetabular fracture treated with spring plate and associated contoured pelvic reconstruction plate.

If both the anterior and posterior components of the fracture are significantly displaced, combined approaches may be required to obtain a reduction. On occasion, with T-shaped fractures as well as other associated fracture types, a separate medial fragment is present. If it is proximal enough to affect stability, a secondary plate or a specialty plate for quadrilateral plate buttress may be necessary (Fig. 4.40).

ANTERIOR COLUMN–POSTERIOR HEMITRANSVERSE FRACTURES

These fractures frequently have minimal displacement of the hemitransverse component and can be treated through the ilioinguinal or anterior intra-pelvic (AIP) approach, combined with the lateral window of the ilioinguinal approach, with typical fixation of the anterior column fracture and separate lag screws from the iliac fossa adjacent to the pelvic brim extending down the posterior column. Fractures with significant posterior displacement or intraarticular comminution with or without impaction may require combined approaches or, if age appropriate, may be considered for a total hip arthroplasty through a Levine approach.

ASSOCIATED BOTH-COLUMN FRACTURES

ABC fractures, by definition, have no articular segments of the acetabulum in continuity with the axial skeleton. They have varying degrees of comminution and can be extremely complex and difficult to treat. Most ABC fractures can be treated through an AIP with a lateral window or ilioinguinal approach (Fig. 4.41), but a staged posterior approach or extensile exposure is required for involvement of the sacroiliac joint, a significant posterior wall fracture, or a segmental posterior column.

While quite varied in presentation, all ABC fractures generally displace in a similar pattern, with the posterior column displaced medially and the anterior column displaced medially and superiorly. This is especially apparent on a true obturator oblique view, taken with the patient tilted toward the

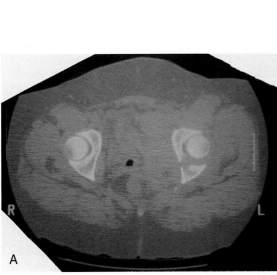

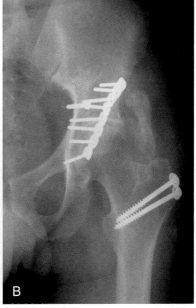

FIGURE 4.35 **A,** Posterior column fracture of acetabulum. **B,** Postoperative radiograph showing definitive fixation and also Brooker grade III heterotopic ossification.

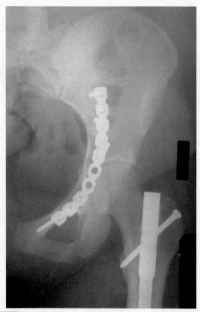

FIGURE 4.36 Fixation of low anterior column fracture with contoured plate along pelvic brim. Note associated femoral shaft fracture fixed with locked intramedullary nail.

intact hemipelvis and displaying what Letournel referred to as the "spur sign."

In general, reduction is begun from the most proximal portion of the fracture and proceeds toward the joint. Each small fragment must be anatomically reduced because a small malreduction in the ilium above the fracture becomes magnified at the level of the joint. Rotational control of the anterior column is critical to obtain an anatomic reduction and should be the first step to reduction. Percutaneous LC2 style screws can be used, in addition to a plate or screw at the iliac crest, to provisionally hold the anterior column before definitive plate fixation.

After reduction of the anterior column, the posterior column is reduced using a Weber or quadrangular clamp from the intrapelvic window. A colinear clamp placed through the lateral window into the lesser sciatic notch can also be used. After reduction of the posterior column, posterior column screws should be placed either alone or through the planned plate fixation.

After provisional fixation, the fracture most often is neutralized with a suprapectineal plate, an infrapectineal plate, or a combination of both. Fixation is as varied as the fracture patterns and the approaches used. More recently, precontoured acetabular plates have become popular because of their ease of use and potentially increased stability; however,

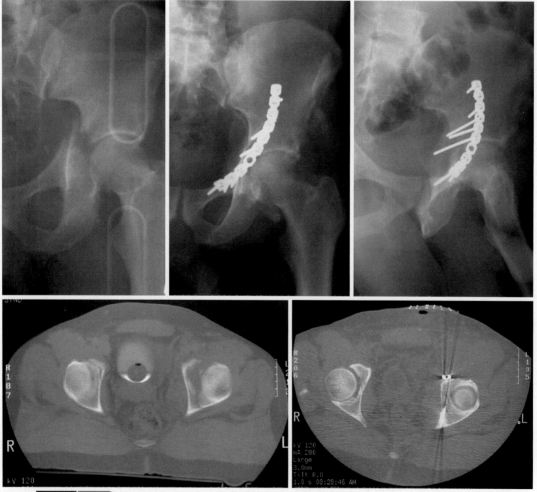

FIGURE 4.37 Transverse acetabular fracture with primarily anterior displacement fixed from anterior ilioinguinal approach.

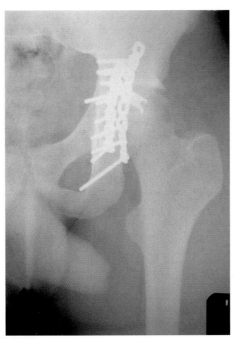

FIGURE 4.38 Posterior column and posterior wall acetabular fracture fixed with two plates. First plate reconstructs posterior column, and second reconstruction plate (supplemental spring plate) fixes posterior wall fragments.

surgeons should be warned that these plates can malreduce the fracture, as they are "one size fits all."

POSTOPERATIVE CARE

Postoperatively, closed suction drainage can be considered; however, evidence has shown that routine use increases hospital length of stay and postoperative transfusion rate without reduction in symptomatic hematoma formation, at least with the Kocher-Langenbeck approach.

Local application of antibiotics may decrease the risk of postoperative infection. The risk of gram-negative infection around the pelvis, acetabulum, and proximal femur is higher and thus both gram-positive and gram-negative pathogens should be covered.

The use of negative pressure wound therapy can be considered, especially in obese patients, but the evidence is controversial at best, and again may increase hospital length of stay when a full-size durable medical equipment unit is used. We prefer to use a low-cost, silver-impregnated standard dressing on all patients undergoing acetabular surgery; however, evidence for the use of silver-impregnated dressings in fracture care is currently lacking, especially around the acetabulum.

Antibiotic therapy should be continued for 24 hours postoperatively and, as above, the risk of gram-negative infection in patients with surgery around the pelvis and acetabulum is higher than in other fracture surgery, and our institution uses a protocol of Zosyn (a combination of piperacillin and tazobactam)

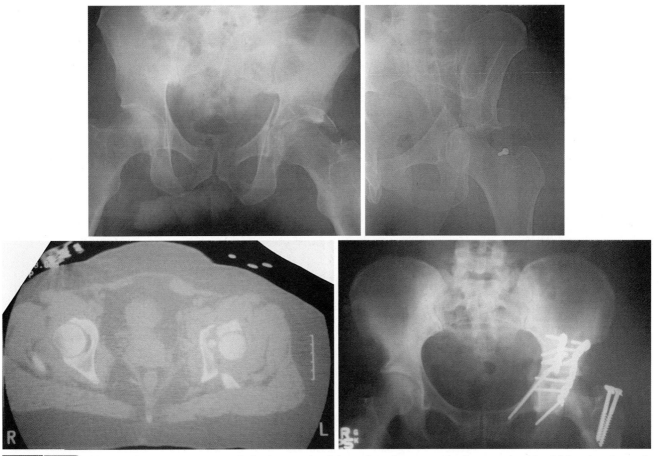

FIGURE 4.39 Transverse posterior wall acetabular fracture fixed through Kocher-Langenbeck approach with additional trochanteric osteotomy.

rather than cefazolin for both preoperative and postoperative prophylaxis.

Passive range of motion of the hip is begun immediately. Touch-down ambulation with crutches or a walker is progressed as tolerated, depending on other injuries. This minimal weight-bearing status is continued for 8 to 12 weeks depending on the displacement and severity of the fracture. Rehabilitation of the abductor muscle group is essential after Kocher-Langenbeck and extensile exposures. Prophylaxis for deep vein thrombosis should be started and prophylaxis for heterotopic ossification may be considered.

OUTCOME AND COMPLICATIONS

Reported overall mortality rates after acetabular fractures range from 0% to 2.5%. In Letournel's classic series, the mortality in patients older than 60 years was 5.7%. A review of data from the National Trauma Data Bank involving 8736 patients with acetabular fractures indicated an overall in-hospital mortality of 1.5%, whereas a meta-analysis of the literature found a mortality rate of 3%.

Letournel's series of 940 patients with acetabular fractures remains the largest published in the literature. Of 569 patients who had ORIF within 21 days of injury, 17% of those observed for at least 1 year had posttraumatic arthritis. After perfect reduction of 418 fractures, the rate of posttraumatic arthritis was 10.2%; and after imperfect reduction of 151 fractures, it was 35.7%. Both-column and transverse posterior wall fractures had worse results than did other associated fracture types, primarily because of imperfect reduction. Posterior wall fractures, although reduced nearly perfectly in 98%, resulted in posttraumatic arthritis in 17%. A study by Tannast, Najibi, and Matta reported a single-surgeon 26-year experience with a cumulative 20-year hip survivorship of 79% after ORIF. Independent negative predictors were nonanatomic fracture reduction, an age of more than 40 years, anterior hip dislocation, postoperative incongruence of the acetabular roof, involvement of the posterior acetabular wall, acetabular impaction, a femoral head cartilage lesion, initial displacement of the articular surface of ≥20 mm, and use of the extended iliofemoral approach. A meta-analysis of multiple studies found an overall incidence of osteoarthritis of 27% in 1211 patients, with incidences of 13% with satisfactory reduction (≤2 mm) and 43% with unsatisfactory reduction. Morbid obesity (body mass index [BMI] > 40) has been described as an impediment to attaining satisfactory reduction by several authors.

One reason for the development of posttraumatic arthritis in some patients with anatomic reductions on

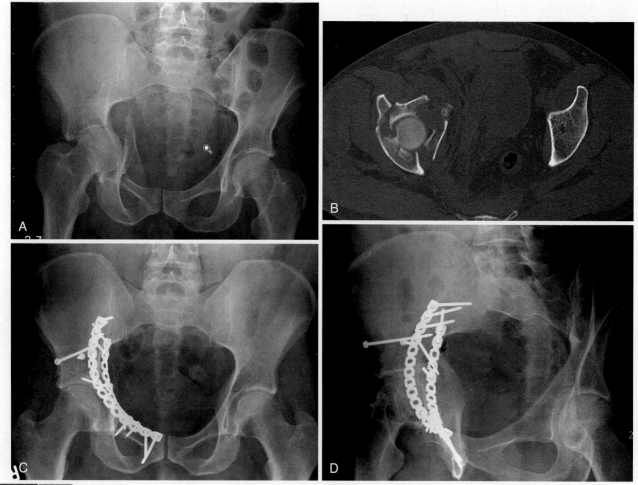

FIGURE 4.40 A and B, Anterior column fracture with quadrilateral surface comminution treated through an ilioinguinal approach with the Stoppa interval used to stabilize the quadrilateral surface (C and D). **SEE TECHNIQUE 4.1.**

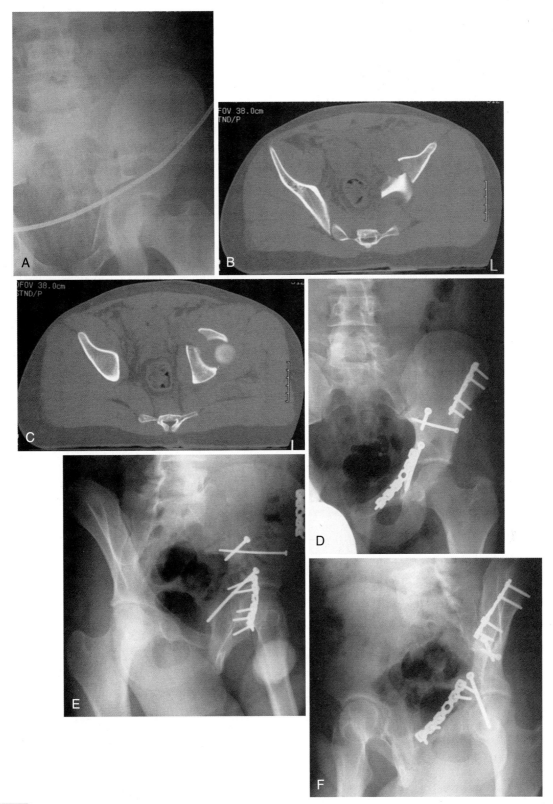

FIGURE 4.41 **A** to **F,** Both-column acetabular fracture treated through ilioinguinal approach with indirect reduction of acetabulum and fixation placed on internal surfaces of pelvis.

plain radiographs is the lack of sensitivity of plain radiographs to detect small incongruencies in the reduction. Moed et al. showed that although anatomic reductions were obtained in 97% of posterior wall fractures when evaluated on plain radiographs, 16% had incongruity of 2 mm or more when measured by CT. Others also have found CT to be more sensitive in showing postoperative gaps and step-offs in the reductions obtained in various fracture patterns and have recommended that postoperative CT be considered for assessment of operative reduction in complex fractures. Jaskolka et al. found that, in five complex acetabular fractures requiring reoperation for malreduction, plain films displayed the malreduction in only one patient while postoperative CT identified the malreduction in all. More recently, Verbeek et al. found that postoperative CT showing more than 5 mm of gap or 1 mm of step displacement was an independent risk factor for late conversion to total hip arthroplasty, reinforcing the importance of anatomic reduction and the potential value of obtaining a postoperative CT scan, not only for surgeon development but also patient prognostication.

Osteonecrosis occurs more frequently after fractures associated with posterior dislocation. Letournel's reported rate of osteonecrosis after posterior dislocation was 7.5%. For other fractures in his series, osteonecrosis occurred in 1.6%. A meta-analysis reported an overall incidence of osteonecrosis of 5.6% in 2010 patients; the incidence was 9% in those with posterior dislocation and 5% in those without a posterior dislocation. Osteonecrosis is radiographically apparent within 2 years of injury in most patients. Osteonecrosis of the posterior wall can be caused by the injury or by excessive surgical dissection, as the only vascular supply of these fragments is through the remaining attachments of the injured posterior capsule of the hip.

Infections are reported to occur in 1% to 5% of patients and may destroy the hip joint, leaving reconstructive options limited. Multiple factors are thought to increase the risk of infection, including higher Injury Severity Score, longer intensive care unit (ICU) stays, larger amount of packed red blood cells transfused, longer operative time, larger estimated operative blood loss, higher BMI, more frequent performance of combined approach, embolization of internal iliac arteries, infection of the urinary tract injury, and a Morel-Lavallée lesion. Obesity, measured by either BMI or waist-hip ratio >1.0 has been shown to increase the rate of multiple complications, including infection. Studies have shown that patients with a BMI of more than 40 have a five times increased risk of infection with acetabular surgery, as well as more frequent overall wound healing complications (46% vs. 12% for patients with indices <40). Incisional wound vacuum closure has been advocated for primary closure of acetabular fracture wounds in obese patients, as mentioned above. Reddix et al. reduced the postoperative deep infection rate from 6.06% to 1.27% by use of an incisional wound vacuum closure in most patients over a 10-year period.

Sciatic nerve palsies because of the initial injury occur in 10% to 15% of patients with acetabular fractures. Sciatic nerve injury because of surgery occurs in 2% to 6% of patients and is more often associated with posterior fracture patterns treated through the Kocher-Langenbeck and extensile exposures. Some authors have proposed intraoperative monitoring of somatosensory evoked potentials as a means of decreasing the incidence of intraoperative sciatic nerve injury, especially with posterior approaches. Other authors, however, have found that, with experience, their rates of iatrogenic nerve injury without monitoring were similar to rates quoted in studies recommending routine monitoring and thus did not recommend intraoperative nerve monitoring. A poll of 181 members of the Orthopaedic Trauma Association (OTA), who commonly perform acetabular surgery, found that only

15% routinely used nerve monitoring during acetabular surgery. There is questionable usefulness of routine monitoring when the operating surgeon is sufficiently experienced. In a report of 14 patients with sciatic nerve injuries, the peroneal component of the sciatic nerve was more often involved than the tibial component and the tibial component had a greater chance of recovery; complete peroneal palsies had the worst prognosis. Functional recovery has been shown in approximately 65% of patients, and function may improve up to 3 years after injury.

Heterotopic ossification (HO) occurs after most extensile approaches, with moderate-to-severe HO occurring in 14% to 50% of patients when no prophylaxis is applied. It occurs after the Kocher-Langenbeck approach in approximately 25% of patients in whom no prophylaxis is used (Fig. 4.42). HO is rare after the ilioinguinal approach unless the external surface of the ilium is stripped. The effectiveness and choice of prophylactic measures to prevent HO remain controversial. Multiple authors have found indomethacin to be effective in decreasing significant HO after acetabular fracture surgery, although this has been called into question by others who found indomethacin to be ineffective in their prospective series. Of concern, Sagi et al. reported a 62% incidence of nonunion in operatively treated acetabular fractures treated with 6 weeks of indomethacin, primarily involving the posterior wall component of fractures. Low-dose irradiation (single dose between 700 and 800 cGy) immediately before surgery or within 72 hours after surgery has been shown to reduce the rate of HO formation. However, surgeons have raised concern about noninfectious wound complications with local radiotherapy. There also is an undetermined risk of late sarcoma formation, which is estimated to be around 1 in 3000. For comparison, the risk of death from bleeding complications related to indomethacin is approximately 1 in 900.

For patients treated with the Kocher-Langenbeck approach, we use debridement of injured gluteus minimus and gemelli, as popularized by Routt et al. More recently, we have had promising results with a thrombin-containing hemostatic matrix applied in the dead space created after muscle debridement.

Thromboembolic complications can be devastating in the postoperative period and the reported risk of pulmonary

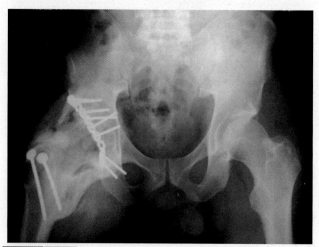

FIGURE **4.42** Brooker grade IV heterotopic ossification occurred despite postoperative irradiation.

embolism ranges from 2% to 6%. Deep vein thrombosis has been reported to occur in 8% to 61% of patients with acetabular fractures; however, this depends on the method used to detect the thrombosis. Venous Doppler ultrasound examination may underestimate the presence of significant clots due to the inability of ultrasound to detect intrapelvic vein thrombosis reliably in comparison to more invasive venographic studies.

Some investigators have shown magnetic resonance venography (MRV) to be more sensitive than venography in detecting clots within the intrapelvic veins and contralateral extremity, detecting asymptomatic deep vein thrombosis in 34% of patients, 49% of which were above the level of the inguinal ligament. Other authors, however, found that MRV and contrast-enhanced CT both had high false-positive rates for detecting deep vein thrombosis when correlated with selective venography and recommended that if either contrast-enhanced CT or MRV is used as a screening test for asymptomatic deep vein thrombosis, correlating selective venography should be used before opting for aggressive prophylactic treatments such as inferior vena cava filters. Slobogean et al. performed a meta-analysis of the available literature involving recommendations for thromboembolic prophylaxis in patients with pelvic and acetabular fractures and could not identify adequate evidence to support one regimen over another.

Our current protocol involves the use of subcutaneous heparin or enoxaparin as well as intermittent compression boots while patients are awaiting surgery. We obtain a preoperative screening duplex Doppler scan in any patient in whom the injury is more than 4 days old and in patients who have not received or have not had well documented administration of prophylaxis, most often due to transfer from an outside facility. We use Greenfield vena cava filters in preoperative patients with confirmed DVT on duplex scan, or pulmonary embolism, and rarely use them in other high-risk groups. Identified high-risk groups include patients older than 60 years, patients with contraindications to anticoagulation, and patients in whom morbid obesity, malignant disease, or a history of prior DVT is a factor. Postoperatively, anticoagulation with enoxaparin alone (30 mg twice daily or 40 mg once daily, unless BMI is over 40) or enoxaparin followed by aspirin (81 mg twice daily) is continued for 6 to 12 weeks, unless it is medically contraindicated.

ACUTE TOTAL HIP ARTHROPLASTY AS TREATMENT OF ACETABULAR FRACTURE

Total hip arthroplasty has been used in older patients for treatment of some acetabular fractures with extremely poor prognoses. Indications tend to be additive, and include intraarticular comminution, full-thickness abrasive loss of the articular cartilage, impaction of the femoral head, impaction of the acetabular dome, associated femoral neck fracture, and preexistent arthritis.

Fractures should be fixed with percutaneous screws, plates, or cables, and fixation then augmented with multiple screw fixation of the ingrowth cup. Unlike in native acetabular fixation, anatomic reduction is not the goal of fixation. Achieving a stable support for the acetabular shell is the goal. A multihole cup alone may not reliably lead to a stable ingrown cup with fracture healing. In their series of 57 patients, Mears and Velyvis found that even with fixation, acetabular shells would routinely subside an average of 3 mm medially and 2 mm vertically during fracture healing and then typically stabilize. They emphasized the avoidance of extensile approaches to minimize the risk of infection. Central to their technique was the use of 2.0-mm cables used in a figure-of-eight configuration for displacement of the quadrilateral surface and percutaneous screws to fix complex anterior column components (Fig. 4.43A to C). Other authors have described use of an acetabular reconstruction ring for fractures with extreme comminution (Fig. 4.44A and B). More recently, the use of a cup-cage construct for reconstruction in the setting of an acetabular fracture has been described; however, the data are limited and the rate of loosening may still be as high as 30%.

For comminuted, nonreconstructable posterior wall fractures, Mears and Velyvis described a useful technique using the femoral head as autograft for defects larger than 40%. Although we have rarely used the figure-of-eight cable

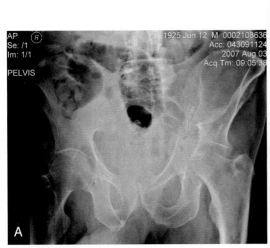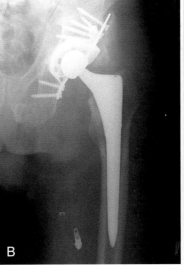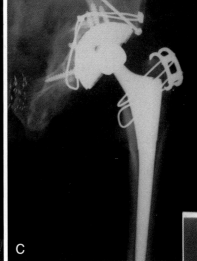

FIGURE 4.43 A and B, Comminuted T-type acetabular fracture treated with figure-8 cable technique described by Mears and Velyvis (C).

technique, we have frequently used a femoral head autograft to reconstruct comminuted posterior walls in older patients when performing acute total hip arthroplasty, with or without transverse fracture components, using the technique as outlined below. We have adhered to the principle of establishing rigid bony fixation, even if not perfectly anatomic, before implantation of a total hip acetabular component, not relying on screw fixation through the cup to contribute significantly to fracture fixation.

FIXATION OF COMMINUTED POSTERIOR WALL FRACTURE WITH OR WITHOUT A TRANSVERSE COMPONENT

TECHNIQUE 4.2

- Position the patient lateral on a flattop radiolucent table using a beanbag or radiolucent positioners.
- Approach the hip through a standard posterolateral hip approach.
- Tag the piriformis and obturator internus separately for easy identification of both greater and lesser sciatic notches and the sciatic nerve.
- Excise any small comminuted fragments of the posterior wall.
- Cut the femoral neck at the appropriate level and carefully remove the femoral head for later use as a bone graft.
- With the femoral head removed, a transverse fracture can be readily reduced and stabilized either with a lag screw placed just anterior to the sciatic notch directly anteromedially or with a percutaneous anterior column screw placed through the gluteus maximus under fluoroscopic control.
- Prepare the femoral head autograft using a female reamer to remove the articular cartilage and cortical bone.
- Gently prepare the posterior wall defect with an acetabular reamer 1 or 2 mm smaller than the female femoral head reamer, while protecting the sciatic nerve with a blunt cobra retractor (Fig. 4.45B).
- Use approximately two thirds of the femoral head with the neck attached to fill the defect and provisionally fix it in position with Kirschner wires placed through the femoral neck still attached to the femoral head autograft (Fig. 4.45C).
- Place a contoured reconstruction plate along the posterior column over the autograft with screws traversing the graft while stabilizing the posterior column (Fig. 4.45D).
- Use a burr to remove the femoral neck and roughly shape the internal contour of the graft to that of the native acetabulum.
- Complete the preparation with acetabular reamers, taking care not to remove subchondral bone (Fig. 4.45E), and place a porous ingrowth cup with multiple screw fixation using fluoroscopy to ensure optimal component positioning in approximately 40 degrees of abduction and 20 degrees of anteversion.

- When cup size allows, we use a 36 mm femoral head and occasionally a posterior lipped liner to minimize posterior dislocation risk, as the posterior capsule is routinely compromised (Fig. 4.45F and G).

POSTOPERATIVE CARE Weight bearing is limited for 6 to 12 weeks depending on the presence and displacement of any transverse or column component. Routine anticoagulation is used for DVT prophylaxis.

Beaulé, Griffin, and Matta revisited a now 80-year-old approach, originally described by Levine as an extension of the well-known Smith-Peterson approach, for use in fixation of displaced anterior column fractures, with or without a posterior hemitransverse component, followed by placement of an acute total hip arthroplasty through an anterior approach. The exposure is extended proximally along the internal iliac fossa for fixation of the anterior column. They described this technique using a fracture table, but it can also be done on a standard operating table with proper positioning to allow hip extension during femoral component preparation, as described by Keggi, Huo, and Zatorski. In patients with a displaced anterior column fracture, in addition to risk factors for early posttraumatic arthritis, the approach allows for definitive fixation and replacement through a single incision (Fig. 4.46).

ANTERIOR APPROACH FOR TOTAL HIP ARTHROPLASTY FOR FRACTURES INVOLVING PRIMARILY THE ANTERIOR WALL AND COLUMN

TECHNIQUE 4.3

(BEAULÉ ET AL.)
- Place the patient supine on a Hana or ProFX fracture table (Orthopedic Systems, Inc., Union City, CA).
- After proper preparing and draping of the pelvis and femoral shaft, make a skin incision along the iliac crest (as in a lateral window), curving it laterally distal to the anterior superior iliac spine, and continuing distally over the tensor fascia lata muscle (as in a Smith-Peterson approach (Fig. 4.47A).
- Carefully release the abdominal musculature from the iliac crest with electrocautery and develop the subperiosteal plane along the inner table of the ilium with a periosteal elevator.
- Release the sartorius and direct head of the rectus with electrocautery.
- Complete the exposure distally by incising the anterior margin of the tensor muscle fascia. This fascia consists of two layers, one of which contains the lateral femoral cutaneous nerve surrounded by a thin layer of fat. The posterior branch of this nerve is always sacrificed, which leaves an area of hypoesthesia.

- Separate the tensor muscle from the rectus femoris. It is important to incise the tensor muscle fascia where it is almost translucent, because going too far medially may lead to loss of the dissection plane.
- Retract the tensor muscle laterally and identify the rectus femoris within the sagittal plane when cutting through its overlying fascial layer.
- Release the reflected head of the rectus and the posterior third of the direct head.
- The next fascial layer lies in the coronal plane and is posterior to the rectus femoris, which is retracted medially. Cut this layer, then isolate and ligate the ascending branch of the lateral circumflex artery.
- Divide the fascia between the rectus femoris to access the plane between the tendon of the gluteus minimus and the hip joint capsule.
- Place a blunt Hohmann retractor under the sheath of the psoas tendon to display full access to the capsule.
- The uppermost fibers of the vastus intermedius muscle and portion of the iliocapsularis muscle take origin from the capsule anteriorly and medially. Elevate these off the anterior capsule with a scalpel and reflect them distally and medially.
- The entire superior, anterior, and inferior portions of the capsule should now be visible from the iliac origin to the femoral insertion.

- Pass a blunt Hohmann retractor laterally and a sharp Hohmann retractor onto the anterior rim of the acetabulum (Fig. 4.47B) then incise the anterior capsule with a T-shaped incision.
- Make the femoral neck osteotomy before attempting fracture reduction.
- Generally, the anterior column fracture extends to the iliac crest and usually is externally rotated in relation to the pelvis. Begin the reduction at the iliac crest to accurately reduce the fracture fragment. The use of a Matta clamp, with one tine on the outer table, will often provide the forces necessary for reduction.
- The other main component of the fracture is the impacted articular surface, usually located posterior-superior-medial in the acetabular fossa.
- Reduce the anterior column fracture first and fix it with a reconstruction plate. Apply the plate in a suprapectineal fashion. Distally, the plate lies over the pectineal eminence and, by being under-contoured, applies compression on the anterior wall/column (Fig. 4.47C).
- Once the acetabular fracture has been accurately reduced and fixed, prepare the acetabular cavity for implantation of the socket. There is no need to reduce the impacted articular surface; remove the cartilage, ligamentum teres, and fat pad with curets and use reamers to prepare only the acetabular rim.

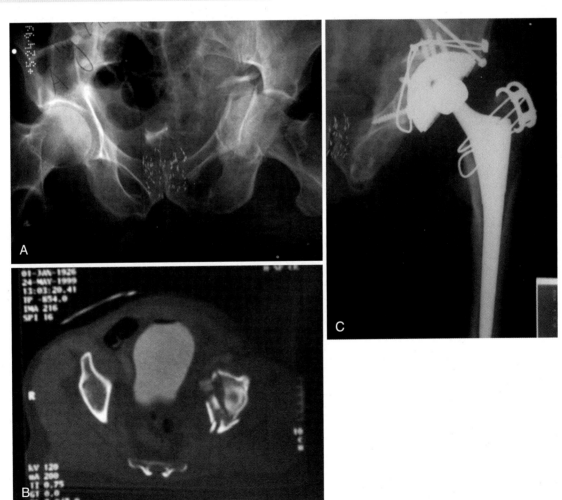

FIGURE 4.44 **A,** Comminuted T-type acetabular fracture treated with a reconstruction ring and primary hip replacement (**B** and **C**).

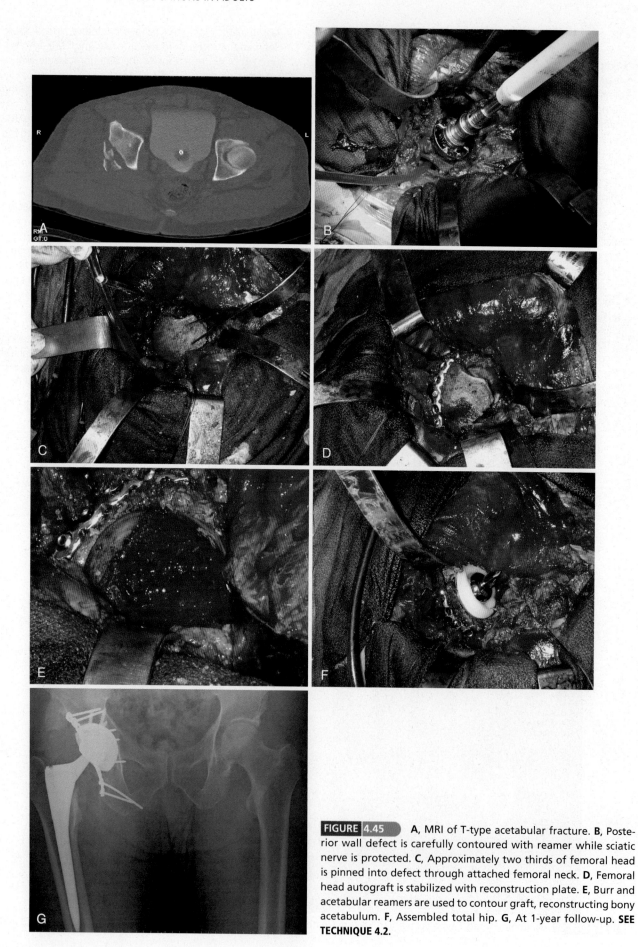

FIGURE 4.45   **A,** MRI of T-type acetabular fracture. **B,** Posterior wall defect is carefully contoured with reamer while sciatic nerve is protected. **C,** Approximately two thirds of femoral head is pinned into defect through attached femoral neck. **D,** Femoral head autograft is stabilized with reconstruction plate. **E,** Burr and acetabular reamers are used to contour graft, reconstructing bony acetabulum. **F,** Assembled total hip. **G,** At 1-year follow-up. **SEE TECHNIQUE 4.2.**

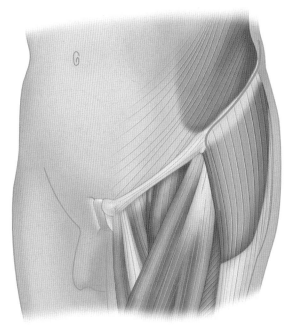

FIGURE 4.46 Levine approach for anterior wall/column acetabular fracture.

- Place morselized bone graft from the femoral head or acetabular reamings into the acetabular cavity to compensate for areas that were not elevated.
- Begin reaming with a size close to the actual implant size, with a final goal of 1 mm of under-reaming.
- Impact the socket in the appropriate amount of abduction and anteversion. Supplemental screw fixation is used to ensure initial socket stability.
- Begin implantation of the femoral component by extending, externally rotating, and adducting the leg using the fracture table in standard anterior approach fashion.
- Verify leg lengths with fluoroscopy: the lesser trochanter is placed at the same level at the most distal aspect of the ischial tuberosity in relation to the nonoperative limb with both legs in neutral abduction-adduction.
- Close the fascial layers sequentially, carefully repairing the proximal abdominal attachments. A double closure should be used for reattachment of the abdominal muscles because this is a high-stress area.

POSTOPERATIVE CARE Weight bearing is limited for 6 to 12 weeks depending on the displacement of any column component. Routine anticoagulation is used for DVT prophylaxis.

COMPLICATIONS OF ACUTE TOTAL HIP ARTHROPLASTY FOR ACETABULAR FRACTURE

The risk of complications after acute total hip arthroplasty for acetabular fractures is not trivial. HO occurs in 6% to 60%, dislocation occurs in 4% to 14%, and the infection rate can be as high as 13%.

TOTAL HIP ARTHROPLASTY FOR POSTTRAUMATIC ARTHRITIS

Total hip arthroplasty for posttraumatic arthritis generally is done in patients younger than those with idiopathic osteoarthritis. In general, it is recommended that only implants that interfere with the placement of the total hip replacement be removed, because posterior column plates can be imbedded in dense scar that can be adherent to the sciatic nerve. Screws that protrude into the bony socket can be removed or recessed with a metal cutting burr from within the socket. Total hip arthroplasty after acetabular fracture (Fig. 4.48) has been found to require longer operative times, have increased blood loss, and more commonly require transfusion compared with total hip arthroplasty for degenerative arthritis. All of these findings were greater in patients who had ORIF of their acetabular fractures compared with patients who had initial nonoperative treatment of their fractures.

Preoperatively, it is prudent to obtain screening tests such as C-reactive protein (CRP) and erythrocyte sedimentation rate (ESR), particularly if there is any history of postoperative drainage or infection after the initial fracture treatment. Intraoperative frozen section at the time of total hip replacement also has been recommended if there is any suspicion of infection. If acute inflammation is evidenced by greater than five white blood cells per high-powered field on microscopic review, debridement with implant removal and placement of a PROSTALAC antibiotic spacer (DePuy, Warsaw, IN) is prudent, with an extended course of intravenous antibiotics before implantation of permanent total hip components.

Romness and Lewallen found that patients younger than 60 years undergoing total hip arthroplasty for posttraumatic arthritis had a 17.2% risk of aseptic loosening at 10 years, compared to 7.7% for those over the age of 60. More recently, Weber and associates found that patients under the age of 50 or those with large residual bony defects were at increased risk of aseptic loosening. Ranawat and colleagues found that a nonanatomic hip center or history of infection increased the risk of revision as well. For patients with compromised acetabular bone stock, Yuan, Lewallen, and Hanssen reported no revisions for loosening at a minimum 5-year follow-up with the use of highly porous tantalum acetabular components. It is our practice to use highly porous, multi-hole acetabular components for all total hip replacements in patients with previous ORIF of the acetabulum. However, patients must be counselled on the increased risk of revision in the posttraumatic setting, with 10-year survivorship at 70% to 97% and 20-year survivorship at only 57%.

PELVIC FRACTURES

Fractures of the adult pelvis, exclusive of the acetabulum, present in a dichotomous distribution of geriatric low-energy trauma, such as ground level falls, or more youthful high-energy trauma that results in significant morbidity and mortality. As is true of fractures of other bones, low-energy trauma to the pelvis generally produces stable fractures that can be treated symptomatically with crutch- or

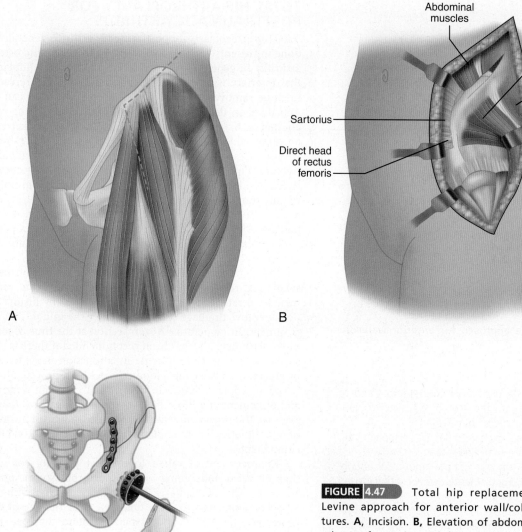

FIGURE 4.47 Total hip replacement through anterior Levine approach for anterior wall/column acetabular fractures. **A,** Incision. **B,** Elevation of abdominal musculature with release of sartorius and direct head of rectus femoris. **C,** After reduction and internal fixation of anterior column, acetabular cavity is prepared. (Redrawn from Beaulé PE, Griffin DB, Matta JM: Levine anterior approach for total hip replacement for the treatment for an acute acetabular fracture, J Orthop Trauma 18:623, 2004.) **SEE TECHNIQUE 4.3.**

walker-assisted ambulation and that can be expected to heal uneventfully in most patients, although this belief is being disputed. High-energy pelvic fractures are often managed operatively, with the treatment method determined by the degree of pelvic stability, in a stepwise treatment algorithm. Although the treatment of the low-energy fractures is briefly discussed, the focus here is on these high-energy injuries, their management in both the resuscitative and reconstructive phases, and their potential complications.

High-energy pelvic fractures result most commonly from roadway accidents, falls from elevation, automobile-pedestrian encounters, and industrial crush injuries. The potential complications of high-energy pelvic fractures include injuries to the major vessels and nerves of the pelvis

(Fig. 4.49) and the major viscera: the intestines/colorectum, the bladder, and the urethra/genitalia. Degloving injuries to the surrounding soft tissues, both open and closed, may accompany these fractures, and complicate their treatment. Reported mortality from severe pelvic fracture ranges from 10% to as high as 50% in some earlier series of open pelvic fractures. Risk factors for increased mortality include the patient's age and injury severity score, associated head or visceral injury, blood loss, hypotension, coagulopathy, and unstable or open pelvic fractures. Mortality in patients with a pelvic injury occurs in a trimodal distribution: death at the scene; death during the first 24 hours, often from hemorrhage or closed-head injury; and late mortality, due to sepsis or multiorgan failure.

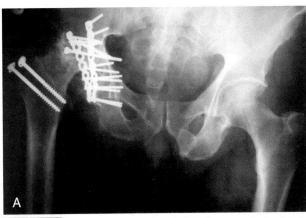 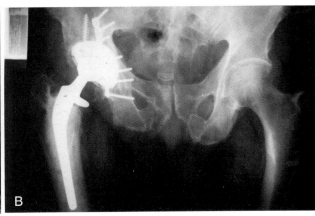

FIGURE 4.48 **A,** Posttraumatic arthritis after acetabular fracture. **B,** After fracture reduction and fixation and total hip arthroplasty.

ANATOMY

The pelvis is composed anteriorly of the ring of the pubic and ischial rami connected with the symphysis pubis. A fibrocartilaginous disc separates the two pubic bodies. Posteriorly, the sacrum and the two innominate bones are joined at the sacroiliac joint by the interosseous sacroiliac ligaments, the anterior and posterior sacroiliac ligaments, the sacrotuberous ligaments, the sacrospinous ligaments, and the associated iliolumbar ligaments (Fig. 4.50A). This ligamentous complex provides stability to the posterior sacroiliac complex, as the sacroiliac joint itself has no inherent bony stability. Tile has compared this relationship of the posterior pelvic ligamentous and bony structures to a suspension bridge, with the sacrum suspended between the two posterior superior iliac spines (Fig. 4.50B).

Pelvic stability is determined by ligamentous structures in various planes. The primary restraints to external rotation of the hemipelvis are the ligaments of the symphysis, the sacrospinous ligament, and the anterior sacroiliac ligaments. Rotation in the sagittal plane is resisted by the sacrotuberous ligament. Vertical displacement of the hemipelvis is controlled by all the mentioned ligamentous structures, but if other ligaments are absent it may be controlled by intact interosseous sacroiliac and posterior sacroiliac ligaments along with the iliolumbar ligament. Frequently, a rotationally unstable hemipelvis may remain vertically stable because of these intact ligamentous structures. This has significant implications in classification, prognosis, and treatment.

RADIOGRAPHIC EVALUATION

The standard radiographic projections required for evaluation of pelvic fractures are an anteroposterior view of the pelvis and 40-degree caudal inlet and 40-degree cephalad outlet views as described by Pennal et al. (Fig. 4.51). The inlet view shows inward or outward rotation of the anterior pelvis as well as anteroposterior displacement of the hemipelvis. The outlet view shows vertical displacement of the hemipelvis as well as superior or inferior rotation of the anterior pelvis, while also serving to better characterize associated sacral fractures and widening or fracture of the anterior pelvis.

CT is an essential part of the evaluation of any significant pelvic injury and allows evaluation of the posterior portion of the pelvic ring that may be poorly visualized on standard radiographs, especially in an obese or osteopenic patient. Before the widespread use of CT, many pelvic fractures were assumed to be purely anterior injuries, as subtle posterior injuries were difficult to identify. Subsequently, CT has long been shown to disclose that isolated anterior injuries remain rare.

Several radiographic signs should be sought as indications of fracture stability. Widening of the symphysis of more than 2.5 cm has been correlated with rupture of the sacrospinous ligament and a rotationally unstable pelvis. Avulsion fractures of the lateral sacrum and ischial spine are additional signs of rotational instability. Widening of the anterior pelvis causes rupture of the anterior sacroiliac ligament, making the sacroiliac joint appear widened on the anteroposterior view. However, as shown by axial CT images, the posterior ligaments of the sacroiliac joint may remain intact, maintaining the vertical stability of the pelvis (Fig. 4.52). The posterior iliac offset, as described by Tonne et al., can also be used to predict pelvic instability. Impacted fractures of the anterior cortex of the sacrum are common with lateral compression (LC) injuries and generally are stable, but a sacral fracture with a gap usually indicates vertical instability. In their review of LC fractures treated nonoperatively, Bruce et al. found that over half (68%) of complete sacral fractures with bilateral rami fractures displaced, while no incomplete sacral fractures with an ipsilateral ramus fracture displaced.

Vertical instability is generally defined as one centimeter or more of cephalad migration of one hemipelvis. In some pelvic injuries, vertical instability is apparent, but if vertical stability is questionable, stress testing can be beneficial. When pelvic stability is questioned, EUA may be helpful. Internal and external rotation of the pelvis may demonstrate rotational instability. In a similar study, Suzuki et al. stressed presumed anteroposterior compression (APC)-I injuries and found that 27% of patients had an occult APC-II injury. Sagi et al. described a stress examination of the pelvic ring using intraoperative dynamic fluoroscopy in which internal and external rotation and push-pull maneuvers were applied to both extremities. Using this method, they identified instability in half of pelvic ring fractures presumed to be stable APC-I injuries. Further, they found that 37% of APC-2 injuries had superior-inferior rotational instability

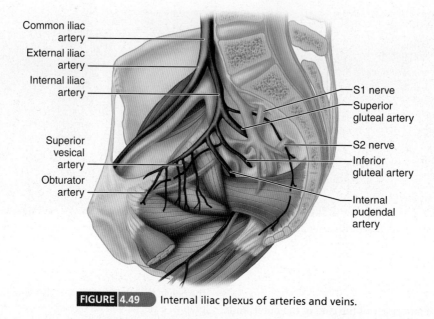

FIGURE 4.49   Internal iliac plexus of arteries and veins.

with axial loading. Under radiographic control, the examiner pushes up on one extremity while pulling down on the other. This maneuver is then reversed, again under radiographic control, and the maximal displacement between the two films is determined. If more than 1 cm of cephalad displacement of a sacral fracture or sacroiliac dislocation is possible with this test, the fracture is vertically unstable. If more than 1 cm of anterior-superior-to-inferior translation is noted, this fracture is believed to have vertical rotational instability indicative of attenuation of the posterior sacroiliac ligaments. This test should be done one time only, with permanent films obtained for accurate measurement of cephalad migration. A quarter, which has a diameter of 2.42 cm, placed on the patient's abdomen can assist with judging movement. Push-pull testing should not be done in acutely injured patients with ongoing hemodynamic instability or in zone II or zone III sacral fractures, in which potential neurologic injury could occur.

CLASSIFICATION

Bucholz, in a classic study of 150 consecutive victims of fatal motor vehicle accidents, found pelvic fractures in 31%. He separated them into three groups: group I had displaced anterior ring injuries with minimally displaced, stable sacral fractures or incomplete tearing of the anterior sacroiliac ligament; group II had anterior injuries associated with a rotational opening of the sacroiliac joint with disruption of only the anterior sacroiliac ligaments, sparing the posterosuperior sacroiliac ligament complex; and group III had complete disruption of the anterior and posterior hemipelvis.

Pennal and associates followed shortly after with a mechanistic classification in which pelvic fractures are described as APC injuries, LC injuries, or vertical shear injuries.

Young and Burgess expanded on the system developed by Pennal et al. In day-to-day communication, the Young and Burgess classification, which, like the Pennal scheme, is based on mechanism, is the most commonly used system. In addition to APC and LC, Young and Burgess added a new category for combined mechanical injuries (see Table 4.1).

One of the original conclusions of their work was that pelvic classification could be used to predict other morbidities in a polytraumatized patient. However, the system fits nicely with the concepts of rotational and vertical stability described by Tile. The AP I (APC type I) and LC I (LC type I) fractures are rotationally and vertically stable (Tile A). The AP II (Fig. 4.53) and LC II (Fig. 4.54) fractures are rotationally unstable but vertically stable (Tile B). The AP III (Fig. 4.55) and often the LC III (Fig. 4.56) fractures are both rotationally and vertically unstable (Tile C). In a subsequent series, LC injuries were the most common injury pattern, accounting for 41%, followed by APC injuries (26%), acetabular fractures (18%), combined mechanism injuries (10%), and vertical shear injuries (5%). Hypovolemic shock and large blood requirements were more common in patients with vertically unstable AP III injuries than in those with vertically stable APC or LC injuries. In the series by Young and Burgess, patients with the most severe LC injuries (type III) had no associated head injuries, whereas those with less severe LC injuries had head injury rates similar to those in patients with other pelvic injury patterns. We find this classification useful in describing and communicating pelvic ring injuries.

Tile soon after developed a system based on the concept of pelvic stability (Box 4.2): A, stable; B, rotationally unstable but vertically stable; and C, rotationally and vertically unstable. Helfet later modified the Tile classification system to align with the AO/OTA fracture and dislocation system, which was originally published in 1996 and has been revised and republished in 2007 and again in 2018. Tile's classification of pelvic ring fractures relates directly to the type of treatment indicated and the prognosis of the injury.

Type A (stable) fractures are further divided into three groups (Fig. 4.57). Type A1 fractures do not involve the pelvic ring, for instance, avulsion fractures of the iliac spines or the ischial tuberosity and isolated fractures of the iliac wing. Type A2 fractures are those that involve a direct blow to the pelvis, such as an iliac wing fracture, without extension into the pelvic ring, known as a Duverney fracture, or an isolated

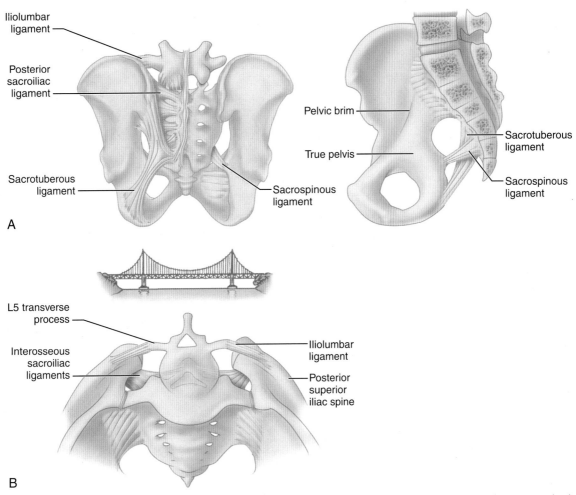

FIGURE 4.50 **A,** Major posterior stabilizing structures of pelvic ring (posterior and sagittal views). **B,** Tile compared relationship of posterior pelvic ligamentous and bony structures to suspension bridge, with sacrum suspended between two posterior superior iliac spines. (From Tile M: Acute pelvic fractures, part I. Causation and classification, *J Am Assoc Orthop Surg* 4:143, 1996.)

injury to the anterior ring without posterior involvement. Type A3 fractures are transverse lesions of the sacrum and coccyx; these are considered spinal injuries rather than pelvic ring disruptions.

Type B fractures are rotationally unstable, but vertically stable. Group B1 fractures often are colloquially referred to as "open book" injuries, as one hemipelvis externally rotates because of injury of the symphysis or a fracture of the anterior ring and, at minimum, attenuation of the anterior sacroiliac ligaments. The posterior injury is widening of the SI joint anteriorly (B1.1) or a sacral fracture with anterior diastasis (B1.2) (Fig. 4.58). The posterior sacroiliac and interosseous ligaments remain intact resulting in external rotational instability, without vertical instability. Tile described stages of this injury. In the first stage, the symphysis separation is less than 2.5 cm and the sacrospinous ligament remains intact. In the second stage, the diastasis is more than 2.5 cm with rupture of the sacrospinous ligament and the anterior sacroiliac ligament. In the third stage, the lesions are bilateral, creating a B3 injury.

Fractures classified as AO/OTA B2 encompass unilateral injuries that are more commonly referred to as Young and Burgess LCI and LCII fracture patterns. The opposite of the B1

fractures, these injuries occur secondary to an internal rotation–type force to the hemipelvis. Subgroup B2.1 fractures are LC injuries with an ipsilateral sacral fracture (Fig. 4.59). Subgroup B2.2 fractures are those LC injuries that, instead of fracturing through the sacrum, result in a rupture of the posterior sacroiliac ligaments or a small avulsion fracture of the ligamentous attachment; internal rotation occurs through the SI joint. Fractures of the subgroup B2.3 are those classified by Young and Burgess as LCII fractures and result in internal rotation through a fracture in the ilium, conversationally known as a "crescent fracture."

Group B3 fractures are like group B1 and B2 fractures, but entail a bilateral injury, rather than a unilateral injury. Subgroup B3.1 injuries are those with bilateral external rotation injuries to the posterior pelvis, classified by Young and Burgess as bilateral APCI or APCII injuries. Subgroup B3.2 are colloquially known as the windswept pelvis, or Young and Burgess LCIII injuries, with internal rotation of one hemipelvis and external rotation of the contralateral hemipelvis. Fractures in subgroup B3.3 are those injuries with bilateral internal rotation (LC-type) injuries and should raise suspicion of the possibility of a transverse sacral fracture and associated spinopelvic dissociation.

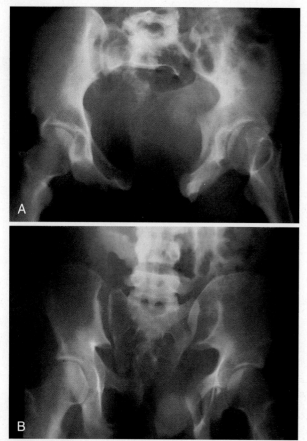

FIGURE 4.51   **A,** Forty-degree caudal inlet view of pelvis. **B,** Forty-degree cephalad outlet view of pelvis.

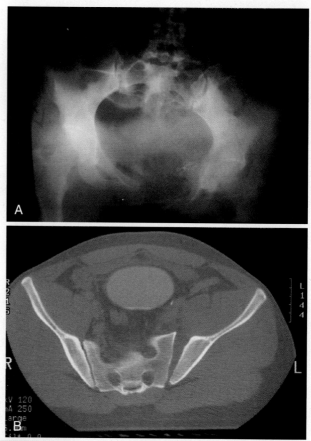

FIGURE 4.52   **A,** Tile type B1 pelvic injury with diastasis of symphysis and anterior widening of sacroiliac joint. **B,** CT scan shows that posterior sacroiliac joint ligaments are intact.

Type C fractures (Fig. 4.60) are unstable both rotationally and vertically. These include vertical shear injuries and anterior compression injuries with disruption of the posterior ligamentous complex. Type C1 fractures include unilateral fractures of the anterior and posterior complex, subdivided by the location of the posterior fracture. Type C2 fractures include bilateral injuries with one hemipelvis vertically stable and the other unstable. Type C3 fractures are bilateral fractures that are both vertically and rotationally unstable.

Sacral fractures have been classified separately by several authors. Currently, the classification used most often is that proposed by Denis, Davis, and Comfort (Fig. 4.61). Classification is divided into three types based on the fracture's relation to the sacral neuroforamina: zone I fractures occur lateral to the neural foramina through the sacral ala (50% of fractures); zone II fractures are transforaminal (34.3% of fractures); zone III fractures occur medial or central to the neural foramina (15.7% of fractures). In the original series of 236 patients, Denis and colleagues found neurologic deficits in 5.9% of patients with zone I fractures, 28.4% of patients with zone II fractures, and 56.7% of patients with zone III fractures. The type of deficit also differed based on location, with zone I fractures most commonly affecting the L5 nerve root, while zone II fractures most often had varying effects on L5-S2, but 18% of those with nerve deficits had bowel or bladder effects as well. Zone III fractures had much more frequent consequences on bowel, bladder, or reproductive organ function, with 76% of those with neurologic deficit suffering such effects. This was

commonly associated (62%) with varying injury to the L5-S2 nerve roots as well.

In a more recent study including 683 patients, Khan et al. found that the frequency of zone I fractures was higher and that of zone II and III fractures was lower than reported by Denis et al. Further, the rate of nerve injury was significantly lower overall at 3.5% compared to 21.6% in the original paper. This decrease was consistent across all zones; however, the trend of increasing frequency of nerve injury with increasing zone was the same as originally reported. This decrease is most likely associated with the increased use of CT for evaluation of trauma patients. In the original paper, Denis et al. diagnosed only 51% of the original fractures during the initial hospital stay, and there is a high likelihood that many minimally displaced fractures were missed and not included in their original study. This is supported by the fact that Khan et al. found that patients with displaced or comminuted fractures and those with transverse fractures extending across the midline had more frequent neurologic insults; these are the fractures that are most likely to be recognized on a pelvic flat-plate radiographic series.

In a study by Nork et al., only 2.9% (13 of 442) of pelvic ring disruptions contained a transverse component crossing the midline; however, these fractures deserve special attention because of the neurologic and biomechanical implications. Roy-Camille and his collaborators were the first to describe a classification for these fractures based on rotation and displacement. Transverse fractures of the sacrum are classified

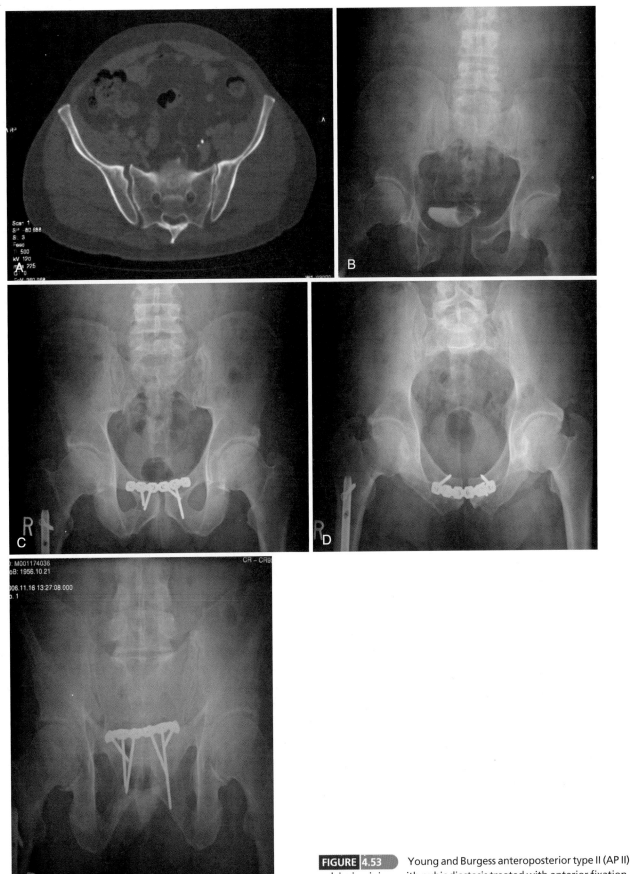

FIGURE 4.53 Young and Burgess anteroposterior type II (AP II) pelvic ring injury with pubic diastasis treated with anterior fixation. **A** and **B,** Preoperative views. **C** to **E,** Postoperative anteroposterior, inlet, and outlet views.

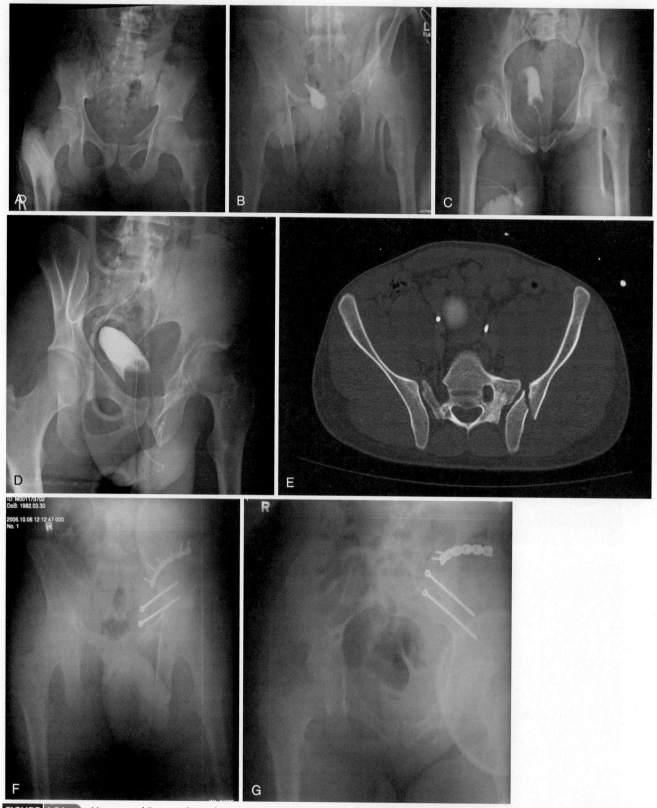

FIGURE 4.54 Young and Burgess lateral compression type II (LC II) pelvic ring injury with posterior crescent fracture. **A** to **D,** Preoperative anteroposterior, oblique, inlet, and outlet views, respectively. **E,** Preoperative CT scan. **F** and **G,** After open reduction and internal fixation with 3.5-mm reconstruction plate with two lag screws in between iliac cortical tables.

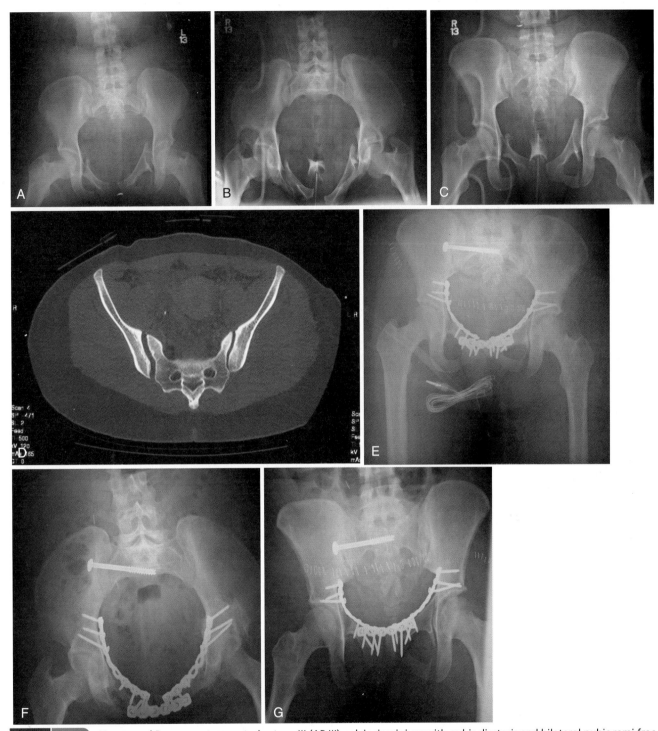

FIGURE 4.55   Young and Burgess anteroposterior type III (AP III) pelvic ring injury with pubic diastasis and bilateral pubic rami fractures. **A-C,** Preoperative anteroposterior, inlet, and outlet views, respectively. **D,** Preoperative CT scan. **E-G,** Postoperative anteroposterior, inlet, and outlet views, respectively.

as zone III injuries in the Denis classification because they involve the spinal canal; however, they are highly variable and should be further subclassified. Generally, the fracture pattern is best described based on the Latin-based letter that the fracture morphology resembles (Fig. 4.62). Critical analysis of the sagittal and coronal reconstructions on CT will best show these injuries. Evaluation of displacement and the sacral level

at which the fracture crosses will play a role. Classification of anterior pelvic ring fractures, as described by Starr et al., is based on the location of the fracture through the superior ramus. The less-known Nakatani classification defines zone I as medial to the obturator foramen, zone III as lateral to the obturator foramen, and zone II between zones I and III. More commonly, fractures lateral to the obturator foramen

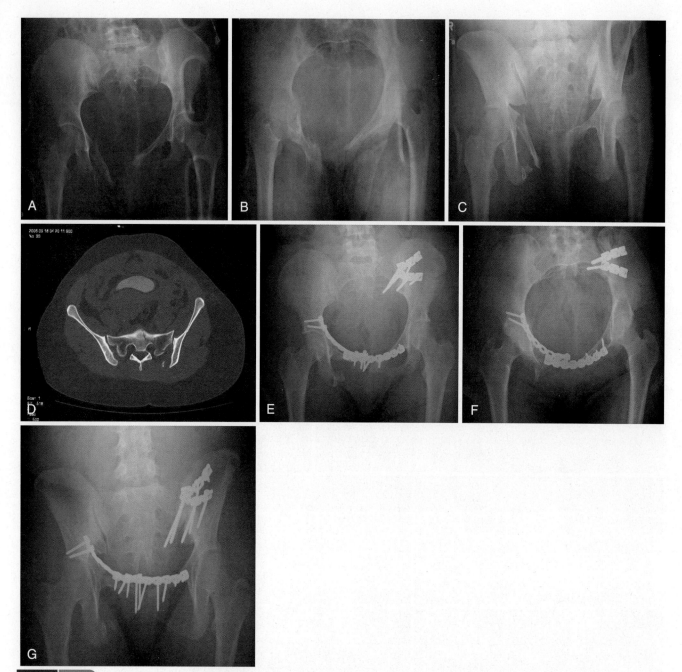

FIGURE 4.56 Young and Burgess lateral compression type III (LC III) injury with marked displacement of the right pubic ramus. Treatment was with open reduction and internal fixation (ORIF) of left sacroiliac joint and ORIF of pubic symphysis and right pubic ramus fractures. **A-C,** Preoperative anteroposterior, inlet, and outlet views, respectively. **D,** Preoperative CT scan. **E-G,** Postoperative anteroposterior, inlet, and outlet views, respectively.

are referred to as pubic root fractures and those medial to the foramen as para-symphyseal fractures.

TREATMENT
■ INITIAL MANAGEMENT
The first hour after a trauma, referred to as the "golden hour" by R. Adams Cowley, whose namesake graces America's first trauma center in Baltimore, is the basis for our current trauma networks and has led to the protocols we use today for rapid transport and treatment of severely traumatized patients.

Acute management of a patient with a pelvic fracture and unrelenting hemorrhage remains a challenge. Because the patient's other injuries generally have a greater effect on outcome than the pelvic fracture, a multidisciplinary approach, with orthopaedic surgeons, general surgeons, and anesthesiologists, is critical to optimizing outcomes.

The initial trauma workup should include chest and pelvic radiographs obtained in the trauma bay, as well as a focused assessment with sonography for trauma (FAST) scan or alternatively a diagnostic peritoneal lavage (DPL),

BOX 4.2

Classification of Pelvic Ring Lesions

Type A: Stable (Posterior Arch Intact)
A1 Avulsion injury
A2 Iliac wing or anterior arch fracture caused by a direct blow
A3 Transverse sacrococcygeal fracture

Type B: Partially Stable (Incomplete Disruption of Posterior Arch)
B1 Open book injury (external rotation)
B2 Lateral compression injury (internal rotation)
B2-1 Ipsilateral anterior and posterior injuries
B2-2 Contralateral (bucket-handle) injuries
B3 Bilateral

Type C: Unstable (Complete Disruption of Posterior Arch)
C1 Unilateral
C1-1 Iliac fracture
C1-2 Sacroiliac fracture-dislocation
C1-3 Sacral fracture
C2 Bilateral, with one side type B, one side type C
C3 Bilateral

From Tile M: Acute pelvic fractures, part I: Causation and classification, *J Am Assoc Orthop Surg* 4:143, 1996.

A-type—stable pelvic ring injuries

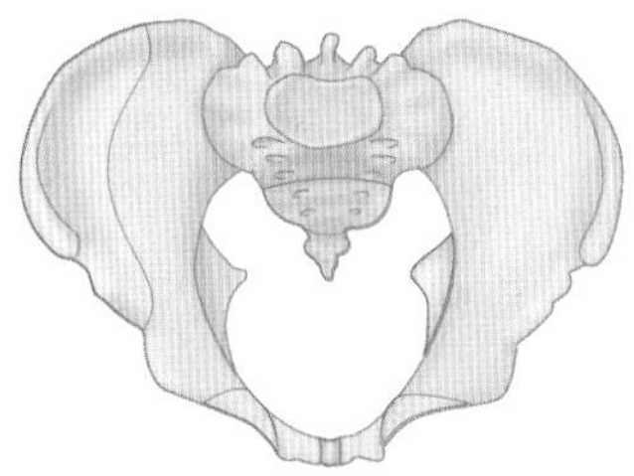

Tile	AO/OTA	Young and Burgess
A1 Avulsion of the innominate bone	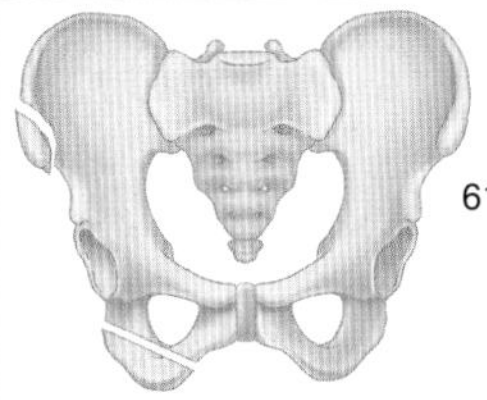 61-A1	n/d
A2 Stable iliac wing fracture or stable, minimally displaced pelvic ring fracture	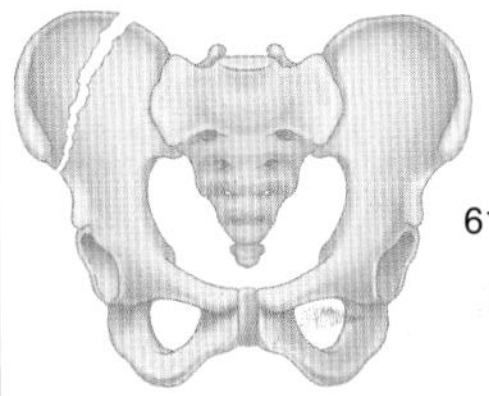 61-A2	(LC I/APC I)
A3 Transverse sacrum or coccygeal fracture	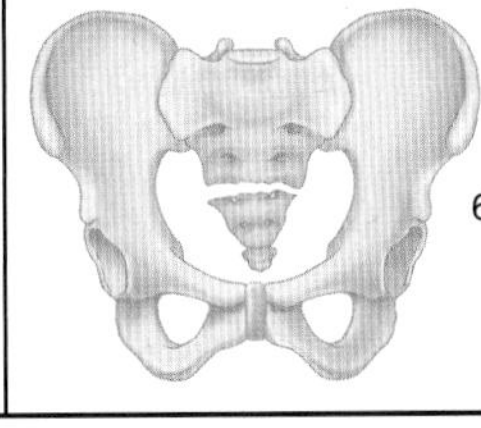 61-A3	n/d

FIGURE 4.57 Type A pelvic ring fractures.

when the patient's body habitus prohibits a FAST. When an unstable pelvic ring injury is identified, we routinely apply a circumferential pelvic binder or sheet (Fig. 4.63). First described in the literature by Routt et al., the technique involves wrapping a bedsheet (or commercially available binder) around the pelvis and greater trochanters. The pelvic volume is manually reduced by one assistant, then two other assistants tighten the sheet. After circumferential tightening, the sheet is clamped. Binding, like external fixation, theoretically reduces pelvic volume, stabilizes raw fracture surfaces, and encourages tamponade. We prefer circumferential pelvic binding to external fixation in the acute resuscitation stage because it is simple, quick, and the necessary items can be quickly attained.

Croce et al. demonstrated a decreased need for transfusions when a pelvic orthotic device was used to apply circumferential pressure in patients with unstable, complex pelvic fractures, but Ghaemmaghami et al. did not find that pelvic binders reduced hemorrhage or mortality associated with pelvic fractures.

The most common error in application is placement of the binding device at the level of the iliac crests rather than centered over the greater trochanters. One study noted inaccurate placement above the level of the greater trochanters to be associated with inadequate fracture reduction. A more recent biomechanical cadaver study found that placement of the binder over the greater trochanter resulted in less motion in all tested planes during bed transfer, log rolling, and elevation of the head of the patient's bed. Although pelvic circumferential compression devices are clinically effective for early fracture reduction, the development of pressure sores are of major concern. Further, use of the device as a reduction tool rather than a fixation device of an already compressed pelvic ring can result in skin sloughing or further soft-tissue injury, and application should be performed by multiple individuals to avoid complication.

Our institution uses a protocol similar to that described by the group at Denver Health (Fig. 4.64). Once stabilized, the patient is taken for advanced imaging of the chest, abdomen, and pelvis. If the patient remains hemodynamically unstable or has a positive FAST examination, he or she should be taken for emergency laparotomy and, if stable afterwards in the controlled environment of the operating room, an external fixator can be applied to maintain stability of the pelvis while allowing access to the abdomen and perineum. A reduction in transfusion requirements has been reported in patients with unstable pelvic fractures who were treated with immediate external fixation compared with those who did not have immediate fixation. Injuries with significant posterior displacement not controlled by anterior external fixation alone may benefit from further stabilization as discussed below.

A patient with a pelvic ring injury, persistent hypotension after circumferential pelvic binding, and a negative FAST examination should be considered for angiography. Hemorrhage frequently results from fracture surfaces and small vessels in the retroperitoneum. Only 5% to 10% of

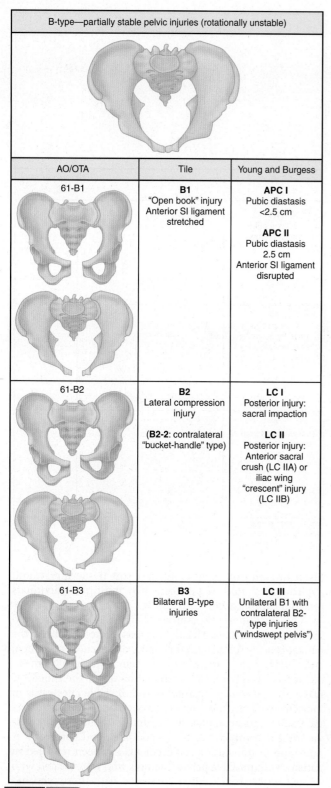

B-type—partially stable pelvic injuries (rotationally unstable)		
AO/OTA	**Tile**	**Young and Burgess**
61-B1	**B1** "Open book" injury Anterior SI ligament stretched	**APC I** Pubic diastasis <2.5 cm **APC II** Pubic diastasis 2.5 cm Anterior SI ligament disrupted
61-B2	**B2** Lateral compression injury (**B2-2**: contralateral "bucket-handle" type)	**LC I** Posterior injury: sacral impaction **LC II** Posterior injury: Anterior sacral crush (LC IIA) or iliac wing "crescent" injury (LC IIB)
61-B3	**B3** Bilateral B-type injuries	**LC III** Unilateral B1 with contralateral B2- type injuries ("windswept pelvis")

FIGURE 4.58 Type B pelvic ring fractures.

patients with pelvic fractures bleed from arterial sources identified by angiography and are treated with embolization. Higher rates of arterial bleeding in the geriatric population have been noted by Henry et al. An algorithm by O'Brien and Dickson (Fig. 4.65) has been proposed; however, the authors recommended that each institution develop its own protocol,

depending on resources and facilities. A recent study demonstrated the institutional problems with angioembolization: patients who were admitted on nights or weekends had long waiting times to the procedure, with a resultant increase in mortality. In addition, angioembolization is not without complications. Matityahu et al. found that bilateral or nondiscriminatory pelvic angioembolism was associated with significant complications (11%), including gluteal muscle necrosis, surgical wound breakdown, and deep infection. Favorable results have been reported with retroperitoneal packing and external fixation. This technique is popular in Europe and has been used in some centers in the United States. Although the technique and algorithm are intriguing, their use requires further investigation in the United States, where the implementation of trauma care is very different.

It is critical to appropriately expose and examine a patient with a pelvic ring injury because open wounds can otherwise easily be missed. Pelvic fractures often communicate through open wounds in the rectum, vagina, or perineum. A rigid sigmoidoscopy or vaginal examination may be necessary if blood is present upon examination. Open pelvic fractures are extremely difficult injuries to manage, with reported mortality rates of up to 50%. If the retroperitoneal space is open, no tamponade effect occurs to prevent excessive bleeding. Sepsis caused by fecal contamination is a major cause of mortality with this injury, and immediate diverting colostomy is indicated in patients with perineal wounds. Faringer et al. anatomically classified open pelvic wounds into zones and recommended selective fecal diversion for patients with open wounds involving the rectum or anus, soft-tissue wounds close to the anus, or large avulsion flaps with associated ischemic pelvic tissue (Fig. 4.66).

Routine vaginal and rectal examinations should be performed in patients with open pelvic fractures because fracture fragments can penetrate these structures, with devastating consequences if timely and appropriate debridement is not performed. External fixation can minimize fracture motion and further soft-tissue injury (Box 4.3).

■ INDICATIONS FOR NONOPERATIVE AND OPERATIVE TREATMENT

Many injuries of the pelvic ring, especially those caused by a low-energy mechanism such as a ground-level fall, can be treated nonoperatively; however, even low-energy mechanisms can lead to fractures with significant instability.

The Tile and AO/OTA classification can provide an initial assessment of stability, and help guide treatment. Both systems define stability based on that of the pelvic ring, and while Type A fractures do not result in pelvic ring instability and can often be managed nonoperatively, there may be circumstances that warrant operative treatment.

AO/OTA A1 fractures are avulsion-type injuries and generally can be treated nonoperatively, unless there is significant displacement that may lead to muscle weakness or displacement that will result in impingement. AO/OTA A2 fractures occur from a direct blow to either the lateral or anterior pelvis and do not cause inherent instability of the pelvic ring. Ilium fractures that involve only the iliac wing and do not extend into the pelvic ring, also known as Duverney fractures, can be treated nonoperatively. However, fractures with significant displacement may require operative fixation, especially in young, high-functioning patients,

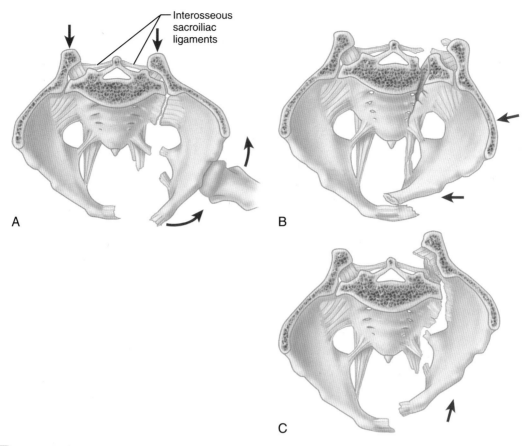

FIGURE 4.59 Tile classification of pelvic fractures based on forces acting on pelvis. **A,** Type B1: External rotation or anteroposterior compression through left femur *(arrows)* disrupts symphysis, pelvis, and anterior sacroiliac ligament until ilium impinges against posterior aspect of sacrum. If force stops at this level, partial stability of pelvis is maintained by interosseous sacroiliac ligaments. **B,** Type B2-1: Lateral compression (internal rotation) force implodes hemipelvis. Rami may fracture anteriorly, and posterior impaction of sacrum may occur, with some disruption of posterior structures, but partial stability is maintained by intact pelvic floor and compression of sacrum. **C,** Type C: Shearing (translational) force disrupts symphysis, pelvic floor, and posterior structures, rendering hemipelvis completely unstable. (From Tile M: Acute pelvic fractures, part I. Causation and classification, J Am Assoc Orthop Surg 4:143, 1996.)

due to the associated muscle attachments and the suggested future effect on function. Similarly, anterior direct blow injuries, often referred to by their mechanism as a "straddle injury," result in either bilateral superior and inferior ramus fractures, or unilateral fractures with injury to the symphysis. While these fractures can occur in isolation, the presence of posterior related injuries often result in the fracture being classified as a different, more unstable, injury. Further, these fractures have a high frequency of urologic injury. AO/OTA A3 fractures are isolated transverse fractures or dislocations of the non–weight bearing portion of the sacrum or coccyx. These fractures are stable because they are outside the weight-bearing pelvis; however, significant displacement can result in neurologic deficit, specifically that of loss of bowel or bladder function, depending on the level of involvement. In fractures with neurologic deficit, early decompression and fixation may be warranted to prevent long-term, cauda equina–like effects.

Historical studies describing the nonoperative treatment of displaced pelvic fractures (Tile types B and C) with traction or a pelvic sling have shown disappointing results, especially in patients with displaced sacral fractures and sacroiliac dislocations. In most reports of these injuries, nearly half of patients had moderate to severe pain after nonoperative treatment.

The significant morbidity associated with nonoperative treatment of displaced, unstable pelvic fractures has led to a more aggressive operative approach. The question of when operative fixation of LC-1 fractures is indicated, however, remains controversial. A survey of 111 members of the OTA found that only 33% of cases showed substantial agreement.

Operative reduction and stabilization have been advocated for rotationally unstable but vertically stable (Tile type B, Young and Burgess type AP II; Figs. 4.53 and 4.59) fractures with a pubic symphysis diastasis of more than 2.5 cm, pubic rami fractures with more than 2 cm displacement, or other rotationally unstable pelvic injuries with significant limb-length discrepancy of more than 1.5 cm or unacceptable pelvic rotational deformity. Traditionally, APCI fractures, those with less than 2.5 cm of symphyseal diastasis, are deemed to be stable and warranted nonoperative management, while those with widening of more than 2.5 cm are deemed unstable and require operative management.

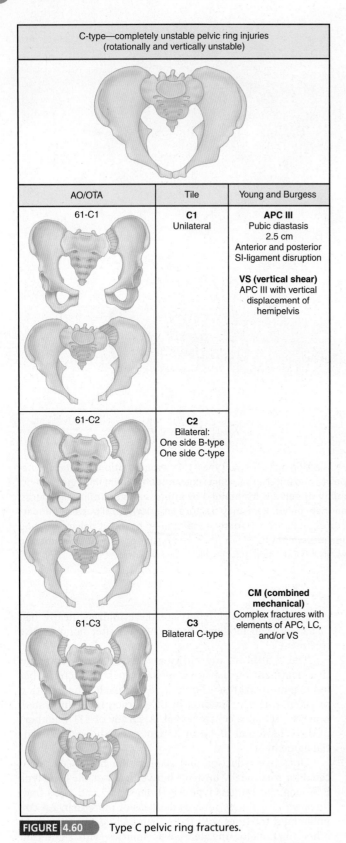

C-type—completely unstable pelvic ring injuries (rotationally and vertically unstable)		
AO/OTA	Tile	Young and Burgess
61-C1	**C1** Unilateral	**APC III** Pubic diastasis 2.5 cm Anterior and posterior SI-ligament disruption **VS (vertical shear)** APC III with vertical displacement of hemipelvis
61-C2	**C2** Bilateral: One side B-type One side C-type	
61-C3	**C3** Bilateral C-type	**CM (combined mechanical)** Complex fractures with elements of APC, LC, and/or VS

FIGURE 4.60   Type C pelvic ring fractures.

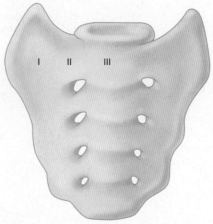

FIGURE 4.61   Denis classification of sacral fractures, in which three zones of injury are differentiated: zone I, sacral ala; zone II, foraminal region; and zone III, spinal canal. Most medial fracture extension is used to classify injury. (From Denis F, Davis S, Comfort T: Sacral fractures: an important problem—retrospective analysis of 236 cases, *Clin Orthop Relat Res* 227:67, 1988.)

The LCI fracture as classified by Young and Burgess includes a variety of fracture patterns and severity. Beckmann et al. attempted to develop a scoring system to predict instability based on radiographic findings (Fig. 4.67 and Table 4.2). Sagi et al. validated the system in a historic cohort of patients who had dynamic fluoroscopic stress of the pelvis and were compared to the operative recommendations of OTA attendees to determine if the radiographic variables were predictive of operative tendency. The validation study determined that a score <7 indicated a propensity for nonoperative treatment with successful radiographic union, a score >9 indicated that a patient may benefit from operative stabilization, and a score of 7 to 9 lacked consensus regarding appropriate treatment and may warrant dynamic stress in the operating room.

Young and Burgess LCII fractures, when minimally displaced, can be treated nonoperatively. However, close monitoring of these fractures is necessary because a fracture through the ilium can be inherently more unstable due to the large muscular attachments to the free segment. Fractures with more than 1 cm of displacement should have operative fixation because of the propensity to vertically displace over time from the muscular attachments.

Type B3 fractures are rotationally unstable fractures with bilateral posterior ring involvement but lacking vertical instability. This group encompasses the bilateral APCII injury, bilateral LCI injury, and a combined variant, the LCIII injury, where there is internal rotation of one hemipelvis (LC type injury) and external rotation of the contralateral hemipelvis (APC type injury). While most of fractures of this type result in instability requiring fixation, some subtle bilateral LC1 or LC3 fractures may warrant nonoperative management based on their anterior ring injury and the patient's functional status and age. As with the LCII fracture, if managed nonoperatively, these fractures should be closely monitored because the risk of late displacement is high.

Type C fractures, as defined by the AO/OTA classification system, generally always require operative intervention. Indications for nonoperative management generally are

However, more recent literature calls into question the use of a single static radiograph and suggests that even APCI may warrant further investigation with dynamic fluoroscopic stress radiographs.

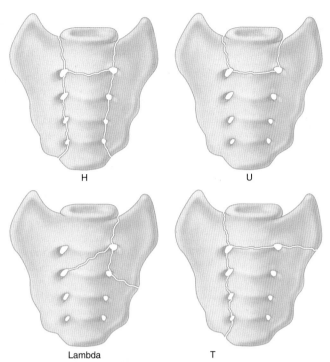

H   U

Lambda   T

FIGURE 4.62 Fracture pattern description based on the Latin-letter that the fracture morphology resembles.

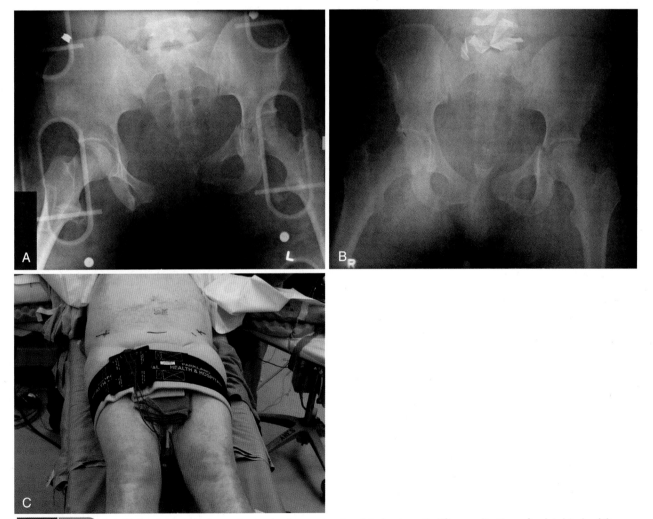

FIGURE 4.63 **A,** Initial anteroposterior radiograph of open-book pelvic fracture. **B,** After application of pelvic binder **(C).**

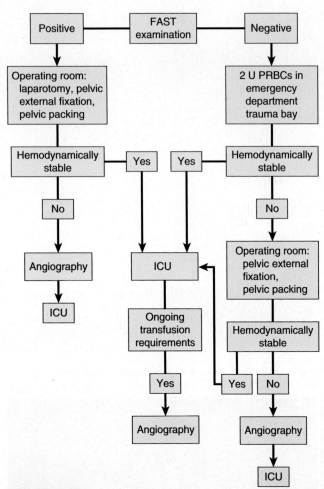

FIGURE 4.64 Algorithm for the treatment of patients with pelvic fracture who present with hemodynamic instability. *FAST*, Focused abdominal sonography for trauma; *PRBCs*, packed red blood cells. (From Hak DJ, Smith WR, Suzuki T. Management of hemorrhage in life-threatening pelvic fracture. *J Am Acad Orthop Surg.* 17:447–457, 2009.)

limited to patient comorbidities or associated injuries that prevent safe presentation to the operating theater.

TIMING OF SURGERY

In patients with a positive FAST examination or persistent hemodynamic instability, emergency pelvic stabilization, with or without pelvic packing, may be warranted. Generally, an external fixator will provide adequate initial stabilization and can be applied expeditiously by an experienced orthopaedic traumatologist. Injuries with significant posterior displacement not controlled by anterior external fixation alone may benefit from an antishock clamp, or C-clamp, type of external fixator applied to the greater trochanters or supraacetabular pelvis, ideally in the operating room (see Technique 4.7). Alternatively, an "antishock iliosacral screw," as described by Gardner and Routt, may offer a safer and less cumbersome substitute.

Timing of definitive management is highly dependent on the patient's overall well-being and resuscitation status. Early works by Bone et al. showed that early treatment of fractures may reduce associated pulmonary complications;

however, Pape et al. provided strong evidence that patients with thoracic trauma, such as pulmonary contusions, had a significantly higher rate of pulmonary complications when undergoing treatment within 24 hours. The concept of "early total care" was developed in the 1980s and was altered based on work by Vallier et al., who described a treatment algorithm known as "early appropriate care" (EAC). EAC is based on early stabilization of pelvic, femoral, acetabular, and spinal fractures after appropriate resuscitation as measured by objective laboratory findings. They found that definitive fixation was safe within 36 hours of injury when resuscitated patients met at least one of the following criteria: venous lactate <4.0 mmol/L, BE ≥ −5.5 mmol/L, or pH ≥7.25. Patients who had EAC had shorter hospital and ICU stays, fewer days spent on ventilator support, and fewer complications.

Our institution uses the criteria developed by Vallier and her partners at MetroHealth in Cleveland. Polytraumatized patients who are hemodynamically unstable and present with chest trauma, a lactate above 4.0 mmol/L, and an unstable pelvic ring are treated with damage-control orthopaedics (DCO) with temporary stabilization of the pelvis as described above. For patients who are hemodynamically stable with chest trauma and a lactate above 4.0 mmol/L, resuscitation is performed in the ICU, and once lactate stabilizes below 4.0 mmol/L, definitive fixation is done unless otherwise prohibited by associated injuries, such as a severe closed head injury. In patients who present with an unstable pelvic ring injury and a lactate below 4.0 mmol/L, operative fixation is done within 24 hours of injury, unless limited by any associated injuries.

CHOICE OF TREATMENT

The goals of treatment of the pelvic ring are no different than for any other bone. After life-saving measures, the goals of definitive treatment follow the AO principles. The aim is to restore length, angulation, and rotation while providing stable fixation to allow early range of motion and allow bony healing, but respecting the surrounding soft tissues and associated soft-tissue injuries.

The treatment options for injuries to the pelvic ring are more varied than for many other injuries. The treating surgeon must have a full understanding of the injury including the associated fractures and dislocations as well as the translational and rotational deformities that are present. This takes expertise and experience to develop, and it is recommended that operative fixation of pelvic ring injuries be performed by an experienced orthopaedic traumatologist with a knowledge of reduction and fixation options and an understanding of the strengths and limitations of each approach or treatment option. Because of the operative proximity to critical nerves and intrapelvic organs, iatrogenic complications can be dire, and with the limited corridors of fixation, there is little room for error.

EXTERNAL FIXATION

Anterior pelvic external fixation is a versatile treatment option that can be used in the acute phase of treatment to provide temporary pelvic stability and allow access to the abdomen and perineum. It also can be used as definitive fixation in some patients or as an adjunct to internal fixation in others. Fractures that involve the iliac wing, the acetabulum, or both usually are contraindications to pelvic external fixation.

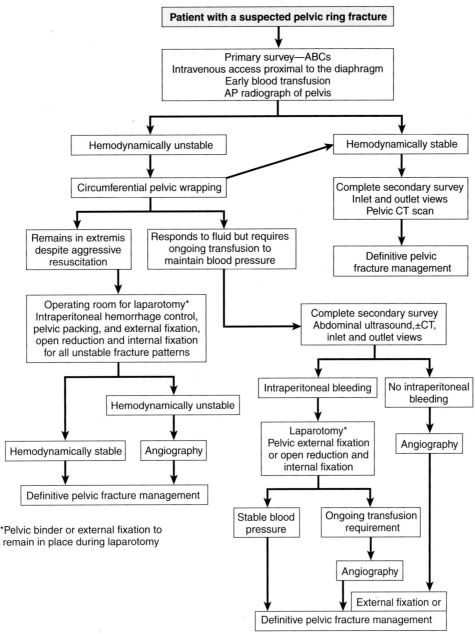

FIGURE 4.65 Initial evaluation and management of patient with pelvic ring fracture. Protocols should be individualized according to resources and facilities. (From O'Brien PJ, Dickson KF: Pelvic fractures: Evaluation and acute management. In Tornetta P III, Baumgaertner M, editors: *Orthopaedic knowledge update, trauma 3*, Rosemont, 2005, American Academy of Orthopaedic Surgeons.)

Options for pin placement for external fixation of the pelvis are the gluteal pillar or supra-acetabular corridor. In the rare circumstance where a fixator is applied to a severely injured patient in the emergency department or in the operating room without fluoroscopy, placement of pins in the supra-acetabular corridor is contraindicated. Pins can be safely placed into the gluteal pillar through a small incision and with direct palpation without the use of fluoroscopy. Placement of two or three pins in each iliac wing will ensure adequate stabilization, as it is common to penetrate the tables of the false pelvis during placement. A simple modular frame that allows abdominal access for exploratory laparotomy or pelvic packing is used.

Supra-acetabular pin placement is more dependent on fluoroscopy but provides improved stability when used in part as definitive treatment. Further, pin placement anteriorly provides better control over the rotational deformity of the pelvis commonly seen in type B fractures, and can be used not only for fixation but also reduction of rotationally unstable injuries. In patients with type C injuries and multiplanar deformity, placement of a supra-acetabular pin on the side of the flexion through the hemipelvis and a gluteal pillar pin on the contralateral side can provide multiplanar deformity correction, as originally described by Routt and Achor (Fig. 4.68).

In patients being managed definitively with an external fixation device, whether alone or in conjunction

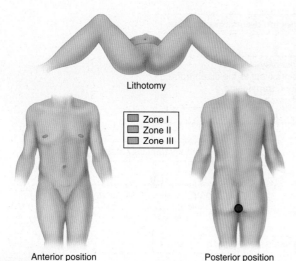

FIGURE 4.66 Three zones of injury that guide decisions regarding need for colostomy in open pelvic fractures, according to Faringer et al. Zone I injuries often require colostomy, whereas diversion is rarely required for zone III wounds. Zone II injuries are diverted selectively, with wounds into subcutaneous fat of anterior groin or medial thigh possibly requiring colostomy. (From Faringer PD, Mullins RJ, Feliciano PD, et al: Selective fecal diversion in complex open pelvic fractures from blunt trauma, *Arch Surg* 129:958, 1994.)

BOX 4.3

Pelvic Damage Control

Closed reduction of the pelvis at admission
External fixation
    Wrapping pelvis with sheets with inner rotation and slight flexion of knees
    External fixator
    Pelvic C-clamp
    Pneumatic antishock garment
Control of hemorrhage
    Pelvic packing
    Angiography
Control of contamination
    Repair of genitourinary and rectal injuries
    Debridement of necrotic tissue in the case of open injury

From Ertel WK: General assessment and management of the polytrauma patient. In Tile M, Helfet DL, Kellam JF, editors: *Fractures of the pelvis and acetabulum*, 3rd ed, Philadelphia, 2003, Lippincott Williams & Wilkins.

---

with internal fixation, placement of the supraacetabular pins can play a major role in a patient's ability to mobilize after surgery. Placement of pins too close to the acetabulum and those headed in a more caudal-to-cranial direction can result in impingement of the device on the patient's thighs and an inability to sit upright. Pin placement should be started as high on the anterior pelvis as allowed by the patient's anatomy and directed in a cranial-to-caudal direction. Pins can be directed just above the greater sciatic notch or can be unicortical in the greater sciatic notch to maximize this angulation. Attachment of the pin to bar clamps above the pins also can help reduce this impingement.

GLUTEAL PILLAR EXTERNAL FIXATION

TECHNIQUE 4.4

- Place the patient supine on a radiolucent table.
- Attempt to attain and maintain reduction with traction or pelvic binders placed distally before placement of the external fixator.
- Palpate the gluteus medius pillar 2 to 4 cm proximal/posterior to the anterior superior iliac spine. This is the widening of bone that allows pin insertion.
- Make an incision perpendicular to the iliac wing.
- Placement of a Kirschner wire along the inner table, when readily available, can provide orientation of the pelvic slope.
- The starting point is along the inner third of the iliac wing. There is significant overlay laterally, and a lateral starting point may exit the outer table. The first pin should be started centrally, from anterior to posterior, within the thickening of the gluteal pillar.
- After drilling a starting point manually, place the pin between the tables by use of sensory feedback to keep the pin within the iliac cortical tables. Aim toward the hip joint to use the column of bone above the acetabulum (Fig. 4.69).
- Place a second and possibly a third pin in a converging pattern.
- Confirm pin placement with fluoroscopy, if available.
- Connect the pin clusters and crossbars.
- Compress the pelvis through pressure on the greater trochanter, then tighten the external fixator.
- In vertically unstable fractures, traction should be used until definitive fracture fixation.

SUPRA-ACETABULAR EXTERNAL FIXATION

TECHNIQUE 4.5

- Palpate and mark the external iliac pulse.
- Palpate the anterior superior iliac spine. The incision will be approximately 1 cm medial and 2 to 3 cm distal to the anterior superior iliac spine. Confirm the proximal-distal starting point on a fluoroscopic iliac oblique view, also commonly referred to as a "teardrop" view (Fig. 4.70).
- Note that the starting point often is on the medial edge of the teardrop because of the slight internal concavity of the supracetabular corridor. We prefer to use a transverse incision, which allows slight adjustment medial to lateral when necessary.
- Gently spread the soft tissues to bone and place a drill with a protective sleeve.

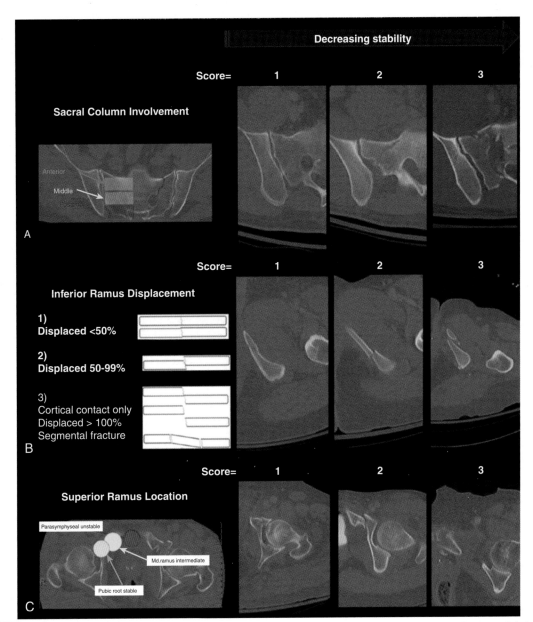

FIGURE 4.67 Beckmann et al. scoring schematic for LC-1 pelvic fractures. Assessing sacral column involvement **(A)**, inferior ramus displacement **(B)**, and superior ramus location **(C)**. See Table 56-2 for scoring criteria. (From Beckmann J, Haller JM, Beebe M, et al: Validated radiographic scoring system for lateral compression type 1 pelvis fractures, *Orthop Trauma* 34:70, 2020.)

- Confirm the anterior inferior iliac spine starting point fluoroscopically on an iliac oblique view. If the tip of the pin has no overlap with bone on the iliac oblique view, the mediolateral starting point is correct. Placement at the superior aspect of the anterior inferior iliac spine will allow optimal caudal trajectory.
- After drilling a starting point, place the pin in bone about 2 to 3 cm heading approximately 25 degrees medially; note that in patients with significant rotational injury this may be highly variable. Attention to the angle of the fluoroscope during the iliac oblique view can give a sense of the angulation needed for pin placement.
- Confirm the caudal to cranial angulation of the pin on the iliac oblique view. Evaluate medial to lateral angu-

lation of the pin on an obturator inlet view. Advance the pin using alternating views to confirm intraosseous placement.
- Based on surgeon preference, advance the pin so the tip impacts but does not exit the sciatic buttress or traverses just above the greater sciatic notch.
- Confirm pin placement on all three views: obturator inlet to assess medial to lateral angulation, iliac oblique to assess caudal to cranial angulation, and obturator outlet to confirm that the pin remains within the supra-acetabular corridor
- An obturator outlet view directly in line with the pin, where the pin is contained within the teardrop of the supra-acetabular corridor, can confirm safe placement.
- Connect the pins to the crossbar.

TABLE 4.2	
LC-1 Fracture Scoring Criteria	
PARAMETER	**POINTS**
SACRAL DISPLACEMENT	
<2 mm	1
≥2 mm	2
DENIS CLASSIFICATION	
Zone 1	1
Zone 2	2
Zone 3	3
SACRAL COLUMNS	
1 column	1
2 columns	2
3 columns	3
INFERIOR RAMUS DISPLACEMENT	
Minimal	1
>50%	2
Complete	3
SUPERIOR RAMUS LOCATION	
Root	1
Mid-ramus	2
Parasymphyseal	3

Scores <7 predict nonoperative treatment recommendation, scores >9 indicate surgical recommendations, and scores 7-9 indicate indeterminate stability that should be further evaluated.
From Beckmann J, Haller JM, Beebe M, et al: Validated radiographic scoring system for lateral compression type 1 pelvis fractures, *J Orthop Trauma* 34:70, 2020.

POSTOPERATIVE CARE If it is used for the definitive treatment of the pelvic fracture, the frame is left in place for 6 to 12 weeks, depending on the fracture type and associated fixation. Pin site care must be meticulous, with peroxide swabs used twice daily to clean away the crusted transudate that often forms. The dressing around the pin site should apply some compression to the skin to minimize motion around the pins. If a pin becomes infected and loose, it should be removed or replaced and the original pin site should be curetted or over-drilled.

ANTERIOR SUBCUTANEOUS INTERNAL FIXATION

The original description of anterior subcutaneous internal fixation was by Kuttner et al. in the German literature in 2009. Vaidya et al. described the modified method and introduced the name "INFIX" in the English literature in 2012. The technique uses US Food and Drug Administration (FDA)-approved devices for spinal surgery, which are

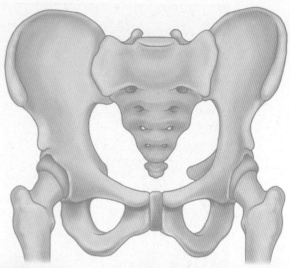

FIGURE 4.68   For type C injuries and multiplanar deformity, placement of supracetabular pin on side of flexion through hemipelvis and gluteal pillar pin on contralateral side can provide multiplanar deformity correction, as originally described by Routt and Achor.

placed in the lower abdominal area through small incisions and span the fractured anterior pelvic ring by interconnecting the left and right hemipelvis, an "off-label" use. Subcutaneous internal fixators for anterior pelvic ring injuries provide the advantages of external fixation while avoiding some of the disadvantages. Cited advantages include minimal soft-tissue dissection, decreased blood loss and postoperative pain, rigid fixation, and increased patient comfort. The low-profile construct allows earlier sitting and mobilization. The biggest disadvantage of subcutaneous internal fixation is that a second operation is required for implant removal.

Cole et al. suggested indications for the use of INFIX that include unstable injuries of the anterior pelvic ring in morbidly obese patients, patients with severe soft-tissue injuries, patients who require prolonged stay in the ICU to reduce the risk of infection and facilitate nursing care, patients with concomitant injuries that may require prone positioning for operative procedures (e.g., spinal fractures), and patients with coagulopathy.

Although there are few clinical reports available, early results have been favorable, with healing at an average of 3 months after surgery with no significant loss of fixation. Vaidya et al. reported a series of 24 patients with rotational or vertically unstable pelvic fractures treated with INFIX. All fractures healed without significant loss of reduction; there were no infections, delayed unions, or nonunions. Vaidya et al. cautioned that it is extremely important that the rod height is just below the skin and that the rod is not impinging on the underlying fascia; this may require longer custom pedicle screws.

Several complications have been noted with the use of INFIX, most frequently lateral femoral cutaneous neurapraxia (30%), which is temporary in most patients, and HO (35%), which is asymptomatic in almost all patients. Reported rates of infection (0% to 12%) and aseptic loosening (0% to 19%) are low.

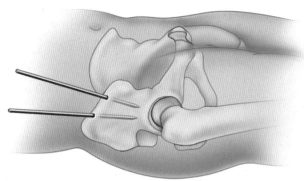

FIGURE 4.69 Pin placement in hemipelvis in relation to body . (From Poka A, Libby EP: Indications and techniques for external fixation of the pelvis, *Clin Orthop Relat Res* 329:54, 1996.) **SEE TECHNIQUE 4.4.**

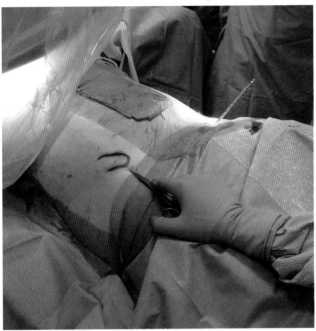

FIGURE 4.70 Starting point for supraacetabular external fixation. **SEE TECHNIQUE 4.5.**

TECHNIQUE 4.6

(VAIDYA ET AL.)

- Position the patient supine on a radiolucent table. Prepare and drape the skin from above the umbilicus to the proximal thigh. Prepare the lower extremity into the field to facilitate reduction techniques.
- If posterior instability is present, correct it first using the standard techniques of iliosacral reduction and screw placement or posterior plating.
- Use fluoroscopic imaging to identify the starting point of the pedicle screw.
- Make a 2- to 3-cm longitudinal incision centered over the anterior interior iliac spine in line with the groin crease (Fig. 4.71A).
- With blunt dissection through the soft tissues, develop the interval between the sartorius and tensor fascia lata muscles to gain access to the anterior inferior iliac spine (Fig. 4.71B).
- Choose a starting point for the supra-acetabular pin just proximal to the insertion of the rectus femoris tendon.

- Place small-fragment Hohmann retractors on either side of the iliac bone at this point. Take care to avoid injury to the lateral femoral cutaneous nerve and violation of the hip joint capsule.
- Once the appropriate starting point is identified, open the cortex with a starting pedicle awl (Fig. 4.71C).
- Use a pedicle finder to establish a corridor between the inner and outer cortices of the ilium, taking care not to penetrate the iliac table. A drill bit can be used instead of the pedicle finder.
- Measure the depth of the hole and select a screw that will sit 15 to 50 mm proud. The height of the screw above the bone depends on the size of the patient. Ideally, the screw head sits at the level of the sartorius muscle or slightly superficial. In some morbidly obese patients, this could be even longer, necessitating custom screws. It is important not to sink the screw below this point because it could lead to compression of the underlying structures by the bar once it is attached.
- Insert a 7- or 8-mm diameter pedicle screw. The length of the screw may vary from 75 to 110 mm, depending on the body habitus of the patient, with at least 60 mm of the screw being intraosseous.
- Precontour a 6-mm titanium rod with an anterior bow (Fig. 4.71D). The curve of the rod is determined by laying it flat on the belly between the two pedicle screws; this area is convex in most individuals. Contour the rod so that it lies slightly above the skin in the center (Fig. 4.71E).
- Cut the rod to the appropriate length, which should be 5 cm longer than the distance between the two pedicle screws.
- Tunnel the rod subcutaneously from one screw to the other, just under the skin and above the sartorius muscle (Fig. 4.71F). The superior border of the "bikini" area (formed by the groin creases on the sides and superiorly by a fold of abdominal tissue) marks the path for the subcutaneous rod.
- Position the rod with the bow anterior to avoid potential compressive complications to the genitourinary or neurovascular structures.
- Connect the rod to both pedicle screws and apply compression or distraction depending on the pelvic deformity (Fig. 4.72).
- Once appropriate reduction is achieved, tighten the pedicle screw caps.
- Trim any excess rod length with a rod cutter.
- Confirm suitable reduction and implant position with fluoroscopic anteroposterior, inlet, and outlet views (Fig. 4.73).

POSTOPERATIVE CARE Toe-touch weight bearing is allowed on the side of the posterior injury and weight bearing as tolerated on the side without a posterior injury. Patients with bilateral posterior pelvic injuries remain non–weight bearing. Weight bearing is begun at 8 to 12 weeks, depending on radiographs, patient comfort, and surgeon preference, and is advanced as tolerated. Implants generally are removed between 3 and 6 months after surgery.

PELVIC CLAMPS

Because in vertically unstable fractures an anteriorly applied external fixator does not control motion in the posterior sacroiliac complex, two pelvic clamps have been developed to help control the posterior pelvis in the resus-

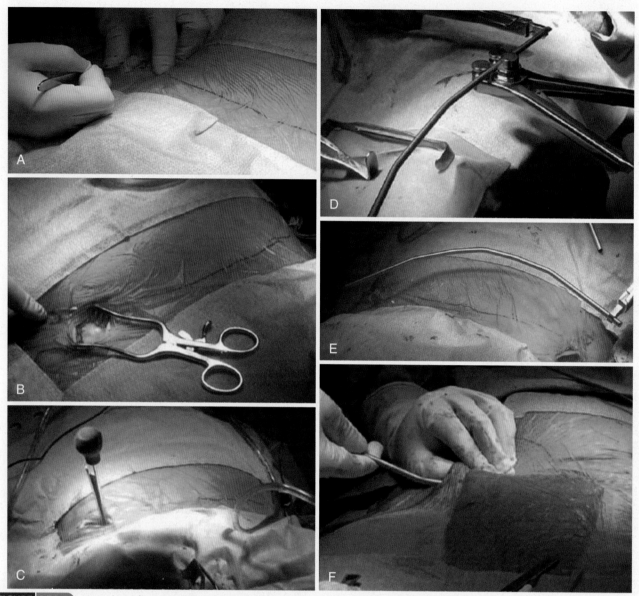

FIGURE 4.71   Anterior subcutaneous internal fixator. **A,** Skin incision. **B,** Blunt dissection of soft tissue. **C,** Starting pedicle awl. **D,** Rod bender in use while rod is held with a rod holder. **E,** Contoured rod. **F,** Rod being tunneled subcutaneously. (From Vaidya R, Colen R, Vigdorchik J, et al: Treatment of unstable pelvic ring injuries with an internal anterior fixator and posterior fixation: initial clinical series, *J Orthop Trauma* 26:1, 2012.) **SEE TECHNIQUE 4.6.**

citation phase: the Ganz C-clamp (Fig. 4.74) and the pelvic stabilizer developed by Browner et al. These devices use large, percutaneously placed pins over the region of the sacroiliac joint posteriorly. We believe that an iliac wing fracture close to the sacroiliac joint is a contraindication to the use of this device, and we use it only as a temporary stabilizing device that should be removed within 5 days if possible.

TECHNIQUE 4.7

(GANZ ET AL.)

- With the patient supine, palpate the posterior superior iliac spine and draw an imaginary line between it and the anterior superior iliac spine. Insert the nail on this line 3 to 4 fingerbreadths anterolateral to the posterior superior iliac spine (Fig. 4.75A). Do not make the entry point too distal to avoid endangering the gluteal vessels or the sciatic nerve.
- Make a generous stab wound over each entry point, insert the Steinmann pins, and make sure the side arm can slide freely (Fig. 4.75B).
- Advance the pins until bone is contacted and then use a hammer to drive the pins approximately 1 cm into the bone (Fig. 4.75C).
- Slide the two side arms medially toward one another until the ends of the threaded bolts, sliding over the pins, contact the bone.

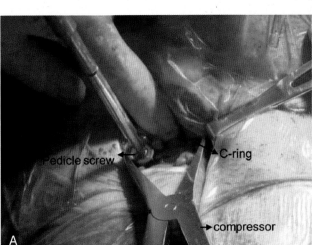
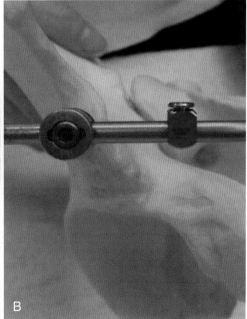

FIGURE 4.72 **A,** C-ring and compression device. **B,** Pedicle screw and C-ring in a Sawbones model. (From Vaidya R, Colen R, Vigdorchik J, et al: Treatment of unstable pelvic ring injuries with an internal anterior fixator and posterior fixation: initial clinical series, *J Orthop Trauma* 26:1, 2012.) **SEE TECHNIQUE 4.6.**

- Drive the threaded bolts inward with a wrench to apply compression to the unstable hemipelvis. This closes the diastasis and stabilizes the posterior pelvic ring (Fig. 4.75D).
- Correct cranial displacement of the hemipelvis by placing traction on the ipsilateral leg before applying compression.
- Correct dorsal displacement by manual traction using the T-handle applied to a Schanz pin placed in the anterior superior iliac spine. Carry out other necessary manipulations in a similar manner.
- Check the reduction maneuvers radiographically, or if other procedures are necessary immediately, obtain a radiograph as soon as possible.
- The device can be applied in an oblique configuration by placing the Steinmann pin on the side of the stable hemipelvis in the anterior superior iliac spine. When the bolt is tightened, one component of the force vector on the unstable side is directed anteriorly, which helps reduce a posteriorly displaced hemipelvis.
- Once the clamp is in place, additional diagnostic or therapeutic procedures can be performed. If a laparotomy is required, rotate the crossbar around the fixed axis of the Steinmann pins away from the abdomen so that it lies distally on the thighs. If a procedure on the proximal femur is required, rotate the crossbar cephalad so that it rests on the abdomen (Fig. 4.75E).
- Leave the clamp in place until definitive internal fixation can be performed. Once the posterior fracture has been exposed and reduction clamps or pins are in place, remove the C-clamp.
- If hemorrhage is not controlled after application of the anterior external fixator or pelvic clamp, angiographic evaluation is indicated. In approximately 10% of patients, a major arterial injury can be identified and treated by embolization. Also consider retroperitoneal packing, as

described by Osborn et al., to control bleeding in these patients.

■ INTERNAL FIXATION OF THE ANTERIOR PELVIS

Anterior internal fixation of the pelvis comes in many forms depending on the injury pattern. The most common form is pubic symphysis plating. In most cases of symphyseal widening there is an associated posterior ligamentous or bony injury, whether clinically or radiographically recognized or not. Anterior plate fixation has progressively changed over the past several decades. Tornetta, Dickson, and Matta reported unacceptably high rates of failure of two-hole symphyseal plating compared to multihole plating. Sagi et al. supported this, showing that two-hole plates failed at a rate of 33% compared to only 12% with multihole plates. Currently, most surgeons advocate a multihole plate for fixation of the symphysis. Internal fixation of the symphysis also has been described using percutaneous crossing screws, although the published outcomes of this technique are limited and there is a risk for iatrogenic injury to the surrounding structures if the surgeon is inexperienced in the technique.

While anterior plating is the most biomechanically advantageous fixation for B1 injuries with failure through the symphysis, many surgeons recommend posterior screw fixation in conjunction with anterior plating. Because of the continued motion at the symphysis during the healing process, implant breakage is common and, when this occurs early enough, malunion may progress. In a study by Avilucea et al., augmentation with percutaneous posterior screw fixation reduced the malunion rate from 36% in the anterior-only group to 1% in the anterior and posterior group.

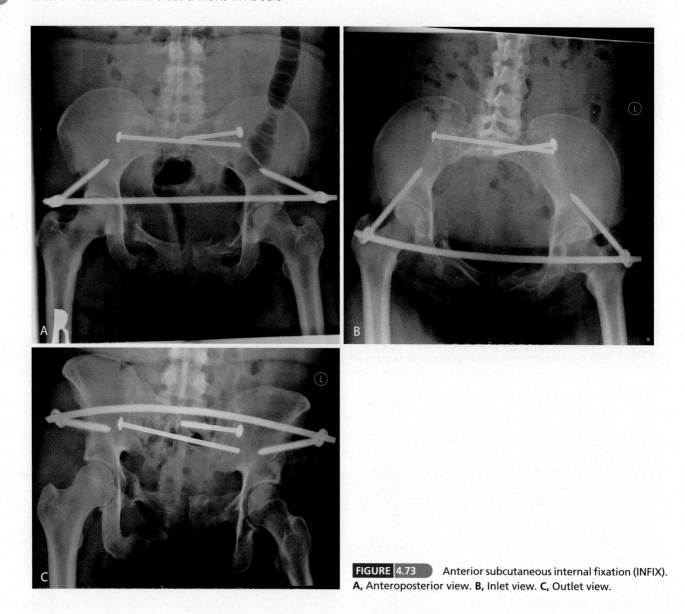

FIGURE 4.73   Anterior subcutaneous internal fixation (INFIX). **A,** Anteroposterior view. **B,** Inlet view. **C,** Outlet view.

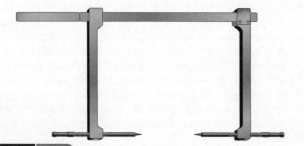

FIGURE 4.74   Ganz "antishock" pelvic fixator for immediate, provisional stabilization of pelvic fractures.

For anterior pelvic ring injuries in which fracture of the ramus occurs, whether from external or internal rotation failure, there are multiple options for definitive treatment. In LC1 patterns, posterior fixation alone may provide enough fixation to prevent the need for anterior fixation, but this is not always the case. In situations requiring fixation of the anterior ring, fracture morphology or patient considerations may dictate treatment. While external fixation of the anterior ring provides adequate resistance to internal and external rotation, this construct provides little stability in rotation or flexion and extension. In this situation, treatment with either a percutaneous screw or open treatment with a plate and screws will increase the stability. Simonian et al. showed that use of a long retrograde ramus screw, one that passed above the anterior acetabulum and engaged the lateral cortex of the ilium, provided fixation similar to a plate along the ramus in external rotation (group B1) injuries. Since that time, the use of percutaneous screw fixation of the rami has grown in popularity. Starr et al. showed that percutaneous screw fixation of the anterior pelvis is best used in patients with pubic root fractures. Nakatani zone III injuries can be treated with an antegrade anterior column screw. While some parasymphyseal (Nakatani zone I) fractures can be treated with retrograde screw fixation, this generally is contraindicated when the fracture extends into the symphysis because of the lack

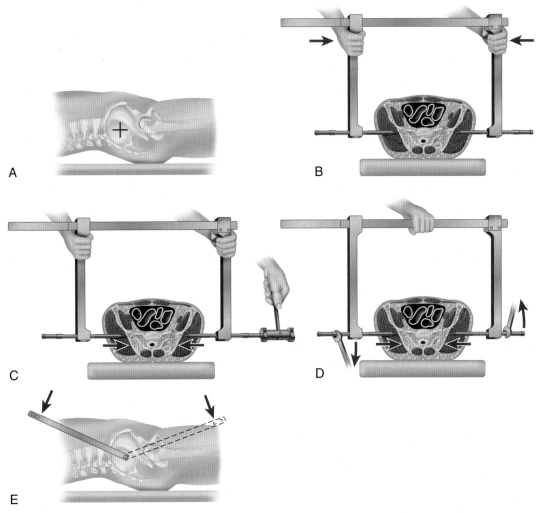

FIGURE 4.75 Application of Ganz fixator (see text). **A,** Nail insertion site. **B,** Steinmann pins are inserted, and free sliding of side arm is ensured. **C,** Pins are driven approximately 1 cm into bone. **D,** Driving threaded bolts inward applies compression to close diastasis and stabilize posterior pelvic ring. **E,** Crossbar can be rotated to allow laparotomy or access to proximal femur. (Courtesy of R. Ganz, MD.) **SEE TECHNIQUE 4.7.**

of bony substance to support the fixation. Zone II injuries can be treated with either an antegrade or retrograde screw; however, retrograde placement may not be possible in obese patients or those with large thighs. In patients who have an anterior corridor that prevents a straight path for a screw or those with larger thighs, the technique can be modified to pass a screw using a retrograde-antegrade-retrograde technique as described by Weatherby et al.

OPEN REDUCTION AND INTERNAL FIXATION OF THE PUBIC SYMPHYSIS

TECHNIQUE 4.8

- Position the patient supine on a radiolucent table.
- Maintain the legs in internal rotation to aid in reductions (Fig. 4.76A).
- Drape the area distal to the pubic tubercles.
- Make a Pfannenstiel incision.
- Incise the rectus longitudinally at the decussation of the fibers. Do not transect the rectus heads.
- Use a malleable retractor in the space of Retzius to protect the bladder (Fig. 4.76B).
- Place narrow sharp Hohmann retractors underneath the rectus and over the pubis to expose the pubic symphysis (Fig. 4.76C and D).
- Place a Weber pointed reduction clamp anteriorly onto the body of the pubis for reduction (Fig. 4.76E and F).
- In fractures with cephalad displacement of the hemipelvis, apply traction. In more severe cases, use pelvic reduction forceps by placing a 4.5-mm screw anteriorly on each side of the symphysis. Use of a plate and nut on the displaced side will allow full mechanical advantage without the risk of screw pull-out (Fig. 4.76G).
- After satisfactory reduction, place a six-hole curved 3-mm reconstruction plate on the superior surface of the symphysis (Fig. 4.76H).
- Eccentrically drill to yield a small amount of compression.

- Confirm reduction and fixation with fluoroscopy.
- For type C injuries for which posterior fixation is not possible, apply a double plate.
- Place a closed suction drain in the space of Retzius.
- In cases of pubic rami fractures in which a Pfannenstiel approach is not enough for ORIF, use a modified AIP or ilioinguinal approach.

■ POSTERIOR APPROACH AND INTERNAL FIXATION

An OTA highlight paper from 2016 showed that in unilateral injuries, an open approach to the posterior pelvis provided no advantage over a closed percutaneous technique. While many surgeons are becoming more aggressive with percutaneous reduction and fixation, familiarity with this approach is paramount. Because neurologic injury occurs with 30% of transforaminal sacral fractures (Denis zone II fractures), some authors advocate ORIF of such fractures with decompression of the involved neural foramina. Transiliac rod fixation has been reported by several authors for sacral disruptions, although there is a risk of neurologic injury with compression of the sacrum (Fig. 4.77). Tension band plating also can be used between the two posterior iliac crests, but is becoming less common (Fig. 4.78).

In patients with highly displaced posterior pelvic fractures or dislocations, a posterior approach may offer the greatest chance to achieve anatomic reduction of the fracture or dislocation, especially in bilateral injuries. In LC2 fractures with a small crescent fragment, the posterior approach may offer a biomechanically advantageous placement of screws and plates. The prone position also offers the ability to decompress the neuroforamina in patients with a neurologic injury or bony fragment within a foramen. However, this approach is not without its disadvantages. In patients who have had embolization of the internal iliac artery or have a large Morel-Lavallée lesion, this approach can be fraught with wound complications.

INTERNAL FIXATION: POSTERIOR APPROACH AND FIXATION OF SACRAL FRACTURES AND SACROILIAC DISLOCATIONS (PRONE)

TECHNIQUE 4.9

(MATTA AND SAUCEDO)
- Position the patient prone on a long radiolucent board to allow anteroposterior, caudal, and cephalad projections with an image intensifier (Fig. 4.79).
- Use a standard posterior vertical incision, 2 cm lateral to the posterior superior iliac spine for sacroiliac dislocations, fracture-dislocations, or sacral fractures.
- Create a full-thickness flap off the gluteus fascia to the midline.

- Reflect the posterior portion of the gluteal muscles from the posterior iliac wing and the gluteus maximus origin from the sacrum (Fig. 4.80A and B).
- Expose the greater sciatic notch to evaluate reduction. For sacral fractures, elevate the multifidus muscles to expose the fracture of the posterior sacral lamina (Fig. 4.80C).
- For sacroiliac dislocations, place pointed reduction forceps from the sacrum to the iliac wing for reduction. Use palpation through the greater sciatic notch as well as direct observation to evaluate the reduction.
- Under image intensifier control, insert screws perpendicular to the iliac wing across the sacroiliac joint into the sacral ala, directing the screws toward the S1 vertebral body. Carefully target the drill bit and screws by multiple anteroposterior, caudal, and cephalad image intensifier projections.
- For sacral fractures, perform reduction in the same manner, checking the reduction with palpation through the greater sciatic notch and observation of the posterior sacral lamina.
- Insert one or two screws into the S1 vertebral body placed from the lateral surface of the iliac wing. If necessary, apply a 3.5-mm reconstruction plate across the posterior sacrum from ilium to ilium as a tension band (Fig. 4.78) just above the greater sciatic notch.
- Suture the gluteal fascia to the sacral spine.
- Close the wounds in the standard manner over suction drains.

▌PERCUTANEOUS ILIOSACRAL SCREW FIXATION OF SACROILIAC DISRUPTIONS AND SACRAL FRACTURES (SUPINE)

Routt et al. described this technique, reported its outcome and complications, and studied the anatomic and radiographic variations of upper sacral morphologic features that affect surgical technique. Their series of articles is essential reading for the trauma surgeon endeavoring to perform this technique. They emphasize the fact that the normal sacral ala has an inclined anterosuperior surface, the sacral alar slope, that extends from proximal-posterior to distal-anterior (Fig. 4.81). Anterior to the sacral ala in this region run the L5 nerve root and the iliac vessels. The cortex of the alar slope forms the superior aspect of the "safe zone" for passage of iliosacral screws into the body of S1. The anterior border is formed by the anterior aspect of the vertebral body, and the posterior and inferior boundary of the safe zone is formed by the foramen of the S1 nerve root.

The sacral alar slope can be estimated on a true lateral fluoroscopic view of the sacrum by identifying the iliac cortical density (ICD), which demarcates the anterior cortical thickening of the iliac portion of the sacroiliac joint (Fig. 4.82). The inclination of the alar slope can be more acute in patients with sacral dysplasia, narrowing the safe zone for screw passage. Routt et al. detected sacral dysplasia in 28 of 80 patients with pelvic fractures evaluated by inlet or outlet and true lateral images. In 94% of nondysplastic upper sacral segments, the ICD coincided with the alar slope as seen on the preoperative CT scan. This makes it a useful radiographic landmark for determining the anterior border of the safe zone (Fig. 4.83). However, 6% of nondysplastic sacral alae displayed an anterior concavity or recession when viewed in the axial plane, projecting the ICD anterior to the alar slope on the true lateral view. Preoperative CT was useful to determine the dimensions of the safe zone and to identify recessed sacral alae (Fig. 4.84). A recessed sacral ala allows for "in-out-in" screws that can injure the L5 nerve root (Fig. 4.85). A thorough evaluation of upper sacral morphologic features must be done to ensure that a safe corridor exists for placement of screws, especially when transiliac transsacral screws are planned for the S1 segment. A dysplastic sacrum can have an atypical sacral alar slope as well as a small corridor, thus placing neural structures at risk (Fig. 4.86).

Transsacral-transiliac fixation allows the use of longer screws with the added advantage of attaining the contralateral cortices of the sacrum and ilium for improved fixation. Transsacral-transiliac fixation should be considered for unstable sacral fractures where typically placed sacroiliac screws would not provide enough fixation in the distal segment and for unstable pure sacroiliac dislocations after a sacroiliac screw has been placed to aid in terminal reduction of the joint. The second screw can then be transsacral-transiliac to improve the overall fixation of the construct. Technical differences between sacroiliac and transsacral-transiliac screws are mainly in the trajectory needed and the corridors required to allow safe placement. Sacroiliac screws are often placed perpendicular to the sacroiliac joint, whereas transsacral-transiliac screws must traverse the entire sacrum without neural compromise and are thus placed in a trajectory parallel to the foramen and parallel to the anterior vertebral cortex (Fig. 4.87).

The surgeon must be familiar with the variations of upper sacral anatomy and fluoroscopic imaging, including the lateral sacral view, must be excellent. Graves and Routt recorded the sagittal plane tilt of the fluoroscope from the vertical required to obtain ideal inlet and outlet views during placement of iliosacral screws (Fig. 4.88). The average degree of tilt required to obtain the ideal inlet view was 25 degrees, and for the ideal outlet view it was 42 degrees.

Routt et al. emphasized that the posterior pelvis must be accurately reduced to allow superimposition of the greater sciatic notches and both ICDs on the true lateral image. With this as a necessary criterion for screw passage, using the ICD as the anterior marker for the safe zone and being aware of anterior sacral recession, no screw placement errors were noted in 51 consecutive patients. Starr and Reinert developed a reduction frame that allows directed forces to be applied to aid in reduction and may allow significant reduction through percutaneous techniques with the patient supine (Fig. 4.89).

PERCUTANEOUS ILIOSACRAL SCREW FIXATION OF SACROILIAC DISRUPTIONS AND SACRAL FRACTURES (SUPINE)

TECHNIQUE 4.10

- Preoperative assessment of the CT including supine measurements of inlet and outlet angulation as well as sacral anatomy is paramount to planning for percutaneous screw fixation of the posterior pelvis.
- Position the patient supine on a radiolucent table. Place a soft support underneath the lumbosacral spine to elevate the patient from the table.
- Place the C-arm fluoroscopy unit opposite the injured hemipelvis.
- Obtain anteroposterior, inlet, outlet, and lateral sacral views to ensure adequate visualization. The position of the inlet and outlet are noted to facilitate changing views throughout the case (Fig. 4.90A and B).
- Reduce the posterior pelvis first. Aids for reduction include traction, Schanz screws in the iliac wings, anterior external fixation frame, and prior anterior pelvic internal fixation.
- On the lateral sacral fluoroscopic view, identify the anterior and posterior aspects of the vertebral body of the first sacral segment. The exact starting point depends on the number of screws planned and the type of injury as well as the patient's pelvic anatomy. In patients with a sacral fracture or

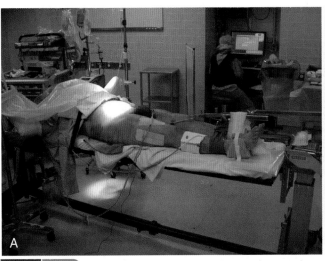
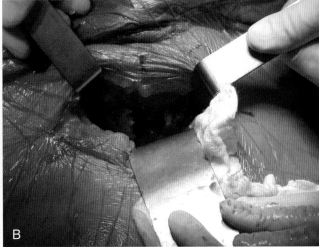

FIGURE 4.76 Anterior internal fixation of pelvic fracture (see text). **A,** Patient positioning. **B,** Retractor placed.

Continued

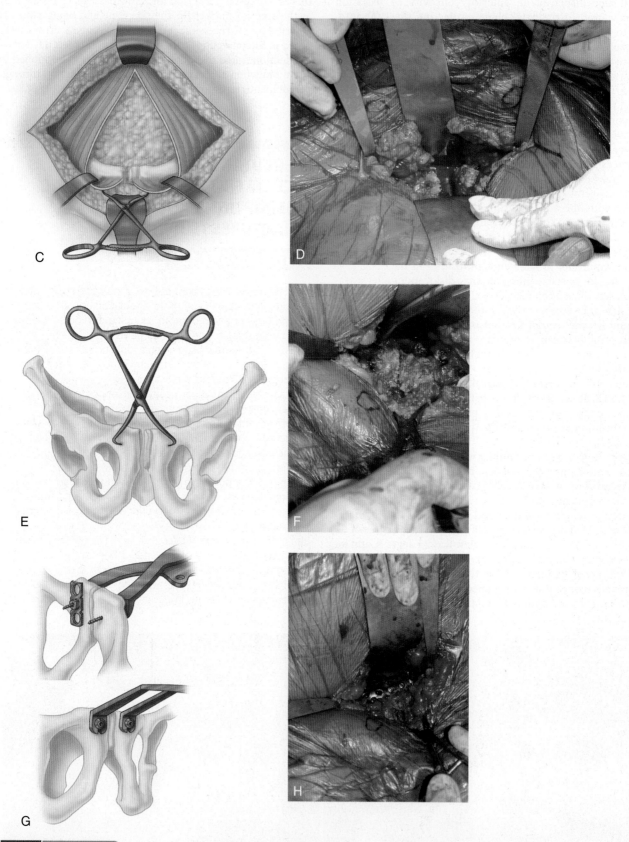

FIGURE 4.76, Cont'd C and D, Type II symphysis diastasis is reduced with Weber clamp placed anterior to rectus muscle. E and F, Points of clamp are placed at same level on pubic body so that with closure, any sagittal plane rotation of symphysis is reduced. G and H, Views from inside and outside pelvis show positioning of Jungbluth clamp with gliding hole and anchoring plate. **SEE TECHNIQUE 4.8.**

isolated anterior widening of the sacroiliac (SI) joint, a transverse screw is more optimal, whereas in patients with anterior and posterior injury to the SI joint, a posterior to anterior and inferior to superior directed screw is optimal.

- Mark the starting point on the skin and make a 1-cm stab incision.
- If used, advance a cannulated guide onto the lateral ilium. (Fig. 4.90C and D).
- On the lateral view, place the tip of the guide on the ideal starting spot and impact it into place with a mallet to prevent slipping (Fig. 4.90E).

- With use of biplanar imagery (inlet and outlet views), adjust the trajectory of the guide to safely enter the first sacral segment (Fig. 4.90F and G).
- Advance the guidewire, confirming safe passage on both the inlet and outlet views (Fig. 4.90H to K).
- Check the lateral sacral view to ensure that the pin is within the sacral body and inferior and posterior to the iliac cortical density (ICD). In a patient with a severely dysmorphic pelvis, the tip of the wire may be just superior to the ICD on this view. Assessment of wire position on the lateral sacral view as it crosses the sacral ala can help confirm safe passage in these patients.
- Measure the screw length.
- Advance the screw over the guidewire; check position on the inlet and outlet views (Fig. 4.90L and M).
- Confirm screw position on anteroposterior, inlet, and outlet views (Fig. 4.90N to P).

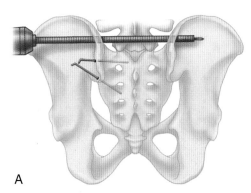

A

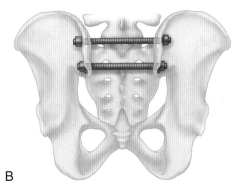

B

FIGURE 4.77 Transiliac rod fixation of sacral fractures. **A,** Large Steinmann pin (8 to 10 mm) is drilled from outer aspect of one ilium through opposite ilium. **B,** Second rod is inserted approximately 1.5 cm distal and parallel to first.

ANTERIOR APPROACH AND STABILIZATION OF THE SACROILIAC JOINT

Simpson et al. described an anterior fixation technique that initially used staples but now uses dynamic compression plates, reconstruction plates, and/or percutaneous sacroiliac screws. They emphasized the proximity of the L5 nerve root to the sacroiliac joint during the exposure. Subsequent cadaver studies have shown that the L4 nerve root and lumbosacral trunk are closer to the sacroiliac joint, particularly in its inferior third, and must be carefully protected.

Iliac wing fractures can be approached through a similar retroperitoneal approach. Reduction is performed with pointed reduction forceps, and fixation is obtained with a 3.5-mm reconstruction plate and lag screw fixation (see Fig. 4.52).

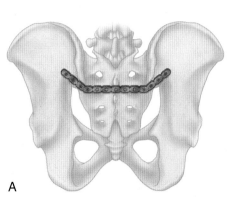

A

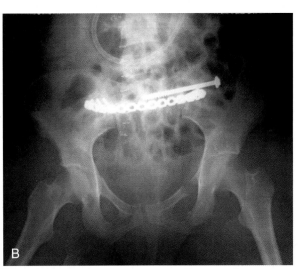

B

FIGURE 4.78 Tension band plating.

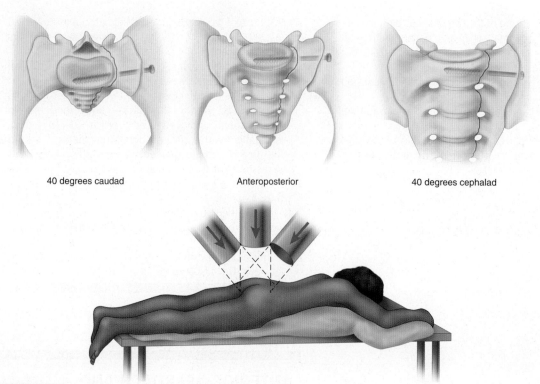

40 degrees caudad

Anteroposterior

40 degrees cephalad

FIGURE **4.79** Posterior screw fixation of sacral fractures and sacroiliac dislocations—patient positioning. Anteroposterior, caudal, and cephalad image intensifier projections show drill bit and screw position. (Redrawn from Matta JM, Saucedo T: Internal fixation of pelvic ring fractures, *Clin Orthop Relat Res* 242:83, 1989; original by Zilbert.) **SEE TECHNIQUE 4.9.**

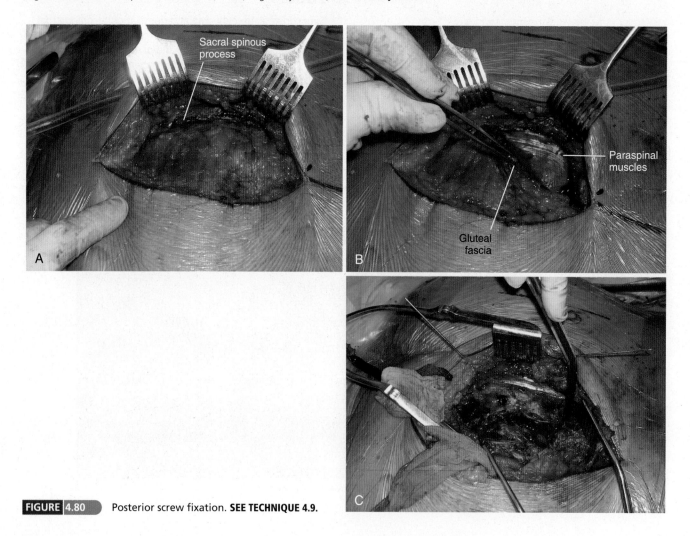

FIGURE **4.80** Posterior screw fixation. **SEE TECHNIQUE 4.9.**

TECHNIQUE 4.11

(SIMPSON ET AL.)

- Place the patient supine with an ipsilateral bump and make the lateral window of an ilioinguinal approach along the anterior iliac crest (Fig. 4.91A). Extend the incision anterior to just anterior to the anterior superior iliac spine. Take care not to release the inguinal ligament during the approach.
- Subperiosteally, dissect the iliacus muscle and medially retract it and the abdominal contents to expose the sacroiliac joint. Take care not to injure the L5 nerve root lying 2 cm to 3 cm medial to the joint.
- Anchor two sharp-tipped Hohmann retractors into the sacral ala to retract the abdominal contents medially. Use careful, intermittent retraction to avoid ilioinguinal or lumbosacral nerve root neuralgias.
- Once the sacroiliac joint has been exposed through retrofascial dissection, manipulate the hemipelvis with a Farabeuf clamp applied to the iliac crest while an assistant manipulates the leg. Distal traction on the leg and internal rotation of the hemipelvis usually are required for reduction. Placement of a Jungbluth clamp with one screw on the sacral ala and one screw on the ilium can assist with reduction, but care must be taken to prevent a block to permanent fixation devices
- Do not debride the cartilaginous surfaces of the joint.
- After reduction, fix the sacral ala to the ilium with two- or three-hole plate and associated screws (Fig. 4.91B). After reduction, further stabilization can also be obtained with sacroiliac screws.
- Close the soft tissues in a layered fashion with special attention to the abdominal musculature to prevent hernia formation.

POSTOPERATIVE CARE When the patient's comfort allows, ambulation is begun with crutches or a walker with touch-down weight bearing on the affected side. For patients with bilateral injuries, bed-to-chair transfers and wheelchair transportation may be warranted when the fractures are highly unstable. Patients generally are allowed to bear weight at 6 to12 weeks after the injury

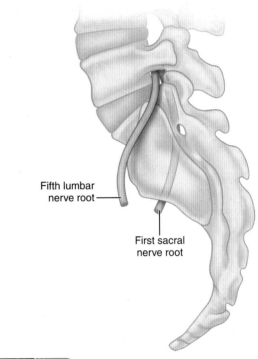

Fifth lumbar nerve root

First sacral nerve root

FIGURE 4.81 Alar slope and locations of fifth lumbar and intraosseous first sacral nerve roots and their relationships with ala.

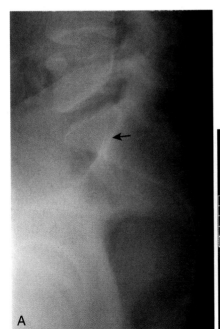

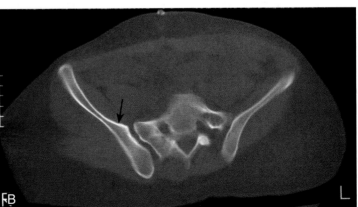

FIGURE 4.82 Iliac cortical density (ICD) can be identified on lateral radiograph **(A)** and CT scan **(B)** for estimation of sacral alar slope.

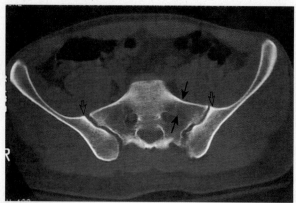

FIGURE 4.83 CT scan confirms narrow safe zone *(solid arrows)* resulting from dysplastic upper sacral segment. Anterior articular surfaces of sacroiliac articulations are noted to be planar bilaterally. Undulating "tongue-in-groove" portions are situated posteriorly. ICD is noted bilaterally *(open arrows)*. (From Chip M, Chip L Jr, Simonian PT, et al: Radiographic recognition of the sacral alar slope for optimal placement of iliosacral screws: a cadaveric and clinical study, *J Orthop Trauma* 10:171, 1996.)

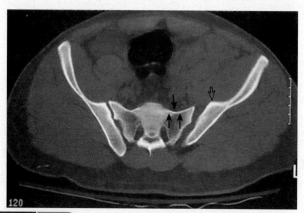

FIGURE 4.84 Recessed sacral ala *(solid arrows)* relative to dense iliac bone adjacent to sacroiliac joint—iliac cortical density (ICD) *(open arrow)*. CT scan best shows these uncommon situations. Nerve roots can be seen surrounded by fat within these recessed alae, especially on uninjured right side of patient. (From Routt MLC Jr, Simonian PT, Agnew SG, et al: Radiographic recognition of the sacral alar slope for optimal placement of iliosacral screws: a cadaver and clinical study, *J Orthop Trauma* 10:171, 1996.)

depending on the fracture pattern and bone quality. In a recent study by Marchand et al., no difference was found in implant failure rates in patients who undertook weight bearing at 6 weeks compared to those who were not allowed to bear weight until 12 weeks. This was a retrospective study, however, and likely incorporated some selection bias by the surgeons involved.

In a review of nearly 13,000 admissions to six major trauma centers in the U.S., 17% of preventable deaths were caused by pulmonary embolism. In patients with pelvic fractures who do not receive prophylaxis, up to 61% will develop DVT and 29% will develop proximal DVT. Chemoprophylaxis against DVT should be initiated immediately after fixation, unless otherwise contraindicated by the patient's history or other injuries. Little evidence exists on the optimal prophylaxis in this patient population. We prefer to keep nonoperatively treated patients on aspirin 81 mg twice daily for 6 weeks or until weight bearing, whichever is later. Operatively treated patients receive low molecular weight heparin (weight based for BMI >40) for 20 days, then transition to aspirin 81 mg twice daily until full weight bearing. Patients who are non–weight bearing bilaterally are kept on low-molecular weight heparin until weight bearing. The Major Extremity Trauma Research Consortium (METRC) is currently enrolling patients in a trial that may help provide greater guidance on the optimal prevention of DVT in these patients (https://clinicaltrials.gov/ct2/show/NCT02984384).

■ OUTCOMES

Historically, the management of pelvic ring injuries was focused on the early stage of care by identification and stabilization of unstable injury patterns that were associated with high mortality because of retroperitoneal hemorrhage and visceral injuries.

Following early resuscitation, skeletal traction was the definitive treatment option for survivors with unstable posterior ring injuries. Prognosis was mixed in this group of patients: 52% incidence of back pain, 38% incidence of pelvic tilt and sitting imbalance, and 32% incidence of limp because of leg-length discrepancy. The risk factors for developing disability because of chronic back pain, malunion, nonunion, and genitourinary and neurologic dysfunction were unclear but common. Several studies sought to define the risk factors for disability to direct care. Most observed that pain and disability were more common with residual posterior ring displacement of more than 10 mm. Although bony posterior ring injuries had an excellent prognosis if they healed in less than 10 mm of displacement, nonanatomic reduction of the sacroiliac joint was tolerated poorly. Most authors noted that, except for rare injury patterns, anterior ring disruption rarely resulted in residual pain and dysfunction

Little evidence exists for the outcomes of avulsion type injuries, but operative fixation generally is recommended in high-functioning patients with more than 1.5 to 2 cm of fracture displacement, with good results in case reports.

Type B fractures have outcomes as variable as their fracture morphology. In open book injuries, loss of reduction and implant failure is variable depending on implant construct. Genitourinary complications are commonly associated with B1 (APC) injuries. Isolated bladder injuries, when recognized early, generally heal without significant issue; however, injuries to the ureter result in a higher rate of complications. These patients also commonly suffer from impotence and dyspareunia well after the bony injury is healed. Tornetta et al. noted excellent results in one of the first series that reported outcomes after operative treatment of type B fractures. At a mean follow-up of 39 months (range, 12 to 84 months), 76% of patients had no limp and 75% had returned to their original jobs.

In a series by Kellam et al., after adequate reduction of type C fractures, only 50% of patients were pain free with no job or lifestyle changes. After inadequate reduction of type C injuries, only 33% of patients returned to their previous

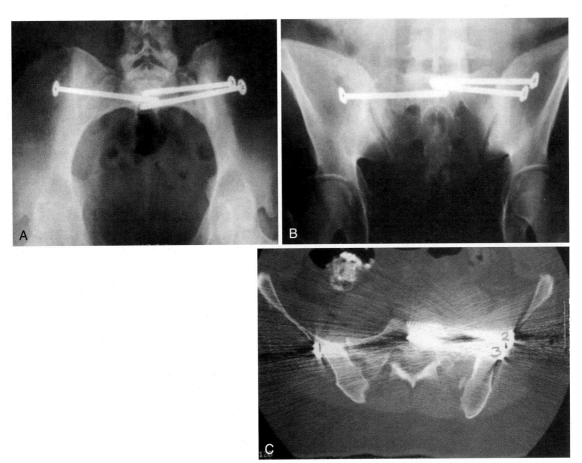

FIGURE 4.85 Screws inserted without use of lateral sacral image and ICD. Screws appear to be intraosseous on inlet (**A**) and outlet (**B**) pelvic radiographs, yet postoperative CT scan (**C**) shows that cephalad anterior no. 2 iliosacral screw on patient's left side is extraosseous. Left L5 nerve root was injured. (From Routt MLC Jr, Simonian PT, Agnew SG, et al: Radiographic recognition of the sacral alar slope for optimal placement of iliosacral screws: a cadaver and clinical study, *J Orthop Trauma* 10:171, 1996.)

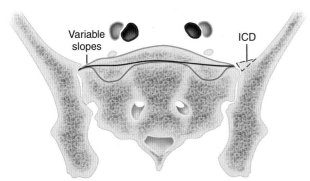

FIGURE 4.86 Variable structure of upper sacrum on outlet views. *ICD,* Iliac cortical density.

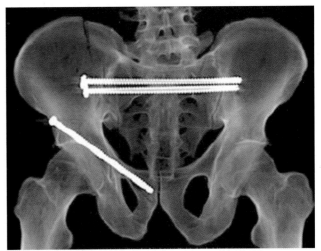

FIGURE 4.87 Y-shaped sacral fracture stabilized percutaneously with two transsacral-transiliac screws. (Courtesy of Dr. ML "Chip" Routt, Jr, University of Texas Health Science Center at Houston, Houston, Texas.)

occupations. For type C fractures that involve the sacroiliac joint, Kellam et al. recommended anatomic reduction of the posterior injury and internal fixation with fusion of the sacroiliac joint. Good results also have been reported with percutaneous iliosacral screw fixation in type C fractures; however, obtaining closed reduction of pure sacroiliac joint dislocations may be difficult and open reduction of the

sacroiliac joint may be necessary before percutaneous screw placement. In a group of patients with vertically unstable pelvic fractures treated with percutaneously placed iliac sacral

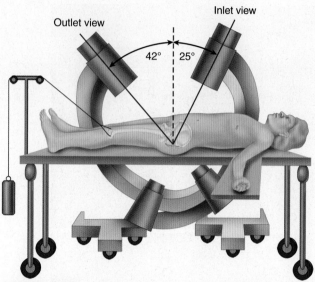

Outlet view Inlet view

42° 25°

FIGURE 4.88 Patient positioning and average angular tilts from perpendicular to achieve ideal inlet and outlet views. (Redrawn from Graves ML, Routt MLC Jr: Iliosacral screw placement: are uniplanar changes realistic based on standard fluoroscopic imaging? *J Trauma* 71:204, 2011.)

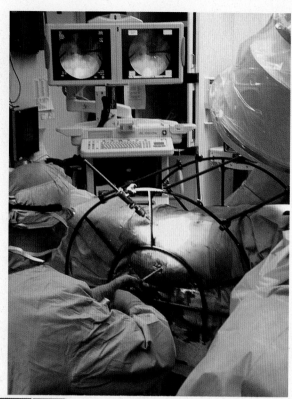

FIGURE 4.89 Starr and Reinert reduction device (see text).

screws, Griffin et al. showed a high rate of failure (13%) in vertical shear fractures through the sacrum. Mullis and Sagi noted poorer outcomes in those with pure sacroiliac dislocations that were mal-reduced than in those with anatomic reductions. Some authors, however, are skeptical that anatomic reduction of type C injuries has a considerable effect on patient outcome. A comparison of results in 80 patients with pelvic fractures, of which 61% were treated with external fixation and 39% were treated nonoperatively, found similar rates of return to previous occupation for Tile types A, B, and C injuries (75% to 81%). The number of patients who perceived pain as the worst sequela of their injury was similar among the three groups, regardless of treatment. Iliosacral screw posterior fixation of Tile type C fractures after open posterior reduction of sacral fractures, fracture-dislocations of the sacroiliac joint, and pure sacroiliac joint dislocations was reported to allow two thirds of patients to return to their preinjury occupations. Associated neurologic injuries compromised the result in 35% of patients. Reduction of the posterior injury to within 10 mm appears to be adequate for functional results, but residual displacement could lead to arthritic changes at longer follow-up.

Because of the high-energy nature and surrounding vital structures, pelvic fractures often are associated with some disability and chronic pain, especially in the more unstable patterns. Holstein et al. showed that older patients with more complex injuries and those who required surgery have a lower quality of life after their injury, highlighting the life-changing event that occurs when a patient suffers a pelvic ring injury.

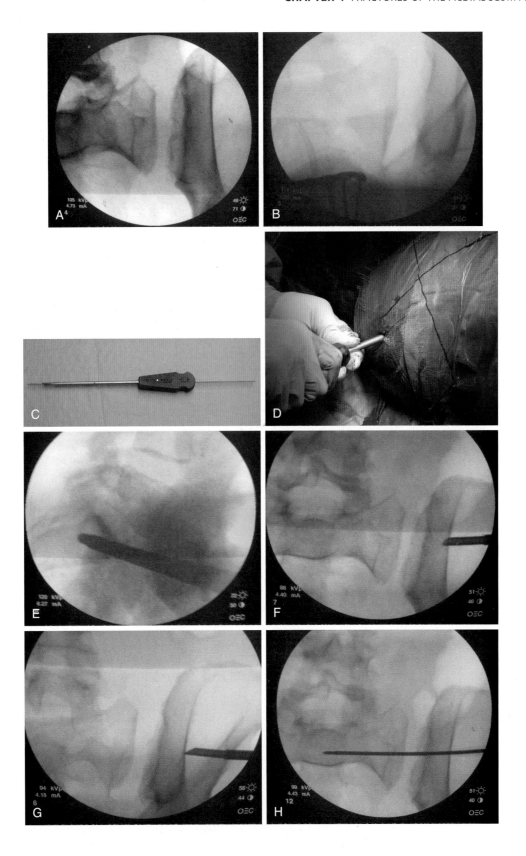

FIGURE 4.90 **A** to **P,** Iliosacral screw fixation. **SEE TEXT AND TECHNIQUE 1.10.**

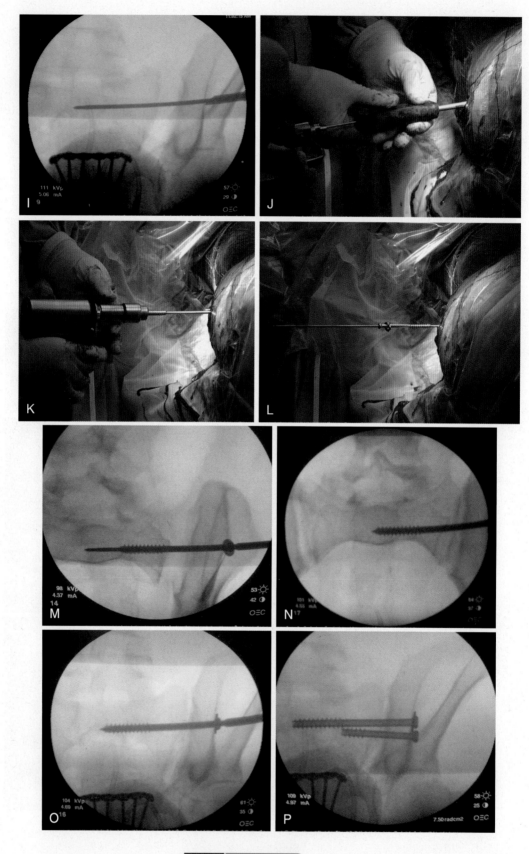

FIGURE 4.90, Cont'd

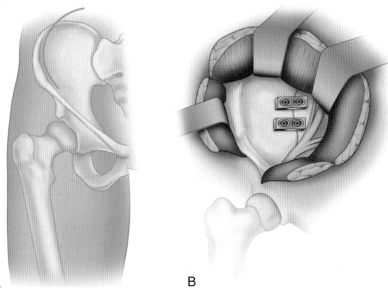

FIGURE 4.91 Anterior approach and stabilization of sacroiliac joint. **A,** Incision for anterior approach. **B,** After reduction, sacral ala is fixed to ilium with two 2-hole dynamic compression plates. **SEE TECHNIQUE 4.11.**

REFERENCES

ACETABULAR FRACTURES

Alfonso NA, Ryan W, Baldini T, et al.: Fixation of transverse acetabular fractures with precontoured plates alone causes fracture malreduction: a biomechanical assessment, *J Orthop Trauma* 34(2):89, 2020.

Archdeacon MT: Comparison of the ilioinguinal approach and the anterior intrapelvic approaches for open reduction and internal fixation of the acetabulum, *J Orthop Trauma* 29(Suppl 2):S6, 2015.

Archdeacon MT, d'Heurle A, Nemeth N, et al.: Is preoperative radiation therapy as effective as postoperative radiation therapy for heterotopic ossification prevention in acetabular fractures? *Clin Orthop Relat Res* 472:3389, 2014.

Archdeacon MT, Kazemi N, Guy P, Sagi HC: The modified Stoppa approach for acetabular fracture, *J Am Acad Orthop Surg* 19:170, 2011.

Awan OA, Sheth M, Sullivan I, et al.: Efficacy of 3D printed models on resident learning and understanding of common acetabular fractures, *Acta Radiol* 26:130, 2019.

Banaszek D, Starr AJ, Lefaivre KA: Technical considerations and fluoroscopy in percutaneous fixation of the pelvis and acetabulum, *J Am Acad Orthop Surg* 27:899, 2019.

Boissonneault AR, Schenker M, Staley C, et al.: Impact of closed suction drainage after surgical fixation of acetabular fractures, *Arch Orthop Trauma Surg* 139:907, 2019.

Burnet NG, Nasr P, Yip G, et al.: Prophylactic radiotherapy against heterotopic ossification following internal fixation of acetabular fractures: a comparative estimate of risk, *Br J Radiol* 87:20140398, 2014.

Carroll EA, Huber FG, Goldman AT, et al.: Treatment of acetabular fractures in an older population, *J Orthop Trauma* 24:637, 2010.

Chakravafrty R, Toossi N, Katsman A, et al.: Percutaneous column fixation and total hip arthroplasty for the treatment of acute acetabular fracture in the elderly, *J Arthroplasty* 29:817, 2014.

Cichos KHG, Mahmoud KH, Spitler CA, et al.: Risk factors for surgical site infection after operative fixation of acetabular fractures: is psoas density a useful metric?, *Clin Orthop Relat Res*, 2020 March 10, [Epub ahead of print].

Cichos KH, Spitler CA, Quade JH, et al.: Do indomethacin or radiation for heterotopic ossification prophylaxis increase the rates of infection or wound complications after acetabular fracture surgery, *J Orthop Trauma*, 2020 April 1, [Epub ahead of print].

Clarke-Jenssen J, Wikerøy AK, Røise O, et al.: Long-term survival of the native hip after a minimally displaced, nonoperatively treated acetabular fracture, *J Bone Joint Surg Am* 98:1392, 2016.

Collinge C, Archdeacon M, Sagi HC: Quality of radiographic reduction and perioperative complications for transverse acetabular fractures treated by the Kocher-Langenbeck approach: prone versus lateral position, *J Orthop Trauma* 25:538, 2011.

Crist BD, Oladeji LO, Khazzam M, et al.: Role of acute negative pressure wound therapy over primarily closed surgical incisions in acetabular fracture ORIF: a prospective randomized trial, *Injury* 48:1518, 2017.

Dailey SK, Archdeacon MT: Open reduction and internal fixation of acetabulum fractures: does timing of surgery affect blood loss and OR time? *J Orthop Trauma* 28:497, 2014.

Daurka JS, Pastides PS, Lewis A, et al.: Acetabular fractures in patients aged > 55 years: a systematic review of the literature, *Bone Joint Lett J* 96-B:157, 2014.

Ding A, O'Toole RV, Castillo R, et al.: Risk factors for early reoperation after operative treatment of acetabular fractures, *J Orthop Trauma* 32:e251, 2018.

Ferguson TA, Patel R, Bhandari M, Matta JM: Fractures of the acetabulum in patients aged 60 years and older: an epidemiological and radiological study, *J Bone Joint Surg* 92B:250, 2010.

Fernicola SD, Elsenbeck MJ, Grimm PD, et al.: Intrasite antibiotic powder for the prevention of surgical site infection in extremity surgery: a systematic review, *J Am Acad Orthop Surg* 28:37, 2020.

Firoozabadi R, Hamilton B, Toogood P, et al.: Risk factors for conversion to total hip arthroplasty after acetabular fractures involving the posterior wall, *J Orthop Trauma* 32:607, 2018.

Firoozabadi R, Stafford P, Routt M: Inguinal abnormalities in male patients with acetabular fractures treated using an ilioinguinal exposure, *Arch Bone Jt Surg* 3:274, 2015.

Furey AJ, Karp J, O'Toole RV: Does early fixation of posterior wall acetabular fractures lead to increased blood loss? *J Orthop Trauma* 27:2, 2013.

Gardner MJ, Chip Routt ML: The antishock iliosacral screw, *J Orthop Trauma* 24:e86–e89, 2010.

Gary JL, Kumaravel M, Gates K, et al.: Imaging comparison of pelvic ring disruption and injury reduction with use of the junctional emergency treatment tool for preinjury and postinjury pelvic dimensions: a cadaveric study with computed tomography, *J Spec Oper Med* 14:30–34, 2014.

Gary JL, Levaivre KA, Gerold F, et al.: Survivorship of the native hip joint after percutaneous repair of acetabular fractures in the elderly, *Injury* 42:1144, 2011.

Gary JL, VanHal M, Gibbons SD, et al.: Functional outcomes in elderly patients with acetabular fractures treated with miminally invasive reduction and percutaneous fixation, *J Orthop Trauma* 26:278, 2012.

Gras F, Marintschev I, Schwarz CE, et al.: Screw- versus plate-fixation strength of acetabular anterior column fractures: a biomechanical study, *J Trauma Acute Care Surg* 72:1664, 2012.

Griffin SM, Sims SH, Karunakar MA, et al.: Heterotopic ossification rates after acetabular fracture surgery are unchanged without indomethacin prophylaxis, *Clin Orthop Relat Res* 471:2776, 2013.

Grimshaw CS, Moed BR: Outcomes of posterior wall fractures of the acetabulum treated nonoperatively after diagnostic screening with dynamic stress examination under anesthesia, *J Bone Joint Surg* 92A:2792, 2010.

Halvorson JJ, Lamonthe J, Martin CR, et al.: Combined acetabulum and pelvic ring injuries, *J Am Acad Orthop Surg* 22:304, 2014.

Hsu JR, Bear RR, Dickson KF: Open reduction internal fixation of displaced sacral fractures: technique and results, *Orthopedics* 33:730, 2010.

Hsu JR, Stinner DJ, Rosenzweig SD, et al.: Is there a benefit to drains with a Kocher-Langenbeck approach? A prospective randomized pilot study, *J Trauma* 69:1222, 2010.

Isaacson MJ, Taylor BC, French BG, Poka A: Treatment of acetabulum fractures through the modified Stoppa approach: strategies and outcomes, *Clin Orthop Relat Res* 472:3345, 2014.

Jabelon T, Perry KJ, Kufera JA: Waist-hip ratio surrogate is more predictive than body mass index of wound complications after pelvic and acetabulum surgery, *J Orthop Trauma* 32:167, 2018.

Jaskolka DN, Di Primio GA, Sheikh AM, Schweitzer ME: CT of preoperative and postoperative acetabular fractures revisited, *J Comput Assist Tomogr* 38:344, 2014.

Jauregui JJ, Clayton A, Kapadia BH, et al.: Total hip arthroplasty for acute acetabular fractures: a review of the literature, *Expert Rev Med Devices* 12:287, 2015.

Jeffcoat DM, Carroll EA, Huber FG, et al.: Operative treatment of acetabular fractures in an older population through a limited ilioinguinal approach, *J Orthop Trauma* 26:284, 2012.

Johnsen NV, Vanni AJ, Voelzke BB: Risk of infectious complications in pelvic fracture urethral injury patients managed with internal fixation and suprapubic catheter placement, *J Trauma Acute Care Surg* 85:536, 2018.

Kazemi N, Archdeacon MT: Immediate full weight bearing after percutaneous fixation of anterior column acetabulum fractures, *J Orthop Trauma* 26:73, 2012.

Khan JM, Marquez-Lara A, Miller AN: Relationship of sacral fractures to nerve injury: is the Denis classification still accurate? *J Orthop Trauma* 31:181, 2017.

Kistler BJ, Smithson IR, Cooper SA, et al.: Are quadrilateral surface buttress plates comparable to traditional forms of transverse acetabular fracture fixation? *Clin Orthop Relat Res* 472:3353, 2014.

Lack WD, Crist BD, Seymour RB, et al.: Effect of tranexamic acid on transfusion: a randomized clinical trial in acetabular fracture surgery, *J Orthop Trauma* 31:526, 2017.

Laflamme GY, Herbert-Davies J, Rouleau D, et al.: Internal fixation of osteopenic acetabular fractures involving the quadrilateral plate, *Injury* 42:1130, 2011.

Lim PK, Stephenson GS, Keown TW, et al.: Use of 3D printed models in resident education for the classification of acetabulum fractures, *J Surg Educ* 75:1679, 2018.

Mani US, DeJesus DE, Ostrum RF: Arthroscopically-assisted removal of retained loose bodies in acute acetabular fractures: a modified technique, *Am J Orthop (Belle Mead NJ)* 42:186, 2013.

Manson TT: Open reduction and internal fixation plus total hip arthroplasty for the acute treatment of older patients with acetabular fracture: surgical techniques, *Orthop Clin North Am* 51:13, 2020.

Manson TT, Perdue PW, Pollack AN, O'Toole RV: Embolization of pelvic arterial injury is a risk factor for deep infection after acetabular fracture surgery, *J Orthop Trauma* 27:11, 2013.

Maracek GS, Routt Jr ML: Percutaneous manip0ulation of intra-articular debris after fracture-dislocation of the femoral head or acetabulum, *Orthopedics* 37:603, 2014.

Masse A, Aprato A, Rollero L, et al.: Surgical dislocation technique for the treatment of acetabular fractures, *Clin Orthop Relat Res* 471:4056, 2013.

Meinberg EG, Agel J, Roberts CS, et al.: Fracture and dislocation classification Compendium-2018, *J Orthop Trauma* 32(Suppl 1):S1, 2018.

Moed BR: The modified Gibson posterior surgical approach to the acetabulum, *J Orthop Trauma* 24:315, 2010.

Moed BR, Miller JR, Tabaie SA: Sequential duplex ultrasound screening for proximal deep venous thrombosis in asymptomatic patients with acetabular and pelvic fractures treated operatively, *J Trauma Acute Care Surg* 72:443, 2012.

Montgomery T, Pearson J, Agarwal A, et al.: Thrombin hemostatic matrix reduces heterotopic ossification in acetabular fractures fixed via the Kocher-Langenbeck approach, *J Orthop Trauma*, 2020 Apr 13, [Epub ahead of print].

Morison Z, Moojen DJF, Nauth A, et al.: Total hip arthroplasty after acetabular fracture is associated with lower survivorship and more complications, *Clin Orthop Relat Res* 474:392, 2016.

Mourad WF, Packianathan S, Shourbaji RA, et al.: A prolonged time interval between trauma and prophylactic radiation therapy significantly increases the risk of heterotopic ossification, *Int J Radiat Oncol Biol Phys* 82:e339, 2012.

Naranje S, Shamshery P, Yadav CS, et al.: Digastric trochanteric flip osteotomy and surgical dislocation of hip in the management of acetabular fractures, *Arch Orthop Trauma Surg* 130:93, 2010.

O'Toole RV, Cox G, Shanmuganathan K, et al.: Evaluation of computed tomography for determining the diagnosis of acetabular fractures, *J Orthop Trauma* 24:284, 2010.

O'Toole RV, Hui E, Chandra A, et al.: How often does open reduction and internal fixation of geriatric acetabular fractures lead to hip arthroplasty? *J Orthop Trauma* 28:148, 2014.

Owen MT, Keener EM, Hyde ZB, et al.: Intraoperative topical antibiotics for infection prophylaxis in pelvic and acetabular surgery, *J Orthop Trauma* 31(11):589, 2017.

Parry JA, Nino S, Khosravani N, et al.: Early operative treatment of acetabular fractures does not increase blood loss: a retrospective review, *J Orthop Trauma* 34:244, 2020.

Porter SE, Graves ML, Maples RA, et al.: Acetabular fracture reductions in the obese patients, *J Orthop Trauma* 25:371, 2011.

Reagan JM, Moed BR: Can computed tomography predict hip stability in posterior wall acetabular fractures? *Clin Orthop Relat Res* 469:2035, 2011.

Reddix Jr RN, Leng XI, Woodall J, et al.: The effect of incisional negative pressure therapy on wound complications after acetabular fracture surgery, *J Surg Orthop Adv* 19:91, 2010.

Ryan W, Alfonso NA, Baldini T, et al.: Precontoured quadrilateral surface acetabular plate fixation demonstrates increased stability when compared with pelvic reconstruction plates: a biomechanical study, *Orthop Trauma* 33(9):e325, 2019.

Ryan SP, Manson TT, Sciadini MF, et al.: Functional outcomes of elderly patients with nonoperatively treated acetabular fractures that meet operative criteria, *J Orthop Trauma* 31:644, 2017.

Sagi HC, Afsari A, Dziadosz D: The anterior intra-pelvic (modified rives-stoppa) approach for fixation of acetabular fractures, *J Orthop Trauma* 24:263, 2010.

Sagi HC, Bolhofner B: Osteotomy of the anterior superior iliac spine as an adjunct to improve access and visualization through the lateral window, *J Orthop Trauma* 29:e266, 2015.

Sagi HC, Dziadosz D, Mir H, et al.: Obesity, leukocytosis, immobilization, and injury severity increase the risk for deep postoperative wound infection after pelvic and acetabular surgery, *J Orthop Trauma* 27:6, 2013.

Sagi HC, Jordan CJ, Barei DP, et al.: Indomethacin prophylaxis for heterotopic ossification after acetabular fracture surgery increases the risk for nonunion of the posterior wall, *J Orthop Trauma* 28:377, 2014.

Schwab JM, Zebrack J, Schmeling GJ, Johnson J: The use of cervical vertebrae plates for cortical substitution in posterior wall acetabular fractures, *J Orthop Trauma* 25:577, 2011.

Siebenrock KA, Keel MJB, Tannast M, et al.: Surgical hip dislocation for exposure of the posterior column, *JBJS Essent Surg Tech* 9:e2, 2019.

Solomon LB, Studer P, Abrahams JM, et al.: Does cup-cage reconstruction with oversized cups provide initial stability in THA for osteoporotic acetabular fractures? *Clin Orthop Relat Res* 473:3811, 2015.

Suzuki T, Morgan SJ, Smith WR, et al.: Postoperative surgical site infection following acetabular fracture fixation, *Injury* 41:396, 2010.

Tannast M, Krüger A, Mack PW, et al.: Surgical dislocation of the hip for the fixation of acetabular fractures, *J Bone Joint Surg* 92B:842, 2010.

Tannast M, Najibi S, Matta JM: Two to twenty-year survivorship of the hip in 810 patients with operatively treated acetabular fractures, *J Bone Joint Surg* 94A:1559, 2012.

Tile M, Helfet DL, Kellam JF, et al.: *Fractures of the pelvis and acetabulum (AO): Principles and methods of management*, ed 4, Thieme, 2015.

Torbert JT, Joshi M, Moraff A, et al.: Current bacterial speciation and antibiotic resistance in deep infections after operative fixation of fractures, *J Orthop Trauma* 29:7, 2015.

Vallier HA, Cureton BA, Ekstein C, et al.: Early definitive stabilization of unstable pelvis and acetabulum fractures reduces morbidity, *J Trauma* 69:677, 2010.

Vaidya R, Waldron J, Scott A, et al.: Angiography and embolization in the management of bleeding pelvic fractures, *J Am Acad Orthop Surg* 26:e68, 2018.

Verbeek DO, van der List JP, Tissue CM, et al.: Predictors for long-term hip survivorship following acetabular fracture surgery: importance of gap compared with step displacement, *J Bone Joint Surg Am* 100:922, 2018.

von Roth P, Abdel MP, Harmsen WS, et al.: Total hip arthroplasty after operatively treated acetabular fracture: a concise follow-up, at a mean of twenty years, of a previous report, *J Bone Joint Surg Am* 97:288, 2015.

Yi C, Hak DJ: Traumatic spinopelvic dissociation or U-shaped sacral fracture: a review of the literature, *Injury* 43:402, 2010.

Yuan BJ, Lewallen DG, Hanssen AD: Porous metal acetabular components have a low rate of mechanical failure in THA after operatively treated acetabular fracture, *Clin Orthop Relat Res* 473:536, 2015.

Ziran BH, Little JE, Kinney RC: The use of a T-plate as "spring plates" for small comminuted posterior wall fragments, *J Orthop Trauma* 25:574, 2011.

PELVIC FRACTURES

Ali AM, Lewis A, Sarraf KM: Surgical treatment of an ischial tuberosity avulsion fracture with delayed presentation, *J Clin Orthop Trauma* 11:S4, 2020.

Avilucea FR, Archdeacon MT, Collinge CA, et al.: Fixation strategy using sequential intraoperative examination under anesthesia for unstable lateral compression pelvic ring injuries reliably predicts union with minimal displacement, *J Bone Joint Surg Am* 100:1503, 2018.

Beckmann JT, Presson AP, Curtis SH, et al.: Operative agreement on lateral compression-1 pelvis fractures. A survey of 111 OTA members, *J Orthop Trauma* 28:681, 2014.

Beckmann J, Haller JM, Beebe M, et al.: Validated radiographic scoring system for lateral compression type 1 pelvis fractures, *Orthop Trauma* 34:70, 2020.

Bonner TJ, Eardley WGP, Newell N, et al.: Accurate placement of a pelvic binder improves reduction of unstable fractures of the pelvic ring, *J Bone Joint Surg* 93B:1524, 2011.

Bruce B, Reilly M, Sims S: Predicting future displacement of nonoperatively managed lateral compression sacral fractures: can it be done? *J Orthop Trauma* 25:523, 2011.

Cole PA, Dyskin EA, Gilbertson JA: Minimally-invasive fixation for anterior pelvic ring disruptions, *Injury* 53:527, 2015.

Eagan M, Kim H, Manson TT, et al.: Internal anterior fixators for pelvic ring injuries: do monaxial pedicle screws provide more stiffness than polyaxial pedicle screws? *Injury* 46:996, 2015.

Fowler TT, Bishop JA, Bellino MJ: The posterior approach to pelvic ring injuries: a technique for minimizing soft tissue complications, *Injury* 44:1780, 2013.

Gardner MJ, Rout Jr ML: Transiliac-transsacral screws for posterior pelvic stabilization, *J Orthop Trauma* 25:378, 2011.

Gaski IA, Barckman J, Naess PA, et al.: Reduced need for extraperitoneal pelvic packing for severe pelvic fractures is associated with improved resuscitation strategies, *J Trauma Acute Care Surg*, 2016, [Epub ahead of print].

Graves ML, Routt Jr MLC: Iliosacral screw placement: are uniplanar changes realistic based on standard fluoroscopic imaging? *J Trauma* 71:204, 2011.

Grewal IS, Starr AJ: What's new in percutaneous pelvis fracture surgery?, *Orthop Clin North Am*, 2020 (in press).

Grimshaw CS, Bledsoe JG, Moed BR: Locked versus standard unlocked plating of the pubic symphysis: a cadaver biomechanical study, *J Orthop Trauma* 26:402, 2012.

Hagen J, Castillo R, Dubina A, et al.: Does surgical stabilization of lateral compression-type pelvic ring fractures decrease patients' pain, reduce narcotic use, and improve mobilization, *Clin Orthop Relat Res* 474:1422, 2016.

Hesse D, Kandmir U, Solberg B, et al.: Femoral nerve palsy after pelvic fracture treated with INFIX: a case series, *J Orthop Trauma* 29:138, 2015.

Heydemann I, Hartline B, Gibson B, et al.: Do transsacral-transiliac screws across uninjured sacroiliac joints affect pain and functional outcomes in trauma patients? *Clin Orthop Relat Res* 474:1417, 2016.

Holstein JH, Pizanis A, Köhler D, et al.: What are predictors for patients' quality of life after pelvic ring fractures? *Clin Orthop Relat Res* 471:2841, 2013.

Khan JM, Marquez-Lara A, Miller AN: Relationship of sacral fractures to nerve injury: is the Denis classification still accurate? *J Orthop Trauma* 31:181, 2017.

Lafaivre KA, Slobogean GP, Ngai JT, et al.: What outcomes are important for patients after pelvic trauma? Subjective responses and psychometric analysis of three published pelvic-specific outcomes instruments, *J Orthop Trauma* 28:23, 2014.

Lindsay A, Tornetta P, Diwan A, et al.: Is closed reduction and percutaneous fixation of unstable posterior ring injuries as accurate as open reduction and internal fixation? *J Orthop Trauma* 30:29, 2016.

Lustenberger T, Wutzler S, Störmann P, et al.: The role of angio-embolization in the acute treatment concept of severe pelvic ring injuries, *Injury* 46(Suppl 4):S33, 2015.

Manson T, O'Toole RV, Whitney A, et al.: Young-Burgess classification of pelvic ring fractures: does it predict mortality, transfusion requirements, and non-orthopaedic injuries? *J Orthop Trauma* 24:603, 2010.

Marchand LS, Working ZM, Rane AA, et al.: Unstable pelvic ring injuries: how soon can patients safely bear weight? *J Orthop Trauma* 33:71, 2019.

Matityahu A, Marmor M, Elson JK, et al.: Acute complications of patients with pelvic fractures after pelvic angiographic embolization, *Clin Orthop Relat Res* 471:2906, 2013.

Mauffrey C, Cuellar 3rd DO, Pieracci F, et al.: Strategies for the management of haemorrhage following pelvic fractures and associated trauma-induced coagulopathy, *Bone Joint Lett J* 96B:1143, 2014.

Meinberg E, Agel J, Roberts C, et al.: Fracture and dislocation classification Compendium–2018, *J Orthop Trauma* 32:(1); Supplement, 2018.

Merriman DJ, Ricci WM, McAndrew CM, Gardner MJ: Is application of an internal anterior pelvic fixator anatomically feasible? *Clin Orthop Relat Res* 470:2111, 2012.

Miller AN, Routt Jr ML: Variations in sacral morphology and implications for iliosacral screw fixation, *J Am Acad Orthop Surg* 20:8, 2012.

Nahm NJ, Como JJ, Wilber JH, et al.: Early appropriate care: definitive stabilization of femoral fractures within 24 hours of injury is safe in most patients with multiple injuries, *J Trauma* 71:175, 2011.

Prasarn ML, Small J, Conrad B, et al.: Does application position of the T-POD affect stability of pelvic fractures? *J Orthop Trauma* 27:262, 2013.

Sagi HC, Coniglione FM, Stanford JH: Examination under anesthetic for occult pelvic ring instability, *J Orthop Trauma* 25:529, 2011.

Scheyerer MJ, Osterhoff G, Wehrle S, et al.: Detection of posterior pelvic injuries in fractures of the pubic rami, *Injury* 43:1326, 2012.

Schiller J, DeFroda S, Blood T: Lower extremity avulsion fractures in the pediatric and adolescent athlete, *J Am Acad Orthop Surg* 25:251, 2017.

Schulman JE, O'Toole RV, Castillo RC, et al.: Pelvic ring fractures are an independent risk factor for death after blunt trauma, *J Trauma* 68:930, 2010.

Schwartz DA, Medina M, Cotton BA, et al.: Are we delivering two standards of care for pelvic trauma? Availability of angioembolization after hours and on weekends increases time to therapeutic intervention, *J Trauma Acute Care Surg* 76:134, 2014.

Sembler Soles GL, Lien J, Tornetta 3rd P: Nonoperative immediate weight bearing of minimally displaced lateral compression sacral fractures does not result in displacement, *J Orthop Trauma* 26:563, 2012.

Service CA, Moses RA, Majercik SD, et al.: Urethral trauma following pelvic fracture from horseback saddle horn injury versus other mechanisms of pelvic trauma, *Urology* 124:260, 2019.

Stover MD, Sims S, Matta J: What is the infection rate of the posterior approach to type C pelvic injuries? *Clin Orthop Relat Res* 470:2142, 2012.

Suzuki T, Morgan SJ, Smith WR, et al.: Stress radiograph to detect true extent of symphyseal disruption in presumed anteroposterior compression type I pelvic injuries, *J Trauma* 69:880, 2010.

Tile M, Helfet DL, Kellam JF, et al.: *Fractures of the pelvis and acetabulum. Principles and methods of management,* ed 4, Stuttgart, 2015, Georg Thieme Verlag, p 978.

Tonne BM, Kempton LB, Lack WD, Karunakar MA: Posterior iliac offset. Description of a new radiological measurement of sacroiliac joint instability, *Bone Joint Lett J* 96B:1535, 2014.

Vaidya R, Colen R, Vigdorchik J, et al.: Treatment of unstable pelvic ring injuries with an internal anterior fixator and posterior fixation: initial clinical series, *J Orthop Trauma* 26:1, 2012.

Vaidya R, Kubiak EN, Bergin PF, et al.: Complications of anterior subcutaneous internal fixation for unstable pelvic fractures: a multicenter study, *Clin Orthop Relat Res* 470:2124, 2012.

Vallier HA, Cureton BA, Ekstein C, et al.: Early definitive stabilization of unstable pelvis and acetabulum fractures reduces morbidity, *J Trauma* 69:677, 2010.

Vallier HA, Cureton BA, Schubeck D: Pregnancy outcomes in women after pelvic ring injury, *J Orthop Trauma* 26:302, 2012.

Vallier HA, Cureton BA, Schubeck D, Wang XF: Functional outcomes in women after high-energy pelvic ring injury, *J Orthop Trauma* 26:296, 2012.

Vallier HA, Moore TA, Como JJ, et al.: Complications are reduced with a protocol to standardize timing of fixation based on response to resuscitation, *J Orthop Surg Res* 10:155, 2015.

Vallier HA, Wang X, Moore TA, et al.: Timing of orthopaedic surgery in multiple trauma patients: development of a protocol for early appropriate care, *J Orthop Trauma* 27:543, 2013.

Wang H, Coppola PT, Coppola M: Orthopedic emergencies: a practical emergency department classification (US-VAGON) in pelvic fractures, *Emerg Med Clin North Am* 33:451, 2015.

Weatherby DJ, Routt ML, Eastman JG: The retrograde-antegrade-retrograde technique for successful placement of a retrograde superior ramus screw, *J Orthop Trauma* 31:e224, 2017.

Yi C, Hak DJ: Traumatic spinopelvic dissociation or U-shaped sacral fracture: a review of the literature, *Injury* 43:402, 2012.

The complete list of references is available online at ExpertConsult.com.

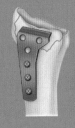

CHAPTER 5

FRACTURES OF THE SHOULDER, ARM, AND FOREARM

Edward A. Perez

CLAVICLE 275
Treatment options 276
  Plate and screw fixation 276
  Intramedullary fixation 279
Lateral clavicular fractures 282

FRACTURES AROUND THE SHOULDER 284
Fractures of the scapula 284
  Treatment options 284
  Glenoid fractures 285
  Scapular body or neck fractures 286
Proximal humeral fractures 286
  Classification 287
  Radiographic evaluation 287
  Nonoperative treatment 287
  Operative treatment 288
  Complications 301

FRACTURES OF THE HUMERAL SHAFT 302
Indications for operative treatment 303
Plate osteosynthesis 303
  Implant choice 304
  Approach 305
  Postoperative care 305

Complications 305
Intramedullary fixation 309

FRACTURES OF THE HUMERAL SHAFT WITH RADIAL NERVE PALSY 311
Periprosthetic humeral shaft fractures 314
Distal humeral fractures 315

FRACTURES, DISLOCATIONS, AND FRACTURE-DISLOCATIONS OF THE ELBOW 321
Fractures of the radial head 321
  Operative treatment 322
Fractures of the coronoid 326
Simple elbow dislocations 327
Fracture-dislocations of the elbow 327
  Treatment 328
"Terrible triad" injuries of the elbow 328
  Treatment 328
  Complications 334
Radial head and neck fractures associated with elbow dislocation 334
Fractures and fracture-dislocations of the olecranon 334

Fractures 334
Fracture-dislocations 336
Fractures of the radial head or neck with dislocation of the distal radioulnar joint (Essex-Lopresti fracture-dislocation) 338
Fractures of the proximal third of the ulna with dislocation of the radial head (Monteggia fracture-dislocation) 338

FRACTURES OF THE SHAFTS OF THE RADIUS AND ULNA 341
Fractures of the distal third of the radius with dislocation of the distal radioulnar joint (Galeazzi fracture-dislocation) 342

FRACTURES OF THE DISTAL RADIUS 343
Classification 344
Assessment of stability 345
Treatment options 346
  Closed treatment 346
  Open reduction and plate fixation 352
Complications 355

Trauma to the upper extremity often presents a difficult challenge for orthopaedic surgeons; whether the problem encountered is a fracture, fracture with dislocation, or severe injury to the soft tissues or neurovascular elements. The ultimate functional results after injuries in the upper extremity often depend as much on the status of the surrounding soft tissues as on the status of the bone. A fracture to the lower extremity may heal with contracture, some loss of motion of the adjacent joints, and other soft-tissue compromise, yet still yield a good functional result, whereas in the upper extremity severe functional impairment often results if fracture healing is accompanied by these sequelae, even though the bone itself has healed satisfactorily. This chapter discusses the surgical management of fractures and fracture-dislocations in the upper extremity and shoulder girdle. Surgeons also must remain continually attentive to soft-tissue injuries.

CLAVICLE

The clavicle is one of the most frequently fractured bones in the body, the fracture most often resulting from a direct blow or a fall on an outstretched arm. Most clavicular fractures heal uneventfully without serious consequences with nonoperative treatment. Historically, the resulting bony prominences have been believed to be preferable to an unsightly scar from open reduction and internal fixation (ORIF). Treatment guidelines were based on Neer and Rowe's two large series that showed nonunion rates of less than 1% in conservatively managed fractures compared with nearly 4% in operatively treated fractures. These results established the concept that union rates and function were excellent with conservative treatment of clavicular fractures and were better than those after operative treatment. More recent studies have questioned union rates, functional recovery, and the morbidity of malunions after conservative treatment. A prospective observational study of 868 patients with clavicular fractures treated nonoperatively found a nonunion rate of 6.2%. Risk factors identified were advanced age, female sex, 100% displacement (lack of cortical contact), and presence of comminution. A meta-analysis including 2144 fractures showed a nonunion rate of 15% for displaced clavicular fractures treated nonoperatively, whereas the nonunion rate for ORIF was only 2% (Table 5.1). Thus, there appears to be a subgroup of patients—those with displaced fractures—who do not do as well as previously thought. Fuglesang et al. reported a 15% nonunion rate with worsening outcome scores in patients with displacement greater than 100%.

These concerns led the Canadian Orthopaedic Trauma Society (COTS) to initiate a multicenter prospective randomized trial to compare nonoperative treatment and plate fixation of displaced clavicular fractures. They concluded that operative treatment resulted in improved functional outcomes and lower rates of malunion and nonunion. Complications occurred in 23 (37%) of 62 patients treated operatively, compared with 31 (63%) of 49 treated nonoperatively (Table 5.2). Since the COTS study, many comparative studies and meta-analyses have been performed comparing operative treatment with nonoperative treatment of midshaft clavicular fractures. Table 5.3 summarizes some of these studies. Woltz et al. confirmed that displacement greater than 100% was associated with a higher nonunion rate, although outcome measures did not differ between treatment types. The authors also published a meta-analysis with similar conclusions. In a separate meta-analysis, Ahmed et al. also confirmed a reduction in nonunion rate with operative fixation of displaced fractures. They noted an improvement in outcome measures; however, as opposed to the study by Woltz et al. and Murray et al. studied the risk of nonunions after nonoperative treatment of displaced clavicular fractures. Smoking, comminution, and fracture displacement were the strongest predictors of nonunion (Table 5.4). This table is used by the author as a guideline when advising patients as to a specific treatment choice.

TREATMENT OPTIONS

Most clavicular fractures still are treated closed. Treatment, however, should not be an "all or nothing" approach; it should be aimed at providing optimal outcomes for individual patients and injuries. Recent reports in the literature have helped to more accurately predict complications after displaced fractures and to allow a frank discussion with the patient to choose the appropriate form of treatment.

Nonoperative treatment consists of the use of a sling for comfort. We rarely use figure-of-eight splinting because of patient discomfort and the lack of proven benefit. Operative management usually consists of ORIF with plates and screws or intramedullary nail fixation. External fixation has been described but rarely is necessary except in unique situations. The relative indications for operative treatment are shown in Box 5.1.

■ PLATE AND SCREW FIXATION

Plating techniques continue to evolve. Newer precontoured plates allow more accurate fitting while maintaining strength; however, complications have been reported with 3.5-mm reconstruction plates, which allow easy contouring but may be too weak to maintain reduction. Currently, the most commonly used technique is superior placement of the plate (Fig. 5.1) or anteroinferior plate placement

---

TABLE 5.1

Results of Nonoperative and Operative Treatment of Acute Midshaft Clavicular Fractures

TREATMENT	% OF NONUNIONS
DISPLACED AND NONDISPLACED FRACTURES	
Nonoperative (1145 fractures)	5.9
Plating (635 fractures)	2.5
Intramedullary pinning (364 fractures)	1.6
All fractures (2144)	4.2
DISPLACED FRACTURES	
Nonoperative (159 fractures)	15
Plating (460 fractures)	2.2
Intramedullary pinning (152 fractures)	2.0
All displaced fractures (771)	4.8

Data from Zlowodzki M, Zelle BA, Cole PA, et al: Treatment of acute midshaft clavicle fractures: systematic review of 2144 fractures. On behalf of the Evidence-Based Orthopaedic Trauma Working Group, *J Orthop Trauma* 19:504, 2005.

TABLE 5.2

Complications and Outcomes After Operative and Nonoperative Treatment of Clavicular Fractures

	OPERATIVE TREATMENT (*N* = 62)	NONOPERATIVE TREATMENT (*N* = 49)
COMPLICATION/ADVERSE EVENT		
Nonunion	2	7
Malunion requiring further treatment	0	9
Wound infection/dehiscence	3	0
Implant irritation requiring removal	5	0
Complex regional pain syndrome	0	1
Surgery for impending open fracture	0	2
Transient brachial plexus symptoms	8	7
Abnormality of AC or SC joint	2	3
Early mechanical failure	1	0
Other	2	2
TOTAL	23 (37%)	31 (63%)
APPEARANCE OF SHOULDER		
"Droopy" shoulder	0	10
Bump and/or asymmetry	0	22
Scar	3	0
Sensitive and/or painful fracture site	9	10
Implant irritation and/or prominence	11	0
Incisional numbness	18	0
Satisfaction with appearance	52 (84%)	26 (53%)
Functional results		

Constant and Disabilities of the Arm, Shoulder and Hand scores approximately 10 points better in operative group at all time points (6, 12, 24, and 52 weeks). *AC*, Acromioclavicular; *SC*, sternoclavicular.
Data from Canadian Orthopaedic Trauma Society: Nonoperative treatment compared with plate fixation of displaced midshaft clavicular fractures: a multicenter, randomized clinical trial, *J Bone Joint Surg* 89A:1, 2007.

because of the safe screw trajectory and less implant irritation (Fig. 5.2). The recent trend of using smaller implants applies also to the clavicle. Evidence exists supporting the use of 2.7-mm compression type plating. The author reserves this technique when 2.7-mm plates are used in a neutralization technique with anatomic reduction and lag screw fixation. A report by Czajka et al. demonstrated a high rate of union with a low rate of soft-tissue irritation with the use of double mini-fragment plate fixation. This technique has become the most frequently used technique by the author (Fig. 5.3). Regardless of the plate placement technique used, meticulous attention is mandatory to preserve the periosteum and avoid injury to the subclavian vessels and lungs; lag screw fixation should be used when possible.

TABLE 5.3

Numbers and Reasons for Secondary Operations

STUDY	PLATE FIXATION	NONOPERATIVE TREATMENT
COTS, 2007	2 nonunion 1 implant failure 3 infection 5 plate removal	7 nonunion 9 malunion
Melean, 2015	4 plate removal	4 nonunion
Mirzatolooei, 2011	1 implant failure 1 infection	
Robinson, 2013	1 nonunion 1 implant failure 1 refracture 1 neurologic complication 2 fracture lateral to plate 10 plate removal	13 nonunion 4 malunion
Virtanen, 2012		1 neurologic complication
Woltz, 2017	1 nonunion 6 implant failure 2 infection 14 plate removal	9 nonunion 1 neurologic complication 1 malunion 1 plate removal*
Total	56	50

*One nonoperatively treated patient developed a nonunion and was treated with secondary plate fixation after 4 months. At 1 year, plate removal was scheduled. This patient was analyzed in the nonoperative group following the intention-to-treat principle.
From Woltz S, Krijnen P, Schipper IB: Plate fixation versus nonoperative treatment for displaced midshaft clavicular fractures, *J Bone Joint Surg Am* 99:1051, 2017.

BOX 5.1

Relative Indications for Primary Fixation of Midshaft Clavicular Fractures

Fracture-Specific
- Displacement >2 cm
- Shortening >2 cm
- Increasing comminution (>3 fragments)
- Segmental fractures
- Open fractures
- Impending open fractures with soft-tissue compromise
- Obvious clinical deformity (usually associated with displacement and shortening)
- Scapular malposition and winging at initial examination

Associated Injuries
- Vascular injury requiring repair
- Progressive neurologic deficit
- Ipsilateral upper extremity injuries/fractures
- Multiple ipsilateral upper rib fractures
- "Floating shoulder"
- Bilateral clavicular fractures

Patient Factors
- Polytrauma with requirement for early upper extremity weight bearing/arm use
- Patient motivation for rapid return of function (e.g., elite sports or self-employed professional)

From McKee MD: Clavicle fractures. In Bucholz RW, Heckman JD, Court-Brown CM, Tornetta P 3rd, editors: *Rockwood and Green's fractures in adults*, 7th ed, Philadelphia, 2010, Lippincott Williams & Wilkins.

TABLE 5.4

"Ready Reckoner" for Estimating the Risk of Nonunion

OVERALL DISPLACEMENT (MM)	NONCOMMINUTED FRACTURE IN NONSMOKER	COMMINUTED FRACTURE IN NONSMOKER	NONCOMMINUTED FRACTURE IN SMOKER	COMMINUTED FRACTURE IN SMOKER
10	2	3	6	10
15	3	6	12	19
20	7	12	23	34
25	14	23	39	52
30	26	39	57	70
40	62	74	86	92

From Murray IR, Foster CJ, Eros A, Robinson CM: Risk factors for nonunion after nonoperative treatment of displaced midshaft fractures of the clavicle, *J Bone Joint Surg Am* 95:1153, 2013.

OPEN REDUCTION AND INTERNAL FIXATION OF CLAVICULAR FRACTURES

TECHNIQUE 5.1

(COLLINGE ET AL., MODIFIED)

ANTEROINFERIOR PLATE AND SCREW FIXATION

- Place the patient supine with a large "bump" placed between the scapulae, allowing the injured shoulder girdle to fall posteriorly, which helps to restore length and increase exposure of the clavicle.
- Make an incision centered over the fracture from the sternal notch to the anterior edge of the acromion (Fig. 5.4A).
- Release the lateral platysma and identify the supraclavicular nerve traversing the anterior aspect of the clavicle.
- Incise the clavipectoral fascia along its attachment to the anterior clavicle and carefully elevate it inferiorly.
- Dissect first along the medial fragment, which usually has flexed up away from the vital infraclavicular structures. For acute fractures, only minimal soft-tissue dissection is needed.
- Reduce the fracture and hold it with bone clamps.
- Use a lag screw if possible for provisional fixation; as an alternative, consider using a mini-fragment screw as provisional fixation to allow perfect contouring of the plate.
- Contour a 3.5-mm plate to fit along the anteroinferior edge of the clavicle. Typically, an eight-hole plate fits well when contoured into an S-shape as viewed on edge (Fig. 5.4B).
- Aim the screws for plate fixation posteriorly and superiorly (Fig. 5.4C). If an oblique fracture is present, a lag screw can be placed either through the plate or directly into the bone at roughly a 90-degree angle to the fracture line.

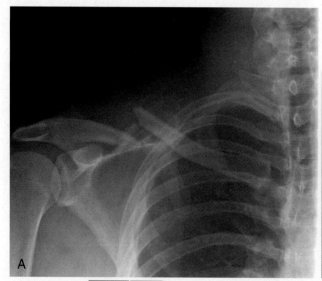
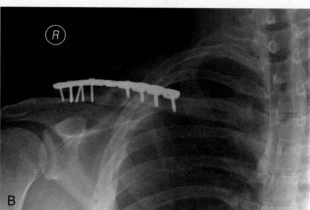

FIGURE 5.1   Clavicular fracture **(A)** fixed with superior plate **(B)**. **SEE TECHNIQUE 5.1.**

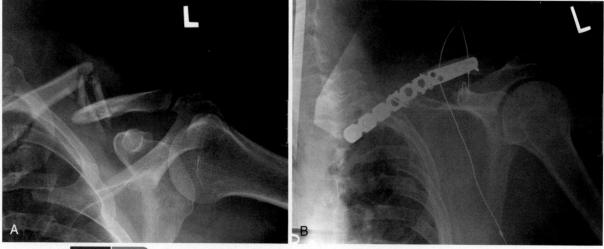

FIGURE 5.2   Clavicular fracture **(A)** fixed with anteroinferior plate **(B)**.

SUPERIOR FIXATION

- For superior fixation, contour the plate to fit the superior edge of the clavicle (see Fig. 5.1). Insert the screws from superior to inferior, taking care to avoid injury to the neurovascular structures.

See also Video 5.1.

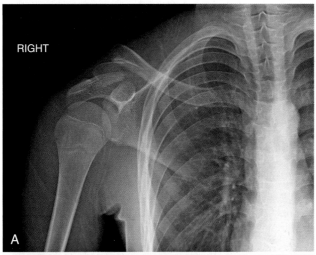

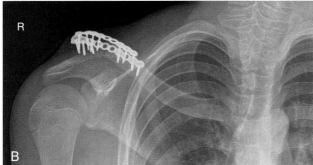

FIGURE 5.3   Dual mini-fragment plate.

POSTOPERATIVE CARE The operated extremity is placed in a sling for comfort. Pendulum and Codman exercises are taught, and the patient is encouraged to use the arm but to avoid heavy lifting, pushing, or pulling. Full return of activities is allowed when fracture healing is present, usually at 2 to 3 months.

■ INTRAMEDULLARY FIXATION

Intramedullary nailing of clavicular fractures has been done for over 50 years, with a variety of devices, including Rockwood pins, Kirschner wires, Küntscher nails, and Rush nails (Fig. 5.5). Suggested advantages of intramedullary fixation include small skin incision, less periosteal stripping, and relative stability to allow callus formation. Frequent complications, such as intrathoracic migration, pin breakage, and damage to underlying structures, however, have limited the use of this technique. A biomechanical study comparing fixation of clavicular osteotomies with 3.5-mm compression plates and 3.8- or 4.5-mm intramedullary pins also showed that plated constructs were superior in resisting displacement. More recently, titanium elastic intramedullary nails have been used, with good results reported in a number of studies. However, reported complication rates have ranged from 9% to 78% with these devices, mainly medial or lateral migration and perforations. Frigg et al. reported a reduction in complications from 60% to 17% with the use of an end cap, converting to open reduction after two failed attempts at closed reduction, using careful manual passage of the nail, obtaining intraoperative oblique radiographs to rule out lateral perforation, and limiting postoperative range of motion to 90 degrees for 6 weeks.

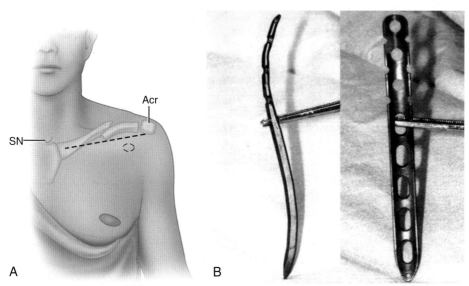

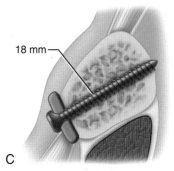

FIGURE 5.4   Open reduction and internal fixation of clavicular fracture. **A,** Incision. **B,** Plate prebent to match normal clavicular anatomy. **C,** Screw placement posteriorly and superiorly. Acr, acromion; SN, sternal notch. **SEE TECHNIQUE 5.1.**

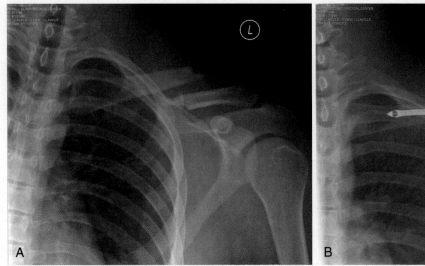
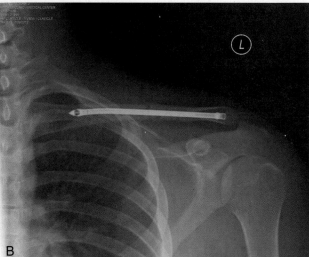

FIGURE 5.5   Clavicular fracture **(A)** treated with intramedullary fixation **(B)**.

INTRAMEDULLARY FIXATION WITH A HEADED, DISTALLY THREADED PIN (ROCKWOOD CLAVICLE PIN)

TECHNIQUE 5.2

- Place the patient in a semi-sitting position on a radiolucent table with an image intensifier on the ipsilateral side. By rotating the image 45 degrees caudal and cephalad, orthogonal views of the clavicle can be obtained.
- Make a 2- to 3-cm incision over the posterolateral corner of the clavicle 2 to 3 cm medial to the acromioclavicular joint. Little subcutaneous fat is in this region, so take care to prevent injury to the underlying platysma muscle.
- Use scissors to free the platysma muscle from the overlying skin; split its fibers in line with the muscle. Take care to prevent injury to the middle branch of the supraclavicular nerve, which usually is found directly beneath the platysma muscle near the midclavicle. Identify and retract the nerve.
- Use a towel clip to elevate the proximal end of the medial clavicle through the incision (Fig. 5.6A).
- Taking care not to penetrate the anterior cortex, attach the appropriate-sized drill to the ratchet T-handle and drill the medullary canal (Fig. 5.6B).
- Remove the drill from the medial fragment, attach the appropriate-sized tap to the T-handle, and tap the medullary canal to the anterior cortex (Fig. 5.6C). Hand tapping is recommended, especially for small patients and smaller-diameter clavicle pins.
- Elevate the lateral fragment through the incision; externally rotating the arm and shoulder helps improve exposure.
- Attach the same-sized drill used in the medial fragment to the ratchet T-handle and drill the medullary canal (Fig. 5.6D).
- Under C-arm guidance, pass the drill out through the posterolateral cortex of the clavicle (Fig. 5.6E). The drill position should be posterior and medial to the acromioclavicular joint, around the level of the coracoid. Allow the

drill to exit no higher than the equator of the posterolateral clavicle.
- Remove the drill from the lateral fragment, attach the appropriate-sized tap to the T-handle, and tap the medullary canal so that the large threads are advanced fully into the canal (Fig. 5.6F). If the tap is a tight fit, consider redrilling with the next larger drill size. Again, hand tapping is recommended.
- While holding the distal fragment with a bone clamp, remove the nuts from the pin assembly and pass the trocar end of the pin into the medullary canal of the distal fragment. The pin should exit through the previously drilled hole in the posterolateral cortex.
- Once the pin exits the clavicle, its tip can be felt subcutaneously. Make a small incision over the palpable tip and spread the subcutaneous tissue with a hemostat (Fig. 5.6G). Place the tip of the hemostat under the tip of the clavicle pin to facilitate its passage through the incision. Then drill the pin out laterally until the large, medial threads start to engage the cortex.
- Attach the Jacobs chuck and T-handle to the end of the pin protruding laterally (take care not to place the chuck over the machined threads, both lateral and medial) and carefully retract the pin into the lateral fragment (Fig. 5.6H). Ensure that the pin is inserted correctly.
- Reduce the fracture and pass the pin into the medial fragment. Advance the pin until all medial threads are across the fracture site. Because the weight of the arm usually pulls the arm down, lifting the shoulder will facilitate pin passage into the medial fragment.
- Place the medial nut on the pin, followed by the smaller lateral nut. Cold weld the two nuts together by grasping the medial nut with a needle driver or needle-nose pliers and tightening the lateral nut against the medial nut with the lateral nut wrench. Use the T-handle and wrench on the lateral nut to medially advance the pin down into the medial fragment until it contacts the anterior cortex. Confirm position with fluoroscopy.
- Break the cold weld between the nuts by grasping the medial nut with a needle driver or pliers and quickly turn-

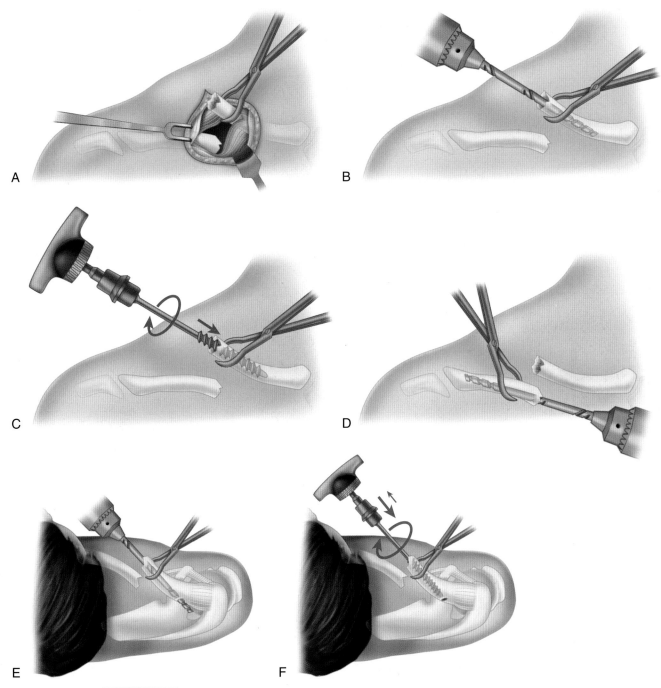

FIGURE 5.6 Intramedullary fixation of clavicular fracture. **A,** Elevation of proximal end of medial clavicle. **B,** Drilling of medullary canal. **C,** Tapping of medullary canal. **D,** Drilling of medullary canal. **E,** Passage of drill out through posterolateral cortex. **F,** Tapping of medullary canal.

ing the lateral nut counterclockwise with the insertion wrench. Advance the medial nut until it against the lateral cortex of the clavicle. Tighten the lateral nut until it engages the medial nut (Fig. 5.6I).

- Use the medial wrench to back out the pin 1 cm or more to expose the nuts from the soft tissue. Ensure that the clavicle threads are still engaged in the cortical bone of the medial fragment.
- Use a side-cutting pin cutter to cut the pin as close to the lateral nut as possible. Readvance the clavicle pin using the lateral nut wrench.

POSTOPERATIVE CARE The arm is placed in a standard sling for comfort, and gentle pendulum exercises are allowed. At 10 to 14 days, sutures are removed and, if healing is seen on radiographs, the sling is discontinued; unrestricted range-of-motion exercises, but no strengthening, resisted exercises, or sports activities are allowed. If radiographs at 6 weeks show union, resisted and strengthening activities are begun. Contact sports (e.g., football, hockey) should be avoided for 12 weeks after surgery. If the fracture is healed at 12 weeks, the pin can be removed.

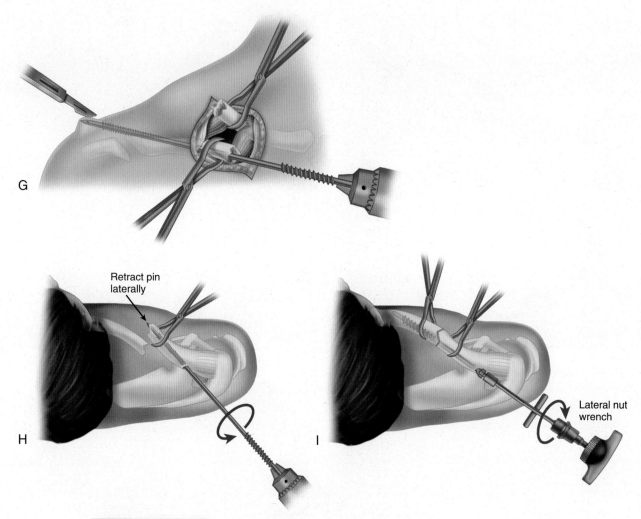

FIGURE 5.6, Cont'd **G,** Incision over tip of intramedullary pin. **H,** Retraction of pin into lateral fragment. **I,** Final position of intramedullary pin. (Redrawn from Lippert S: Rockwood clavicle pin surgical technique, Warsaw IN, DePuy.) **SEE TECHNIQUE 5.2.**

LATERAL CLAVICULAR FRACTURES

Neer described five types of lateral clavicular fractures (Table 5.5 and Fig. 5.7). Types I and II are lateral to the coracoclavicular ligaments and are inherently stable. Type II fractures occur just medial to the coracoacromial ligaments (type IIa) or occur with rupture of the ligaments (type IIb). The trapezius can be a deforming force and cause displacement of type II fractures. Treatment is still controversial, with good results reported with both operative and nonoperative treatment, even with malunions. The challenge is to obtain secure fixation in the lateral segments. Anatomic locking plates have improved fixation in the distal segment (Fig. 5.8) Other strategies include plating over to the acromion to gain greater fixation, supplementing fixation with sutures from the clavicle to the coracoid (Fig. 5.9), and using subacromial hook-plates (Figs. 5.10 and 5.11). High rates of union (95% or higher) and good shoulder function have been reported with the use of hook-plates, but patient discomfort and acromial osteolysis generally require plate removal as soon as union occurs. The author uses hook plates only in rare circumstances and recommends judicious use.

TABLE 5.5

Neer Classification of Lateral Clavicular Fractures

TYPE	DESCRIPTION
I	Coracoclavicular ligaments intact, attached to medial segment
II	Coracoclavicular ligaments detached from medial segment, but trapezoid intact to distal segment
IIa	Both conoid and trapezoid attached to distal segment
IIb	Conoid is torn
III	Intraarticular extension into acromioclavicular joint

Recently, Yagnik et al. reported a combination of cortical button fixation with coracoclavicular ligament reconstruction for distal clavicular fracture repair. Fractures united in all patients with low complication rates (Fig. 5.12).

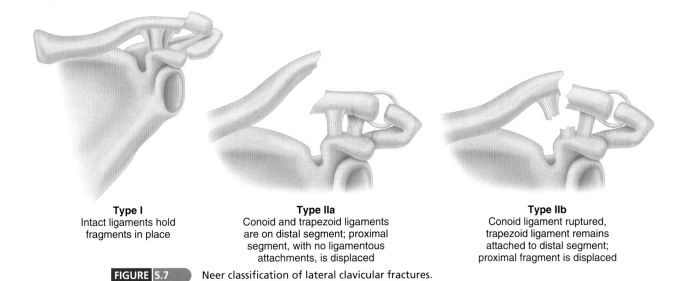

Type I
Intact ligaments hold
fragments in place

Type IIa
Conoid and trapezoid ligaments
are on distal segment; proximal
segment, with no ligamentous
attachments, is displaced

Type IIb
Conoid ligament ruptured,
trapezoid ligament remains
attached to distal segment;
proximal fragment is displaced

FIGURE 5.7   Neer classification of lateral clavicular fractures.

DISTAL CLAVICULAR FRACTURE REPAIR WITH CORACOCLAVICULAR LIGAMENT RECONSTRUCTION AND CORTICAL BUTTON FIXATION

TECHNIQUE 5.3

(YAGNIK ET AL.)
- After administration of a regional interscalene block and general anesthesia, place the patient in a modified beach-chair position.
- Make a 5-cm vertical incision 2 to 3 cm medial to the acromioclavicular joint, with the base of the incision at the proximal aspect of the coracoid. Carefully incise the deltotrapezial fascia in line with the clavicle to facilitate closure over the implants at the end of the procedure.
- Bluntly dissect the medial and lateral soft tissues adjacent to the coracoid for later passage of the sutures and graft around the coracoid.
- Prepare a 7 × 240-mm semitendinosus allograft, tapering the ends of the graft using a whip stitch (No. 2 nonabsorbable suture). Both ends of the graft should easily pass through the 6-mm tunnel.
- Using a coracoid passer, shuttle a strong passing suture through the instrument and under the coracoid and then shuttle two different-colored suture tapes and allograft around the coracoid.
- Using a 2.4-mm drill, create a bicortical hole for the suture tape as close to the fracture site as possible, preserving 5 mm of bone laterally to prevent iatrogenic fracture through this drill hole.
- Create a second tunnel for the graft with a 6.0-mm cannulated reamer over a 2.4-mm guide wire at least 15 mm medial to the first tunnel.
- Shuttle the two suture tapes through the lateral tunnel before the graft so that they lie posterior to the graft.

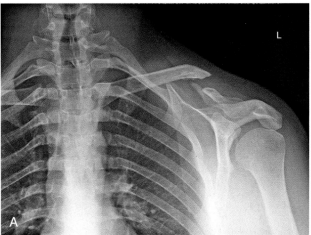

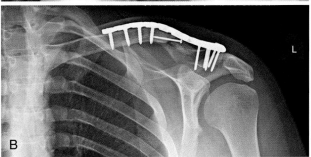

FIGURE 5.8   Anatomic locking plate.

- Pass both ends of the graft through the 6-mm tunnel using a second shuttle suture (Fig. 5.13A).
- Pass four limbs of the colored suture tape through a cortical button and tie, reducing the medial fragment to the lateral fragment.
- Tension the graft and insert a 5.5 × 10-mm PEEK interference screw, then cut the ends of the graft (Fig. 5.13B).
- Pass the free ends of the suture tape through the anterior deltotrapezial fascia in a horizontal mattress fashion.

- Tie the sutures, repair the deltotrapezial fascia to the clavicle, bury the knots to minimize soft-tissue irritation, and close the incision in the standard fashion.

POSTOPERATIVE CARE The arm is placed in a sling to minimize tension on the repair for 4 to 6 weeks. Passive range of motion is started immediately after surgery. After 4 to 6 weeks, patients begin active and active-assisted range of motion exercises, with strengthening exercises at 8 weeks. Patients may return to full activity and sports around 4 months.

FRACTURES AROUND THE SHOULDER
FRACTURES OF THE SCAPULA

Fractures of the scapula account for 3% to 5% of all fractures about the shoulder, are most often caused by high-energy trauma, and are frequently associated with multiple trauma

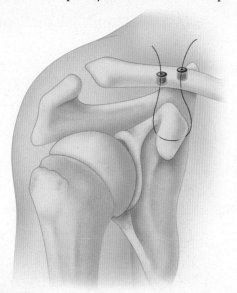

FIGURE 5.9 Supplemental suture fixation from clavicle to coracoid over the acromion for lateral clavicular fracture.

(approximately 90% of patients with scapular fractures have associated injuries). Treatment of scapular fractures has traditionally been described as "benign neglect" and, like clavicular fractures, most scapular fractures do well with conservative management. Although outcomes are generally good, not all scapular fractures heal uneventfully and there has been a resurgence of interest in determining which patients would benefit from operative treatment. In their systematic review of the literature concerning scapular fractures, Zlowodzki et al. found that of the total 520 fractures reported, 82% had good-to-excellent functional results. Almost all scapular body fractures were treated nonoperatively, with 86% good-to-excellent results; scapular neck and isolated glenoid fractures were most often treated operatively (83%), with good-to-excellent results in 76% and 82%, respectively. Although the numbers of specific fractures were small, the overall results after operative treatment were better than those after nonoperative treatment in all types (Table 5.6). Lantry et al. also reported a systematic review of operative treatment of scapular fractures in which good-to-excellent functional results were found in approximately 85% of patients. In contrast, in their comparison of 31 displaced scapular fractures treated operatively to 31 treated nonoperatively (matched by age, occupation, and sex), Jones and Sietsema found that all fractures healed with no differences in return to work, pain, or complications. Dienstknecht et al. reported that a meta-analysis of the literature indicated that operatively treated scapular fractures had better radiographic results and more pain-free results, whereas nonoperatively treated patients had significantly better range of motion. Although the literature is still lacking in sufficient evidence to formulate concrete treatment guidelines, these two reviews emphasize that most scapular fractures do well, but criteria for deciding which fractures are at risk for poor outcomes are still evolving. Recent reports by Schroder et al. and Tatro et al. continue to support operative treatment in widely displaced scapular fractures with high functional outcomes and low complication rates.

■ TREATMENT OPTIONS

Almost all scapular body and neck fractures are still treated nonoperatively. We immobilize the shoulder for 2 to 3 weeks and begin an active-assisted range-of-motion protocol when pain permits. An active range-of-motion program is then

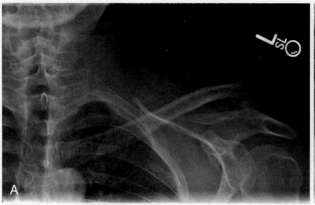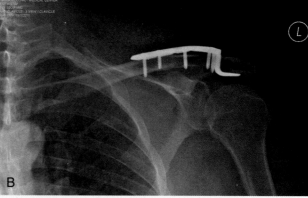

FIGURE 5.10 Clavicular fracture **(A)** fixed with hook plate **(B)**.

begun, and strengthening exercises are allowed when fracture healing is confirmed clinically and radiographically.

The mobility of the shoulder is predictive of function in many patients with a scapular fracture; however, there is still a small group of patients in whom ORIF probably is indicated. The goal of treatment is to preserve shoulder function by avoiding malalignment, arthrosis, scapulothoracic dyskinesis, and impingement pain (Table 5.7).

▮ GLENOID FRACTURES

Glenoid fractures should be treated as all other intraarticular fractures, and reduced and stabilized when significant (>4 mm) displacement exists through the articular surface that leads to joint subluxation or incongruency. Anavian et al. reported that, of 33 patients with complex and displaced intraarticular glenoid fractures, 87% were pain free and 90%

returned to preinjury levels of work or activity after operative treatment. The operative approach of choice is the Judet or modified Judet (see Technique 1.94). Additional anterior approaches occasionally are needed.

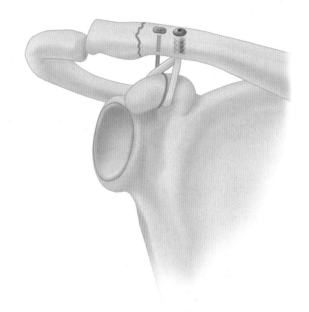

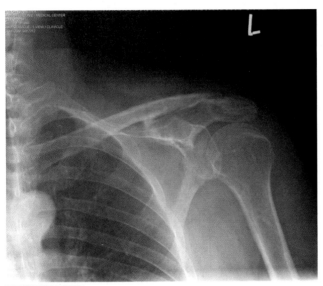

FIGURE 5.11 Healed clavicular fracture after plate removal.

FIGURE 5.12 Distal clavicle repair using combination of cortical button fixation and coracoclavicular ligament reconstruction. (Redrawn from Yagnik GP, Jordan CJ, Narvel RR, Hassan RJ, Porter DA: Distal clavicle fracture repair: clinical outcomes of a surgical technique utilizing a combination of cortical button fixation and coracoclavicular ligament reconstruction, *Orthop J Sports Med* 7(9):2325967119867920, 2019.)

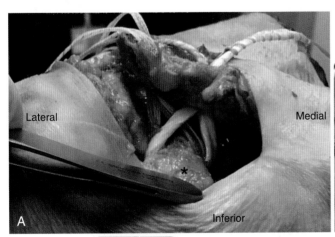

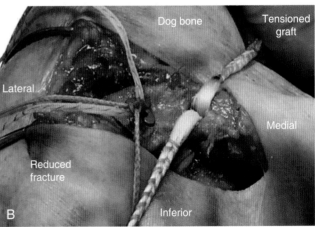

FIGURE 5.13 **A,** Distal clavicular fracture with suture tapes passed through laterally based tunnel and allograft passed through medial tunnel. Asterisk indicates coracoid process. **B,** Final construct demonstrates reduction with suture tapes tied over cortical button and graft tensioned with interference screw. Graft is passed anterior to suture tapes. (From Yagnik GP, Jordan CJ, Narvel RR, Hassan RJ, Porter DA: Distal clavicle fracture repair: clinical outcomes of a surgical technique utilizing a combination of cortical button fixation and coracoclavicular ligament reconstruction, *Orthop J Sports Med* 7(9):2325967119867920, 2019.). **SEE TECHNIQUE 5.3.**

TABLE 5.6

Results of Operative and Nonoperative Treatment of Scapular Fractures

FRACTURE TYPE	OPERATIVE: EXCELLENT/GOOD	NONOPERATIVE: EXCELLENT/GOOD
Glenoid only	82% (45/55)	67% (6/9)
Neck with or without other associated scapular fractures (excluding glenoid)	92% (23/25)	79% (110/140)
Acromion and/or coracoid (with/without associated scapular fractures)	88% (7/8)	77% (80/104)
Body only (including spine)	100% (2/2)	86% (6/7)

Data from Zlowodzki M, Bhandari M, Zelle BA, et al: Treatment of scapula fractures: systematic review of 520 fractures in 22 case series, *J Orthop Trauma* 20:230, 2006.

TABLE 5.7

Indications for Surgical Treatment of a Scapular Fracture

INDICATION	CRITERION
INTRAARTICULAR FRACTURE Articular step-off Percentage of glenoid affected Glenohumeral articulation	≥4-5 mm ≥20% Unstable despite closed reduction
EXTRAARTICULAR Glenopolar angle Lateral border offset Angulation Translation	≤20° ≥20 mm ≥45° ≥100%

From Furey MJ, McKee MD: Fractures of the clavicle and scapula, *AAOS OKU: Trauma* 5:241, 2016.

■ SCAPULAR BODY OR NECK FRACTURES

Fractures of the scapular body or neck that are so significantly displaced that malunion and pain are of concern should be considered for operative treatment. Medialization of the glenoid has been questioned by Zuckerman et al., who recommended evaluation of lateralization of the scapular border. CT evaluation also found that in patients with glenoid neck fractures, pure medial translation of the glenoid relative to the axial skeleton was rare; instead, there was typically a component of shortening of the scapular width combined with lateralization of the scapular body. Treatment decisions should be based on the amount of displacement. Some authors use the glenopolar angle as a criterion for determining treatment. This angle is formed by a line drawn from the inferior pole of the glenoid fossa up to the superior pole and a second line drawn from the superior pole of the glenoid fossa down through the inferiormost angle of the scapular body (Fig. 5.14). The normal glenopolar angle ranges from 30 to 45 degrees. Anavian et al. suggested that three-dimensional CT is more reliable than plain radiography in the evaluation of extraarticular scapular fracture displacement.

Cole et al. listed several criteria for operative treatment of scapular fractures:

- A 15 to 20 mm lateral border offset (lateralization).
- Forty degrees of scapular body angulation, as measured on a scapular-Y view.
- Glenopolar angle of 20 degrees or less and greater than 60 degrees.

- Scapular body fracture with injury to the clavicle or clavicle-acromion complex.

These decision-making criteria have not yet been shown to produce improved outcomes; the surgeon's skill level and patient issues should contribute to the decision for operative treatment. We generally favor conservative treatment, but this is an active treatment decision and not "benign neglect" (Fig. 5.15).

PROXIMAL HUMERAL FRACTURES

Use adequate radiograms to understand the traumatic lesion, be careful denying older patients effective treatment, use a safe and simple surgical approach, know the options for internal fixation, recognize the value of prosthetic replacement, avoid technical pitfalls, and thoughtfully supervise the postoperative patient care.— *R.H. Cofield (1988)*

Cofield's summary of treatment of proximal humeral fractures is an indication of the difficulty of treating these injuries—from first evaluation to final outcome. Much controversy and confusion still exist, and no single treatment protocol or algorithm has been proved to be universally effective. As indicated by Cofield, areas still in question include radiographic diagnosis, operative or nonoperative treatment, consideration of patient age in treatment decision making, surgical approach, fracture fixation or hemiarthroplasty, type of internal fixation, and rehabilitation protocol. Numerous authors have suggested that nonoperative treatment may be preferable for two-, three-, and four-part proximal humeral fractures in elderly patients, but pain and loss of function have been reported in high percentages of patients after this treatment approach. Several more recent reports, however, have indicated that the functional results of operative treatment are not significantly better than the results of nonoperative treatment in elderly patients, although radiograph results may be superior. Court-Brown et al. reported good or excellent results in 81% of impacted valgus fractures in elderly patients treated nonoperatively, and in a comparison of operative and nonoperative treatment of displaced two-part fractures, these authors found similar results in the two treatment groups. In one of the largest studies to date (PROFHER), with 231 patients, the authors were unable to show superiority of operative or nonoperative treatment using the Oxford Shoulder Score as the primary outcome. A 5-year follow-up study of the PROHFER study again was unable to show any advantage of operative treatment over nonoperative treatment. Although there are many

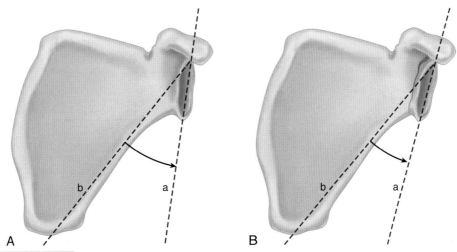

FIGURE 5.14 Normal **(A)** and abnormal **(B)** glenopolar angle. Angle is measured between line connecting most cranial with most caudal point of glenoid cavity (*a*) and line connecting most cranial point of glenoid cavity with most caudal point of scapular body (*b*). Normal glenopolar angle ranges from 30 to 45 degrees.

limitations of the PROHFER studies, it certainly demonstrates some of the difficulty in treatment of patients with proximal humeral fractures. A meta-analysis by Beks et al. confirmed the PROHFER finding of no difference between operative and nonoperative treatment. In a study of the geographic incidence and treatment variation of common fractures in elderly patients, Sporer et al. found large variations in the percentage of proximal humeral fractures treated operatively, ranging from 6.4% to 60%; in eight regions of the United States, at least 40% were treated operatively, whereas in 35 regions, fewer than 20% were treated operatively. The fact that 10 different fixation techniques were evaluated for a single fracture type (fractures of the surgical neck of the humerus) is further indication of the complexity of treating proximal humeral fractures. Interestingly, one study showed a higher rate of operative treatment of proximal humeral fractures among upper extremity surgeons compared with trauma surgeons. In another study by LaMartina et al., experienced shoulder surgeons agreed on treatment plans only 63% of the time, demonstrating the difficulty in devising and evaluating treatment plans.

■ CLASSIFICATION

The most commonly used classification system for proximal humeral fractures is that of Neer (Fig. 5.16). Although limited reliability, reproducibility among observers, and consistency by the same observer at different times have been cited as limitations of the Neer system, it remains useful in guiding treatment. Classification is based on the four-part anatomy of the proximal humerus: the humeral head, the lesser and greater tuberosities, and the proximal humeral shaft. The criterion for displacement is more than 1 cm of separation of a part or angulation of 45 degrees. Displaced three-part and four-part fractures markedly alter the articular congruity of the glenohumeral joint and have the highest likelihood of disrupting the major blood supply to the proximal humerus (Fig. 5.17). Osteonecrosis is most likely after displaced four-part fractures.

■ RADIOGRAPHIC EVALUATION

An anteroposterior view of the shoulder in the plane of the scapula, a lateral view of the scapula (Y view) (Fig. 5.18), and a supine axillary view (Fig. 5.19) are necessary in all patients initially to evaluate a proximal humeral fracture. If the amount of displacement of the humeral head or tuberosity fragments is unclear on radiographs, an axial CT scan with 2-mm sections is indicated (Fig. 5.20).

■ NONOPERATIVE TREATMENT

Nonoperative treatment can obtain a functional, painless extremity in most proximal humeral fractures. The range of motion of the shoulder joint accommodates moderate angular deformity without significant functional loss. Neer described acceptable angulation as less than 45 degrees and less than 1 cm of displacement. Although these criteria are not absolute, they do provide a guide. An elderly, infirm patient can tolerate functional loss better than a young, active patient. The first step in treatment decision-making is to determine if displacement (<66%) and angulation (varus is poorly tolerated) are acceptable for a particular patient; the second is to determine if the humeral head and shaft move as a unit. If both of these conditions are present, the fracture is stable and in an acceptable position. A sling is used for comfort, and a physical therapy regimen with pendulum exercises is started, usually within 1 week. If the humeral head and shaft do not move as a unit, physical therapy can be delayed for 2 to 4 weeks in patients who are poor surgical candidates because of age, low functional demands, or comorbidities that preclude participation in rehabilitation. In young, active patients, early operative fixation should be considered. Generally, the longer the period of immobilization, the longer the period of therapy, and the greater the disability. A randomized controlled trial involving 74 patients with impacted proximal humeral fractures found that early (within 72 hours of injury) passive mobilization was safe and more effective in restoring function than conventional immobilization (3 weeks) followed by physical therapy. Another study, however, pointed out that fracture settling continues to occur with conservative treatment.

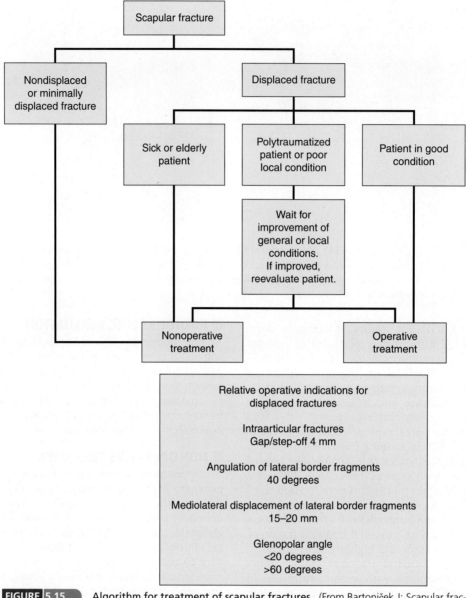

FIGURE 5.15   **Algorithm for treatment of scapular fractures.** (From Bartoniček J: Scapular fractures. In Tornetta P, Ricci W, Court-Brown CM, et al., editors: *Rockwood and Green's Fractures in Adults,* ed 9, Philadelphia, 2020, Wolters Kluwer, p. 996.)

■ OPERATIVE TREATMENT

The decision that operative treatment is appropriate is complicated by the numerous and varied techniques described for fixation of proximal humeral fractures. Generally, fracture displacement is used as the indicator of stability. The goal is restoration of proximal humeral anatomy with stable fixation that allows early functional range of motion. Chronic malunions and nonunions that are subsequently treated surgically are associated with poor outcomes. Consequently, it is imperative to recreate the normal proximal humeral anatomy with respect to tuberosity reduction and the head-neck relationship. Indications for operative treatment include displaced two-part surgical neck fractures, displaced (>5 mm) greater tuberosity fractures, displaced three-part fractures, and displaced four-part fractures in young patients. The type of fixation (transosseous suture fixation, percutaneous pinning, intramedullary nailing, or plate fixation) used depends on the patient's age, activity level, and bone quality; the fracture type

and associated fractures; and the surgeon's technical ability (Table 5.8). Age alone has been shown both to be predictive of failure and to have no association with failure. In their series of 154 fractures with proximal humeral fractures treated with plating, Boesmueller et al. found that the risk of screw cut-out was four times higher in patients over the age of 60 years and the overall risk for complications was three times higher than in younger patients.

Before surgery is considered, it is important to determine if the blood supply and bone quality are adequate. The Hertel radiographic criteria for perfusion of the humeral head (Fig. 5.21) can be used to predict ischemia: metaphyseal extension of the humeral head of less than 8 mm and medial hinge disruption of more than 2 mm are predictive of ischemia. The combination of metaphyseal extension of the humeral head, medial hinge disruption of more than 2 mm, and an anatomic neck fracture pattern has a 97% positive predictive value for humeral head ischemia. According

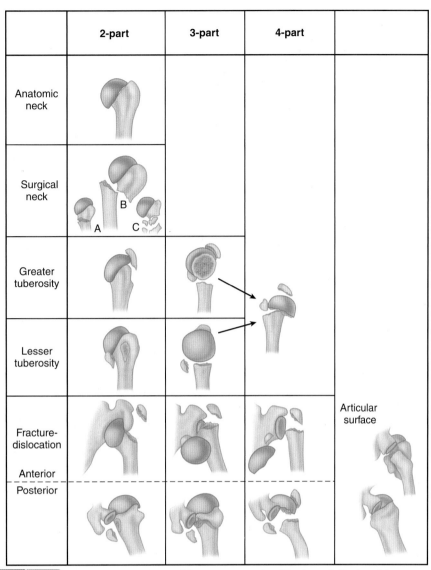

	2-part	**3-part**	**4-part**	
Anatomic neck				
Surgical neck	A B C			
Greater tuberosity				
Lesser tuberosity				
Fracture-dislocation Anterior Posterior				Articular surface

FIGURE 5.16 Neer's terminology of four-segment classification of displaced fractures and fracture-dislocations relates pattern of displacement (two-part, three-part, or four-part) and key segment displaced. In each two-part pattern, segment named is one displaced. Two-part surgical neck fractures are impacted *(A)*, unimpacted *(B)*, and comminuted *(C)*. All three-part patterns have displacement of shaft segment, and displaced tuberosity identifies type of three-part fracture. In four-part pattern, all segments are displaced. Fracture-dislocations are identified by anterior or posterior position of articular segment. Large articular surface defects require separate recognition.

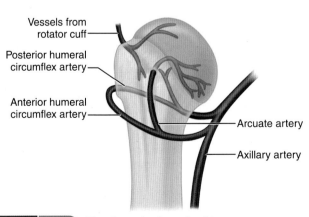

Vessels from rotator cuff

Posterior humeral circumflex artery

Anterior humeral circumflex artery

Arcuate artery

Axillary artery

FIGURE 5.17 Blood supply of proximal humerus.

to the AO/ASIF classification system, extraarticular type A fractures have an intact vascular supply, whereas type B fractures have a possible injury to the vascular supply and type C articular fractures have a high probability of osteonecrosis. The cortical thickness of the humeral diaphysis has been suggested to be a reliable and reproducible predictor of bone mineral density and the success of internal fixation. The combined cortical thickness is the average of the medial and lateral cortical thickness at two levels (Fig. 5.22). Generally, a cortical thickness of less than 4 mm precludes internal fixation because adequate screw purchase cannot be obtained; sling immobilization, transosseous suture, or hemiarthroplasty may be better options. Spross et al. and Newton et al. also demonstrated that the quality of the bone was associated with late cut-out.

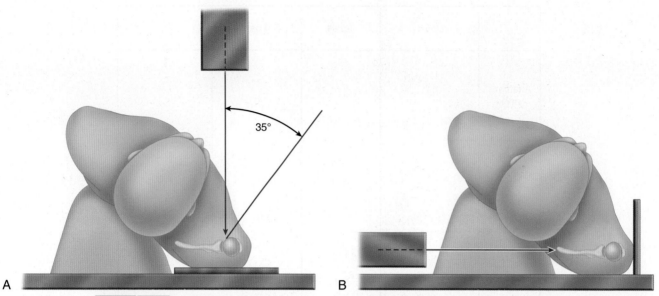

A

B

FIGURE 5.18 Special radiographic view perpendicular to plane of scapula to show glenohumeral joint in profile **(A)** and parallel to plane of scapula to show anterior and posterior displacement **(B)**.

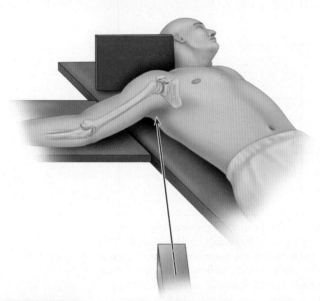

FIGURE 5.19 Method of obtaining axillary view of glenohumeral joint. This exposure can be obtained with patient prone, supine, or standing. Minimal abduction of injured arm is required to determine anteroposterior relationships.

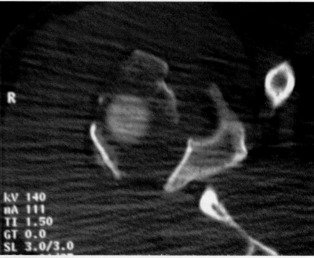

FIGURE 5.20 CT scan of humeral head-splitting fracture.

Transosseous suture fixation techniques are well defined in the orthopaedic literature. Park et al. reported 78% excellent results in patients with two-part and three-part proximal humeral fractures treated with suture fixation. The use of strong nonabsorbable suture provides the advantage of incorporating the rotator cuff insertion to increase fixation in patients with poor bone quality (Fig. 5.23). The level of soft-tissue dissection is not extensive, and relatively low rates of osteonecrosis have been reported with this technique. Concerns include the ability of the patient to move the shoulder joint and loss of reduction secondary to a nonrigid construct. More recently, Dimakopoulos et al. reported good results in 188 displaced proximal humeral fractures treated

with transosseous fixation (Fig. 5.24). They suggested as advantages of this technique less surgical soft-tissue dissection, a low rate of humeral head osteonecrosis, fixation sufficient to allow early passive joint motion, and the avoidance of bulky and expensive implants.

Percutaneous pinning has the advantage of avoiding further damage to the soft-tissue envelope and the blood supply to the humeral head (Figs. 5.25 and 5.26). It also is a relatively inexpensive technique, and several series have reported good results in two-part, three-part, and valgus-impacted four-part fractures. The procedure is technically challenging and requires a satisfactory closed reduction, adequate bone stock, minimal comminution (particularly of the tuberosities), an intact medial calcar, and a compliant patient. In their series of 74 older patients (average age, 71 years), Calvo et al. demonstrated that reduction was associated with satisfactory outcome. However, if satisfactory closed reduction cannot be obtained, another form

TABLE 5.8		
Advantages and Disadvantages of Techniques Used to Treat Displaced Fractures of the Proximal Humerus		
TECHNIQUE	**ADVANTAGES**	**DISADVANTAGES**
Nonoperative treatment	Function as good as operative treatment for many fractures Low risk of infection and other operative complications	Malunion inevitable: ▪ Cuff dysfunction/stiffness more likely ▪ Later salvage surgery more difficult Risk of nonunion increased
Minimally invasive techniques	Reduced injury to soft-tissue envelope Lower risk of infection	Steep learning curve Risk of axillary nerve/vascular injury Less stable fixation
Intramedullary nailing	More stable fixation technique in osteoporotic bone Minimal dissection required for insertion	Rotator cuff dysfunction after anterograde insertion Poor results in multipart fractures High rate of late implant removal
Open reduction and plate fixation	Anatomic fracture reduction possible ▪ Improved functional outcome ▪ Later revision easier Most stable fixation in multipart fractures ▪ Rigid implants ▪ Adjuvant bone grafting possible	Open surgical approach required: ▪ Increased risk of infection ▪ Increased risk of osteonecrosis
Hemiarthroplasty	Risk of nonunion, osteonecrosis, symptomatic malunion avoided Low reoperation rate	Poor functional outcome Late arthroplasty complications difficult to treat in elderly patients

From Robinson CM: Proximal humerus fractures. In Bucholz RW, Heckman JD, Court-Brown CM, Tornetta P 3rd, editors: *Rockwood and Green's fracture in adults*, ed 7, Philadelphia, 2010, Lippincott Williams & Wilkins.

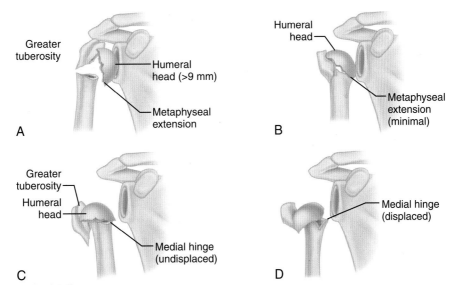

FIGURE 5.21   Hertel radiographic criteria for perfusion of humeral head. **A,** Metaphyseal extension of humeral head of more than 9 mm. **B,** Metaphyseal extension of humeral head less than 8 mm. **C,** Undisplaced medial hinge. **D,** Medial hinge of more than 2-mm displacement.

of reduction and fixation should be used. Loss of fixation, pin track infections, and axillary nerve injuries are common complications. Terminally threaded Schanz pins and bicortical pins inserted from the greater tuberosity to the medial humeral shaft add stability to the overall construct.

Percutaneous pinning is contraindicated for fractures with metaphyseal comminution.

Intramedullary nailing (see Technique 5.4) provides more stable fixation than percutaneous pinning, although less than locked plate fixation. The Polarus nail (Accumed, Portland,

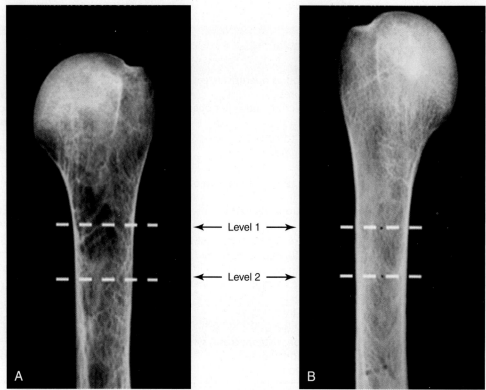

FIGURE 5.22 Two levels used to measure cortical thickness of humeral diaphysis. Level 1, most proximal aspect of humeral diaphysis, is at level in which endosteal borders of medial and lateral cortices are parallel. Level 2 is 20 mm distal to level 1. Examples of patients with low bone mineral density **(A)** and high bone mineral density **(B)**. (From Tingart MS, Apprelexa M, von Stechow D, et al: The cortical thickness of the proximal humeral diaphysis predicts bone mineral density of the proximal humerus, *J Bone Joint Surg* 85B:611, 2003. Copyright British Editorial Society of Bone and Joint Surgery.)

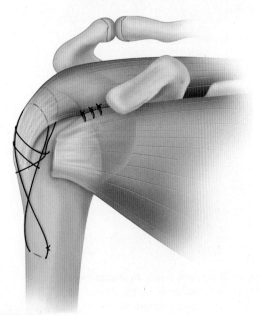

FIGURE 5.23 Transosseous nonabsorbable sutures incorporate rotator cuff to increase fixation and help control tuberosity fragments.

OR) has been shown to provide more biomechanical stability than pin fixation, and good clinical outcomes have been reported with this device. Newer nail designs with polyaxial screws have more stability than earlier designs, and the addition of polyethylene bushings may increase stability and prevent screw back-out (Fig. 5.27). Insertion of an intramedullary nail into the proximal humerus violates the rotator cuff, which can lead to postoperative shoulder pain. The advantages of the technique include preservation of the soft tissues and the theoretical biomechanical properties of intramedullary nails. A comminuted lateral cortex fracture or fractures involving the tuberosities may be a contraindication to intramedullary nailing. A recent randomized controlled trial demonstrated that complications were fewer with a straight nail design compared with a curvilinear design. A systematic review by Wong et al. reported satisfactory results in displaced two- and three-part proximal humeral fracture treatment with intramedullary nails. Sun et al. compared locking plates with intramedullary nails in displaced proximal humeral fractures in a systematic review and meta-analysis and demonstrated similar performance between the two fixation types.

Plate-and-screw constructs provide the most stable fixation of the three fixation methods (Fig. 5.28). Locked plates add stability, especially in osteoporotic bone. An open reduction and rigid fixation allow accurate reduction and stabilization of the tuberosities, which is important because malunion of the tuberosities is poorly tolerated and is associated with poor outcomes in posttraumatic reconstructive shoulder arthroplasty. A prospective randomized trial by Zhu et al. found that at 1-year follow-up patients treated with locking plates had better outcomes than those treated with locked

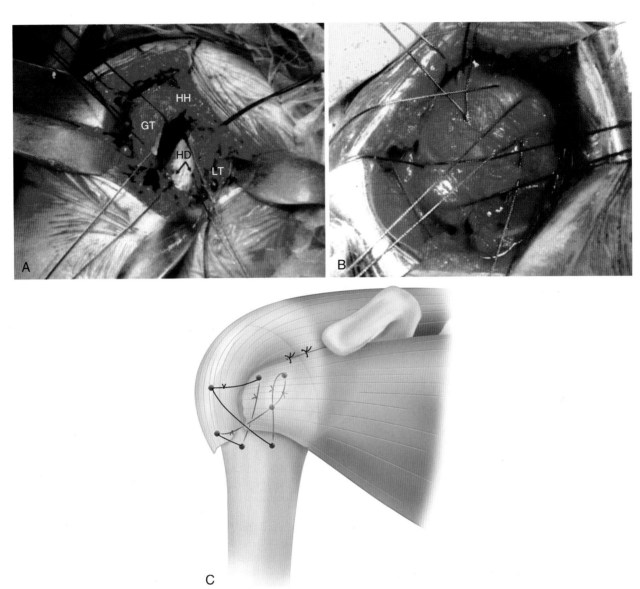

FIGURE 5.24 Transosseous fixation of displaced proximal humeral fracture. **A,** Sutures placed through drill holes in medial and lateral aspects of humeral diaphysis (HD). Black arrows (just below HD) indicate drill holes in diaphysis. *GT,* Greater tuberosity; *LT,* lesser tuberosity; *HH,* humeral head. **B,** Just before tying of knots there is adequate reduction and balance of involved rotator cuff tendons. Fracture site has been closed, and both tuberosities have been placed below articular margin of humeral head. Note cruciate configuration of sutures. **C,** Final suture configuration. (From Dimakopoulos P, Panagopoulos A, Kasimatis G: Transosseous suture fixation of proximal humeral fractures: surgical technique, *J Bone Joint Surg* 91A[Suppl 2, pt 1]:8, 2009.)

intramedullary nailing, but at 3-year follow-up outcomes were equal. The locking nail group had a significantly lower complication rate (4%) than the locking plate group (13%). Konrad et al. also reported similar outcomes in three-part proximal humeral fractures treated with intramedullary nailing (58 fractures) or plate fixation (153 fractures).

Historically, plate fixation of the proximal humerus has been fraught with complications, with malunion and nonunion caused by poor fixation in the humeral head (Fig. 5.29). In addition, extensive soft-tissue dissection increases the possibility of osteonecrosis of the humeral head, leading to a painful and functionally limited shoulder joint. The development of locked proximal humeral plates was expected

to improve treatment of these complex injuries greatly. The advantage of ORIF with a locked plate is an ability to reduce the fracture fragments into an anatomic position and stabilize them rigidly to allow early motion. Numerous outcome studies are now available because the locked proximal humeral plate has been widely used for more than 10 years; however, as was pointed out in a Cochrane review, there is little level I or II evidence. A recent randomized controlled trial comparing locked plating with conservative treatment of three-part and four-part fractures in elderly patients found no difference in outcomes at 1-year follow-up. Despite the lack of a large body of supporting literature, the locked proximal humeral plate is considered by most fracture surgeons to be a great

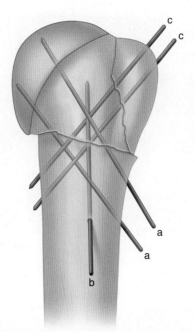

FIGURE 5.25 Placement of percutaneous pins for fracture fixation. Two are passed through lateral aspect of shaft, just above deltoid insertion (*a*), and one is placed through anterior cortex (*b*); if greater tuberosity is fractured and displaced, two pins are inserted retrograde (*c*) to reduce and repair this fracture component.

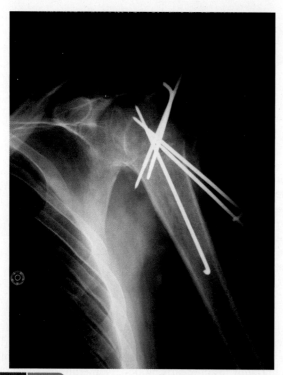

FIGURE 5.26 Two-part proximal humeral fracture stabilized with percutaneous pins.

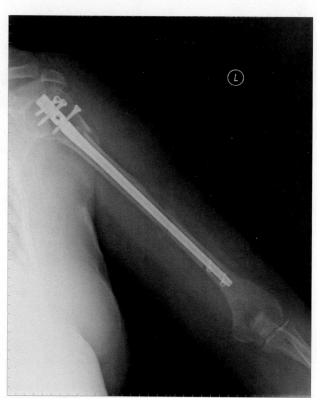

FIGURE 5.27 Fixation of segmental proximal humeral fracture with locked intramedullary nail.

improvement in the management of proximal humeral fractures, and it has become the implant of choice for these fractures. Schnetzke et al. reported 98 patients treated with locked plating and concluded that anatomic reduction significantly improved outcomes.

Much attention has been focused on the medial side of the metaphyseal injury. Gardner et al. called attention to this by documenting the importance of the inferior screw behaving as a medial calcar substitution. Biomechanical studies have confirmed this importance, and Jung et al. confirmed it clinically by identifying medial comminution and insufficient medial support (no cortical or screw support) as independent risk factors for loss of reduction in 17 (7%) of 252 proximal humeral fractures. As an alternative to medial calcar screws, fracture site impaction adds stability by impacting the humeral head onto the humeral shaft. As modified by Torchia, valgus impaction osteotomy (Fig. 5.30A-D) appears promising, although no large series have been reported. In a biomechanical study, Weeks et al. found that fracture impaction increased the ability of the locking plate to withstand repetitive varus loading and was biomechanically superior to locking plate fixation alone. Gardner et al. described the use of a fibular strut graft to provide medial column support. Although promising, the technique also is demanding, and further randomized trials are needed to confirm its efficacy. Kim et al. noted improvement using a fibular strut graft versus inferomedial screws in conjunction with locking plates in four-part fractures, but there was no advantage noted in three-part fractures. In a systematic review, Saltzman et al. found satisfactory results when fibular strut grafts were used for augmentation.

Some issues with open reduction and locked plating include the extensive exposure required for plate application that carries a risk of damage to neurovascular structures, especially the ascending branch of the lateral circumflex artery. The complication and reoperation rates do remain high with this technique. Screw perforation through the humeral head

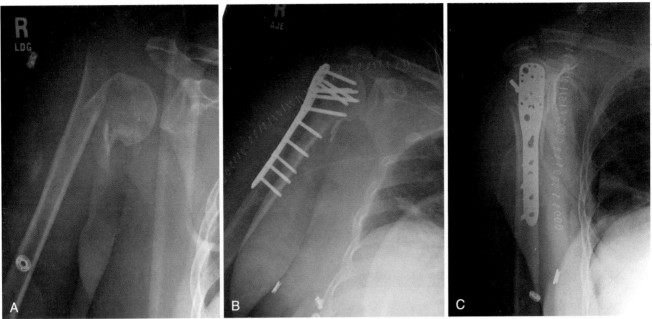

FIGURE 5.28 **A,** Displaced two-part surgical neck fracture with extension between greater and lesser tuberosities. **B** and **C,** After locking plate fixation. Note screw in inferior head because of medial comminution. **SEE TECHNIQUE 5.5.**

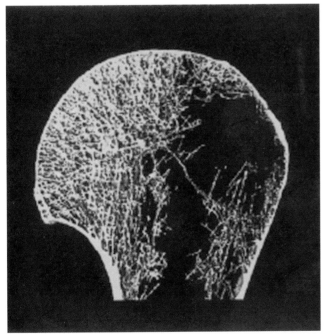

FIGURE 5.29 Micro-CT study of cancellous trabecular bone in humeral head shows marked porosity in greater tuberosity region and densest bone just underneath humeral head. (From Meyer DC, Fucentese SF, Koller B, et al: Association of osteopenia of the humeral head with full-thickness rotator cuff tears, *J Shoulder Elbow Surg* 13:333, 2004.)

is the most frequently reported complication. Perforation can occur as cutout from fracture settlement or from poor initial technique. Calcium phosphate cement augmentation has been shown to decrease this complication. Other complications include arthrofibrosis, impingement, malunion, nonunion, osteonecrosis, infection, and hardware failure. Poor outcomes are associated with initial varus displacement of three- and four-part fractures.

In an attempt to decrease complications with plate fixation, Gardner et al. used an anterolateral acromial (Mackenzie) approach in which the axillary nerve is identified and protected, anterior dissection near the critical blood supply is avoided, substantial muscle retraction is minimized, and the lateral plating zone is directly accessed (see Technique 5.6). Laflamme et al. reported no axillary nerve injuries and no loss of reduction in fractures treated with percutaneous humeral plating through two minimal incisions (a lateral deltoid split and a more distal shaft incision). As our understanding of the anatomy of the proximal humerus and our instruments improve, less invasive techniques appear promising. Electrophysiologic findings in a study by Westphal et al., however, revealed a 10% axillary nerve injury rate.

FIXATION OF SPECIFIC FRACTURE TYPES

- *Two-part greater tuberosity fractures* have historically been treated operatively when displacement is greater than 1 cm; however, Rath et al. reported satisfactory outcomes after nonoperative treatment of 69 fractures with less than 3 mm of displacement. Many authors have suggested that the shoulder has little tolerance for displacement of the tuberosities and have advocated operative treatment for displacement of more than 5 mm because of functional loss and complications secondary to impingement. Usually these fractures are stabilized with transosseous sutures (Fig. 5.31; see also Fig. 5.23) or occasionally with screws in larger fragments. The rotator interval also must be repaired.
- *Two-part surgical neck fractures* with displacement do poorly with nonoperative treatment. Closed reduction and percutaneous pinning have been reported to be successful

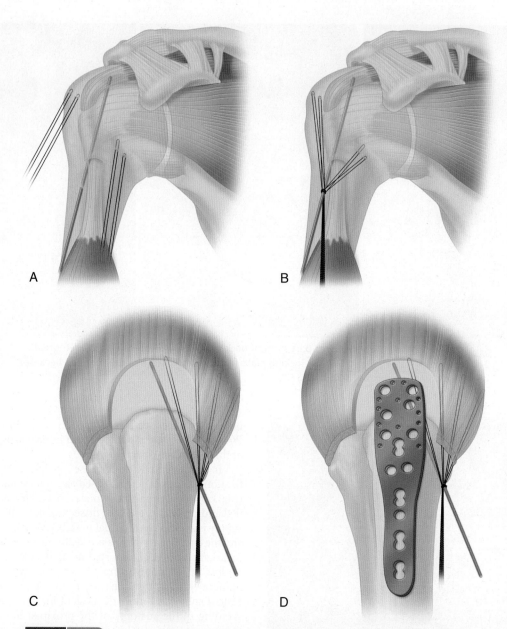

FIGURE 5.30   Fixation of proximal humeral fracture after valgus impaction osteotomy. **A,** Long Steinmann pin is placed from shaft into head segment. **B,** Traction sutures are tensioned and tied to pin. Tensioning sutures pulls head segment out of varus. **C,** Lateral view of proximal humerus after provisional fixation; note that position of pin and sutures allows unobstructed access for definitive fixation with precontoured locking plate **(D).** (Redrawn from Torchia ME: Technical tips for fixation of proximal humeral fractures in elderly patients, *Instr Course Lect* 59:553, 2010, with permission from the Mayo Foundation of Medical Education and Research, Rochester, MN.)

in fractures that are reducible and are not comminuted. Complications such as loss of fixation, pin migration, infection, and malunion have made rigid intramedullary nailing our preferred technique, however, for fractures that can be reduced closed and for segmental fractures (see Fig. 5.27). The violation of the rotator cuff is offset by the advantages of decreased soft-tissue violation and decreased blood loss compared with ORIF. Widely displaced fractures, fractures with comminution, and irreducible fractures are stabilized with a locked-plate construct (see Fig. 5.28). Improved proximal fixation of these systems has increased stability so

that immediate postoperative range of motion is allowed. For extremely osteopenic patients, Banco et al. described a "parachute" technique, which included a valgus impaction osteotomy and tension-band fixation incorporating transosseous sutures (Fig. 5.32). Union was obtained in all 14 elderly patients, and patient satisfaction and function were excellent.

- *Three-part proximal humeral fractures* in elderly patients with osteopenic bone may require hemiarthroplasty, but for most of these fractures plate fixation is the preferred procedure. Realignment of the head and shaft, combined with reduction of the tuberosity, gives the best chance

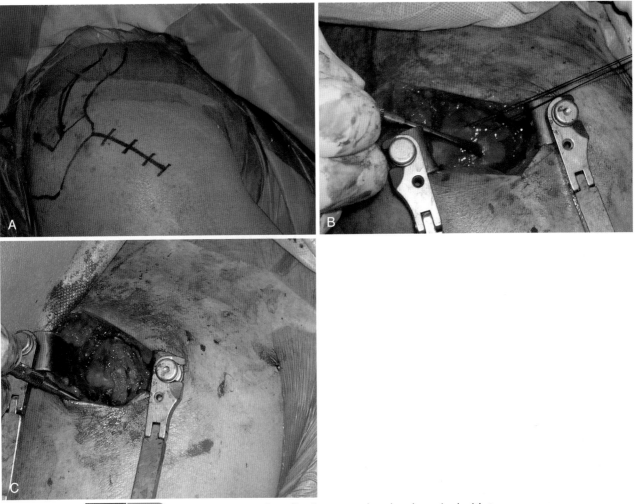

FIGURE 5.31 **A** to **C,** Greater tuberosity fracture reduced and repaired with transosseous sutures.

for a good outcome. The rigid fixation provided by locking plates allows early range of motion, one of the goals of operative treatment.

■ *Four-part proximal humeral fractures* treated nonoperatively generally have poor outcomes; however, poor bone quality makes fixation difficult, and the vascular insult to the articular surface increases the risk of osteonecrosis of the humeral head. Osteonecrosis alone does not lead to a poor outcome if the anatomic relationships of the humeral head, tuberosities, and shaft are reestablished. Wijgman et al. reported osteonecrosis in 22 (37%) of 60 patients with three-part and four-part proximal humeral fractures treated with T-plates or cerclage wires, but 17 of the 22 patients had good or excellent functional outcomes. In young, active patients, open reduction and plate fixation usually are successful if soft-tissue stripping is kept to a minimum to avoid further damage to the humeral head blood supply. Rigid fixation with locking plates currently is our procedure of choice for four-part proximal humeral fractures in young, active patients. Initial varus displacement has been shown to be associated with poor outcomes, as have varus malreductions.

Successful closed reduction and percutaneous pinning have been reported, but we have no experience with this technique for four-part fractures. Hemiarthroplasty is a viable option in elderly patients with low functional demands.

INTRAMEDULLARY NAILING OF A PROXIMAL HUMERAL FRACTURE

TECHNIQUE 5.4

■ Position the patient on a radiolucent table with the thorax "bumped" 30 to 40 degrees. Place the image intensifier unit on the opposite side of the table from the surgeon; rolling the unit back allows an adequate anteroposterior view (Fig. 5.33A,B), and rolling it forward allows an adequate lateral view of the shoulder and humerus (Fig. 5.33C,D).

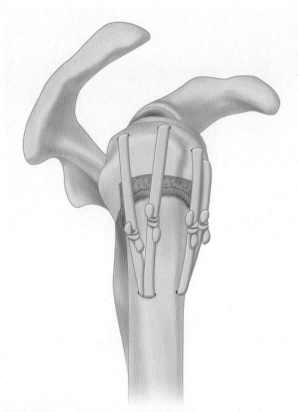

FIGURE **5.32** Parachute technique using valgus impaction osteotomy and tension-band fixation incorporating transosseous sutures.

- Make an incision diagonally from the anterolateral corner of the acromion, splitting the deltoid in line with its fibers in the raphe between the anterior and middle thirds of the deltoid (Fig. 5.34). To protect the axillary nerve, avoid splitting the deltoid more than 5 cm distal to the acromion.
- Under direct observation, incise the rotator cuff in line with its fibers. Use full-thickness sutures to protect the cuff from damage during reaming of the humeral canal.
- Use a threaded pin as a "joystick" in the posterior humeral head to derotate the head into a reduced position (Fig. 5.35A,B).
- Place the initial guidewire posterior to the biceps tendon and advance it under fluoroscopic guidance into the appropriate position as shown on anteroposterior and lateral views (Fig. 5.35C).
- Carefully advance the proximal reamer, protecting the rotator cuff.
- Use the reduction device to reduce the fracture and pass the bead-tipped guidewire.
- With sequentially larger reamers, ream the humerus to the predetermined diameter, usually 1.0 to 1.5 mm larger than the nail diameter.
- When reaming is completed, pass the nail down the humeral canal, avoiding distraction of the fracture (Fig. 5.36); ensure that the nail is below the articular surface of the humeral head.
- With the use of the outrigger device, insert the proximal locking bolts (see Fig. 5.35D). Carefully spread the soft tissues to avoid injury to the axillary nerve.

- Repair the rotator cuff with full-thickness sutures under direct observation (Fig. 5.37).
- Confirm reduction and screw placement and length on anteroposterior and lateral fluoroscopy images.
- Early rehabilitation is begun with active-assisted range-of-motion exercises.

OPEN REDUCTION AND INTERNAL FIXATION OF PROXIMAL HUMERAL FRACTURES

TECHNIQUE 5.5

- Position the patient on a radiolucent table with a bean-bag "bump" holding the shoulder and thorax 30 to 40 degrees off the table. Place the C-arm on the opposite side of the table from the surgeon; rolling the unit back allows an adequate anteroposterior view (see Fig. 5.33A,B), and rolling it forward allows an adequate lateral view of the shoulder and humerus (see Fig. 5.33C,D).
- Make a deltopectoral approach to the proximal humerus.
- Release the anterior portion of the deltoid to expose the fracture site.
- If necessary, use a threaded pin as a joystick in the posterior humeral head to derotate the head into a reduced position (see Fig. 5.35). Sutures placed through the rotator cuff tendon (supraspinatus) also can be helpful for mobilization (see Fig. 5.23).
- For three-part or four-part fractures, place sutures into the rotator cuff tendons attached to the displaced tuberosity to aid in reduction (Fig. 5.38).
- For simpler fracture patterns, reduce the fracture and provisionally fix it with Kirschner wires; confirm reduction with fluoroscopy. If medial comminution is present, check to ensure that a varus malreduction has not occurred.
- Place the plate onto the greater tuberosity, posterior to the biceps tendon, and provisionally fix it in place with Kirschner wires; confirm correct plate position with fluoroscopy. A plate placed too far proximally may cause impingement, and a plate placed too close to the biceps tendon may damage the anterior humeral circumflex artery.
- Place two locking screws through the plate holes into the humeral head segment and one or two screws into the shaft. Confirm subchondral placement of the proximal screws and the quality of the reduction with fluoroscopy; this is easier with the fluoroscopy unit on the opposite side of the table from the surgeon.
- When accurate reduction is confirmed, insert remaining screws under direct fluoroscopic guidance.
- For fractures with medial comminution, fix the plate to the proximal segment with screws and reduce the shaft

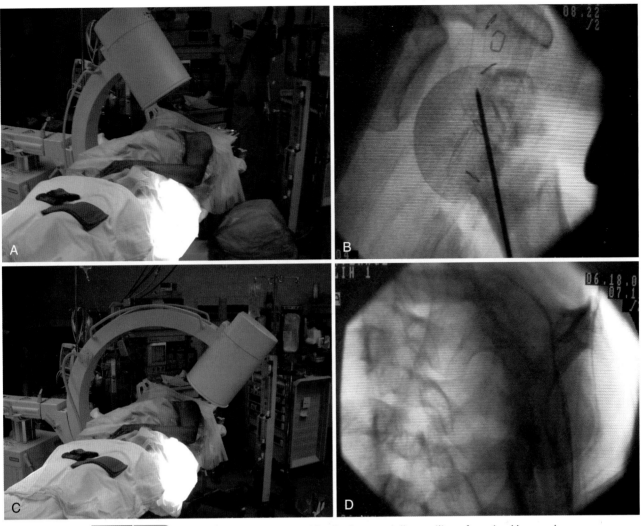

FIGURE 5.33 Placement of image intensifier for intramedullary nailing of proximal humeral fracture (**A** and **C**). Rolling unit back (**A**) allows anteroposterior view (**B**), whereas rolling it forward (**C**) allows lateral view (**D**) of shoulder and humerus. **SEE TECHNIQUES 5.4, 5.5, AND 5.9.**

segment to the plate. This helps avoid varus malposition, which is associated with higher failure rates. Screw fixation into the inferomedial humeral head also adds stability for fractures with medial comminution (see Fig. 5.28B).

■ In three-part or four-part fractures, sutures inserted into the supraspinatus and subscapularis tendons aid in controlling the fracture fragments (see Fig. 5.38).

■ Reduce the tuberosities to the articular surface and to each other with pins or sutures or both (Fig. 5.39); Observation or palpation through the rotator interval may aid in reduction of the lesser tuberosity to the humeral head. Often there is a small segment of articular surface with the lesser tuberosity that is a key to reduction. Fluoroscopy is helpful during difficult proximal humeral reconstruction.

■ Fix the plate in the same manner as for a two-part fracture. Rotator cuff sutures can be incorporated into the plate for added stability.

■ Confirm reduction and screw placement on anteroposterior and lateral fluoroscopy images.

POSTOPERATIVE CARE An early rehabilitation program is begun with active-assisted range-of-motion exercises.

ANTEROLATERAL ACROMIAL APPROACH FOR INTERNAL FIXATION OF PROXIMAL HUMERAL FRACTURE

TECHNIQUE 5.6

(GARDNER ET AL.; MACKENZIE)

■ Position the patient in either the beach chair or supine semilateral position.

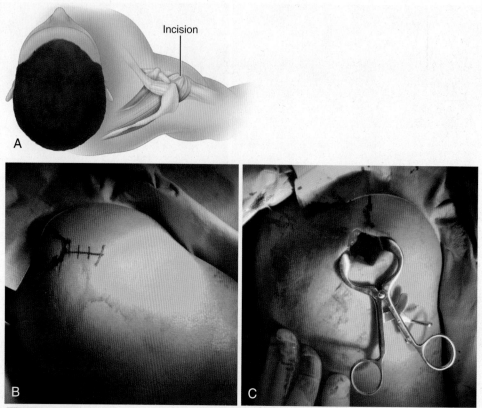

FIGURE 5.34 Entry portal for intramedullary nailing of proximal humeral fracture. **A,** Diagonal incision from anterolateral corner of acromion splits deltoid in line with its fibers in raphe between anterior and middle thirds. **B,** Location of incision. **C,** Establishment of portal. **SEE TECHNIQUES 5.4 AND 5.9.**

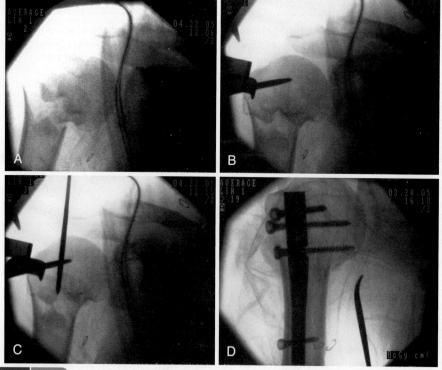

FIGURE 5.35 Intramedullary nailing of proximal humeral fracture. **A,** Two-part surgical neck fracture. **B,** Threaded pin used as "joystick" to reduce fracture. **C,** Placement of initial guidewire. **D,** After nail insertion and placement of locking screws. **SEE TECHNIQUES 5.4 AND 5.5.**

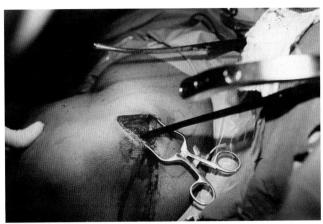

FIGURE 5.36 Antegrade insertion of humeral nail for fixation of proximal humeral fracture. **SEE TECHNIQUE 5.4.**

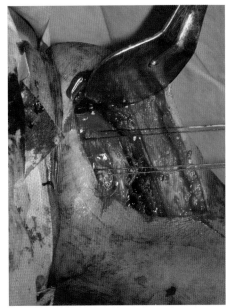

FIGURE 5.38 Open reduction and internal fixation of proximal humeral shaft fracture. Sutures placed in rotator cuff can be used to assist reduction of tuberosities. **SEE TECHNIQUE 5.5.**

lary nerve to a level where the axillary nerve overlies the junction of the head and shaft of the plate (Fig. 5.40B). While positioning the plate, be sure to stay on the "bare spot" on the lateral cortex posterior to the bicipital groove (Fig. 5.40C) to avoid the humeral head penetrating vessels.
- Secure the plate to the humeral shaft through the lower soft-tissue window distal to the axillary nerve.
- After thorough irrigation, close the raphe and deltoid fascial layers with absorbable sutures. Place a suction drain and close the subcutaneous tissue in layers.

POSTOPERATIVE CARE Postoperative care is the same as that after Technique 5.5.

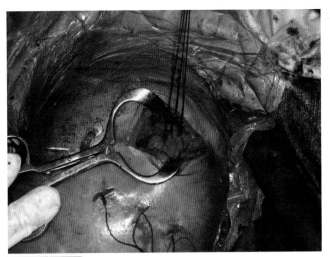

FIGURE 5.37 Repair of rotator cuff after nail insertion. **SEE TECHNIQUE 5.4.**

- Make a 10-cm skin incision from the palpable anterolateral edge of the acromion distally in line with the fibers of the deltoid.
- Identify the deltoid fascia and anterior deltoid raphe between the anterior middle heads of the deltoid (Fig. 5.40A) and split the raphe in line with its fibers for several centimeters. For maximal exposure, split the deltoid up to the margin of the acromion but do not split it distally more than 5 cm from its origin to avoid damage to the axillary nerve. To prevent damage to the axillary nerve from too-distal dissection, place a stay suture at the inferior border of the deltoid raphe.
- If the nerve is in proximity to a fracture line, gently explore it. If it is tethered or incarcerated in the fracture, gently free it.
- Reduce the fracture fragments with indirect reduction techniques, working within the tuberosity fracture lines if present. If extension of the subdeltoid interval anteriorly is necessary, take care to handle the soft tissues carefully.
- With the fracture reduced and the axillary nerve protected, slide the plate from proximal to distal under the axil-

■ COMPLICATIONS

The most common complication of proximal humeral fractures is loss of motion (stiffness). Early physical therapy is associated with improved motion, but many patients do not recover full motion even with early physical therapy. Impingement from high-riding tuberosities or subacromial scarring also can limit motion. Nonunion also is fairly common, but nonunion rates have been decreasing with the use of new technologies such as locking plates and improved intramedullary nails. Malunion can result from unstable or delayed fracture fixation, patient factors, and poor surgical technique. In older patients with limited functional demands, malunion generally is well tolerated, but it may be debilitating in younger patients because of poor shoulder function, impingement, or rotator cuff tears. Osteonecrosis is relatively uncommon after nondisplaced or unoperated two-part and three-part fractures; functional outcome is improved if the proximal humeral anatomy has been restored. The presence of osteonecrosis does not always result in a poor outcome; osteonecrosis

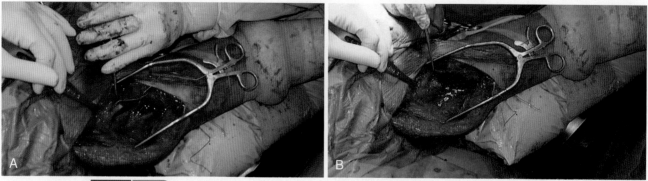

FIGURE 5.39 Open reduction and internal fixation of proximal humeral shaft fracture (see text). **A** and **B**, Sutures used for reduction and fixation of tuberosity fragments. **SEE TECHNIQUE 5.5.**

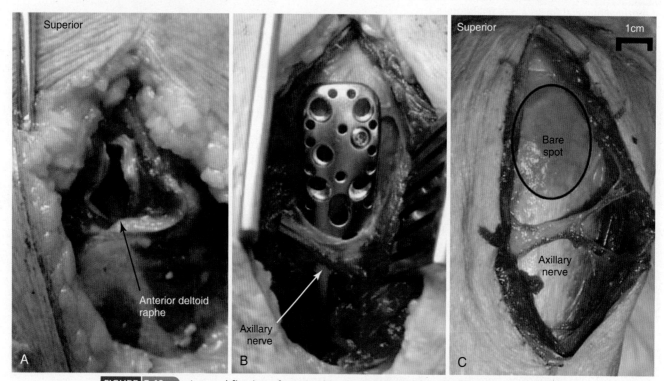

FIGURE 5.40 Internal fixation of proximal humeral fracture through anterolateral acromial approach. **A**, Raphe between anterior and middle head of deltoid is developed. **B**, With axillary nerve protected, plate is slid deep to nerve. **C**, "Bare spot" on lateral humerus posterior to bicipital groove; plate position here avoids humeral head penetrating vessels. (From Gardner MJ, Voos JE, Wanich T, et al. Vascular implications of minimally invasive plating of proximal humerus fractures. *J Orthop Trauma* 2006;20:602-607). **SEE TECHNIQUE 5.6.**

may be evident radiographically but cause minimal symptoms. Because late hemiarthroplasty has poorer results than early hemiarthroplasty, it is important to be sure that ORIF can adequately stabilize four-part fractures and restore humeral anatomy before this option is chosen.

FRACTURES OF THE HUMERAL SHAFT

Fractures of the humeral shaft account for approximately 3% of all fractures; most can be treated nonoperatively. Charnley stated, "It is perhaps the easiest of the major long bones to treat by conservative methods." The range of motion afforded by the shoulder and elbow joints, coupled with a tolerance for small amounts of shortening, allow radiographic imperfections that cause minimal functional deficit and are well tolerated by the patient. Historically, methods of conservative treatment have included skeletal traction, abduction casting and splinting, Velpeau dressing, and hanging arm cast, each with its own advantages and disadvantages.

Functional bracing has essentially replaced all other conservative methods and has become the "gold standard" for nonoperative treatment because of its ease of application, adjustability, allowance of shoulder and elbow motion, relatively low cost, and reproducible results. Initially popularized by Sarmiento in 1977, the functional brace works on the principles of the hydraulic effect of the brace, active contraction of the muscles, and beneficial effect of gravity. Union rates of 77% to 100% have been reported with this technique (Papasoulis et al. 2010). In a randomized controlled trial comparing minimally invasive plate osteosynthesis and functional bracing, Matsunaga et al. reported a 15% nonunion rate with functional bracing. Driesman et al. reported 84 consecutive patients with diaphyseal humeral fractures managed nonoperatively. Within 6 months 87% of fractures healed. They noted that a mobile humeral shaft fracture at the 6-week follow-up visit was a predictor of nonunion with 82% sensitivity and 99% specificity. This author counsels patients appropriately as to risk of developing a nonunion if fracture site variability exists at 6 weeks. We currently use a coaptation splint or hanging arm cast for the first 7 to 10 days to allow pain to subside and then convert to a prefabricated functional brace. The use of a sling is discouraged to avoid varus and internal rotation deformities. Pendulum exercises are started early, and use of the extremity is encouraged as tolerated, avoiding active shoulder abduction. The brace is worn until the patient is pain free and there is radiographic evidence of union. Skin maceration is a concern, so daily hygiene is stressed. Morbid obesity may increase the risk of varus deformities; however, these deformities are more of a cosmetic issue than a functional issue and often are not evident in an obese arm. Shields et al. showed no correlation between residual deformity and functional outcome scores.

A nonrandomized study by Jawa et al. compared outcomes in 21 distal-third diaphyseal fractures treated with functional bracing to those of 19 treated with plate-and-screw fixation. Operative treatment resulted in more predictable alignment and faster healing but was associated with more complications, such as iatrogenic nerve injury, loss of fixation, and infection. Plate-and-screw fixation was done in two patients initially treated with bracing because of concerns about alignment. Complications associated with bracing included skin breakdown and malunion. The advantages, disadvantages, and risks of both nonoperative and operative treatment should be discussed with the patient before a decision is made.

We reserve the use of a hanging arm cast for patients in whom compliance or finances preclude the use of a functional brace. Guidelines for acceptable reduction include less than 3 cm of shortening, angulation of less than 20 degrees, and rotation of less than 30 degrees. In a series of 32 patients with humeral shaft fractures treated nonoperatively, Shields et al. found that residual angular deformity ranging from 0 to 18 degrees in the sagittal plane and from 2 to 27 degrees in the coronal plane had no correlation with patient-reported outcomes.

INDICATIONS FOR OPERATIVE TREATMENT

The choice of operative treatment for a humeral shaft fracture depends on multiple factors. McKee divided the indications for operative treatment into three categories: (1) fracture indications, (2) associated injuries, and (3) patient indications (Box 5.2). Some indications are more absolute than others. Failure of conservative treatment, pathologic fracture, displaced intraarticular extension, vascular injury, and brachial

---

BOX 5.2

Indications for Primary Operative Treatment of Humeral Shaft Fractures

Fracture Indications
- Failure to obtain and maintain adequate closed reduction
  Shortening >3 cm
  Rotation >30 degrees
  Angulation >20 degrees
- Segmental fracture
- Pathologic fracture
- Intraarticular extension (shoulder joint, elbow joint)

Associated Injuries
- Open wound
- Vascular injury
- Brachial plexus injury
- Ipsilateral forearm fracture
- Ipsilateral shoulder or elbow fracture
- Bilateral humeral fractures
- Lower extremity fracture requiring upper extremity weight bearing
- Burns
- High-velocity gunshot injury
- Chronic associated joint stiffness of elbow or shoulder

Patient Indications
- Multiple injuries, polytrauma
- Head injury (Glasgow Coma Scale score = 8)
- Chest trauma
- Poor patient tolerance, compliance
- Unfavorable body habitus (morbid obesity, large breasts)

From McKee MD: Fractures of the shaft of the humerus. In Bucholz RW, Heckman JD, Court-Brown CM, editors: *Rockwood and Green's fractures in adults*, ed 6, Philadelphia, 2006, Lippincott Williams & Wilkins.

---

plexus injury almost always require surgery. Other conditions, such as minimally displaced segmental fractures and obesity, are only relative indications. Our most common indication for operative treatment is early mobilization of patients with polytrauma. Treatment decisions must take all factors into consideration, tailoring the treatment to the specific patient.

The goal of operative treatment of humeral shaft fractures is to reestablish length, alignment, and rotation with stable fixation that allows early motion and ideally early weight bearing on the fractured extremity. Options for fixation include plate osteosynthesis, intramedullary nailing, and external fixation. External fixation generally is reserved for high-energy gunshot wounds, fractures with significant soft-tissue injuries, and fractures with massive contamination. Suzuki et al. suggested that immediate external fixation with planned conversion to plate fixation within 2 weeks is a safe and effective strategy for treatment of humeral shaft fractures in selected patients with multiple injuries or severe soft-tissue injuries that preclude early plate fixation; however, two of their 17 patients, both with open fractures, developed deep infections after conversion from external fixation to plating.

PLATE OSTEOSYNTHESIS

Plate osteosynthesis remains the gold standard of fixation for humeral shaft fractures. Plating can be used for fractures with proximal and distal extension and for open fractures. It provides enough stability to allow early upper extremity weight bearing in polytrauma patients and produces minimal shoulder or elbow morbidity, as shown by Tingstad et al. Numerous reports in the literature cite high union rates, low complication rates, and rapid return to function after plate fixation of humeral shaft fractures. Five large series (Foster et al., McKee et al., Vander Griend et al., Bell et al., and Tingstad et al.) including 361 fractures had an average union rate of 96.7%.

A prospective, randomized comparison of plate fixation and intramedullary nail fixation of humeral shaft fractures found no significant differences in the function of the shoulder and elbow, but shoulder impingement occurred more often with intramedullary nailing, and a second surgical procedure was required in more patients with intramedullary nails than with a plate. Another study comparing antegrade intramedullary nailing with plating found that although patients had slightly more shoulder pain after intramedullary nailing than after plating, there was no difference in shoulder joint function except for flexion, which was better in patients with plating. A meta-analysis of the literature that included 155 patients found that reoperation and shoulder impingement were significantly more common after intramedullary nailing than after compression plating. In their updated meta-analysis, Heineman et al. concluded that the data were insufficient to show superiority of either technique. Gottschalk et al., however, noted that although complication rates in regard to infection and nerve palsies were significantly lower in intramedullary nailing compared with ORIF with plates (3.1% compared with 7.8%, and 1.5% compared with 3.0%, respectively), mortality was higher with intramedullary nailing (4.9% vs. 0.7%, respectively), and intramedullary nailing had significantly more pathologic fractures than open reduction with plate fixation (26.8% compared with 1.5%, respectively).

■ IMPLANT CHOICE

The most commonly used plate for fixation of humeral shaft fractures is the broad, 4.5-mm, limited-contact dynamic compression plate (Fig. 5.41); occasionally, a narrow, 4.5- or 3.5-mm, limited-contact dynamic compression plate is used for smaller bones. The distal metaphyseal-diaphyseal transition zone may require dual 3.5-mm, limited-contact dynamic compression plates (Fig. 5.42) or newer plates designed specifically for the metaphysis. For spiral or oblique fractures, the ideal construct consists of a lag screw with a neutralization plate, whereas transverse fractures are ideally suited for a compression plating technique. In these fractures, attaining provisional reduction with a lag screw, Kirschner wire, or mini-fragment plate (Eglseder technique) allows direct observation of the reduction and a relatively simple plate application on the reduced humeral shaft (Fig. 5.43); we believe this also limits periosteal stripping by clamps.

Comminuted fractures may require a bridge plating technique. Anatomic reduction of each fracture fragment is unnecessary. Attaining correct alignment, rotation, and length without disrupting the soft-tissue attachments to the comminuted fragments often leads to successful healing. Livani et al. reported 15 patients with bridge plating done through two small incisions proximal and distal to

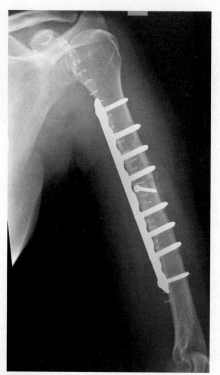

FIGURE **5.41** Anterior plating of humeral shaft fracture with limited-contact dynamic compression plate in neutralization mode with lag screw.

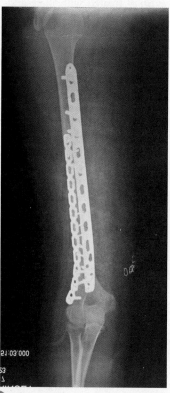

FIGURE **5.42** Dual plating of distal metaphyseal-diaphyseal humeral shaft fracture.

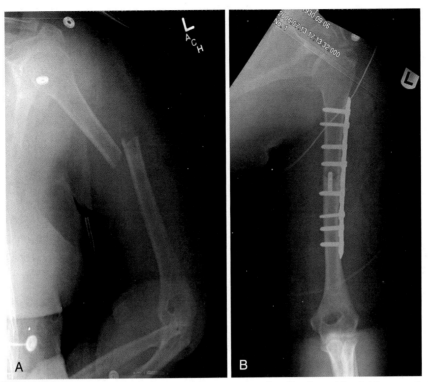

FIGURE 5.43   **A,** Displaced humeral shaft fracture. **B,** After fixation with mini-fragment plate (Eglseder technique) and compression plating.

the fracture; all fractures united within 12 weeks except for a grade III open fracture with an associated brachial plexus injury.

In patients with poor bone quality, longer implants should be used to improve stability (Fig. 5.44). Locking plates and screw augmentation with methyl methacrylate have been reported to add more stability to the construct. Generally, at least eight cortices (four screws) above and below the fracture are necessary to avoid screw pullout. The length of the plate is as important as the number of screws. More screws and longer plates for a greater working length of the implant may be needed for instability caused by poor bone quality or fracture comminution. We reserve the use of locking screws for poor bone quality and short segments.

APPROACH

Numerous approaches can be used for plate fixation of the humerus. Fractures of the middle or proximal third usually are best approached through an anterolateral approach (brachialis-splitting approach). A posterior approach (triceps-splitting or modified posterior approach) is best for fractures that are midshaft or extend into the distal third of the humerus (Fig. 5.45). Gerwin, Hotchkiss, and Weiland described a modified posterior approach in which the triceps is reflected medially off the lateral intermuscular septum (see Technique 5.7). This approach exposes an average 10 cm more of the humeral shaft than the standard posterior approach. Less frequently, a direct lateral or anteromedial approach may be appropriate. A recent study using this approach showed high union rates and low complications.

POSTOPERATIVE CARE

Postoperatively, range of motion of the shoulder and elbow is begun within the first week and weight bearing usually is allowed if fixation is stable. A biomechanical study found that both large (4.5-mm) and small (3.5-mm) plate constructs would experience plastic deformation during bilateral crutch weight bearing in patients weighing 50 kg (~110 lb) or more. The large construct was not predicted to fail with loads of 90 kg (almost 200 lb) or less, whereas the small-fragment construct was predicted to fail in patients weighing 70 kg (approximately 150 lb) or more.

COMPLICATIONS

The most frequently reported complication after plate fixation of humeral shaft fractures is radial nerve palsy. Primary radial nerve injury ranges from 4% to 22%; iatrogenic or secondary injury has been reported to be 0 to 10% (Chang and Ilyas et al.) and is more common in ORIF techniques. Gausden et al.'s report on a single series of a triceps-reflecting approach for ORIF demonstrated a 4% secondary nerve injury rate in a single experienced trauma surgeon's practice. When using an anterolateral (brachialis-splitting) approach, it is essential to ensure that the nerve is not under the implant during plate application to avoid iatrogenic radial nerve injury. Posteriorly, soft-tissue tethers on the radial nerve can lead to iatrogenic injury in posterior approaches. This can be remedied by adequate soft-tissue release off the radial nerve. Infection is reported to occur after 1% to 2% of closed humeral fractures and 5% of open fractures. Refractures occur in approximately 1% of patients. Nonunion of humeral shaft fractures is infrequent. Treatment of nonunion is discussed in chapter 7.

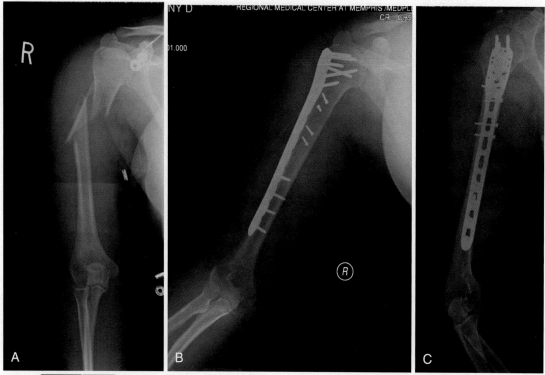

FIGURE 5.44   **A,** Segmental shaft fracture with extension into proximal humerus. **B** and **C,** Long plate used to obtain secure fixation.

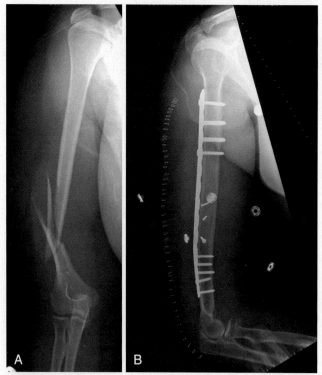

FIGURE 5.45   **A,** Fracture of distal third of humeral shaft. **B,** After plate fixation through posterior triceps-splitting approach.

OPEN REDUCTION AND INTERNAL FIXATION OF THE HUMERAL SHAFT THROUGH A MODIFIED POSTERIOR APPROACH (TRICEPS-REFLECTING)

TECHNIQUE 5.7

- Place the patient in a lateral decubitus position.
- Use a wide proximal preparation and drape to allow for the use of a sterile tourniquet.
- Make an incision from the tourniquet to the tip of the olecranon in line with the humerus (Fig. 5.46A).
- Carry dissection down to the triceps fascia, incise the fascia, and carry the dissection laterally to the intermuscular septum (Fig. 5.46B).
- Identify the lower lateral brachial cutaneous nerve and follow it proximally where it meets the radial nerve as it pierces the septum (Fig. 5.46C). This usually is at the level of the tourniquet. Release the tourniquet.
- Identify the radial nerve.
- Dissect the triceps muscle proximally off the intermuscular septum.
- Free the radial nerve proximally, distally, anteriorly, and posteriorly, including incision of the lateral intermuscular septum for 3 cm to allow mobilization of the nerve (Fig. 5.46D).
- Incise the triceps off the periosteum to expose the humerus; preserve as much of the periosteum as possible.
- Proximally, reflect the posterior border of the deltoid anteriorly if needed for exposure.

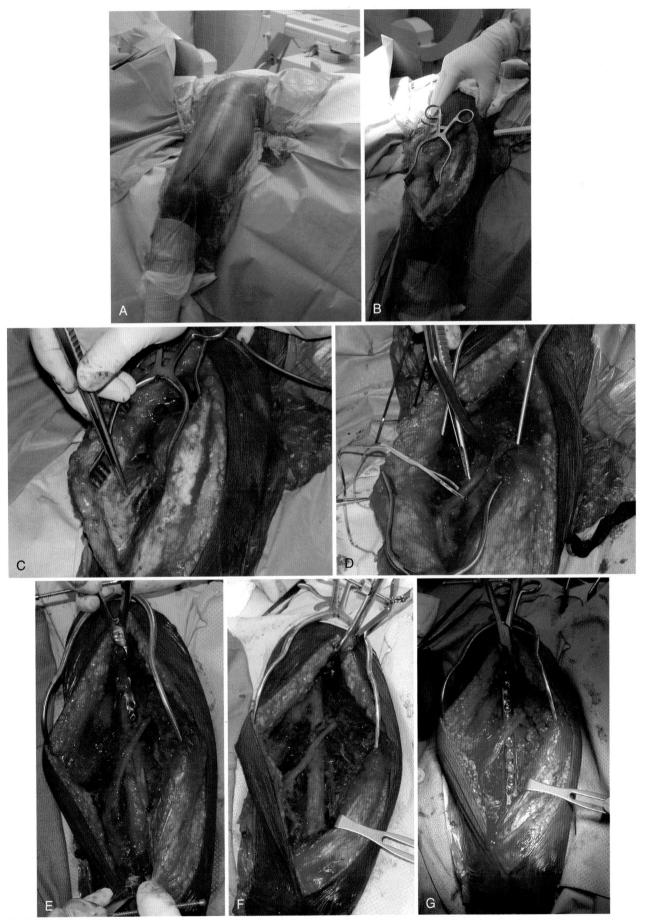

FIGURE 5.46 Open reduction and internal fixation of humeral shaft fracture through modified (triceps-reflecting) posterior approach. **A,** Incision. **B,** Incision of fascia to expose intramuscular septum. **C,** Identification of lateral brachial cutaneous nerve. **D,** Mobilization of radial nerve. **E,** Bone clamp used to control fragments. **F,** After debridement, fixation with lag screw. **G,** After plate application. **SEE TECHNIQUE 5.7.**

- Place a single bone clamp in the proximal and distal fragments, far away from the fracture, to control the fragments and reflect the triceps (Fig. 5.46E). Avoid circumferential stripping of the soft tissues with the clamp.
- After debridement of the fracture site, insert a lag screw for provisional fixation (Fig. 5.46F). Alternatively, for transverse fractures where lag screw fixation is difficult, a compression plating technique can be used, or a minifragment plate (Eglseder technique) can be used for provisional fixation, followed by plate fixation.
- Perform large-fragment plating in neutralization, compression, or bridge-plating mode (Fig. 5.46G).
- Confirm alignment of the humerus and reduction of the fragments with fluoroscopy.
- Perform routine skin closure over a drain.

MINIMALLY INVASIVE PLATE OSTEOSYNTHESIS

Minimally invasive plate osteosynthesis has been shown to be a successful technique in other anatomic areas of the body, particularly the femur and tibia. The theoretical advantages in the upper extremity are (1) less soft-tissue damage, (2) avoidance of shoulder pain as seen with intramedullary nailing, and (3) secondary bone healing. Case reports of minimally invasive plate osteosynthesis of the humeral shaft was first described by Fernández Dell'Oca in 2002, but the first small series was described by Livani and Belangero. They reported 14 of 15 successful unions with this technique. Since then numerous case series, comparative studies, randomized controlled trials, systematic reviews, and meta-analyses have been reported. The data suggest that minimally invasive plate osteosynthesis of the humeral shaft has low nonunion rates, low complication rates, and minimal shoulder problems. On the other hand, this technique is technically challenging and is subject to a learning curve. Surgeons skilled at minimally invasive plate osteosynthesis in other long bones should be able to adopt the technique swiftly. However, surgeons with minimal skills in minimally invasive techniques need to be careful, and should consider a gradual transition from full open to minimally invasive plate osteosynthesis. Box 5.3 outlines basic minimally invasive plate osteosynthesis principles. Tetsworth et al. have written an excellent state-of-the-art review paper on this subject.

TECHNIQUE 5.8

(APIVATTHAKAKUL ET AL.; TETSWORTH ET AL.)

- Place the patient supine on a radiolucent table, with the elbow in mild flexion to relax the biceps and mark the incisions (Fig. 5.47A,B).
- Through a deltopectoral approach, make a proximal incision inferiorly, using the biceps groove and pectoralis tendon as landmarks, and expose the proximal diaphysis immediately lateral to the biceps tendon (Fig. 5.47C,D).

BOX 5.3

Basic Minimally Invasive Plate Osteosynthesis Principles

1. Thorough knowledge of upper extremity anatomy
2. Awareness of at-risk structures, notably the radial nerve
3. Skilled at indirect reduction techniques
4. Understanding of a functional reduction: length, alignment, and rotation
5. Techniques of plate provisional fixation that allows assessment of reduction and plate placement
6. A good understanding of relative stability and secondary bone healing

---

- Begin the distal incision 1 to 2 cm proximal to the antecubital crease and extend it proximally for 4- to 5-cm in the midline (see Fig. 5.47C).
- Identify the interval between the biceps and brachialis laterally and retract the biceps medially. Protect the lateral antebrachial cutaneous nerve beneath (Fig. 5.47E).
- Split the brachialis longitudinally by blunt dissection to bone. Keep the forearm supinated to protect the radial nerve in the distal portion of the approach.
- Obtain provisional fracture reduction under fluoroscopic control and develop a submuscular extraperiosteal tunnel, connecting the two incisions (see Fig. 5.47C).
- Insert a locking compression plate (Fig. 5.47F). If the patient depends on the operated limb for ambulation (polytraumatized patient with lower extremity fractures that limit mobilization), a narrow 4.5-mm plate is used. Align the proximal segment of the plate and use a single unlocked screw to reduce the plate to the anterior humeral cortex. The plate can be precontoured to achieve the most anatomic reduction (Fig. 5.47G and H).
- Augment fixation with two additional locked screws, using the plate to assist with reduction. Then align the distal segment of the plate, checking fracture reduction with fluoroscopy. Correct any malalignment at this time; rotation may be the most difficult to judge correctly.
- Manually compress the fracture site to limit distraction that may result in delayed union.
- After provisional fixation, assess rotation by directly comparing rotational excursion with the opposite limb.
- Reduce the plate to the distal humerus with a single unlocked cortical screw and augment with two additional locked screws.

POSTOPERATIVE CARE A sling is used for comfort for the first 2 weeks postoperatively. Range of motion of the shoulder and elbow (active and assisted) is encouraged immediately without restrictions and gradually increased with emphasis placed on full elbow extension. Minor functional limitations are placed on the arm until solid bridging is noted radiographically, and patients can return to unrestricted activity at 4 to 6 months (Fig. 5.48).

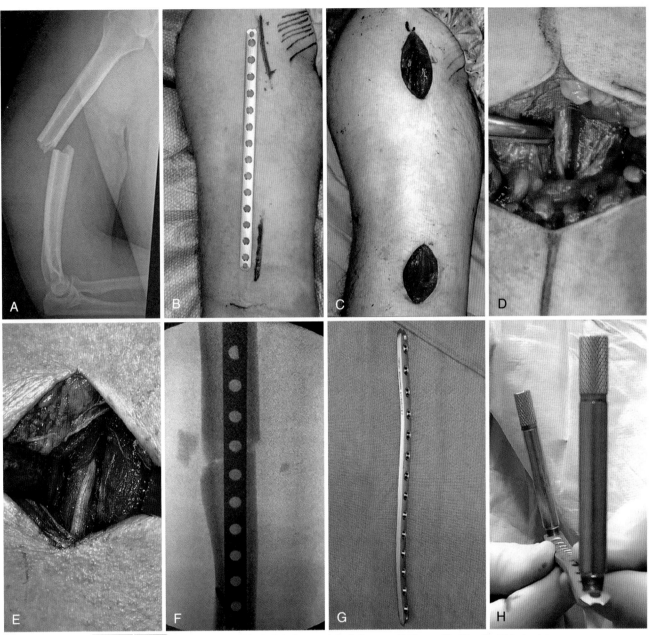

FIGURE 5.47   **A,** Closed midshaft right humeral shaft fracture. **B,** Planned incision for 14-hole plate. **C,** Two incisions on anterior arm connected by a submuscular extraperiosteal tunnel. **D,** Proximal 4- to 5-cm incision at level of pectoralis major insertion, with cephalic vein preserved. **E,** Distal 4- to 5-cm incision proximal to antecubital crease; lateral antebrachial cutaneous nerve identified beneath biceps. **F,** Provisional reduction and alignment after plate insertion. **G,** Plate contoured to match normal anterior humeral cortical surface. **H,** Plate internally rotated 15 to 20 degrees through its midportion, consistent with normal anatomy.   (From Tetsworth K, Hohmann E, Glatt V: Minimally invasive plate osteosynthesis of humeral shaft fractures: current state of the art, *J Am Acad Orthop Surg* 26:252, 2018.) **SEE TECHNIQUE 5.8.**

INTRAMEDULLARY FIXATION

The success of intramedullary nailing in the lower extremities led to an initial enthusiasm for intramedullary nailing of the humeral shaft. Although there are many reports in the literature of good results with nailing techniques, problems with insertion site morbidity and union rates have dampened the original enthusiasm for this mode of treatment. Shoulder pain has been reported after antegrade intramedullary nailing in 16% to 37% of patients in more recent studies, and Bhandari et al. found that reoperation and shoulder impingement were significantly more common after intramedullary nailing than after plate fixation. A systematic review by Zhao et al. found no differences in union rate, infections, or iatrogenic injury to the radial nerve. The risk of shoulder complications, however, was higher. Confounding variables, such as flexible or rigid nails;

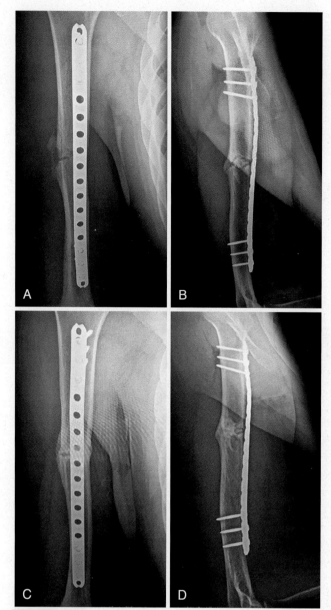

FIGURE 5.48 **A** and **B,** Eight weeks postoperatively demonstrating early callus formation with minor varus alignment. **C** and **D,** One year postoperatively demonstrating mature bridging callus. (From Tetsworth K, Hohmann E, Glatt V: Minimally invasive plate osteosynthesis of humeral shaft fractures: current state of the art, *J Am Acad Orthop Surg* 26:252, 2018.) **SEE TECHNIQUE 5.8.**

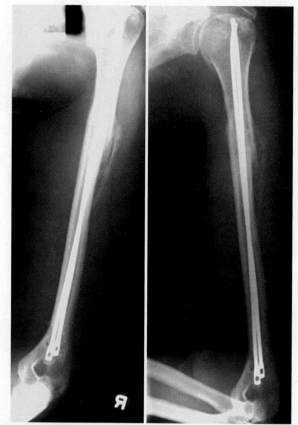

FIGURE 5.49 Humeral shaft fracture treated by closed intramedullary nailing with multiple flexible intramedullary (Ender) nails.

antegrade or retrograde insertion; and lateral, anterolateral, or extraarticular portal for antegrade insertion, make conclusions difficult to interpret. A large well-controlled trial is needed.

Early flexible nails, such as Rush and Enders, provided little axial or rotational stability and required additional forms of stabilization (cerclage wiring or prolonged immobilization) in comminuted or unstable fractures (Fig. 5.49). Even with additional stabilization, the resulting construct generally was not stable enough to allow early motion or weight bearing in multiply injured patients with concomitant lower extremity injuries. The development of locking nails improved stability and rotational control but results still did not reach the successful outcomes obtained in lower extremity fractures.

Because nail sizes were limited, reaming was required for insertion of most locked nails, and fracture distraction was a problem, especially in small medullary canals. Newer nails come in smaller sizes (7, 8, or 9 mm) to fit smaller bones and can be inserted with or without reaming.

An antegrade approach is most commonly used for intramedullary nail fixation of humeral shaft fractures in adults. The specific portal placement is controversial, however. Traditionally, a midacromial lateral incision was used, which tends to place the nail through the posterior humeral head. In addition, the incision through the rotator cuff is not in line with the fibers of the tendon (see Fig. 5.34). An anterolateral starting portal is in line with the humeral medullary canal, and the incision is in line with the fibers of the rotator cuff. Several authors have postulated that shoulder pain after antegrade nailing is caused by the transverse incision through the rotator cuff. Alternatives to antegrade humeral nailing (e.g., plate osteosynthesis) should be considered in patients who have preexisting shoulder pathology or who require upper extremity weight bearing for ambulation (paraplegic or amputee patients).

Because of the frequency of shoulder pain after antegrade insertion, retrograde insertion has been advocated to avoid this complication; however, retrograde insertion has been associated with distal humeral fracture propagation. The traditional starting point for retrograde humeral nailing is in the midline, 2 cm above the olecranon fossa. More recently, insertion through the superior aspect of the olecranon fossa has been recommended. Proposed advantages of the olecranon fossa site include an increase in the effective working length of the distal fracture segment and straight alignment with the medullary canal; however, biomechanical studies have shown less resistance to torque and a reduction in load-to-failure with this approach compared with the more superior portal.

Although flexible humeral nails have been successful in obtaining fracture union, insertion site morbidity and their suitability for only the most stable fracture patterns have limited their use. A cadaver study found that the axillary nerve is at significant risk during insertion of the interlocking and tension screws of a titanium flexible humeral nail; blunt dissection through the deltoid, direct observation of the humeral cortex, and use of a soft-tissue sleeve during predrilling and placement of the screws can help prevent this complication.

Newer self-locking expandable nails are reported to be easier to insert, while providing bending and torsional stiffness equal to that of locked nails. Few clinical studies are available to allow evaluation of these nails. Franck et al. described the use of an expandable nail (Fixion; Disc-o-Tech, Herzliya, Israel) for fixation of 25 unstable humeral shaft fractures in elderly patients with osteoporotic bone; all fractures healed without complications. Stannard et al. used a flexible locking nail (Synthes, Paoli, PA) inserted through an extraarticular antegrade or retrograde portal for fixation of 42 humeral shaft fractures, with healing in 39; 86% had full range of motion, and 90% had no pain. Five complications occurred in four patients: two nonunions, two hardware failures, and one wound infection. All complications occurred in patients whose fractures were fixed with 7.5-mm nails, and the authors recommended that flexible nails should be used with caution in medullary canals with a diameter of 8 mm or less. The technique is technically demanding.

Currently, we prefer rigid, locked nails inserted through an antegrade approach when intramedullary nailing is indicated, such as for segmental fractures (see Fig. 5.27), for proximal-to-middle third junction fractures, for pathologic fractures, for fractures with poor soft-tissue coverage, for fractures in obese patients, and for fractures in certain patients with polytrauma (Fig. 5.50A-C). We use an anterolateral incision with direct inspection and repair of the rotator cuff. Iatrogenic radial nerve injury has been reported, and care must be taken during fracture reduction, reaming, nail insertion, and locking screw placement. Intramedullary nailing is contraindicated in patients with very narrow medullary canals.

- Position the patient on a radiolucent table with the thorax "bumped" 30 to 40 degrees. Place the image intensifier unit on the opposite side of the table from the surgeon (see Fig. 5.33); rolling the unit back allows an adequate anteroposterior view, and rolling it forward allows an adequate lateral view of the shoulder and humerus.
- Make an incision diagonally from the anterolateral corner of the acromion, splitting the deltoid in line with its fibers in the raphe between the anterior and middle thirds of the deltoid (see Fig. 5.34). To protect the axillary nerve, avoid splitting the deltoid more than 5 cm distal to the acromion.
- Under direct observation, incise the rotator cuff in line with its fibers (see Fig. 5.34). Use full-thickness sutures to protect the cuff from damage during reaming of the humeral canal.
- Place the initial guidewire posterior to the biceps tendon and advance it under fluoroscopic guidance into the appropriate position as shown on anteroposterior and lateral views (see Fig. 5.33).
- Carefully advance the proximal reamer, protecting the rotator cuff.
- Use the reduction device to reduce the fracture and pass the bead-tipped guidewire (Fig. 5.50E and F). With sequentially larger reamers, ream the humerus to the predetermined diameter, usually 1.0 to 1.5 mm larger than the nail diameter (Fig. 5.50G). With fractures of the middle third of the shaft, a small incision can be made at the fracture site to ensure manually that the radial nerve is not entrapped in the fracture before reduction and reaming.
- When reaming is complete, pass the nail down the humeral canal, avoiding distraction of the fracture; ensure that the nail is below the articular surface of the humeral head.
- With the use of the outrigger device, insert the proximal locking bolts (Fig. 5.50H). Carefully spread the soft tissues to avoid injury to the axillary nerve.
- Place the distal interlocking screws in an anterior-to-posterior direction to avoid the radial nerve. Make a 4- to 5-cm incision anteriorly to expose the biceps musculature; bluntly split the muscle to avoid iatrogenic damage to the brachial artery.
- Repair the rotator cuff with full-thickness sutures.
- Confirm reduction and screw length on anteroposterior and lateral fluoroscopy images (Fig. 5.50I).
- Begin an early rehabilitation program with active-assisted range-of-motion exercises.

ANTEGRADE INTRAMEDULLARY NAILING OF HUMERAL SHAFT FRACTURES

TECHNIQUE 5.9

- Carefully evaluate preoperative radiographs (Fig. 5.50D) to ensure that the diaphyseal diameter is adequate to accommodate the intramedullary nail; if the diameter is too small, plate fixation is indicated.

FRACTURES OF THE HUMERAL SHAFT WITH RADIAL NERVE PALSY

The radial nerve is the nerve most frequently injured with fractures of the humeral shaft because of its spiral course across the back of the midshaft of the bone and its relatively fixed position in the distal arm as it penetrates the lateral intermuscular septum anteriorly (Fig. 5.51). Usually the radial nerve injury is a neurapraxia, with recovery rates of 100% in low-energy injuries and up to 71% in high-energy

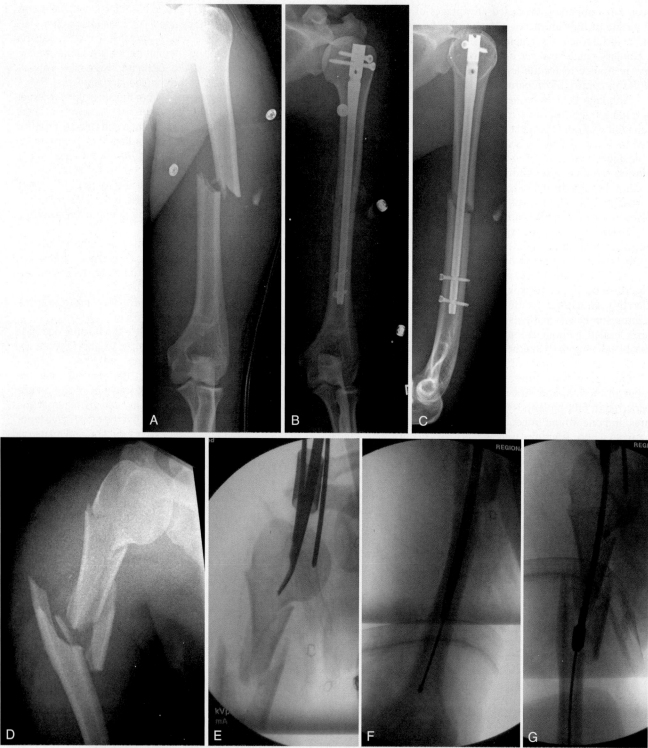

FIGURE 5.50 Intramedullary nailing of humeral shaft fracture (see text). **A,** Segmental shaft fracture in patient with multiple trauma. **B** and **C,** After fixation with intramedullary nail. **D,** Transverse shaft fracture. **E** and **F,** Reduction device is used to reduce fracture. **G,** Reaming is done to 1.0 to 1.5 mm larger than nail diameter.

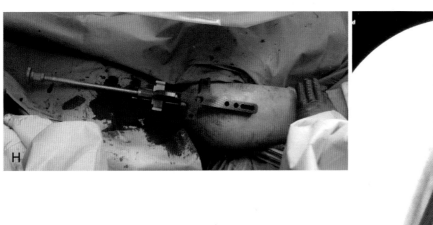
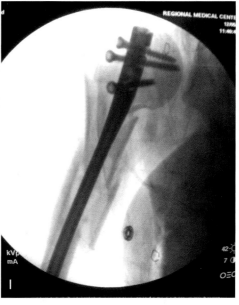

FIGURE 5.50, Cont'd **H,** Outrigger device is used for insertion of proximal locking bolts.**I,** Reduction and screw placement confirmed with fluoroscopy. (**D-I** courtesy Thomas A. Russell, MD, Memphis, TN.) **SEE TECHNIQUE 5.9.**

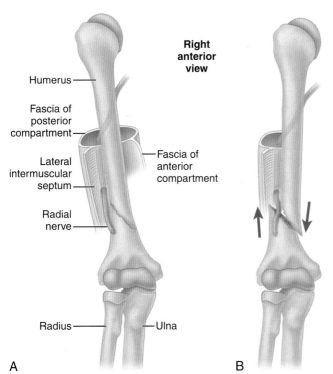

FIGURE 5.51 Entrapment of radial nerve between fragments in spiral fracture of distal third of humerus. **A,** Nerve is least mobile as it passes through lateral intermuscular septum in distal third of arm. **B,** Oblique fracture is typically angulated laterally, and distal fragment is displaced proximally. Radial nerve, fixed to proximal fragment by lateral intermuscular septum, is trapped between fragments when closed reduction is attempted.

open injuries; Bumbasirevic et al. reported recovery in 94% of 16 open fractures. Although it is possible for the nerve to be severed by the sharp edge of a bone fragment, this rarely occurs. We treat the fractured humeral shaft in the usual nonoperative manner, support the wrist and fingers with a dynamic splint, and reserve exploration of the nerve for instances when function has not returned in 3 to 4 months and the fracture has healed. Because the nerve usually is only bruised or stretched, function can be expected to return spontaneously. Routine exploration of the nerve would subject many patients to an unnecessary operation and might increase the frequency of complications. Early exploration and repair of a severed nerve have not been proved to produce any better results than repair at a later date.

If radial nerve palsy occurs with an open fracture of the humeral shaft, the nerve should be explored at the time of the irrigation and debridement of the wound. If it is found intact, only watchful waiting is required while the fracture heals. Early exploration is required if evidence suggests that the radial nerve is impaled on a bone fragment or is caught between the fragments. Advances in ultrasonography have been useful in diagnosing entrapped and lacerated radial nerves. If this diagnostic tool proved to be reproducible in large numbers of patients, the indications for nerve exploration would be more specifically defined.

In patients with radial nerve palsy for whom operative treatment of a humeral shaft fracture is indicated, the nerve should be explored at the time of fracture fixation. Shao et al. reviewed 21 scientific articles that included 4517 humeral shaft fractures and found an overall prevalence of radial nerve palsy of almost 12% ($n = 532$). Radial nerve palsy was most frequent with fractures of the middle and middle-distal humeral shaft and was more common

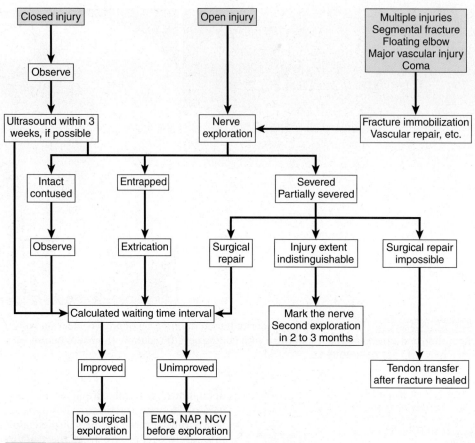

FIGURE 5.52 Treatment algorithm for radial nerve palsy associated with humeral shaft fracture. *EMG*, Electromyogram; *NAP*, nerve axonal physiology; *NCV*, nerve conduction velocity. (From Shao YC, Harwood P, Grotz MR, et al: Radial nerve palsy associated with fractures of the shaft of the humerus: a systematic review, *J Bone Joint Surg* 87B:1647, 2005.)

with transverse and spiral fractures than with oblique or comminuted fractures. Overall, recovery occurred in 88%. Complete transection of the radial nerve usually occurs with open fractures of the humerus and requires nerve repair or grafting; most nerve palsies that occur with a closed fracture recover without treatment. Based on their review, Shao et al. developed an algorithm for the treatment of radial nerve palsy associated with humeral shaft fractures (Fig. 5.52).

PERIPROSTHETIC HUMERAL SHAFT FRACTURES

Periprosthetic humeral shaft fractures after shoulder or elbow arthroplasty are rare but can be difficult to treat. Poor bone stock from osteoporosis, osteomalacia, or rheumatoid arthritis is the major contributing factor, and a variety of fracture patterns can result from low-energy direct blows, minor twisting injuries, "same level" falls, or intraoperative technical errors. Fractures around humeral arthroplasties may occur at the tuberosity level, the metaphysis, or the upper diaphysis around the stem or distal to the stem tip. Fractures around the humeral component of total elbow arthroplasties also can occur at any level from the medial or lateral column to proximal to the stem tip.

Stable postoperative fractures without component loosening can be treated conservatively with immobilization.

Stable fractures with component loosening require revision immediately or after fracture healing if still painful. Unstable fractures with or without component loosening require operative fixation with or without component revision. If revision is necessary, the general principles of revision arthroplasty should be followed. Bone quality determines the need for supplemental allograft, strut grafts, methyl methacrylate cement, or autogenous bone grafts. Most patients requiring either hemiarthroplasty or total shoulder arthroplasty or elbow arthroplasty have age-related osteoporosis.

When treating unstable periprosthetic humeral shaft fractures with well-fixed components, we have found the following guidelines helpful as outlined by Cameron and Iannotti: (1) displaced tuberosity fractures should be repaired with wire or heavy suture, and associated rotator cuff tears should be treated; and (2) unstable diaphyseal fractures around or below the prosthesis require ORIF. Cerclage wire or limited screw fixation is unsatisfactory. A heavy plate with proximal cerclage wires and distal screws is preferred. At least four proximal cables and four distal screws, engaging eight cortices, are necessary. We recommend using 2-mm cables instead of the usual 1.6-mm cables. An anatomic reduction is necessary for union, and bone grafting the fracture site should be considered.

When poor bone quality is present, fixation can be supplemented with methyl methacrylate cement. Cement should be kept out of the fracture site. If severe osteopenia is present, we recommend adding a full-thickness cortical allograft strut applied with additional cables 90 degrees to the plate-cable-screw construct. Autograft bone should be applied to the fracture site. We do not believe that a well-fixed, good functional shoulder or elbow arthroplasty should be revised to a long-stem implant just to repair a postoperative shaft fracture. Results with revision shoulder and elbow arthroplasty are not as satisfactory as primary arthroplasty. Instead, we believe every effort should be made to achieve primary fracture union.

Intraoperative fractures during shoulder arthroplasty can be avoided by careful attention to detail and respect for osteopenic bone. Intraoperative fractures should be repaired at the time of surgery by internal fixation or revision to a longer stem implant.

The general treatment principles of periprosthetic humeral fractures around the humeral component of total elbow arthroplasties are as just outlined. Fractures of the medial or lateral column with a firmly seated implant can be treated with immobilization. Union of a column fracture is unnecessary for a good functional outcome.

DISTAL HUMERAL FRACTURES

Fractures of the distal humerus remain a challenging problem despite advances in technique and implants. These injuries often involve articular comminution, and many occur in older patients with osteoporotic bone. Joint function often is compromised because of stiffness, pain, and weakness. Rarely is a "normal" elbow the outcome after these fractures, but outcomes have been improved with advances in implant technology, surgical approaches, and rehabilitation protocols, with good to excellent results reported in approximately 87% of patients. Most distal humeral fractures in adults must be treated operatively, in contrast to fractures of the proximal humerus or humeral shaft. Nonoperative treatment with the "bag of bones" technique may be reasonable in an elderly patient with significant medical comorbidities. Desloges et al. reported good to excellent subjective outcomes with this technique in 13 of 19 low-demand elderly patients. Alternatively, Shannon et al. have reported the shock-trauma experience of treating elderly patients with comminuted distal humeral fracture with ORIF. Fractures united in all 16 patients in their series, with only an 18% reoperation rate.

Both ORIF and total elbow arthroplasty have been reported to obtain good outcomes in lower-demand patients. In their meta-analysis, Githens et al. found that total elbow arthroplasty and ORIF produced similar functional scores, although there was an insignificant trend toward more complications and reoperations after open reduction. The many variables that must be considered in choosing treatment include fracture patterns, comminution, bone quality, surgeon experience (with total elbow arthroplasty and/or ORIF), underlying arthrosis, and patient comorbidities, making it imperative to individualize treatment according to patient and fracture characteristics.

The complexity of distal humeral fractures in adults is reflected in the attempts at classifying the variety of

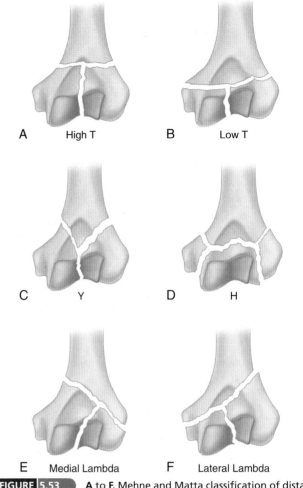

FIGURE 5.53 **A to F,** Mehne and Matta classification of distal humeral fractures.

injuries possible in this location. The AO/OTA classification, if all subgroup classifications are used, defines 61 types, although the three kinds of articular involvement are the most commonly used designations: A, extraarticular; B, partially articular; and C, completely articular. A more recent classification system suggested by Jupiter and Mehne is simpler: it describes only 25 types. This classification system is based on the "two-column" and "tie-arch" concepts of elbow stability. Mehne and Matta described complex bicolumnar distal humeral fractures according to the configuration formed by the fracture lines (Fig. 5.53): high or low T-fractures, Y-fractures, H-fractures, and medial and lateral L-fractures. We generally prefer to use the Jupiter classification system because it has been useful for preoperative planning.

The goal of treatment is anatomic restoration of the joint surface with stable internal fixation that allows early motion. Lateral or medial column fractures (AO/OTA type B) (Fig. 5.54) usually can be reduced through a direct approach and fixed with simple buttress plating. Intraarticular fractures (AO/OTA type C) vary greatly. Generally, the lower the transverse component, the more difficult is attaining stable fixation. Likewise, the greater the comminution, the more difficult is attaining an anatomic reduction.

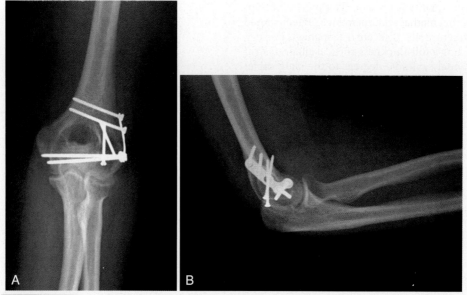

FIGURE 5.54 **A** and **B,** Isolated lateral condylar fracture fixed with lag screw and minifragment buttress plate.

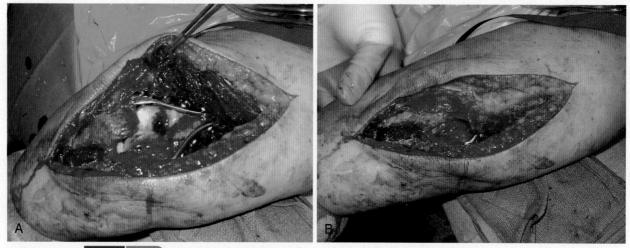

FIGURE 5.55 **A** and **B,** Plate application through triceps-reflecting approach.

A variety of approaches have been described for reduction and fixation of distal humeral fractures (Table 5.9). Most commonly, a posterior approach with an olecranon osteotomy has been used (see Technique 5.10), but concerns about healing and symptomatic implants have led to more frequent use of a triceps-reflecting (Bryan-Morrey [Fig. 5.55] or triceps-reflecting anconeus pedicle [Fig. 5.56]) approach, as advocated by Bryan and Morrey and O'Driscoll, or a triceps-splitting (Campbell [Fig. 5.57]) approach, as advocated by McKee et al. The best fracture exposure is provided by an olecranon osteotomy approach. As more familiarity is gained with fracture patterns and reduction techniques, a triceps-reflecting or triceps-splitting approach may be selected to reduce complications. Sharma et al. reported in a systematic review that functional outcomes did not differ based on the approach used. With all posterior approaches, the ulnar nerve must be carefully dissected without excessive stripping and can be transposed anterior to the medial epicondyle at the end of the procedure. More recent reports have questioned the benefit of nerve transposition, noting that the frequency of ulnar neuritis in patients with ulnar nerve transposition was almost four times that in patients without transposition. Wiggers et al. found ulnar neuropathy in 17 (16%) of 107 patients, 16 of whom had columnar fractures. Only one patient with a capitellar or trochlear fracture developed ulnar neuropathy. These authors suggested that it was not the ulnar nerve transposition alone that placed the ulnar nerve at risk, but rather it was the additional handling of the ulnar nerve

TABLE 5.9

Surgical Approaches Used for Treatment of Fractures of the Distal Humerus

	SURGICAL APPROACH	INDICATIONS	CONTRAINDICATIONS	ADVANTAGES	DISADVANTAGES
POSTERIOR	Olecranon osteotomy	ORIF for fractures involving columns and articular surface	TER	Good access to posterior articular surfaces for reconstruction	Nonunion and failure of fixation of osteotomy Poor anterior access to capitellum
	Triceps-splitting	ORIF/TER for fractures involving columns and articular surface	Previous olecranon osteotomy approach Patients at increased risk for healing problems	Avoids complications associated with olecranon osteotomy	Poor access to articular surface for internal fixation Risk of triceps detachment
	Triceps-reflecting	Fractures requiring TER	ORIF Previous olecranon osteotomy approach Patients at risk for healing problems	Avoids complications associated with olecranon osteotomy	Risk of triceps detachment
	Triceps-detaching	ORIF/TER for fractures involving columns and articular surface	Previous olecranon osteotomy approach Patients at risk for healing problems	Avoids complications associated with olecranon osteotomy	Poor access to articular surfaces for internal fixation Risk of triceps detachment
MEDIAL		Medial epicondylar fractures Medial column fractures			Lateral column inaccessible
	Koher	Lateral column fractures Lateral epicondylar fractures Capitellar fractures	Suspected more complex articular surface fracture	Radial nerve protected	Medial column inaccessible
LATERAL	Koeber				Risk of injury to radial nerve Medial column inaccessible
	Jupiter	Complex articular surface fractures	Significant involvement of the columns		Medial column inaccessible
ANTERIOR	Henry	Vascular injury	Requirement for plate fixation of columns or articular surface reconstruction	Good access to brachial artery	Limited access to columns

ORIF, Open reduction and internal fixation; *TER*, total elbow replacement.
Modified from Robinson CM: Fractures of the distal humerus. In: Bucholz RW, Heckman JD, Court-Brown CM, editors: *Rockwood and Green's fractures in adults*, ed 6, Philadelphia, 2006, Lippincott Williams & Wilkins.

during reduction of a columnar fracture and application of a medial plate.

The standard plating technique calls for plates to be placed at orthogonal angles (90-90 plating) (Fig. 5.58). Studies have shown that direct medial and lateral plating is biomechanically sound (Fig. 5.59), and clinical reports have confirmed stable fixation and high rates of union with parallel (180-degree) plating. Sanchez-Sotelo et al. listed several principles for distal humeral fracture fixation that we have incorporated into our treatment protocol (Box 5.4). Small osteochondral fragments can be fixed with headless screws, countersunk mini-fragment screws, or absorbable screws (Fig. 5.60). In a recent meta-analysis,

Shih et al. concluded that parallel plating may provide improved axial stiffness. These authors suggested that either orthogonal or parallel plating performed well will almost always lead to successful union. However, many confounding variables, such as locked versus nonlocked plating, screw size, or hybrid plates that are placed posterior but incorporate a lateral "tub" make a direct inference from the data difficult.

Reconstruction of the distal humerus can be done according to two strategies: (1) reduction and fixation of the articular surfaces followed by attachment to the humeral shaft; or (2) reduction and fixation of the medial or lateral condyle to the shaft, then reconstruction of the

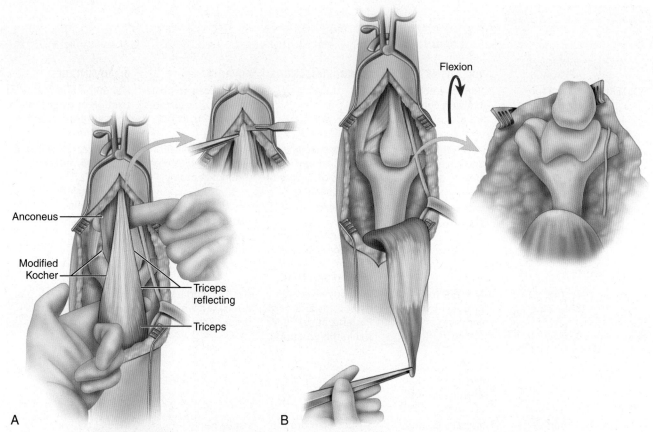

Anconeus

Modified
Kocher

Triceps
reflecting

Triceps

Flexion

A

B

FIGURE **5.56** Triceps-reflecting anconeus pedicle approach. **A,** Modified Kocher lateral approach is combined with medial triceps-reflecting approach. **B,** Access to distal humerus is similar to that provided by olecranon osteotomy.

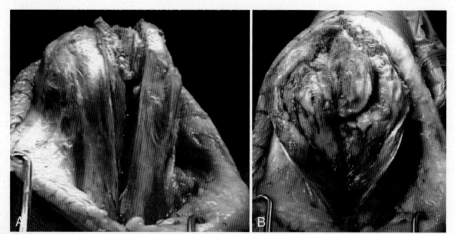

FIGURE **5.57** Triceps-splitting approach to distal humerus. **A,** Triceps split. **B,** Split extended to transcutaneous border of ulna. (From Frankle MA: Triceps split technique for total elbow arthroplasty, *Tech Shoulder Elbow Surg* 3:23, 2002.)

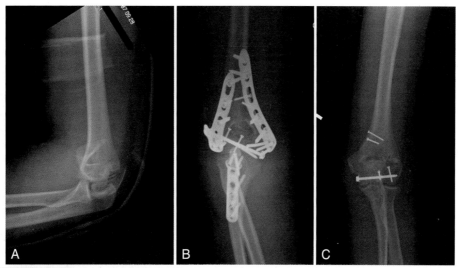

FIGURE 5.58   **A,** Supracondylar fracture with intraarticular extension. **B,** Fixation with 90-90 locked plates through olecranon osteotomy approach. **C,** After removal of symptomatic implants.

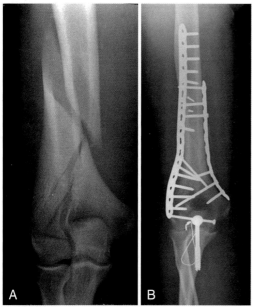

FIGURE 5.59   **A,** Distal humeral fracture with intraarticular extension. **B,** After direct medial and lateral plate fixation.

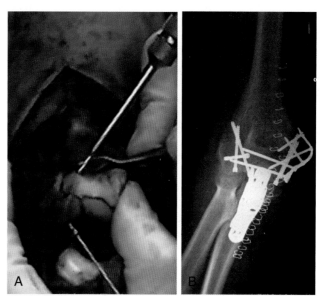

FIGURE 5.60   **A,** Fixation of small osteochondral fragment with absorbable screw. **B,** Very distal intercondylar fracture fixed with headless screws and minifragment buttress plating through olecranon osteotomy approach.

articular surface (advantageous when the articular surface is comminuted), followed by reduction and fixation of the contralateral condyle. Care must be taken not to narrow the trochlea with a lag screw when there is bone loss because this would not allow the arm to sit properly. Because the area for screws is limited in the distal segment, provisional fixation can be used at the joint, with definitive

fixation screws passing through the plate to ensure that the screws in the distal segment contribute to the overall stability of the construct (see Fig. 5.60). Newer plates that are precontoured or 3.5-mm compression plates are preferable to one third tubular and 3.5-mm reconstruction plates

Technical Objectives for Fixation of Distal Humeral Fractures

- Every screw should pass through a plate.
- Each screw should engage a fragment on the opposite side that is also fixed to a plate.
- As many screws as possible should be placed in the distal fragments.
- Each screw should be as long as possible.
- Each screw should engage as many articular fragments as possible.
- Plates should be applied such that compression is achieved at the supracondylar level for both columns.
- Plates used must be strong enough and stiff enough to resist breaking or bending before union occurs at the supracondylar level.

From Sanchez-Sotelo J, Torchia ME, O'Driscoll SW: Principle-based internal fixation of distal humerus fractures, *Tech Hand Upper Extremity Surg* 5:179, 2001.

because of fatigue failure in the latter group in fractures with metaphyseal comminution. For low-type fractures, additional mini-fragment plates may provide added fixation (see Fig. 5.60). Locking plates have been shown to provide added stability and may allow earlier rehabilitation. Poly-axial screws have been demonstrated to have a biomechanical advantage over locking screws in poor bone stock.

If the goal of stable fixation that allows early motion is met, rehabilitation can begin within 3 days of surgery. Waddell et al. showed that disabling stiffness develops if the elbow is immobilized for more than 3 weeks. Supervised physical therapy sessions are scheduled three times a week, along with a daily home exercise program. Dynamic flexion and extension splinting is prescribed when early motion goals are not obtained. Tunali et al. noted that increased fracture severity and delay to surgery were predictors of postoperative arthrofibrosis.

Union rates for distal humeral fractures have improved significantly over the years. The most frequent complication is stiffness, which often requires a second procedure. McKee et al. reported an average motion arc of 108 degrees, 74% strength compared with the opposite side, and a mean DASH (Disability of the Arm, Shoulder, and Hand) score of 20 (0 = perfect and 100 = complete disability) in 25 patients at an average 3 years after medial and lateral plate fixation of intraarticular distal humeral fractures. Other complications include ulnar neuropathy, posttraumatic arthritis, osteonecrosis, and symptomatic implants (see Fig. 5.58). Wound complications are more frequent with open fractures and fractures in which a plate was used for olecranon fixation. It has been estimated that one in eight patients with operative fixation of a distal humeral fracture eventually requires a second procedure. Many complications can be avoided by the appropriate choice of procedure and meticulous attention to technical details.

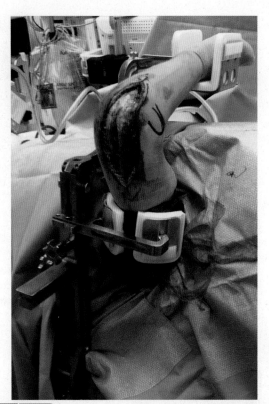

FIGURE 5.61 Arm holder (Elbow LOC, Symmetry Medical, Warsaw, IN) helps with arm positioning during surgery. **SEE TECHNIQUE 5.10.**

OPEN REDUCTION AND INTERNAL FIXATION OF THE DISTAL HUMERUS WITH OLECRANON OSTEOTOMY

TECHNIQUE 5.10

- Position the patient in the lateral decubitus position. A prone or supine position also can be used. An advantage of the supine position is improved anterior exposure of the joint, which is helpful with very low fractures and fractures with anterior comminution. Fixation of the fracture with extension into the shaft can be difficult to reduce with the patient supine. When the supine position is chosen, we use an arm holder (Elbow LOC, Symmetry Medical Inc., Warsaw, IN) to assist with arm positioning (Fig. 57.61).
- Prepare and drape the entire forequarter to allow placement of a sterile tourniquet on the proximal arm.
- Make a midline incision, with or without a curve over the tip of the olecranon, and develop full-thickness flaps medially and laterally.
- Dissect the ulnar nerve free from the medial edge of the triceps and from the medial epicondyle. Preserve the vascular structures that supply the ulnar nerve (Fig. 57.62A).
- Laterally, dissect the triceps off the lateral intermuscular septum. Incise the interval between the triceps and anconeus muscles to expose the joint. Alternatively, preserve the anconeus innervation by using the interval between

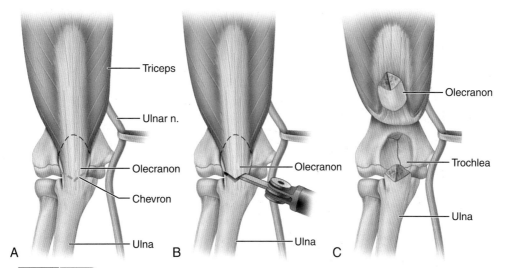

FIGURE 5.62 Olecranon osteotomy approach. **A,** Olecranon osteotomy is marked in shape of shallow V or chevron. **B,** Thin-blade oscillating saw is used to start osteotomy. **C,** Osteotomized proximal olecranon fragment is elevated proximally; ulnar nerve is isolated, mobilized, and protected. **SEE TECHNIQUE 5.10.**

the anconeus and the extensor carpi radialis brevis and elevating the anconeus with the triceps.

- Ensure that the medial and lateral olecranon articular surface can be seen.
- Predrill the holes for olecranon fixation before making the osteotomy. We routinely use plate fixation.
- Make a distally oriented chevron osteotomy with an oscillating saw directed toward the sulcus of the articular surface of the olecranon (Fig. 5.62B). Use an osteotome to complete the osteotomy carefully. If the osteotomy is forcefully wedged open with the osteotome, a large cartilaginous flap can be created inadvertently.
- Raise the triceps with the proximal olecranon and direct the triceps musculature off the humerus, preserving the periosteum (Fig. 5.62C).
- Debride the fracture edges to clean surfaces.
- Use threaded Kirschner wires as joysticks to manipulate the medial and lateral condyles.
- If the articular fracture is simple, reduce the fracture with the joysticks and a Weber clamp and insert Kirschner wires for provisional fixation (Fig. 5.63A).
- Plate the column with the better key to reduction first, then the opposite column (Fig. 5.63B).
- If the articular fracture is complex and either the medial or lateral condyle has a good key to reduction with the shaft, reduce the condyle to the shaft. A countersunk mini-fragment (2-mm or 2.4-mm) lag screw can be used for provisional fixation because its low profile does not interfere with plate positioning. Alternatively, a plate can be placed along the column with provisional unicortical screws distally.
- Reconstruct the articular surface "around the clock," provisionally fix the reconstructed fragments, and reduce the remaining condyle to the shaft and apply plate fixation.
- Use headless screws, mini-fragment screws, or absorbable screws for fixation of articular comminution (see Fig. 5.63B).
- Either 90-90 or medial and lateral plates are acceptable (Fig. 5.63C).
- Evaluate every screw to ensure that it does not cross the articular surface.

- Repair the olecranon osteotomy, consider transposing the ulnar nerve, and close the incision in layers over closed suction drainage.

POSTOPERATIVE CARE The elbow is splinted in extension. The drain is removed 2 days after surgery, and range of motion is begun 3 days after surgery. No bracing is used.

FRACTURES, DISLOCATIONS, AND FRACTURE-DISLOCATIONS OF THE ELBOW

FRACTURES OF THE RADIAL HEAD

Radial head fractures can occur in isolation or as part of a more complex elbow dislocation (see "terrible triad" section, later) or Essex-Lopresti injury. When confirmed that the fracture is in isolation, the goal of treatment is a pain-free, stable arc of motion in flexion-extension and pronation-supination. The Mason classification system is widely used to describe these fractures (Fig. 5.64). Most radial head fractures are treated conservatively (Mason types I and II). However, Motisi et al. noted an increase in the rate of radial head fixation. Nonunion and fracture displacement are rare. Stiffness, however, can be a complication. If the patient has no block to range of motion, a sling and immediate use (as pain allows) predictably yields good results. Lindenhovius et al. reported that results of operative treatment at long-term (22-year) follow-up demonstrated no appreciable advantage over the reported long-term results of nonoperative treatment. Of 49 patients with Mason type II fractures (2 to 5 mm of displacement), Akesson et al. reported that 80% were pain free and had ranges of motion similar to the noninjured extremity after primary nonoperative treatment. Those with poor results improved with delayed radial head resection. More recently, Duckworth et al. reported excellent

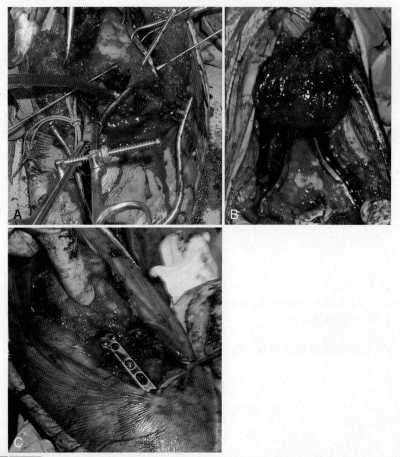

FIGURE 5.63 Open reduction and internal fixation of distal humerus through olecranon osteotomy approach. **A,** Threaded Kirschner wires used as joysticks for fracture reduction. **B,** After plate application. **C,** After plate fixation of olecranon osteotomy. **SEE TECHNIQUE 5.10.**

results with nonoperative treatment of 100 Mason types I and II fractures. Overall elbow stability must be confirmed before treating Mason type III fractures conservatively; careful evaluation may reveal a Mason type IV fracture. Egol et al. reported that nondisplaced or minimally displaced radial head and neck fractures do not need formal physical therapy and good outcomes can be achieved with a home exercise program. Critical to making the decision about operative treatment is determining that (1) the injury is isolated and not part of a complex dislocation and (2) there is no block to flexion-extension or pronation-supination.

■ OPERATIVE TREATMENT

Displaced Mason types II and III fractures that are part of an elbow dislocation pattern (Mason type IV) or have a limitation to motion require operative treatment.

▍TREATMENT OF MASON TYPE II FRACTURES

ORIF is the usual form of treatment for these injuries when surgery is indicated. The use of mini-fragment screws, with or without a buttress plate placed in the "safe zone" (area of radial head that does not articulate with the ulna [Fig. 5.65]), has had good results. Also partial resection of the radial head has been shown to provide satisfactory results. If the remaining

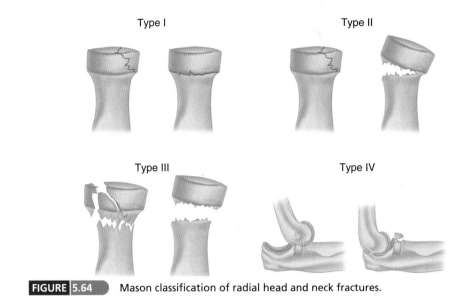

Type I   Type II

Type III   Type IV

FIGURE 5.64   Mason classification of radial head and neck fractures.

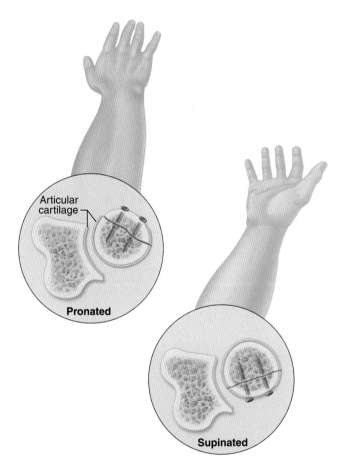

FIGURE 5.65   "Safe zone" (area of radial head that does not articulate with ulna) for placement of fixation. **SEE TECHNIQUE 5.11.**

articular surface is small, resection with radial head replacement is necessary as a primary stabilizer of the elbow in a complex fracture-dislocation. If the elbow is stable, resection without replacement has shown good results. Newer techniques with headless compression screws, such as cross-screw

fixation and the tripod technique, have shown good promise (Fig. 5.66).

TREATMENT OF MASON TYPE III FRACTURES

These fractures often are part of a more severe injury and may occur with elbow dislocation and other injuries about the elbow. They are less frequently appropriate for ORIF than are type II fractures. Radial head resection may be a good option for isolated fractures in elderly patients, but it has been associated with variable results in younger patients. Undiagnosed concomitant injuries likely play a role in long-term outcome. Long-term arthrosis, valgus elbow instability, and longitudinal forearm instability have led many to avoid radial resection in younger patients. In one group of five patients, however, satisfactory results were reported at 16- to 21-year follow-up, and Faldini et al. described good results in 36 of 42 patients an average of 18 years after radial head excision. Before resection of the radial head, elbow and forearm instability must be ruled out. Lópiz et al. also concluded that resection had fewer complications than radial head replacement in fractures with instability.

ORIF can be done with good results in selected patients; Ikeda et al. reported greater strength and better function in 15 patients with ORIF than in 13 patients with radial head resection for Mason type III fractures. The ideal fracture for ORIF has three or fewer fragments, each of which is large enough to accept a screw for fixation, with minimal metaphyseal bone loss. Otherwise, excision or replacement should be considered. Prosthetic replacement with metallic implants has provided good results at short-term follow-up. Sun, Duan, and Li, in a meta-analysis that included 138 patients with ORIF and 181 with radial head arthroplasty, found a significantly higher satisfaction rate, better elbow scores, shorter operation time, and lower incidence of nonunion at short- and medium-term follow-up in those with prosthetic replacement. However, in a cohort of military patients, Kusnezov et al. found a higher rate of implant failure. The surgical technique can be challenging, with the main complication being overstuffing of the radiocapitellar

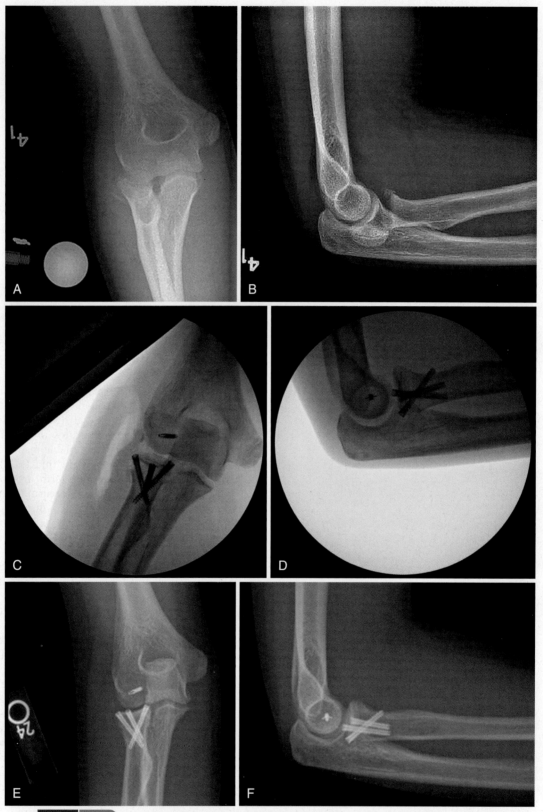

FIGURE 5.66   **A** and **B,** Anteroposterior and lateral radiographs of right elbow demonstrating initial transverse metaphyseal radial head fracture with posterior displacement and rotation of fragment. **C** and **D,** Anteroposterior and lateral views intraoperatively under image fluoroscopy after tripod fixation of fracture and lateral collateral ligament repair. **E** and **F,** Anteroposterior and lateral radiographs 5 months after surgery, demonstrating well-healed fracture without implant complications. (From Lipman MD, Gause TM, Teran VA, Chhabra AB, Deal DN: Radial head fracture fixation using tripod technique with headless compression screws, *J Hand Surg Am* 43(6):575.e1-e6, 2018.)

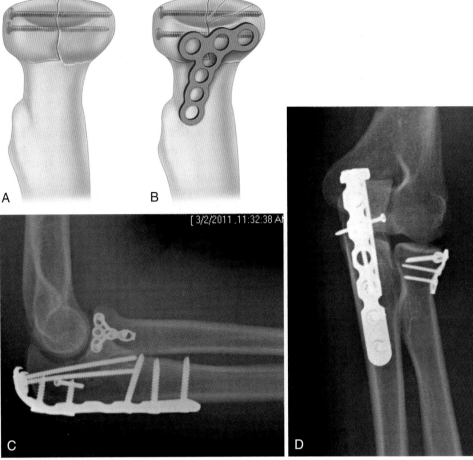

FIGURE 5.67 Open reduction and internal fixation of radial head fractures. **A,** Mason type II fracture stabilized with two small screws. **B to D,** Mason type III fracture stabilized with plate and screws. **SEE TECHNIQUE 5.11.**

joint, leading to erosion, pain, and decreased motion. The primary advantage of prosthetic replacement is maintenance of the radiocapitellar relationship for elbow stability and longitudinal radioulnar stability.

The Kocher approach has long been the mainstay for surgical approaches to the radial head. Many surgeons, including the author, now use the Kaplan approach. Barnes et al. concluded that the Kaplan approach affords significantly greater visibility compared with the Kocher approach.

OPEN REDUCTION AND INTERNAL FIXATION OF RADIAL HEAD FRACTURE

TECHNIQUE 5.11

- Expose the radial head and neck with a Kocher or Kaplan approach.

- Take care to preserve the lateral collateral ligament. In "terrible triad" injuries, the ligament will be reattached at the end of the procedure.

MASON TYPE II FRACTURE

- Reduce the partial fracture, taking care not to disrupt the periosteum; tamps, dental picks, or Freer elevators can be used as needed.
- Stabilize the reduction with one or two small screws (Fig. 5.67A). Occasionally, a buttress plate can be useful if the apex of the fracture is comminuted and a large defect remains under the articular segment.
- If reliable fixation cannot be obtained (as with fracture-dislocations), consider radial head replacement.

MASON TYPE III FRACTURES

- If needed for improved exposure, release the origin of the lateral collateral ligament; this will be repaired at the end of the procedure.
- Reduce and provisionally fix the articular surface with Kirschner wires. Occasionally, removing the fragments and assembling them on the back table may facilitate reduction.

- Protect the posterior interosseous nerve by pronating the forearm.
- Apply a small plate along the lateral surface of the proximal radius with the wrist in neutral (safe zone) (see Fig. 5.65) and secure it with lag screws as needed (Fig. 5.67B-D).
- Bone graft the defect if needed.
- Check pronation and supination of the forearm.

POSTOPERATIVE CARE
The arm is placed in a molded posterior plaster splint at 90 degrees. At 3 to 7 days, the splint is removed and the arm is supported in a sling. At about that time, active and active-assisted exercises are begun. The patient should discontinue the sling at 3 weeks, gradually increasing the exercises as tolerated. Forceful manipulation of the elbow is never permitted.

FRACTURES OF THE CORONOID

Coronoid fractures occur in 10% to 15% of elbow dislocations. They historically were classified into three types, as described by Regan and Morrey: type I, fracture of the intraarticular tip of the coronoid (no long-term instability); type II, fracture involving half or less of the coronoid (may significantly affect ulnohumeral stability); and type III, fracture involving more than half of the coronoid process (often associated with posterior instability) (Fig. 5.68). More recently, the classification system developed by O'Driscoll et al. (Table 5.10 and Fig. 5.69) has been shown to more reliably predict associated injuries and guide treatment decisions (Fig. 5.70).

Because a coronoid fracture fragment may appear small on a lateral radiograph or may be confused with a radial fracture, CT is recommended when a coronoid fracture is suspected.

Displaced coronoid fractures should be reduced and stabilized with fixation. Careful assessment is mandatory to ensure that the coronoid fracture is not part of a more serious injury (see later section on "terrible triad" injuries). Sutures can be used for fixation of small coronoid fracture fragments (Fig. 5.71A) and lag screws can be used for larger fragments (Fig. 5.71B). In a cadaver study, Huh et al. demonstrated more extensive exposure of the anteromedial coronoid and proximal ulna with a flexor carpi ulnaris-splitting approach compared with an over-the-top approach. A distinct type of coronoid fracture, fracture of the anteromedial facet (Fig. 5.72), occurs from a varus force to the elbow and, if left untreated, can result in posteromedial rotary instability. Repair of the lateral collateral ligament and ORIF of the coronoid are recommended (Fig. 5.73). Chan et al. reported functional and radiographic outcomes of select patients with anteromedial coronoid fractures treated nonoperatively. All 10 patients in their study achieved bony union without radiographic arthrosis and no recurrent instability. They noted that nonoperative treatment is feasible in small, minimally

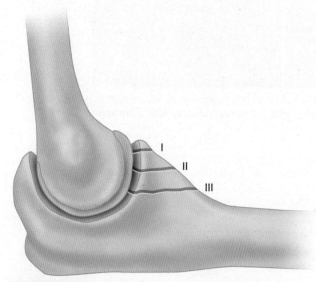

FIGURE 5.68 Regan and Morrey classification of fractures of coronoid process.

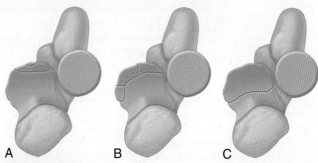

FIGURE 5.69 Classification of coronoid fracture based on fragmentation pattern (O'Driscoll et al.). **A,** Type 1, transverse fracture at tip of coronoid process. **B,** Type 2, fracture of anteromedial facet of coronoid process. **C,** Type 3, fracture of the base of coronoid process.

TABLE 5.10

Coronoid Fracture Classification (O'Driscoll et al.)

FRACTURE	SUBTYPE	DESCRIPTION
Type I: Tip	1	≤2 mm coronoid bony height (i.e., flake fracture)
	2	>2 mm coronoid height
Type II: Anteromedial	1	Anteromedial rim
	2	Anteromedial rim + tip
	3	Anteromedial rim + sublime tubercle (± tip)
Type III: Basal	1	Coronoid body and base
	2	Transolecranon basal coronoid fracture

displaced fractures with no evidence of elbow subluxation; the elbow joint must be congruent and demonstrate a stable range of motion to a minimum 30 degrees of extension.

SIMPLE ELBOW DISLOCATIONS

Simple elbow dislocations are dislocations of the ulnohumeral radiocapitellar joints. They are termed "simple" because there is no associated fracture. Treatment is almost always conservative, with a closed reduction after a thorough neurovascular examination. The propensity to redislocate is evaluated after reduction and noted. Radiographs should confirm a concentric reduction. Initially the elbow is splinted in 90 degrees of flexion, and range of motion is begun at 5 to 10 days after injury if the elbow is stable after reduction. More unstable injuries may require splinting for up to 2 or 3 weeks with a protected range-of-motion program or ligamentous repair. In their series of nearly 5000 simple elbow dislocations, Modi et al. found that 2.3% required stabilization surgery at a median of 1 month and 1.2% required soft-tissue release at a median of 9 months after injury (Fig. 5.74)

FRACTURE-DISLOCATIONS OF THE ELBOW

Fracture-dislocations of the elbow usually result from a fall on the outstretched hand with a shearing component to the injury, and fractures of the radial head, radial neck, or coronoid process, or combinations of these, occur as the proximal ulnar-radial complex is driven posteriorly. Valgus-directed stress can result in avulsion of the medial epicondyle, which is much more common in adolescents. The medial collateral ligament and lateral collateral ligamentous complex are invariably torn.

Posterior fracture-dislocations of the elbow in adults usually are treated surgically because the fracture and ligamentous components of the injury make most of these dislocations unstable. Fracture of the coronoid process or radial head or both can render the elbow significantly unstable after reduction (Fig. 5.75). Untreated injury to the collateral ligamentous complex and medial collateral ligament after repair of the osseous component of the injury can leave residual instability. Lengthy immobilization greatly increases stiffness, and open reduction and stable fixation should be done to allow early motion.

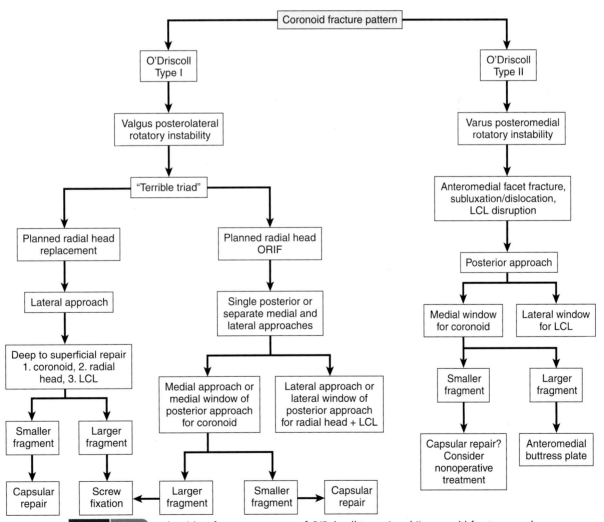

FIGURE 5.70 Algorithm for management of O'Driscoll types I and II coronoid fractures and associated injuries. *ORIF*, Open reduction internal fixation; *LCL*, lateral collateral ligament. (From Manidakis N, Sperelakis I, Hackney R, Kontakis G: Fractures of the ulnar coronoid process, *Injury* 43:989, 2012.)

■ TREATMENT

Closed reduction should be done as soon as possible. Radiographs often are necessary after reduction to define the osseous injury completely. Three-dimensional CT may be necessary to identify all of the components of this injury. The elbow should be carefully moved through a flexion-extension arc of motion. Subluxation or impending dislocation at 30 degrees or more from full extension indicates instability, and surgical stabilization is required. In the rare situation of a stable, concentric reduction, the patient can be started on early active exercises at 2 to 3 weeks, with close follow-up; if subluxation or spontaneous redislocation occurs, the elbow is surgically stabilized.

"TERRIBLE TRIAD" INJURIES OF THE ELBOW

Originally described by Hotchkiss, the "terrible triad" consists of an elbow dislocation in conjunction with fractures of the radial head and coronoid. Historically, poor outcomes led to the designation of this combination of injuries as "terrible." The essential lesion is disruption of the lateral collateral ligament with progression to the medial structures (Fig. 5.76). The lateral collateral ligament injury occurs as an avulsion of its origin, along with a variable amount of common extensor musculature, from the lateral distal humerus, leaving the typical bare-spot appearance of the distal humerus (Fig. 5.77B). The injuries to the radial head and coronoid vary in fragment size and complexity.

Early studies reporting elbow dislocations and fracture-dislocations indicated that triad injuries have uniformly poor outcomes, with Ring et al. reporting fair and poor results in four of their eight patients. However, excellent or good results were reported in 70% of 105 patients in four studies (Pugh et al., Egol et al., Forthman et al., and Lindenhovius et al.). McKee et al. reported good-to-excellent results in 78% of 36 "terrible triad" injuries treated with a standardized surgical protocol (Box 5.5), and Lindenhovius et al. reported good-to-excellent results in 15 (83%) of 18 patients. Mathew et al. also developed a surgical management algorithm for "terrible triad" fractures (Fig. 5.78). More recent reports by Fitzgibbons et al. and Gupta et al. continue to confirm excellent results after these injuries.

■ TREATMENT

A number of surgical approaches to the elbow have been described, and the best approach for treatment of "terrible triad" injuries remains controversial. The choice of approach depends primarily fracture pattern, type of instability, soft-tissue injury, and surgeon experience. A direct lateral approach or a midline incision with subcutaneous flaps to the Kocher interval usually is used; the latter allows a second interval medially if necessary. The fixation strategy usually is from deep to superficial as seen from the lateral approach (coronoid to anterior capsule to radial head to lateral collateral ligament to common extensor origin). Regardless of the approach selected, every effort should be made to operate through the traumatized planes and minimize surgical dissection.

Coronoid fixation depends on the size of the fragment. Small tip avulsions usually are reduced and fixed with sutures through holes drilled in the posterior olecranon. This effectively anchors the anterior capsule to the coronoid. Larger fragments are stabilized with lag screws from the posterior olecranon. Coronoid fixation is more easily observed when the radial head injury necessitates excision and replacement. The need for coronoid fixation has been questioned lately, first in a biomechanical study by Beingessner et al. and then in a clinical study by Papatheodorou et al. who noted excellent outcomes without coronoid fixation in triad injuries in which (1) the radial head was repaired or replaced, (2) the lateral ulnar collateral ligament was repaired, and (3) intraoperative fluoroscopic confirmed a concentric stable elbow.

Management of the radial head fracture is determined by the ability to obtain a reduction and whether the quality of the bone allows the reduction to be maintained. If the fracture cannot be reduced and stabilized adequately, replacement with a metal prosthesis is indicated. Although this decision is made early in the treatment process, we generally place the radial head prosthesis after fixation of the coronoid fracture because removal of the radial head provides good exposure of the coronoid fragment.

After coronoid and radial head stabilization or replacement, the lateral collateral ligament is reattached to its origin, as is the common extensor origin. Reestablishment of the soft-tissue restraints adds greatly to the overall stability in the elbow joint. If residual instability exists after fracture fixation and collateral ligament repair, a hinged external fixator can be used to maintain stability. However, it becomes more challenging after fracture of the radial head. For this reason, the author usually repairs or stabilizes the coronoid fragment. Orbay et al. reported a technique utilizing a new device known as internal joint stabilizer. Essentially, the device functions as an internal, low-profile, hinged fixator that allows for elbow motion while maintaining elbow stability. A more recent multicenter series by Orbay et al. reported outcomes of 24 elbows that had recurrent instability with elbow fracture or dislocation, or both, treated with an internal joint stabilizer. Stability was maintained in 23 of 24, with the only loss of concentric reduction in a coronoid-deficient elbow. We have used internal joint stabilizers with success at our institution and always have one available when treating these injuries.

In an assessment of risk of subluxation or dislocation, Zhang et al. advised that "terrible triad" injuries treated after 2 weeks might benefit from ancillary fixation to limit subluxation (i.e., cross-pinning, external fixation, or internal joint stabilizer).

STABILIZATION OF "TERRIBLE TRIAD" ELBOW FRACTURE-DISLOCATION

TECHNIQUE 5.12

(MCKEE ET AL.)

- Place the patient supine with the arm on a hand table and make a direct lateral approach to the elbow (see Fig. 5.77A). Alternatively, if a posterior approach is chosen, place the patient in the lateral position with the affected side up and arm lying over a bolster, draped free. This position also is used if placement of a hinged external fixator or a separate medial approach is anticipated.

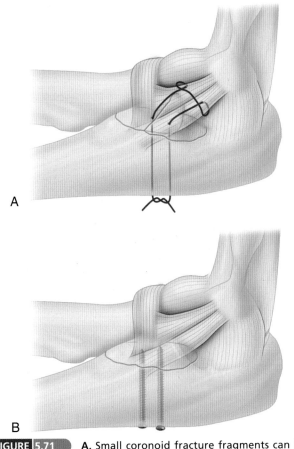

FIGURE 5.71 **A,** Small coronoid fracture fragments can be fixed with sutures. **B,** Lag screws can be used for larger fragments.

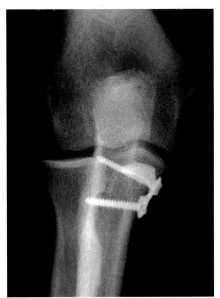

FIGURE 5.73 Plate fixation of anteromedial coronoid fracture. (From Steinmann SP: Coronoid process fractures, *J Am Acad Orthop Surg* 16:519, 2008.)

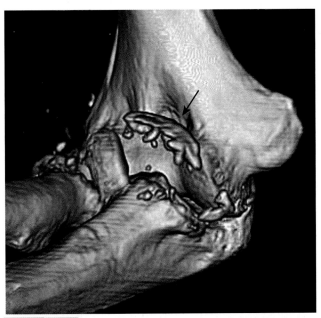

FIGURE 5.72 Three-dimensional CT scan of anteromedial coronoid fracture; *arrow* indicates fracture fragment. (From Steinmann SP: Coronoid process fractures, *J Am Acad Orthop Surg* 16:519, 2008.)

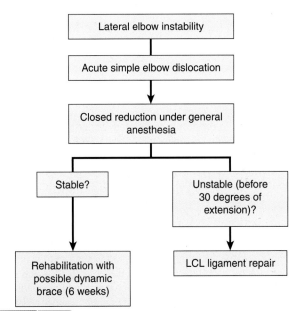

FIGURE 5.74 Algorithm for management of acute simple elbow dislocations and chronic lateral ligament injuries. LCL, Lateral collateral ligament. (From Tashjian RZ, Wolf BR, van Riet RP, Steinmann SCP: The unstable elbow: current concepts in diagnosis and treatment, *AAOS Instr Course Lect* 65:55, 2016.)

- Identify the "bare spot" left by stripping of the lateral collateral ligament complex from the posterolateral aspect of the lateral condyle. Take care to work through any soft-tissue disruption created by the trauma (with proximal and distal surgical extension as required), preserving intact structures as much as possible.
- Tag the detached lateral ligament complex for repair. Also tag the common extensor origin if it is disrupted.
- Inspect the coronoid to determine fracture pattern and severity; view of the coronoid is enhanced by removing an irreparably damaged radial head (which occurs in 60% of these injuries).
- If a large fragment (type II or III coronoid fracture) is found, reduce it and place one or two small-fragment (3.0- or 3.5-mm) lag screws from the posterior surface of the ulna. Insert a guidewire from the dorsal surface of the ulna and check its exit point from the coronoid process visually; reduce the fragment under direct vision.
- Larger coronoid fragments can be fixed with plates designed specifically for the coronoid (Fig. 5.79), but this requires a direct medial approach to the coronoid.
- For comminuted fractures, attempt to fix the largest fragment possible (typically the articular portion) to restore the anterior buttress of the coronoid and prevent posterior subluxation of the elbow joint.
- Type I coronoid fracture fragments are too small to be fixed with screws. Repair them by placing lasso-type sutures around the fragment and the attached anterior capsule and tying the sutures to the base of the coronoid through drill holes made with an eyed Kirschner wire (Fig. 5.77B).
- Evaluate the radial fracture. If there are one or two fragments, reduce them and hold the reduction with small reduction forceps while inserting small Kirschner wires for temporary fixation. Insert small fragment screws (e.g., Herbert screws) and countersink them below the articular surface (Fig. 5.77C).
- If fracture comminution (three or more fragments), impaction, cartilage damage, or an associated radial neck fracture indicates that a stable anatomic reduction is not feasible, excise the radial head.
- Insert the trial components from a metal modular radial prosthesis and move the elbow through a range of motion to determine the size that best restores joint stability, then insert the definitive components.
- Once fracture fixation is completed, repair the detached lateral ligament complex with nonabsorbable sutures placed either through drill holes in the bone or with suture anchors (Fig. 5.77D).
- Before closure, examine the elbow for stability and confirm concentric reduction with no observed posterior or posterolateral subluxation or dislocation through an arc of flexion-extension from 20 to 130 degrees.
- If residual posterior or posterolateral instability is evident, check the quality of the reduction and fixation of the coronoid fracture and radial head and placement of the lateral ligament repair sutures. If these appear satisfactory, options are to repair any disrupted medial structures (medial collateral ligament and flexor pronator mass) or apply a hinged external fixator or an internal joint stabilizer (Fig. 5.80).
- Close the skin and subcutaneous tissue in standard fashion and apply a well-padded posterior splint with the elbow in the most stable position, typically at 90 degrees of flexion and full pronation.

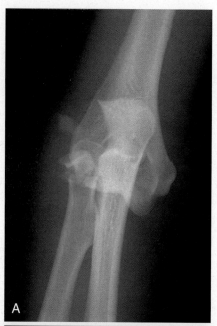

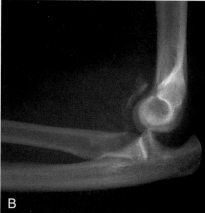

FIGURE 5.75   Fracture-dislocation of elbow. **A,** Posterior fracture-dislocation with irreparable radial head and neck fractures. Type II coronoid fracture is not apparent. This patient's injuries were bilateral and almost identical. **B,** One elbow has redislocated in posterior splint at 90 degrees of elbow flexion. Large radial head fragment and coronoid fracture are readily apparent. Coronoid fracture had to be repaired to provide stability before radial head could be excised.   (From Crenshaw AH: Adult fractures and complex joint injuries of the elbow. In Stanley D, Kay NRM, editors: *Surgery of the elbow: practical and scientific aspects,* London, 1998, Arnold.)

POSTOPERATIVE CARE The splint is left in place for 1 to 10 days, depending on the stability obtained and other associated injuries. In most patients, range-of-motion exercises are started on the first postoperative day. Active and active-assisted exercises are allowed for recruitment of muscle groups that act as dynamic stabilizers (flexor-pronator mass and common extensor origin). Full forearm rotation is allowed with the elbow flexed 90 degrees. Unrestricted shoulder and wrist exercises are encouraged. Typically, patients should avoid the terminal 30 degrees of extension (the most unstable position) for 4 weeks.

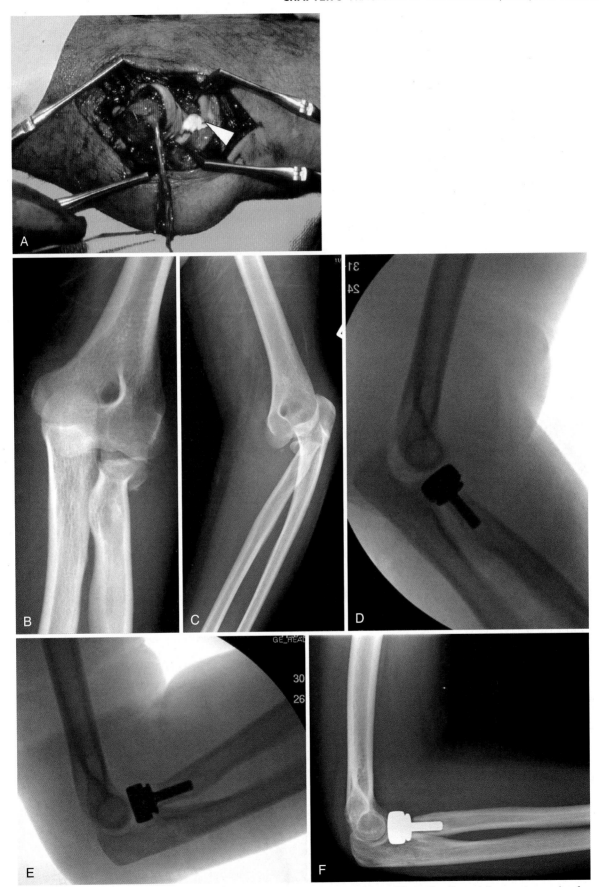

FIGURE 5.76 **A,** "Terrible triad" elbow injury. There is characteristic stripping of lateral collateral ligament complex from distal humerus. Portion of common extensor origin/lateral ligament complex is hanging down from bare lateral condyle. Coronoid fragment is trapped in joint *(arrowhead).* Defect in radial head can be seen behind coronoid fragment. **B** and **C,** Radiographic images of "terrible triad" injury. **D,** After radial head resection, instability was still present. **E,** After coronoid suture repair, minor subluxation was still present. **F,** Stability was obtained with repair of coronoid and lateral collateral ligament. (**A** from Pugh DM, Wild LM, Schemitsch EH, et al: Standard surgical protocol to treat elbow dislocations with radial head and coronoid fractures, *J Bone Joint Surg* 86A:1122, 2004.)

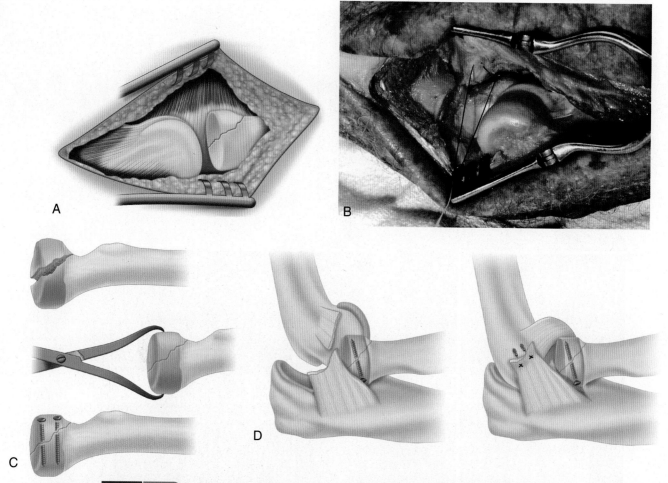

FIGURE 5.77 Treatment of "terrible triad" elbow injury. **A,** Lateral approach. **B,** Anterior capsule captured by nonabsorbable sutures and secured through drill holes in fracture bed of coronoid. **C,** Reduction and fixation with two countersunk screws. **D,** Avulsed lateral ligamentous complex repaired to lateral condyle. (From McKee MD, Pugh DM, Wild LM, et al: Standard surgical protocol to treat elbow dislocations with radial head and coronoid fractures, *J Bone Joint Surg* 87A(Suppl 1, Pt 1):22, 2005.) **SEE TECHNIQUE 5.12.**

INTERNAL JOINT STABILIZATION FOR ELBOW INSTABILITY

Orbay et al. described the use of a low-profile elbow joint stabilizer to prevent redislocation while bone and other structures are healing in patients with difficult elbow instability (Fig. 5.80A). Notable distal humeral or proximal ulnar bone loss may be a contraindication. The joint stabilizer can typically be removed in 3 to 4 months.

TECHNIQUE 5.13

(ORBAY ET AL.)

- The approach and incision depend on the individual case (Fig. 5.80B).
- Approach the extensor carpi radialis brevis and extensor digitorum communis (Kaplan interval), which splits the common extensors 50:50.
- Elevate the origin of the extensor carpi radialis longus, brachialis, and anterior capsule from the anterior humerus to improve access to the elbow. The avulsed origin of the lateral collateral ligament and the common extensors will be reattached at the end of the procedure.

- Treat any fractures of the coronoid, radial head, olecranon, and distal humerus.
- To apply the internal elbow joint stabilizer, find the axis of ulno-humeral rotation. Two points in the line define this axis: the lateral point and the medial point. Locate visually the lateral point first at the geometric center of the dome of the capitellum or the center of a circle that fits the curvature of the articular surface as seen from the lateral view. Mark this point on the bone surface (Fig. 5.80C). To locate the medial point on the axis, use a centering guide that consists of a metallic arc of 240 degrees that is inserted over the waist of the trochlea and pushed medially until it self-aligns on the medial trochlear expansion (Fig. 5.80D, E). Apply varus stress to the elbow to see the trochlea during placement.
- Under fluoroscopy and using the centering guide insert a 1.5-mm guidewire toward the medial cortex. Avoid drilling through the medial cortex to avoid ulnar nerve injury. Use of an oscillating drill increases safety.
- After measuring the length of the axis pin, drill over the Kirschner wire using a 2.7-mm cannulated drill to create the axis pin track. Confirm that the Kirschner wire is not in contact with the lateral aspect of the capitellum before drilling because this can displace the axis guide and lead to incorrect placement of the axis pin.

■ Position the base plate at the most proximal aspect of the ulna, taking care to avoid placing screws into the articular surface. The base plate has a sliding slot that can be used to adjust positioning under fluoroscopic imaging.

■ After securing the baseplate, connect the boom to the axis pin, with the head of the locking screw near the axis pin eyelet facing proximally. Secure the boom arm with a counter-torque device while tightening the axis pin to prevent deformation. It is easier to assemble the axis pin to the boom before its insertion onto the humerus.

■ Insert the connecting boom and axis pin into the humerus and into the base plate clamp simultaneously to facilitate the internal joint stabilization assembly.

■ Before tightening the two locking screws on the boom arm, ensure that the elbow is reduced concentrically by placing the hand over the head of the patient. This removes torsional stresses across the elbow joint by placing the shoulder in the position of neutral resting tension of the humeral rotators (Fig. 5.80F).

■ Apply a reducing compressive force on the proximal ulna in line with the humeral shaft and inspect the reduction visually before locking the reduction by tightening both the gold boom locking screw and the purple base plate locking screw (Fig. 5.80G).

■ Confirm that reduction is maintained through full range of motion using fluoroscopic imaging (Fig. 5.80H).

BOX 5.5

Principles of Operative Treatment of "Terrible Triad" Fracture-Dislocations of the Elbow

■ Restore coronoid stability through fracture fixation (type II or III) or through anterior capsular repair (type I).
■ Restore radial head stability through fracture fixation or replacement with a metal prosthesis.
■ Restore lateral stability through repair of the lateral collateral ligament complex and associated so-called secondary constraints such as the common extensor origin and/or the posterolateral capsule.
■ Repair the medial collateral ligament in patients with residual posterior instability.
■ Apply a hinged external fixator when conventional repair does not establish sufficient joint stability to allow early motion.

From Pugh DMW, Wild LM, Schemitsch EH, et al: Standard surgical protocol to treat elbow dislocations with radial head and coronoid fractures, *J Bone Joint Surg* 86A:1122, 2004.

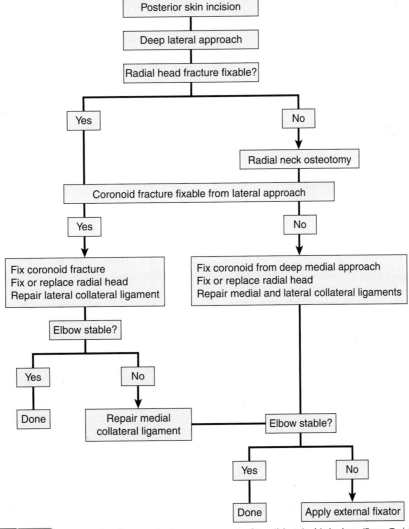

FIGURE 5.78 Algorithm for surgical management of terrible triad injuries. (From Tashjian RZ, Wolf BR, van Riet RP, Steinmann SCP: The unstable elbow: current concepts in diagnosis and treatment, AAOS *Instr Course Lect* 65:55, 2016.)

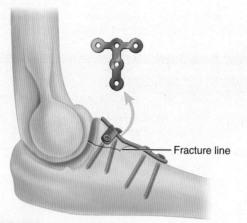

Fracture line

FIGURE 5.79 Plate fixation of coronoid process. **SEE TECHNIQUE 5.12.**

■ COMPLICATIONS

Complications of elbow fracture-dislocations include infection, synostosis, arthrofibrosis, symptomatic hardware, and residual instability. Anatomic reduction of intraarticular fractures is necessary to prevent arthritic changes. Loss of extension to some degree is expected.

Ectopic calcification is relatively common, including calcium deposition in the collateral ligaments and capsule; most reports indicate an occurrence of less than 20%. Shukla et al., however, found a 43% rate of heterotopic ossification in operatively treated fracture-dislocations, with about half of these requiring surgical intervention, and Foruria et al. reported that in 20% of 130 elbows heterotopic ossification was associated with clinically relevant motion deficits.

Heterotopic ossification can cause almost complete ankylosis of the elbow if severe enough (Fig. 5.81). It is common after fracture-dislocations and can be seen on radiographs 3 to 4 weeks after injury. Its severity seems to be associated with the magnitude of the injury and the length of immobilization, as well as to a longer time to surgical treatment.

RADIAL HEAD AND NECK FRACTURES ASSOCIATED WITH ELBOW DISLOCATION

Treatment of radial head and neck fractures associated with elbow dislocations is controversial. The radial head, similar to the coronoid process, is an important stabilizer of the elbow joint. ORIF of radial head fractures is preferable to excision if the radial head is salvageable. If the radial head cannot be preserved, use of a metallic radial head implant after excision of the radial head is controversial but should be used in most "terrible triad" injuries if instability is still present after the medial and lateral collateral ligaments and flexor-pronator mass have been repaired. Complications include loosening and revision. Watters et al. reported good short-term results with radial head replacement. The goal of surgical intervention is a stable elbow, and, if necessary, all structures should be repaired to achieve this.

FRACTURES AND FRACTURE-DISLOCATIONS OF THE OLECRANON
■ FRACTURES

Fractures of the olecranon can be caused either by direct trauma, such as falling on the tip of the elbow, or by indirect trauma, such as falling on a partially flexed elbow with indirect forces generated by the triceps muscle avulsing the

olecranon. These fractures were classified by Schatzker based on fracture pattern and mechanical considerations as to the type of internal fixation required for repair (Fig. 5.82).

The goal of treatment of olecranon fractures is restoration of function without pain. With displaced fractures, loss of active extension is common. Anatomic reduction and stable internal fixation are vital for both function and prevention of arthrosis. Implementation of an early range-of-motion program will decrease the chances of posttraumatic arthrofibrosis making stable internal fixation that will tolerate motion mandatory. Nondisplaced or minimally displaced fractures with maintenance of active extension can be treated nonoperatively. The elbow is splinted in 90 degrees of flexion for 3 to 4 weeks, followed by gentle passive motion with progression to active-assisted and then active motion.

Complications stem from the subcutaneous border of the olecranon in the form of wound complications and symptomatic implants. In addition, the distraction forces across the fracture from flexion or active extension may contribute to nonunion.

Most olecranon fractures are displaced and require surgery. As in all surgically treated fractures, an appropriate preoperative evaluation and plan are necessary. The correct treatment must be chosen for each fracture to ensure a successful outcome. Critical to management is recognition of concurrent elbow injuries and dislocations.

▌TREATMENT

Excision of the olecranon and triceps advancement are not often necessary because reduction and internal fixation usually are achievable. Excision of the proximal fragment with suture fixation of the triceps into the distal olecranon has been reported to be successful in low-demand and infirm patients, patients with severe nonreconstructable proximal comminution, or for revision after failed fixation. Recent biomechanical data suggest that posterior rather than anterior attachment of the triceps on the olecranon leads to greater triceps strength. Nonoperative treatment also is a reasonable option in our elderly population. Duckworth et al. reported a randomized trial of operative versus nonoperative treatment of olecranon fractures in the elderly. The overall low number of patients in their study makes the results difficult to interpret. This was secondary to the study being aborted because of an unacceptably high rate of complications in the operative arm. Challenges in this population include poor bone quality and questionable soft-tissue envelope, as well as difficulty in participating in a rehabilitation protocol. The author has had satisfactory results with nonoperative treatment.

The tension-band wiring technique has been purported to create compression at the articular end of an olecranon fracture when the dorsal cortex is tensioned under flexion of the elbow; however, biomechanical studies have not been able to demonstrate the conversion of tensile forces to compression forces. Tension-band wiring has been proved to be a useful technique in simple transverse olecranon fractures without comminution. It is contraindicated in fractures that are oblique, comminuted, or distal to the sigmoid notch. The procedure is fraught with complications, most commonly symptomatic implants that require removal, which is required in up to 80% of patients in some reports. Poorer outcomes have been noted in patients with elbow instability and fractures of the coronoid and radial head.

Kirschner wires have historically been used to anchor the tension band. Risks of this technique include injury to the neurovascular structures in the forearm. Use of an

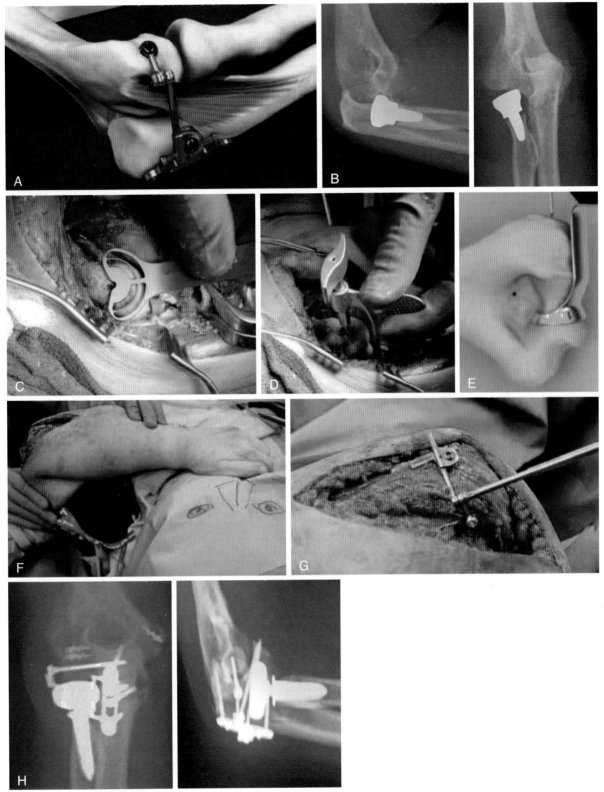

FIGURE 5.80 **A,** Internal elbow joint stabilizer. **B,** Terrible triad injury with coronoid deficiency and overstuffed radial head. **C,** Locating point where axis of elbow flexion-extension exits capitellum using guide. **D** and **E,** Using centering guide along curvature of medial trochlear axis of ulnohumeral rotation is identified. Centering guide is pushed against medial trochlear expansion to locate center point **(E).** Kirschner wire is inserted through guide and advanced into humerus, stopping short of medial cortex **(D).** **F,** For optimal congruent reduction, humerus placed in vertical position. With elbow in 90 degrees of flexion, ulna is pressed against humerus. Rotational stress is eliminated by placing hand over mouth. **G,** Tightening of connecting joints. **H,** Repaired terrible triad, with elbow full reduced and supported by internal joint stabilizer. Fixation of coronoid graft with compression screws and replacement of overstuffed radial head. (Courtesy Dr. Jorge Orbay, MD.)

intramedullary screw in conjunction with the tension band has been recommended, and transcortical rather than intramedullary placement of the Kirschner wires has been reported to increase stability and decrease complications.

We infrequently use the tension-band technique for displaced olecranon fractures because of the high complication and reoperation rates compared with other techniques. Its main advantages are low cost and minimal space occupation in patients with poor soft tissues.

Plate fixation has the advantage of maintaining fixation in fractures with comminution, distal fractures, and complex fracture-dislocations. Typically used in neutralization mode, the plating technique allows lag screw fixation of the olecranon and/or coronoid to anatomically reconstruct the proximal ulna (Figs. 5.83 to 5.85). The plate then provides the overall stability needed to obtain union and initiate an early range-of-motion program to promote maximal function.

The most frequently cited disadvantage of plate fixation has been symptomatic hardware problems. More recent reports, however, refute this. Newer precontoured plates are lower in profile, provide more screw options for the proximal segment, have locking screw capabilities, and can contain a bend to match the proximal ulnar anatomy for extended fractures (Fig. 5.86). These plates have produced favorable results in up to 80% of patients, and biomechanical testing found that they provide significantly greater compression than tension bands in the treatment of transverse olecranon fractures. Reconstruction plates and one third tubular plates have been used with some success, but we do not recommend them. De Giacomo et al. evaluated the use of precontoured locked plates. Their results showed 100% union, but a third of patients had symptomatic implants, with 10% choosing implant removal. Wound complications are the biggest concern with plate fixation because the proximal ulna has a compromised soft-tissue envelope in addition to being placed in tension with elbow flexion. Duckworth et al. performed a prospective randomized trial comparing plate versus tension-band wiring. Functional outcomes were similar at 1 year, with the tension-band group experiencing a significantly higher hardware removal rate. They warned that deep infection occurred almost exclusively in the plate fixation group. Their study did not use locked plates.

Of interest, Wellman et al. reported successful biomechanical testing of mini-fragment plates for olecranon fractures. The lower-profile nature of these implants may help with soft-tissue complications.

▦ FRACTURE-DISLOCATIONS

Olecranon fracture-dislocations typically occur as anterior or posterior dislocations. In anterior dislocation the distal humerus implodes through the olecranon (transolecranon fracture-dislocation). There is an ulnohumeral dislocation, whereas the proximal radioulnar joint is preserved, as are the collateral ligaments. Varying in complexity, comminution can be extensive and the coronoid can be involved. We routinely treat these injuries with anatomic reconstruction of the articular surface and plate fixation. The coronoid is reduced and stabilized with lag screws, followed by articular reduction with provisional fixation and/or lag screw fixation and then plate fixation spanning the entire injury (Figs. 5.87 and 5.88).

Posterior dislocations are ulnohumeral and radioulnar and can be considered variants of Bado type II Monteggia fracture-dislocations. Coronoid fractures, radial head fractures, and lateral collateral ligament injuries are common, and these injuries are similar to "terrible triad" injuries. These challenging injuries require accurate diagnosis, an understanding of the multiple injuries present, and a sound treatment plan for a successful outcome. Beingessner et al. reported good outcomes in 16 patients with a fragment-specific surgical protocol: (1) repair or replacement of the

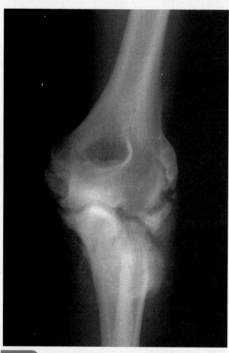

FIGURE 5.81 Extensive heterotopic ossification after fracture-dislocation of elbow and radial head excision.

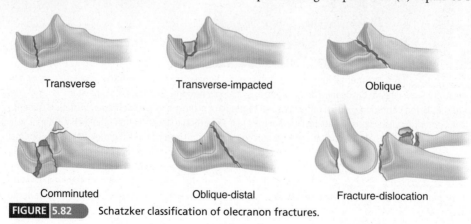

Transverse   Transverse-impacted   Oblique

Comminuted   Oblique-distal   Fracture-dislocation

FIGURE 5.82 Schatzker classification of olecranon fractures.

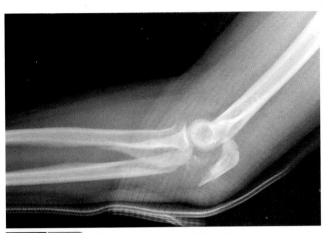

FIGURE 5.83 Olecranon fracture-dislocation.

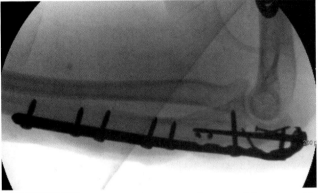

FIGURE 5.84 Fixation of olecranon fracture-dislocation with lag screw and plate.

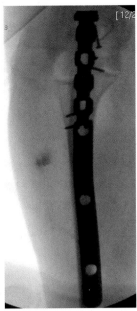

FIGURE 5.85 Fixation of olecranon fracture-dislocation with lag screw and plate.

radial head; (2) reduction of the ulnar shaft, including the anterior oblique cortical fragment if present; (3) reduction and stabilization of the coronoid process with either screws or transosseous sutures; (4) reduction and fixation of the olecranon process to the ulnar shaft and definitive fixation of the ulnar shaft component; (5) repair of osseous ulnar insertion of the medial collateral ligament and/or lateral collateral ligament; and (6) repair of the humeral origin of the lateral collateral ligament.

OPEN REDUCTION AND INTERNAL FIXATION OF OLECRANON FRACTURE

TECHNIQUE 5.14

- Position the patient supine or in the lateral decubitus position.
- Make a posterior skin incision from the tip of the olecranon to an adequate distance distally to secure fixation.
- Dissect out and protect the ulnar nerve if necessary in more complex injuries.
- Carefully debride the fracture edges, making sure to preserve the periosteum and soft-tissue attachments to comminuted fragments.

SIMPLE FRACTURES

- Inspect the articular surface and reduce the fracture with pointed tenaculums (Fig. 5.89A).
- Insert Kirschner wire provisional fixation, out of the plane where the plate will sit; consider lag screw fixation if possible (Fig. 5.89B).
- Position the plate (ideally precontoured for the olecranon) over the proximal fragment on top of the triceps insertion.
- Place the proximal screw in intramedullary fashion to cross the fracture site if possible.
- Use an adequate number of screws proximally and distally.
- Confirm reduction and screw passage with fluoroscopy.
- Close the wound in layers and splint the elbow in extension with an anterior plaster slab.

COMMINUTED OR COMPLEX FRACTURES

- Sequentially reduce and stabilize with small lag screws one fracture fragment at a time. If a large anterior oblique fragment is present, stabilize it to the shaft. This will help stabilize the elbow joint and facilitate sequential reduction.
- Where use of lag screws is not possible, use provisional Kirschner wires.
- Reduce impacted subchondral segments and stabilize them with Kirschner wires, with or without supporting bone graft.
- Reduce the proximal segment and provisionally fix it with Kirschner wires.
- Apply the plate. If fixation is questionable because of the size or quality of the bone, consider using locked screws.
- Confirm reductions and screw placement on fluoroscopy.

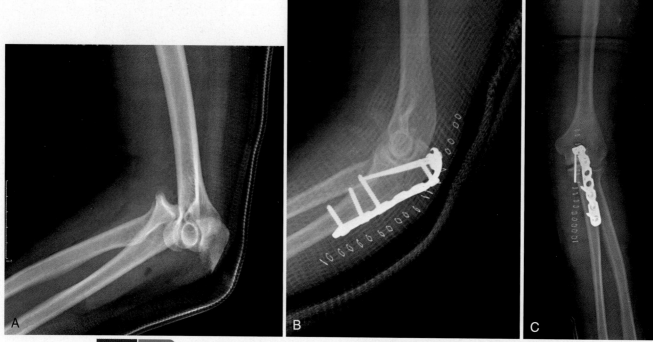

FIGURE 5.86 A, Olecranon fracture-dislocation, B and C, Fixation with low-profile plate.

■ Close the wound in layers and apply a splint with the elbow in extension.

POSTOPERATIVE CARE The splint is worn for 2 to 5 days; if the elbow is stable, protected range-of-motion exercises are begun and advanced as tolerated.

FRACTURES OF THE RADIAL HEAD OR NECK WITH DISLOCATION OF THE DISTAL RADIOULNAR JOINT (ESSEX-LOPRESTI FRACTURE-DISLOCATION)

A hard fall on the outstretched hand can result in a fracture of the radial head or neck, disruption of the distal radioulnar joint, and tearing of the interosseous membrane for a considerable distance proximally (Fig. 5.90). The tethering effect of the proximal radial-oriented fibers of the interosseous membrane is lost; if the radial head is resected, rapid proximal migration of the radius can occur, resulting in wrist pain from ulnar carpal impingement and elbow pain from radiocapitellar impingement. Disruption of the distal radioulnar joint must be recognized early, before radial migration occurs. When migration has occurred, late reconstruction often is unsatisfactory (Fig. 5.91). Schnetzke et al. reported "deteriorated" outcomes with late diagnosis. Pain in the distal radioulnar joint with a displaced fracture of the radial head or neck should alert the surgeon to the possibility of this injury combination. ORIF of the proximal radial fracture and pinning of the distal radioulnar joint should be performed; the pin is left in place for 6 weeks. Edwards and Jupiter advised replacement of the radial head if the radial head fracture cannot be repaired. Pinning of the

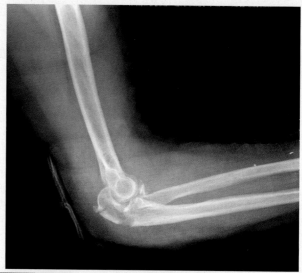

FIGURE 5.87 Olecranon fracture-dislocation.

distal radioulnar joint is still needed to allow healing of the interosseous membrane.

FRACTURES OF THE PROXIMAL THIRD OF THE ULNA WITH DISLOCATION OF THE RADIAL HEAD (MONTEGGIA FRACTURE-DISLOCATION)

The combination of injuries known as a Monteggia fracture-dislocation is an often treacherous condition to treat. According to Watson-Jones, "No fracture presents so many problems, no injury is beset with greater difficulty, no treatment is characterized by more general failure." This combination of fracture of the ulna with dislocation of the proximal end of the radius with or without fracture of the radius

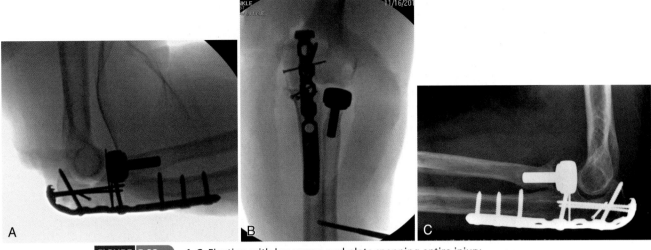

FIGURE 5.88   A-C, Fixation with lag screws and plate spanning entire injury.

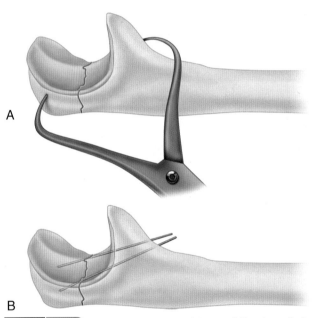

FIGURE 5.89   Open reduction and internal fixation of olecranon fracture. **A,** Reduction with bone tenaculum. **B,** Kirschner wires for provisional fixation. **SEE TECHNIQUE 5.14.**

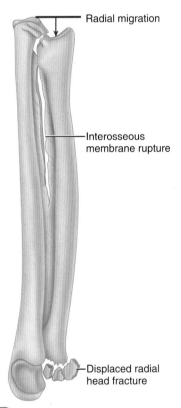

FIGURE 5.90   Essex-Lopresti fracture-dislocation (see text).

usually can be treated conservatively in children but routinely requires open reduction in adults.

Bado suggested classification into four types (Fig. 5.92): type 1, fracture of the middle or proximal third of the ulna with anterior dislocation of the radial head and characteristic apex anterior angulation of the ulna; type 2, fracture of the middle or proximal third of the ulna (the apex usually is posteriorly angulated) with posterior dislocation of the radial head and often a fracture of the radial head; type 3, fracture of the ulna just distal to the coronoid process with lateral dislocation of the radial head; and type 4, fracture of the proximal or middle third of the ulna, anterior dislocation of the radial head, and fracture of the proximal third of the radius below the bicipital tuberosity. In all series, type 1 far exceeds all others in frequency, although children's injuries are included in most series. Several mechanisms of injury probably exist,

including direct blows to the ulnar aspect of the forearm and a fall with hyperpronation or hyperextension, with the strong supinating force of the biceps pulling the radial head anteriorly as the fracture of the ulna is produced by the compression forces of the fall.

Historically, treatment of this injury, especially of the dislocation of the radial head, has been controversial. Early reports stated that all Monteggia fracture-dislocations could be treated nonoperatively, whereas later investigations determined that the best results were obtained when open reduction of the radial head with repair or reconstruction of the annular ligament was done with internal fixation of the ulna. A report by

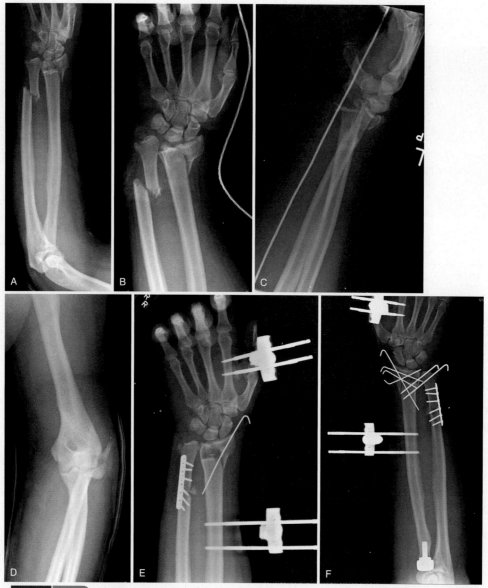

FIGURE **5.91** **A** to **D,** Essex-Lopresti fracture-dislocation. **E,** After external fixation, radial shortening is evident. **F,** Revision with radial head prosthesis restored radial length.

Boyd and Boals of 159 Monteggia-type injuries recommended rigid internal fixation of the fractured ulna with either a compression plate or a medullary nail and closed reduction of the radial head. Good results in approximately 80% of patients were reported with this treatment protocol. A better understanding of the injury and an awareness of the necessity of treating associated pathologic processes have led to better outcomes. Ring and Jupiter reported 83% good and excellent results with open reduction and stable fixation. Poor results are most frequent in Bado type 2 fractures, which are more complex injuries with elbow dislocations and fractures of the coronoid and radial head and greater soft-tissue compromise.

Monteggia fracture-dislocations with associated radial head fracture can pose a difficult problem. Reynders et al. recognized early resection of the radial head as contributing to delayed union or nonunion of the ulnar fracture by allowing increased angular forces on the ulnar fracture fixation. They recommended that radial head fractures be repaired, replaced

with an implant, or left in place until union of the ulnar fracture. Ring and Jupiter recommended radial head replacement for comminuted radial head fractures.

Although closed treatment is usual in children, Monteggia injuries in adults require surgical intervention. Anatomic ORIF of the ulna with stable fixation almost always (90%) allows closed reduction of the radial head dislocation. Continued radiocapitellar instability most frequently is caused by malreduction of the ulna. Comminution of the ulnar fracture can make anatomic reduction difficult. An apex-dorsal malreduction can force the radial head posteriorly. Jupiter and Kellam recommended a dorsal plate in this situation. We also have noted that with more proximal fractures, plate contouring must match the proximal ulnar bow. A straight (uncontoured) plate will malreduce the fracture and prevent the radial head from remaining reduced.

When continued radial head subluxation or dislocation persists despite anatomic reduction of the ulnar fracture, the radiocapitellar joint must be exposed and inspected. Often the annular ligament, capsule, and soft tissue (even the posterior interosseous nerve) is interposed and must be removed. Hamaker et al. from the Maryland Shock-Trauma unit reported a series of 121 adult Monteggia fractures. They noted that in 17% of patients the radial head was not reducible and that annular ligament entrapment was the cause, necessitating an open reduction. The radiocapitellar joint can be exposed by extending the approach to a Boyd-Thompson approach or using a Kocher approach. Reconstruction of the annular ligament rarely is necessary. We routinely use 3.5-mm limited-contact dynamic compression plates for ulnar fixation. If comminution is present, we attempt to reduce and fix the fracture with small-diameter screws in all fragments possible, with the goal of obtaining an anatomic reduction that will produce a stable radiocapitellar joint. For more proximal injuries, we find that precontoured olecranon plates facilitate stable fixation. A thorough fluoroscopic evaluation of the radiocapitellar joint is critical after ulnar fixation. Any subluxation noted should prompt reevaluation of the ulnar reduction or consideration of exploration of the radiocapitellar joint for tissue interposition.

Complications of Monteggia fractures include arthrofibrosis, synostosis, nonunion, malunion, infection, and neurologic injury. In 20 patients with Monteggia variant injuries, Egol et al. found that nine had fair or poor outcomes at 2-year follow-up; overall, 7 had heterotopic ossification, 14 had arthritic changes on radiographs, and 8 had required revision surgery.

FRACTURES OF THE SHAFTS OF THE RADIUS AND ULNA

The relationship between the radius and ulna in the forearm is critical for function, especially pronation and supination. This relationship is so critical that the forearm has been called a "functional joint." Malunited fractures can impair this functional joint, with resulting impairment of pronation and supination. Abe et al. recently evaluated malunions of the forearm with three-dimensional CT scans to further understand the pathoanatomy and plan the appropriate reconstruction. It is important to reestablish length, alignment, and rotation for the forearm to maintain its dynamic function.

Operative treatment is indicated for almost all both-bone forearm fractures in adults. The goal is to reestablish the anatomic relationship between the radius and ulna with rigid fixation. There is almost no role for closed treatment except in the most infirm patients, and, although intramedullary nailing of the forearm has its indications, the most common form of stabilization is plate-and-screw fixation. Anderson's landmark report in 1975 from this clinic reported excellent or satisfactory results in 86% of patients, with union rates of 98% and 96% of the radius and ulna, respectively. Chapman et al. reported similar results with 3.5-mm plates. These and other reports in the literature establish that ORIF of the radius and ulna predictably leads to bony union and good results.

We routinely use plate fixation for both-bone forearm fractures in adults (Fig. 5.93). The volar approach of Henry is used in all but the most proximal fractures of the radius, in which a dorsal Thompson approach is used. Limited-contact dynamic compression 3.5-mm plates are most commonly used. If a butterfly fragment is present, lag screw fixation (with 2.4- or 2.7-mm screws) is used to obtain anatomic reduction, followed by application of a neutralization plate. For transverse or short oblique fractures, a compression plating technique is used. For distal ulnar fractures or proximal radial fractures where a 3.5-mm plate may be too large, 2.7-mm plates and locking screws can be used to lower the profile of the fixation while providing rigid stabilization.

Open fractures with relatively minimal contamination are treated with thorough debridement, irrigation, and immediate ORIF. With grossly contaminated injuries, after thorough debridement and irrigation, splinting or temporary external fixation is used, with repeat debridement and irrigation followed by ORIF if the appearance of the tissue bed is satisfactory. The use of antibiotic-impregnated polymethylmethacrylate beads is considered for grossly contaminated fractures. If the soft-tissue wounds preclude the use of internal fixation, intramedullary nails are used to minimize the zone of injury and exposure to metallic implants. Auld et al. noted that the risk of compartment syndrome increased with the higher-energy variants of the AO/OTA classification, with group C fractures having a 33% compartment syndrome rate.

Isolated ulnar fractures can pose a treatment dilemma in deciding between operative and nonoperative treatment. Although most heal uneventfully without surgery, Coulibaly et al. recommended operative treatment of proximal-third fractures because of progressive displacement; they also recommended surgery if 50% displacement and more than 8 degrees of angulation were present, as both are markers of stability.

Historically, intramedullary nailing of forearm fractures has had poor outcomes with earlier devices such as Kirschner wires and Rush rods. The Sage nail addressed the issue of radial bow, allowing improved motion and a decreasing the rate of nonunion. The ForeSight nail (Smith and Nephew, Memphis, TN), an interlocking nail that can be contoured to recreate the radial bow, has had satisfactory results in many studies. Despite the satisfactory outcomes with modern intramedullary nailing, the outcomes of open reduction and plate fixation remain superior. We reserve the use of intramedullary nails for injuries in which the soft-tissue envelope is so traumatized that safe plate application is not possible. The risks of decreased range of motion and decreased union rates are offset by the risk to limb salvage. Often, an intramedullary nail can be used for one bone (usually the ulna) with plate fixation of the other (usually the radius) to limit soft-tissue complications. We also use this technique for segmental ulnar fractures.

For intramedullary nailing of forearm fractures **see Video 5.2.**

OPEN REDUCTION AND INTERNAL FIXATION OF BOTH-BONE FOREARM FRACTURES

TECHNIQUE 5.15

- After evaluation of the radiographs, plan the sequence of fixation:

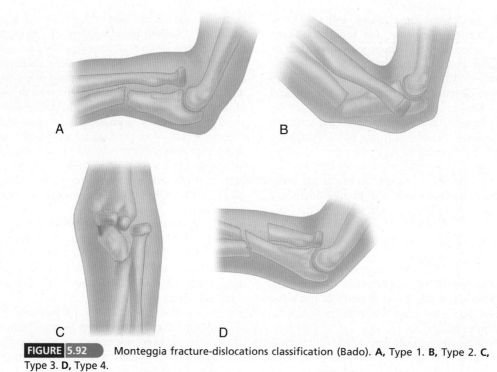

FIGURE 5.92 Monteggia fracture-dislocations classification (Bado). **A,** Type 1. **B,** Type 2. **C,** Type 3. **D,** Type 4.

If anatomic reduction is possible, begin with fixation of the radius.

If both fractures are extensively comminuted, begin with fixation of the radius.

If the radius is comminuted and the ulnar fracture is simpler, reduce and stabilize the ulna first.

■ For most fractures, make a volar Henry approach to the distal radius (Fig. 5.94A). If a fracture requires fixation proximal to the biceps tuberosity, make a dorsal Thompson approach (see Technique 1.117).

■ Preserve the periosteum along the proximal and distal segments (Fig. 5.94B, C).

■ Debride the fracture edges of hematoma and debris.

■ Assess the necessity for lengthening; options for attaining length include chemical paralysis, distraction using a screw in the radial shaft and a lamina spreader, and soft-tissue releases if the fracture has been in a shortened position for an extended period of time.

■ For transverse fractures, apply a 3.5-mm limited-contact compression plate. If there is a butterfly fragment, stabilize it with 2.0- or 2.4-mm lag screws before plate application (Figs. 5.95 and 5.96).

■ For oblique fractures, reduce the fracture and stabilize it with a 2.0-, 2.4-, or 2.7-mm lag screw, followed by a 3.5-mm limited-contact neutralization plate.

■ For extensively comminuted fractures, use a bridge plate at the appropriate length. If the span of the plate is longer than 6 or 7 holes, adding a lateral contour to the plate will help match the radial bow.

■ After fixation of the radial fracture, approach the ulna through the interval between the flexor carpi ulnaris and the extensor carpi ulnaris (Fig. 5.94D, E). The plating strategies used for the radius are applicable to the ulnar fracture. We attempt to avoid direct ulnar placement of the plate because of prominent hardware irritation.

■ The volar or distal aspect of the ulna is chosen for dissection based on which aspect of the ulna has more traumatic dissection. Take care to preserve the periosteum.

■ After both the radius and ulna are stabilized, confirm adequate reduction and fixation with fluoroscopy (Fig. 5.97).

■ Close the wounds in standard fashion.

POSTOPERATIVE CARE Typically, only a soft dressing is necessary. Splinting is used if the elbow or wrist joint is involved or if fixation is questionable. Range-of-motion exercises are begun 3 to 7 days after surgery; heavy lifting is avoided until fracture healing is evident.

FRACTURES OF THE DISTAL THIRD OF THE RADIUS WITH DISLOCATION OF THE DISTAL RADIOULNAR JOINT (GALEAZZI FRACTURE-DISLOCATION)

The combination of fracture of the distal or middle third of the shaft of the radius and dislocation of the distal radioulnar joint was called "the fracture of necessity" by Campbell. Similar to Monteggia fracture-dislocations, Galeazzi fracture-dislocations often go unrecognized. Isolated fractures of the radial shaft are rare; more often there is some involvement of the distal radioulnar joint. Dislocation of the distal radioulnar joint at the time of injury should be suspected with a displaced fracture of the distal third of the shaft of the radius. Radiographic findings that suggest a distal radioulnar joint injury include (1) fracture at the base of the ulnar styloid; (2) widening of the distal radioulnar joint on the anteroposterior view; (3) dislocation of the ulna relative to the radius on a true lateral view of the wrist; and (4) more than 5 mm of shortening of the radius relative to the ulna when compared with the contralateral wrist.

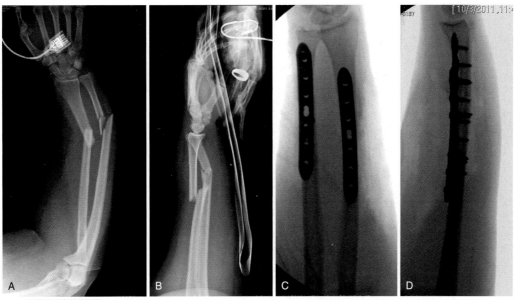

FIGURE 5.93 **A** and **B,** Both-bone forearm fracture. **C** and **D,** Fixation with plates and screws.

Galeazzi fracture-dislocations have been classified based on the direction of radial displacement (Fig. 5.98).

Treatment with closed reduction and cast immobilization has a high rate of unsatisfactory results. Open reduction of the radial shaft fracture through an anterior Henry approach (see Technique 1.114) and internal fixation with a 3.5-mm AO dynamic compression plate is the treatment of choice in adults (Figs. 5.99 and 5.100). Rigid anatomic fixation of the radial shaft fracture generally reduces the distal radioulnar joint dislocation. The forearm should then be splinted in the position of greatest stability, usually supination, for 6 weeks, although recent reports have indicated that immobilization in neutral for 2 weeks is just as effective. If this joint is still unstable, it should be temporarily transfixed with two Kirschner wires (four cortices to allow for removal in case of breakage) with the forearm in supination (Fig. 5.101). The Kirschner wires are removed after 6 weeks, and active forearm rotation is begun. Alternatively, the ulnar styloid can be fixed or the soft tissue of the triangular fibrocartilage complex can be repaired (Fig. 5.102). The radial shaft fracture usually is too distal to allow fixation with an intramedullary device. An irreducible distal radioulnar joint usually indicates soft-tissue interposition and requires open treatment. In a 7-year follow-up of 40 patients with distal radioulnar joint instability after radial shaft fracture fixation, Korompilias et al. found that instability was significantly more frequent with type I fractures than with type II or III fractures. They suggested that the location of the radial fracture can serve as a predictor of instability after fracture fixation.

FRACTURES OF THE DISTAL RADIUS

... will at some remote period again enjoy perfect freedom in all of its motions and be completely exempt from pain.

Abraham Colles, 1814

The management of distal radial fractures has changed significantly since Colles's proclamation in 1814. Although

distal radial fractures account for up to 20% of all fractures treated in emergency departments, many are not "completely exempt from pain" after treatment. More than 1000 peer-reviewed studies have been published on the subject, yet there is no consensus on which treatment is superior or firm guidelines for treatment decisions. Many confounding variables exist, all of which are somewhat controversial: the level to which the anatomy is restored, the quality of the bone, the emergence of new techniques and devices, the experience and ability of the surgeon, and outcomes in older populations.

The desire for anatomic restoration of the distal radial joint often is the rationale for operative treatment. Many studies have associated as little as 1 mm of incongruity of the articular surface with worse outcomes, whereas other reports have found no association between radiographic arthrosis and outcomes. Complicating matters further is the fact of a bimodal distribution of patients: do the young and the elderly fare differently? Multiple reports indicate that older, low-demand patients tend to tolerate incongruity, deformity, and malunion well; however, Madhok et al. noted that in elderly patients treated nonoperatively 26% reported functional impairment. Essentially, we know that elderly patients will tolerate more displacement (and closed treatment) than younger patients, but some still have poor outcomes. What is unknown is who would benefit from operative anatomic restoration. High-demand patients represent only a small percentage in most series and, although most patients do well, restoration of the distal radial anatomy is believed to be essential to minimize the complications of arthrosis and functional impairment in these patients.

Bone quality also is a confounding variable in trying to determine the best treatment for a particular patient. Bone quality is directly related to the ability to obtain and maintain reduction. In patients with poor bone quality, low-energy trauma may produce significant displacement and comminution, indicating that osteoporosis should be included in classification systems for distal radial fractures.

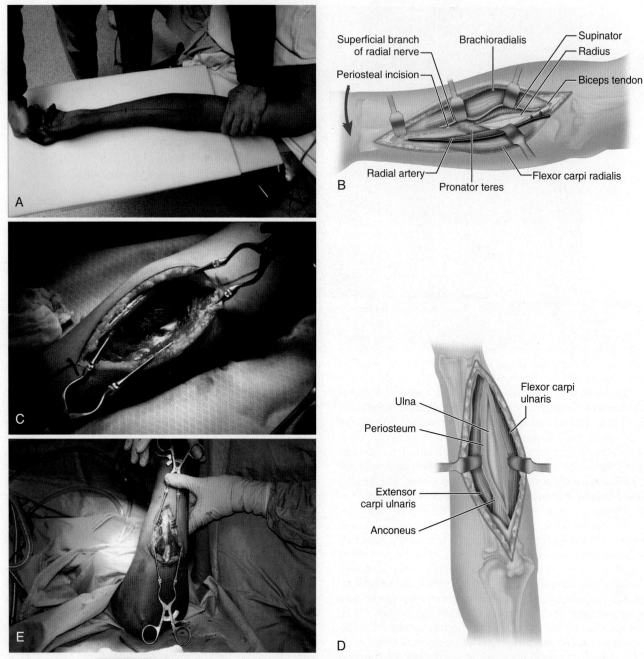

FIGURE 5.94 Open reduction and internal fixation of both-bone forearm fractures. **A,** Volar approach. **B** and **C,** Deep dissection. **D** and **E,** Approach to ulna. **SEE TECHNIQUE 5.15.**

One constant in the recent literature is that the specific technique is not as important as attaining anatomic reduction. Both clinical outcome and biomechanical studies demonstrate that maintenance of palmar tilt (normally 11 degrees), of ulnar variance (normally −2 mm), and of radial height (normally 12 mm) is the most important factor in obtaining good results. Numerous techniques are available (e.g., closed reduction and percutaneous pinning, external fixation, dorsal plating, volar locked plating, intramedullary nailing), each with its specific complications and learning curve (Table 5.11).

Because of the unanswered questions concerning the treatment of distal radial fractures in a heterogeneous group of patients, treatment must be individualized for each patient based on expectations, demand level, age, bone quality, fracture characteristics, and surgeon experience and ability.

CLASSIFICATION

More than 20 classification systems have been proposed for distal radial fractures. As with most fracture classifications, the intraobserver and interobserver agreement rates usually are only moderate at best. These classifications can, however, help in understanding the fracture and conceptualizing some of the challenges in treatment. Gartland and Werley's system emphasized metaphyseal comminution, intraarticular extension, and fragment displacement. Frykman added

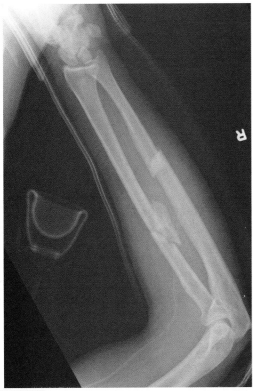

FIGURE 5.95 Both-bone forearm fracture. **SEE TECHNIQUE 5.15.**

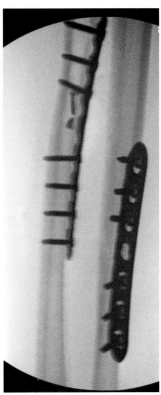

FIGURE 5.97 Reduction and plate placement confirmed on fluoroscopy. **SEE TECHNIQUE 5.15.**

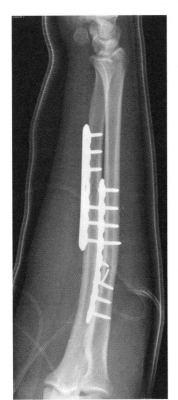

FIGURE 5.96 Fixation of both-bone forearm fracture with lag screws and plate. **SEE TECHNIQUE 5.15.**

involvement of the radioulnar and radiocarpal joints to assessment of intraarticular and extraarticular involvement, and Melone evaluated the four major fracture components. Fernandez based his classification system on mechanism of injury (Table 5.12).

ASSESSMENT OF STABILITY

Most distal radial fractures are treated with immobilization after closed reduction; unfortunately, many of these fractures lose reduction or the initial reduction was not acceptable and outcomes are poor. LaFontaine et al. identified five factors indicative of instability: (1) initial dorsal angulation of more than 20 degrees (volar tilt); (2) dorsal metaphyseal comminution; (3) intraarticular involvement; (4) an associated ulnar fracture; and (5) patient age older than 60 years. Other suggested indicators of instability include volar tilt, dorsal angulation, comminution, and initial shortening. Goldwyn et al. suggested that traction radiographs can aid in treatment decision-making. There are no definitive criteria or guidelines to guide treatment decision making, and a number of factors must be considered in developing a treatment plan, including initial injury characteristics, alignment after reduction, patient age, bone quality, patient demand, and expected outcome. If closed treatment is chosen for a fracture with questionable stability, close monitoring is advised. It is important to note any change in the reduction over a series of radiographs that indicate instability or displacement and to change treatment when necessary. Fractures that are considered to be potentially unstable should be evaluated with serial radiographs until fracture healing results in stability.

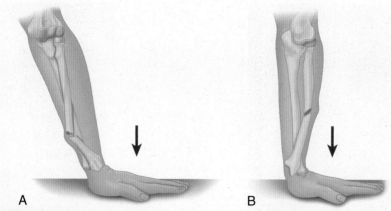

FIGURE 5.98   Classification of Galeazzi fracture based on direction of radial displacement. **A,** Type I, apex volar, fractures are caused by axial loading of forearm in supination, which results in dorsal displacement of radius and volar dislocation of distal ulna. **B,** Type II, apex dorsal, fractures are caused by axial loading of forearm in pronation, resulting in anterior displacement of radius and dorsal dislocation of distal ulna.

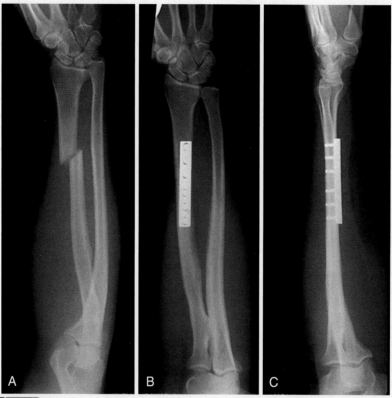

FIGURE 5.99   **A,** Galeazzi fracture-dislocation. **B** and **C,** After fixation with 3.5-mm AO dynamic compression plate and screws. Temporary stabilization of distal radioulnar joint with transverse Kirschner wire was unnecessary.

TREATMENT OPTIONS
■ CLOSED TREATMENT

Stable fractures can be successfully treated with closed reduction and immobilization, initially with a splint followed by a cast, and weekly radiographic evaluation for 3 weeks. Significant changes in radial length, palmar tilt, or radial inclination should prompt consideration of operative treatment. In infirm and low-demand patients, closed treatment often is appropriate even with factors that are indications for operative

treatment in more active patients. In a prospective randomized trial comparing nonoperative treatment with volar locking plate fixation in 73 patients aged 65 years or older, Arora et al. found no differences in range of motion or level of pain at 1-year follow-up; although grip strength was better in those treated operatively, anatomic reconstruction did not improve patients' ability to perform daily living activities. Egol et al. also found that minor limitations in wrist range of motion and diminished grip strength after nonoperative treatment

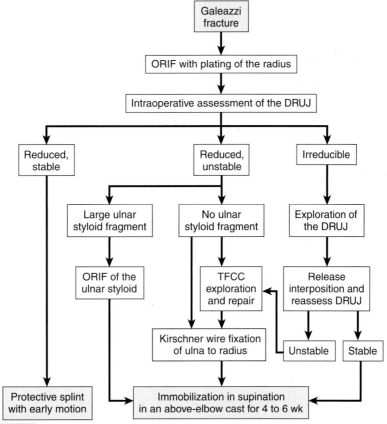

FIGURE **5.100**   Treatment algorithm for Galeazzi fractures in adults. *ORIF*, Open reduction internal fixation; *DRUJ*, distal radioulnar joint; *TFCC*, triangular fibrocartilage complex.

did not limit functional recovery in 90 patients older than the age of 65 years. In their systematic review and meta-analysis, Chen et al. determined that although operative management resulted in better radiographic outcomes and grip strength, there was no significant difference in pain, function, or range of motion, and major complications were significantly more frequent in those treated operatively.

PERCUTANEOUS PINNING

Percutaneous pinning after closed reduction is useful for distal radial fractures with metaphyseal instability or simpler intraarticular displacement. An anatomic reduction must be obtained first, and then stability is provided by the Kirschner wires. Usually the first pins are placed from the radial styloid across to the medial radial metaphysis and diaphysis. We generally use at least two pins and confirm adequate reduction on anteroposterior and lateral views. The lunate facet can then pinned into position if needed. Intrafocal pins (Kapandji technique) can be added to provide a dorsal buttress. A number of studies have reported success with this technique. Glickel et al. reported good long-term outcomes with closed reduction and percutaneous pinning of all but the most complex injuries. Three recent randomized controlled trials comparing volar locking plates and closed reduction with percutaneous pinning of distal radial fractures failed to show an advantage to the use of volar locking plates.

Percutaneous pinning tends to work better when placed in subchondral bone, where bone quality and density usually are better. Splint or cast immobilization usually is necessary after percutaneous pinning. Some complications related to the technique of percutaneous pinning include tendon tethering, injury, or rupture; pin migration; nerve injury; and pin site infections.

CLOSED REDUCTION AND PERCUTANEOUS PINNING OF DISTAL RADIAL FRACTURE

TECHNIQUE 5.16

(GLICKEL ET AL.)

- After sterile preparation and draping, place the thumb and index fingers in finger traps for longitudinal traction (typically 10 lb). Manipulate and reduce the fracture (Fig. 5.103A).
- Evaluate the reduction fluoroscopically; if adequate, proceed with percutaneous pinning. If the reduction is not anatomic, or if there is severe comminution, alternative techniques such as ORIF may be indicated.
- Make a 1.5-cm incision longitudinally, beginning at the radial styloid and proceeding distally (Fig. 5.103B).

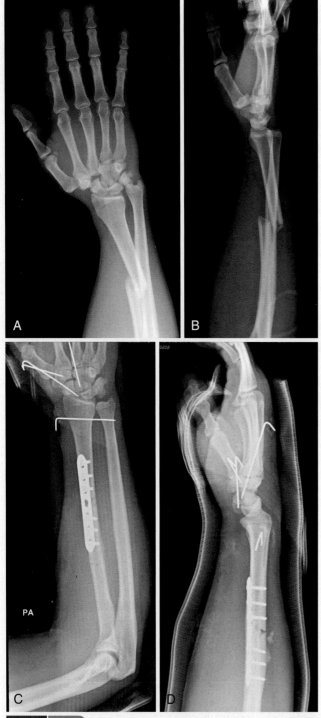

FIGURE 5.101 **A** and **B,** Galeazzi fracture-dislocation. **C** and **D,** Fixation of radius with dynamic compression plate; fixation of distal radioulnar joint with Kirschner wires.

- Identify the branches of the superficial radial nerve, mobilize them with blunt dissection, and retract them.
- Identify the first extensor compartment and place two 1.6-mm (0.062-inches) Kirschner wires in succession from the radial styloid across the fracture site to engage the ulnar cortex of the radius proximal to the fracture. Place these wires either dorsal or volar to the first extensor compartment, depending on fracture pattern and anatomic variations.

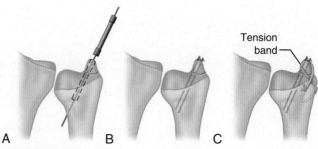

FIGURE 5.102 Open reduction and internal fixation of ulnar styloid fracture with lag screw **(A)**, pins **(B)**, and tension band technique **(C)**. (Adapted from Katolik LI, Trumble T: Distal radioulnar joint dysfunction, *J Am Soc Surg Hand* 5:8, 2005.)

- Place one 1.6-mm Kirschner wire percutaneously 90 degrees orthogonally to these wires, starting at the dorsal rim of the distal radius just distal to the Lister tubercle. Confirm the correct starting point with fluoroscopy and drive the wire in a proximal and volar direction across the fracture site to engage the volar cortex of the radius proximal to the fracture (Fig. 5.103C).
- If there is marked dorsal comminution, a second dorsal pin can be placed either into the dorsal rim of the distal radius or used as an intrafocal pin. If there is marked radial comminution and prereduction radial translation, an additional buttress pin can be placed into the radial aspect of the fracture and driven into the proximal ulnar cortex of the radius. A crossed-pin configuration, in which the pins are placed from the distal ulnar radial cortex and passed to engage the intact cortex radially, also may be helpful (Fig. 5.103D).
- Place additional wires as necessary to secure additional fracture fragments.
- Bend and cut the wires, leaving them superficial to the skin. Close the radial styloid incision with interrupted absorbable sutures. Apply a sugar-tong splint.

POSTOPERATIVE CARE The splint is worn for 2 weeks to control rotation and minimize irritation at the pin sites, and then a soft arm cast is applied. The cast and pins are removed at between 5 and 6 weeks depending on the fracture pattern, the patient's age and bone quality, and the extent of healing seen on radiographs. When healing is confirmed by lack of tenderness over the fracture and radiographic evidence of bridging callus across the fracture, supervised hand therapy is begun, including wound care and 1 to 2 weeks of splinting. As edema and pain decrease, soft-tissue and joint mobilization protocols are instituted and active and active-assisted range-of-motion exercises are begun. Functional use and activities are strongly encouraged by 8 to 10 weeks after surgery.

EXTERNAL FIXATION

External fixation can be useful as primary or adjunctive treatment in certain distal radial fractures. The external fixator neutralizes the axial load placed on the distal radius by physiologic activity of the forearm musculature. It can be placed in a bridging or nonbridging (does not cross the wrist joint) technique, with or without supplemental stabilization. Linear traction typically does not

TABLE 5.11

Radiographic Criteria for Acceptable Reduction of Distal Radial Fracture

CRITERION	NORMAL	ACCEPTABLE
Ulnar variance (radial length)	±2 mm comparing level of lunate facet to ulnar head	No more than 2 mm of shortening relative to ulnar head
Radial height	12 mm	????
Palmar (lateral) tilt	11 degrees of volar tilt	Neutral
Radial inclination	20 degrees as measured from lunate facet to radial styloid	No less than 10 degrees
Intraarticular step or gap	None	Less than 2 mm of either

fully restore volar tilt; however, neutral tilt is acceptable, and Wei et al. reported good results with external fixation when satisfactory reduction is obtained. Because external fixation alone can allow shortening and loss of reduction over time, supplemental fixation with percutaneous Kirschner wires is often used. The fixator is then used to neutralize the Kirschner wires. We rarely apply definitive external fixation without the use of supplemental Kirschner wires. The addition of a graft also can be useful with external fixation.

External fixation has been reported by several authors to obtain good results in distal radial fractures. In a comparison to cast treatment in 46 patients 65 years of age or older, Aktekin et al. found that wrist extension, ulnar deviation, palmar tilt, and radial height were better in those treated with external fixation. In a similar comparison to ORIF, better grip strength and range of motion, as well as fewer malunions, were found with internal fixation. A meta-analysis of comparative clinical trials concluded that ORIF yields significantly better functional outcomes, forearm supination, and restoration of volar tilt while external fixation results in better grip strength and wrist flexion. The quality of the reduction appears to be the determining factor in outcome. Two studies comparing volar locking plates to external fixation by Grewal et al. and Williksen et al. did not show conclusively that volar locking plates obtained superior results.

Nonbridging external fixation consists of a distal pin cluster inserted into the distal fragment without crossing the wrist joint. McQueen has reported on this technique for fractures that demonstrate enough distal bone to accept the external fixator pins. In extraarticular fractures, the results have been excellent. Despite the number of reports of its successful use, external fixation has not become an often used technique for distal radial fracture fixation.

There are a variety of spanning and nonspanning external fixation devices available, and the techniques of application differ slightly according to the specific device chosen.

EXTERNAL FIXATION OF FRACTURE OF THE DISTAL RADIUS

TECHNIQUE 5.17

SPANNING EXTERNAL FIXATION
- With the use of brachial block or general anesthesia, prepare and drape the upper extremity and apply a tourni-

quet to the arm. Reduce the fracture manually or with the aid of sterile finger traps or traction device (see Fig. 5.103A).
- Make a 2- to 3-cm incision over the dorsoradial aspect of the index metacarpal base and use blunt dissection with scissors to expose the metacarpal. Take care to preserve and reflect the branches of the dorsal radial sensory nerve.
- Place a soft-tissue protector on the metacarpal and insert 3-mm self-tapping half-pins at a 30- to 45-degree angle dorsal to the frontal plane of the hand and forearm. Confirm pin position and length with fluoroscopy.
- Make a 4-cm skin incision 8 to 10 cm proximal to the wrist joint and just dorsal to the midline.
- With blunt dissection, expose the superficial branches of the lateral antebrachial cutaneous nerve and the radial sensory nerve, the latter of which exits in the midforearm from the investing fascia between the brachioradialis and extensor carpi radialis longus (Fig. 5.104A).
- Insert two 3-mm half-pins, 1.5 cm apart, through a soft-tissue protector between the radial wrist extensors at a 30-degree angle dorsal to the frontal plane of the forearm (Fig. 5.104B). The pins should just perforate the medial cortex of the radius. Confirm pin position and length with fluoroscopy.
- Irrigate and close both incisions with 4-0 nylon sutures.
- Apply the selected external fixation frame according to the manufacturer's instructions. For relatively stable fractures and when using Kirschner wires for augmentation of the fixation, a simple single-bar frame usually is sufficient (Fig. 5.105); more complex fixators allow independent palmar carpal translation to adjust volar tilt.

NONSPANNING EXTERNAL FIXATION
- If nonspanning external fixation is chosen for a minimally comminuted extraarticular or simple articular fracture in a patient with good bone stock, insert the proximal pins as described earlier.
- Insert the distal pins into the distal fragment. Place a radial-sided pin through a small dorsal radial incision between the wrist extensors in the radial half of the distal fragment. Direct the pin dorsal palmar, parallel to the joint surface in the sagittal plane.
- Insert a second pin in the ulnar aspect of the distal fragment through a limited incision between the fourth and fifth extensor compartments. Also direct this pin dorsal

TABLE 5.12

Classification of Distal Radial Fractures

GARTLAND AND WERLEY (1951)

Group 1	Simple Colles fracture
Group 2	Comminuted Colles fracture, undisplaced intraarticular fragment
Group 3	Comminuted Colles fracture, displaced intraarticular fragment

FRYKMAN (1967)

Group 1	Extraarticular without fracture of the distal ulna
Group 2	Extraarticular with fracture of the distal ulna
Group 3	Intraarticular involving the radiocarpal joint without fracture of the distal ulna
Group 4	Intraarticular involving the radiocarpal joint with fracture of the distal ulna
Group 5	Intraarticular involving the distal radioulnar joint without fracture of the distal ulna
Group 6	Intraarticular involving the distal radioulnar joint with fracture of the distal ulna
Group 7	Intraarticular involving both radiocarpal and distal radioulnar joints without fracture of the distal ulna
Group 8	Intraarticular involving both radiocarpal and distal radioulnar joints with fracture of the distal ulna

MELONE (1986)

Type 1	Undisplaced, minimal comminution, stable
Type 2	Unstable, displacement of medial complex, moderate-to-severe comminution
Type 3	Displacement of medial complex as a unit plus an anterior spike
Type 4	Wide separation or rotation of the dorsal fragment and palmar fragment rotation

FERNANDEZ (1987)

Type 1	*Bending*: One cortex of the metaphysis fails because of tensile stress; opposite cortex with some comminution
Type 2	*Shearing:* Fracture of the joint surface
Type 3	*Compression:* Fracture of the joint surface with impaction of subchondral and metaphyseal bone, intraarticular comminution
Type 4	*Avulsion:* Fracture of the ligament attachments of the ulnar and radial styloid process, radiocarpal fracture-dislocation
Type 5	*Combination:* High-velocity injuries

COONEY (1990) UNIVERSAL CLASSIFICATION

Type I	Extraarticular, undisplaced
Type 2	Extraarticular, displaced
Type 3	Intraarticular, undisplaced
Type 4	Intraarticular, displaced

MODIFIED AO

Type A	Extraarticular

Type B	Partial articular
	    B1–radial styloid fracture
	    B2–dorsal rim fracture
	    B3–volar rim fracture
	    B4–die-punch fracture

Type C	Complete articular

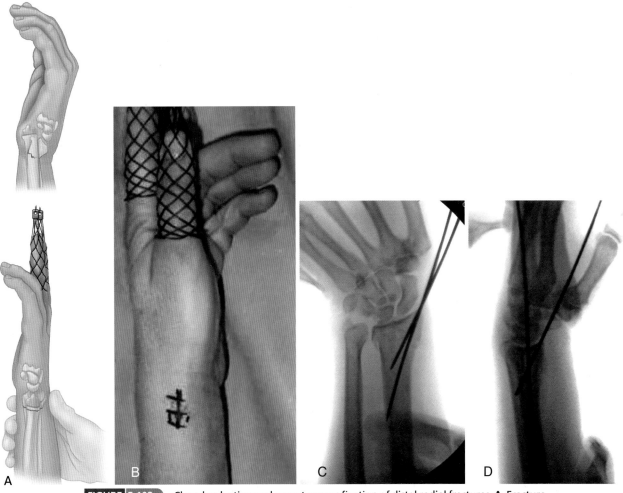

FIGURE 5.103   Closed reduction and percutaneous fixation of distal radial fractures. **A,** Fracture reduction. Suspension from finger allows disimpaction of the fracture, followed by pressure applied with thumb over distal fragment. **B,** Longitudinal incision. **C,** Percutaneous pinning confirmed fluoroscopically. **D,** Crossed pin configuration. (From Wolfe SW: Distal radius fractures. In Wolfe SW, Hotchkiss RN, Pederson WC, Kozin SH, editors: *Green's operative hand surgery*, ed 6, Philadelphia, 2011, Elsevier.) **SEE TECHNIQUES 5.16 AND 5.17.**

palmar, but aim it slightly obliquely from the ulnar to radial side to engage the palmar ulnar cortex of the distal fragment.

- Use the distal pins as "joysticks" to reduce the fracture and restore volar tilt.
- Assemble the pins with separate clamps and rods to create a triangular frame.

AUGMENTED EXTERNAL FIXATION

- For all but minimally comminuted extraarticular fractures, augmentation of the external fixation is recommended to provide additional support to individual fracture fragments and increase stability.
- For unstable fractures without depressed articular fragments, introduce 0.045- or 0.0625-inch Kirschner wires into the fracture fragments; a crossed configuration can be used to increase stability (Fig. 5.106A,B). Drive one or two pins through the radial styloid fragment and one through the dorsal ulnar fragment into the radial shaft to produce maximal stability. Pins should pierce the ulnar cortex of the radius but not penetrate into the ulnar shaft.

- Cut off the pins 1 cm external to the skin margin and bend them at an acute angle.
- Apply the external fixator according to manufacturer's instructions (Fig. 5.106C,D). Some fixators have components to accommodate the Kirschner wires.

POSTOPERATIVE CARE The wrist remains immobilized in a supinated position with a sugar-tong splint for 10 days until pain and swelling have subsided. This promotes stability of the distal radioulnar joint and facilitates resumption of full supination. The external fixator frame usually is removed at 6 weeks; any supplemental pins are kept in place for 8 weeks. Active and passive finger motion is begun as soon as the anesthesia wears off and is encouraged the entire time the frame is in place. Supination and pronation of the forearm are begun at the first postoperative visit. Supervised hand therapy is recommended for patients who are unwilling or unable to mobilize their fingers and forearm independently.

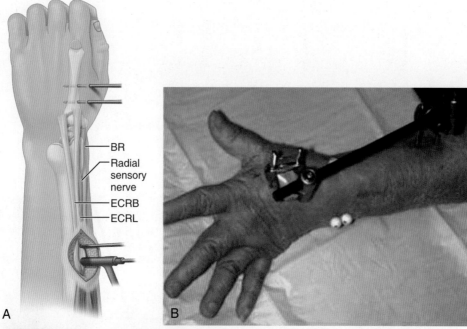

FIGURE 5.104   **A,** Two 3-mm half-pins introduced into base or second metacarpal and two into distal radius. *BR,* brachioradialis; *ECRB,* extensor carpi radialis brevis; *ECRL,* extensor carpi radialis longus. **B,** Single-bar frame for external fixation of distal radial fracture. (From Wolfe SW: Distal radius fractures. In Wolfe SW, Hotchkiss RN, Pederson WC, Kozin SH, editors: *Green's operative hand surgery,* ed 6, Philadelphia, 2011,Elsevier.) **SEE TECHNIQUE 5.17.**

■ OPEN REDUCTION AND PLATE FIXATION
▌DORSAL PLATING

Most distal radial fractures result in an apex-volar angulation with dorsal cortical comminution. First-generation dorsal plate designs were a logical solution but were fraught with complications secondary to tendon dysfunction and rupture, which prompted a move to fixed-angle volar plating techniques after the development of angle-stable screws. There is still a role for dorsal plating, and newer lower-profile designs may decrease complications. In certain situations, such as dorsal die-punch fractures or fractures with displaced dorsal lunate facet fragments, a dorsal approach with a low-profile fragment-specific plate appears to work well. At this time, most of our dorsal plating is done with a fragment-specific technique, often in conjunction with other forms of fixation.

▌VOLAR PLATING

The popularity of locked volar distal radial plate fixation continues to prompt development of new devices. Capo et al. demonstrated the biomechanical superiority of volar plating over dorsal and radioulnar dual-column plating, and several clinical studies have reported better functional results with volar plating than with dorsal plating, external fixation, and percutaneous pinning; however, a complication rate of approximately 15% also has been reported with volar plating, primarily problems with tendon ruptures and tenosynovitis from prominent screws. Screw penetration of the radiocarpal joint occurred in 11 of 40 patients described by Knight et al. A low-profile volar plate produced no tendon ruptures in 95 patients reported by Soong et al. Precise volar plate placement on the metaphyseal area of the distal radius may lessen the problems of flexor tendon irritation and eventual rupture (Fig. 5.107). In their series of 122 patients with distal radial fractures treated with volar locking plates, Roh et al. identified an increase in age and a decrease in bone mineral density as important risk factors for delayed functional recovery up to 12 months after surgery; fracture severity and high-energy trauma were associated with decreased functional outcomes up to 6 months after surgery. Wadsten et al., in a multicenter cohort study, showed that volar and dorsal comminution predicted later displacement. Volar comminution was the strongest predictor of displacement.

VOLAR PLATE FIXATION OF FRACTURE OF THE DISTAL RADIUS

TECHNIQUE 5.18

(CHUNG et al.)

- Make an 8-cm incision over the forearm between the radial artery and the flexor carpi radialis. Extension of the incision distally at the wrist crease in a V-shape may provide wider exposure of the fracture and help prevent scar contracture. The distal incision does not need to cross into the palm (Fig. 5.108A).
- Carry the incision to the sheath of the flexor carpi radialis (Fig. 5.108B). Open the sheath and incise the forearm deep fascia to expose the flexor pollicis longus.

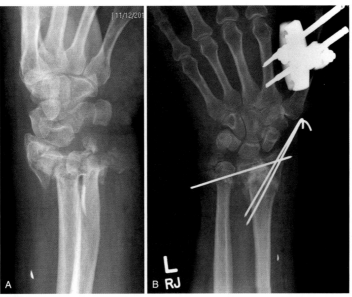

FIGURE 5.105 **A,** Fracture of distal radius. **B,** External fixation with supplemental percutaneous Kirschner wire fixation. **SEE TECHNIQUE 5.17**.

- Place an index finger into the wound and gently sweep the flexor pollicis longus ulnarly. Partially detach the flexor pollicis longus muscle belly from the radius to gain full exposure of the pronator quadratus (Fig. 5.108C).
- Make an L-shaped incision over the radial styloid along the radial border of the radius to expose the pronator quadratus and use a Freer elevator to elevate it from the radius (Fig. 5.108D). The entire fracture line across the distal radius is now fully exposed (Fig. 5.108E).
- Insert a Freer elevator or small osteotome into the fracture line to serve as a lever to reduce the fracture. Insert the elevator or osteotome across the fracture line all the way to the dorsal cortex to allow disimpaction and reduction of the distal fragment. Apply finger pressure to the dorsal cortex to reduce the dorsal fragments.
- With a displaced radial styloid fracture, the brachioradialis may prevent reduction by pulling on the radial styloid. To relieve the deforming force, the brachioradialis can be transacted or detached from the distal radius.
- If necessary, use a Kirschner wire to temporarily fix the distal fragment to the proximal fragment. This usually is not necessary because distal traction should maintain reduction while the volar plate is placed.
- Disimpact and reduce the fracture through capsuloligamentotaxis achieved by an assistant through finger traction. After successful fracture reduction, position the volar plate under fluoroscopic guidance and insert a screw into the oblong or gliding hole first to allow proximal-distal adjustment (Fig. 5.108F). Use a 2.5-mm drill bit to drill into the center of the oblong hole and insert a self-tapping 3.5-mm screw.
- Confirm proper placement of the volar plate with mini-C-arm fluoroscopy. If necessary, shift the plate proximally or distally to provide the best placement for the distal screws.
- Use a 2.0-mm drill bit to drill the distal holes. Measure the holes for screw length and insert smooth locking screws. Use a screw that is 2 mm shorter than the measured length to avoid having a prominent distal screw perfo-

rate the dorsal cortex; typically, 20- to 22-mm screws are optimal, except for screws directed into the radial styloid, which are significantly shorter. Threaded screws may gain better bone dorsally; however, pegs may be sufficient when bone quality is poor.
- Once the first screw is inserted, distal traction on the fingers can be released because the fracture usually is appropriately reduced and fixed (Fig. 5.108G).
- Because of the fixed-angle design, the screws may perforate into the radiocarpal joint if the plate is placed too far distally. Obtain fluoroscopic views tangential to the subchondral bone in both the coronal and sagittal planes to assess for intraarticular penetration. Adjust the plate or screws, or both as indicated.
- After placement of the distal screws, place the remaining proximal screws (Fig. 5.108H).
- Reattach the pronator quadratus with braided absorbable sutures. Note that the pronator will not be able to cover the entire plate; the distal portion should be covered when possible to reduce flexor tendon-plate contact. For better purchase, the pronator quadratus can be sutured to the edge of the brachioradialis (Fig. 5.108I).
- If the ulnar styloid is fractured and displaced, making the distal radioulnar joint unstable, fix the styloid with one or two percutaneous Kirschner wires (Fig. 5.109). A volar approach may be helpful to obtain ulnar styloid reduction. Smaller fragments usually do not require surgical management; however, if the distal radioulnar joint is unstable after fixation of the radial fracture, styloid fragments can be excised and the peripheral rim of the triangular fibrocartilage complex anchored to the ulnar styloid base with nonabsorbable braided suture through drill holes or a bone anchor.
- Close the wound in layers and apply a splint.

POSTOPERATIVE CARE At 1 week, the sutures are removed and active wrist motion is begun when there is confidence in fracture stability. A removable Orthoplast (Northcoast Medical, Gilroy, CA) splint is worn for 6 weeks. Most

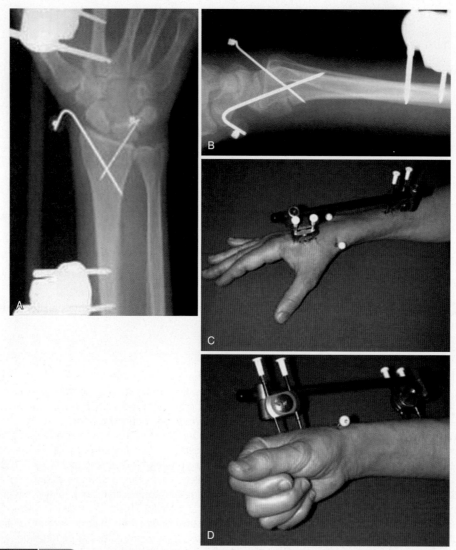

FIGURE 5.106 **A** and **B,** Crossed-pin augmentation with external fixation **(C** and **D)** of distal radial fracture. (From Wolfe SW: Distal radius fractures. In Wolfe SW, Hotchkiss RN, Pederson WC, Kozin SH, editors: *Green's operative hand surgery*, ed 6, Philadelphia, 2011, Elsevier.) **SEE TECHNIQUE 5.17.**

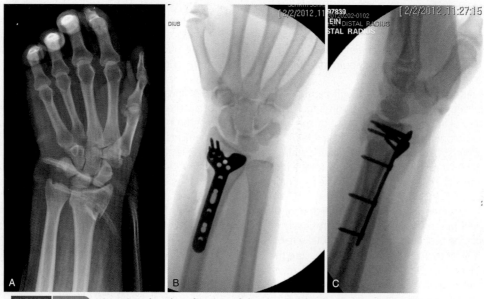

FIGURE 5.107 **A** to **C,** Volar plate fixation of distal radial fracture.

patients are given a home therapy program, but elderly patients may require twice-a-week supervised home therapy. Brehmer and Husband found in a prospective randomized controlled study that an accelerated rehabilitation protocol, which emphasizes motion immediately postoperatively and initiates strengthening at 2 weeks after volar open reduction and internal fixation, results in an earlier return to function than a standard rehabilitation protocol.

DISTRACTION PLATE FIXATION

As an alternative to external fixation of highly comminuted fractures of the distal radius, Burke and Singer described the use of a distraction plate as an internal fixator. The plate is applied to the dorsal surface of the hand, wrist, and distal forearm using three small incisions. External fixation pin site problems are avoided, and the plate can remain in place as long as necessary for union. Secondary bone grafting procedures also are done more easily without an overlying external fixator. Ruch et al. reported good-to-excellent outcomes in 90% of 22 patients using this technique, and Richard et al. reported good results in 33 patients over the age of 60 years.

TECHNIQUE 5.19

(BURKE AND SINGER AS MODIFIED BY RUCH ET AL.)

- Make a 4-cm longitudinal incision over the dorsal aspect of the long finger metacarpal shaft. Expose the bone by retracting the long finger extensor tendon.
- Make a second 4-cm dorsal incision at least 4 cm above the comminuted segment of the radius and expose the bone.
- Make a third 2-cm dorsal incision over the Lister tubercle, exposing the extensor pollicis longus tendon.
- Pass a 12- to 16-hole, 3.5-mm plate from the distal incision in a proximal direction using the plane between the extensor tendons (fourth dorsal compartment) and the joint capsule and periosteum. Mobilize the extensor tendons if necessary.
- Secure the plate to the long finger metacarpal shaft with three bicortical 3.5-mm screws.
- Under fluoroscopic guidance, apply distal traction to obtain normal radial length. With the hand in 60 degrees of supination, secure the plate to the radius with a bone clamp.
- Confirm that full rotation of the forearm is possible and then secure the plate with three bicortical 3- to 5-mm screws (Fig. 5.110).
- Reduce and fix diaphyseal fragments to the shaft with interfragmentary screws if possible.
- Elevate the lunate fossa through the middle incision.
- Insert a 3.5-mm screw through the plate and under the elevated lunate fossa to serve as a buttress.
- Percutaneously pin other fragments to stabilize the articular surface using Kirschner wires.

- Place bone graft into the defects through the middle incision using autograft, allograft, or bone graft substitute.
- Assess the stability of the distal radioulnar joint. If it is unstable, immobilize the wrist in a sugar-tong splint.

POSTOPERATIVE CARE Finger and other joint upper extremity exercises are begun immediately. If a splint was applied, it should be removed at 3 weeks. Percutaneous Kirschner wires should be removed at 6 weeks. Activities of daily living are allowed, but lifting should be restricted to 5 lb. When union is achieved, the distraction plate is removed and range-of-motion exercises are begun.

▎FRAGMENT-SPECIFIC OPEN REDUCTION AND INTERNAL FIXATION OF COMMINUTED DISTAL RADIAL FRACTURES

Recognizing the pitfalls of Kirschner wire fixation and plate and screw fixation when used alone for repair of comminuted intraarticular distal radial fractures, Medoff developed a wrist fixation system that combines both methods for stable reconstruction of the distal radius. Five potential fracture fragments are possible, especially in osteopenic bone: radial column, dorsal cortical wall, dorsal ulnar split, volar rim, and the central intraarticular fragment (Fig. 5.111). Radial styloid Kirschner wire fixation does not prevent settling or radial drift of the distal radial fracture fragments (Fig. 5.112). Thin metaphyseal cortical bone, especially in osteopenic bone, does not hold screws well, and conventional plates cannot be applied easily on the dorsal aspect of the distal radius because of plate thickness, potential irritation, and eventual rupture of the dorsal wrist tendons.

The addition of a small buttress plate to a radial styloid pin prevents collapse and radial migration of the distal radius (Fig. 5.113). The radial styloid pin now has two fixation points—the first through the distal end of the plate and the second through the intact medial radial cortex.

The dorsal ulnar fragment is stabilized with an ulnar pin-plate of a similar design. This pin-plate maintains the length of the ulnar column and reduction of the distal radioulnar joint (Fig. 5.114). Wire-form implants are used to stabilize the dorsal cortical wall, the intraarticular fragment, and any structural bone graft used to support the articular fragment. Three different wire-form implants are used, depending on the fracture fragments present (Fig. 5.115). The volar rim–lunate facet fragment is secured with a low-profile buttress plate similar to that used for repair of volar Barton fractures (Fig. 5.116).

Medoff reported 20 good-to-excellent results in 21 patients with intraarticular comminuted distal radial fractures treated with the TriMed system (TriMed Inc., Valencia, CA). We have had similar good results (Fig. 5.117).

COMPLICATIONS

The type and frequency of complications of the distal radius vary greatly among reported series. In their literature review, McKay et al. found overall complication rates ranging from 6% to 80% and rates of posttraumatic arthritis that ranged from 7% to 65% (Table 5.13). Jupiter and Fernandez identified malunion with an intraarticular or extraarticular deformity as the most frequent complication. The reported incidence of distal radial malunion is approximately 17%. It is

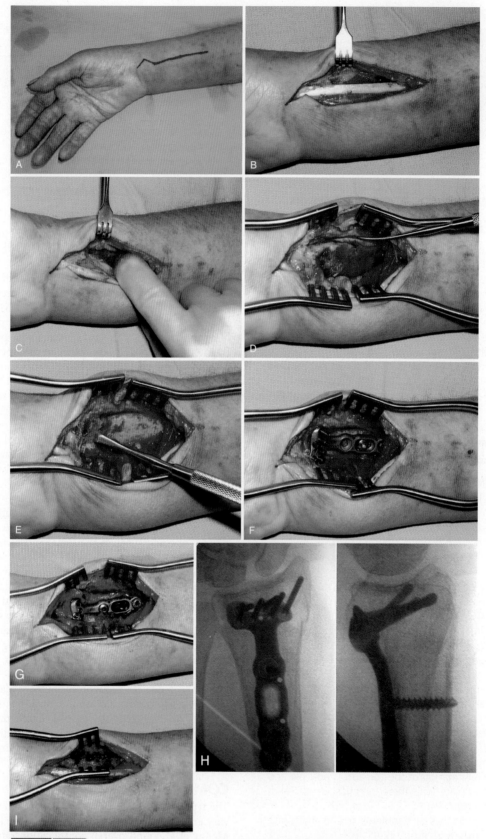

FIGURE 5.108 Volar plate fixation of distal radial fracture. **A,** Skin incision. **B,** Incision carried to flexor carpi radialis sheath. **C,** Flexor pollicis longus muscle belly is partially detached from radius to expose pronator quadratus. **D,** Freer elevator is used to elevate pronator quadratus from radius. **E,** Fracture line is exposed. **F,** Volar plate positioned, insertion of first screw. **G,** Insertion of second screw after release of distal traction on fingers. **H,** Remaining proximal screws are placed. **I,** Pronator quadratus sutured to edge of brachioradialis. **SEE TECHNIQUE 5.18.**

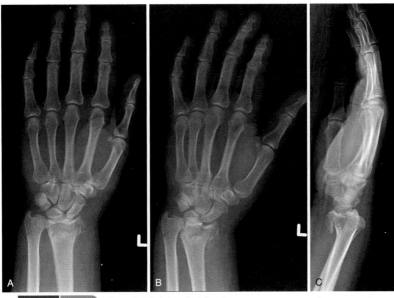

FIGURE 5.109   **A** to **C,** Distal radial fracture.

more common after nonoperative than operative treatment. The most common deformity after extraarticular distal radial fracture is shortening, rotation of the distal fragment, loss of volar tilt, and loss of ulnar inclination. Osteotomies and other operative procedures for the treatment of wrist problems after distal radial fracture are discussed in other chapter.

Other less frequently reported complications include nonunion, implant complications, tendon rupture or scarring, and neurologic injuries. Nonunion of distal radial fractures is uncommon, occurring in less than 1% of patients, and is more frequent after operative treatment than nonoperative treatment. Factors suggested to predispose to nonunion include open comminuted fractures, infections, pathologic lesions, soft-tissue interposition, inadequate fixation, excessive distraction with an external fixator, and a concomitant fracture of the distal ulna.

Tendon complications are most frequent after locked volar plating when the plate is placed too distal or off the bone or when screws that are too long are used, resulting in impingement on the traversing flexor tendons. Prominence of the volar plate at the watershed line, where the flexor tendons lie closest to the bone and plate, also has been implicated as a cause of flexor tendon rupture from abrasion. Flexor tendon ruptures have been reported in up to 12% of patients with locked volar plating. In a series of 96 distal radial fractures treated with volar plating, complications were identified in 23%; the frequency of complications decreased with increased surgeon experience. A systematic literature review of unstable distal radial fractures in elderly patients (60 years or older) identified rupture or adhesion of the flexor pollicis longus tendon, extensor pollicis longus, or both as the most common major complication requiring surgery after volar locked plating. In a comparison of younger (20 to 40 years of age) and older (60 years or older) patients treated with volar locking plates, Chung et al. found no increase in complication rates in older patients. Hanel et al. reported 16 complications (12%) in 144 fractures treated with dorsal distraction plates, noting that patients whose plates were left in place for longer than 16 weeks had an overall complication rate of 21%,

compared with a complication rate of 8.5% in those plates that were removed earlier. Rhee et al. listed several measures to avoid tendon injuries, including placement of volar plates proximal to the watershed line, closure of the pronator quadratus over a volar plate, and use of shorter unicortical screws or smooth pegs with volar plates. A dorsal tangential view of the wrist is helpful to detect screw penetration to the dorsal cortex during volar plating.

Compartment syndrome associated with distal radial fractures is rare, occurring in approximately 1% of patients, primarily younger patients with high-energy injuries. Complex regional pain syndrome (CRPS) occurs most commonly in elderly patients and those with psychological or psychiatric conditions and has been reported in 8% to 35% of patients with distal radial fractures. A randomized, controlled, multicenter study involving 416 patients with 427 distal radial fractures determined that vitamin C (500 mg daily) can reduce the prevalence of CRPS, and this was listed as having "adequate evidence to support a moderately strong endorsement" in the recent AAOS clinical practice guidelines for distal radial fractures.

The median nerve is the most frequently injured (0% to 17%), followed by the radial and ulnar nerves, primarily because of its close proximity to the fracture and its confinement within the carpal canal. Mild carpal tunnel syndromes occur in up to 20% of patients, but most resolve without treatment. Acute carpal tunnel syndrome requiring immediate release is most likely after high-energy, severely comminuted fractures. Late median neuropathy may be associated with malunion, residual palmar displacement, nerve impingement by callus formation, or prolonged immobilization with the wrist in flexion and ulnar deviation. Injury to the radial and ulnar nerves is less common (0% to 10%). Immobilization with the wrist in excessive flexion (more than 20 degrees) and ulnar deviation should be avoided because this increases carpal tunnel pressure.

Regardless of the management strategy chosen for distal radial fractures, complications can occur even when appropriate care is delivered. The sequelae of specific complications may be lessened by prompt and problem-specific intervention.

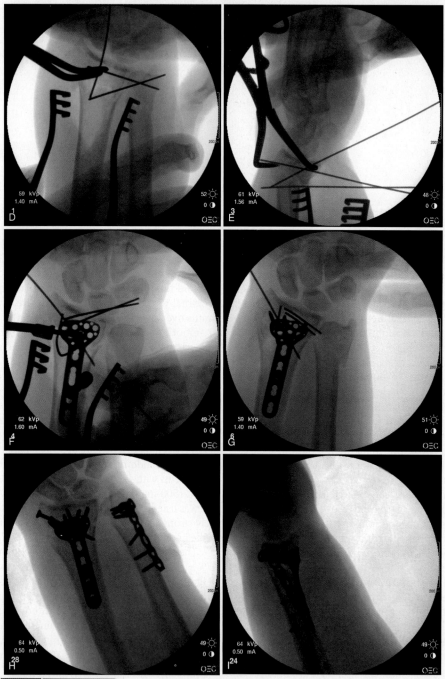

FIGURE 5.109, Cont'd **D** and **E,** Reduction and placement of Kirschner wires for provisional fixation. **F** and **G,** Plate application. **H** and **I,** Plate in place after removal of Kirschner wires. **SEE TECHNIQUE 5.18.**

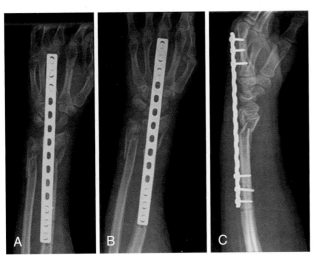

FIGURE 5.110   **A to C,** Distraction plate internal fixator. (From Ruch DS, Ginn TA, Yang CC, et al: Use of a distraction plate for distal radial fractures with metaphyseal and diaphyseal comminution, *J Bone Joint Surg* 87A:945, 2005.) **SEE TECHNIQUE 5.19.**

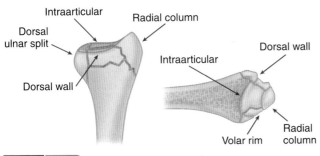

FIGURE 5.111   Distal radial fracture elements.

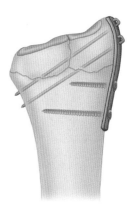

FIGURE 5.113   Radial pin-plate provides transstyloid Kirschner wires with two-point fixation, enhancing stability. Plate adds radial buttress to radial column and helps resist dorsal torque on radial column fracture. (Redrawn from Dr. R. Medoff.)

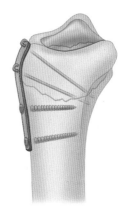

FIGURE 5.114   Ulnar pin-plate. Application of ulnar pin-plate for stabilization of dorsal ulnar split fragment. By proper contouring, plate can close gaps in sagittal plane.

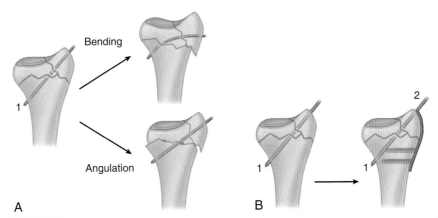

FIGURE 5.112   **A,** Transstyloid Kirschner wire has only single point of fixation. Minor bending of wire or angulation at site of purchase may result in significant loss of position of radial column fracture. **B,** By adding second point of constraint, pin-plate greatly enhances Kirschner wire fixation. In addition, pin-plate adds buttress to radial column fragment.

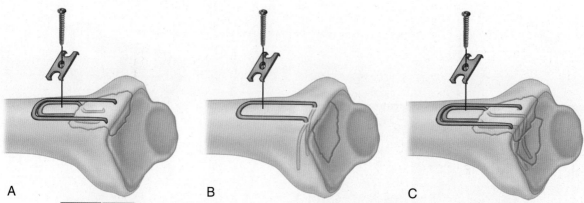

A   B   C

FIGURE 5.115 **A,** Small fragment clamp. Dorsal cortical wall fragment stabilized by small fragment clamp that provides pinch-type grip with extraosseous and endosteal wire form. **B,** Buttress pin. Intraarticular fragments are stabilized by providing peripheral cortical reconstruction around fragment and adding endosteal buttress, as shown here. **C,** Small fragment clamp/buttress pin combines function of small fragment clamp and buttress pin into single device to provide simultaneously stabilization of dorsal wall fragment and intraarticular component.

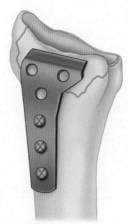

FIGURE 5.116 L-plate provides volar buttress to volar rim of lunate facet, yet allows fixation to subcutaneous radial side of proximal fragment.

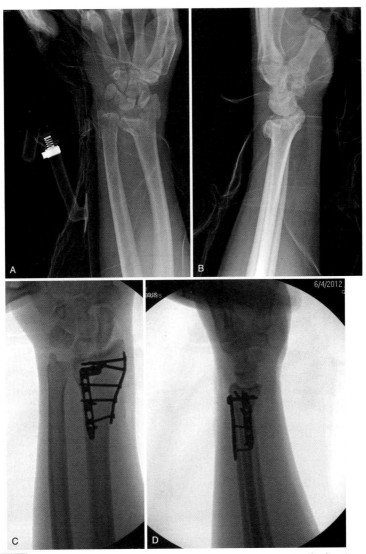

FIGURE 5.117 **A** and **B,** Distal radial fracture. **C** and **D,** Fragment-specific fixation.

TABLE 5.13

Complications After Fracture of Distal Radius

COMPLICATION	INCIDENCE (%)	NO. OF STUDIES*
Arthritis/arthrosis	7-65	4
Loss of motion	0-31	10
Implant complications	1.4-26	14
Nerve compression/neuritis	0-17	11
Osteomyelitis	4-9	2
Dupuytren contracture	2-9	4
Persistent pain/pain syndromes (CRPS)	0.3-8	11
Tendon (rupture, lag, trigger, tenosynovitis)	0-5	3
Delayed union/nonunion	0.7-4	4
Radioulnar (synostosis, disturbance)	0-1.3	2

*Number of studies from which frequencies were determined to calculate incidence.
CRPS, Complex regional pain syndrome.
Data from McKay SC, MacDermid JC, Roth JH, Richards RS: Assessment of complications of distal radius fractures and development of a complication checklist, *J Hand Surg* 26A:916, 2001.

REFERENCES

CLAVICLE AND SCAPULA

Ahmed AF, Salameh M, Al Khatib N, et al.: Open reduction and internal fixation versus nonsurgical treatment in displaced midshaft clavicle fractures: a metaanalysis, *J Orthop Trauma* 32:e276, 2018.

Ahrens PM, Garlick NI, Barber J, Tims EM: The Clavicle Trial Collaborative Group: the clavicle trial. A multicenter randomized controlled trial comparing operative with nonoperative treatment of displaced midshaft clavicle fractures, *J Bone Joint Surg Am* 99:1345, 2017.

Anavian J, Conflitti JM, Khanna G, et al.: A reliable radiographic measurement technique for extra-articular scapular fractures, *Clin Orthop Relat Res* 469:3371, 2011.

Anavian J, Gauger EM, Schroder LK, et al.: Surgical and functional outcomes after operative management of complex and displaced intra-articular glenoid fractures, *J Bone Joint Surg* 94:645, 2012.

Anavian J, Khanna G, Plocher EK, et al.: Progressive displacement of scapula fractures, *J Trauma* 69:156, 2010.

Assobhi JEH: Reconstruction plate versus minimal invasive retrograde titanium elastic nail fixation for displaced midclavicular fractures, *J Orthop Traumatol* 12:185, 2011.

Bachoura A, Deane AS, Kamineni S: Clavicle anatomy and the applicability of intramedullary midshaft fracture fixation, *J Shoulder Elbow Surg* 21:1384, 2012.

Bachoura A, Deane AS, Wise JN, Kamineni S: Clavicle morphometry revisited: a 3-dimensional study with relevance to operative fixation, *J Shoulder Elbow Surg* 22:e15, 2013.

Banerjee R, Waterman B, Padalecki J, Robertson W: Management of distal clavicle fractures, *J Am Acad Orthop Surg* 19:392, 2011.

Bartonicek J, Fric V: Scapular body fractures: results of operative treatment, *Int Orthop* 35:747, 2011.

Cole PA, Gauger EM, Herrera DA, et al.: Radiographic follow-up of 82 operatively treated scapula neck and body fractures, *Injury* 43:327, 2012.

Cole PA, Gauger EM, Schroder LK: Management of scapular fractures, *J Am Acad Orthop Surg* 20:130, 2012.

Cole PA, Dugarte AJ: Posterior scapula approaches: extensile and modified Judet, *J Orthop Trauma* 32(8):s10, 2018.

Cole PA, Gilbertson JA, Cole PA: Functional outcomes of operative management of scapula fractures in a geriatric cohort, *J Orthop Trauma* 31:e1, 2017.

Czajka CM, Kay A, Gary JL, et al.: Symptomatic implant removal following dual mini-fragment plating for clavicular shaft fractures, *J Orthop Trauma* 31:236, 2017.

Dienstknecht T, Horst K, Pishnamaz M, et al.: A meta-analysis of operative versus nonoperative treatment in 463 scapular neck fractures, *Scand J Surg* 102:69, 2013.

Dimitroulias A, Molinero KG, Krenk DE, et al.: Outcomes of nonoperatively treated displaced scapular body fractures, *Clin Orthop Relat Res* 469:1459, 2011.

Duan X, Zhong G, Cen S, et al.: Plating versus intramedullary pin or conservative treatment for midshaft fracture of clavicle: a meta-analysis of randomized controlled trials, *J Shoulder Elbow Surg* 20:1008, 2011.

Ferran NA, Hodgson P, Vannet N, et al.: Locked intramedullary fixation vs plating for displaced and shortened mid-shaft clavicle fractures: a randomized clinical trial, *J Shoulder Elbow Surg* 19:783, 2010.

Fox HM, Ramsey DC, Thompson AR, et al.: Neer type-II distal clavicle fractures: a cost-effectiveness analysis of fixation techniques, *J Bone Joint Surg Am*, 2019. https://doi.org/10.2106/JBJS.19.00590.

Frigg A, Rillmann P, Perren T, et al.: Intramedullary nailing of clavicular midshaft fractures with the titanium elastic nail: problems and complications, *Am J Sports Med* 37:352, 2009.

Frigg A, Rillmann P, Ryf C, et al.: Can complications of titanium elastic nailing with end cap for clavicular fractures be reduced? *Clin Orthop Relat Res* 469:3356, 2011.

Fuglesang HF, Flugsrud GB, Randsborg PH, et al.: Radiological and functional outcomes 2.7 years following conservatively treated completely displaced midshaft clavicle fractures, *Arch Orthop Trauma Surg* 136(1):17, 2016.

Furey MJ, McKee MD: Fractures of the clavicle and scapula, AAOS orthopaedic knowledge update, *Trauma* 5:244, 2016.

Gauger EM, Cole PA: Surgical technique: a minimally invasive approach to scapula neck and body fractures, *Clin Orthop Relat Res* 469:3390, 2011.

Good DW, Lui DF, Leonard M, et al.: Clavicle hook plate fixation for displaced lateral-third clavicle fractures (Neer type II): a functional outcome study, *J Shoulder Elbow Surg* 21:1045, 2012.

Goudie EB, Clement ND, Murray IR, et al.: The influence of shortening on clinical outcome in healed displaced midshaft clavicular fractures after nonoperative treatment, *J Bone Joint Surg Am* 99:1166, 2017.

Harvey E, Audigé L, Herscovici Jr D, et al.: Development and validation of the new international classification for scapula fractures, *J Orthop Trauma* 26:364, 2012.

Hill BW, Jacobson AR, Anavian J, Cole PA: Surgical management of coracoid fractures: technical tricks and clinical experience, *J Orthop Trauma* 28:e114, 2014.

Houwert RM, Wijdicks FJ, Steins Bisschop C, et al.: Plate fixation verus intramedullary fixation for displaced mid-shaft clavicle fractures: a systematic review, *Int Orthop* 36:579, 2012.

Jain S, Altman GT: Lateral clavicle fractures, *J Hand Surg Am* 36A:1213, 2011.

Jarvis NE, Halliday L, Sinnott M, et al.: Surgery for the fractured clavicle: factors predicting nonunion, *J Shoulder Elbow Surg* 27:e155, 2018.

Jeray KJ, Cole PA: Clavicle and scapula fracture problems: functional assessment and current treatment strategies, *Instr Course Lect* 60:51, 2011.

Hsu KH, Tzeng YH, Chang MC, Hiang CC: Comparing the coracoclavicular loop technique with a hook plate for the treatment of distal clavicle fractures, *J Shoulder Elbow Surg* 27(2):224, 2018.

Hulsmans MH, van Heijl M, Houwert RM, et al.: Surgical fixation of midshaft clavicle fractures: a systematic review of biomechanical studies, *Injury Int J Care Injured* 49:753, 2018.

Jones CB, Sietsema DL: Analysis of operative versus nonoperative treatment of displaced scapular fractures, *Clin Orthop Relat Res* 469:3379, 2011.

Kleweno CP, Jawa A, Wells JH, et al.: Midshaft clavicular fractures: comparison of intramedullary pin and plate fixation, *J Shoulder Elbow Surg* 20:1114, 2011.

Lambotte A: *Chirurgie operatoire des fractures*, Paris, 1913, Masson & Cie.

Lewis S, Argintar E, Jahn R, et al.: Intra-articular scapular fractures: outcomes after internal fixation, *J Orthop* 10:188, 2013.

Liu HH, Chang CH, Chia WT, et al.: Comparison of plates versus intramedullary nails for fixation of displaced midshaft clavicular fractures, *J Trauma* 69:E82, 2010.

McKee MD: Clavicle fractures in 2010: sling/swathe or open reduction and internal fixation? *Orthop Clin North Am* 41:225, 2010.

McKnight B, Heckmann N, Hill JR, et al.: Surgical management of midshaft clavicle nonunions is associated with a higher rate of short-term complications compared with acute fractures, *J Shoulder Elbow Surg* 25:1412, 2016.

Millett PJ, Hurst JM, Horan MP, Hawkins RJ: Complications of clavicle fractures treated with intramedullary fixation, *J Shoulder Elbow Surg* 20:86, 2011.

Mudd CD, Quigley KJ, Gross LB: Excessive complications of open intramedullary nailing of midshaft clavicle fractures with the Rockwood Clavicle Pin, *Clin Orthop Relat Res* 469:3364, 2011.

Murray LR, Eros A, Robinson CM: Risk factors for nonunion after nonoperative treatment of displaced midshaft fractures of the clavicle, *J Bone Joint Surg* 95:1153, 2013.

Noguchi T, Mautner JF, Duncan SFM: Dorsal plate fixation of scapular fracture, *J Hand Surg Am* 42(10):843, 2017.

Nourian A, Dhaliwal S, Vangala S, Vezeridis PS: Midshaft fractures of the clavicle: a meta-analysis comparing surgical fixation using anteroinferior plating versus superior plating, *J Orthop Trauma* 31(9):461, 2017.

Oh JH, Kim SH, Lee JH, et al.: Treatment of distal clavicle fracture: a systematic review of treatment modalities in 425 fractures, *Arch Orthop Trauma Surg* 131:525, 2011.

Patterson JM, Galatz L, Streubel PN, et al.: CT evaluation of extra-articular glenoid neck fractures: does the glenoid medialize or does the scapula lateralize? *J Orthop Trauma* 26:360, 2012.

Payne DE, Wray WH, Ruch DS, et al.: Outcome of intramedullary fixation of clavicular fractures, *Am J Orthop (Belle Mead NJ)* 40:E99, 2011.

Pizanis A, Tosounidis G, Braun C, et al.: The posterior two-portal approach for reconstruction of scapula fractures: results of 39 patients, *Injury* 44:1630, 2013.

Pulos N, Yoon RS, Shetye S, et al.: Anteroinferior 2.7-mm versus 3.5-mm plating of the clavicle: a biomechanical study, *Injury* 47(8):1642, 2016.

Rijal L, Sagar G, Joshi A, Joshi KN: Modified tension band for displaced type 2 lateral end clavicle fractures, *Int Orthop* 36:1417, 2012.

Schroder LK, Gauger EM, Gilbertson JA, Cole PA: Functional outcomes after operative management of extra-articular glenoid neck and scapular body fractures, *J Bone Joint Surg Am* 98:1623, 2016.

Serrano R, Borade A, Mir H, et al.: Anterior-inferior plating results in fewer secondary interventions compared to superior plating for acute displaced midshaft clavicle fractures, *J Orthop Trauma* 31:468, 2017.

Seyhan M, Kocaoglu B, Kiyak G, et al.: Anatomic locking plate and coracoclavicular stabilization with suture endo-button technique is superior in the treatment of Neer type II distal clavicle fractures, *Eur J Orthop Surg Traumatol* 25(5):827, 2015.

Shin SJ, Ko YW, Lee J, Park MG: Use of plate fixation without coracoclavicular ligament augmentation for unstable distal clavicle fractures, *J Shoulder Elbow Surg* 25(6):942, 2016.

Smekal V, Irenberger A, Attal RE, et al.: Elastic stable intramedullary nailing is best for mid-shaft clavicular fractures without comminution: results in 60 patients, *Injury* 42:324, 2011.

Tatro JM, Gilbertson JA, Schroder LK, Cole PA: Five to ten-year outcomes of operatively treated scapular fractures, *J Bone Joint Surg Am* 100:871, 2018.

Tiren D, van Bemmel AJ, Swank DJ, van der Linden FM: Hook plate fixation of acute displaced lateral clavicle fractures: mid-term results and a brief literature overview, *J Orthop Surg Res* 7(2), 2012.

Woltz S, Krijnen P, Schipper IB: Mid-term patient satisfaction and residual symptoms after plate fixation for nonoperative treatment for displaced midshaft clavicular fractures, *J Orthop Trauma* 32:e435, 2018.

Woltz S, Krijnen P, Schipper IB: Plate fixation versus nonoperative treatment for displaced midshaft clavicular fractures, *J Bone Joint Surg Am* 99:1051, 2017.

Woltz S, Stegeman SA, Krijnen P, et al.: Plate fixation compared with nonoperative treatment for displaced midshaft clavicular fractures. A multicenter randomized controlled trial, *J Bone Joint Surg Am* 99:106, 2017.

Wu K, Chang CH, Yang RS: Comparing hook plates and Kirschner tension band wiring for unstable lateral clavicle fractures, *Orthopedics* 34, 2011:e718.

Zuckerman SL, Song Y, Obremskey WT: Understanding the concept of medialization in scapula fractures, *J Orthop Trauma* 26:350, 2012.

Yagnik GP, Brady PC, Zimmerman JP, et al.: A biomechanical comparison of new techniques for distal clavicular fracture repair versus locked plating, *J Shoulder Elbow Surg* 28(5):982, 2019.

Yagnik GP, Jordan CJ, Narvel RR, et al.: Distal clavicle fracture repair: clinical outcomes of a surgical technique utilizing a combination of cortical button fixation and coracoclavicular ligament reconstruction, *Orthop J Sports Med* 7(9):2325967119867920, 2019.

PROXIMAL HUMERUS

Bae JH, Oh JK, Chon CS, et al.: The biomechanical performance of locking plate fixation with intramedullary fibular strut graft augmentation in the treatment of unstable fractures of the proximal humerus, *J Bone Joint Surg* 93:937, 2011.

Bahrs C, Kühle L, Blumenstock G, et al.: Which parameters affect medium- to long-term results after angular stable plate fixation for proximal humeral fractures? *J Shoulder Elbow Surg* 24:727, 2015.

Bai L, Fu Z, An S, et al.: Effect of calcar screw use in surgical neck fractures of the proximal humerus with unstable medial support: a biomechanical study, *J Orthop Trauma* 28:452, 2014.

Beks RB, Ochen Y, Frima H, et al.: Operative versus nonoperative treatment of proximal humeral fractures: a systematic review, meta-analysis, and comparison of observational studies and randomized controlled trials, *J Shoulder Elbow Surg* 27:1526, 2018.

Bell JE, Leung BC, Spratt KF, et al.: Trends and variation in incidence, surgical treatment, and repeat surgery of proximal humeral fractures in the elderly, *J Bone Joint Surg* 93A:121, 2011.

Boesmueller S, Wech M, Gregori M, et al.: Risk factors for humeral head necrosis and non-union after plating in proximal humeral fractures, *Injury* 47:350, 2016.

Boileau P, Pennington SD, Alami G: Proximal humeral fractures in younger patients: fixation techniques and arthroplasty, *J Shoulder Elbow Surg* 20(Suppl 2):S47, 2011.

Brorson S, Frich LH, Winther A, Hrobjartsson A: Locking plate osteosynthesis in displaced 4-part fractures of the proximal humerus: a systematic review of benefits and harms, *Acta Orthop* 82:475, 2011.

Cadet ER, Ahmad CS: Hemiarthroplasty for three- and four-part proximal humerus fractures, *J Am Acad Orthop Surg* 20:17, 2012.

Capriccioso CE, Zuckerman JD, Egol KA: Initial varus displacement of proximal humerus fractures results in similar function but higher complication rates, *Injury* 47:909, 2016.

Castoldi F, Bonasia DE, Blonna D, et al.: The stability of percutaneous fixation of proximal humeral fractures, *J Bone Joint Surg* 92A(Suppl 2):90, 2010.

Catalano 3rd L, Dowling R: Valgus impacted fracture of the proximal humerus, *J Hand Surg Am* 36A:1843, 2011.

Chow RM, Begum F, Beaupre LA, et al.: Proximal humeral fracture fixation: locking plate construct ± intramedullary fibular allograft, *J Shoulder Elbow Surg* 21:894, 2012.

Clavert P, Adam P, Bevort A, et al.: Pitfalls and complications with locking plate for proximal humerus fractures, *J Shoulder Elbow Surg* 19:489, 2010.

Clement ND, Duckworth AD, McQueen MM, Court-Brown CM: The outcome of proximal humeral fractures in the elderly: predictors of mortality and function, *Bone Joint Lett J* 96B:870, 2014.

Corbacho B, Duarte A, Keding A, et al.: Cost effectiveness of surgical versus non-surgical treatment of adults with displaced fractures of the proximal humerus: economic evaluation alongside the PROFHER trial, *Bone Joint Lett J* 98B:152, 2016.

Dilisio MF, Nowinski RJ, Hatzidakis AM, Fehringer EV: Intramedullary nailing of the proximal humerus: evolution, technique, and results, *J Shoulder Elbow Surg* 25, 2016:e130.

Egol KA, Sugi MT, Ong CC, et al.: Fracture site augmentation with calcium phosphate cement reduces screw penetration after open reduction-internal fixation of proximal humeral fractures, *J Shoulder Elbow Surg* 21:741, 2012.

Euler SA, Petri M, Venderley MB, et al.: Biomechanical evaluation of straight antegrade nailing in proximal humeral fractures: the rationale of the "proximal anchoring point", *Int Orthop* 41(9):1715, 2017.

Farmer KW, Wright TW: Three- and four-part proximal humerus fractures: open reduction and internal fixation versus arthroplasty, *J Hand Surg Am* 35A:2010, 1881.

Fjalestad T, Hole MØ, Hovden IA, et al.: Surgical treatment with an angular stable plate for complex displaced proximal humeral fractures in elderly patients: a randomized controlled trial, *J Orthop Trauma* 26:98, 2012.

Foruria AM, de Gracia MM, Larson DR, et al.: The pattern of the fracture and displacement of the fragments predict the outcome in proximal humeral fractures, *J Bone Joint Surg* 93B:378, 2011.

Foruria AM, Marti M, Sanchez-Sotelo J: Proximal humeral fractures treated conservatively settle during fracture healing, *J Orthop Trauma* 29:e24, 2014.

Gavaskar AS, Chordary N, Abraham S: Complex proximal humeral fractures treated with locked plating utilizing an extended deltoid split approach and a shoulder strap incision, *J Orthop Trauma* 27:73, 2013.

Gavaskar AS, Tummala NC: Locked plate osteosynthesis of humeral head-splitting fractures in young adults, *J Shoulder Elbow Surg* 24:908, 2015.

Grawe B, Le T, Lee T, Wyrick J: Open reduction and internal fixation (ORIF) of complex 3- and 4-part fractures of the proximal humerus: does age really matter? *Geriatr Orthop Surg Rehabil* 3:27, 2012.

Haasters F, Siebenbürger G, Helfen T: Complications of locked plating for proximal humeral fractures – are we getting any better? *J Shoulder Elbow Surg* 25:3296, 2016.

Hagerman MG, Jayakumar P, King JD, et al.: The factors influencing the decision making of operative treatment for proximal humeral fractures, *J Shoulder Elbow Surg* 24:e21, 2015.

Handoll HH, Keding A, Corbacho B, et al.: Five-year follow-up results of PROFHER trial comparing operative and non-operative treatment of adults with as displaced fracture of the proximal humerus, *Bone Joint Lett* 99B:383, 2017.

Handoll HH, Ollivere BJ, Rollins KE: Interventions for treating proximal humeral fractures in adults, *Cochrane Database Syst Rev* 12:CD000434, 2012.

Hardeman F, Bollars P, Donnelly M, et al.: Predictive factors for functional outcome and failure in angular stable osteosynthesis of the proximal humerus, *Injury* 43:153, 2012.

Harmer LS, Crickard CV, Phelps KD, et al.: Surgical approaches to the proximal humerus: a quantitative comparison of the deltopectoral approach and the anterolateral acromial approach, *J Am Acad Orthop Surg* 2(6):e017, 2018.

Hatzidakis AM, Shevlin MJ, Fenton DL, et al.: Angular-stable locked intramedullary nailing of two-part surgical neck fractures of the proximal part of the humerus: a multicenter retrospective observational study, *J Bone Joint Surg* 93A:L2172, 2011.

Hauschild O, Konrad G, Audige L, et al.: Operative versus non-operative treatment for two-part surgical neck fractures of the proximal humerus, *Arch Orthop Trauma Surg* 133:1385, 2013.

Hinds RM, Garner MR, Tran WH, et al.: Geriatric proximal humeral fracture patients show similar clinical outcomes to non-geriatric patients after osteosynthesis with endosteal fibular strut allograft augmentation, *J Shoulder Elbow Surg* 24:889, 2015.

Hirschmann MT, Fallegger B, Amsler F, et al.: Clinical longer-term results after internal fixation of proximal humerus fractures with a locking compression plate (PHILOS), *J Orthop Trauma* 25:286, 2011.

Inauen C, Platz A, Meier C, et al.: Quality of life after osteosynthesis of fractures of the proximal humerus, *J Orthop Trauma* 27:e74, 2013.

Iyengar JJ, Devcic Z, Sproul RC, Feeley BT: Nonoperative treatment of proximal humerus fractures: a systematic review, *J Orthop Trauma* 25:612, 2011.

Jung SW, Shim SB, Kim HM, et al.: Factors that influence reduction loss in proximal humerus fracture surgery, *J Orthop Trauma* 29:276, 2015.

Katthagen JC, Schwarze M, Meyer-Kobbe J, et al.: Biomechanical effects of calcar screws and bone block augmentation on medial support in locked plating of proximal humeral fractures, *Clin Biomech (Bristol, Avon)* 29:735, 2014.

Kennedy J, Feerick E, McGarry P, et al.: Effect of calcium triphosphate cement on proximal humeral fracture osteosynthesis: a finite element analysis, *J Orthop Surg (Hong Kong)* 21:167, 2013.

Kennedy J, Molony D, Burke NG, et al.: Effect of calcium triphosphate cement on proximal humeral fracture osteosynthesis: a cadaveric biomechanical study, *J Orthop Surg* 21:173, 2013.

Kim DS, Lee DH, Chun YM, Shin SJ: Which additional augmented fixation procedure decreases surgical failure after proximal humeral fracture with medial comminution: fibular allograft or inferomedial screws? *J Shoulder Elbow Surg* 27:1852, 2018.

Klement MR, Nickel BT, Bala A, et al.: Glenohumeral arthritis as a risk factor for proximal humerus nonunion, *Injury* 47(Suppl):S36, 2016, 7.

Königshausen M, Kübler L, Godry H, et al.: Clinical outcome and complications using a polyaxial locking plate in the treatment of displaced proximal humerus fractures: a reliable system? *Injury* 43:223, 2012.

Konrad G, Audigé L, Lambert S, et al.: Similar outcomes for nail versus plate fixation of three-part proximal humeral fractures, *Clin Orthop Relat Res* 470:602, 2012.

Konrad G, Bayer J, Hepp P, et al.: Open reduction and internal fixation of proximal humeral fractures with use of the locking proximal humerus plate: surgical technique, *J Bone Joint Surg* 92A(Suppl 1 Pt):85, 2010.

Kralinger F, Blauth M, Goldhahn J, et al.: The influence of local bone density on the outcome of one hundred and fifty proximal humeral fractures treated with a locking plate, *J Bone Joint Surg* 96:1026, 2014.

Krappinger D, Bizzotto N, Riedmann S, et al.: Predicting failure after surgical fixation of proximal humerus fractures, *Injury* 42:1283, 2011.

LaMartina J, Christmas KN, Simon P, et al.: Difficulty in decision making in the treatment of displaced proximal humerus fractures: the effect of uncertainty on surgical outcomes, *J Shoulder Elbow Surg* 27:470, 2018.

Lopiz Y, Garcia-Coiradas J, Garcia-Fernandez C, Marco F: Proximal humerus nailing: a randomized clinical trial between curvilinear and straight nails, *J Shoulder Elbow Surg* 23:369, 2014.

Lange M, Brandt D, Mittlmeier T, Gradl G: Proximal humeral fractures: non-operative treatment versus intramedullary nailing in 2-,3- and 4-part fractures, *Injury* 47(Suppl 7):S14, 2016.

Maier D, Jaeger M, Izadpanah K, et al.: Current concepts review. Proximal humeral fracture treatment in adults, *J Bone Joint Surg* 96:251, 2014.

Matassi F, Angeloni R, Carulli C, et al.: Locking plate and fibular allograft augmentation in unstable fractures of proximal humerus, *Injury* 43:1939, 2012.

Menendez ME, Ring D: does the timing of surgery for proximal humeral fracture affect inpatient outcomes? *J Shoulder Elbow Surg* 23:1257, 2014.

Murray IR, Amin AK, White TO, Robinson CM: Proximal humeral fractures: current concepts in classification, treatment and outcomes, *J Bone Joint Surg* 93B:1, 2011.

Neuhaus V, Bot AG, Swellengrebel CH, et al.: Treatment choice affects inpatient ad verse events and mortality in older aged in patients with an isolated fracture of the proximal humerus, *J Shoulder Elbow Surg* 23:800, 2014.

Neviaser AS, Hettrich CM, Beamer BS, et al.: Endosteal strut augment reduces complications associated with proximal humeral locking plates, *Clin Orthop Relat Res* 469:3300, 2011.

Neviaser AS, Hettrich CM, Dines JS, Lorich DG: Rate of avascular necrosis following proximal humerus fractures treated with a lateral locking plate and endosteal implant, *Arch Orthop Trauma Surg* 131:1617, 2011.

Newton AW, Selvaratnam V, Pydah SK, Nixon MF: Simple radiographic assessment of bone quality is associated with loss of surgical fixation in patients with proximal humeral fractures, *Injury* 47(4):904, 2016.

Nolan BM, Kippe MA, Wiater JM, Nowinski GP: Surgical treatment of displaced proximal humeral fractures with a short intramedullary nail, *J Shoulder Elbow Surg* 20:1241, 2011.

Obert L, Saadnia R, Tournier C, et al.: Four-part fractures treated with a reversed total shoulder prosthesis: prospective and retrospective multicenter study. Results and complications, *Orthop Traumatol Surg Res* 102:279, 2016.

Ockert B, Siebenbürger G, Kettler M, et al.: Long-term functional outcomes (median 10 years) after locked plating for displaced fractures of the proximal humerus, *J Shoulder Elbow Surg* 23:1223, 2014.

Ogawa K, Kobayashi S, Ikegami H: Retrograde intramedullary multiple pinning through the deltoid "V" for valgus-impacted four-part fractures of the proximal humerus, *J Trauma* 71:238, 2011.

Okike K, Lee OC, Makanji H, et al.: Factors associated with the decision for operative versus no-operative treatment of displaced proximal humerus fractures in the elderly, *Injury* 44:448, 2013.

Olerud P, Ahrengart L, Ponzer S, et al.: Hemiarthroplasty versus nonoperative treatment of displaced 4-part proximal humeral fractures in elderly patients: a randomized controlled trial, *J Shoulder Elbow Surg* 20:1025, 2011.

Olerud P, Ahrengart L, Ponzer S, et al.: Internal fixation versus nonoperative treatment of displaced 3-part proximal humeral fractures in elderly patients: a randomized controlled trial, *J Shoulder Elbow Surg* 20:747, 2011.

Olerud P, Ahrengart L, Söderqvist A, et al.: Quality of life and functional outcome after a 2-part proximal humeral fracture: a prospective cohort study on 50 patients treated with a locking plate, *J Shoulder Elbow Surg* 19:814, 2010.

Osterhoff G, Hoch A, Wanner GA, et al.: Calcar comminution as prognostic factor of clinical outcome after locking plate fixation of proximal humeral fractures, *Injury* 43:1651, 2012.

Petrigliano FA, Bezrukov N, Gamardt SC, SooHoo NE: Factors predicting complication and reoperation rates following surgical fixation of proximal humeral fractures, *J Bone Joint Surg* 96:1544, 2014.

Ponce BA, Thompson KJ, Raghava P, et al.: The role of medial comminution and calcar restoration in varus collapse of proximal humeral fractures treated with locking plates, *J Bone Joint Surg* 95:e113, 2013.

Rangan A, Handoll H, Brealey S, et al.: Surgical vs nonsurgical treatment of adults with displaced fractures of the proximal humerus: the PROFHER randomized clinical trial, *J Am Med Assoc* 313:1037, 2015.

Rath E, Alkrinawi N, Levy O, et al.: Minimally displaced fractures of the greater tuberosity: outcome of non-operative treatment, *J Shoulder Elbow Surg* 22:e8, 2013.

Reitman RD, Kerzhner E: Reverse shoulder arthroplasty as treatment for comminuted proximal humeral fractures in elderly patients, *Am J Orthop (Belle Mead NJ)* 40:458, 2011.

Robertson TA, Granade CM, Hunt Q, et al.: Nonoperative management versus reverse shoulder arthroplasty for treatment of 3- and 4-part proximal humeral fractures in older adults, *J Shoulder Elbow Surg* 26(6):1017, 2017.

Robinson CM, Amin AK, Godley KC, et al.: Modern perspectives of open reduction and plate fixation of proximal humerus fractures, *J Orthop Trauma* 25:618, 2011.

Robinson CM, Wylie JR, Ray AG, et al.: Proximal humeral fractures with a severe varus deformity treated by fixation with a locking plate, *J Bone Joint Surg* 92B:672, 2010.

Röderer G, Erhardt J, Graf M, et al.: Clinical results for minimally invasive locked plating of proximal humerus fractures, *J Orthop Trauma* 24:400, 2010.

Röderer G, Erhardt J, Kuster M, et al.: Second generation locking plating of proximal humerus fractures—a prospective multicentre observational study, *Int Orthop* 35:425, 2011.

Ruchholtz S, Hauk C, Lewan U, et al.: Minimally invasive polyaxial locking plate fixation of proximal humerus fractures: a prospective study, *J Trauma* 71:1737, 2011.

Saltzman BM, Erickson BJ, Harris JD, et al.: Fibular strut graft augmentation for open reduction and internal fixation of proximal humerus fracture, *Orthop J Sports Med* 4(7):2325967116656829, 2016.

Sanders RJ, Thissen LG, Teepen JC, et al.: Locking plate versus nonsurgical treatment for proximal humeral fractures: better midterm outcome with nonsurgical treatment, *J Shoulder Elbow Surg* 20:1118, 2011.

Schnetzke M, Bockmeyer J, Porschke F, et al.: Quality of reduction influences outcome after locked-plate fixation of proximal humeral type-C fractures, *J Bone Joint Surg Am* 98:1777, 2016.

Schulte LM, Matteini LE, Neviaser RJ: Proximal periarticular locking plates in proximal humeral fractures: functional outcomes, *J Shoulder Elbow Surg* 20:1234, 2011.

Shields E, Sundem L, Childs S, et al.: The impact of residual angulation on patient reported functional outcome scores after nonoperative treatment for humeral shaft fractures, *Injury* 47:914, 2016, compared with.

Soliman OA, Koptan WM: Four-part fracture dislocations of the proximal humerus in young adults: results of fixation, *Injury* 44:442, 2013.

Sosef N, van Leerdam R, Ott P, et al.: Minimal invasive fixation of proximal humeral fractures with an intramedullary nail: good results in elderly patients, *Arch Orthop Trauma Surg* 130:605, 2010.

Spross C, Zeledon R, Zdravkovic V, Jost B: How bone quality may influence intraoperative and early postoperative problems after angular stable open reduction-internal fixation of proximal humeral fractures, *J Shoulder Elbow Surg* 26:1566, 2017.

Sproul RC, Iyengar JJ, Devcic Z, Feeley BT: A systematic review of locking plate fixation of proximal humerus fractures, *Injury* 42:408, 2011.

Sun Q, Ge W, Li G, et al.: Locking plates versus intramedullary nails in the management of displaced proximal humeral fractures: a systematic review and meta-analysis, *Int Orthop* 42(3):641, 2018.

Theopold J, Weihs K, Marqua ß, et al.: Detection of primary screw perforation in locking plate osteosynthesis of proximal humerus fracture by intraoperative 3D fluoroscopy, *Arch Orthop Trauma Surg* 137:1491, 2017.

Torchia ME: Technical tips for fixation of proximal humeral fractures in elderly patients, *Instr Course Lect* 59:553, 2010.

Torrens C, Corrales M, Vila G, et al.: Functional and quality-of-life results of displaced and nondisplaced proximal humeral fractures treated conservatively, *J Orthop Trauma* 25:581, 2011.

Visser CPJ, Tavy DLJ, Coene LNJEM: Letter to the editor regarding Westphal T et al: "Axillary nerve lesions after open reduction and internal fixation of proximal humeral fractures through an extended lateral deltoid-split approach: electrophysiological findings" *J Shoulder Elbow Surg* 26:e364, 2017.

Wallace MJ, Bledsoe G, Moed BR, et al.: Relationship of cortical thickness of the proximal humerus and pullout strength of a locked plate and screw construct, *J Orthop Trauma* 26:222, 2012.

Weeks CA, Begum E, Beaupre LA, et al.: Locking plate fixation of proximal humeral fractures with impaction of the fracture site to restore medial column support: a biomechanical study, *J Shoulder Elbow Surg* 22:1552, 2013.

Werner BC, Griffin JW, Yang S, et al.: Obesity is associated with increased postoperative complications after operative management of proximal humerus fractures, *J Shoulder Elbow Surg* 24:593, 2015.

Westphal T, Woischnik S, Adolf D, et al.: Axillary nerve lesions after open reduction and internal fixation of proximal humeral fractures through an extended lateral deltoid-split approach: electrophysiological findings, *J Shoulder Elbow Surg* 26:464, 2017.

Wild JR, DeMers A, French R, et al.: Functional outcomes for surgically treated 3- and 4-part proximal humerus fractures, *Orthopedics* 34:e629, 2011.

Wong J, Newman JM, Gruson KI: Outcomes of intramedullary nailing for acute proximal humerus fractures: a systematic review, *J Orthop Traumatol* 17(2):113, 2016.

Wu CH, Ma CH, Yeh JJ, et al.: Locked plating for proximal humeral fractures: differences between the deltopectoral and deltoid-splitting approaches, *J Trauma* 71:1364, 2011.

Yang H, Li Z, Zhou F, et al.: A prospective clinical study of proximal humerus fractures treated with a locking proximal humerus plate, *J Orthop Trauma* 25:11, 2011.

Yüksel HY, Yilmaz S, Aksahin E, et al.: The results of nonoperative treatment for three- and four-part fractures of the proximal humerus in low-demand patients, *J Orthop Trauma* 25:588, 2011.

Zhu Y, Lu Y, Shen J, et al.: Locking intramedullary nails and locking plates in the treatment of two-part proximal humeral surgical neck fractures: a prospective randomized trial with a minimum of three years of follow-up, *J Bone Joint Surg* 93A:159, 2011.

HUMERAL SHAFT

An Z, He X, Jiang C, Zhang C: Treatment of middle third humeral shaft fractures: minimal invasive plate osteosynthesis versus expandable nailing, *Eur J Orthop Surg Traumatol* 22:193, 2012.

An Z, Zeng B, He X, et al.: Plating osteosynthesis of mid-distal humeral shaft fractures: minimally invasive versus conventional open reduction technique, *Int Orthop* 34:131, 2010.

Bumbasirevic M, Lesic A, Bumbasirevic V, et al.: The management of humeral shaft fractures with associated radial nerve palsy: a review of 117 cases, *Arch Orthop Trauma Surg* 130:519, 2010.

Chang G, Ilyas AM: Radial nerve palsy after humeral shaft fractures. The case for early exploration and a new classification to guide treatment and prognosis, *Hand Clin* 34:105, 2018.

Davies G, Yeo G, Meta M, et al.: Case-match controlled comparison of minimally invasive plate osteosynthesis and intramedullary nailing for the stabilization of humeral shaft fractures, *J Orthop Trauma* 30:612, 2016.

Driesman AS, Fisher N, Karia R, et al.: Fracture site mobility at 6 weeks after humeral shaft fracture predicts nonunion without surgery, *J Orthop Trauma* 31(12):657, 2017.

Esmailiejah AA, Abbasian MR, Safdari F, Ashoori K: Treatment of humeral shaft fractures: minimally invasive plate osteosynthesis versus open reduction and internal fixation, *Trauma Mon* 20:e26271, 2015

Gausden EB, Christ AB, Warner SJ, et al.: The triceps-sparing posterior approach to plating humeral shaft fractures results in a high rate of union and low incidence of complications, *Arch Orthop Trauma Surg* 136:1683, 2016.

Gosler MW, Testroote M, Morrenhof JW, Janzing HM: Surgical versus non-surgical interventions for treating humeral shaft fractures in adults, *Cochrane Database Syst Rev* (1)CD008832, 2012.

Gottschalk MB, Carpenter W, Hiza E, et al.: Humeral shaft fracture fixation. Incidence rates and complications as reported by American Board of Orthopaedic Surgery Part II Candidates, *J Bone Joint Surg Am* 98:e71, 2016.

Heineman D, Poolman RW, Nork SE, et al.: Plate fixation or intramedullary fixation of humeral shaft fractures: an updated meta-analysis, *Acta Orthop* 81:216, 2010.

Hohmann E, Glatt V, Tetsworth K: Minimally invasive plating versus either open reduction and plate fixation or intramedullary nailing of humeral shaft fractures: a systematic review and meta-analysis of randomized controlled trials, *J Shoulder Elbow Surg* 25:1634, 2016.

Hollister AM, Saulsbery C, Odom JL, et al.: New technique for humerus shaft fracture retrograde intramedullary nailing, *Tech Hand Up Extrem Surg* 15:138, 2011.

Idoine JD, French BG, Opalek JM, DeMott L: Plating of acute humeral diaphyseal fractures through an anterior approach in multiple trauma patients, *J Orthop Trauma* 26:9 2012.

Kim JW, Oh CW, Byun YS, et al.: A prospective randomized study of operative treatment for noncomminuted humeral shaft fractures: conventional open plating versus minimal invasive plate osteosynthesis, *J Orthop Trauma* 29:189, 2015.

Kobayashi M, Watanabe Y, Matsushita T: Early full range of shoulder and elbow motion is possible after minimally invasive plate osteosynthesis for humeral shaft fractures, *J Orthop Trauma* 24:212, 2010.

Liang K, Wang L, Lin D, Chen Z: Minimally invasive plating osteosynthesis for mid distal third humeral shaft fractures, *Orthopedics* 36:e1025, 2013

López-Arévalo R, de Llano-Temboury AQ, Serrano-Montilla J, et al.: Treatment of diaphyseal humeral fractures with the minimally invasive percutaneous plate (MIPPO) technique: a cadaveric study and clinical results, *J Orthop Trauma* 25:294, 2011.

Matsunaga FT, Tamaoki MJS, Matsumoto MH, et al.: Minimally invasive osteosynthesis with a bridge plate versus a functional brace for humeral shaft fractures. A randomized controlled trial, *J Bone Joint Surg Am* 99:583, 2017.

Nachef N, Bariatinsky V, Sulimovic S, et al.: Predictors of radial nerve palsy recovery in humeral shaft fractures: a retrospective review of 17 patients, *Orthop Traumatol Surg Res* 103:177, 2017.

Oh CW, Byun YS, Oh JK, et al.: Plating of humeral shaft fractures: comparison of standard conventional plating versus minimally invasive plating, *Orthop Traumatol Surg Res* 98:54, 2012.

Papasoulis E, Drosos GI, Ververidis AN, Verettas DA: Functional bracing of humeral shaft fractures, A review of clinical studies, Injury, 41:e21, 2010.

Patel R, Neu CP, Curtiss S, et al.: Crutch weightbearing on comminuted humeral shaft fractures: a biomechanical comparison of large versus small fragment fixation for humeral shaft fractures, *J Orthop Trauma* 25:300, 2011.

Qiu H, Wei Z, Liu Y, et al.: A Bayesian network meta-analysis of three different surgical procedures for the treatment of humeral shaft fractures, *Medicine (Baltim)* 95:e5454, 2016

Scolaro JA, Voleti P, Makani A, et al.: Surgical fixation of extra-articular distal humerus fractures with a posterolateral plate through a triceps-reflecting technique, *J Shoulder Elbow Surg* 23:251, 2014.

Shields E, Sundem L, Childs S, et al.: The impact of residual angulation on patient-reported functional outcome scores after nonoperative treatment for humeral shaft fractures, *Injury* 47:914, 2016.

Shin SJ, Sohn HS, Do NH: Minimally invasive plate osteosynthesis of humeral shaft fractures: a technique to aid fracture reduction and minimize complications, *J Orthop Trauma* 26:585, 2012.

Suzuki T, Hak DJ, Stahel PF, et al.: Safety and efficiency of conversion from external fixation to plate fixation in humeral shaft fractures, *J Orthop Trauma* 24:414, 2010.

Tetsworth K, Hohmann E, Glatt V: Minimally invasive plate osteosynthesis of humeral shaft fractures: current state of the art, *J Am Acad Orthop Surg* 26:652, 2018.

Updegrove GF, Mourad W, Abboud JA: Humeral shaft fractures, *J Shoulder Elbow Surg* 27:e87, 2018.

Wang C, Li J, Li Y, et al.: Is minimally invasive plating osteosynthesis for humeral shaft fracture advantageous compared with the conventional open technique? *J Shoulder Elbow Surg* 24:1741, 2015.

Yu BF, Liu LL, Yang GJ, et al.: Comparison of minimally invasive plate osteosynthesis and conventional plate osteosynthesis for humeral shaft fracture: a meta-analysis, *Medicine (Baltim)* 95:e4955, 2016

Zhao JG, Wang J, Wang C, Kan SL: Intramedullary nail versus plate fixation for humeral shaft fractures, *Medicine (Baltim)* 94:e599, 2015.

Ziran BH, Kinney RC, Smith WR, Preacher G: Sub-muscular plating of the humerus: an emerging technique, *Injury* 41:1047, 2010.

DISTAL HUMERUS

Antuna SA, Laakso RB, Barrera JL, et al.: Linked total elbow as treatment of distal humerus fractures, *Acta Orthop Belg* 78:465, 2012.

Burg A, Berenstein M, Engel J, et al.: Fractures of the distal humerus in elderly patients treated with a ring fixator, *Int Orthop* 35:101, 2011.

Burkhart KJ, Nijs S, Mattyasovszky SG, et al.: Distal humerus hemiarthroplasty of the elbow for comminuted distal humeral fractures in the elderly patient, *J Trauma* 71:635, 2011.

Chen G, Liao Q, Luo W, et al.: Triceps-sparing versus olecranon osteotomy for ORIF: analysis of 67 cases of intercondylar fractures of the distal humerus, *Injury* 42:366, 2011.

Chen RC, Harris DJ, Leduc S, et al.: Is ulnar nerve transposition beneficial during open reduction internal fixation of distal humerus fractures? *J Orthop Trauma* 24:391, 2010.

Desloges W, Faber KJ, King GJW, Athwal GS: Functional outcomes of distal humeral fractures managed nonoperatively in medically unwell and lower-demand elderly patients, *J Shoulder Elbow Surg* 24:1187, 2015.

Egol KA, Tsai P, Vazquez O, Tejwani NC: Comparison of functional outcomes of total elbow arthroplasty vs plate fixation for distal humerus fractures in osteoporotic elbow, *Am J Orthop* 40:67, 2011.

Erpelding JM, Mallander A, High R, et al.: Outcomes following distal humeral fracture fixation with an extensor mechanism-on approach, *J Bone Joint Surg* 94A:548, 2012.

Foruria AM, Lawrence TM, Augustin S, et al.: Heterotopic ossification after surgery for distal humeral fractures, *Bone Joint Lett J* 96B:1681, 2014.

Frattini M, Soncini G, Corradi M, et al.: Mid-term results of complex distal humeral fractures, *Musculoskelet Surg* 95:205, 2011.

Galano GJ, Ahmad CS, Levine WN: Current treatment strategies for bicolumnar distal humerus fractures, *J Am Acad Orthop Surg* 18:20, 2010.

Githens M, Yao J, Sox AH: Bishop J: open reduction and internal fixation versus total elbow arthroplasty for the treatment of geriatric distal humerus fractures: a systematic review and meta-analysis, *J Orthop Trauma* 28:481, 2014.

Got C, Shuck J, Biercevicz A, et al.: Biomechanical comparison of parallel versus 90-90 plating of bicolumn distal humerus fractures with intra-articular comminution, *J Hand Surg Am* 37:2512, 2012.

Huang JI, Paczas M, Hoyen HA, Vallier HA: Functional outcome after open reduction internal fixation of intra-articular fractures of the distal humerus in the elderly, *J Orthop Trauma* 25:259, 2011.

Hungerer S, Wipf F, von Oldenburg G, et al.: Complex distal humerus fractures—comparison of polyaxial locking and nonlocking screw configurations—a preliminary biomechanical study, *J Orthop Trauma* 28:130, 2014.

Kaiser T, Brunner A, Hohendorff B, et al.: Treatment of supra- and intra-articular fractures of the distal humerus with the LCP distal humerus plate: a 2-year follow-up, *J Shoulder Elbow Surg* 20:206, 2011.

Kudo T, Hara A, Iwase H, et al.: Biomechanical properties of orthogonal plate configuration versus parallel plate configuration using the same locking plate system for intra-articular distal humeral fractures under radial or ulnar column axial load, *Injury* 47(10):2071, 2016.

Lawrence TM, Ahmadi S, Morrey BF, Sánchez-Sotelo J: Wound complications after distal humerus fracture fixation: incidence, risk factors, and outcome, *J Shoulder Elbow Surg* 23:258, 2014.

Manst P, Nouaille Degorce H, Bonnevialle N, et al.: Total elbow arthroplasty for acute distal humeral fractures in patients over 65 years old—results of multicenter study in 87 patients, *Orthop Traumatol Surg Res* 99:779, 2013.

Min W, Ding BC, Tejwani NC: Comparative functional outcome of AO/OTA type C distal humerus fractures: open injuries do worse than closed fractures, *J Trauma Acute Care Surg* 72:E27, 2012.

Min W, Ding BC, Tejwani NC: Staged versus acute definitive management of open distal humerus fractures, *J Trauma* 71:944, 2011.

Muhldofer-Fodor M, Bekler H, Wolfe VM, et al.: Paratricipital-triceps splitting "two-window" approach for distal humerus fractures, *Tech Hand Up Extrem Surg* 15:156, 2011.

Nauth A, McKee MD, Ristevski B, et al.: Distal humeral fractures in adults, *J Bone Joint Surg* 93A:686, 2011.

Paryavi E, O'Toole RV, Frisch HM, et al.: Use of 2 column screws to treat transcondylar distal humeral fractures in geriatric patients, *Tech Hand Up Extrem Surg* 14:209, 2010.

Popovic D, King GJ: Fragility fractures of the distal humerus: what is the optimal treatment? *J Bone Joint Surg* 94B:16, 2012.

Prasarn ML, Ahn J, Paul O, et al.: Dual plating for fractures of the distal third of the humeral shaft, *J Orthop Trauma* 25:57 2011.

Puchwein P, Wildburger R, Archan S, et al.: Outcome of type C (AO) distal humeral fractures: follow-up of 22 patients with bicolumnar plating osteosynthesis, *J Shoulder Elbow Surg* 20:631, 2011.

Sela Y, Baratz ME: Distal humerus fractures in the elderly population, *J Hand Surg Am* 40:599, 2015.

Shannon SF, Wagner ER, Houdek MT, et al.: Osteosynthesis of AO/OTA 13-C3 distal humeral fractures in patients older than 70 years, *J Shoulder Elbow Surg* 27:291, 2018.

Sharma S, John R, Dhillon MS, Kishore K: Surgical approaches for open reduction and internal fixation of intra-articular distal humerus fractures in adults: a systematic review and meta-analysis, *Injury* 49:1381, 2018.

Shih CA, Su WR, Lin WC, T TW: Parallel versus orthogonal plate osteosynthesis of adult distal humerus fractures: a meta-analysis of biomechanical studies, *Int Orthop* 43:449, 2019.

Swellengrebel HJC, Saper D, Yi P, et al.: Nonoperative treatment of closed extra-articular distal humeral shaft fractures in adults: a comparison of functional bracing and above-elbow casting, *Am J Orthop (Belle Mead NJ)* 47(5), 2018. https://doi:12788/ajo.2018.0031.

Tunali O, Erşen A, Pehlivanoğlu T, et al.: Evaluation of risk factors for stiffness after distal humerus plating, *Int Orthop* 42(4):92, 2018.

Varecka TF, Myeroff C: Distal humerus fractures in the elderly population, *J Am Acad Orthop Surg* 25:673, 2017.

Vazquez O, Rutgers M, Ring DC, et al.: Fate of the ulnar nerve after operative fixation of distal humerus fractures, *J Orthop Trauma* 24:395, 2010.

Wiggers JK, Brouwer KM, Helmerhorst GT, Ring D: Predictors of diagnosis of ulnar neuropathy after surgically treated distal humerus fractures, *J Hand Surg Am* 37:1168, 2012.

Woods BI, Rosario BL, Siska PA, et al.: Determining the efficacy of screw and washer fixation as a method for securing olecranon osteotomies used in the surgical management of intraarticular distal humerus fractures, *J Orthop Trauma* 29:44, 2015.

Zalavras CG, Vercillo VT, Jun BJ, et al.: Biomechanical evaluation of parallel versus orthogonal plate fixation of intra-articular distal humerus fractures, *J Shoulder Elbow Surg* 20:12, 2011.

Zhang C, Zhong B, Luo CF: Comparing approaches to expose type C fractures of the distal humerus for ORIF in elderly patients: six years clinical experience with both the triceps-sparing approach and olecranon osteotomy, *Arch Orthop Trauma Surg* 134:803, 2014.

Zumstein MA, Raniga S, Flueckiger R, et al.: Triceps-sparing extra-articular step-cut olecranon osteotomy for distal humeral fractures: an anatomic study, *J Shoulder Elbow Surg* 26:1620, 2017.

ELBOW DISLOCATION; FOREARM FRACTURE; RADIAL HEAD, CORONOID, OLECRANON FRACTURE

Antuna SA, Sanchez-Marquez JM, Barco R: Long-term results of radial head resection following isolated radial head fracture in patients younger than forty years old, *J Bone Joint Surg* 92A:558, 2010.

Atesok KI, Jupiter JB, Weiss AP: Galeazzi fracture, *J Am Acad Orthop Surg* 19:623, 2011.

Barnes LF, Lombardi J, Gardner TR, et al.: Comparison of exposure in the Kaplan versus the Kocher approach in the treatment of radial head fractures, *Hand (N Y)* 14(2):253, 2019.

Bauer AS, Lawson BK, Bliss RL, Dyer GSM: Risk factors for posttraumatic heterotopic ossification of the elbow: case-control study, *J Hand Surg Am* 37A:1422, 2012.

Behnke NMK, Redjal HR, Nguyen VT, Zinar DM: Internal fixation of diaphyseal fractures of the forearm: a retrospective comparison of hybrid fixation versus dual plating, *J Orthop Trauma* 26:611, 2012.

Beingessner DM, Nork SE, Agel J, Viskontas D: A fragment-specific approach to type IID Monteggia elbow fracture-dislocations, *J Orthop Trauma* 25:414, 2011.

Beutel BG: Monteggia fractures in pediatric and adult populations, *Orthopedics* 35:138, 2012.

Bot AGJ, Dornberg JN, Lindenhovius ALC, et al.: Long-term outcomes of fractures of both bones of the forearm, *J Bone Joint Surg* 93A:527, 2011.

Chan K, Faber KJ, King GJW, Athwal GS: Selected anteromedial coronoid fractures can be treated nonoperatively, *J Shoulder Elbow Surg* 25:1251, 2016.

Coulibaly MO, Jones CB, Sietsema DL, Schildhauer TA: Results of 70 consecutive ulnar nightstick fractures, *Injury* 46:1359, 2015.

De Giacomo AF, Tornetta P, Sinicrope BJ, et al.: Outcomes after plating of olecranon fractures: a multicenter evaluation, *Injury* 47:1466, 2016.

Della Rocca GJ, Beuerlein MJ: Fractures and dislocations of the elbow. In Schmidt AH, Teague DC, editors: *Orthopaedic knowledge update: trauma 4*, Rosemont, IL, 2010, American Academy of Orthopaedic Surgeons.

Ditsios K, Boutsiadis A, Papadopoulos P, et al.: Floating elbow injuries in adults: prognostic factors affecting clinical outcomes, *J Shoulder Elbow Surg* 22:74, 2013.

Duckworth AD, Clement ND, McEachan JE, et al.: Prospective randomized trial of non-operative versus operative management of olecranon fractures in the elderly, *Bone Joint Lett J* 99-B:964, 2017.

Duckworth AD, Clement ND, White TO, et al.: Plate versus tension-band wire fixation for olecranon fractures. A prospective randomized trial, *J Bone Joint Surg Am* 99:1261, 2017.

Duckworth AD, Wickramasinghe NR, Clement ND, et al.: Long-term outcomes of isolated stable radial head fractures, *J Bone Joint Surg* 96:1716, 2014.

Duckworth AD, Wickramasinghe NR, Clement ND, et al.: Radial head replacement for acute complex fractures. What are the rate and risk factors for revision or removal? *Clin Orthop Relat Res* 472:2136, 2014.

Edwards SG, Argintar E, Lamb J: Management of comminuted proximal ulna fracture-dislocations using a multiplanar locking intramedullary nail, *Tech Hand Up Extrem Surg* 15:106, 2011.

Egol KA, Haglin JM, Lott A, et al.: Minimally displaced, isolated radial head and neck fractures do not require forma physical therapy, *J Bone Joint Surg* 100:648, 2018.

Faldini C, Nanni M, Leonetti D, et al.: Early radial head excision for displaced and comminuted radial head fractures: considerations and concerns at long-term follow-up, *J Orthop Trauma* 26:236, 2012.

Fantry A, Sobel A, Capito N, et al.: Biomechanical assessment of locking plate fixation of comminuted proximal olecranon fractures, *J Orthop Trauma* 32:e445, 2018.

Fitzgibbons PG, Louie D, Dyer GSM, et al.: Functional outcomes after fixation of "terrible triad" elbow fracture dislocation, *Orthopedics* 37:e373, 2014.

Foruria AM, Augustin S, Morrey BF, Sánchez-Sotelo J: Heterotopic ossification after surgery for fractures and fracture-dislocations involving the proximal aspect of the radius or ulna, *J Bone Joint Surg* 95:e66, 2013.

Garrigues GE, Wray 3rd WH, Lindenhovius AL, et al.: Fixation of the coronoid process in elbow fracture-dislocations, *J Bone Joint Surg* 93A:1873, 2011.

Giannicola G, Polimanti D, Bullitta G, et al.: Critical time period for recovery of functional range of motion after surgical treatment of complex elbow instability: prospective study on 76 patients, *Injury* 45:540, 2014.

Giannoulis FS, Sotereanos DG: Galeazzi fractures and dislocations, *Hand Clin* 23:153, 2007.

Grassman JP, Hakimi M, Gehrmann SV, et al.: The treatment of the acute Essex-Lopresti injury, *Bone Joint Lett J* 96B:1385, 2014.

Gupta A, Barei D, Khwaja A, Beingessner D: Single-staged treatment using a standard protocol results in functional motion in the majority of patients with a terrible triad elbow injury, *Clin Orthop Relat Res* 472:2075, 2014.

Hamaker M, Zheng A, Eglseder WA, Pensy RA: The adult Monteggia fracture: patterns and incidence of annular ligament incarceration among 121 cases at a single institution over 19 years, *J Hand Surg Am* 43(1):85. e1-85.e6, 2018

Hopf JC, Berger V, Krieglstein CF, et al.: Treatment of unstable elbow dislocations with hinged elbow fixation—subjective and objective results, *J Shoulder Elbow Surg* 24:250, 2015.

Huh J, Krueger CA, Medvecky MJ, Hsu JR: Medial elbow exposure for coronoid fractures: FCU-split versus over-the-top, *J Orthop Trauma* 27:730, 2013.

Iannuzzi NP, Paez AG, Parks BG, Murphy MS: Fixation of Regan-Morrey type II coronoid fractures: a comparison of screws and suture lasso technique for resistance to displacement, *J Hand Surg Am* 42(1):e11, 2017.

Iordens GIT, Den Hartog D, Van Lieshout EMM, et al.: Good functional recovery of complex elbow dislocations treated with hinged external fixation: a multicenter prospective study, *Clin Orthop Relat Res* 473:1451, 2015.

Jeon IH, Sanchez-Sotelo J, Zhao K, et al.: The contribution of the coronoid and radial head to the stability of the elbow, *J Bone Joint Surg* 94:86, 2012.

Klug A, Gramlich Y, Buckup J, et al.: Excellent results and low complication rate for anatomic polyaxial locking plates in comminuted proximal ulna fractures, *J Shoulder Elbow Surg* 27:2198, 2018.

Korompilias AV, Lykissas MG, Kostas-Agnantis IP, et al.: Distal radioulnar joint instability (Galeazzi type injury) after internal fixation in relation to the radius fracture pattern, *J Hand Surg Am* 36A:847, 2011.

Kupperman ES, Kupperman AI, Mitchell SA: Treatment of radial head fractures and need for revision procedures at 1 and 2 years, *J Hand Surg Am* 43:241, 2018.

Kusnezov N, Eisenstein E, Dunn JC, et al.: Operative management of unstable radial head fractures in a young active population, *Hand* 13(4):473, 2018.

Lanting BA, Ferreira LM, Johnson JA, et al.: The effect of radial head implant length on radiocapitellar articular properties and load transfer within the forearm, *J Orthop Trauma* 28:348, 2014.

Leigh WB, Ball CM: Radial head reconstruction versus replacement in the treatment of terrible triad injuries of the elbow, *J Shoulder Elbow Surg* 21:1336, 2012.

Li SL, Lu Y, Wang MY: Is cross-screw fixation superior to plate for radial neck fractures? *Bone Joint Lett J* 97-B(6):830, 2015.

Lipman MD, Gause TM, Teran VA, et al.: Radial head fracture fixation using tripod technique with headless compression screws, *J Hand Surg Am* 43:575.3e1, 2018.

Lópiz Y, González A, García-Fernández C, et al.: Comminuted fractures of the radial head: resection or prosthesis? *Injury* 47S3:S29, 2016.

Lovy AJ, Levy I, Keswani A, et al.: Outcomes of displaced olecranon fractures treated with olecranon sled, *J Shoulder Elbow Surg* 27:393, 2018.

Marmor M, Amano K, Yamamoto A, et al.: Acute shortening versus bridging plate for highly comminuted olecranon fractures, *Am J Orthop Sept/Oct* E330, 2017.

Marsh JP, Grewal R, Faber KJ, et al.: Radial head fractures treated with modular metallic radial head replacement, *J Bone Joint Surg* 98:527, 2016.

Modi CS, Wasserstein D, Mayne IP, et al.: The frequency and risk factors for subsequent surgery after a simple elbow dislocation, *Injury* 46:1156, 2015.

Motisi M, Kurowicki J, Berlund DD, et al.: Trends in management of radial head and olecranon fractures, *Open Orthop J* 11:239, 2017.

Neumann M, Nyffeler R, Beck M: Comminuted fractures of the radial head and neck: is fixation to the shaft necessary? *J Bone Joint Surg* 93B:223, 2011.

Nijs S, Graeler H, Bellemans J: Fixing simple olecranon fractures with olecranon osteotomy nail (OleON), *Oper Orthop Traumatol* 23:438, 2011.

Obly N, Reid J: Tripod fixation of radial neck fractures, *J Bone Joint Surg Br* 93-B(Suppl II):187, 2011.

Orbay JL, Mijares MR: The management of elbow instability using an internal joint stabilizer: preliminary results, *Clin Orthop Relat Res* 472:2049, 2014.

Orbay JL, Ring D, Kachooei AR, et al.: Multicenter trial of an internal joint stabilizer for the elbow, *J Shoulder Elbow Surg* 26(1):125, 2017.

Papatheodorou LK, Rubright JH, Heim KA, et al.: Terrible triad injuries of the elbow: does the coronoid always need to be fixed? *Clin Orthop Relat Res* 472:2084, 2014.

Park SM, Lee JS, Jung JY, et al.: How should anteromedial coronoid facet fracture be managed? A surgical strategy based on O'Driscoll classification and ligament injury, *J Shoulder Elbow Surg* 24:74, 2015.

Park MJ, Pappas N, Steinberg DR, Bozentka DJ: Immobilization in supination versus neutral following surgical treatment of Galeazzi fracture-dislocations in adults: case series, *J Hand Surg Am* 37A:528, 2012.

Paschos NK, Mitsionis GI, Vasilladis HS, Georgoulis AD: Comparison of early mobilization protocols in radial head fractures, *J Orthop Trauma* 27:134, 2013.

Potini VC, Ogunro S, Henry PDG, et al.: Complications associated with hinged external fixation for chronic elbow dislocations, *J Hand Surg Am* 40:730, 2015.

Rhyou IH, Kim KC, Lee JH, Kim SY: Strategic approach to O'Driscoll type 2 anteromedial coronoid facet fracture, *J Shoulder Elbow Surg* 23:924, 2014.

Ring D, Bruinsma WE, Jupiter J: Complications of hinged external fixation compared with cross-pinning of the elbow for acute and subacute instability, *Clin Orthop Relat Res* 472:2044, 2014.

Schnetzke M, Porschke F, Hoppe K, et al.: Outcome of early and late diagnosed Essex-Lopresti injury, *J Bone Joint Surg Am* 99:1043, 2017.

Schulte LM, Meals CG, Neviaser RJ: Management of adult diaphyseal both-bone forearm fractures, *J Am Acad Orthop Surg* 22:437, 2014.

Shimura H, Nimura A, Nasu H, et al.: Joint capsule attachment to the coronoid process of the ulna: an anatomic study with implications regarding the type 1 fractures of the coronoid process of the O'Driscoll classification, *J Shoulder Elbow Surg* 25:1517, 2016.

Shukla DR, Pillai G, McAnany S, et al.: Heterotopic ossification formation after fracture-dislocations of the elbow, *J Shoulder Elbow Surg* 24:333, 2015.

Sun H, Duan J, Li F: Comparison between radial head arthroplasty and open reduction and internal fixation in patients with radial head fractures (modified Mason type III and IV): a meta-analysis, *Eur J Orthop Surg Traumatol* 26:283, 2016, compared with.

Tashjian RZ, Wolf BR, van Riet RP, Steinmann SP: The unstable elbow: current concepts in diagnosis and treatment, *AAOS Instr Course Lect* 65:55, 2016.

Van Riet RP: Assessment and decision-making in the unstable elbow: management of simple dislocations, *Shoulder Elbow* 9(2):136, 2017.

Venouziou AI, Papatheodorou LK, Weiser RW, Sotereanos DG: Chronic Essex-Lopresti injuries: an alternative treatment method, *J Shoulder Elbow Surg* 23:861, 2014.

Watters TS, Garrigues GE, Ring D, Ruch DS: Fixation versus replacement of radial head in terrible triad: is there a difference in elbow stability and prognosis? *Clin Orthop Relat Res* 472:2128, 2014.

Wellman DS, Tucker SM, Baxter JR, et al.: Comminuted olecranon fractures: biomechanical testing of locked versus minifragment non-locked plate fixation, *Arch Orthop Trauma Surg* 137:1173, 2017.

Yoon A, King GJ, Grewal R: Is ORIF superior to nonoperative treatment in isolated displaced partial articular fractures of the radial head? *Clin Orthop Relat Res* 472:2105, 2014.

Yoon RS, Tyagi V, Cantlon MB, et al.: Complex coronoid and proximal ulna fractures are we getting better at fixing these? *Injury* 47:2053, 2016.

Zhang D, Tarabochia M, Janssen S, et al.: Risk of subluxation or dislocation after operative treatment of terrible triad injuries, *J Orthop Trauma* 30:660, 2016.

DISTAL RADIAL FRACTURE

Abe S, Murase T, Oka K, et al.: In vivo three-dimensional analysis of malunited forearm diaphyseal fractures with forearm rotational restriction, *J Bone Joint Surg Am* 100:e113, 2018.

Aktekin CN, Altay M, Gursoy C, et al.: Comparison between external fixation and cast treatment in the management of distal radius fractures in patients aged 65 years and older, *J Hand Surg Am* 35:86, 2010.

Arora R, Lutz M, Deml C, et al.: A prospective randomized trial comparing nonoperative treatment with volar locking plate fixation for displaced and unstable distal radial fractures in patients sixty-five year of age and older, *J Bone Joint Surg* 93A:2146, 2011.

Auld TS, Hwang JS, Stekas N, et al.: The correlation between the OTA/AO classification system and compartment syndrome in both bone forearm fractures, *J Orthop Trauma* 31:606, 2017.

Bales JG, Stern PJ: Treatment strategies of distal radius fractures, *Hand Clin* 28:177, 2012.

Beumer A, Lindau TR, Adlercreutz C: Early prognostic factors in distal radius fractures in a younger than osteoporotic age group: a multivariate analysis of trauma radiographs, *BMC Musculoskelet Disord* 14:170, 2013.

Brehmer JL, Husband JB: Accelerated rehabilitation compared with a standard protocol after distal radial fractures treated with volar open reduction and internal fixation. A prospective, randomized, controlled study, *J Bone Joint Surg* 96:1621, 2014.

Chan YH, Foo TL, Yeo CJ, Chew WY: Comparison between cast immobilization versus volar locking plate fixation of distal radius fractures in active elderly patients, the Asian prospective, *Hand Surg* 19:19, 2014.

Chappuis J, Bouté P, Putz P: Dorsally displaced extra-articular distal radius fractures fixation: dorsal IM nailing versus volar plating. A randomized controlled trial, *Orthop Traumatol Surg Res* 97:471, 2011.

Chen Y, Chen X, Li Z, et al.: Safety and efficacy of operative versus nonsurgical management of distal radius fractures in elderly patients: a systematic review and meta-analysis, *J Hand Surg Am* 41:404, 2016.

Cherubino P, Bini A, Marcolli D: Management of distal radius fractures: treatment protocol and functional results, *Injury* 41:1120, 2010.

Chou YC, Chen AC, Chen CY, et al.: Dorsal and volar 2.4-mm titanium locking plate fixation for AO type C3 dorsally comminuted distal radius fractures, *J Hand Surg Am* 36A:974, 2011.

Costa ML, Achten J, Parsons NR, et al.: Percutaneous fixation with Kirschner wires versus volar locking plate fixation in adults with dorsally displaced fracture of distal radius: randomised controlled trial, *BMJ* 349:g4807, 2014.

Cui Z, Pan J, Yu B, et al.: Internal versus external fixation for unstable distal radius fractures: an up-to-date meta-analysis, *Int Orthop* 35:1333, 2011.

Daneshvar P, Chan R, MacDermid J, Grewal R: The effects of ulnar styloid fractures on patients sustaining distal radius fractures, *J Hand Surg Am* 39:1915, 2014.

Diaz-Garcia RJ, Chung KC: Common myths and evidence in the management of distal radius fractures, *Hand Clin* 28:127, 2012.

Diaz-Garcia RJ, Oda T, Shauver MJ, Chung KC: A systematic review of outcomes and complications of treating unstable distal radius fractures in the elderly, *J Hand Surg Am* 36A:824, 2011.

Dzaja I, MacDermid JC, Roth J, Grewal R: Functional outcomes and cost estimation for extra-articular and simple intra-articular distal radius fractures treated with open reduction and internal fixation versus closed reduction and percutaneous Kirschner wire fixation, *Can J Surg* 56:378, 2013.

Egol KA, Walsh M, Romo-Cardoso S, et al.: Distal radial fractures in the elderly: operative compared with nonoperative treatment, *J Bone Joint Surg* 92A:1851, 2010.

Eichenbaum MD, Shn EK: Nonbridging external fixation of distal radius fractures, *Hand Clin* 26:381, 2010.

Ekrol I, Duckworth AD, Ralston SH, et al.: The influence of vitamin C on the outcome of distal radial fractures: a double-blind, randomized controlled trial, *J Bone Joint Surg* 96:1451, 2014.

Fujitani R, Omokawa S, Akahane M, et al.: Predictors of distal radioulnar joint instability in distal radius fractures, *J Hand Surg Am* 36A:2011, 1919.

Gofton W, Liew A: Distal radius fractures: nonoperative and percutaneous pinning treatment options, *Hand Clin* 26:43, 2010.

Goldwyn E, Pensy R, O'Toole RV, et al.: Do traction radiographs of distal radial fractures influence fracture characterization and treatment? *J Bone Joint Surg* 94:2055, 2012.

Grewal R, MacDermid JC, King GJ, Faber KJ: Open reduction and internal fixation versus percutaneous pinning with external fixation of distal radius fractures: a prospective, randomized clinical trial, *J Hand Surg Am* 36A:1899, 2011

Gyuricza C, Carlson MG, Weiland AJ, et al.: Removal of locked volar plates after distal radius fractures, *J Hand Surg Am* 36A:982, 2011.

Hakimi M, Jungbluth P, Windolf J, Wild M: Functional results and complications following locking palmar plating on the distal radius: a retrospective study, *J Hand Surg Eur* 35:283, 2010.

Hanel DP, Ruhlman SD, Katolik LI, Allan CH: Complications associated with distraction plate fixation of wrist fractures, *Hand Clin* 26:237, 2010.

Hull P, Baraza N, Gohil M, et al.: Volar locking plates versus K-wire fixation of dorsally displaced distal radius fractures—a functional outcome study, *J Trauma* 70:E125, 2011.

Hussain A, Nema SK, Sharma D, et al.: Does operative fixation of isolated fractures of ulna shaft results in different outcomes than non-operative management by long arm cast? *J Clin Orthop Trauma* 9S:S86, 2018.

Ilyas AM, Jupiter JB: Distal radius fractures—classification of treatment and indications for surgery, *Hand Clin* 26:37, 2010.

Jeudy J, Steiger V, Boyer P, et al.: Treatment of complex fractures of the distal radius: a prospective randomized comparison of external fixation versus locked volar plating, *Injury* 43:174, 2012.

Jupiter JB, Marent Huber M, LCP Study Group: Operative management of distal radial fractures with 2.4-millimeter locking plates: a multicenter prospective case series. Surgical technique, *J Bone Joint Surg* 92A(Suppl 1 Pt 1):96, 2010.

Karantana A, Downing ND, Forward DP, et al.: Surgical treatment of distal radial fractures with a volar locking plate versus conventional percutaneous methods. A randomized controlled trial, *J Bone Joint Surg* 95:1737, 2013.

Kitay A, Swanstrom M, Schreiber JJ, et al.: Volar plate position and flexor tendon rupture following distal radius fracture fixation, *J Hand Surg Am* 38:1091, 2013.

Knight D, Hajducka C, Will E, McQueen M: Locked volar plating for unstable distal radial fractures: clinical and radiological outcomes, *Injury* 41:184, 2010.

Kodama N, Imai S, Matsusue Y: A simple method for choosing treatment of distal radius fractures, *J Hand Surg Am* 38:1896, 2013.

Kural C, Sungu I, Kaya I, et al.: Evaluation of the reliability of classification systems used for distal radius fractures, *Orthopedics* 33:801, 2010.

Landgren M, Jerrhag D, Tägil M, et al.: External or internal fixation in the treatment of non-reducible distal radial fractures, *Acta Orthop* 82:610, 2011.

Lattmann T, Meier C, Dietrich M, et al.: Results of volar locking plate osteosynthesis for distal radial fractures, *J Trauma* 70:1510, 2011.

Lee YS, Wei TY, Cheng YC, et al.: A comparative study of Colles' fractures in patients between fifty and seventy years of age: percutaneous K-wiring versus volar locking plating, *Int Orthop* 36:789, 2012.

Lichtman DM, Bindra RR, Boyer MI, et al.: Treatment of distal radius fractures, *J Am Acad Orthop Surg* 18:180, 2010.

Lichtman DM, Bindra RR, Boyer MI, et al.: American Academy of Orthopaedic Surgeons clinical practice guideline on the treatment of distal radius fractures, *J Bone Joint Surg* 93A:775, 2011.

Lutz K, Yeoh KM, MacDermid JC, et al.: Complications associated with operative versus nonsurgical treatment of distal radius fractures in patients aged 65 years and older, *J Hand Surg Am* 39:1280, 2014.

Martineau PA, Berry GK, Harvey EJ: Plating for distal radius fractures, *Hand Clin* 26:61, 2010.

Matschke S, Marent-Huber M, Audigé L, et al.: The surgical treatment of unstable distal radius fractures by angle stable implants: a multicenter prospective study, *J Orthop Trauma* 25:312, 2011.

Matschke S, Wentzensen A, Ring D, et al.: Comparison of angle stable plate fixation approaches for distal radius fractures, *Injury* 42:385, 2011.

Meyer C, Chang J, Stern PJ, et al.: Complications of distal radial and scaphoid fracture treatment, *Instr Course Lect* 63:113, 2014.

Moriya K, Saito H, Takahashi Y, Ohi H: Locking palmar plate fixation for dorsally displaced fractures of the distal radius: a preliminary report, *Hand Surg* 16:263, 2011.

Neidenbach P, Audigé L, Wilhelmi-Mock M, et al.: The efficacy of closed reduction in displaced distal radius fractures, *Injury* 41:592, 2010.

Nishiwaki M, Tazaki K, Shimizu H, Ilyas AM: Prospective study of distal radial fractures treated with an intramedullary nail, *J Bone Joint Surg* 93A:1436, 2011.

Ozer K, Toker S: Dorsal tangential view of the wrist to detect screw penetration to the dorsal cortex of the distal radius after volar fixed-angle plating, *Hand (N Y)* 6:190, 2011.

Patel VP, Paksima N: Complications of distal radius fracture fixation, *Bull NYU Hosp Jt Dis* 68:112, 2010.

Payandeh JB, McKee MD: External fixation of distal radius fractures, *Hand Clin* 26:55, 2010.

Rampoldi M, Paolmbi D, Tagliente D: Distal radius fractures with diaphyseal involvement: fixation with fixed angle volar plate, *J Orthop Traumatol* 12:137, 2011.

Rhee PC, Dennison DG, Kakar S: Avoiding and treating perioperative complications of distal radius fractures, *Hand Clin* 28:185, 2012.

Rhee SH, Kim J, Lee YH, et al.: Factors affecting late displacement following volar locking plate fixation for distal radial fractures in elderly female patients, *Bone Joint Lett J* 95B:396, 2013.

Richard MJ, Katolik LI, Hanel DP, et al.: Distraction plating for the treatment of highly comminuted distal radius fractures in elderly patients, *J Hand Surg Am* 37A:948, 2012.

Richard MJ, Wartinbee DA, Riboh J, et al.: Analysis of the complications of palmar plating versus external fixation for fractures of the distal radius, *J Hand Surg Am* 36A:1614, 2011.

Riddick AP, Hickey B, White SP: Accuracy of the skyline view for detecting dorsal cortical penetration during volar distal radius fixation, *J Hand Surg Eur* 37:407, 2012.

Roh YH, Lee BK, Noh JH, et al.: Factors delaying recovery after volar plate fixation of distal radius fractures, *J Hand Surg Am* 39:1465, 2014.

Roth KM, Blazar PE, Earp BE, et al.: Incidence of displacement after nondisplaced distal radial fractures in adults, *J Bone Joint Surg* 95:1398, 2013.

Ruckenstuhl P, Brnhardt GA, Sadoghi P, et al.: Quality of life after volar locked plating: a 10-year follow-up study of patients with intra-articular distal radius fractures, *BMC Musculoskelet Disord* 15:250, 2014.

Schwarz AM, Hohenberger GM, Weiglein AH, et al.: Avoiding radial nerve palsy in proximal radius shaft plating – a cadaver study, *Injury* 48S5:A23, 2017.

Soong M, Earp BE, Bishop G, et al.: Volar locking plate implant prominence and flexor tendon rupture, *J Bone Joint Surg* 93A:328, 2011.

Soong M, van Leerdam R, Guitton TG, et al.: Fracture of the distal radius: risk factors for complications after locked volar plate fixation, *J Hand Surg Am* 36A:3, 2011.

Souer JS, Ring D, Jupiter J, et al.: Comparison of intra-articular simple compression and extra-articular distal radial fractures, *J Bone Joint Surg* 93A:2093, 2011.

Tan V, Bratchenk W, Nourbakhsh A, Capo J: Comparative analysis of intramedullary nail fixation versus casting for treatment of distal radius fractures, *J Hand Surg Am* 37A:460, 2012.

Tarallo L, Mugnai R, Zambianchi F, et al.: Volar plate fixation for the treatment of distal radius fractures: analysis of adverse events, *J Orthop Trauma* 27:740, 2013.

Turner RG, Faber KJ, Athwal GS: Complications of distal radius fractures, *Hand Clin* 26:85, 2010.

Wadsten MA, Sayed-Noor AS, Englund E, et al.: Cortical comminution in distal radial fractures can predict the radiological outcome. A cohort multicenter study, *Bone Joint Lett J* 96B:978, 2014.

Ward CM, Kuhl TL, Adams BD: Early complications of volar plating of distal radius fractures and their relationship to surgeon experience, *Hand* 6:185, 2011.

Wei DH, Poolman RW, Bhandari M, et al.: External fixation versus internal fixation for unstable distal radius fractures: a systematic review and meta-analysis of comparative clinical trials, *J Orthop Trauma* 26:386, 2012.

Weinberg DS, Park RJ, Boden KA, et al.: Anatomic investigation of commonly used landmarks for evaluating rotation during forearm fracture reduction, *J Bone Joint Surg* 98:1103, 2016.

White BD, Nydick JA, Karsky D, et al.: Incidence and clinical outcomes of tendon rupture following distal radius fractures, *J Hand Surg Am* 37:2035, 2012.

Williksen JH, Frihagen F, Hellund JC, et al.: Volar locking plates versus external fixation and adjuvant pin fixation in unstable distal radius fractures: a randomized, controlled study, *J Hand Surg Am* 38:1469, 2013.

Yu YR, Makhni MC, Tabrizi S, et al.: Complications of low-profile dorsal versus volar locking plates in the distal radius: a comparative study, *J Hand Surg Am* 36A:1135, 2011.

The complete list of references is available online at ExpertConsult.com.

CHAPTER 6

MALUNITED FRACTURES

A. Paige Whittle

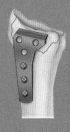

FOOT	372	Femoral malunion in children	398	Proximal third of the ulna with
Phalanges of the toes	372	Trochanteric region of the femur	400	anterior dislocation of the radial head
Metatarsals	372	Subtrochanteric osteotomy for		(Monteggia fracture) 414
Tarsals	373	coxa vara and rotational		Synostosis between the radius
Talus	373	deformities	401	and the ulna 415
Malunion of the talar neck	373	Cervicotrochanteric region of the		Shafts of the radius and ulna in
Malunion of the talar body	374	femur	401	adults 416
Calcaneus	374	**ACETABULUM**	402	Forearm malunions with distal
ANKLE	381	**PELVIS**	402	radioulnar joint instability 418
Arthrodesis for malunited fractures		Three-stage reconstruction for		Shaft of the ulna 419
of the ankle	384	pelvic malunions	403	**DISTAL RADIUS** 419
TIBIA	384	**SCAPULA**	403	Clinical evaluation 419
Shafts of the tibia and fibula	384	**CLAVICLE**	405	Radiographic evaluation 420
condyles of the tibia	392	Midshaft malunions of the clavicle	405	Operative treatment 420
Inverted-Y fractures of the		**HUMERUS**	409	Extraarticular malunion with
tibial condyles	394	Proximal humerus	409	dorsal angulation 422
Fracture of the intercondylar		Evaluation	410	Osteotomy and grafting of the
eminence of the tibia	394	Treatment	410	radius 422
PATELLA	394	Humeral shaft	412	Extraarticular malunion with
FEMUR AND HIP	394	Middle third	413	volar angulation 424
Condyles of the femur	394	Distal humerus	413	Intraarticular malunions 428
Lateral femoral condyle	394	**FOREARM**	413	Salvage procedures 429
Medial femoral condyle	395	Proximal third of the radius and ulna	413	Distal radioulnar joint incongruity
Both femoral condyles	395	Radial head	413	and arthrosis 430
Supracondylar femur	395	Radial neck	414	**CARPUS** 433
Femoral shaft	395	Olecranon	414	**HAND** 433

A malunited fracture is one that has healed with the fragments in a nonanatomic position. Whether the deformity is unsightly or not it can impair function in several ways: (1) an abnormal joint surface can cause irregular weight transfer and arthritis of the joint, especially in the lower extremities; (2) rotation or angulation of the fragments can interfere with proper balance or gait in the lower extremities or positioning of the upper extremities; (3) overriding of fragments or bone loss can result in perceptible shortening; and (4) the movements of neighboring joints can be blocked. Malunions, by strict definition, commonly are the rule in the closed treatment of fractures; however, they frequently are compatible with function. A malunited fracture becomes surgically significant only when it impairs function.

Malunions generally are caused by either inaccurate reduction or ineffective immobilization during healing. Most malunions could be prevented by skillful treatment of fresh fractures; however, malunion sometimes occurs despite the most expert treatment. Malunion may develop in patients with multiple trauma in whom treatment of more life-threatening injuries takes precedence. Especially in patients with head injuries, displacement can occur later and result in deformity and disability after the patient regains mobility.

When treating malunions, the following facts must be considered. Of the four characteristics that determine the acceptability of fracture reduction, the first in importance is alignment, the second is rotation, the third is restoration of normal length, and the fourth and least important is the actual position of the fragments. A slight deformity can be seriously disabling when a malunion involves a joint or is near one. If malunion causes only slight disability, function sometimes cannot be improved enough to justify surgery; however, a rotational deformity can be so disabling that surgery is required. Deformity of axial alignment in children younger than 9 years old may correct spontaneously with growth, especially if it is near a joint and in the plane of its motion. An offset in an epiphysis usually also corrects itself spontaneously in a child if the physis has not been injured.

Analysis of the deformity should take into consideration that most deformities can be resolved into one plane with regard to anteroposterior and varus or valgus deformity. Ries and O'Neill developed a trigonometric analysis of deformity and designed a graph to determine the true maximal deformity on the basis of the true anteroposterior and lateral radiographic views (Fig. 6.1). Other trigonometric analyses of angulation osteotomies also have been reported.

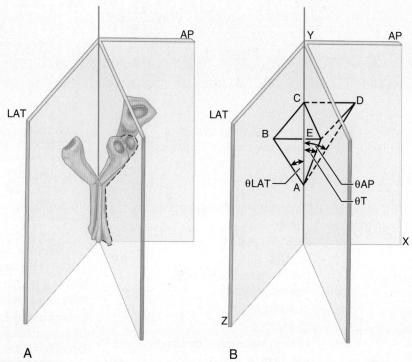

FIGURE 6.1 Ries and O'Neill method for determining bony deformity from anteroposterior and lateral radiographs. **A,** Tibial fracture angulated in plane between anteroposterior *(AP)* and lateral *(LAT)* planes. **B,** Angles formed by tibial fracture. *CAD* is the angle shown on anteroposterior view, *CAB* is the angle shown on lateral view, and *CAE* is the angle in the true plane *(T)* of deformity. (Redrawn from Ries M, O'Neill D: A method to determine the true angulation of long bone deformity, *Clin Orthop Relat Res* 218:191, 1987.)

The objective of surgery for malunion is to restore function. Although improving the appearance of the part may be equally important to the patient, surgery rarely is justified for cosmetic reasons alone. Operative treatment of malunion of most fractures should not be considered until 6 to 12 months after the fracture has occurred. In intraarticular fractures, surgery may be required sooner if satisfactory function is to be restored. When considering surgery, the degree of osteoporosis and soft-tissue atrophy must be evaluated, and a decision must be made whether early surgery would be preferable to active rehabilitation of the part followed by the surgery. Corrective surgery at the site of malunion is not always feasible. In some instances, a compensatory procedure may be necessary to restore function; in others, pain may be the predominant symptom and may require fusion of a joint.

Ilizarov pioneered work on intercalary limb regeneration with the use of circular external fixation techniques and various hinged constructs. These developments make possible the simultaneous restoration of alignment, rotation, and length. These techniques require a thorough understanding of frame design and construction, intensive patient counseling, and intensive physical therapy. Impressive results have been reported in some of the most challenging situations, especially infected nonunions and bone loss problems. Circular fixation techniques have a definite role in malunion surgery for the restoration of length and when previous infection has made conventional

open reduction techniques inappropriate. Detailed instruction and experience with these techniques are necessary, however, before they can be used for reconstruction of complex malunions. Three-dimensional modeling can be useful in preoperative planning for various bone and joint malunions.

FOOT
PHALANGES OF THE TOES
Malunion of fractures of the phalanges of the toes rarely causes enough disability to justify surgery. A deformity that causes pain can be corrected easily, however, through a lateral or dorsal incision that does not injure the tendons. Osteotomy and alignment of the fragments may be sufficient. For complete correction, however, wide resection may be required; this can be done with impunity because skillful movements of the toes are not needed.

METATARSALS
If malunion of the neck or shaft of a metatarsal is disabling, the fragments almost always are angulated toward the plantar surface of the foot, producing an osseous mass on the sole; if the fracture was severely comminuted, the mass may simulate a tumor. Surgery should not aim to restore perfect apposition and alignment but only to correct angulation so that weight bearing does not cause painful pressure on the sole of the foot.

CORRECTION OF METATARSAL ANGULATION

TECHNIQUE 6.1

- Make an incision on the dorsum of the forefoot parallel with the shaft of the affected bones; often one skin incision provides access to two bones.
- Expose the old fractures and divide them with a small osteotome. In some instances, a wedge of bone must be removed to permit elevation of the fragments, but resection must not be extensive enough to result in nonunion.
- Raise the fragments into a slightly overcorrected position by pressing from below and forcibly flexing the toes.
- Fix the fragments with an intramedullary pin as described for fresh fractures.

POSTOPERATIVE CARE A cast is applied from the tibial tuberosity to the toes; the bottom of the cast should be well molded to maintain the overcorrected position. At 3 weeks, any intramedullary pin or pins and the cast are removed and a walking boot cast is applied; a felt pad is inserted beneath the fractures to hold the toes in plantarflexion. At 6 weeks, the cast is replaced by a sturdy shoe fitted with an arch support and metatarsal pad.

TARSALS

Malunion of the tarsals except the talus and calcaneus can be discussed together. Because most fractures in this region are caused by violent trauma, several bones may be involved and perhaps severely comminuted and one or more of the tarsal joints may be dislocated. The distal fragment or fragments usually are displaced dorsalward, and sometimes the bones overlap slightly; in these instances, the distal fragment produces a prominence on the dorsum of the foot and the proximal fragment beneath forms a mass on the sole. Occasionally, lateral movements of the foot can be preserved to some extent by osteotomy through the old fracture and reduction of the fragments. Even when resection of the articular surfaces is unnecessary, however, lateral movements usually are lost. Partial or total resection and arthrodesis of one or more of the tarsal joints frequently are required, not only to correct the position of the bones but also to relieve pain and prevent traumatic arthritis. Because lateral movements often are already partially or completely lost, arthrodesis that entirely eliminates lateral motion does not add much to the disability, especially in young people. When the subtalar joint is not involved, its motion should be preserved by fusing only the midtarsal joints.

Unless deformity and pain are severe, operations for malunion in this area are not advisable until weight bearing has been tried for 6 to 12 months.

CORRECTION OF TARSAL MALUNION

TECHNIQUE 6.2

- Make an incision either lateral to the extensor tendons on the dorsum of the foot or middorsally in line with the third metatarsal; reflect the periosteum and expose the old fracture.
- If the injury is only a few months old, divide the bones with an osteotome at the fracture; if the fragments overlap excessively, remove a small section from each.
- Using a bone skid or periosteal elevator, lever the fragments into position.
- The reduction usually is stable; if desired, however, bone staples or crossed Kirschner wires can be used to maintain apposition.
- If malunion has been present for several months or years, the tarsus may be completely fused and the old fracture line may be invisible; in these instances, osteotomize the bones without regard to joints or to the possible site of the old fracture. If the deformity is severe, reduction is impossible without wide resection of the bones.
- If the malunion has caused tenosynovitis of the extensor tendons and dorsal contracture of the toes, the deformities can be corrected later by an operation for claw toes.

POSTOPERATIVE CARE With the foot at a right angle to the leg, a plaster cast is applied from the toes to just below the knee. After 1 week, radiographs are made through the cast to confirm the position. At 2 weeks, the cast and sutures are removed, the foot is inspected, and, if necessary, any residual deformity is corrected with the patient under general anesthesia. A short leg cast is applied and is worn for 1 month. Impressions for arch supports are made, and a walking boot cast is applied; the cast is well molded beneath the metatarsal necks and the longitudinal arch and is worn for 4 weeks. The cast is removed, and the patient is instructed in foot and toe exercises; the arch supports are worn for 4 to 6 months.

TALUS

Malunion of a fracture of the talus is always seriously disabling. The neck, body, or both may be involved in the malunion and can produce an irregularity of the ankle joint or the subtalar or talonavicular joint.

■ MALUNION OF THE TALAR NECK

Malunited fractures of the neck of the talus are analogous to intracapsular fractures of the neck of the femur in that they often impair circulation and can cause degeneration or even osteonecrosis of the talar head or body and consequent irregularity of one or more of the articular surfaces. Union may occur with the distal fragment in rotation or in lateral or medial deviation, producing a varus or valgus deformity. Treatment of varus malunion of the talar neck has been limited to triple arthrodesis, with unpredictable results. Shortening of the lateral column or lengthening of the medial column to correct forefoot rotation also has been suggested. A talar neck osteotomy at the apex of the deformity with a rhomboid-shaped autogenous tricortical iliac crest bone graft impacted into the osteotomy to maintain correction can be performed; however, care must be taken to preserve the extraosseous blood supply to the talus to prevent osteonecrosis. When the body of the talus is avascular, treatment is as described in other chapter. A triple arthrodesis with resection of suitable wedges of bone may be necessary to correct heel inversion and forefoot varus.

A malunited fracture of the base of the neck or of the anterior part of the body, with dorsal displacement of the distal fragment, may painfully block the ankle joint anteriorly. Excision of the protruding part of the bone may restore ankle motion, although traumatic arthritis may develop eventually. If symptoms of traumatic arthritis are incapacitating, ankle arthrodesis is indicated.

■ MALUNION OF THE TALAR BODY

Fractures of the body of the talus, although rare, often unite in malposition. Disability is extreme when the fracture involves the subtalar or ankle joint or both.

Arthrodesis or talectomy is the preferred treatment. If an articular surface of the talus is grossly distorted, and the bone is viable and is not infected, arthrodesis is the procedure of choice. When the superior and inferior articular surfaces of the talus are irregular, posterior arthrodesis of the ankle, including the subtalar joint, is preferable. When the body is nonviable, calcaneotibial arthrodesis is indicated because motion in the midtarsal joints can be preserved.

Traumatic arthritis may be limited to the ankle joint or to the subtalar joint. In these instances, ankle arthrodesis or subtalar fusion may be indicated. Good results have followed subtalar fusion without arthrodesis of the midtarsal joints.

Occasionally, a malunited comminuted fracture of the body or neck of the talus can be treated by pantalar arthrodesis. Pantalar and calcaneotibial arthrodeses are difficult and extensive operations.

For open fractures complicated by infection and draining sinuses and sequestration of the talus, talectomy has been recommended in the past. The technique of excision of the talus is similar to that described for tuberculosis of this bone. To preserve limb length, we have used Ilizarov circular fixation techniques and bone segment transport after corticotomy of the distal tibia to facilitate calcaneotibial arthrodesis, especially after loss of the talar body from open fractures or sepsis. This technique requires a compliant patient, radical debridement of the infected bone, and appropriate antibiotic therapy.

CALCANEUS

Pain and disability often persist after fractures of the calcaneus even though the original injury was treated skillfully; this is especially likely if the patient's occupation requires walking over rough ground. Deformities associated with nonoperative management of calcaneal fractures include heel widening, subtalar incongruity, loss of calcaneal height (decreased Böhler angle), and varus alignment. Heel widening can lead to subfibular impingement and dysfunction of the peroneal tendons. Decreased calcaneal height results in a more horizontally oriented talus, which causes anterior tibiotalar impingement, decreased dorsiflexion, and decreased push-off strength. Impaired calcaneal cuboid motion can occur from overhang of the anterolateral calcaneal wall. Varus deformity leads to excessive stress on the lateral foot, whereas subtalar incongruity causes posttraumatic arthrosis.

Because pain after calcaneal fractures may improve for 1 to 2 years after injury, surgical treatment usually is deferred

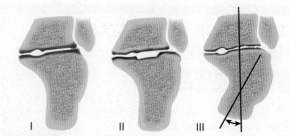

FIGURE 6.2   Three types of calcaneal malunions: *I,* large lateral wall exostosis, no subtalar arthritis; *II,* large lateral wall exostosis, significant subtalar arthritis; and *III,* lateral exostosis, significant subtalar arthritis, calcaneal body malalignment of more than 10 degrees of hindfoot varus.

as long as the patient is making progress in rehabilitation. If a patient's function fails to progress during this time, however, surgical intervention is warranted. Preoperative evaluation should include analysis of the location of the pain. Lateral pain usually is caused by lateral wall impingement or peroneal tendinitis, whereas more circumferential pain likely is caused by subtalar arthrosis. Anterior ankle pain may be caused by impingement. Posterior ankle pain may be caused by a posterior calcaneal bone spike behind the facet. An injection of 1% lidocaine into the subtalar joint may be helpful in differentiating the origin of the pain. Operative treatment may consist of osteotomy, arthrodesis, or resection of a prominence of the calcaneus laterally to free the peroneal tendons, or a combination of these techniques. A laterally based opening wedge osteotomy for extraarticular malunited fractures has been reported with good results for patients with a symptomatic heel valgus before the onset of subtalar arthritis. If arthrodesis is considered, having the patient wear a limited motion, double upright brace or prefabricated walking boot for 8 weeks can be useful in predicting the success of the procedure.

Although smoking is not an absolute contraindication to surgical management, smoking increases the incidence of nonunion after subtalar arthrodesis and the likelihood of wound complications. Smokers should be encouraged to quit preoperatively and be counseled about potential complications.

Radiographic evaluation includes standard lateral and lateral weight-bearing radiographs and views of the calcaneus. A Broden view can provide information about the subtalar joint; however, a CT scan most accurately shows alignment and subtalar congruity. CT scans are obtained in the transverse and coronal planes.

Stephens and Sanders used CT to identify three types of calcaneal malunions (Fig. 6.2) and to develop treatment guidelines (Table 6.1). Using these guidelines in 26 malunions, they obtained 18 excellent, five good, and three fair results. Although outcomes deteriorated as the complexity of the malunions increased, significant clinical improvement was obtained in even the most severe deformities. In a follow-up study, Clare et al. reported that the extensile lateral approach allowed adequate decompression of the peroneal tendons, bone block arthrodesis, and calcaneal osteotomy all through the same incision, which is not possible with other proposed approaches (Gallie, Ollier). Ninety-three percent of the arthrodeses united, all feet were plantigrade, and 93% were in neutral or valgus alignment. Twenty-four percent

TABLE 6.1	
Guidelines for Treatment of Calcaneal Malunions	
Type I	Lateral exostectomy through extensile L-shaped lateral incision
Type II	Lateral exostectomy plus subtalar arthrodesis using resected exostosis as graft
Type III	Lateral exostectomy plus subtalar arthrodesis plus calcaneal osteotomy

Adapted from Stephens HM, Sanders R: Calcaneal malunions: results of prognostic computed tomography classification system, *Foot Ankle Int* 17:395, 1996.

had delayed healing, but only one deep infection occurred, and no free-tissue transfers were necessary. A nonsignificant trend toward increased nonunion and wound problems was noted in smokers, and mild residual pain was present in 64% of patients, usually lateral in location. There were no implant failures, which the authors attributed to using large (7.3 or 8.0 mm) titanium screws placed with a lag technique.

Flemister et al. found that outcomes were similar regardless of the reconstructive procedure—lateral calcaneal closing wedge osteotomy, bone block arthrodesis, in situ fusion—but malunion and nonunion were more frequent after bone block procedures (15%) than after in situ fusions (5%). They recommended in situ fusion, unless anterior ankle impingement requires a more complicated bone block fusion.

If the subtalar joint alone is involved, enough bone is resected to correct the weight-bearing alignment and the joint is arthrodesed. If the midtarsal joints also are involved, a triple arthrodesis (subtalar, talonavicular, and calcaneocuboid) is advisable. Romash described a reconstructive osteotomy of the calcaneus with subtalar arthrodesis for malunited calcaneal fractures with satisfactory results. According to him, the reconstructive osteotomy, which re-creates the primary fracture, allows repositioning of the tuberosity to narrow the heel, alleviates impingement, and returns height to the heel; the subtalar arthrodesis alleviates the symptoms of posttraumatic arthritis. Good or excellent results also have been reported with subtalar distraction realignment arthrodesis using lateral decompression, medial subtalar capsulotomy, and distraction and realignment of the subtalar joint with a tapered wedge bone graft (Fig. 6.3). The lateral approach has several advantages over the Gallie-type posterolateral approach, including less soft-tissue dissection, good view of the subtalar joint, easier access to the medial subtalar capsule and sustentaculum tali, and decreased risk of damage to the sural nerve.

Several bone block fusion techniques to restore heel height and improve talar inclination have been described with union rates of 80% to 100% with no varus malunions. However, one study reported good results in only seven of 14 patients, and another study reported varus malunions of the arthrodesis in four of 15 patients. Trnka et al. reported 29 complications after subtalar bone block arthrodesis. Four of the five nonunions in their series were in patients in whom allografts were used, and they cautioned against allograft use. Bone block fusion rather than in situ fusion has been recommended for patients with loss of heel height; however, satisfactory results have been reported even with loss of heel height using subtalar arthrodesis without interpositional bone grafting. Distraction arthrodesis should

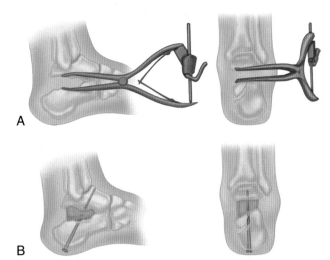

FIGURE 6.3 Subtalar distraction realignment arthrodesis for calcaneal malunions. **A,** Subtalar distraction with lamina spreader. **B,** Subtalar distraction arthrodesis with anterior wedge bone graft and cannulated screw.

be considered only for patients with less than 10 degrees of ankle dorsiflexion and disabling pain. For a severe crushing fracture of the calcaneus, either fresh or malunited, triple arthrodesis has been recommended because there is not only derangement of the subtalar joint but also a subluxation of the calcaneocuboid and talonavicular joints caused by depression of the sustentaculum tali. With subtalar fusion alone, the head and neck of the talus are left projecting forward without support and form a constant lever in weight bearing that interferes with fusion. According to Conn, triple arthrodesis is preferable to subtalar fusion because the talonavicular, calcaneocuboid, and subtalar joints have a reciprocal action and because triple arthrodesis does not add to the disability since little midtarsal motion remains after the original injury. Others, however, believe that triple arthrodesis has no advantage in most patients with calcaneal malunions. We believe that unless the midtarsal joints are involved, arthrodesis should be limited to the subtalar joint; motion in the midtarsal joints may increase with activity and should be preserved.

POSTERIOR SUBTALAR ARTHRODESIS

Gallie advised arthrodesis of the subtalar joint from the posterior aspect because the procedure is simpler than the one usually employed (Fig. 6.4); however, it does not allow correction of varus or valgus position of the calcaneus or of any other deformity of the foot. According to Gallie, a mild valgus position of the heel usually can be disregarded. His operation is not suitable if the primary deformity is one of varus because excessive weight would be borne on the head of the fifth metatarsal and cause a painful callus.

TECHNIQUE 6.3

(GALLIE)

■ With the patient prone, make a longitudinal incision along the lateral border of the Achilles tendon for 6 to

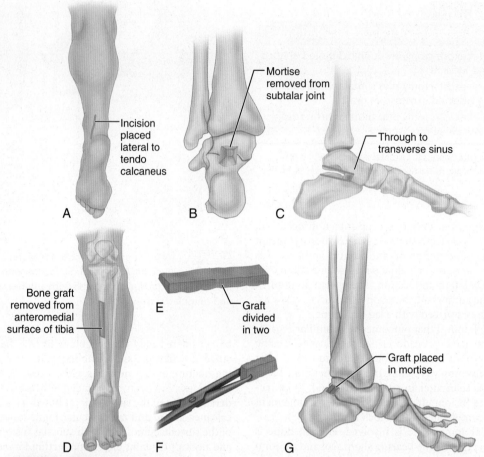

FIGURE 6.4 Gallie subtalar fusion for malunited fracture of calcaneus. **A,** Line of skin incision. **B** and **C,** Mortise removed from subtalar joint, extending from posterior surface to transverse sinus. **D–G,** Tibial grafts inserted to fill mortise.

8 cm and incise transversely the posterior capsule of the ankle and of the subtalar joint.

- Locate the subtalar joint by medial and lateral motions of the calcaneus.
- Probe the subtalar joint to determine its general direction and cut a mortise in the calcaneus and talus approximately 1.3 cm wide, 0.6 cm deep, and as far distally as the sinus tarsi.
- Flex the knee and remove a graft 6.2 cm long × 1.3 cm wide from the anteromedial surface of the proximal tibia. Divide the graft into two parts and bevel one end of each.
- Pack cancellous bone into the depth of the mortise. With their cortical surfaces apposed, drive the two grafts into the mortise. If the grafts are of the proper size, their cancellous surfaces press snugly against the lateral walls of the mortise. Strips of cancellous bone from the ilium probably are preferable to the tibial grafts used by Gallie; they are packed tightly into the cavity.
- Close only the subcutaneous and skin layers over a suction drain.
- Apply a bulky dressing followed by a short leg cast.

DISTRACTION ARTHRODESIS

TECHNIQUE 6.4

(CARR ET AL.)

- Place the patient in the lateral decubitus position with the affected side up. Prepare and drape the posterior iliac crest.
- Under tourniquet control, make a longitudinal posterolateral Gallie-type approach to the subtalar joint. There should be no horizontal extension of this incision to avoid undue tension on the wound.
- Expose the lateral calcaneal wall subperiosteally and excise it to a more normal width (lateral wall decompression). This step should ensure peroneal and fibular decompression.
- Identify the subtalar joint and apply a femoral distractor with half-pins in the medial subcutaneous tibia and medial calcaneus. The medial application helps to correct hindfoot varus.

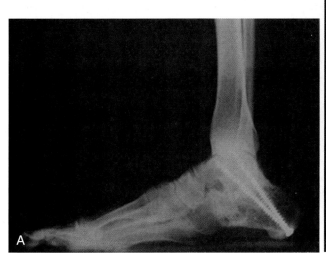
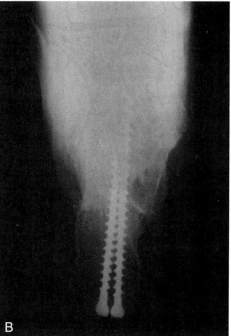

FIGURE 6.5 **A** and **B,** Distraction arthrodesis. (From Robinson JF, Murphy GA: Arthrodesis as salvage for calcaneal malunions, *Foot Ankle Clin* 7:107, 2002.) **SEE TECHNIQUE 6.4.**

- Apply distraction and denude the posterior subtalar joint to subchondral bone. Use a lamina spreader to aid in subtalar joint exposure.
- Correct any heel varus or valgus by manipulation.
- Obtain intraoperative radiographs to ensure correction of the lateral talocalcaneal angle (normally 25 to 45 degrees). A weight-bearing view of the opposite foot obtained preoperatively is helpful in confirming a normal talocalcaneal angle.
- Measure the subtalar joint gap and harvest an appropriately sized tricortical posterior iliac crest bone graft. A block 2.5 cm in height may be required for severe deformity. Two separate pieces may be required to fill the gap completely and help prevent late collapse into varus or valgus.
- After inserting the graft, release the distraction forces.
- Insert two fully threaded, 6.5-mm AO cancellous screws through stab incisions in the heel to fix the calcaneus and the talus firmly. Two screws provide rigid fixation and help prevent rotatory movements around the axis of subtalar motion. Fully threaded screws are used to help prevent late collapse (Fig. 6.5).
- Obtain final radiographs to confirm position before wound closure.

POSTOPERATIVE CARE The drain is removed at 24 hours. The foot is elevated for 72 hours, and the cast is not bivalved if the neurovascular status remains satisfactory. Crutch walking without weight bearing is allowed. At 2 weeks, the cast and sutures are removed and a well-molded short leg nonwalking cast is applied and worn 4 weeks. Active toe exercises are encouraged during this time. During the first 6 weeks, if patient compliance concerning weight bearing is questionable, a long leg cast with the knee bent is applied. At 6 weeks, a short leg walking cast is applied and weight bearing to tolerance is allowed. Radiographs of

the arthrodesis are obtained at 6 and 12 weeks. Usually a leather lace-up shoe with a rigid shank can be worn after 12 weeks, in conjunction with a leather lace-up ankle corset to control edema for another 4 to 6 weeks. The patient should be informed preoperatively that swelling around the hindfoot may persist for 6 to 9 months after surgery.

RESECTION OF LATERAL PROMINENCE OF CALCANEUS

According to Kashiwagi, pain in malunited fractures of the calcaneus sometimes is caused by changes around the peroneal tendons. The tendons may be buried in callus, caught by bony fragments, affected by adhesions, or displaced superiorly by a bony prominence. Kashiwagi recommended peroneal tomography to show changes around the tendons and their sheaths (Fig. 6.6). If pain is caused by such changes, he advised freeing the tendons and sheaths, resecting the bony prominence laterally, and, if necessary, subtalar arthrodesis.

TECHNIQUE 6.5

(KASHIWAGI, MODIFIED)

- Make a Kocher incision, but extend its distal half one fingerbreadth superior to the sole of the foot and end it at the base of the fifth metatarsal.
- Identify the peroneus longus and brevis tendons, and, without opening their sheaths, deepen the incisions to the lateral surface of the calcaneus 0.6 cm inferior to the peroneus longus tendon. Extend the dissection superiorly next to the bone and deep to the tendons, separating the peroneal retinaculum from the bone.

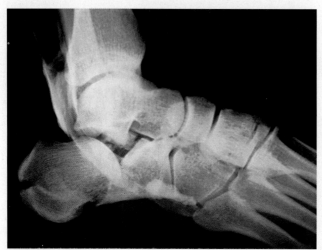

FIGURE 6.6 Peroneal tenogram in acute fracture of calcaneus. Peroneal sheaths fail to fill with contrast medium opposite laterally displaced fragment of calcaneus. (Courtesy Daiji Kashiwagi, MD.)

- Retract the tendons superiorly over the tip of the lateral malleolus. Free the origin of the extensor digiti brevis from the calcaneus and retract it superiorly also. The lateral surface of the calcaneus is exposed, including the lateral aspect of the subtalar and calcaneocuboid joints.
- With a wide osteotome, make a sagittal osteotomy through the calcaneus extending from the calcaneocuboid joint anteriorly to the tuberosity of the bone posteriorly and from the subtalar joint superiorly to the plantar surface inferiorly.
- Discard the bone resected. The lateral side of the calcaneus should now consist of a vertical wall, all excessive bone lateral to the subtalar joint and inferior to the lateral malleolus having been removed.
- The lateral aspects of the subtalar and calcaneocuboid joints are now exposed; if necessary, arthrodese these joints.
- Replace the peroneal tendons and sheaths inferior to the lateral malleolus and suture the peroneal retinaculum to the plantar fascia.
- Close the wound.
- With the knee flexed 30 degrees, apply a long leg cast.

POSTOPERATIVE CARE At 10 to 14 days, the cast and sutures are removed. If the operation includes an arthrodesis, a short leg walking cast is applied and the postoperative care is the same as for triple arthrodesis.

CORRECTION OF CALCANEAL MALUNION THROUGH EXTENSILE LATERAL APPROACH

TECHNIQUE 6.6

(CLARE ET AL.)
- Place the patient in the lateral decubitus position on a beanbag, with the normal leg down and in front of the injured extremity.

- Place a thigh tourniquet. Prepare and drape the leg and exsanguinate the extremity with the use of an Esmarch bandage. Inflate the tourniquet to 350 mm Hg.
- Make a lateral extensile incision over the calcaneus and raise a full-thickness subperiosteal flap. The vertical limb of the incision should be just anterior to the Achilles tendon and posterior to the sural nerve, allowing the nerve to be elevated with the full-thickness flap posteriorly. Avoid violation of the nerve at the terminal portion of the horizontal limb of the incision.
- Place three 1.6-mm Kirschner wires, one in the distal fibula, one in the talar neck, and the third in the cuboid, for retraction of the peroneal tendons and the subperiosteal flap.
- Carefully free the lateral wall of the calcaneus of all adjacent soft tissue as far distally as the calcaneocuboid articulation. In all three types of calcaneal malunions, the lateral wall exostosis must be resected.
- Place a Hohmann retractor on the plantar aspect of the calcaneus and one on the anterior process of the calcaneus, and perform an exostectomy using a thin-bladed AO osteotomy saw (Synthes USA, Paoli, PA). Starting posterior, angle the saw blade slightly medially relative to the longitudinal axis of the calcaneus, leaving more residual bone plantarly and providing decompression of the area of impingement in the subfibular region (Fig. 6.7A). Do not violate the talofibular joint.
- Continue the exostectomy to the level of the calcaneocuboid joint because the residual overhang of the lateral wall often results in an osseous block to motion of this joint. Remove the overhang and the lateral fourth of the distal aspect of the calcaneus because articulation of this lateral portion with the cuboid is almost always arthritic.
- Complete the exostectomy distally with an osteotome to avoid saw blade damage to the cuboid and remove the fragment en bloc (Fig. 6.7B). The excised lateral wall fragment should be maintained as a single fragment, if possible, for later use as a bone block autograft in type II and type III malunions.
- In type II and type III calcaneal malunions, attention is directed to the subtalar joint. If it is arthritic, perform a subtalar arthrodesis. Place a lamina spreader within the joint and debride the remaining articular surface using a sharp periosteal elevator or osteotome.
- Prepare the inferior talar and superior calcaneal osseous surfaces with a 2.5-mm drill bit, creating multiple perforations within the subchondral bone for vascular ingrowth.
- With the lamina spreader fully expanded within the subtalar joint posteriorly, verify by fluoroscopy how much height needs to be obtained. The talar head should align anatomically with the navicular, indicating restoration of the medial column, the normal angle of talar declination, and the talocalcaneal angle.
- When alignment is confirmed radiographically, measure the dimensions of the defect with a ruler, allowing the autograft bone block to be contoured to match the defect. If the joint is excessively tight medially, place lamina spreaders in the sinus tarsi and the posterior facet of the subtalar joint. A femoral distractor placed medially is not used because it is cumbersome and not as effec-

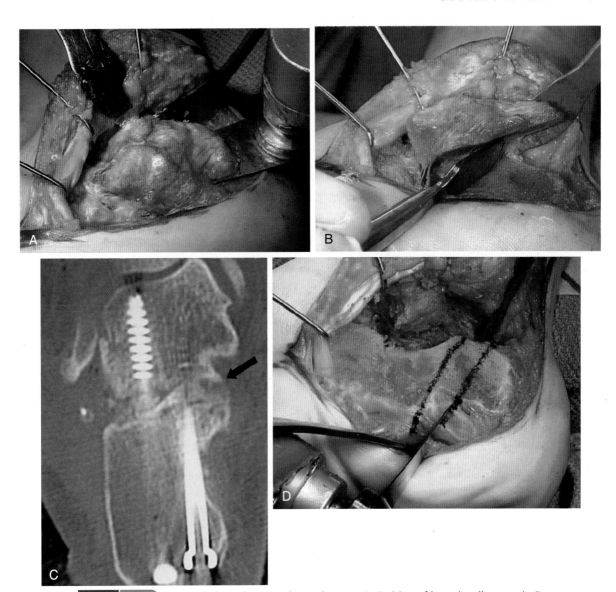

FIGURE 6.7 Extensile lateral approach to calcaneus. **A,** Excision of lateral wall exostosis. **B,** En bloc removal of lateral wall exostosis. **C,** CT scan showing excised lateral wall used as autograft bone block. **D,** Completion of Dwyer-type calcaneal osteotomy for type III calcaneal malunion with severe varus malalignment of hindfoot. (From Clare MP, Lee WE, Sanders R: Intermediate to long-term results of a treatment protocol for calcaneal fracture malunions, *J Bone Joint Surg Am* 87A:963, 2005.) **SEE TECHNIQUE 6.6.**

tive as direct intraarticular distraction. Avoid incising the deltoid ligament from inside the subtalar joint because this renders the joint unstable and overdistraction of the graft may result.

- Place the previously excised lateral wall fragment within the joint as an autograft bone block (Fig. 6.7C). This bone can be folded over on itself to obtain more height if need-

ed, but it should fill the subtalar joint because the height of the lateral calcaneus (and the graft) usually is equal to the width of the posterior facet. Additional cancellous allograft chips may be placed in the debrided sinus tarsi to assist fusion.

- If a subtalar arthrodesis alone is needed (type II malunion), place fixation at this point. With the subtalar joint held in neutral to slight valgus alignment, place two terminally threaded 3.2-mm guide pins percutaneously from the posterior plantar edge of the calcaneus, and advance across the subtalar joint perpendicular to the plane of the posterior facet and into the talar dome. Angle the guide pin in a divergent fashion into the talar dome for increased stability. Avoid placing a pin in the lateral aspect of the ankle joint.

- Obtain fluoroscopic anteroposterior and mortise images of the ankle and obtain an axial radiograph of the calcaneus to verify correct pin placement and hindfoot alignment.
- If more stable fixation is required, place a third guide pin from the plantar margin of the anterior process of the calcaneus into the distal aspect of the talar neck and head for more stable fixation. Avoid violating the talonavicular joint.
- Place large fragment, partially threaded (7.3 or 8 mm) cannulated screws in lag mode for definitive fixation.
- In patients with a type III malunion, correction of axial malalignment also is necessary. Because rotation of the midfoot in the coronal plane around an anteroposterior axis (pronation-supination) would not correct a malpositioned calcaneal tuberosity healed in varus or valgus, a calcaneal osteotomy is performed before placement of the fixation for subtalar arthrodesis. For varus malalignment, perform a Dwyer lateral closing wedge osteotomy posterior to the posterior facet (Fig. 6.7D). Use a medial displacement calcaneal osteotomy with rotation for valgus malalignment.
- When the osteotomy is completed, insert the guide pins in the manner described earlier. In this way, the osteotomy and the fusion can be compressed simultaneously. If bone is removed during the closing wedge osteotomy, it can be used as graft material as well.
- Remove the Kirschner wires and examine the tendons for dislocation. In many ankles with obvious preoperative tendon subluxation, removal of the exostosis allows the tendons to fall back behind the fibula and no further treatment is needed. The peroneal tendon sheath should be entered distally with a Freer elevator, however, to evaluate sheath stenosis proximally.
- If stenosis is found, incise the sheath over a length of 2 to 3 cm along the undersurface of the subperiosteal flap so that a tenolysis can be performed.
- If a peroneal tendon dislocation is identified, reconstruct the superior peroneal retinaculum through a small separate incision in the flap.
- Place a deep drain exiting at the proximal tip of the vertical limb of the incision and close the subperiosteal flap in a layered fashion.
- Pass interrupted 0 Vicryl sutures in the deep layers of the subperiosteal flap, angling such that the flap is advanced to the apex of the incision.
- Clamp the sutures until all deep sutures have been placed. When completed, hand-tie the sutures sequentially, starting at the proximal and distal ends and working toward the apex of the incision.
- Close the subcuticular layer in a similar fashion with interrupted 2-0 Vicryl. Close the skin with 3-0 nylon suture, starting at the ends and progressing toward the apex. If height restoration prevents wound closure, the vertical limb of the incision can be extended proximally to allow the flap to shift and rotate downward, with the proximal wound being left open to granulate.

POSTOPERATIVE CARE Patients with type I malunions are kept non–weight bearing until the incision has healed, and physical therapy with early range-of-motion activities and gait training with full weight bearing is initiated thereafter, usually by 3 weeks. Patients with type II and type III malunions are kept non–weight bearing with the leg in a cast for 12 weeks (with cast changes every 4 to 6 weeks). This is followed by progression of weight bearing and the initiation of physical therapy after radiographic evidence of union of the subtalar fusion mass is confirmed.

CORRECTION OF VALGUS MALUNION OF EXTRAARTICULAR CALCANEAL FRACTURE

For malunited extraarticular fractures, Aly described a laterally based opening wedge osteotomy for symptomatic valgus calcaneal deformity in 34 patients. He obtained good or excellent results in 91% and poor results in 9% at a mean follow-up of 56.2 months. The mean AOFAS hindfoot and ankle score improved from 57 preoperatively to 90 postoperatively. In the patients with poor results, bilateral fractures and subtalar arthritis contributed to their gait abnormality and restricted hindfoot motion.

TECHNIQUE 6.7

(ALY)
- Approach the calcaneus through an oblique lateral incision. Protect and retract the superficial branches of the peroneal nerve.
- Identify the sustentaculum tali by probing over the dorsum of the exposed calcaneus.
- Shave the lateral border of the widened calcaneus. Incise the periosteum in line with the planned osteotomy, starting laterally approximately 2.5 cm proximal to the calcaneocuboid joint in the interval between the middle and posterior facets of the subtalar joint.
- Make a lateral to medial oblique osteotomy. The osteotomy line should be made slightly oblique from proximal-lateral to distal-medial. The required depth of the osteotomy should be estimated from the preoperative calcaneal axial radiographs.
- Open the osteotomy with a large osteotome. Preserve the periosteum of the medial calcaneus to prevent medial displacement of the posterior fragment.
- Take a suitable tricortical bone graft from the posterior iliac crest and place it into the osteotomy site and add the bone shavings.
- Through a posterior approach, place one cannulated screw through the long axis of the calcaneus.

POSTOPERATIVE CARE Postoperatively, the patient is kept non–weight bearing in a cast for 6 weeks and then

arthritis, another cadaver study found that 2 mm or more of shortening or lateral displacement and 5 degrees or more of external rotation increase contact pressures significantly in the posterolateral and midlateral quadrants of the talar dome, and a corresponding decrease in the contact pressures was noted in the medial quadrants of the talar dome. Anatomic reduction of pronation-lateral rotation fractures of the lateral malleolus was recommended to diminish the risk of posttraumatic arthritis.

Osteotomies to correct uncomplicated deformities caused by recently malunited fractures of the ankle usually are satisfactory, but displacement of the talus within the ankle mortise for more than 3 months may result in pathologic changes in the articular cartilage, with a diminished potential for satisfactory outcome with osteotomy. Some authors, however, have reported improvement in patients with adequate surgery after displacement of more than 3 months. Nevertheless, all agree that when the deformity has been of short duration and has been corrected with minimal trauma to the articular surfaces, good function usually can be obtained if the normal weight-bearing alignment of the lower extremity and the normal relationships between the articular surfaces of the tibia, the fibula, and the talus are restored (Fig. 6.8). Displacement and residual tilt of the talus have been associated with poor results, as have inaccurate reduction and poor surgical technique.

Osteotomies have been less successful in treating bimalleolar malunions associated with moderate-to-severe arthritis. An osteotomy can restore weight-bearing alignment of the ankle, but pain and swelling can persist because of arthritic deterioration. Some authors recommend realignment osteotomies as the initial treatment of all symptomatic ankle malunions, regardless of the age of the patient, time from initial injury, severity of malunion, or presence of arthritic changes. However, although arthritis is not a contraindication to osteotomy, chondral damage has been found to be indicative of a poor result. Ankle arthrodesis or ankle arthroplasty should be considered in patients with severe arthritic changes and severely impaired function or in patients who remain significantly symptomatic after osteotomy. It is important to remember that walking on rough ground is difficult after arthrodesis, especially if the subtalar joint is secondarily fibrosed or ankylosed. Complications as high as 30% have been reported after ankle arthrodesis, including nonunion and malunion.

Paley et al. treated malunion after ankle arthrodesis with Ilizarov reconstruction. They concluded that the Ilizarov apparatus can simultaneously treat the foot deformity, length discrepancy, and infection, achieving a solid union and plantigrade foot. However, 20 major complications that required surgery occurred during treatment and seven occurred after frame removal, four of which required additional surgery.

There are three requirements for the anatomic restoration of the ankle joint: (1) a perfectly equidistant and parallel joint space; (2) a fibular spike in its normal position pointing exactly to the level of the distal tibial subchondral bone, indicating that the length of the fibula is correct; and (3) a normal contour at the lateral part of the articular surface of the talus in continuity as an unbroken curve to the recess of the distal fibula where the peroneal tendons lie.

Up to 78% good results have been reported with fibular osteotomy and lengthening for ankle malunion. The criteria for osteotomy include radiographic confirmation

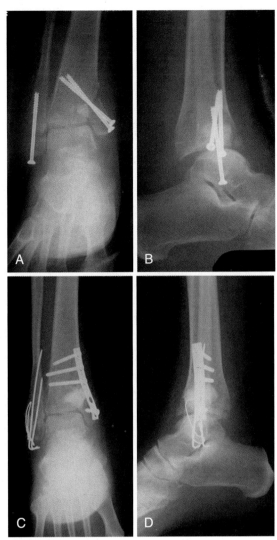

FIGURE 6.8 **A** and **B,** Malunion of bimalleolar ankle fracture fixed with interfragmentary screws in elderly patient. **C** and **D,** Revision fixation with one third tubular buttress plate and hydroxyapatite grafting of medial malleolus and tension band fixation of lateral malleolus.

placed in a walking cast for an additional 6 weeks. Thereafter, the patient may wear normal shoes.

ANKLE

Occasionally, malunion occurs after the most accurate reduction of closed ankle fractures or more commonly after "stable" injuries that displace with widening of the mortise because of syndesmotic disruption. Malunion also can develop if fixation of the fibula is inadequate and the fibula is allowed to shorten and rotate. Disability from a malunited ankle fracture can be so extreme that relief can be obtained only by surgery. Even a minor varus or valgus deformity of the joint produces an abnormal weight-bearing alignment and posttraumatic arthritis. Although one cadaver study suggested that factors other than the magnitude of normal contact stresses are of greater importance in the pathogenesis of posttraumatic

of malunion (Fig. 6.9), a demonstrable joint space on anteroposterior and mortise views, and remaining articular cartilage covering the tibial plafond and the talus. Contraindications include ankylosis, loss of bone stock, and severe degenerative arthritis.

Operations to correct malunited ankle fractures are (1) osteotomy of the fractured fibula or medial malleolus or both with restoration of fibular length and internal fixation of the osteotomies, (2) supramalleolar osteotomy when only realignment of the lower extremity is required, and (3) arthrodesis of the ankle with or without supramalleolar osteotomy. Although a variety of malunions can occur, the procedures described here can be modified to treat most malunions.

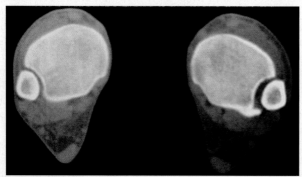

FIGURE 6.9 CT scan of occult malunion. Right ankle *(left)* is normal; left ankle *(right)* shows widening of distal tibiofibular joint, indicating fibular shortening and external rotation of lateral malleolus. (From Yablon IG, Leach RE: Reconstruction of malunited fractures of the lateral malleolus, *J Bone Joint Surg Am* 71A:521, 1989.)

OSTEOTOMY FOR BIMALLEOLAR FRACTURE

TECHNIQUE 6.8

- Make a longitudinal lateral incision over the old fibular fracture, curving slightly anteriorly at its distal end.
- With an osteotome or oscillating saw, make either a transverse or an oblique osteotomy of the fibula at the area of the old fracture.
- Excise scar tissue between the fibula and tibia to allow correct positioning of the fibula in the notch. Length and rotation of the fibula can be restored with the technique described by Weber.
- Attach a five-hole or six-hole, 3.5-mm dynamic compression plate to the distal fibular fragment with two screws (Fig. 6.10A). Before plate application, make a small recess in the distal fibula so that the plate is not prominent. Place the plate slightly posterior on the distal fragment to allow internal rotation of the fragment. Correct the rotation of the distal fragment by internally rotating it 10 degrees.
- Attach the articulated tensioning device from an AO small fragment system to the proximal end of the plate (Fig. 6.10B). Apply distraction until the distal fibula is reduced anatomically to its articulations with the tibia and talus.
- Confirm the reduction with radiographs or fluoroscopy.
- If a transverse osteotomy has been made, fill the gap created by distraction with a small wafer of corticocancellous bone from the medial tibial metaphysis above the medial malleolus (Fig. 6.10C).

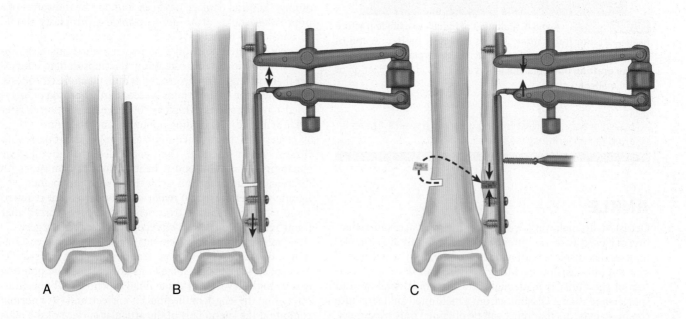

FIGURE 6.10 Technique of fibular lengthening (see text). **A,** Five-hole plate is secured to fibula with two distal screws, and osteotomy is made. **B,** Lengthening is obtained with distraction device. **C,** Corticocancellous graft from tibia is placed in osteotomy, and compression is applied; remaining screws are inserted to attach plate to fibula. **SEE TECHNIQUE 6.8.**

- Change the AO tensioning device to the compression mode and apply compression to the osteotomy site. Attach the plate to the proximal fibula using three 3.5-mm cortical screws. Yablon and Leach recommended the addition of a syndesmosis screw if the interosseous membrane is detached during the fibular dissection. In very distal fractures, it may be necessary to stabilize the fibula with transfixing Kirschner wires.
- Alternatively, Ward et al. described the use of the small AO distractor to restore fibular length and rotation. Expose the fibula, resect scar tissue, and osteotomize the fibula as previously described.
- Insert two 2.5-mm partially threaded pins in the anterior distal fibular fragment in 10 degrees of external rotation.
- Correct rotation of the distal fragment and insert two 2.5-mm pins into the proximal fibula in the same plane.
- Attach the small AO distractor and distract the fibula until it is anatomically aligned.
- Fill the gap with bone graft and apply compression with the distractor.
- Apply a one third tubular plate to stabilize the fibula.

CORRECTION OF DIASTASIS OF THE TIBIA AND FIBULA

Operations for diastasis of the tibia and fibula should allow a shift of the talus medially and repositioning of the lateral malleolus. Yablon and Leach reported that a more extensive dissection usually is necessary to restore anatomic alignment in fibular malunion associated with lateral shift of the talus.

TECHNIQUE 6.9

- Make a fibular osteotomy and rotate it distally 180 degrees to allow removal of an adequate amount of scar from the area of syndesmosis.
- Make a second incision over the anterior aspect of the medial malleolus and excise scar tissue between the medial malleolus and talus.
- Reduce the talus and place a Steinmann pin from the tibia into the talus to hold the reduction temporarily while the fibula is reduced and plated, as described for bimalleolar malunions.
- If the medial malleolus also has united in a poor position, make a second longitudinal incision just proximal to its base and drive an osteotome from above through four fifths of the diameter of the medial malleolus distally and laterally. Make this osteotomy through the medial part of the tibia just above the old fracture to obtain a broader bony surface. Refracture the bone by forcefully adducting the foot.
- Stabilize the medial malleolus with parallel small fragment lag screws and Kirschner wires as necessary.
- If a gap has been created by reduction of the medial malleolus, insert bone graft to prevent future collapse. Use

a small fragment one third tubular plate as a buttress if necessary.
- Obtain intraoperative radiographs to confirm anatomic reduction of the ankle.

POSTOPERATIVE CARE A cast is applied over padding from the tibial tuberosity to the toes with the foot in neutral position. The cast is changed in 2 weeks, the sutures are removed, and a cast is reapplied and worn for 10 to 12 weeks. If stable fixation is obtained in a compliant patient, a removable cast brace that does not allow rotation can be substituted to allow controlled physical therapy. An ankle brace with a medial T-strap and an arch support may be necessary for an additional 10 to 12 weeks and can be worn for 3 to 6 months after difficult reconstructions. Physical therapy should be used to restore the soft tissues and encourage strengthening of the bone.

SUPRAMALLEOLAR OSTEOTOMY

Occasionally, a malunion of the distal tibia and fibula occurs in which the normal tibiotalar relationships are retained but the ankle is in valgus or varus. A supramalleolar osteotomy is recommended for this malunion. Opening wedge, closing wedge, or dome osteotomies can be used. Because dome osteotomies do not sacrifice length to gain correction of the deformity, they may be preferred in malunions associated with shortening. Dome osteotomies are more effective, however, in correcting deformity in the frontal (varus-valgus) plane than in the sagittal (flexion-extension) plane. A properly positioned wedge osteotomy can be used to correct multiplanar deformities. Closing wedge osteotomies provide broad bony surfaces for healing but cause some shortening of the extremity. Opening wedge osteotomies maintain length, but bone grafting is required to fill the gap created. The Ilizarov method of gradual deformity correction with distraction osteogenesis also can be used.

TECHNIQUE 6.10

- To create a dome osteotomy, expose the distal tibia through an anterolateral Henry approach.
- Use a 3.2-mm drill bit to create a series of holes in the distal tibial metaphysis in the shape of an arc, convex superiorly. The medial and lateral edges of the arc should be 1.0 to 1.5 cm proximal to the ankle joint, and the height of the arc should be 1.0 to 1.5 cm (Fig. 6.11A).
- Through the same incision or a separate lateral incision, expose the fibula and make an osteotomy at the same level as the tibial osteotomy. If the fracture has healed in varus, resect 1 to 3 cm of the fibula to correct the deformity. If the fracture has healed in valgus, make an oblique osteotomy of the fibula. Use an oscillating saw to connect the holes drilled anteriorly, medially, and laterally in the tibia.
- With fluoroscopic control, insert a 4-mm or 5-mm threaded pin transversely from medial to lateral into the distal tibial

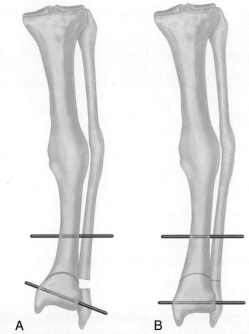

FIGURE 6.11 Supramalleolar osteotomy. **A,** Dome osteotomy is created 1.0 to 1.5 cm proximal to ankle joint. Threaded pins are inserted parallel to ankle and knee joint lines. **B,** Osteotomy is completed, and pins are brought parallel to correct varus or valgus deformity. **SEE TECHNIQUE 6.10.**

fragment parallel to the joint line. Keep the pin out of the joint, the osteotomy site, and the neurovascular bundle.

- Insert a second 4-mm or 5-mm bicortical threaded pin 6 to 10 cm proximal to the osteotomy and parallel to the knee joint.
- With an osteotome, complete the tibial osteotomy through the posterior cortex. Correct varus or valgus deformity by making the pins parallel (Fig. 6.11B).
- If complete reduction is not obtained, it may be necessary to resect more of the fibula or to release more soft tissue, including the interosseous membrane.
- When the reduction is acceptable, connect the pins with an external fixator bar and apply compression. Additional external fixation pins can be placed in the tibia and talus.
- Alternatively, if the soft-tissue coverage is adequate, stabilize the osteotomy with a 3.5-mm dynamic compression plate and remove the two external fixation pins. The fibula also can be stabilized with a one third tubular plate if desired. Bone grafting is left to the surgeon's discretion.
- An opening or closing wedge osteotomy can be made in the following manner. Through a lateral longitudinal incision, expose and osteotomize the fibula as previously described to correct either varus or valgus deformity.
- Through the same incision, expose the lateral surface of the tibia 1.3 cm proximal to the joint line and drive a wide osteotome transversely almost through the bone; carry out a manual osteoclasis. Insert cancellous iliac bone, or use a wedge-shaped graft taken from the shaft of the tibia into the lateral side of the osteotomy to pack it open.
- Stabilize the osteotomy with an external fixator applied in the standard fashion with pins through the tibia and talus.

- If the fractures have healed in varus position, a closing wedge osteotomy of the tibia can be made in a similar fashion or internal fixation with a plate and screws can be used in conjunction with autogenous iliac bone grafts.
- Close the wound in layers and apply a bulky dressing if an external fixator has been used.
- If not, apply a cast from the tibial tuberosity to the toes.

POSTOPERATIVE CARE If casting was used, the cast and the sutures are removed at 2 weeks and then a new cast is reapplied. Weight bearing is not permitted for 6 weeks. If external fixation was used, it is removed at 6 to 8 weeks, and a short leg walking cast is applied. Weight bearing is progressed as tolerated, and the cast is removed when the osteotomies have healed (12 to 16 weeks after surgery). Rehabilitation of the lower extremity is begun by physical therapy.

ARTHRODESIS FOR MALUNITED FRACTURES OF THE ANKLE

Arthrodesis is indicated as a primary procedure in the following types of malunited fractures of the ankle:

1. Malunited bimalleolar fractures, with or without significant deformity, in which radiographs show definite traumatic arthritic changes to be the cause of persistent pain and disability (Fig. 6.12)
2. Malunited trimalleolar fractures of long duration with posterior and proximal dislocation of the talus
3. Malunited fractures in which the deformity cannot be completely corrected by conservative reconstruction or in which such extensive surgery is required for correction that arthritic changes in the ankle are inevitable

When malalignment is marked, it should always be corrected by osteotomy at the time of arthrodesis; otherwise, a foot strain can be severely disabling later. This additional procedure does not materially complicate the operation or delay recovery. See other chapter for techniques of arthrodesis of the ankle.

TIBIA

SHAFTS OF THE TIBIA AND FIBULA

In malunions of the shafts of the tibia and fibula, the degree of deformity that requires surgery is not clearly defined. It is widely believed that angular deformities of the tibial shaft cause alterations in the contact pressures of the knee and ankle joints and predispose them to the development of osteoarthritis. Clinical series with long-term follow-up have not always supported this hypothesis, however. One study found that the ankle joint is more affected than the knee and that the location of the fracture is significant. Poorer functional ankle scores were correlated with the degree of malalignment and the proximity of the deformity to the ankle joint. Varus deformities were more poorly tolerated than were valgus deformities. A later study found just the opposite, that symptoms at the knee were correlated with arthritic changes, whereas symptoms at the ankle were not. In addition, no relationship was shown between the location of the fracture and development of osteoarthritis of the knee or ankle. Rotational deformity also was not associated with arthritic changes.

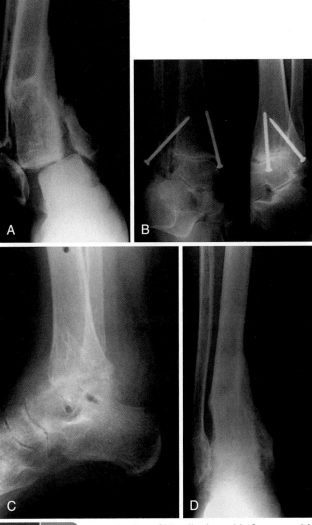

FIGURE 6.12 **A,** Malunion of bimalleolar ankle fracture with preexisting malunion of distal tibia. **B,** Correction of malunion was achieved; however, arthritis developed, causing pain and disability. **C** and **D,** Tibiotalar arthrodesis was performed using compression clamps. Ankle is now painless and stable.

Milner et al. determined that fracture malunion did not cause a higher incidence of ankle and subtalar arthritis ipsilateral to the fracture. There was a trend toward a higher prevalence of medial compartment osteoarthritis of the knee in patients with varus malalignment of the limb, and shortening of 10 mm or more correlated with subjective complaints of knee pain. Although osteoarthritis occurred more frequently on the side of the fracture, factors other than malalignment were believed to contribute more to the development of osteoarthritis.

The degree of acceptable deformity noted by various authors is extremely variable. Surgery has been recommended for valgus deformity of more than 12 degrees, varus deformity of more than 6 degrees, external rotation deformity of more than 15 degrees, or internal rotation deformity of more than 10 degrees. Shortening of 2 cm or less usually is well tolerated with shoe modifications, but more than 2.5 cm of shortening can cause significant disability.

When surgery is considered for correction of a tibial malunion, the degree of the deformity, the patient's symptoms, the condition of the injured extremity, and the functional demands of the patient all must be taken into account. Disability from malunion of the tibial shaft is produced mainly by rotational deformity, lateral and posterior bowing, and usually some degree of shortening. Often a resulting contracture of the Achilles tendon causes an equinus deformity of the foot. Symptoms may include ankle, knee, or back pain; gait disturbances; and a cosmetically unacceptable deformity. The limb must be evaluated for a history of neurologic or vascular injury, adequacy of soft-tissue coverage, and presence of infection. With a history of vascular injury, preoperative arteriograms can be helpful in determining the operative approach. If soft tissues in the area of the planned operative site are poor, a simultaneous rotation or vascularized free tissue transfer flap may be necessary to promote bone healing and prevent wound complications. In a patient with a previous infection, preoperative indium-labeled white blood cell scans, gallium scans, or technetium scans can help to determine the activity of the infection. It is generally desirable to treat the infection before osteotomy for malunion. Equinus contractures should be corrected by lengthening the Achilles tendon.

When planning an osteotomy, the amount of angular and rotational deformity, leg-length discrepancy, and translation must be determined. Simple opening wedge, closing wedge, or dome-shaped osteotomies can be used to correct relatively small degrees of malunion; however, closing wedge osteotomies can create additional shortening and opening wedge osteotomies often require bone grafting. Oblique osteotomies can be used to correct multiplanar deformities. These osteotomies provide broad surface areas for healing, and lengthening can be obtained by sliding the osteotomy distally. Angular deformities in the frontal (varus-valgus) and sagittal (flexion-extension) planes can be resolved into a uniplanar deformity in an oblique plane (Fig. 6.13). The degree of maximal deformity is greater than the angular measurements on either anteroposterior or lateral radiographs. The plane of maximal deformity can be found by rotating the leg under fluoroscopy until the maximal degree of deformity is seen. A radiograph taken at 90 degrees to this plane should show no deformity. The oblique osteotomy should be made perpendicular to the plane of maximal deformity. Rotational deformity can be evaluated with CT or clinically by measuring the intermalleolar angle. Preoperative planning should include drawings of the injured and uninjured extremities, the site and configuration of the planned osteotomy, and the type of internal fixation device to be used. To prevent neurologic complications, somatosensory evoked potentials should be used during correction of a severe deformity, especially if lengthening is involved. Although the osteotomy usually is performed at the site of the old fracture, a supramalleolar osteotomy (see Technique 6.10) may be preferable if the previous fracture has been slow to heal, is covered with poor soft tissue, or contains extremely dense sclerotic bone. Russell et al. described a clamshell osteotomy for treatment of complex nonunions of the tibial or femoral diaphysis and noted that it is especially helpful in malunions that have a long malaligned segment.

Satisfactory alignment after osteotomy is difficult to maintain without some type of internal fixation, such as a compression plate or intramedullary nail or external

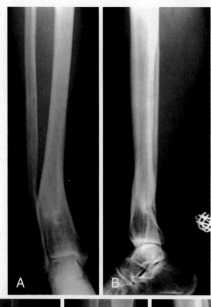

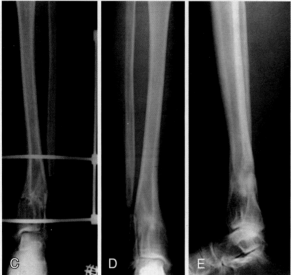

FIGURE 6.13 **A** and **B,** Varus malunion of distal tibia. **C,** Osteotomy of tibia and fibula with reduction maintained by external fixator. **D** and **E,** Tibial union obtained with normal alignment; asymptomatic nonunion of fibular osteotomy persists.

fixation. If an intramedullary nail is used, the medullary canal must be opened at both ends of the old fracture, and any gaps created by the osteotomy should be filled with cancellous bone. Reamed, locked intramedullary nailing has been recommended for stabilization of osteotomies made to correct tibial malunions. We prefer to use statically locked nails to increase the stability of the osteotomy. The limited incisions used for the osteotomy are closed after opening of the medullary canals in both fragments and passing of the reaming guidewire but before reaming and nail insertion. Static locking can be converted to dynamic locking in several weeks if needed to promote healing. If a large amount of soft-tissue stripping is necessary to correct the deformity, fixation methods other than intramedullary nailing are preferable because intramedullary reaming often devascularizes the exposed bone segment further. A history of previous external fixation,

especially if associated with pin track infection, also is a relative contraindication to intramedullary nailing because of an increased risk of infection.

Oblique tibial osteotomies stabilized with dynamic compression plates and lag screws have been advocated for the treatment of multiplanar tibial deformities with good results (Fig. 6.14). Sanders et al. recommended this technique for tibial shaft deformities that require less than 2.5 cm of lengthening. Contraindications to this procedure include inadequate soft-tissue coverage and active infection. The inability to restore full length, delayed union, plate failure, infection, vascular injury, and wound dehiscence are possible complications.

Osteotomies for infected tibial malunions and malunions associated with a poor soft-tissue envelope may be best treated by the Ilizarov technique of corticotomy and gradual correction of deformity with a ring and wire fixator to correct tibial malunions. This technique is described in chapter 2.

OBLIQUE TIBIAL OSTEOTOMY

TECHNIQUE 6.11

(SANDERS ET AL.)

- Place a tourniquet on the proximal part of the thigh. Prepare and drape both legs so that they can be compared after correction.
- If axial lengthening is planned, place electrodes for measurement of somatosensory evoked potentials.
- Under fluoroscopic control, insert a 6-mm Schanz pin in the proximal tibial metaphysis absolutely parallel to the proximal tibial articular surface (Fig. 6.15A). Similarly, place a 6-mm Schanz pin in the distal tibial metaphysis absolutely parallel to the tibial plafond.
- If lengthening is planned, or if the fibula interferes with correction of the tibia, make an oblique fibular osteotomy, ideally at the level of the proposed site of the tibial osteotomy.
- Exsanguinate the leg with a pressure bandage, inflate the tourniquet to 300 mm Hg (39.99 kPa), and remove the pressure bandage.
- Make a standard anterior extensile incision to expose the tibia.
- Identify the area of malunion and subperiosteally dissect all soft tissue from the area. Place Hohmann retractors to protect the neurovascular structures.
- Sculpt the bone to remove excess callus while the tibia is still intact; save the bone that is removed to be used later as a local graft.
- Place a femoral distractor (Synthes USA, Paoli, PA) on the Schanz pins, with the universal joint locked, leaving the rotational joint open (Fig. 6.15B). Make the tibial osteotomy with a single cut perpendicular to the plane of maximal deformity (see Fig. 6.15B). If lengthening is not needed, hold the saw at an angle of 30 to 45 degrees in the coronal plane to allow enough bone on either side of the cut to overlap and be lagged together.

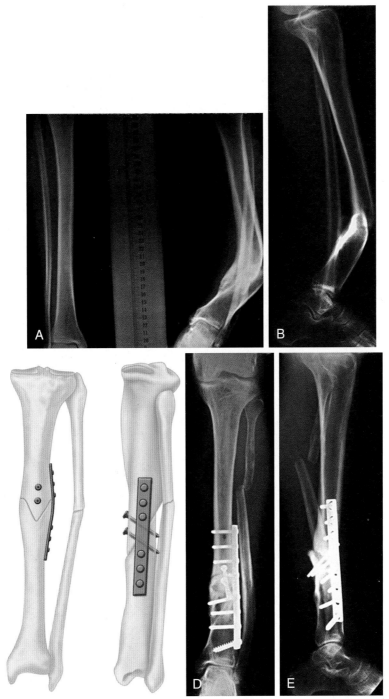

FIGURE 6.14   **A,** Multiplane osteotomy of tibia for diaphyseal malunion. **B,** Severe deformity: 45 degrees of varus, 50 degrees of anterior bowing, 15 degrees of internal rotation, 1.4 cm of shortening, and distal tibiofibular synostosis. **C–E,** After osteotomy, correction of deformity. Lateral view shows minimal overcorrection in sagittal plane. (From Johnson EE: Multiplane correctional osteotomy of the tibia for diaphyseal malunion, *Clin Orthop Relat Res* 215:223, 1987.)

- If more lengthening is needed, the exact amount, in millimeters, to be obtained from axial lengthening already has been determined by preoperative planning. Obtain this length by decreasing the angle between the osteotomy and the axis of the tibia in the coronal plane so that the bones can slide apart lengthwise at the cut while remaining in contact. The angle of the cut in the coronal plane is determined preoperatively and is marked on the bone with a marking pen and angle templates from the angled blade plate instrument set (Synthes USA, Paoli, PA). Rotate the saw to this angle in the coronal plane and make the tibial cut accordingly. Cuts made at angles of less than 20 degrees to the coronal axis are impossible to perform.

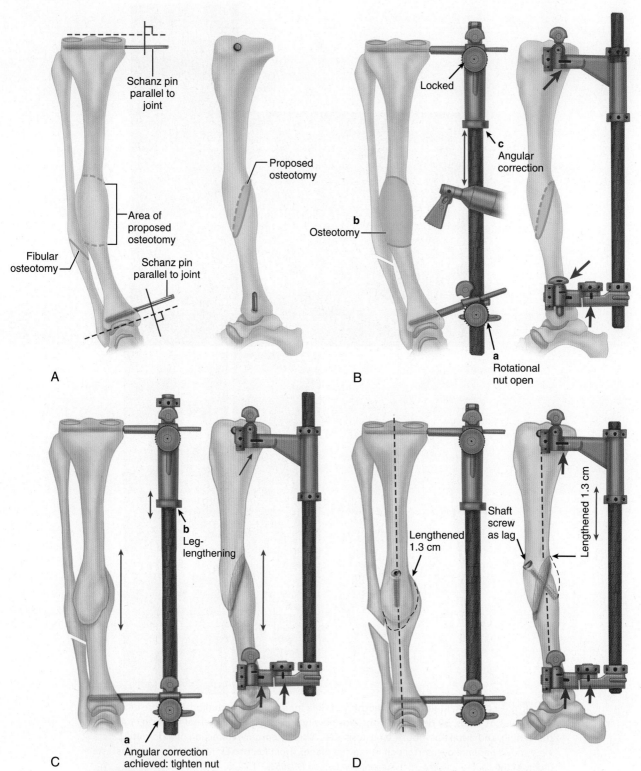

FIGURE 6.15 Oblique osteotomy for tibial malunion (see text). **A,** Anterior and lateral views showing placement of Schanz pins parallel to planes of proximal and distal joints and to site of proposed osteotomy. **B,** Anterior view *(left)* after femoral distractor has been applied; rotational joint *(a)* is left open to allow lateral angular correction. Oblique osteotomy *(b)* is made to correct varus angulation and procurvatum; axial correction occurs as nut *(c)* is turned to lengthen distractor. Lateral view *(right)*. Markings on distractor indicate angular correction has not been obtained. **C,** After angular correction is obtained, rotational joint is locked and further lengthening of distractor results in pure axial lengthening. Markings *(right)* now indicate that angular correction has been obtained. **D,** Anterior and lateral views after correction; lag screw has been inserted perpendicular to osteotomy.

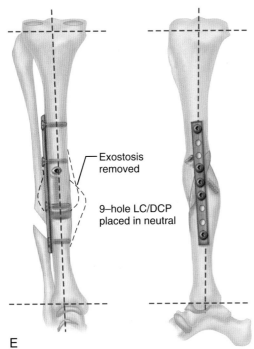

Exostosis
removed

9–hole LC/DCP
placed in neutral

E

FIGURE **6.15, Cont'd** **E,** Final result with neutralization plate in place. (From Sanders R, Anglen JO, Mark JB: Oblique osteotomy for the correction of tibial malunion, *J Bone Joint Surg* 77A:240, 1995.) **SEE TECHNIQUE 6.11.**

- As the femoral distractor is lengthened, the lengthening translates into angular correction. Leaving the rotational joint open (see Fig. 6.15B) allows simultaneous correction of the multiplanar deformity by rotating the two tibial segments around an axis perpendicular to the cut surface. Continue this correction until the two Schanz pins are parallel (Fig. 6.15C).
- If the cut is not perfect, additional bone can be shaved from the cut surfaces to correct alignment.
- If axial lengthening is not required, place a lag screw perpendicular to the cut surface and tighten it. If axial lengthening is required, use a clamp (bone reduction forceps with pointed tips) to hold the two cut surfaces together until the angular correction has been obtained and then lock the rotational joint of the distractor. Additional lengthening of the distractor now lengthens the tibia axially. Gently loosen the bone clamp, but hold it in place to allow sliding in the axial plane while preventing translation and loss of angular correction. If somatosensory evoked potentials change before axial lengthening is completed, stop the lengthening and reverse it until the potentials return to baseline.
- When lengthening is completed, tighten the clamp, lock the distractor joints, and obtain anteroposterior and lateral radiographs. Superimpose these radiographs on the preoperative drawings and on the radiograph of the normal leg and make modifications as needed.
- When the alignment and length are satisfactory, place a lag screw perpendicularly across the osteotomy (Fig. 6.15D).

- Contour a narrow 4.5-mm dynamic compression plate and place it as a neutralization plate (Fig. 6.15E).
- Shave the bone and place the bone shavings as grafts around the osteotomy as needed.
- If an equinus contracture developed as the bone was lengthened, perform a Z-lengthening of the Achilles tendon.
- Remove the distractor, close the wound over a drain, and apply a bulky dressing and a below-knee posterior splint.

POSTOPERATIVE CARE Range of motion of 0 to 90 degrees is begun immediately after surgery in a continuous passive motion machine. The patient is allowed out of bed on the first postoperative day. The drain is removed when less than 10 mL of drainage occurs in an 8-hour period, usually by the second day after surgery. The dressing is removed at 3 days, and if the wound appears satisfactory, a below-knee non–weight-bearing fiberglass cast is applied and touch-down weight bearing is allowed. The sutures are removed at 10 to 14 days, and the cast is changed. At 10 to 12 weeks, the cast is removed and a removable tibial brace is fitted. If bridging trabeculae across the osteotomy are visible on anteroposterior and lateral radiographs, partial weight bearing is allowed and is progressed as tolerated. Gait-training, range-of-motion, and strengthening exercises are begun. At the end of 16 weeks, if the tibial osteotomy seems to be healed clinically and radiographically, the brace is discontinued and activities of daily living and full weight bearing are encouraged. The patient is examined every 6 months for 2 years. The plate is removed if requested by the patient because of pain but not before 12 months after surgery.

CLAMSHELL OSTEOTOMY

Russell et al. described a clamshell osteotomy in 10 patients for treatment of complex femoral and tibial diaphyseal malunions, in which the malunited segment is transected perpendicular to the normal diaphysis proximally and distally and the transected segment is wedged open by osteotomy much like opening a clamshell. An intramedullary rod is used to anatomically align the proximal and distal segments of the diaphysis. Pires et al. expanded the use of the clamshell osteotomy to facilitate intramedullary nailing in acute fractures of long bones with preexisting deformity. Contraindications for this technique include an unsuitable soft-tissue sleeve for open exposure, a metaphyseal malunion, intramedullary osteomyelitis, absent medullary canal, morbid obesity, open physes, and lengthening of the tibia by more than 3 cm. We have not used this technique.

TECHNIQUE 6.12

(RUSSELL ET AL.)
- Position the patient supine with both lower extremities included in the operative field. A tourniquet is not used.

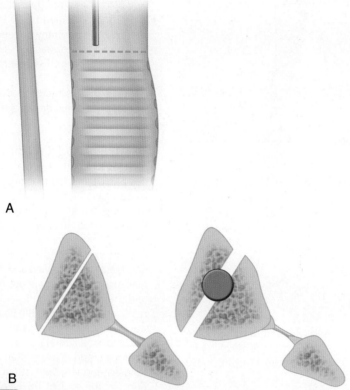

A

B

FIGURE 6.16 Clamshell osteotomy as described by Russell et al. **A,** Kirschner wire placed proximal to malunion. **B,** Plane of longitudinal portion of the clamshell osteotomy for tibia. Plane is approximately parallel to medial face of tibia. **SEE TECHNIQUE 6.12.**

- Make a lateral incision along the fibular shaft at the planned level of the proximal transverse component of the tibial osteotomy. Perform a fibular oblique osteotomy to obtain complete freedom in repositioning the tibia after the osteotomy.
- Use a transpatellar or medial parapatellar tendon entrance to the previously defined safe zone for the tibial rod starting point. Take care to ensure an appropriate entrance angle into the proximal tibial segment. Open the proximal tibial segment with a threaded wire over which an opening reamer is passed. No attempt is made to ream the proximal tibia at this time.
- To expose the osteotomy site, make a longitudinal incision over the anterior compartment one fingerbreadth lateral to the tibial crest along the proposed longitudinal osteotomy site.
- Translate the anterior compartment musculature posteriorly to allow for an extraperiosteal exposure of the lateral aspect of the malunited segment. Only the anterolateral portion of the tibia is exposed.
- With radiographic guidance, localize the positions of the proximal and distal transverse osteotomies and place a Kirschner wire perpendicular to the anatomic axis to guide the osteotomies (Fig. 6.16A).
- Create the clamshell component of the osteotomy parallel to the medial tibial face, beginning just posterior to the anterolateral subcutaneous prominence of the tibia and aiming in a posteromedial direction (Fig. 6.16B).

- Use a 3.5-mm drill bit to create the path for the longitudinal osteotomy with the goal of creating a bicortical uniform plane of stress risers (Fig. 6.17). Only osteotomy of the near cortex is accomplished with an osteotome using the drill holes as a guide. Use a sagittal saw to create the transverse proximal and distal osteotomies.
- Split the far cortex of the osteotomized segment parallel to the medial face with the use of an osteotome and laminar spreader. Separate the longitudinal osteotomy of the intercalary segment with a laminar spreader; the posterior cortex is hinged on the periosteal sleeve. If the posteromedial cortex does not open easily, then use an osteotome to cut the posteromedial cortex and then the laminar spreader to open the osteotomy.
- Place the limb over a radiolucent triangle and pass the guidewire from the proximal tibial segment through the osteotomized segment into the distal segment with the aid of fluoroscopic guidance. Measure the length of the guidewire. Make sure the entrance angle and the ending point in the distal segment are in the center of the tibia on both the anteroposterior and lateral fluoroscopic images.
- Before reaming, the anterior muscular compartment is allowed to drape over the cortex to preserve the bone fragments produced by subsequent reaming at the osteotomy sites. Ream the proximal and distal segments until cortical

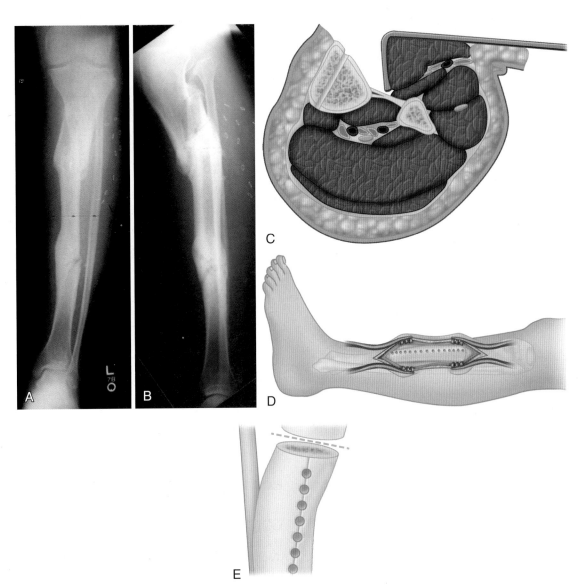

FIGURE **6.17** Clamshell osteotomy as described by Russell et al. **A,** Anteroposterior standing radiograph of lower extremity, showing shortened tibia with medially translated distal tibial segment and varus malunion at inferior end of intercalary segment. **B,** Lateral radiograph demonstrating marked deformity of tibia highlighted by marked posterior translation and apex posterior angulation at superior end of intercalary segment. **C,** Tibial clamshell osteotomy with soft tissues included. Anterolateral muscular sleeve is being retracted posteriorly, exposing lateral aspect of tibia. Osteotomy is initiated 3 to 5 cm posterior to anterolateral tibial prominence and angled posteromedially and parallel to subcutaneous surface of tibia. **D,** Surgical exposure for tibial osteotomy. Anterolateral muscular envelope retracted posteriorly. Transverse osteotomies are denoted by *blue lines,* and *circles* represent drill holes. **E,** Lateral view showing osteotomy parallel to anteromedial surface of tibia. (**A** to **D** from Russell GV, Graves ML, Archdeacon MT, et al: The clamshell osteotomy: a new technique to correct complex diaphyseal malunions: surgical technique, *J Bone Joint Surg Am* 92A[Suppl 1 pt 2]:158, 2010; **E** redrawn from Pires RE, Gausden EB, Sanchez GT, et al: Clamshell osteotomy for acute fractures in the malunion setting: a technical note, *J Orthop Trauma* 32(10):e415, 2018.) **SEE TECHNIQUE 6.12.**

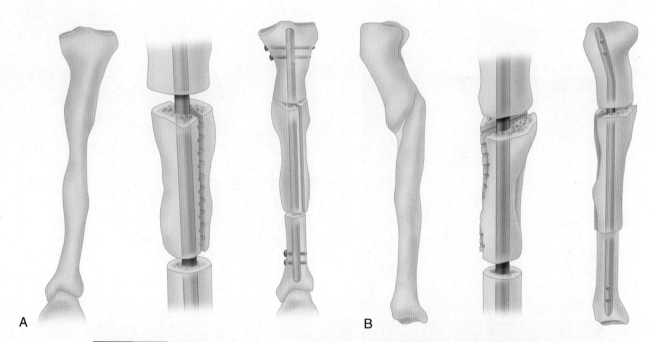

FIGURE 6.18 **A,** Deformity correction in coronal plane. **B,** Sagittal plane. (Redrawn from Russell GV, Graves ML, Archdeacon MT, et al: The clamshell osteotomy: a new technique to correct complex diaphyseal malunions: surgical technique, *J Bone Joint Surg* 92A[Suppl 1 pt 2]:158, 2010.) **SEE TECHNIQUE 6.12.**

chatter is noted. The reaming should result in a deposit of bone fragments at the osteotomy gap sites.

- Push the reamer through the clamshell segment to protect the neurovascular structures and to avoid binding against the osteotomized fragments. Continue reaming in 0.5-mm increments until cortical chatter is obtained. A tibial rod measuring 1 mm less in diameter than the final reamer is selected.

- Pass the rod and accomplish proximal interlocking. Remove the jig from the proximal aspect of the tibial nail and remove the limb from the triangle and place it flat on the operating table.

- The sagittal and coronal plane corrections have been accomplished at this point and only length and rotation need to be corrected (Fig. 6.18). Have an assistant apply manual traction or use a femoral distractor or an external fixator to correct length and rotation. Place the distal interlocking bolts with the use of fluoroscopic guidance.

- Retract the anterior compartment posteriorly from the lateral part of the tibia to inspect the osteotomy site. Fill the gaps with the bone fragments left from reaming. For gaps of more than 1 cm, demineralized bone matrix or autogenous bone graft can be used. Make sure that there is no space left between the osteotomy fragments and the intact proximal or distal parts of the tibia.

- Loosely approximate the fascia over the anterior compartment. However, if there is concern that excessive swelling may cause a compartment syndrome, do not close the anterior compartment.

- Close the extensile approach with the use of the Allgöwer modification of the Donati technique with careful soft-tissue handling.

POSTOPERATIVE CARE Monitor the patient for signs of compartment syndrome. Intravenous cephazolin is ad-

ministered for 24 hours postoperatively. The patient may begin touch-toe weight bearing on the first postoperative day using crutches. Russell et al. recommended prophylactic heparin until the patient is discharged from the hospital. Weight bearing is advanced as the osteotomy healing progresses with full weight bearing allowed by 12 weeks (Fig. 6.19).

CONDYLES OF THE TIBIA

If a fracture of a tibial condyle heals with moderate-to-severe displacement, the change in position of its weight-bearing surface produces an increase in the joint space, a relaxation of some of the knee ligaments, a valgus or varus weight-bearing alignment, and frequently some rotational deformity. Any such displacement must be corrected if a severe disability from traumatic arthritis is to be avoided. The procedure of choice for this type of malunion varies with the kind of fracture and the exact source of the disability. Before surgery, the lateral instability might seem to indicate that a ligament should be repaired; yet after correction of the bony deformity, the joint usually is stable.

If the disability is caused mainly by axial malalignment after depression of a condyle, the weight-bearing surfaces of the tibia usually do not need to be disturbed. Rather, a transverse subcondylar osteotomy combined with the insertion of a graft and internal fixation is indicated; this procedure is especially appropriate when the patient is of middle age, the malunion is of long duration, and the lateral displacement is not severe. In other instances, an oblique osteotomy through the old fracture is possible; the depressed condyle is elevated and fixed with a buttress plate and screws, and the defect is filled with bone grafts. This procedure is applicable to young patients after a fairly recent fracture. Sometimes the

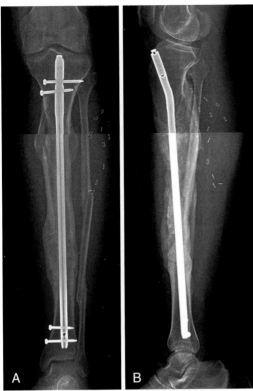

FIGURE 6.19 Anteroposterior **(A)** and lateral **(B)** radiographs 1 year after surgery, demonstrating healed osteotomy with restoration of tibial length and alignment. (From Russell GV, Graves ML, Archdeacon MT, et al: The clamshell osteotomy: a new technique to correct complex diaphyseal malunions: surgical technique, *J Bone Joint Surg* 92A[Suppl 1 pt 2]:158, 2010.) **SEE TECHNIQUE 6.12.**

deformity of the condyle and the degeneration of the articular cartilage are so severe that reconstruction is impractical; an arthrodesis or arthroplasty is then usually indicated.

- Fill the wedge-shaped or cuneiform space created by the osteotomy with bone grafts. Make an anterior incision 7.5 cm long and 5 cm distal to the first incision and expose the shaft of the tibia; remove a free cortical graft to serve as a wedge (usually 1.9 cm wide and about 3.8 cm long). Set the graft on edge and, using an inlay, drive it tightly into the space beneath the lateral condyle. Insert around this graft cancellous bone from the opening in the tibia and a few shavings from the surface of the bone. No undue lateral motion should be possible after the procedure. A full-thickness iliac graft provides more stability, but removal of such a graft increases the complexity of the operation.
- Stabilize the osteotomy as for a fresh fracture with a T-plate as a buttress.
- Confirm the reduction with intraoperative radiographs.
- A similar procedure can be used for malunited fractures of the medial condyle.
- If the weight-bearing surface was comminuted at the time of fracture, elevation of only the depressed fragments produces a refracture through its articular surface and the fragments can be difficult to hold in position; even attempts to pry them into position usually lead only to crushing rather than to correction of the deformity.

POSTOPERATIVE CARE The knee is held in extension and immobilized in a cast from the toes to the groin. At 2 weeks, the cast is removed and radiographs are obtained. If satisfactory stability of the osteotomy is obtained by internal fixation, range-of-motion exercises are begun. A cast brace can be worn if further protection is needed until the osteotomy has united. Union may be solid at 8 weeks, but direct weight bearing should not yet be allowed, lest the depression recur. Walking is permitted with crutches, and weight bearing is increased as tolerated, but the crutches must not be discarded for 1 month. Weight bearing and undue strain must be prevented until union of the grafted area is absolutely solid.

SUBCONDYLAR OSTEOTOMY AND WEDGE GRAFT FOR MALUNION OF LATERAL CONDYLE

TECHNIQUE 6.13

- Begin an incision over the anterolateral aspect of the knee 2.5 cm proximal to the joint and extend it distally parallel with the shaft of the tibia for 7.5 cm.
- Make an inverted-L–shaped incision across the lateral condyle and down the crest of the tibia; detach the origin of the extensor muscles and dissect the muscles subperiosteally from the bone.
- Completely divide the bone by a transverse osteotomy at a point immediately distal to the tibial tuberosity.
- Using a broad osteotome as a lever, tilt the upper fragment proximally and angulate the distal shaft medially; the normal transverse plane of the tibial condyles and the normal alignment of the extremity are largely restored.

OSTEOTOMY AND INTERNAL FIXATION OF THE LATERAL CONDYLE

TECHNIQUE 6.14

- Expose the operative field as just described except that the incision must extend proximally far enough to expose the knee joint.
- Examine the lateral meniscus, and if it is torn, treat it as described in other chapter.
- Dissect all scar tissue from between the tibia and the condylar fragment and denude their surfaces as far distally as possible.
- Refracture the fragment at its base by inserting an osteotome in a proximal and medial direction.
- Sever the soft-tissue attachments only at the line of fracture or as necessary to mobilize the fragment.
- Drill a Knowles pin or Schanz screw into the fragment to use first as a lever to aid in reduction.

- Drill a Kirschner wire into the fragment across the fracture and into the opposite tibial condyle.
- Fix the fracture using AO techniques as for a fresh fracture.
- Fill any residual defect with cancellous bone. Because in this type of fracture some bone substance is lost, perfect apposition and contour cannot be restored.
- A similar procedure can be used for the medial condyle.

POSTOPERATIVE CARE With the knee extended, a plaster cast is applied from the toes to the groin. If satisfactory stability has been achieved at 2 weeks, the cast is removed and a cast brace is substituted to begin controlled range-of-motion exercises. Walking also is permitted with crutches and a cast brace. If consolidation of bone is sufficient 12 weeks after surgery, the crutches and cast brace can be discarded.

■ INVERTED-Y FRACTURES OF THE TIBIAL CONDYLES

Malunited Y-shaped fractures or malunited fractures of both condyles are approached from both sides and are corrected by the method of osteotomy and internal fixation for malunion of a single condyle described previously. The operation is extensive and usually should be chosen only as a preliminary procedure to restore the contour of the condyles for a future arthroplasty. Practical function rarely can be expected, unless the deformity is corrected within a few months after injury; even then, osteoporosis may make replacement of the fragments difficult.

■ FRACTURE OF THE INTERCONDYLAR EMINENCE OF THE TIBIA

Malunion of displaced fractures of the intercondylar eminence of the tibia can severely restrict knee extension because of impingement of the malunited fragment on the femoral intercondylar notch. Arthroscopic or open removal of the fragment, debridement, and open anatomic reduction and fixation have been recommended for treatment of this malunion. In patients with functionally stable anterior cruciate ligaments, arthroscopic notchplasty, in which the femoral notch is enlarged with a power burr until it can accommodate the prominent intercondylar eminence and allow full knee extension, can be performed. Panni et al. recommended as sparing a notchplasty as possible to achieve full extension. Arthroscopic notchplasty is described in other chapter.

PATELLA

The symptoms of a malunited fracture of the patella are similar to those of advanced chondromalacia. Disability is proportionate to the amount of irregularity of the articular surface of the patella and of the roughening of the contiguous surface of the femur. For even a relatively recent malunion, patellectomy usually is the procedure of choice (see chapter 2).

FEMUR AND HIP
CONDYLES OF THE FEMUR

Malunion of one or both femoral condyles, as of the tibial condyles, distorts the articular surface of the knee; frequently, however, it produces a much more severe disability than does one of a tibial condyle. Malunion of the lateral femoral condyle can produce external rotation, flexion, and valgus deformities of the knee; malunion of the medial condyle produces internal rotation, flexion, and varus deformities.

■ LATERAL FEMORAL CONDYLE

OPEN REDUCTION AND INTERNAL FIXATION
TECHNIQUE 6.15

- Approach the joint through a lateral incision beginning 10 cm proximal to the knee and extending distally to 2.5 cm distal and slightly anterior to the head of the fibula.
- Incise the iliotibial band, but avoid the peroneal nerve that passes over the head of the fibula.
- Incise the vastus lateralis muscle and retract it anteriorly to expose the old fracture.
- Open the capsule and synovial membrane so that the interior of the joint can be seen during reduction of the fracture.
- Divide the bone as near the plane of the old fracture as possible, but protect the peroneal nerve.
- Grasp the condyle with bone-holding forceps and place it in its normal position; drill two Kirschner wires through the fragment into the medial condyle, the wires crossing each other at an angle of 30 degrees. The wires should protrude through the opposite cortex.
- Make two-plane radiographs to verify the position of the wires and of the fragment, then fix the fragment with AO cancellous screws.
- To expose a malunited fracture of the posterior part of the lateral condyle, use the same lateral incision but carry the dissection posteriorly.
- Expose the biceps tendon and peroneal nerve and retract them laterally and posteriorly.
- Incise the posterolateral part of the capsule and expose the malunited fragment. The fragment always is displaced proximally and usually can be refractured from above downward.
- After the fragment is freed, place it in position with a towel clip and fix it securely with two AO cancellous screws. If fixation is not sufficiently rigid, a buttress plate can be added.
- Close the incision in routine fashion and apply a plaster cast from the toes to the groin with the knee in extension.

POSTOPERATIVE CARE At 2 weeks, the cast is removed, a cast brace is applied, and active and passive exercises and physical therapy are begun; if fixation is firm, exercises can be done with overhead pulleys. An elevated shoe is fitted on the opposite side, and walking with crutches is permitted; however, weight bearing is not allowed until union is complete, usually at 8 weeks or more after surgery. Free motion of the knee in the brace is allowed at 10 to 12 weeks. The reduction can be partially lost unless every precaution is taken to preserve it.

▣ MEDIAL FEMORAL CONDYLE

Malunion of fractures of the medial femoral condyle can be corrected by the same procedure described for malunion of the lateral condyle. The exposure is as described previously. When the distal femoral physis is involved in a child, growth of the distal femur can be disturbed.

Sasidharan et al. described an osteotomy to treat a malunited medial Hoffa fracture (coronal intraarticular fracture of the posterior femoral condyle). In their technique, the fracture was approached through a medial parapatellar arthrotomy, with the leg in a lazy figure-of-four position. A Hohmann retractor was placed adjacent to the posterior aspect of the medial femoral condyle at the junction to the femoral shaft. The authors emphasized meticulous dissection on the posterior surface of the medial femoral condyle to avoid injury to the superior medial genicular artery, which is its primary blood supply, as this can lead to osteonecrosis of the medial femoral condyle. They also stressed preserving the femoral attachment of the medial collateral ligament and posterior oblique ligament when making the intraarticular osteotomy, as well as maintaining an awareness of the origin of the posterior cruciate ligament. The authors noted that posterior capsular contracture increases the difficulty of the procedure. In their patient, two Steinmann pins were placed on the medial aspect of the medial femoral condyle and used as joysticks to aid in reduction. The reduced condyle was stabilized with two partially threaded 4.0-mm screws placed in an anterior to posterior direction, with countersinking of the screw heads (headless screws of a similar size is another option). The authors advised immobilization in a cylinder cast for 2 weeks postoperatively followed by motion. The patient was kept non–weight bearing for 2 months. At 3-month follow-up, the patient was full weight bearing with a congruous articular surface on CT scan. Knee range of motion had improved from 20 to 80 degrees preoperatively to 5 to 110 degrees postoperatively. At latest follow-up, he had pain at the extreme of flexion.

▣ BOTH FEMORAL CONDYLES

Malunion of fractures of both condyles with marked displacement rarely should be corrected by open reduction of each condyle as just described, unless it is of short duration and is in a young patient. When there is a varus or valgus deformity, the extremity should be realigned by an osteotomy through the metaphysis. When the contour of the joint is irregular enough to impair function and cause pain (Figs. 6.20 and 6.21), arthroplasty or arthrodesis may be indicated.

SUPRACONDYLAR FEMUR

Supracondylar femoral malunions are infrequently reported. If a malunion is associated with an angular deformity of the medial condyle and shortening, treatment may become challenging. Wu described a one-stage surgery using antegrade intramedullary nailing in 19 patients with supracondylar femoral fracture malunion associated with varus deformity and shortening of the medial condyle. Sixteen fractures healed without additional surgery at a median period of 4.5 months. Complications included nonunion in one patient and deep infection in one patient. No malunions or neurovascular injuries occurred, and the amount of lengthening obtained was 2.0 to 3.5 cm.

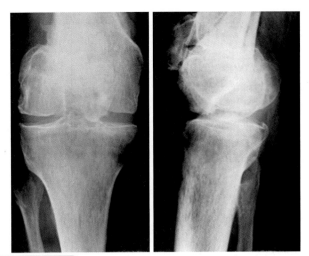

FIGURE 6.20 Malunited comminuted fracture of both condyles of femur 1 year after injury. Knee motion was markedly limited and painful.

FEMORAL SHAFT

Malunions of femoral shaft fractures are much less common with the increased popularity of interlocking intramedullary nailing procedures. Malunions after closed treatment are the rule, but become significant only if they result in shortening of more than 2.5 cm, are angulated more than 10 degrees, or are internally or externally rotated to the point that the knee cannot be aligned with forward motion during gait. Although many authors define rotational malunion as 10 degrees or more of axial malalignment, many of these do not produce symptoms (0% in < 10 degrees; 12% in 10 to 15 degrees; and up to 38% in >15 degrees).

Malunions of the femur can cause disturbances in gait and posture, which can cause abnormal stresses on the knee and spine. Whether femoral shaft fracture malunion leads to the development of knee osteoarthritis has not been well established. Phillips et al., in a study of 62 patients with femoral shaft fractures, found no significant association between malunion, the WOMAC scores, and the presence of clinical or radiographic osteoarthritis at 22 years' follow-up. When corrective surgery is planned, the patient's overall medical condition, functional demands, and severity of symptoms should be considered. The extent of angular deformity and shortening, degree of bony consolidation, and condition of the neurovascular structures and soft tissues also must be determined. Preoperative evaluation should include long, weight-bearing radiographs of the involved and uninvolved extremities for comparison. Femoral osteotomies in adults, especially osteotomies that involve acute lengthening, are associated with numerous complications, including infection, nerve palsies, hardware failure, and nonunion. Detailed preoperative planning is essential to select the optimal operative procedure and to avoid complications. Cancellous bone grafting usually is necessary to improve healing.

Malunions of the femoral shaft from the lesser trochanter to within 5 cm of the intercondylar notch of the femur at the knee can be treated by several methods. In adults with aseptic malunions and good soft tissues, osteotomy, fixation with an interlocking intramedullary nail, and autogenous iliac bone grafting result in a high percentage of unions and offer the advantage of early mobilization with weight bearing

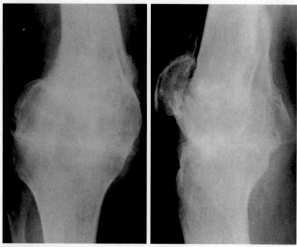

FIGURE 6.21   Same patient as in Fig. 6.20, 3.5 months after compression arthrodesis. Knee is painless.

without the need for external immobilization (Fig. 6.22). This approach requires sophisticated instrumentation, image intensification equipment, an appropriate fracture table, and skill in the use of interlocking intramedullary nails. In children, for whom nonoperative treatment of femoral fractures is the standard of care, osteotomy combined with traction and casting can yield satisfactory results. The femur can be divided through the plane of the malunion with a reciprocating or oscillating saw, or the plane of malunion can be outlined with holes drilled close together and division of the bone completed with a small chisel. For patients who do not fulfill the aforementioned criteria, the options are open reduction and internal fixation with broad dynamic compression plates and screws with autogenous iliac bone grafting or external fixation with the Ilizarov technique.

Malunions of the femoral shaft with angulation and rotation but with end-to-end apposition of the fragments often are the result of bearing weight before union has become completely solid (Fig. 6.23). If the malunion is of short duration and has occurred after nonoperative treatment, it can be broken up manually, and the overlapping and angulation can be corrected by skeletal traction or graduated distraction with an external fixation assembly; in these instances, care must be taken not to produce paralysis of the sciatic nerve or one of its branches with the traction. Most malunions of the femoral shaft that require surgery should be fixed internally at the time of such surgery and should be grafted when securing apposition has required extensive periosteal stripping.

For malunion of the proximal third of the femoral shaft, especially of the subtrochanteric region, a cephalomedullary interlocking nail (reconstruction nail), a conventional interlocking nail, or compression hip screws suitable for fixing a subtrochanteric fracture can be used (Fig. 6.24). Distal femoral malunions also can be stabilized with a conventional interlocking intramedullary nail, a dynamic condylar compression plate, or a blade plate.

Various osteotomies can be used depending on the deformity. Opening or closing wedge osteotomies can be used for axial corrections and transverse osteotomy to correct rotational deformity. A one-stage femoral lengthening using a Z-step osteotomy stabilized with an intramedullary nail has been reported (Fig. 6.25) with good results in selected patients. The defects

were filled with corticocancellous bone. Reported complications have included femoral nerve palsies, infection, nonunion, and loss of length. Extensive scarring and a history of infection, nerve injury, or previous bone graft are considered contraindications to this procedure. The successful use of oblique osteotomy with intramedullary nailing and autogenous bone grafting also has been reported as has oblique osteotomy using plate osteosynthesis and autogenous bone grafting. Complications with the use of plates included infection; persistent deformity; plate avulsion, loosening, or fracture; and nonunion. Chiodo et al. used an oblique osteotomy combined with closing wedges to correct coronal, transverse, and sagittal plane deformities in six femoral malunions. All six femurs had varus (average 22 degrees) and antecurvatum (average 23 degrees) deformities, and two had internal rotation deformities (10 degrees and 15 degrees). All that had at least 10 degrees of varus had medial knee pain. Limb-length discrepancy averaged 1.8 cm. Fixation was performed with 4.5-mm lag screws and 4.5-mm plates in five malunions and a 95-degree blade plate in one. All patients improved clinically, and all osteotomies healed. Average postoperative limb-length discrepancy was within 0.5 cm, and axial limb alignment was within 10 degrees of the contralateral side. The authors stated that plate fixation of femoral osteotomies for malunion may be preferred in cases in which the femoral canal is distorted or the fracture is in the distal part of the femur.

Any operation for a malunited femoral fracture in an adult is easier with the patient on a fracture table. The affected extremity should be draped into the sterile field, and the footpiece should be covered with sterile drapes. Although the old fracture can be seen clearly in the radiographs, the ends of the fragments may be covered with so much callus that even after extensive stripping of soft tissues the exact plane of fracture can be difficult to recognize at surgery. To aid in identifying the fracture and in placing the osteotomy properly, a Kirschner wire or small pin can be drilled through the bone in what appears to be the plane of fracture, and the relative positions of the wire and the fracture are checked by radiographs or image intensifier. Alternatively, the thickened part of the bone can be divided by a long oblique osteotomy, producing a larger area for apposition of the fragments after length and alignment have been restored.

Occasionally, internal fixation devices are fractured and deformed when the patient experiences a new injury. This situation frequently is difficult because the deformed internal fixation device must be removed first before the new fracture can be definitively fixed. If not corrected acutely, malalignments can cause pain and joint deformity.

OSTEOTOMY FOR FEMORAL MALUNION

TECHNIQUE 6.16

- After determining preoperatively the site of osteotomy, expose the area of malunion through an appropriate anterolateral or lateral incision.
- Incise the periosteum longitudinally for a distance of 6 to 8 cm if interlocking nail techniques are to be used over the area of maximal deformity.

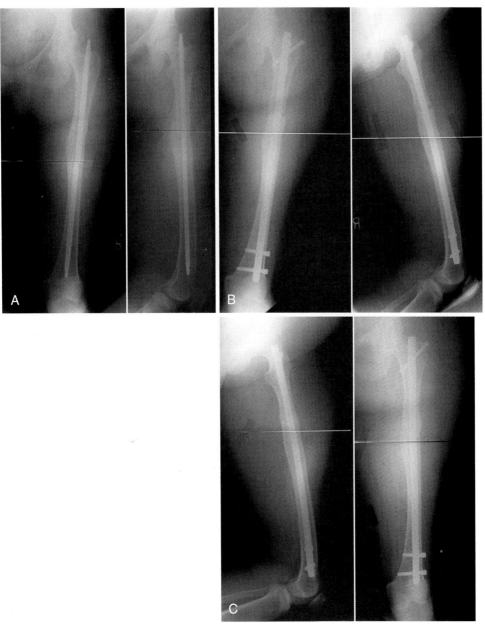

FIGURE 6.22   **A,** Rotational malunion of femur after unlocked intramedullary nailing. **B,** Correction of malunion with proximal femoral derotational osteotomy and locked nailing. **C,** Healed osteotomy.

- Divide the bone transversely with a reciprocating motor saw, or, if preferable, drill several holes transversely through the bone and divide it in the plane of the holes with an osteotome to form broad, even surfaces for maximal apposition. Drilling the holes not only ensures that the osteotomy is transverse but also, because the femur is often exceedingly dense, saves time and decreases the effort required of the surgeon.
- Correct the deformity by manual force.
- Open the medullary canal of both fragments.
- In adults, the reduction is unstable, especially in the proximal half of the femur, and end-to-end apposition and proper alignment of the fragments can be maintained with certainty only by internal fixation. Use an interlocking intramedullary nail within the levels ordinarily indi-

cated for intramedullary nailing of fresh fractures of the femoral shaft (see chapter 2).
- Alternatively, the fragments can be fixed with a compression plate. With either type of fixation, cancellous grafts should be placed at the osteotomy.

For a severe deformity of long duration, an operation in two stages may be necessary. In the first stage, union is broken up in an oblique plane by osteotomy; length is restored after surgery by skeletal traction or by external fixation distraction. In the second stage, satisfactory apposition and alignment are obtained, the fragments are fixed internally with an intramedullary nail or a large compression plate, and bone grafts are placed around the osteotomy medially and posteriorly.

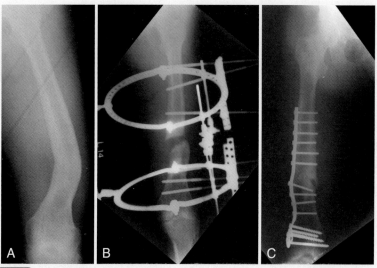

FIGURE 6.23 **A,** Distal femoral fracture with 30-degree varus malunion. **B,** External fixation was used to correct deformity before plating. **C,** After osteotomy and plating.

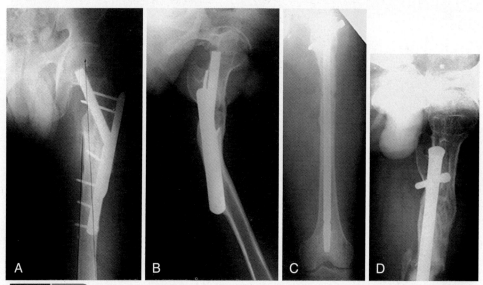

FIGURE 6.24 **A** and **B,** Malunion of subtrochanteric fracture with severe internal rotational deformity. **C** and **D,** Corrective osteotomy, implant removal, and fixation with proximal interlocking Grosse-Kempf medullary nail.

When alignment is satisfactory but overlapping is excessive, experience and mature judgment are required to determine which malunions should be treated surgically, but the following general principles usually can be applied. In young children, overlapping that results in final shortening of more than 3.8 cm usually should be corrected. In young adults, surgery usually is indicated when the overlap is more than 3.8 cm, but the operation is difficult, union may be delayed after surgery, and impairment of function of the knee and of the vascular and nerve supplies of the extremity is possible. When osteoporosis is marked, the patient should bear weight before surgery until it has at least partially disappeared and pain and swelling have ceased.

■ FEMORAL MALUNION IN CHILDREN

Angular deformity has been reported to occur in 40% of children with femoral shaft fractures, although it usually remodels with growth. In children younger than 13 years, malunion of 25 degrees in any plane remodels enough to give normal alignment of joint surfaces. If significant angular deformity is present after fracture union, corrective osteotomy should be delayed for at least 1 year, unless the deformity is severe enough to impair function. The ideal osteotomy corrects the deformity at the site of fracture. In juvenile patients, metaphyseal osteotomy of the proximal or distal femur may be preferable, however. In adolescents with midshaft deformities, diaphyseal osteotomy and fixation with an interlocking intramedullary nail are preferable. Although rotational deformity

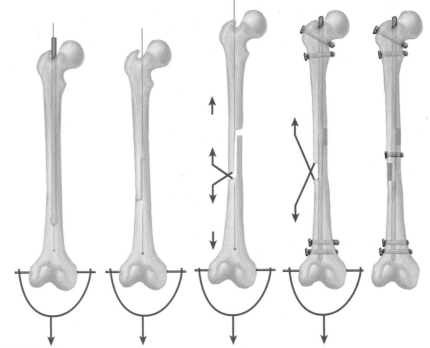

FIGURE 6.25   One-stage femoral lengthening: reaming, Z-shaped osteotomy, lengthening, static locked medullary nailing, transverse screws, and bone grafts.

does not remodel significantly, it usually is well tolerated and rarely requires treatment.

Complications of femoral shaft fractures in children, including malunion, are discussed in other chapter. Osteotomies for correction of varus and valgus deformities and leg-length discrepancy are described in other chapters.

OSTEOTOMY FOR FEMORAL MALUNION IN CHILDREN

TECHNIQUE 6.17

- Expose the malunion through an appropriate lateral or anterolateral incision.
- Inspect the old fracture carefully and compare it with the radiograph so that the osteotomy can be placed as near to the fracture as possible. Usually the proximal fragment is located lateral and anterior to the distal one, and it can be identified easily if the malunion is of only 6 to 12 months' duration.
- Incise the periosteum and strip it from the lateral, anterior, and posterior surfaces of the proximal fragment.
- Use a reciprocating motor saw to separate the fragments through the plane of union, or, if desired, outline the plane of union with a motor-driven drill and divide the bone with a narrow osteotome by connecting the holes. With either method of osteotomy, proceed cautiously to avoid injuring important nerves and vessels on the medial side of the femur. If union is far advanced, an oblique osteotomy can be made without regard to the plane of fracture.

- Resect 0.6 to 1.3 cm of bone from each fragment with a saw. This resection is made for several reasons: (1) the ends of the fragments usually are sclerotic and should be resected back to comparatively normal bone; (2) the surfaces formed permit more stable and accurate apposition; and (3) apposing the fragments is less difficult and recurrence of deformity is less likely when the malunion has been of long duration and the soft tissues otherwise would be under too much tension.
- Apposing and firmly interlocking the fragments may be possible; apply a plate for fixation. If the deformity is severe, apposing the fragments may be impossible without too much stripping of soft tissues and without resection of too much bone from the ends of the fragments. In this instance, external fixation may be preferable. In older children and adolescents, an intramedullary nail usually is preferred for fixation.

If adequate radiography or equipment for interlocking intramedullary nailing techniques or internal fixation is unavailable or cannot be used, older techniques can provide good results (Fig. 6.26). Malunions of the femoral shaft with angulation but little, if any, rotation can be treated by osteotomy and osteoclasis. Ferguson et al. described a two-stage osteotomy that can be used in the femur, tibia (Fig. 6.27), or other long bone. A rectangular segment consisting of one half the width of the bone is removed from the concave side of the deformity; this segment is cut into small chips and is packed back into the defect. About 3 weeks later, the osteotomy is completed on the convex side of the deformity by removing a wedge opposite the middle of the first defect. The second stage is not done until sufficient callus has formed at the first defect; if necessary, additional

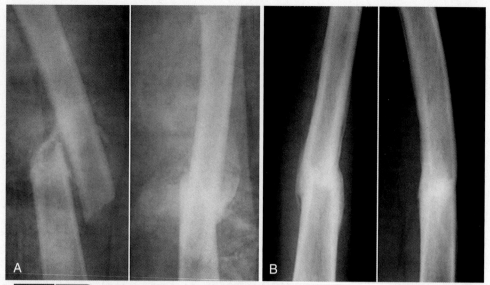

FIGURE 6.26 **A,** Malunited fracture of femur with overlapping of fragments in 11-year-old boy. **B,** Five months after open reduction, insertion of Kirschner wire through distal femur and application of spica cast incorporating wire. Length of limb and function of knee were regained.

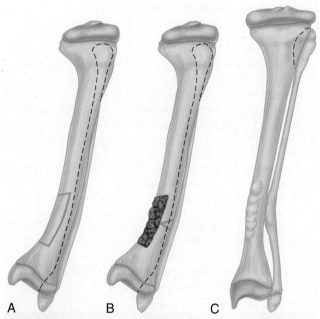

FIGURE 6.27 Ferguson, Thompson, and King two-stage osteotomy. **A,** Segment of bone resected from medial half of tibia *(blue lines)* and cut into chips for grafting. **B,** Grafts placed in defect to complete first stage. Second stage is delayed until sufficient callus has formed across defect. Varus deformity is corrected by resecting wedge of bone laterally *(blue lines).* **C,** Deformity has been corrected, and union is solid.

grafts are placed over the first defect before the osteotomy is completed.

Moore described a method of correcting deformity of a long bone (including malunited fractures) in which about three fourths of the circumference of the bone is divided with an osteotome at the level of maximal deformity; the rest of the bone is broken by manual osteoclasis (Fig. 6.28). Irwin used a similar method for trochanteric osteotomy that also

can be used for joints ankylosed in a position of deformity, genu valgum or varum, coxa vara, cubitus varus, and other deformities.

Malunions that occur in patients with fibrous dysplasia are complicated by poor fixation with plates and screws in the pathologic bone. We have found that reconstruction with an intramedullary nail is helpful in this situation because it effectively splints the entire femur, avoiding delayed angulation and stress fractures at the ends of the implant.

TROCHANTERIC REGION OF THE FEMUR

Varus malunion is the most common deformity after intertrochanteric fracture and leads to limb shortening; abductor muscle imbalance; limp; and hip, back, and knee pain. Malunited fractures in the trochanteric region can be divided into two types: (1) malunions with internal or external rotation, coxa vara, and shortening of about 2.5 cm and (2) malunions with internal or external rotation, severe coxa vara, and shortening of 5 cm or more. In malunions of the first type, rotation and coxa vara are corrected by a subtrochanteric osteotomy and no attempt is made to reduce the shortening other than by angulating the bone at the osteotomy. Malunions of the second type are treated by a procedure similar to that described subsequently for malunited cervicotrochanteric fractures with extreme overriding.

Bartonicek et al. reported their results with a valgus intertrochanteric osteotomy by removal of a lateral wedge, lateral displacement of the femoral shaft, and fixation with a 120-degree blade plate. Fourteen of 15 osteotomies healed uneventfully, and there were no infections, osteonecrosis, or osteoarthritis at an average follow-up of 5.5 years. All patients were satisfied with the result, and Harris hip scores improved from an average of 73 preoperatively to 92 postoperatively. Indications for surgery were greater than 2 cm of shortening, a limp, gluteal muscle imbalance, and pain in the hip and lumbar spine.

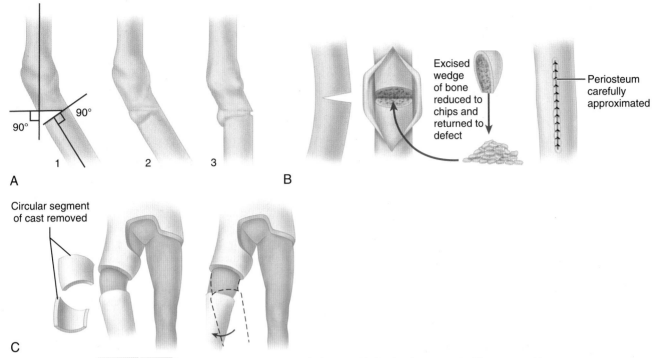

FIGURE 6.28   Moore osteotomy-osteoclasis. **A,** *1,* Wedge has been resected from normal bone distal to malunion, leaving cortex on concave side of deformity intact; proximal cut is perpendicular to long axis of proximal fragment, and distal cut is perpendicular to that of distal fragment. *2,* Grafts have become consolidated with early callus. *3,* Deformity has been corrected by manual osteoclasis. **B,** Detail of technique. Wedge of bone is removed and is cut into chips that are placed back into defect; periosteum is carefully sutured. **C,** At 3 to 4 weeks after surgery, section of cast is removed and deformity is corrected manually. Cast is repaired with plaster.

■ SUBTROCHANTERIC OSTEOTOMY FOR COXA VARA AND ROTATIONAL DEFORMITIES

The routine technique for this procedure, useful in treating many conditions, is described in other chapter. Variations are described under the discussions of compensatory trochanteric osteotomy for malunited slipped proximal femoral epiphysis and congenital coxa vara.

CERVICOTROCHANTERIC REGION OF THE FEMUR

Cervicotrochanteric fractures occur at the junction of the trochanter and femoral neck. Posteriorly, the fracture is always outside the capsule of the hip because the posterior part of the capsule does not cover the distal third of the neck; anteriorly, the fracture can be just inside the capsule or can extend a short distance within it. Unless fractures in this region are treated properly, malunion is inevitable; usually coxa vara of 90 degrees, external rotation of the distal fragment, and about 5 cm of shortening are the deformities. In children, the shortening may be slight at the time of union but increase with growth and ultimately may be 7.5 cm, even though the physis is not affected; this increase in discrepancy seems to be caused by the partial disability of the extremity that results in insufficient stimulation of the physes by normal activity. After the deformity has been corrected, maintaining the position is especially difficult in children; the likelihood of maintaining satisfactory alignment and securing normal function is much more favorable in young adults. In the elderly,

subtrochanteric osteotomy alone is used to correct the deformity; even though length is only partially restored, function is improved.

CORRECTION OF CERVICOTROCHANTERIC MALUNION

TECHNIQUE 6.18

- Expose the malunion, the trochanters, and the proximal 5 cm of the femoral shaft through a curved lateral incision between the tensor fasciae latae and gluteus medius muscles.
- Because of the external rotation, the fractured surface of the greater trochanter faces anteromedially. A wedge-shaped space with its base anterior is present between the fragments and usually is filled with fibrous tissue. Excise this fibrous tissue down to normal bone and divide the osseous union posteriorly with an osteotome.
- Appose the bone surfaces and correct the deformity by abducting and internally rotating the distal fragment while marked traction is applied to the leg.
- Tenotomize the adductors if necessary to obtain enough abduction of the distal fragment.
- Apply traction through the fracture table or a femoral distractor and confirm reduction of the neck-shaft angle

with image intensification or anteroposterior radiographs of the hip.

- If the normal angle between the shaft and the neck has been restored, fix the fracture with a compression screw or some other type of nail by a technique similar to that described for trochanteric fractures (see chapter 3). For children, a pediatric compression hip screw is preferable because it is much easier to insert into the hard bone of the femoral neck and head. The capital femoral physis should be avoided if possible.

POSTOPERATIVE CARE If complete correction has been secured, and the fracture was fixed internally in a child, a cast should be applied and worn for at least 8 weeks; even with the most careful treatment after surgery, decrease in the angle between the neck and femoral shaft is fairly common even after union seems to be solid. In children, the results of this operation usually are disappointing because only moderate improvement in position may be secured; efficient treatment of fresh cervicotrochanteric fractures is crucial. In young adults, function is much improved but rarely, if ever, is the angle between the neck and shaft or the length of the limb restored completely.

Fractures of the femoral head occur infrequently, and malunion has rarely been reported. Yoon et al. described three femoral head malunions after posterior hip dislocation with Pipkin type I fracture of the femoral head that had been treated with closed reduction and traction. Symptoms included limp and limited hip motion. All patients were treated with resection of the protruding bony prominence inferiorly followed by immediate full weight bearing and range-of-motion exercises. Results were excellent in all patients, with nearly full range of motion achieved postoperatively without pain. The authors stated that malunion should be suspected in patients with limited hip motion after femoral head fractures. Sontich and Cannada reported a femoral head avulsion fracture (Pipkin type I) that was malunited to the acetabulum. An excellent result was obtained after surgical debridement.

ACETABULUM

Usually, malunions of the pelvis in which correction is justified are those involving the acetabulum. Even with modern methods of treatment, malunion of fractures of the acetabulum with central dislocation of the femoral head still occurs; also, traumatic arthritis usually develops after comminuted fractures of the acetabulum. The treatment of either of these conditions varies with the severity of the injury, the deformity, the disability, and the age and health of the patient. When hip motion is limited and painful, and depending on the patient's occupation, arthrodesis or total hip arthroplasty may be indicated. The treatment of fractures of the acetabular rim with dislocation of the hip is similar to that described in chapter 4.

The following elements should be considered before attempting acetabular reconstruction: (1) the location and condition of the different segments of the acetabular articular surface and of the bony columns supporting them, (2) the amount of wear of the femoral head, (3) the degree of

osteoarthritis, and (4) the existence of osteonecrosis. This type of surgery should be attempted only by surgeons experienced in the surgical treatment of acute acetabular and pelvic fractures.

PELVIS

A pelvic nonunion does not always cause pain, but pain occurs frequently with severe malunions, most commonly from malunion of the sacroiliac complex. Symptoms also can be caused by an internal rotational deformity or leg-length discrepancy. Impingement on the bladder by a displaced superior pubic ramus can cause urinary frequency.

Late correction of a pelvic deformity is more difficult, less successful, and associated with a higher incidence of complications than management of acute pelvic fractures. Therefore, initial reduction and stabilization of pelvic injuries is of utmost importance to prevent malunion and nonunion.

Indications for surgical treatment of pelvic malunions include pain, instability, sitting imbalance, limb shortening, and vaginal wall impingement. Pelvic tilt fractures that cause erosion into the perineum from a displaced fracture of the superior pubic ramus and severely shortened and internally rotated pelvic malunions also justify surgical correction. Cosmetic deformities secondary to limb shortening and malrotation also may be present. Cranial displacement of the hemipelvis of 1 cm or more may lead to leg-length discrepancy, sitting imbalance, a characteristic cosmetic deformity, and sacral prominence that can cause pain while sitting or lying supine. Patients with leg-length discrepancy but no other symptoms related to the pelvis can be treated with standard methods of limb-length equalization. In addition to pelvic osteotomy and fixation, several operations for leg-length equalization exist. For severe shortening and internal rotation, a two-stage correction, with a period of skeletal traction after the osteotomy to minimize neurologic complications has been reported. For chronic sacroiliac pain not relieved by conservative treatment, arthrodesis is the treatment of choice.

Patient selection is important. Patients must have realistic expectations, accept known risks (loss of reduction, nerve or vascular injury, persistent nonunion, and significant blood loss), and be compliant with 3 to 5 months of restricted weight bearing. Anatomic reduction of the pelvic deformity frequently is impossible. Posterior pelvic pain usually is caused by nonunion, instability, or malreduction, and correction of these problems provides pain relief in most patients. Posterior pelvic pain of uncertain etiology or pain caused by old neurologic injury is less likely to be improved by surgery. Posterior pelvic pain also may be caused by concomitant lumbar injuries, which should be evaluated if present. In a study of 437 malunions, Kanakaris et al. reported that treatment in most patients is effective, with union rates averaging 86%, pain relief 93%, and patient satisfaction 79%. However, the return to a preinjury level of activity was reported in only 50%.

Pelvic malunions are assessed radiographically with anteroposterior, 45-degree internal and external oblique, and 40-degree caudal and cephalad views. A pelvic CT scan also should be obtained, and three-dimensional CT reconstruction is helpful if it is available. Right and left single-leg standing anteroposterior pelvic radiographs are useful for detecting instability. Limb shortening is evaluated on the anteroposterior pelvic views by comparing the cranial displacement of the acetabular roof with the contralateral side. A line perpendicular to the midline of the sacrum is used to make the comparative measurements. Radiographic evaluation provides information about the extent of fracture union and the nature of the deformity. Deformities often are complex and involve multiple planes.

Operative correction of pelvic deformity is difficult and should be undertaken only by surgeons experienced in pelvic surgery. Each pelvic malunion is unique and requires individualized plans and techniques for operative reduction and stabilization.

Nonunions without significant deformity can be treated with a one-stage or two-stage procedure with risks similar to those of acute fracture surgery. A three-stage procedure is recommended for malunited or malaligned fractures to provide the maximal amount of deformity correction. Anterior structures are approached with the patient supine, whereas posterior deformities are corrected with the patient prone.

THREE-STAGE RECONSTRUCTION FOR PELVIC MALUNIONS

Patients are placed on a radiolucent operating table, and fluoroscopy is used to guide osteotomy, reduction, and fixation. A Judet traction table is useful in some cases.

In the first stage, the deformed anterior pelvic structures are osteotomized and anterior nonunions are mobilized. The patient is repositioned prone for the second stage. Posterior pelvic deformities are osteotomized or mobilized, the pelvis is reduced, and posterior structures are internally fixed. Wounds are closed between each stage. In the third stage, the patient is returned to a supine position, the initial wound is reopened, the anterior reduction is completed, and internal fixation is applied. The procedure also can be done in the opposite order: (1) mobilizing the posterior pelvis first; (2) mobilizing, reducing, and internally fixing the anterior pelvis; and (3) completion of reduction and fixation of the posterior pelvis. Osteotomies should be made at the old injury sites when possible. Correction of cranial displacement is made easier by dividing the attachment of the sacrospinous and sacrotuberous ligaments to the sacrum. External fixators can be used intraoperatively to aid in reduction. Anterior structures are stabilized by plate fixation, and plates or large iliosacral screws or both are used for posterior fixation. Old deformities often are resistant to correction and may require stronger fixation than is commonly used in acute fractures to prevent loss of reduction.

In one study, 36 of 37 patients had stable unions of the pelvic ring. The overall incidence of complications was 19% (persistent nonunion, loss of reduction, neurologic injury, vascular injury, and persistent pain), and no infections were reported. Rousseau et al. reported a prone-supine, two-stage procedure in eight patients with 10-months' follow-up. The surgery consisted of opening the sacroiliac joint and cutting the sacrotuberous and sacrospinous ligaments through a posterior approach; in a second stage, the pubic symphysis and the anterior aspect of the sacroiliac joint were released through an ilioinguinal approach to achieve reduction and then osteosynthesis of the pubic symphysis and sacroiliac joint, including bone graft harvesting and grafting. Anatomic reduction was achieved in six of eight patients. In the two patients without anatomic reduction, mechanical problems from leg-length inequality persisted. Complications included one bladder injury, one nosocomial infection in the postoperative period, three motor deficits with footdrop, and a possible nonunion.

SCAPULA

With few exceptions, fractures of the scapular body and neck continue to be treated nonoperatively. In a review of 520 scapular fractures by Zlowodzki et al., 82% had good or excellent functional results. Although most patients do well, there recently has been increased interest in identifying which fractures are likely to develop a symptomatic malunion. Parameters that have been evaluated include the degree of medial and lateral displacement of the glenoid on the anteroposterior radiograph, angulation of the scapular body as measured on the scapular Y radiograph, and the glenopolar angle as measured on the anteroposterior scapular view (normal 30 to 45 degrees). The degree of angular deformity and displacement causing functional impairment has not been precisely defined.

In an analysis of 113 scapular fractures, Ada and Miller noted subacromial pain, decreased range of motion, and weakness with overhead activities in patients with displaced scapular neck fractures. They recommended surgical reduction and stabilization of scapular fractures, with more than 9 mm of glenoid medialization, or 40 degrees of angulation. Romero et al. reported that patients with fractures having significant rotational deformity of the glenoid neck (quantified as a glenopolar angle of less than 20 degrees) had poor functional results. Operative criteria developed by Cole et al. include medial and lateral displacement of 2 cm or more, scapular body angulation of 45 degrees, and glenopolar angle of 22 degrees or less. Despite these recommendations, there are currently no studies confirming the superiority of operative treatment in this subset of scapular fractures.

There have been a few reports describing surgical management of symptomatic scapular malunions. Moreover, favorable outcomes have been achieved. Success depends on appropriate patient selection and the surgeon's familiarity with the anatomy and surgical techniques. Cole et al. evaluated the functional outcome in five patients with extraarticular malunions of the scapular neck or body treated with osteotomy, reduction, plate osteosynthesis, and bone graft performed through a posterior Judet approach. One ipsilateral clavicular malunion also was repaired. Preoperatively, all patients complained of chronic pain, decreased range of motion, weakness, and unsatisfactory cosmetic deformity of the involved shoulder. All patients had marked deformity of the scapula on radiographs. None were able to perform their usual occupation. Radiographic deformity was a mean of 3.0 cm (range 1.7 cm to 4.2 cm) of medial or lateral displacement, 25 degrees of angulation (range 10 to 40 degrees) on scapular Y view, and a glenopolar angle of 25 degrees (range 19 to 29 degrees). Preoperative evaluation included a true anteroposterior scapular radiograph, scapular Y, and axillary lateral views, anteroposterior radiograph of the uninvolved shoulder, and CT scan with 3D reconstruction. The mean time from injury to surgery was 15 months (range 8 to 41 months). There were no intraoperative complications. The mean estimated blood loss was 569 mL (range 350 to 1125 mL). The mean follow-up was 39 months (range 18 to 101 months). All osteotomies united. All patients were pain free and highly satisfied with the result. Four of the five returned to their preinjury occupation and activities. Patients had statistically significant increases in forward flexion and abduction shoulder range

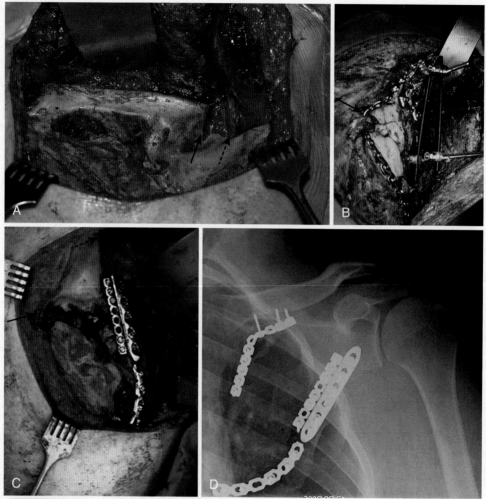

FIGURE 6.29 Cole osteotomy and reorientation of scapular neck. **A,** Posterior Judet approach and surgical exposure of scapular nonunion. Note scapular deformity *(solid arrow)*. Dashed arrow shows neurovascular bundle at spinoglenoid notch. **B,** Small external fixator used to maintain desired reduction at lateral border of scapula. Solid arrow shows superomedial angle. **C,** After corrective osteotomy and anatomic reduction, a 3.5-mm dynamic compression plate and a 2.7-mm reconstruction plate with conventional or locking screws are used for fixation. Solid arrow points out superomedial angle and dashed arrow the spinoglenoid notch. **D,** Thirty-two-month postoperative anteroposterior radiograph showing complete scapular healing in anatomic alignment with no evidence of hardware loosening. **SEE TECHNIQUE 6.19.** (From Cole PA, Talbot M, Schroder LK, Anavian J: Extra-articular malunions of the scapula: a comparison of functional outcome before and after reconstruction, *J Orthop Trauma* 25:649, 2011.) **SEE TECHNIQUE 6.19.**

of motion, and improved Disabilities of the Arm, Shoulder and Hand (DASH) and Short Form (SF)-36 scores. One patient developed asymptomatic heterotopic ossification.

OSTEOTOMY AND REORIENTATION OF SCAPULAR NECK

TECHNIQUE 6.19

(COLE ET AL.)

- Place the patient in the lateral decubitus position, leaning slightly prone on a beanbag. Position the arm on an arm board abducted and in 90 degrees forward flexion. Prepare the shoulder, neck, and posterior hemithorax allowing access and manipulation of the shoulder.
- Through a posterior Judet approach, elevate the infraspinatus and teres minor muscles off the vertebral scapular border and retract the neurovascular pedicle that courses through the spinoglenoid notch. Take care to protect these structures. Using a large Deaver and Hohmann retractor, expose the scapular neck and body taking care not to damage the nerve or vessel (Fig. 6.29A).
- Carry out osteotomies along the original fracture pattern with a sagittal saw or an osteotome through multiple drill holes. Remove any ectopic bone encountered and store in saline solution for later use as bone graft. Use a laminar spreader to complete the osteotomies.

- Once the primary fracture patterns are recreated, further debride the osteotomy sites to better delineate the true fracture lines, thereby allowing anatomic realignment of the fragments. Reduce the fragments by placing a 4-cm Schanz pin into the glenoid neck and another in the lateral border distal to the osteotomy. A small external fixator with the aid of multiple reduction clamps may be necessary to obtain anatomic alignment and compression at the fracture sites (Fig. 6.29B).
- Apply a 3.5-mm dynamic compression plate spanning the osteotomy site at the inferior glenoid neck or lateral border and fix with conventional or locking screws. Supplement this lateral fixation by applying a second 2.7-mm reconstruction plate at the angle formed by the medial extent of the acromial spine and the medial border (Fig. 6.29C) and secure with conventional or locking screws. If the fracture extends down into the inferior angle of the scapular body, an additional reconstruction plate may be necessary.
- Mix the ectopic bone extracted from the malunion site during the osteotomies with other autogenous bone and with 20 to 30 mL platelet-rich plasma. Use this to fill large defects in the scapula.
- Close the wound over a suction drain. Manipulate the shoulder to break apart longstanding adhesions and scar tissue.

POSTOPERATIVE CARE Patients are placed in a sling for comfort. Early physical therapy is initiated after the first postoperative visit, with passive and active-assisted range-of-motion exercises for a period of 1 month followed by active range-of-motion and repetition exercises for 1 month. Resistance and strengthening exercises with 3- to 5-lb weights are begun at 2 months, and all restrictions can be removed at 3 months (Fig. 6.29D).

CLAVICLE

Most fractures of the clavicle are treated nonoperatively and frequently heal with some degree of deformity. It is generally believed that clavicular malunions are tolerated well in most patients and cause no significant functional limitations. In some patients, however, malunion of the clavicle is painful or results in functional deficits. Shortening of 15 mm or more has been shown to cause discomfort and dysfunction of the shoulder girdle, and 20 mm of shortening after closed treatment of displaced middle-third clavicular fractures has been associated with poor results. A cadaver study showed that shortening combined with caudal displacement leads to functional deficits in abduction, particularly overhead motion. A vector model was devised to calculate the position of the glenoid fossa in relation to the position of the clavicle, which could be used for planning open reduction and fixation. Symptoms include rapid fatigability, thoracic outlet syndrome, difficulty wearing over-the-shoulder straps, weakness, pain, and cosmetic deformity of a droopy, "driven-in," or ptotic shoulder. The malunions that usually are disabling are malunions of the medial or lateral third of the bone. Angular deformity and shortening can alter the position of the glenoid fossa, which may affect glenohumeral mobility and scapular rotation.

In some patients with thoracic outlet syndrome after clavicular malunion, excising the bony prominence that is compressing the brachial plexus relieves symptoms.

Several investigators have recommended osteotomy and plate fixation for symptomatic clavicular nonunions. McKee et al. reported 15 patients with malunions of the clavicle after nonoperative management who actively sought treatment for persistent complaints. Indications for surgery were chronic pain, weakness, and thoracic outlet syndrome not responsive to conservative management for at least 1 year after injury. No osteotomies were performed for cosmesis alone. Preoperative shortening averaged 2.9 cm (range 1.6 to 4.0 cm). Functional scores improved in all patients. In 12 patients with preoperative pain and weakness, symptoms resolved in eight and improved in four patients. In 11 patients with preoperative neurologic complaints, symptoms resolved in seven, improved in three, and were unchanged in one. Of 13 patients who regarded the cosmetic appearance of their shoulder as unacceptable preoperatively, 12 were satisfied with postoperative cosmesis. There was one hypertrophic scar. Complications included one loss of fixation that resulted in nonunion. There were no cases of infections, neurovascular injury, or wound breakdowns. Two plates were removed electively. Overall, 14 of 15 patients were satisfied after surgery. No intercalary bone grafts were used in this series. The authors' current radiographic criteria for osteotomy and plating for symptomatic clavicular malunions include malunions with substantial shortening (<1 cm, usually 2 to 3 cm), angular deformity greater than 30 degrees, or translation greater than 1 cm. Contraindications include inadequate soft-tissue coverage, active infection, asymptomatic malunion, noncompliant patient, or severely osteopenic or pathologic bone. Patients with associated nonunion of the clavicle also require bone grafting. Other authors also have reported osteotomy and plating of clavicular nonunions with good functional and cosmetic results. The osteotomy corrects scapular winging secondary to medial and forward displacement of the shoulder. Rosenberg et al. noted that although a solid union is obtained after reduction and plating with bone grafting, patients can remain functionally impaired. Only six of their 13 patients returned to their previous professional and recreational activities. Smekal et al. described corrective osteotomy in symptomatic clavicular malunions using an elastic stable intramedullary nail with good cosmetic and functional outcomes in five patients. For fractures of the lateral third of the clavicle with rupture of the coracoclavicular ligaments, a procedure similar to that described for acromioclavicular dislocations is indicated (see chapter 8).

MIDSHAFT MALUNIONS OF THE CLAVICLE

OSTEOTOMY AND PLATE FIXATION

TECHNIQUE 6.20

- Determine the amount of length to be gained clinically and radiographically preoperatively. If the clinical shortening is substantially greater than the observed radiographic shortening, an intercalary bone graft may be required to compensate for the absolute bone loss.

- Place the patient in a "beach-chair" semisitting position, with a small pad behind the shoulder blade and the involved upper extremity tucked into the side. Drape the opposite iliac crest if desired.
- Administer general anesthesia.
- Make an oblique incision along the superior surface of the clavicle (Fig. 6.30A).
- Raise the skin and subcutaneous tissue as a flap and identify the underlying myofascia. This layer is raised as contiguous flaps and is preserved so that later a two-layered closure can be achieved over the plate (Fig. 6.30B and C).
- Identify the malunion site and plan the corrective osteotomy (Fig. 6.30D). It is possible to identify the malunited position of the proximal and distal fragments in most pa-

tients. In some patients, a correction must be performed with an oblique sliding osteotomy through an extensively remodeled malunion.
- Use a combination of osteotomes and a microsagittal saw cooled continually with irrigation throughout the cutting to re-create the original fracture line (Fig. 6.30E and F).
- Hold the proximal and distal fragments with reduction forceps and realign the clavicle (Fig. 6.30G). As little soft-tissue dissection as possible should be used to allow correct repositioning and apposition of the proximal and distal fragments.
- Reestablish the medullary canal with a 3.5-mm drill bit in each fragment. If absolute bone loss has occurred, a bone graft can be used.

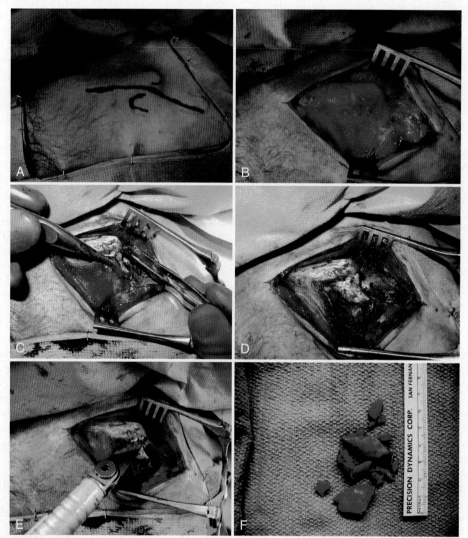

FIGURE 6.30 A-M, Osteotomy and plate fixation of malunited clavicular fractures. See text. (From McKee MD, Wild LM, Schemitsch EH: Midshaft malunions of the clavicle: surgical technique, *J Bone Joint Surg* 86A:37, 2005.) **SEE TECHNIQUE 6.20.**

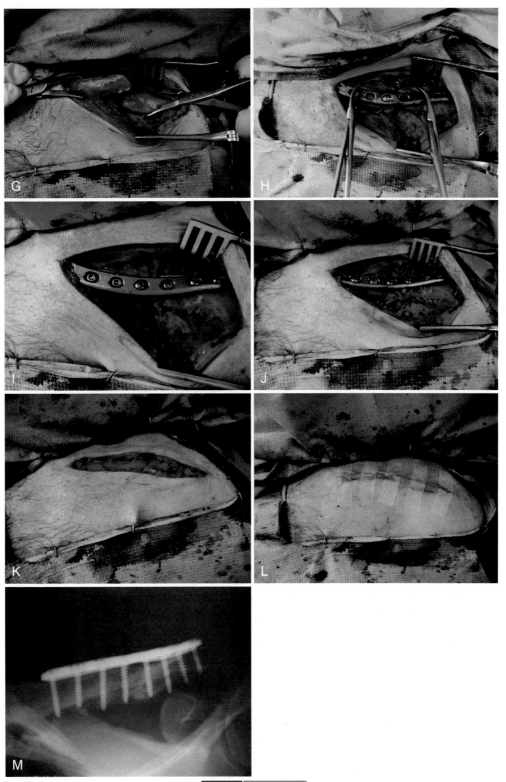

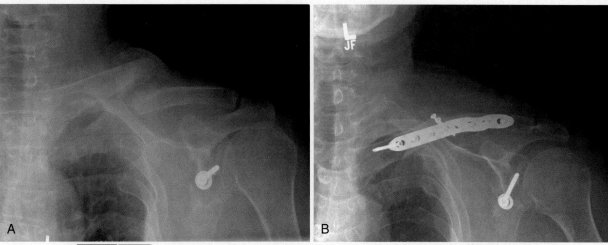

FIGURE 6.31 **A,** Midshaft clavicular malunion with significant shortening. **B,** Clavicular length and alignment restored after osteotomy, plating, and bone grafting. **SEE TECHNIQUE 6.20.**

- Make a small notch with the saw in each fragment before the osteotomy to make it possible to measure the degree of lengthening achieved.
- Rotate the distal fragment anteriorly so that its flat superior surfaces face anteriorly rather than superiorly.
- Correct the malrotation by redirecting the flat superior surface of the distal fragment superiorly, creating similar clavicular surfaces on both sides of the osteotomy. Avoid the underlying neural and vascular structures and make no attempt to explore or decompress the brachial plexus.
- After approximation of the proximal and distal fragments, temporarily fix the osteotomy site with a 2-mm Kirschner wire.
- Apply a 3.5-mm limited contact dynamic compression plate with a minimum of six holes (range, six to 10 holes) (Fig. 6.30H and I).
- Contour this plate to the S-shaped clavicle. Use of anatomic plates contoured to fit the clavicle saves time because extensive intraoperative contouring is not required and their low-profile anatomic shape minimizes prominence especially medially, whereas a straight plate tends to project anteriorly. Because the osteotomy is typically transverse, apply the plate in the compression mode to maximize compression.
- Smooth the bone ends with a rongeur and pack morselized callus around the osteotomy site (Fig. 6.30J).
- Close the wound in layers with the use of No. 1 absorbable sutures for the myofascia, No. 2-0 absorbable sutures for the subcutaneous tissue, and clips or a subcuticular stitch for the skin (Fig. 6.30K and L). Place the arm in a conventional sling postoperatively.

POSTOPERATIVE CARE The patient begins pendulum exercises immediately postoperatively and active-assisted motion at 2 weeks. At 4 weeks, if radiographs show no loss of reduction (Fig. 6.30M), full active and passive motion is initiated and the patient is weaned from the sling. Resistive and strengthening activities are allowed when radiographs reveal union, typically at 6 to 8 weeks (Fig. 6.31).

OSTEOTOMY AND ELASTIC INTRAMEDULLARY NAILING OF MIDSHAFT CLAVICULAR FRACTURE

TECHNIQUE 6.21

(SMEKAL ET AL.)
- Place the patient in a slightly upright "beach-chair" position and administer general anesthesia.
- With the involved limb draped freely, palpate the hump at the malunion site and make an oblique incision of 5-cm length above the Langer skin lines.
- Incise the periosteum sharply and separate the delto-trapezial muscle attachment subperiosteally as an intact layer. Expose the deformity over a distance of 5 cm.
- Determine the osteotomy plane under fluoroscopic control (Fig. 6.32A). Using a fine-bladed saw, perform the osteotomy, separating the two main original fracture fragments.
- Hold the proximal and distal fracture fragments with reduction clamps and reopen the medullary canal on both sides with a 2.7-mm drill under fluoroscopic guidance. Make a small skin incision (1 to 2 cm) above the sternal end of the clavicle. Open the anterior cortex with a 2.7-mm drill and insert a 2.5-mm nail (TEN, Synthes, West Chester, PA).
- The distal fragment is always caudal and malrotated with the superior surface facing anteriorly. Realign the clavicle by lifting and derotating the distal fragment. Freshen the osseous surfaces and insert the nail into the lateral fragment under fluoroscopic control (Fig. 6.32B). This prevents perforation of the cortex of the distal fragment.
- Cut the inserted nail back to the medial insertion point as short as possible to prevent medial skin irritation. Smooth the bone ends with a rongeur and suture the periosteal layers.

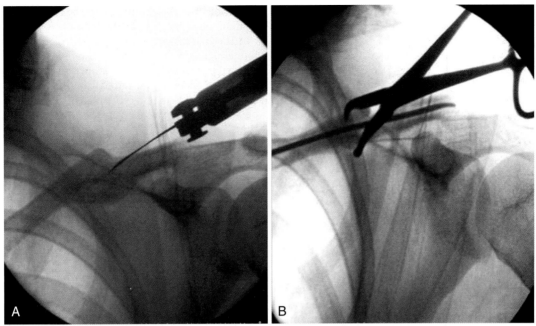

FIGURE 6.32 **A,** Determination of osteotomy plane using fluoroscopy. **B,** Insertion of nail under fluoroscopic control. (From Smekal V, Deml C, Kamelger F, et al: Corrective osteotomy in symptomatic midshaft clavicular malunion using elastic stable intramedullary nails, *Arch Orthop Trauma Surg* 130:681, 2010.) **SEE TECHNIQUE 6.21.**

HUMERUS
PROXIMAL HUMERUS

Malunion of a fracture of the proximal humerus can result from inadequate operative reduction, loss of operative reduction, or nonoperative treatment of a displaced fracture. Disruption of the normal anatomic relationships between the tuberosities, the humeral head, and the humeral shaft can limit the range of motion and decrease the strength of the shoulder. Bony abnormalities can include displacement of the tuberosity, articular surface incongruity, and malalignment of an articular segment, often in combination. Soft-tissue pathologic findings may include capsular contracture, tears of the rotator cuff, and neurologic injury.

Each of the structures that may be involved in a proximal humeral fracture—the humeral head and articular fragment, the greater and lesser tuberosities, and the humeral shaft—has its own tendinous insertions that pull a free fracture fragment in a predictable direction, resulting in a characteristic deformity. Two-part fractures of the surgical neck may heal in varus and anterior angulation. The humeral shaft displaces anteromedially because of the pull of the pectoralis major, and the proximal fragment is abducted by the rotator cuff. Considerable deformity in the region of the surgical neck may be compatible with satisfactory function, especially in the elderly. If the deformity is great enough, however, varus alignment of the humeral head and anterior displacement of the distal fragment can lead to loss of forward flexion and abduction severe enough to require surgery. With two-part fractures that involve the greater tuberosity, the tuberosity may be displaced posteriorly and superiorly because of the forces exerted by the supraspinatus, teres minor, and infraspinatus muscles. A malunion of this type of fracture can cause limitation of abduction and external rotation and may lead to subacromial impingement. Two-part fractures of the lesser tuberosity may displace medially owing to the pull of the subscapularis. Function usually is not significantly impaired, but in some patients the fragment can impinge on the coracoid, limiting internal rotation or elevation. In three-part fractures with displacement of the greater tuberosity and surgical neck, the head fragment is internally rotated by the action of the subscapularis inserting on the intact lesser tuberosity. The shaft displaces anteromedially, and the greater tuberosity displaces posterosuperiorly. Malunions of this kind can cause severe impairment because of the loss of abduction and rotation. Three-part fractures that involve the lesser tuberosity and surgical neck are characterized by external rotation and abduction of the articular segment because of the pull of the rotator cuff muscles on the intact greater tuberosity. A malunion in this position causes pain and severe limitation of motion, especially internal rotation. Malunions of three-part fractures are difficult to treat because they can be complicated by contractures of the deforming muscles, subluxation, posttraumatic arthritis, or osteonecrosis. Malunions of four-part fractures and fracture-dislocations are especially difficult because of the frequent presence of articular incongruity, muscular contractions, adhesions, osteonecrosis, and, sometimes, neurologic injury. Fractures involving the anatomic neck in particular can be associated with osteonecrosis and posttraumatic arthritis.

Currently, there is no universally accepted classification of proximal humeral malunions. Beredjiklian et al. described a classification system in which malunions were categorized based on the osseous and soft-tissue abnormalities: type I, malposition of the greater or lesser tuberosity of more than 1 cm; type II, intraarticular incongruity or step-off of the articular surface of more than 5 mm; and type III, rotational malalignment of the articular segment by more than

45 degrees in the coronal, sagittal, or axial plane. Soft-tissue abnormalities were categorized as soft-tissue contracture, rotator cuff tear, and impingement. In their 39 patients, only eight (21%) had malunions without any associated soft-tissue abnormality.

■ EVALUATION

A thorough history and careful physical examination are essential in the evaluation of a patient with a proximal humeral malunion. Determining the mechanism, associated injuries, and treatment of the initial fracture is important, especially the type of hardware that was used so that appropriate equipment for hardware removal is available. Range-of-motion evaluation, especially passive range of motion, can indicate the presence and severity of soft-tissue contractures. Active and passive ranges of motion are measured in all planes of movement. Potential causes of decreased range of motion include capsular contracture, extracapsular contracture, impingement, pain, and rotator cuff tears. Limited passive range of motion often indicates a soft-tissue contracture. External rotation should be checked with the arm at the side and at 90 degrees of abduction. A classic, but not pathognomonic, sign of malunion of the greater tuberosity is absence of external rotation with the arm maximally abducted. The integrity of the infraspinatus, teres minor, and supraspinatus should be determined by evaluation of external rotation strength, the Gerber lift-off test, and opposed abduction at 90 degrees. Instability is evaluated by provocative maneuvers, such as the drawer or shift test, load test, anterior apprehension test, posterior stress test, and sulcus test (see other chapter for a detailed description of stability evaluation). Instability may be elicited by these provocative tests; however, in most patients, stiffness limits their effectiveness.

The exact nature of a soft-tissue pathologic process is difficult to determine clinically. Intraoperative assessment of the soft tissues is mandatory if surgery is chosen. Because many patients with proximal humeral malunions have neurologic deficits, function of the axillary, suprascapular, and musculocutaneous nerves should be documented preoperatively. Electromyography and nerve conduction studies may be helpful to determine the pattern of nerve injury and the likelihood of recovery of nerve function.

Radiographic studies should include anteroposterior, lateral, axillary, and Y-scapular views; supplemental internal and external rotational anteroposterior views can provide additional information. CT can help determine the three-dimensional spatial relationships between the malunited tuberosities, head, and shaft fragments. Because it provides a clear image of the glenohumeral articular surface, CT also can help evaluate articular congruity. Three-dimensional CT reconstructions can be used to create models and patient-specific guides to be used in preoperative planning and during surgery.

MRI can provide information about the integrity of the rotator cuff and the presence of early osteonecrosis of the humeral head.

■ TREATMENT

Nonoperative management of proximal humeral malunions may be indicated for patients with low activity levels and minimal pain who are able to remain independent with limited use of a single upper extremity and for patients with medical conditions that would make surgery too risky or that would prohibit postoperative rehabilitation.

The indications for surgical correction of proximal humeral malunions are severe pain or loss of function or both that have not responded to nonoperative treatment consisting of physical therapy, nonsteroidal antiinflammatory drugs, and corticosteroid injections. The patient also must be deemed to be an operative candidate on the basis of overall health and functional demands.

Operative procedures for the treatment of proximal humeral malunions include (1) acromioplasty, osteotomies of the tuberosities or surgical neck, and soft-tissue reconstruction if the blood supply to the humeral head is maintained and the articular surface is preserved; (2) hemiarthroplasty or total shoulder arthroplasty if there is extensive damage to the articular surface or osteonecrosis of the humeral head; and (3) arthrodesis, rarely, if a severe neurologic deficit or previous infection is present.

▌ ACROMIOPLASTY AND OSTEOTOMY

If pain and impingement are the primary complaints, and loss of motion is minimal, Siegel and Dines recommended excision of bony prominences and lysis of adhesions. Beredjiklian et al. found that a delay in the operative treatment of proximal humeral malunions had a negative effect on outcome. In their study, 16 (84%) of 19 patients who were treated less than 1 year after injury had satisfactory outcomes compared with 11 (55%) of 20 who were treated more than 1 year after injury. These authors also emphasized the necessity of adequate treatment of all osseous and soft-tissue abnormalities.

Beredjiklian et al. stated that acromioplasty is indicated for greater tuberosity fractures with 1.0 to 1.5 cm of displacement. In their series, two such greater tuberosity malunions were treated with arthroscopic acromioplasty. Martinez et al. reported arthroscopic acromioplasty, detachment of the rotator cuff, tuberoplasty of the greater tuberosity, and repair of the rotator cuff in eight patients with malunion of the greater tuberosity. Two patients reached full activity level, five had only slight functional restriction, and one had mild limitation in activities of daily living. Arthroscopy also can be helpful in assessing intraarticular and soft-tissue abnormalities and in treating capsular contractures and subacromial or subcoracoid impingement. One case of arthroscopic debridement has been described for a malunited lesser tuberosity that caused a bony block to rotation.

Beredjiklian et al. recommended osteotomy and reduction of the tuberosity for greater tuberosity fractures with more than 1.5 cm of displacement. Treatment of malunion of two-part greater tuberosity fractures is similar to that of acute fractures. Open reduction and internal fixation through an anterosuperior approach with the patient in a modified "beach-chair" position has been described.

There is little in the literature regarding the treatment of varus malunions of two-part surgical neck fractures of the proximal humerus. In patients with a symptomatic surgical neck malunion with an intact rotator cuff and congruous articular surface, joint-preserving surgery is indicated. In varus deformities, the subacromial space is decreased as the greater tuberosity becomes closer to the coracoacromial arch. The lever arm of the supraspinatus tendon and the sliding surface of the humeral head and the glenoid are likewise decreased. These anatomic changes can cause impairment of active forward flexion and abduction and pain from impingement. Such functional limitations may be unacceptable to young patients or active older patients. Some investigators recommend release of soft-tissue contractures and removal of bony prominences for less severe deformities. Benegas et al. and others described a closing wedge valgus osteotomy for the treatment of varus malunions of the proximal humerus. In Benegas et al.'s series, proximal humeral angles ranged from 98 to 107 degrees (normal, 130 to 140 degrees). The osteotomy is performed through a deltopectoral approach and stabilized with a T-shaped plate and 4.5-mm screws. Contraindications to this procedure are massive rotator cuff tears; significant arthritic changes, including avascular necrosis; multiple angular deformities; infection; and nerve injury involving the shoulder girdle. Benegas et al. reported their results in five patients with an average age of 53 years (range 25 to 73 years). All osteotomies united; range of motion, flexion strength, and function improved in all patients; and all patients were satisfied with the results. There were no neurologic injuries. Two patients had mild pain, and one manual laborer was unable to return to previous employment. One patient had postoperative bleeding from the surgical site requiring reexploration, and two patients subsequently had hardware removal because of impingement-related pain. Ranalletta et al. described using three-dimensional CT scanning to fabricate a patient-specific guide before multiplanar osteotomy for a patient with proximal humeral malunion.

▌ARTHROPLASTY

Some three-part and most four-part and humeral head-splitting malunions are treated best by arthroplasty, as are malunions with severe articular damage, avascular necrosis, arthritic changes, significant osteoporosis, inadequate bone stock, or rotator cuff insufficiency. The choice between hemiarthroplasty and total shoulder arthroplasty is based on the integrity of the rotator cuff and the condition of the glenoid articular surface. Prosthetic replacement for proximal humeral malunions seems to have less satisfactory results than arthroplasty done for acute fracture or glenohumeral arthritis. Distorted bony and soft-tissue anatomy makes arthroplasty particularly demanding in this situation. Although pain relief has been reported in 75% to 85% of patients with late reconstruction, functional outcome generally is less favorable because of long-standing stiffness. Reverse total shoulder arthroplasty has a role in the treatment of proximal humeral malunions with concomitant rotator cuff insufficiency and/or tuberosity malunions. In patients with infection or severe neurologic deficit, arthrodesis is recommended.

Antuna et al. reported the long-term results of 50 shoulder arthroplasties (either total shoulder or hemiarthroplasty) performed for humeral malunions causing moderate to severe pain and functional impairment. Indications for arthroplasty included articular step-off, osteonecrosis, and secondary degenerative arthritis. Thirty-five of the 50 patients had nonoperative treatment of their fracture initially. Additional procedures included acromioplasty, trimming of the greater tuberosity, distal clavicular excision, biceps tenodesis, Z-lengthening of the pectoralis major, transfer of the pectoralis minor to the lesser tuberosity, and osteotomy of the tuberosities for exposure or implant placement.

Significant pain relief was achieved in most patients, although 11 had moderate-to-severe pain postoperatively. Pain relief was less complete in patients who had previous operative treatment, patients with osteonecrosis, and patients who had an arthroplasty within 2 years of the initial injury. Active elevation and internal and external rotation were significantly improved. Patients who required tuberosity osteotomy and patients who had operative treatment of the initial fracture had poorer motion. In those who had greater tuberosity osteotomy, nonunion, malunion, or resorption occurred in 41%. All patients with nonunion or resorption had poor results. Overall, 50% had excellent or satisfactory results by Neer's criteria. Complications included anterior instability, partial brachial plexus palsy, and intraoperative humeral fracture complicated by deep infection.

Antuna et al. stressed that concomitant soft-tissue abnormalities must be treated. Contractures limiting motion require capsular release from the humeral neck or glenoid rim. Rotator cuff injuries should be repaired when necessary. Acromioplasty should be performed if superior displacement of the greater tuberosity leads to impingement. They agreed with Neer that malposition of the humeral component is sometimes acceptable to avoid osteotomy. They reported no increase in loosening of the humeral component with slight varus or valgus position. If the greater tuberosity is displaced more than 1.5 cm, it is often necessary to reposition it. When osteotomies are performed, a tuberosity fragment large enough to accommodate reattachment with heavy nonabsorbable sutures is necessary to facilitate osseous healing. Results were comparable to cases without tuberosity osteotomies when bony union occurred.

Mansat et al. and Boileau et al. reported similar results for arthroplasty in the treatment of sequelae of proximal humeral fractures. In Mansat et al.'s series of 28 patients, 85% had slight or no pain and 64% had satisfactory results by Neer's criteria. All three patients with greater tuberosity osteotomies had unsatisfactory results. Results were better in patients with an intact rotator cuff and in those with acromial-humeral distances of greater than 8 mm. In the study of Boileau et al., 42% of 71 patients had good and excellent results and 27% had complications (four diaphyseal fractures, one metaphyseal fracture, two deep infections, one reoperation for acromioplasty, and one failure of fixation of the greater tuberosity). No patient who had a greater tuberosity osteotomy had greater than 90 degrees of active elevation. The authors believed that devascularization of the greater tuberosity led to nonunion, migration, and resorption and thus to subsequent poor results. Jacobson et al., however, found no negative functional impact from tubercle osteotomies in 95 patients with proximal humeral malunions treated with anatomic total shoulder arthroplasties. However, lack of tuberosity healing was noted on radiographs in 11 of 31 patients. Most patients had pain relief and improved function, but 16.8% of patients had complications. Severe instability was the most common complication, occurring in 9.5% of patients. Revision was required in 10.5% of patients.

Boileau et al. recognized the often unsatisfactory results of unconstrained anatomic total shoulder arthroplasty for proximal humeral malunions with associated tuberosity malunions and proposed reverse total shoulder arthroplasty as the solution. Raiss et al. reported a multicenter retrospective series of 42 reverse total shoulder arthroplasties performed

Effect of Proximal Humeral Fracture Type on Anatomic Shoulder Arthroplasty

BOILEAU CLASSIFICATION	DESCRIPTION	EFFECT ON ANATOMIC SHOULDER ARTHROPLASTY
INTRACAPSULAR, IMPACTED	Cephalic collapse or osteonecrosis	Possible w/o osteotomy of tuberosities
Type 1	of the humeral head	Possible w/o osteotomy of tuberosities
Type 2	Locked dislocation or fracture-dislocation	
EXTRACAPSULAR, DISPLACED	Surgical neck nonunions	Osteotomy of tuberosities sometimes
Type 3	Tuberosity malunions	necessary
Type 4		Osteotomy of tuberosities necessary

Modified from: Raiss P, Edwards TB, Collin P, et al: Reverse shoulder arthroplasty for malunions of proximal part of the humerus (type-4 fracture sequelae), *J Bone Joint Surg Am* 98:893, 2018.

for these difficult proximal humeral malunions (Boileau et al. type IV; Table 6.2) between 2000 and 2010. The average age was 68 years, the average time from fracture to surgery was 5.1 years, and average follow-up was 4 years. The average Constant score increased from 19.7 to 54.9. Shoulder flexion and external fixation were both significantly increased. Shoulder flexion increased from an average of 53 degrees to 120 degrees. Shoulder external rotation increased from -5.4 degrees to 8.5 degrees. There were no significant differences in function between patients initially treated surgically compared to those treated nonoperatively. Internal rotation did not improve. Results were very good in 43%, good in 15%, satisfactory in 10%, and unsatisfactory in 2%. Four patients (9.5%) had complications. One patient had an intraoperative humeral fracture treated at the time of surgery, one young patient had a traumatic dislocation and infection, one patient sustained a periprosthetic fracture below the stem after a fall, and another patient had aseptic loosening of the humeral and glenoid components 13 years after arthroplasty. Martinez et al. studied 44 patients with sequelae of proximal humeral fractures treated with reverse total shoulder arthroplasty. The average Constant score improved from 28 to 58, flexion increased from 40 to 100 degrees, and external rotation increased from 15 to 35 degrees. Dislocations occurred in 13.6% of patients and required revision of the polyethylene liner or conversion to hemiarthroplasty. Results were unsatisfactory in 13.6% of patients.

CLOSING WEDGE VALGUS OSTEOTOMY FOR VARUS MALUNION OF PROXIMAL HUMERUS

TECHNIQUE 6.22

(BENEGAS ET AL., MODIFIED)
- Preoperatively obtain external rotation anteroposterior radiographs of both shoulders to determine the length of the base of the bone wedge to be removed (Fig. 6.33).

- Place the patient in the "beach-chair" position with a sandbag between the scapula and spine.
- Make an incision over the anterolateral aspect of the shoulder beginning at the lateral third of the clavicle and extending distally 10 cm in line with the anterior border of the deltoid muscle.
- Separate the deltoid and pectoralis major muscles while protecting the cephalic vein.
- If exposure is insufficient, divide the attachment of the deltoid to the clavicle and turn the muscle laterally.
- Remove excess callus from the bone.
- Expose the area immediately below the greater tuberosity, which will be the lateral base of the closing wedge osteotomy. Divide the bone using an osteotome and remove a wedge of the previously calculated size with the apex at the medial surgical neck. Use a bone skid to lever the fragments into normal position.
- Stabilize the osteotomy with a T-shaped plate and 4.5-mm screws. Benegas et al. recommended a locking compression plate system. A proximal humeral locking plate as described in chapter 5 provides more optimal fixation.
- Perform an acromioplasty if necessary to treat persistent impingement.

POSTOPERATIVE CARE A shoulder abduction brace may be applied if needed to counteract muscle spasm. If stability is satisfactory, a sling and swathe can be used instead. Codman range-of-motion exercises can be started between 2 and 8 days. Active range of motion is allowed as fracture consolidation occurs, usually at 6 weeks postoperatively. Protection with the abduction brace or a sling between exercise sessions is continued for 2 more weeks.

HUMERAL SHAFT

In malunions of the proximal third of the humeral shaft, the bone usually is angulated medially and either anteriorly or posteriorly; the medial angulation makes it impossible to touch the elbow to the chest. Shoulder motion usually is limited in abduction and external rotation.

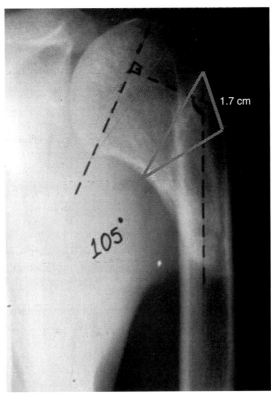

FIGURE 6.33   Calculation of bone wedge osteotomy. (From Benegas E, Filho AZ, Filho AAF, et al: Surgical treatment of varus malunion of the proximal humerus with valgus osteotomy, *J Shoulder Elbow Surg* 16:55, 2007.) **SEE TECHNIQUE 6.22.**

CORRECTION OF PROXIMAL THIRD HUMERAL MALUNION

TECHNIQUE 6.23

- Expose the fracture through an anterolateral incision 7.5 cm long centered over the apex of the angulation.
- Extensive stripping of the periosteum is unnecessary.
- Divide the bone with an osteotome or reciprocating motor saw through the apex of the angulation and correct the deformity.
- Fix the fragments with a 4.5-mm compression plate. A proximal humeral locking plate may provide more optimal fixation.
- Place cancellous grafts around the osteotomy.

POSTOPERATIVE CARE The extremity is immobilized on an abduction humeral brace or sling. Shoulder and elbow range of motion are initiated in the first postoperative week.

MIDDLE THIRD

Unless angulation is severe, malunion of the middle third of the humeral shaft rarely requires correction because shortening, rotation deformity, and angulation of this bone impair function less than when the femur is similarly affected. The

same principles are used in correcting this malunion as in malunions of other long bones: the deformity is corrected by osteotomy, and a compression plate is applied; and because the fragments otherwise often fail to unite, cancellous grafts are placed around the osteotomy (or, if desired, an onlay bone graft can be used).

DISTAL HUMERUS

Malunions of the distal humerus can develop after the following fractures: (1) supracondylar fractures (more common in children), (2) T-fractures of the condyles, (3) fractures of the distal condylar articular surface, and (4) fractures of the condyles. Although cubitus varus deformity has long been considered merely a cosmetic deformity, more recent reports have associated it with ulnar nerve dislocation, ulnar neuropathy, snapping of the medial head of the triceps, secondary distal humeral or lateral condylar fracture, osteonecrosis of the distal humeral epiphysis, joint ganglia, and even osteoarthritis.

Cubitus varus deformity after childhood elbow fracture has been linked to elbow instability in adulthood (up to 51 years later in one study). O'Driscoll et al. reported that lateral elbow pain typically occurred before symptoms of instability. Physical findings included obvious cubitus varus, tenderness over the lateral collateral ligament complex and the common extensor tendon, and a prominent tendon of the medial head of the triceps. Signs of posterolateral rotatory instability included a positive posterolateral rotatory apprehension test and positive lateral pivot shift and posterolateral rotatory drawer signs. Several patients also had dislocation (snapping) of a portion of the medial head of the triceps and the ulnar nerve and ulnar neuropathy. With cubitus varus, the mechanical axis, the olecranon, and triceps line of pull are all displaced medially. The repetitive external rotation torque on the ulna that results can stretch the lateral collateral ligament complex and lead to posterolateral rotatory instability. The abnormal mechanics of the elbow also may predispose the elbow to injury during a fall.

Surgical treatment may consist of reconstruction of the lateral collateral ligament and osteotomy, ligament reconstruction alone, osteotomy alone, or total elbow arthroplasty. For a severe deformity (>15 degrees) and high functional demands, O'Driscoll et al. recommended osteotomy combined with ligament reconstruction.

FOREARM
PROXIMAL THIRD OF THE RADIUS AND ULNA

Malunions of the proximal third of the radius and ulna can be classified as follows: (1) malunions of the radial head, (2) malunions of the radial neck, (3) malunions of the olecranon, (4) malunions of the proximal third of the ulna with anterior dislocation of the proximal radius (Monteggia fracture), and (5) malunions with synostosis between the radius and ulna.

■ RADIAL HEAD

Malunion of the radial head with only mild deformity may not be disabling. If symptoms are caused by a small abnormal prominence of bone, resecting the prominence may relieve them. Severe deformity can cause pain and limit pronation and supination; occasionally, it also can limit flexion or extension of the elbow. It should be treated by excising the radial head as described for fresh fractures (see chapter 5). All loose fragments of bone, any excess bone, the scar tissue, the periosteum, and the remnants of the annular ligament should be excised carefully to help prevent the formation of new bone in the region. Use of the extremity is begun gradually as soon as the wound has healed.

In a few patients, excising the radial head results in complete restoration of function; the result frequently is disappointing, however, and the patient should be informed in advance of this possibility. Reported complications of radial excision include loss of grip strength, wrist pain, distal radial ulnar joint instability, and valgus instability of the elbow. Rosenblatt et al. reported five intraarticular osteotomies of the head of the radius in patients with symptomatic healed displaced articular fractures. The average Mayo Elbow Performance Index Score improved significantly from 74 before to 88 after osteotomy, with four patients having a good or excellent result. Prosthetic radial head replacement should be considered for patients with radial head malunions associated with distal radioulnar joint pain or instability or laxity of the medial collateral complex of the elbow.

■ RADIAL NECK

Most radial neck fractures can be treated successfully with nonoperative methods; however, symptomatic malunions occasionally occur. A malunited radial neck fracture can cause pain, crepitance, elbow laxity, limitation of elbow flexion and extension, and limitation of forearm pronation and supination. It is desirable to maintain radial length and restore the congruity of the radiocapitellar articulation if the articular cartilage remains in good condition because of the potential for adverse sequelae after radial head excision. Corrective osteotomy of the radial neck should be considered for symptomatic malunions.

CORRECTION OF RADIAL NECK MALUNION

TECHNIQUE 6.24

(INHOFE AND MONEIM, MODIFIED)
- Expose the proximal radius and radiocapitellar joint through a posterolateral approach.
- Debride the joint of inflamed synovium. Inspect the articular cartilage of the capitellum and proximal radius.
- If the extent of arthritic changes does not preclude a good result, make an osteotomy in the proximal radius approximately 1.5 cm from the articular surface using a small motorized oscillating saw, while protecting the soft tissues.
- Alternatively, an osteotome can be used to divide the bone.
- Realign the proximal radius, restoring the congruity of the radiocapitellar joint, and fix the osteotomy with two Herbert screws directed from proximal to distal. Kirschner wires or minifragment lag screws (2 or 2.7 mm) are alternative methods of fixation. If hardware is placed through the articular surface of the proximal radius, recess the screw head below the surface of the cartilage.

- Place bone graft at the osteotomy site. Bone graft can be obtained from the lateral epicondyle of the humerus.
- Repair the annular ligament and lateral collateral ligament at the time of wound closure.

POSTOPERATIVE CARE The elbow is immobilized in midflexion and midsupination for 2 weeks, after which a removable splint or functional orthosis is applied and progressive active range-of-motion exercises are begun. External support can be discontinued when healing of the osteotomy is secure.

■ OLECRANON

In malunion of the olecranon, osteotomy and realignment of the fragments should not be attempted because the operation almost always increases the disability, but function of the elbow can be improved considerably by excising the deformed part of the bone. It has been repeatedly shown that a large part of the olecranon can be excised without causing much disability of the elbow. The part that can be excised is determined as follows. A lateral radiograph of the elbow is made with the joint flexed to 90 degrees. A line is drawn through the center of the longitudinal axis of the humerus and across the joint. At least 0.3 cm of olecranon should project posterior to this line; this much of the olecranon is enough to prevent anterior subluxation of the proximal ulna. The rest of the olecranon can be excised, and the triceps muscle is reattached accurately and firmly to the proximal ulna.

■ PROXIMAL THIRD OF THE ULNA WITH ANTERIOR DISLOCATION OF THE RADIAL HEAD (MONTEGGIA FRACTURE)

If a Monteggia fracture unites in poor position, the deformity often is so disabling that almost any reconstruction is worth a trial. At 1 year or more after injury, the joint will have become so damaged that it may be impossible to restore elbow function to near normal.

OSTEOTOMY AND FIXATION OF MONTEGGIA FRACTURE MALUNION

TECHNIQUE 6.25

- Expose the radial head and the malunion of the ulna through a single incision, or make two incisions as follows.
- Make a posterolateral incision 5 cm long, and free the dislocated radial head from all of its attachments.
- Divide the neck of the radius just proximal to the bicipital tuberosity.
- Drill several holes transversely through the bone at the level of the anticipated osteotomy, complete the division of the bone with double-action bone cutting forceps while rotating the radial shaft, and smooth the end of the bone with a small rongeur.

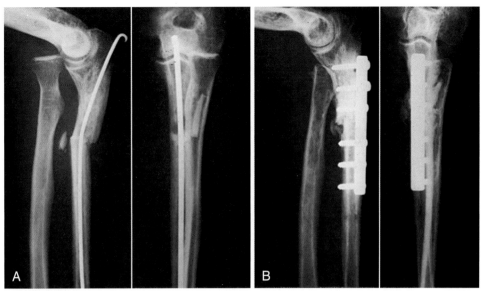

FIGURE 6.34 **A,** Malunited fracture of shaft of ulna and dislocation of proximal radius (Monteggia fracture). **B,** Four months after removal of medullary nail, osteotomy of ulna, and application of compression plate; radial head was excised, fragmented, and used for grafting ulna. Motion of elbow and forearm is excellent. **SEE TECHNIQUE 6.25.**

- Make a second incision 7.5 cm long over the posterior aspect of the ulna and divide the bone as near the old fracture as possible.
- Align the fragments properly and fix them with a compression plate (Fig. 6.34); place autogenous cancellous bone around the osteotomy.
- Apply a long arm cast with the elbow at 90 degrees and the forearm in neutral rotation.

POSTOPERATIVE CARE A cast is worn until union is solid, usually at about 12 weeks, and active exercises are then begun.

We have had satisfactory results in children with malunited Monteggia fractures treated by osteotomy of the ulna, reduction of the radial head, and fixation with Kirschner wires to maintain the reduction until the bone and soft tissues have healed.

■ SYNOSTOSIS BETWEEN THE RADIUS AND THE ULNA

Synostosis between the radius and the ulna may develop at the proximal radioulnar joint after severely comminuted fractures in this region. Jupiter and Ring classified proximal radioulnar synostosis into three types: A, synostosis at or distal to the bicipital tuberosity; B, synostosis involving the radial head and the proximal radioulnar joint; and C, synostosis contiguous with bone extending across the elbow to the distal aspect of the humerus. In their 17 patients (18 synostoses), operative resection of the synostosis gave good results in 16 patients (17 limbs). The only recurrence of synostosis was in a patient with a closed head injury. They found that the ultimate range of motion was not affected by any of the variables generally cited as contributing factors—size and location of the synostosis, severity of initial trauma, use of a free nonvascularized fat graft, and especially time between injury

and excision. Excision 6 to 12 months after initial injury did not increase the risk of recurrence, and although not statistically significant, patients with earlier resections had better motion than patients treated later.

Although historically a delay in operative treatment for 6 to 12 months after injury has been recommended, Jupiter and Ring suggested that early resection is preferable because of its potential ability to limit the degree of soft-tissue contracture and the overall period of severe disability. No adjunctive radiotherapy or nonsteroidal antiinflammatory drugs were used in their patients, and they questioned the need for these prophylactic measures and the necessity of using interpositional fat to prevent recurrence. Other authors also have observed better results with fewer complications after early excision of the synostosis mass with or without interposition material.

Although the most common and most direct treatment of proximal radioulnar synostosis is resection of the synostosis, creation of a pseudarthrosis of the radius distal to the synostosis has been used to restore forearm rotation. Kamineni et al. reported that resection of a 1-cm thick section of the proximal part of the radial shaft provided a safe and reliable method of improving forearm rotation in six of their seven patients. At almost 7-year follow-up, forearm rotation had improved from an average fixed pronation of 5 degrees to an average arc of motion of 98 degrees and re-ankylosis had occurred in only one patient, who also was the only patient in whom resection was done proximal to the bicipital tuberosity. Kamineni et al. noted that the single technical factor that seemed to influence results positively was the application of bone wax at the resection site. They recommended this procedure as a simple, safe alternative to synostosis resection in patients who have a proximal radioulnar synostosis that (1) is too extensive to allow a safe and discrete resection, (2) involves the articular surface, and (3) is associated with an anatomic deformity. They also emphasized that this technique should not be considered an alternative to removal of the synostosis when it is technically possible to excise a discrete bridge of bone.

RESECTION OF PROXIMAL PART OF RADIAL SHAFT

TECHNIQUE 6.26

(KAMINENI ET AL.)

- With the patient supine and under general anesthesia, apply and inflate a tourniquet.
- Bring the affected arm across the patient's chest and have an assistant stabilize it in this position.
- Make a Kocher approach to the proximal radius.
- When the interval between the anconeus and the extensor carpi ulnaris is entered, direct the dissection toward the ulnar shaft and the synostosis; follow the synostosis to its distal margin by elevating the supinator from the radius.
- With a power saw, resect a 1-cm section of the radial shaft either proximal or distal to the bicipital tuberosity as dictated by the extent of the synostosis.
- Examine the range of motion of the forearm and, if needed, gently manipulate the forearm.
- Cover the transected bone ends with bone wax and bridge the interval between bone ends with absorbable gelatin sponge (Gelfoam; Upjohn, Kalamazoo, MI).
- Release the tourniquet, secure hemostasis, and close the exposure in layers over a single suction drain.

POSTOPERATIVE CARE Continuous passive motion therapy can be used for 48 hours after surgery if desired. The postoperative rehabilitation program used by Kamineni et al. involves a two-component splint to achieve static pronation-supination splinting. The first component spans from the arm to the forearm, and the second component consists of an inner shell that wraps the distal part of the forearm and wrist like a gauntlet. A Velcro strap is used to rotate the forearm and wrist alternatively to the maximal attainable amounts of pronation and supination. For the first 3 weeks, the program proceeds as follows: full supination at night, active and passive motion for 1 hour on rising in the morning, full pronation until noon, removal of the splint for 1 hour at lunch, full supination until dinner, removal of the splint for 1 hour at dinner, full pronation during the evening, and removal of the splint for 1 hour until bedtime. After 3 weeks, the periods in which the splint is not worn are progressively increased. Patients are evaluated every 3 weeks, and the program is modified as needed. If motion is not maximal at 3 months, the splint is worn at night in the position in which it is most needed until no further progress is being made. The specific regimen varies from patient to patient.

SHAFTS OF THE RADIUS AND ULNA IN ADULTS

Malunion of both-bone fractures of the forearm occasionally causes functional deficits severe enough to warrant surgical correction. Malrotation, angulation with encroachment on the interosseous space between the radius and ulna, and loss of the radial bow all have been associated with loss of motion and compromised functional outcomes. Malunited forearm fractures may lead to disturbances of the distal radioulnar joint, and arthritis of the proximal radioulnar joint has been reported after long-standing (>20 years) malunions.

Cadaver studies have shown insignificant reduction in forearm rotation with a 10-degree angular deformity, whereas a 20-degree angulation has been shown to result in loss of pronation and supination. With 15 degrees of total deformity, forearm motion was reduced by more than 27% except in distal-third fractures. Failure to restore the proper magnitude and location of the radial bow has been correlated with reduced forearm rotation and grip strength.

The decision to operate on a forearm malunion should be based on an individual's functional limitations and physical demands, rather than on the degree of radiographic deformity. Indications for surgery are loss of motion, distal radioulnar joint instability, and unacceptable cosmetic appearance. Restoring proper skeletal alignment in the forearm may not improve functional deficits caused by soft-tissue injury or prolonged immobilization; these factors also must be considered. In addition, the patient should be aware of potential complications, such as delayed union and nonunion, infection, loss of motion, radial nerve paresthesias, wrist pain, and instability of the distal radioulnar joint. Malunions are corrected by osteotomies of one or both bones of the forearm, correction of the deformity in all planes, compression plating, and bone grafting (Fig. 6.35). Operative treatment of forearm malunions is more likely to improve forearm motion significantly if done within the first year after injury. After 1 year, the soft-tissue contractures and scarring may limit the amount of motion that can be obtained.

Trousdale and Linscheid retrospectively reviewed the results of osteotomy and plating in 27 patients with forearm malunions treated at the Mayo Clinic over a 15-year period. Most of the initial injuries occurred from falls during childhood and adolescence and originally were treated by closed methods. The average age at the time of correction of the deformity was 19 years. Of these 27 patients, 19 patients sustained fractures of both bones of the forearm, and eight patients sustained isolated fractures of the radius. Twenty patients had corrective osteotomies of the radius, two patients had corrective osteotomies of the ulna, and five patients required corrective osteotomies of the radius and ulna. Indications for surgery included loss of motion, instability of the distal radioulnar joint, and cosmesis. No information about the magnitude of the deformities was reported.

Patients treated for loss of motion within 12 months of the original injury gained an average of 79 degrees of rotation (range 20 to 160 degrees), and those treated more than 12 months after injury gained an average of only 30 degrees additional rotation (range, 25 to 95 degrees). The results of the patients treated for distal radioulnar joint instability are discussed later in this chapter. Complications occurred in 48% of patients treated more than 1 year after surgery and included loss of motion (three patients), heterotopic ossification along the interosseous membrane (one patient), delayed union (one patient), subluxation of the ulnar head (one patient), and refracture after plate removal (one patient). Complications in the group treated earlier were mild wrist pain (two patients), a single postoperative infection, and a retained drain. Nagy et al. reported 17 patients who were operated on for

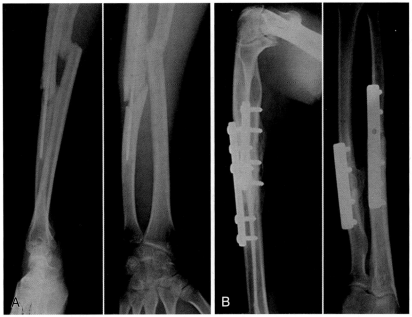

FIGURE 6.35 **A,** Malunion of shaft of radius and nonunion of shaft of ulna. **B,** Solid union and normal alignment 6 months after osteotomy of radius, fixation of both bones by compression plates, and application of iliac grafts.

symptomatic malunion. They found improvement in range of motion in all patients, but the overall improvement range was much better in patients with a supination deficit than a pronation deficit.

OSTEOTOMY AND PLATING FOR FOREARM MALUNION

TECHNIQUE 6.27

(TROUSDALE AND LINSCHEID, MODIFIED)

- Preoperatively, record the amount of forearm pronation and supination and elbow flexion and extension.
- Evaluate the stability of the distal and proximal radioulnar joints by manual stress palmarly and dorsally.
- Obtain full-length anteroposterior, lateral, and pronation and supination radiographs of the involved forearm and the contralateral forearm for comparison.
- Assess the relative lengths of the radius and ulna and identify the site and magnitude of the deformity.
- CT with both forearms in maximal pronation and supination is useful for evaluating rotational deformities. Cross-sectional cuts proximal and distal to the fracture are compared with the uninjured side. The proximal fragment usually is supinated relative to the distal fragment because of the insertion of the supinator and biceps proximally and the insertion of the pronator teres and pronator quadratus distally.
- Determine whether one or both bones of the forearm are significantly malaligned. If only one bone is malunited, osteotomy of only the involved bone is done.

- If both bones are malaligned, osteotomy, realignment, and stabilization of the more severely deformed bone are done first. If the radius is more severely malaligned than the ulna and realignment of the radius produces smooth forearm rotation with passive manipulation, the ulna does not require osteotomy. If both bones are equally malaligned, it is preferable to osteotomize and correct the ulna first to establish proper forearm alignment and then osteotomize the radius to conform to the ulna. In some patients, osteotomy of both bones may be required to allow proper realignment of the forearm.
- Expose the radius through a 10- to 15-cm longitudinal anterior Henry approach centered over the malunion site.
- Expose the ulna (if necessary) through a 10- to 15-cm longitudinal subcutaneous approach between the extensor carpi ulnaris and flexor carpi ulnaris. Minimize dissection in the interosseous space between the radius and ulna to decrease the risk of heterotopic ossification and synostosis.
- Determine the type of osteotomy required to restore alignment in all three planes. If the deformity is in one plane, a uniplanar osteotomy is sufficient. If the deformity is complex as determined on preoperative radiographs, a multiplanar osteotomy is necessary.
- Make the osteotomy according to preoperative plans at the apex of the deformity by dividing the bone with a small motorized oscillating saw.
- Alternatively, the plane of the osteotomy can be outlined with drill holes and the bone can be divided with an osteotome. Use a drill or hand reamer to reestablish the medullary canal in both fragments if this can be accomplished without excessive soft-tissue stripping.
- After the osteotomy is made, correct rotation and angulation and clamp a plate to each fragment.

- Assess the reduction clinically and radiographically and make adjustments as necessary.
- Additional contouring of the plate often is necessary, especially to restore the radial bow. A 3.5-mm dynamic compression plate long enough to provide six cortices of fixation proximal and distal to the osteotomy is preferred. If there is a short proximal radial fragment, it may be impossible to obtain more than four cortices of fixation without risking injury to the radial nerve.
- After alignment of the bone and contouring of the plate are satisfactory, provisionally fix the plate to the bone with screws on both sides of the osteotomy.
- Reassess the reduction radiographically and evaluate flexion and extension of the elbow and pronation and supination of the forearm to ensure that correction of the malunion has improved passive range of motion.
- If alignment seems satisfactory and significant motion has been restored, place the remaining screws through the plate, ideally with at least six cortices of fixation proximal and distal to the osteotomy.
- If the ulna has been osteotomized and realigned first, but the radius remains significantly deformed, restricting motion, correct radial alignment with the same procedure as described for the ulna. Sometimes osteotomies of both bones are required before either can be realigned properly.
- After realignment, close bony apposition at the osteotomy is not always possible. Place autogenous cancellous bone grafts in any bone gaps and in patients with any risk factors for delayed union or nonunion.

POSTOPERATIVE CARE A posterior splint is applied after surgery. The splint usually is removed in 3 or 4 days if fixation is secure, and active and active-assisted range-of-motion exercises of the hand, wrist, forearm, elbow, and shoulder are begun as tolerated. In some patients, temporary use of a removable orthosis is required. Normal activities can be resumed after healing of the osteotomies is solid (usually 4 months); plates are not routinely removed in adults.

■ FOREARM MALUNIONS WITH DISTAL RADIOULNAR JOINT INSTABILITY

Malunions of fractures of the radial shaft or both bones of the forearm can cause instability in the distal radioulnar joint. This problem occurs most frequently with fractures located in the distal third of the forearm. A corrective osteotomy of the deformed bone is sometimes all that is necessary to restore stability to the distal radioulnar joint. In other cases, capsular imbrication and temporary transfixion of the distal radioulnar joint may be required.

Trousdale and Linscheid treated six patients with forearm malunions and associated instability of the distal radioulnar joint. In three patients, stability of the distal radioulnar joint was obtained by osteotomy and plating of the bony deformity alone, and the other three patients required additional reconstruction of the distal radioulnar joint. A stable wrist was obtained in five of the six patients, but four lost some forearm motion (range 25-degree loss to 25-degree gain). Three patients had complications: one, mild instability of the ulna; one, mild wrist pain; and one, pain in the radial nerve distribution.

CORRECTION OF FOREARM MALUNION WITH DISTAL RADIOULNAR JOINT INSTABILITY

TECHNIQUE 6.28

(TROUSDALE AND LINSCHEID, MODIFIED)
- Preoperative planning, osteotomy, realignment, and fixation of the malaligned forearm bones are done as described in Technique 6.27.
- After the plate is applied, evaluate the stability of the distal radioulnar joint using palmar and dorsal stress of the ulna. If instability is present, imbricate the palmar capsule of the distal radioulnar joint with 3-0 or 4-0 nonabsorbable sutures placed in a horizontal mattress fashion to shorten and tighten this structure.
- With the forearm supinated, stabilize the distal radioulnar joint with one or two 0.062-inch Kirschner wires inserted through the ulna and radius just proximal to the distal radioulnar joint.

POSTOPERATIVE CARE After skin closure, an above-elbow splint is applied with the forearm in supination. Sutures are removed at approximately 2 weeks, and a second above-elbow cast or splint is applied with the forearm in supination. At 6 weeks, the cast or splint is removed, Kirschner wires are removed if they have been used, and range-of-motion exercises are begun.

DRILL OSTEOCLASIS

Blackburn et al. reported good results using drill osteoclasis in 10 of 12 patients, and they recommended this as an alternative to open osteotomy in children. They cited as advantages the lack of a second operation to remove the plate and screws and the elimination of the possibility of refracture through screw holes.

TECHNIQUE 6.29

(BLACKBURN ET AL.)
- After administration of a general anesthetic, prepare and drape the extremity.
- Make a 0.5-cm stab incision at the site of the malunion.
- Insert a 3.2-mm drill guide to the bone and drill several holes in the radius; repeat the same steps for the ulna.
- Perform a manual osteoclasis.
- Apply a long arm, above-elbow cast.

POSTOPERATIVE CARE The cast is worn for 3 to 6 weeks. The progress of union is monitored radiographically at weekly intervals until callus is seen. The cast is removed when union is apparent clinically and radiographically.

■ SHAFT OF THE ULNA

An operation for malunion of the ulna alone rarely is necessary; if it is necessary, the principles described for malunion of the radial shaft can be followed.

DISTAL RADIUS

Despite improvements in treatment since the early 1980s, malunion remains a common cause of residual disability after distal radial fractures. Modern investigators have not confirmed Colles' observation in 1814 that the deformity will persist, but that the wrist eventually will "enjoy perfect freedom in all its motions and be completely exempt from pain." Not all distal radial malunions are symptomatic, especially malunions in elderly patients with low functional demands. In such patients, no further treatment is indicated. Posttraumatic wrist deformities in younger, active patients may be sufficiently disabling, however, to warrant surgical correction. In one study malunion was found to be associated with higher arm-related disability regardless of age.

Fracture characteristics and initial treatment contribute to the development of a malunion. Malunion can be caused by failure to achieve or maintain an accurate reduction or by inadequate duration or type of immobilization. Reduction is most difficult to obtain and maintain in fractures with marked comminution (especially fractures involving the articular surface), severe osteoporosis, or disruption of the distal radioulnar ligaments. Age also may be a factor in the development of malunion. In a study of 200 patients comparing distal radial fractures in patients at different ages, Hollevoet found that older patients had more malunions. The mean age of patients with malunions was 60 years, whereas the mean age of patients without malunions was 51 years. Efforts have been made to reduce the incidence of malunion by refining the indications and techniques for surgical management of acute distal radial fractures (see chapter 5).

Malunions of the distal radius may be associated with extraarticular deformities, intraarticular malalignment, distal radioulnar joint incongruity or instability, or a combination of these features. Extraarticular deformities include shortening and excessive dorsal or volar tilt of the distal radial articular surface. Radiographic measurement of alignment of an intact distal radius shows an average of 22 to 23 degrees of radial inclination, 11 to 12 mm of radial height, 11 to 12 degrees of volar tilt, and ± 2 mm of ulnar variance.

No absolute radiographic criteria define a significant distal radial malunion; however, several investigators have identified parameters that are likely to be associated with a poor functional outcome, including intraarticular incongruity in the radiocarpal joint of more than 2 mm, a 1- to 2-mm step-off at the distal radioulnar joint, dorsal angulation of more than 20 degrees and radial inclination of less than 10 degrees, and the loss of sagittal tilt of 20 to 30 degrees. More than 10 degrees of dorsal tilt leads to decreased wrist flexion, and 6 mm of radial shortening causes dysfunction of the distal radioulnar joint. Fernandez observed that fractures with more than 25 or 30 degrees of angulation in the frontal or sagittal plane or 6 mm or more of radial shortening were likely to become

TABLE 6.3

Radiographic Criteria for Acceptable Healing of Distal Radial Fractures

CRITERION	ACCEPTABLE MEASUREMENT
Radioulnar length	Radial shortening of < 5 mm at distal radioulnar joint compared with contralateral wrist
Radial inclination	Inclination on posteroanterior film ≥ 15 degrees
Radial tilt	Sagittal tilt on lateral projection between 15-degree dorsal tilt and 20-degree volar tilt
Articular incongruity	Incongruity of intraarticular fracture ≤ 2 mm at radiocarpal joint

Modified from Graham TJ: Surgical correction of malunited fractures of the distal radius, *J Acad Orthop Surg* 5:270, 1997.

symptomatic. He also noted that patients with constitutional joint laxity may develop midcarpal instability with a dorsal tilt of only 10 to 15 degrees. One study reported significant changes to distal radioulnar joint mechanics as well as ligament lengthening with malunion of the distal radius, which may contribute to the dysfunction associated with these injuries.

Laboratory studies showed that 20 to 30 degrees of dorsal tilt altered the force distribution across the radiocarpal joint, and this degree of deformity should be considered a prearthritic condition. Based on clinical and laboratory studies, Graham developed radiographic criteria for the acceptable healing of distal radial fractures (Table 6.3). These criteria should be used only as guidelines because of individual variations in preinjury anatomy and because some patients tolerate a greater degree of deformity than others. Significant articular incongruity and radial shortening are more consistently correlated with the development of symptoms than are other measurements.

CLINICAL EVALUATION

Pain, stiffness, weakness, and cosmetic deformity are common complaints in patients with distal radial malunions. Pain may be localized to the radiocarpal joint or distal radioulnar joint or both. Carpal instability patterns causing midcarpal pain may occur after dorsally tilted malunions (Fig. 6.36) (dorsal intercalated segment instability patterns) or diepunch fractures of the lunate facet (Fig. 6.37) (volar intercalated segment instability patterns). Decreased wrist flexion is typical of dorsally tilted malunions, and extension is limited with volarly tilted malunions. Loss of radial inclination can cause impaired ulnar deviation. Malunited Smith fractures and incongruity at the distal radioulnar joint lead to decreased pronation and supination, with supination affected more. Grip strength is impaired because of a combination of pain and altered wrist mechanics. Symptoms of median nerve compression may result from a dorsally tilted malunion that increases pressure within the carpal tunnel. Attritional ruptures of extensor tendons (most commonly the extensor pollicis longus) and, less frequently, of flexor tendons also have been reported.

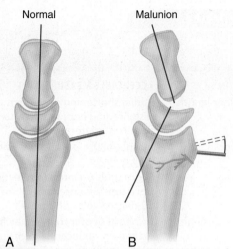

Normal　　　　Malunion

A　　　　　　　B

FIGURE 6.36　**A,** Normal radiocarpal and intercarpal alignment in sagittal plane. **B,** Dorsal tilting of radius may produce carpal collapse pattern similar to that in dorsal intercalated segment instability but without interosseous ligament disruption or secondary midcarpal instability. (From Graham TJ: Surgical correction of malunited fractures of the distal radius, *J Acad Orthop Surg* 5:270, 1997.)

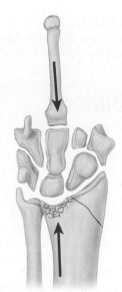

FIGURE 6.37　Die-punch fracture of lunate facet may produce volarly tilted malunion similar to volar intercalated segment instability.

Evaluation of distal radial malunions should include a detailed history and physical examination. The site of the pain (radiocarpal joint, distal radioulnar joint, midcarpal joint), intensity of the pain, and precipitating factors all should be noted. Mechanical symptoms should be distinguished from dystrophic pain. Range of motion in flexion, extension, radial and ulnar deviation, and pronation and supination should be measured. The stability of the distal radioulnar joint is assessed. Grip strength measurements of the affected and the uninjured wrists are helpful to determine the degree of weakness and can be used to assess functional recovery after surgery. The integrity of the soft tissues and degree of scar formation also should be noted.

RADIOGRAPHIC EVALUATION

Plain anteroposterior and lateral radiographs of both wrists in neutral rotation are obtained to determine the nature and degree of deformity, to detect carpal subluxation and instability patterns, and to evaluate the quality of the bone. The uninjured wrist can be used as a template for surgical reconstruction if an osteotomy is chosen. The degree of correction necessary in the sagittal, coronal, and axial planes and the size and shape of the bone graft necessary to obtain the desired correction can be determined.

CT is helpful to evaluate the potential for congruity of the distal radioulnar joint (axial views) and the condition of the articular surface. Malunions of the ulnar styloid also are well delineated by CT. MRI or arthrography can be used to evaluate the integrity of the triangular fibrocartilage complex and intercarpal ligaments.

OPERATIVE TREATMENT

Indications for surgical intervention in a distal radial malunion include pain and functional deficits severe enough to interfere significantly with daily activities. Deformity of the

distal radius, distal radioulnar joint, or both, or arthrosis of the radiocarpal joint or distal radioulnar joint also should be identified on radiographic studies. Operative treatment seldom is indicated for minimally symptomatic patients despite radiographic or cosmetic deformity. One possible exception is a young, active patient (<40 years old) with a deformity that is likely to become symptomatic with time (articular step-off of > 2 mm, carpal instability, >20 to 30 degrees of dorsal angulation, incongruent distal radioulnar joint). Surgery is contraindicated in patients with active reflex sympathetic dystrophy syndrome.

Reflex sympathetic dystrophy syndrome, also known as complex regional pain syndrome, is a distressing complication that often occurs after fractures around the wrist. In its early stages, this condition is characterized by extreme swelling of the soft tissues, exquisite tenderness to pressure, and pain on motion. Later, definite circulatory changes occur in the soft tissues and bone; the skin gradually becomes purplish and cold and perspires excessively. Even later, the joints of the fingers and wrist become increasingly stiff; even the shoulder and elbow can be affected secondarily from voluntary immobilization of the extremity in one position. Radiographs may show mottled decalcification or osteoporosis of the bones in late stages, but 30% of patients have no radiographic abnormalities. Three-phase delayed image bone scanning has been reported to be helpful in the diagnosis of reflex sympathetic dystrophy syndrome. Kozin et al. suggested that an abnormal bone scan in any of the three phases correlated with reflex sympathetic dystrophy syndrome, whereas Mackinnon and Holder indicated that only abnormalities in the third phase (regular bone scan) correlated with it. Reflex sympathetic dystrophy syndrome must be treated before surgery for malunion. No treatment is entirely satisfactory; treatment consisting of minimal immobilization with active and passive exercises, sympathetic blocks, and occupational and physical therapy seems to be as effective as any other treatment. Until symptoms and findings are relatively static or definite improvement is apparent, surgery usually should be delayed.

TABLE 6.4

Guidelines for Treatment of Distal Radioulnar Joint in Radial Malunions

RADIUS PARAMETERS INDICATED	RADIOULNAR LENGTH	DRUJ REDUCIBLE BY RADIAL OSTEOTOMY	POTENTIAL FOR DRUJ CONGRUITY	RECONSTRUCTION
Unacceptable	Unacceptable	Yes	Yes	DRO
Acceptable	Unacceptable	Yes	Yes	US
Unacceptable	Unacceptable	No	Yes	DRO plus US or two-stage reconstruction
Unacceptable	Unacceptable	No	No	DRO plus DRUJ ablation

DRO, Distal radial osteotomy; *DRUJ,* distal radioulnar joint; *US,* ulnar shortening.
Modified from Graham TJ: Surgical correction of malunited fractures of the distal radius, *J Acad Orthop Surg* 5:270, 1997.

Procedures used to treat malunions of the distal radius fall into three general categories: (1) procedures that correct the deformity of the distal radius (intraarticular and extraarticular osteotomies), (2) procedures that treat the pathologic process of the distal radioulnar joint (ulnar shortening, hemiresection arthroplasty, Sauvé-Kapandji procedure, Darrach resection of the distal ulna), and (3) salvage procedures (limited or total wrist arthrodesis, arthroplasty, proximal row carpectomy). These procedures can be used alone or in combination, depending on the specific deformity, functional demands, and degree of arthritic changes present in a particular patient (Table 6.4).

Distal radial osteotomy and bone grafting are most often indicated in young, active patients with a significant radial deformity, good bone quality, good soft tissues, and minimal arthritic changes. Distal radial osteotomy alone often corrects distal radioulnar joint incongruence. In patients with remaining incongruity, an ulnar shortening osteotomy also is indicated. Lengthening of the distal radius more than 6 mm usually is impossible with distal radial osteotomy alone, and a concomitant ulnar shortening osteotomy often is needed in patients with more than 6 mm of radial shortening. If the distal radioulnar joint is arthritic or irreducible, a Bowers hemiresection arthroplasty or Sauvé-Kapandji distal radioulnar arthrodesis with pseudarthrosis should be done. Long-term results after osteotomy have shown that wrist alignment is maintained; however, some instability or symptomatic wrist arthritis may occur.

An ulnar shortening osteotomy alone can be used to correct incongruence of the distal radioulnar joint if the radial deformity is minor. Resection of the distal ulna is another relatively simple technique that is useful in providing pain relief and improving motion in many patients with distal radial malunions. The technique is technically easier than radial osteotomy and bone grafting and does not have the danger of nonunion or recurrence of deformity. The distal radial deformity is not corrected, however, and radiocarpal symptoms may persist. Other potential complications include instability of the distal ulna and loss of grip strength.

The primary indications for resection of the distal ulna are malunions in older patients with a significant ulnar variance, arthritis of the distal radioulnar joint, or as a salvage procedure after failed reconstruction of the distal radioulnar joint. Salvage procedures (wrist fusions) are indicated for symptomatic fractures with marked intraarticular comminution or severe radiocarpal or intercarpal degenerative changes for which conservative treatment has failed.

Carpal tunnel release sometimes is indicated either alone or in combination with other procedures. Dorsally displaced malunions decrease the space within the carpal tunnel, which can impair the excursion of the flexor tendons of the fingers or compress the median nerve. Division of the deep transverse carpal ligament in this situation improves function in the hand and wrist.

Several types of fixation methods have been evaluated in the literature with comparable results. Fixed-angle volar plating with bone grafting provides stable fixation after corrective osteotomy and allows early mobilization. Tarng et al. used a 2.4-mm locking palmar plate without autologous bone grafting and noted that there was sufficient stability without the need for cast immobilization. Range of motion of the wrist was restored early. Intramedullary nailing has been reported to reliably correct deformity and produce good functional outcomes. A benefit of using an intramedullary nail is its percutaneous insertion, minimizing soft-tissue irritation. Distraction osteogenesis with the use of external fixation is an alternative to plating and has the benefit of not requiring plate removal and a second surgical procedure. Lubahn et al. reported that 17 of 20 patients healed uneventfully with this technique. Complications have included pin track infection and extensor pollicis longus rupture. Sammer et al., in a prospective study of five patients, found that although distraction osteogenesis was useful in improving the anatomy and function in distal radial malunions that required correction in multiple planes, a substantial amount of residual impairment remained in all domains of the Michigan Hand Outcomes Questionnaire, including activities of daily living; function cannot be expected to return to baseline.

The use of bone graft also has been an area of study in the literature. Ozer et al. found no significant differences in clinical or statistical outcomes between patients who had locked volar plating without bone grafting and those who had locked volar plating with allograft bone. Abramo et al. used bone graft substitute with a buttress pin and plate system and reported minor loss of correction. They thought that a more rigid fixation system might be necessary with this type of bone graft substitute. Other authors have investigated whether precise preoperative planning of the size and shape of the corticocancellous bone graft restores alignment better than other grafting techniques, but they found no differences. Viegas described a modification that would

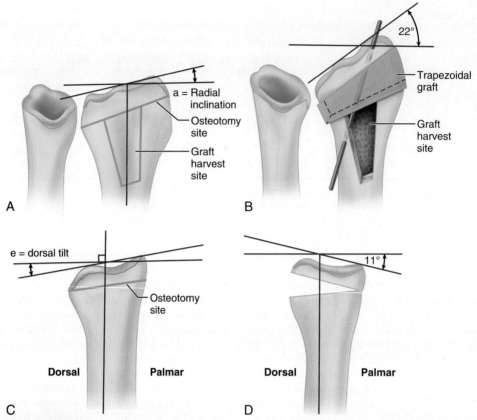

FIGURE 6.38 Trapezoidal osteotomy of distal radius. **A,** Preoperative posteroanterior view with decreased radial inclination; osteotomy and trapezoidal graft site are outlined. **B,** Postoperative posteroanterior view shows normal radial tilt and single "caging" pin. **C,** Abnormal dorsal tilt of radial articular surface reverses all loads across carpals and does not tolerate loading in active patients. **D,** Postoperative lateral view shows restoration of 11 degrees of palmar tilt before insertion of graft.

minimize or eliminate the need for bone grafting. The technique uses a volar and dorsal approach for an angled step-cut osteotomy, release of the extensor retinaculum, and volar plating. The dorsally extruded fracture fragments are mobilized and used as a dorsal strut graft to span the opening wedge osteotomy. Obert et al. used a costal cartilage graft harvested from the eighth rib to be placed in the epiphyseal-metaphyseal defect. Although costal cartilage grafts have been used in maxillofacial surgery, this was the first report of their use in intraarticular malunion. They reported results comparable to other grafts.

EXTRAARTICULAR MALUNION WITH DORSAL ANGULATION
■ OSTEOTOMY AND GRAFTING OF THE RADIUS

Osteotomy and grafting most commonly are indicated for malunited Colles fractures in patients younger than 45 years old. Age should not be used as an absolute criterion, however. Older patients with good bone quality and high functional demands also may be considered for an osteotomy. Fernandez obtained satisfactory results with an opening wedge metaphyseal osteotomy combined with reinsertion of a graft and internal fixation with a plate and screws when no degenerative changes were present in the radiocarpal and intercarpal joints and when the preoperative range of motion of the wrist was adequate. Some patients benefited from the addition of a Bowers arthroplasty to the radial osteotomy. The evaluation

and treatment of distal radioulnar joint incongruity are discussed in more detail in the section on distal radioulnar joint arthrosis. Watson and Castle reported success with an osteotomy technique using a trapezoidal graft obtained from the dorsal radius (Fig. 6.38). Contraindications to radial osteotomy include active reflex sympathetic dystrophy, acceptable function despite deformity, poor soft-tissue envelope, severe osteopenia, and advanced radiocarpal or intercarpal arthritis.

The role of timing of osteotomy for distal radial malunions has received attention more recently. It is well recognized that some patients regain adequate function despite residual deformity. Traditionally, osteotomy has not been done unless a patient has persistent pain and functional limitations after fracture healing and rehabilitation. Delaying corrective surgery until a patient is proved to be symptomatic may adversely affect the overall result. Prolonged angular deformity and shortening can produce altered loading of the articular surface, maladaptation of the soft tissues (capsule, ligaments), and dysfunction of the distal radioulnar joint. One comparison study showed no differences in outcomes between an early treatment group and a late treatment group; however, the overall time of disability was significantly shorter in the early group and the procedures were technically easier.

Fracture lines were more easily identified, congruity of the distal radioulnar joint was more easily restored, and soft-tissue contractures were easier to correct. Although early intervention may lead to unnecessary surgery in some patients,

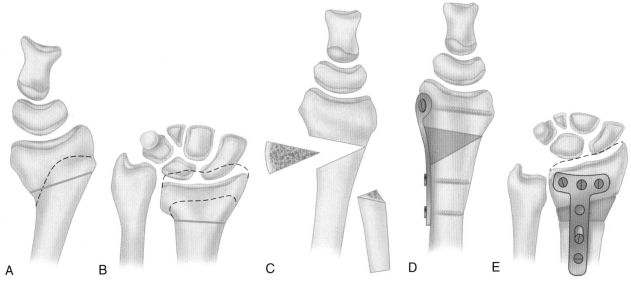

FIGURE 6.39 Fernandez technique of osteotomy and grafting of distal radius. **A** and **B,** Site of osteotomy is marked. **C,** Osteotomy is opened dorsally, and graft is prepared. **D** and **E,** Graft is inserted and plate applied. **SEE TECHNIQUE 6.30.**

early reconstruction of distal radial malunions should be considered in young patients with high functional demands who have unfavorable radiographic parameters.

Wada et al. reviewed opening and closing wedge osteotomy techniques in 42 patients with extraarticular distal radial malunions and found that radial closing wedge osteotomy and ulnar shortening without bone grafting produced better results in terms of restoration of ulnar variance, the extension-flexion arc of wrist motion, and the Mayo wrist score, although complications were similar to those observed with opening wedge osteotomy.

Flinkkilä et al. did not recommend performing distal radial osteotomy for treatment of malunion in patients with mild symptoms. They examined their results in 45 patients with an average follow-up of 5.7 years and found that restoration of normal anatomy did not correlate with subjectively good results. Most patients received a dorsal opening wedge osteotomy and iliac crest bone graft stabilized with a plate. Good or satisfactory results were achieved in 33 of 45 patients. Seven patients had grade 2 osteoarthritis preoperatively. The distal radioulnar joint was not treated at the initial surgery. Overall, 12 patients required 19 additional surgeries; six were for distal radioulnar joint instability, and four were for osteoarthritis. Loss of supination and ulnar deviation correlated with an unsatisfactory result.

OPENING WEDGE METAPHYSEAL OSTEOTOMY WITH BONE GRAFTING AND INTERNAL FIXATION WITH PLATE AND SCREWS

TECHNIQUE 6.30

(FERNANDEZ)

- For a malunited Colles fracture, make a straight distal radial incision parallel to the long axis of the radius, begin-ning 2 cm distal to Lister's tubercle and extending 8 cm proximally into the forearm.
- Expose the radius between the extensor carpi radialis brevis and extensor digitorum communis after mobilizing and protecting the extensor pollicis longus tendon. Subperiosteally, expose the radius to allow adequate seating of the buttress plate.
- Mark the site of osteotomy approximately 2.5 cm proximal to the wrist joint with an osteotome (Fig. 6.39A and B).
- Insert a Kirschner wire 4 cm proximal to the osteotomy site and perpendicular to the long axis of the radius.
- Insert a second Kirschner wire into the distal portion of the radius so that the angle subtended by it and the first Kirschner wire is equal to the angle of deformity in the sagittal plane.
- Confirm that the cut in the sagittal plane is parallel to the joint surface.
- Make the osteotomy and open it dorsally until the two Kirschner wires are parallel to restore the normal volar tilt of 5 to 10 degrees to the distal radial articular surface. Restoration of radial length is accomplished by opening the osteotomy on the radial side until the gap corresponds to the distance measured on the preoperative drawing (Fig. 6.39B to D).
- Stabilize the fragments with an oblique Kirschner wire.
- Obtain a bone graft from the ilium and trim it to fit the dorsal radial bone defect. Insert the bone graft and tamp it into place. Any pronation or supination of the distal fragment should be corrected before introducing the graft by rotating it around the long axis of the radius.
- Contour a small T-plate to fit the radius perfectly and stabilize it with two screws in each fragment (Fig. 6.39D and E). This should offer enough stability to allow motion soon after surgery.
- If the fixation is unstable, increase the number of screws in each fragment or add an additional oblique lag screw in the radial styloid across the osteotomy and into the cortex of the proximal radial fragment.

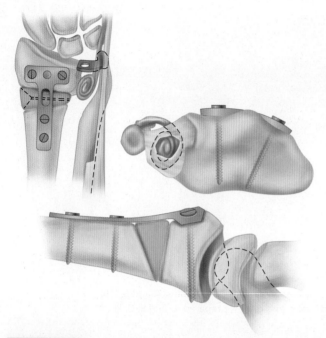

FIGURE 6.40 Bowers arthroplasty with "anchovy" interposition of extensor carpi ulnaris. **SEE TECHNIQUE 6.30.**

- If the distal radioulnar joint is arthritic, a Bowers arthroplasty is added using a graft from the extensor carpi ulnaris (Fig. 6.40); if it is not arthritic but remains incongruent, an ulnar shortening osteotomy is done (see Technique 6.36).
- Close the wound in layers and apply a sugar-tong splint.

POSTOPERATIVE CARE The wrist is immobilized in a volar plaster splint until the soft tissues heal. At 2 weeks, range-of-motion exercises are begun under the supervision of a physical therapist. No lifting work is allowed until the osteotomy has healed radiographically.

EXTRAARTICULAR MALUNION WITH VOLAR ANGULATION

Fractures of the distal radius that unite with excessive volar inclination (Smith fractures) are less common than dorsally displaced malunions. Frequent sequelae of these malunions include decreased grip strength, decreased wrist extension, and cosmetic deformity owing to increased volar inclination, decreased radioulnar inclination, and the resultant ulnar deviation of the wrist. In addition, radial shortening and the characteristic pronation of the distal fragment cause incongruence and instability of the distal radioulnar joint. As a result, forearm rotation (especially supination) is limited and the distal ulna may impinge on the ulnar portion of the carpus. These deformities can cause pain and eventually arthrosis of the radiocarpal and particularly the distal radioulnar joint. Most researchers reported that volarly angulated malunions that were symptomatic initially were treated either nonoperatively or with internal fixation.

Volar opening wedge osteotomy of the distal radius, with bone grafting and plating for symptomatic malunited Smith

fractures has been advocated. The procedure is similar to the dorsal osteotomy described by Fernandez for dorsally angulated fractures. Additional procedures on the ulnar side of the wrist sometimes are necessary to correct distal radioulnar joint dysfunction. Indications for osteotomy are pain or functional deficits, rather than the extent of the deformity. Goals of the procedure are to reduce pain, improve motion, and correct deformity. Contraindications to the procedure are the same as the contraindications for the dorsal osteotomy. Shea et al. reported 72% satisfactory results with this technique at short-term follow-up with improvement in radiographic parameters, wrist extension, forearm supination, and grip strength. Persistent pain in the distal radioulnar joint and restricted motion were noted in 6%.

VOLAR OSTEOTOMY

TECHNIQUE 6.31

(SHEA ET AL.)

- Obtain anteroposterior and lateral radiographs of the contralateral wrist to determine normal degrees of radioulnar and volar inclination. The goals are to restore the articular alignment of the distal radius to within 5 degrees of that on the contralateral side in the frontal and sagittal planes and to restore the articular congruity of the distal radioulnar joint.
- Plan the osteotomy so that it is transverse in the frontal plane and oblique in the sagittal plane. Locate the osteotomy as close as possible to the apex of the deformity. The shape of the corticocancellous graft is trapezoidal in the frontal plane and wider on the radial side to restore radioulnar inclination (Fig. 6.41A). The planned graft is triangular in the sagittal plane with the apex placed dorsally.
- Position the patient supine.
- Prepare and drape the involved arm and contralateral iliac crest after general endotracheal anesthesia has been induced.
- Use a volar approach between the tendon of the flexor carpi radialis and the radial artery, using the distal extent of the Henry approach.
- Use a pneumatic tourniquet to reduce bleeding.
- Elevate the pronator quadratus from the radial aspect of the distal radius and protect surrounding soft tissue with small Hohmann retractors.
- Drill a smooth 0.062- or 0.045-inch Kirschner wire into the radial shaft proximal to the site of the osteotomy and perpendicular to the long axis of the radius (Fig. 6.41B). Control the degree of planned correction in the sagittal plane by drilling a 0.062-inch Kirschner wire into the distal fragment in the predetermined angle of the deformity. Use these wires to help evaluate the correction of the deformity after the osteotomy.
- Use a small external fixator frame with one pin placed in the radial diaphysis to maintain the corrected alignment before placement of the bone graft, plate, and screws (Fig. 6.41C).

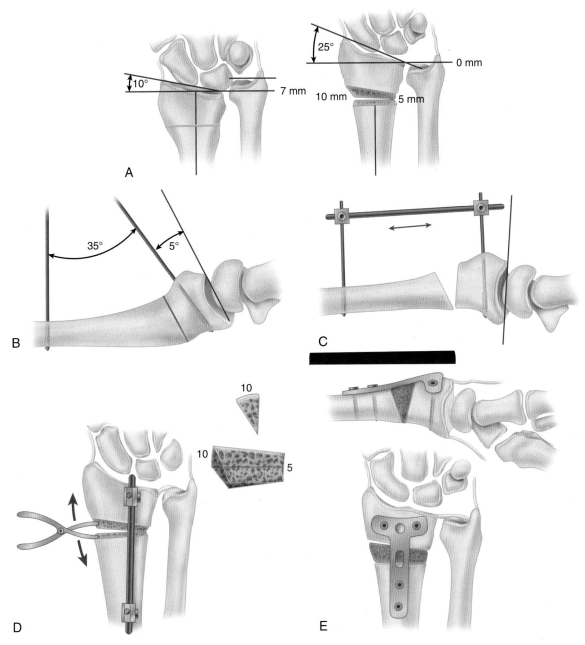

FIGURE 6.41   Volar osteotomy for malunited distal radial fracture (see text). **A,** Preoperative planning. **B,** Kirschner wire drilled into radial shaft proximal to osteotomy site. **C,** Small external fixator used to maintain corrected alignment. **D,** Osteotomy wedged open with lamina spreader. **E,** Iliac graft inserted and osteotomy stabilized with T-plate. (From Fernandez DL: Malunion of the distal radius: current approach to management, *Instr Course Lect* 42:99, 1993.) **SEE TECHNIQUE 6.31.**

- Create the osteotomy with a sagittal saw, preferably at the site of the original fracture.
- Wedge open the osteotomy with a small lamina spreader clamp (Fig. 6.41D). Preserve the dorsal periosteum. This type of osteotomy corrects 10 mm of radial shortening.
- If lengthening of more than 10 mm is necessary, perform a Z-lengthening of the brachioradialis tendon and transect the dorsal periosteal sleeve. In this situation, the graft needed is trapezoidal in the frontal and sagittal planes. The resulting construct is less stable than if the dorsal periosteum is left intact.

- Obtain and contour the corticocancellous iliac crest graft with the dimensions determined according to the preoperative plan.
- Insert the graft and stabilize the osteotomy with a 3.5-mm angled T-shaped plate (Fig. 6.41E).
- The pronation deformity of the distal radial fragment tends to be corrected when the flat surface of the plate used to secure the osteotomy is applied to the volar aspect of the radius.
- Assess the distal radioulnar joint reduction.
- Perform an ulnar shortening osteotomy if normal ulnar variance cannot be restored with the distal radial

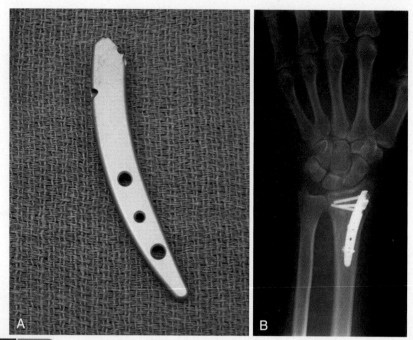

FIGURE 6.42 **A,** Intramedullary nail implant. **B, In vivo.** (From Ilyas AM, Reish MW, Beg TM, Thoder JJ: Treatment of distal radius malunions with an intramedullary nail, *Tech Hand Up Extr Surg* 13:30, 2009.)

osteotomy and interposition of corticocancellous iliac crest graft.
- Perform an arthroplasty of the distal radioulnar joint if there is residual articular incongruity of that joint despite a more normal alignment and length of the distal radial fragment or if there is residual loss of passive rotation of the forearm intraoperatively after stable fixation of the osteotomy.

POSTOPERATIVE CARE The wrist is supported with a volar splint for 2 weeks, unless lengthening of 10 mm or more is necessary, in which case a below-elbow cast is worn for 6 weeks. Exercises and activities of daily living are encouraged after the external support has been removed. Activities against resistance and manual labor are not permitted until union has been confirmed radiographically, rarely before 8 weeks. The plate and screws are removed only if requested by the patient.

INTRAMEDULLARY FIXATION

Ilyas et al. reported a technique of intramedullary fixation after corrective osteotomies for treatment of extraarticular distal radial malunions. The implant (MICRONAIL; Wright Medical, Memphis, TN) (Fig. 6.42) is low profile and sits completely within the medullary canal of the distal radius. Unlike a locking plate that can be used for reduction, the distal radius requires reduction before insertion of the intramedullary nail. Three interlocking nails are placed through the distal implant in a divergent pattern. Two 2.7-mm bicortical interlocking screws are placed in a dorsal to volar direction, locking in the length and rotation. The indication for this procedure includes a distal radial deformity of more than 15 degrees radial inclination, 4 mm loss of radial length, 4 mm ulnar variance, and 15 degrees dorsal or 20 degrees volar lateral tilt. The intramedullary nail should not be used in intraarticular fractures or in patients with active infections. Ilyas et al. used this fixation in more than 10 patients without any soft-tissue or hardware complications. We have not used this technology.

TECHNIQUE 6.32

- Prepare the arm in a standard fashion. Use a hand table, tourniquet, and image intensifier.
- Make a 3-cm dorsal longitudinal incision extending from Lister's tubercle proximally to over the radial shaft. Carry sharp dissection through the skin only. Perform blunt dissection to the level of the extensor retinaculum. Identify and release the extensor pollicis longus tendon and transpose it radially. Develop the interval between the pollicis longus tendon and the extensor digitorum communis, exposing the malunion site. Debride the overlying hypertrophied tissue.
- Perform the osteotomy at the malunion site using an oscillating saw or osteotome. For dorsally malunited fractures, use an osteotome to free the distal radius and hinge the dorsally malunited fracture on the intact volar cortex with a laminar spreader. If the cortex is not intact or if there is shortening of the distal radius with overlap of the volar cortices, take the osteotomy through both the dorsal and volar cortices circumferentially. Maximize mobilization of the distal radial fragment and release the surrounding soft tissue, in particular the brachioradialis.

- After the distal radial fragment is freed, restore the radial length, radial inclination, and lateral tilt. Fix the provisional reduction with a 0.062-inch Kirschner wire placed dorsally along the ulnar column and then assess reduction. Volar tilt cannot be further corrected with the intramedullary nail, so it must be corrected and provisionally fixed before insertion of the nail. After insertion of the intramedullary nail, further height and inclination can be obtained.
- For nail insertion, make a 3-cm incision over the radial styloid, and with blunt dissection develop the interval between the first and second dorsal compartments. Identify and protect the branches of the radial sensory nerves. Place an additional 0.062-inch Kirschner wire into the radial styloid in the bare spot between the first and second dorsal compartments. Place a cannulated reamer over the Kirschner wire. Do not violate the articular surface of the radiocarpal joint or distal radial ulnar joint. Enter the distal radius with a starting awl and a broach and sequentially ream with the osteotomy held reduced.
- When selecting the actual implant, downsizing the nail proximally allows for further manipulation and reduction of the radius. Attach the implant to the aiming jig and place it into the broached path through the radial styloid. Place three divergent locking screws through the aiming jig directed into the subchondral bone of the distal radius. Remain subchondral to optimize purchase and avoid penetration of the articular surface or injury to the superficial radial sensory nerve.
- If necessary, the final position can be optimized by manipulation through the handle of the aiming jig that is still attached to the intramedullary nail within the distal radial fragment.
- Place bone graft into the dorsal defect.
- Place the proximal locking screws using the locking jig over the dorsum of the distal radius through the first incision, fixing the position of the osteotomy.
- Close the wound in the standard fashion and apply a plaster volar splint with the metacarpophalangeal joints and fingers left free.

POSTOPERATIVE CARE The splint is left in place for 10 to 14 days. The sutures are removed, and a removable splint is applied. Gentle range of motion is started.

EXTERNAL FIXATION

Plate and screw fixation of distal radial malunions may be complicated by prominent hardware, late extensor tendon rupture, and need for subsequent hardware removal. To avoid these potential complications, Melendez advocated a technique of opening wedge osteotomy, bone grafting, and external fixation for symptomatic extraarticular distal radial malunions. The external fixator used does not span the wrist and allows early motion. Melendez reported his results in seven patients, all of whom had significant radiographic deformities and pain associated with lifting or axial loading of the wrist and forearm rotation. A Darrach procedure also was done in two patients with radial shortening of 8 mm. All osteotomies healed at an average 7.5 weeks. Pain was reduced, mobility was increased, and radiographic parameters were significantly improved in all patients. Postoperative motion was an average of 88% of that of the contralateral wrist. Five complications occurred in three patients. Two patients with pin site infections were treated with local irrigation and cephalosporin. One patient developed a wound dehiscence at the distal pin site that required early fixator removal at 5 weeks and cast placement. One patient required remanipulation of the osteotomy, and one patient developed a transient radial nerve paresthesia. Contraindications to this technique include osteoporosis, more than 8 mm of radial shortening, intraarticular malunions, and malunions associated with radiocarpal or midcarpal arthritis.

TECHNIQUE 6.33

(MELENDEZ)
- Approach the wrist through a longitudinal radial incision.
- Incise the retinaculum over the first dorsal compartment and retract the tendons dorsally.
- Insert small guiding needles into the subcutaneous tissue to help view the direction in which the pins should be drilled. Use an image intensifier to guide pin placement. Drill the first pin into the distal radius in a radial-to-ulnar direction, parallel to the articular surface, starting in the groove of the first dorsal compartment. Insert the second pin dorsal to the tendons of the first dorsal compartment, aiming radially to ulnarly and paralleling the articular surface. The extensor tendons of the first dorsal compartment and sensory branch of the radial nerve lie between the two pins.
- Open the osteotomy site using traction or a lamina spreader.
- Using the Orthofix (Orthofix SRL, Verona, Italy) minifixator as a template, insert the two proximal pins into the proximal radius.
- Adjust the position of the osteotomy using the ball joint and distraction mechanism.
- Use image intensification to ensure proper position.
- Harvest a block of corticocancellous iliac crest bone graft, fashion it to fit the osteotomy gap, and place it into the osteotomy site.
- Close the skin. Make relaxing incisions around the pin sites.
- Apply a removable wrist splint.

POSTOPERATIVE CARE Active finger motion is encouraged, and pin site care instructions are given. Patients are seen weekly for the first 2 weeks. After suture removal, active range of motion of the wrist is encouraged. A removable wrist splint is used between exercise sessions. After 2 weeks, patients are evaluated clinically and radiographically until the osteotomy has healed and the external fixator is removed in the office.

Shin and Jones reported using provisional stabilization of the osteotomy with the Agee WristJack external fixation device (Hand Biomechanics Laboratory, Sacramento, CA) to facilitate plate application with minimal interference from the distal pins. They cite several benefits over other small external fixation devices in that its gear mechanism confers stable distraction of the distal radius and facilitates positioning of the distal fragment. Bone graft can be shaped to precisely fit the defect. The fixator also can be maintained after surgery to supplement internal fixation.

INTRAARTICULAR MALUNIONS

Intraarticular malunions of the distal radius frequently lead to functional disability. Intraarticular incongruity of 2 mm or more was associated with poor results and a likelihood of posttraumatic arthritis. It is preferable to prevent malunions through aggressive initial management of intraarticular distal radial fractures. Surgical treatment of intraarticular distal radial malunions can be broadly grouped into procedures aimed at preventing posttraumatic arthritis (intraarticular osteotomies) and salvage procedures (limited carpal arthrodesis, total wrist arthrodesis, proximal row carpectomy, wrist denervation, and wrist arthroplasty).

Intraarticular osteotomies are indicated in young, active patients with high functional demands, more than 2 mm of articular step-off, and no evidence of posttraumatic arthritis. An additional indication is volar or dorsal subluxation of the radiocarpal joint. Because these procedures are technically demanding, they are recommended only for malunions with simple intraarticular fracture patterns, such as radial styloid fractures, Barton fractures, and dorsal die-punch fractures. Contraindications to intraarticular osteotomy include advanced osteoarthritis, massive articular comminution, poor bone quality, low functional demands, poor soft-tissue coverage, and reflex sympathetic dystrophy.

Preoperative evaluation should include tomography or CT with 1-mm cuts to characterize the malunion more precisely. Three-dimensional reconstruction, when available, also can be useful. If the condition of the articular cartilage is uncertain, wrist arthroscopy can be done. Optimally, intraarticular osteotomies are done within 6 weeks after injury, when fracture lines are more easily identified. With large articular step-offs, arthritis may develop within the first year, and the wrist may become unsalvageable if osteotomy is delayed too long. Intraarticular malunions frequently are associated with other pathologic conditions (extraarticular malunions, distal radioulnar joint dysfunction, scapholunate ligament injury), which also should be treated at the time of surgery.

There are few reports in the literature concerning the results of intraarticular osteotomy for intraarticular distal radial malunions, and long-term outcome is uncertain. Two- and 3-year outcomes in small series report good or excellent results in most patients. Ruch et al. noted that early intraarticular osteotomy significantly improved grip strength and range of motion of the wrist. Marx and Axelrod reported excellent results in one patient and good results in three patients, and all were satisfied with the result.

In a multicenter study, Ring et al. reported 23 intraarticular distal radial malunions treated with corrective osteotomy, with an average follow-up of 38 months. The indication in 14 patients was dorsal or volar subluxation of the radiocarpal joint, and 17 patients had at least 2 mm of articular incongruity. Six patients had combined intraarticular and extraarticular malunions. Malunions were corrected an average of 6 months after the initial injury. Fixation was performed with screws alone in seven patients, Kirschner wire fixation alone in two patients, and plate and screw fixation in 14 patients. Seventeen patients required autogenous bone grafting. All osteotomies healed with an average postoperative incongruity of 0.4 mm, and there was no osteonecrosis. Six patients had grade I arthrosis preoperatively, and 10 had postoperative arthrosis (eight grade I, two grade II). Dorsal implants were removed in seven patients, whereas no volar implants were removed. Five patients required other procedures at a later date (one partial wrist arthrodesis, three procedures for distal radioulnar joint dysfunction, and one tendon transfer for extensor pollicis longus rupture). Using the Fernandez and the Gartland and Werley criteria, 83% had good or excellent results. Grip strength averaged 83% of the opposite side, flexion averaged 56 degrees, and extension averaged 56 degrees. The authors asserted that this procedure cannot restore a normal wrist but can improve wrist function and delay arthritis in a healthy, active patient.

OSTEOTOMY FOR INTRAARTICULAR MALUNION

TECHNIQUE 6.34

(MARX AND AXELROD)

- If the articular malunion is located dorsally, approach the distal radius through a longitudinal incision between the third and fourth extensor compartments. Continue the dissection through the third compartment and reflect the extensor tendons ulnarly without violating the fourth compartment. Continue the exposure distally into the dorsal wrist capsule.
- Expose the distal radial articular surface with a T-shaped incision. If the intraarticular malunion is located volarly (malunited volar Barton fracture), approach the distal radius through a palmar incision in the interval between the flexor carpi radialis and the radial artery. The articular surface is seen through the fracture site, preserving the volar radiocarpal ligaments.
- Use a dull instrument to distinguish between hyaline cartilage and fibrocartilage; fibrocartilage feels softer.
- Carefully remove the fibrocartilage to appreciate the articular step.
- Identify the metaphyseal scar to re-create the primary extraarticular fracture.
- Pass two or three small (0.062-inch) Kirschner wires along the plane of the fracture, beginning at the extraarticular component and exiting within the joint to ensure that the correct plane is identified.
- Confirm Kirschner wire placement radiographically.
- Make the osteotomy through the old fracture site into the joint using a 3- or 4-mm wide osteotome. Monitor reduction with direct vision and radiographs. Intraoperative fluoroscopy is useful.

- Provisionally stabilize the osteotomy with Kirschner wires.
- Use lag screws or a dorsal buttress plate for definitive fixation. The small 2.0- and 2.7-mm plate designs may be useful.
- If the osteotomy creates a large metaphyseal defect, fill the void with autogenous iliac crest bone graft.
- Extraarticular malunions, if present, are corrected before definitive fixation. If scapholunate instability is present, treat it with a ligament repair if the injury is recent or a reconstructive procedure if the injury is old. Any pathologic process in the distal radioulnar joint that is not corrected by the radial osteotomy alone requires further treatment.

POSTOPERATIVE CARE A light volar plaster splint is worn until suture removal. A removable plastic volar splint is worn for 6 weeks. Range of motion of the hand and wrist are encouraged immediately postoperatively. Strenuous activities are avoided until solid union (usually at least 3 months).

■ SALVAGE PROCEDURES

Symptomatic comminuted intraarticular fractures and distal radial malunions that develop posttraumatic arthritis should be treated with salvage procedures. The treatment chosen depends on the severity of pain and functional limitations and the functional demands of the patient. Denervation of the wrist has been recommended as a palliative procedure in patients with low physical demands who have persistent pain despite conservative treatment (splinting, antiinflammatory medications).

Total wrist arthrodesis is the treatment of choice in young patients with strenuous physical demands who have advanced arthritic changes in the radiocarpal and midcarpal joints of the dominant hand. A stable, painless wrist can be achieved; however, motion is sacrificed. Because of discrepancy in length between the radius and ulna, or because of traumatic arthritis in the distal radioulnar joint, the distal ulna usually should be resected at the time of arthrodesis. Total wrist arthrodesis can be used as a salvage procedure when other surgical treatment options have failed. This technique is described in other chapter.

If posttraumatic arthritis is limited to the radiocarpal joint, and the midcarpal joints are spared, a partial wrist arthrodesis may be effective. Pain is reduced, stability is improved, and some wrist motion is retained through the midcarpal joints. If the entire radiocarpal joint is involved, a radioscapholunate fusion is preferred. If arthritis is isolated to the lunate facet after a die-punch type of injury, a radiolunate arthrodesis can be done. This more limited arthrodesis preserves more motion than a total wrist or radioscapholunate fusion but has narrow indications. Saffar reported the results of radiolunate fusion in 11 patients with high functional demands. Arthritis was limited to the lunate facet, and no patient had degenerative changes in the midcarpal joints. Pain was reduced in all patients, and grip strength improved from an average of 45% of the uninjured wrist preoperatively to 57% postoperatively. Motion was preserved, with patients achieving an average of 33 degrees of flexion, 39 degrees of extension, 17 degrees of radial deviation, and 29 degrees of ulnar deviation. Nonunion

was reported in one patient; eight patients returned to their preinjury occupation, and two patients returned to lighter work. Long-term results are unknown; however, no progression of degenerative arthritis was seen at an average follow-up of 28.5 months.

RADIOLUNATE ARTHRODESIS
TECHNIQUE 6.35

(SAFFAR)
- Approach the wrist through a dorsal incision. Assess the status of the cartilage, especially over the head of the capitate.
- Excise the remaining articular cartilage from the lunate fossa and proximal lunate.
- Apply manual distraction to regain normal carpal height and allow the scaphoid to return to its normal alignment.
- Harvest a corticocancellous graft from the iliac crest.
- Create a trough in the dorsomedial aspect of the distal radius and in the dorsal lunate.
- Interpose the corticocancellous graft to restore the normal carpal height and disimpact the carpus from the radius. The dorsal aspect of the graft must be at the level of the dorsal radius to avoid impeding the glide of the extensor tendons. Pack surplus cancellous bone between the radius and lunate. Alternatively, a graft can be fashioned from the distal radius and slid distally to cover the lunate.
- Stabilize the graft with two screws, one through the graft and the palmar surface of the radius and the other through the graft and the palmar aspect of the lunate. Alternatively, a plate or staples can be used. Kirschner wire fixation alone is not recommended.
- Perform additional procedures as necessary to treat distal radioulnar joint pathologic processes.

POSTOPERATIVE CARE A volar splint is applied and is replaced after 4 days with a cast. Cast immobilization is maintained until union occurs. Progressive range-of-motion and strengthening exercises are done daily for the next 2 months.

Proximal row carpectomy is a motion-preserving procedure that has limited indications for salvage of distal radial malunions. This procedure is contraindicated in patients with a step-off between the scaphoid and lunate fossae and in patients with destruction of the articular cartilage of the lunate facet. In the unusual case in which the cartilage of the proximal capitate and the lunate facet are intact and degenerative arthritis is limited to the radial side of the wrist, proximal row carpectomy is an option; this procedure is described in other chapter. Total wrist arthroplasty also can be used as a salvage procedure for symptomatic distal radial malunions but is preferably restricted to patients without heavy functional demands. This procedure is described in other chapter.

DISTAL RADIOULNAR JOINT INCONGRUITY AND ARTHROSIS

Positive ulnar variance or protrusion of the ulna distal to its normal articulation with the ulnar notch of the radius and consequent impingement on the carpus can be caused by numerous conditions; three of the most common are malunited Colles fracture, malunion or nonunion of the radius, and cessation or abnormality of growth of the distal radius. This discrepancy in length can be treated in one of three ways: (1) the length of the radius can be restored, (2) the ulna can be shortened, or (3) the distal ulna can be resected either partially (hemiresection arthroplasty) or entirely (Darrach procedure).

Dysfunction of the distal radioulnar joint is a frequent source of persistent complaints after distal radial malunions. Characteristic symptoms include pain, decreased forearm rotation, decreased grip strength, and instability. Symptoms can be caused by malunion of fractures into the sigmoid notch, injuries to the triangular fibrocartilage complex, and palmarly displaced malunions of ulnar styloid fractures. In addition, studies have shown that significant extraarticular deformities of the distal radius adversely affect distal radioulnar joint function.

Radioulnar arthrosis has been found to be more common than radiocarpal arthrosis. Approximately 70% of the patients who developed radioulnar arthritis require surgical intervention. Deterioration of the distal radioulnar joint is believed to be caused by shortening and angular deformities of the distal radius. In a cadaver study, radial shortening produced the most profound changes, decreased radial inclination and dorsal tilt led to moderate changes, and dorsal displacement caused minimal changes in joint kinematics. Only 6 mm of radial shortening has been shown to cause distal radioulnar joint dysfunction. A biomechanical analysis showed that increasing ulnar variance by 2.5 mm dramatically increases the load borne by the distal ulna. Indications for surgical correction and preoperative evaluation are discussed in the earlier section on Colles fracture malunion.

Surgical procedures to correct distal radioulnar joint dysfunction can be grouped into two major categories: procedures that preserve the distal radioulnar joint and procedures that ablate it. Joint-preserving procedures afford a more anatomic reconstruction and better preservation of joint kinematics. Many investigators have recommended preservation of the distal radioulnar joint when the joint can be congruously reduced and arthritic changes are minimal. Joint-preserving procedures consist of radial and ulnar osteotomies alone or in combination. An ulnar shortening osteotomy alone is indicated if the radial deformity is not severe (<10 degrees of abnormal angulation in the frontal and sagittal planes), there is unacceptable positive ulnar variance, and the distal radioulnar joint is reducible. In addition to restoring joint congruity and unloading the ulnar side of the wrist, ulnar shortening tightens the triangular fibrocartilage complex and stabilizes the distal ulna.

If the radial deformity is unacceptable, a distal radial osteotomy alone frequently realigns the distal radioulnar joint, especially if radial shortening is 6 mm or less. If a positive ulnar variance remains after distal radial osteotomy, an ulnar shortening procedure can be done as well. If pain in the distal

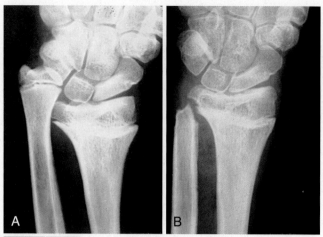

FIGURE 6.43 **A,** Disproportion in length of radius and ulna secondary to injury of distal radial physis. **B,** After resection of distal end of ulna. Unless child is approaching end of growth period, Milch cuff resection would be preferable.

radioulnar joint persists after joint-preserving procedures, an ablative procedure can be done at a later date.

Ulnar shortening also may be indicated after distal radial growth arrest. If the discrepancy in length is the result of abnormality or cessation of growth of the distal radial physis, the ulna is relatively lengthened and may impinge on the carpus (Fig. 6.43). The stability provided by the distal ulna should be preserved, especially in growing children. Instead of resecting the distal ulna with its physis, a segment of the ulnar shaft can be resected, shortening the ulna enough to allow its head to articulate with the ulnar notch of the radius. If prevention of further growth of the distal ulna is desirable, the resection may include the distal ulnar physis. Usually a segment is removed about 2.5 cm proximal to the head of the ulna and long enough to correct the discrepancy in length of the two bones.

ULNAR SHORTENING OSTEOTOMY

TECHNIQUE 6.36

(MILCH)
- Expose the distal ulna through a medial incision 6.3 to 7.5 cm long.
- With a Gigli saw, resect a segment of bone long enough to correct the discrepancy (Fig. 6.44).
- Appose and align the fragments properly and fix them with a wire loop (in adults especially, fixation is more secure if the bone is step-cut and the fragments are fixed with a screw).

POSTOPERATIVE CARE A long arm cast is applied and is worn for 6 to 8 weeks. Union is then usually solid and active exercises can be started.

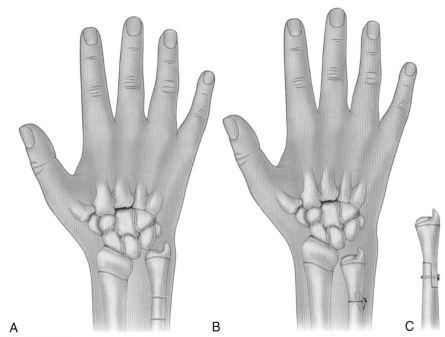

FIGURE 6.44 Milch cuff resection of ulna. **A,** *Shaded area* indicates bone to be resected. **B,** Ends of ulna apposed, correcting disproportion in length of radius and ulna. **C,** More stable fixation secured by step-cut procedure and fixation with one screw. **SEE TECHNIQUE 6.36.**

Ablative procedures are indicated if arthritis of the distal radioulnar joint is advanced or if the joint cannot be reduced by distal radial or ulnar osteotomies. This can be done alone or in combination with distal radial osteotomies. There are three types of ablative procedures: complete ablation of the distal ulna (Darrach procedure), partial resection of the distal ulna (Bowers and Watson arthroplasties), and distal radioulnar joint fusion with proximal ulnar pseudarthrosis (Sauvé-Kapandji procedure).

RESECTION OF THE DISTAL ULNA

Distal ulnar resection was recommended in the past to treat most painful conditions involving the distal radioulnar joint. The distal ulna was first resected by Darrach at the suggestion of Dwight in 1910. The operation originally was done for an old dislocation of the distal ulna associated with a fracture of the distal radius. Since then, it has been used alone or in combination with other procedures for several conditions. Darrach noted that after resection, new bone within the sutured periosteal envelope usually formed to some extent, varying from a mild excrescence on the distal end of the ulna to almost complete osseous union with the styloid process, but the head of the ulna never re-formed. Rotary motions of the forearm usually are restored, and pain is relieved within a few weeks after surgery.

The Darrach procedure also may be useful for some malunions and nonunions of the radial shaft with distal radioulnar joint incongruity. In nonunions of the radius or malunions with overlapping of the fragments without fracture of the ulna, radial shortening produces a derangement of the articular surfaces of the distal radioulnar joint.

If shortening is marked, the joint can become dislocated secondarily. If the malunion or nonunion is of long duration, the soft tissues may have contracted so much that the length of the radius cannot be restored at surgery, even after the fragments have been thoroughly mobilized. Rather than attempting to bridge the defect and restore the length of the radius, resecting the distal ulna (see earlier) and grafting the shortened radius with the two fragments in apposition may be the best alternative.

The Darrach procedure also has disadvantages. Resection of the distal ulna results in loss of the ulnar support of the carpus and alters axial loading characteristics of the wrist. Peterson and Adams and others have noted that decreased grip strength, pain, and instability of the ulnar stump (usually caused by excessive resection) all are potential complications. Coulet et al. found that ulnar resection after distal osteotomy of the radius was limited in correcting the deformity and increasing mobility and grip strength. After resection, pain caused by ulnar tilt of the wrist from instability of the distal ulnar stump was noted; cartilage damage and ulnar deviation (more than 5 mm) also were noted.

If the ulna has been resected at a level proximal to the pronator quadratus, the distal ulna may subluxate dorsally on pronation and cause pain and disability; if the disability warrants surgery, a tendon graft can be looped around the ulna and the tendon of the flexor carpi ulnaris (Bunnell). The tendon graft is joined to itself by a removable running suture of stainless steel wire (Fig. 6.45). The flexor carpi ulnaris holds the ulna anteriorly.

The Darrach procedure is most commonly recommended for symptomatic distal radioulnar joint problems in patients who are elderly, are debilitated, or have low functional demands. The Darrach procedure also is used to salvage other failed distal radioulnar joint procedures.

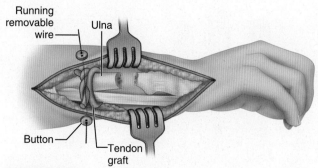

FIGURE 6.45 Bunnell technique for restoring stability of distal ulna after too much bone has been resected (see text).

TECHNIQUE 6.37

(DARRACH)

- Expose the distal ulna through a medial longitudinal incision.
- Incise the periosteum longitudinally and reflect it from the distal ulna with care to avoid otherwise perforating it (Fig. 6.46A).
- About 2.5 cm proximal to its distal end, drill holes transversely through the ulna and complete the division of the bone with bone-biting forceps (Fig. 6.46B and C). Lift the distal fragment outside the wound.
- Divide the capsule of the joint close to the articular cartilage; divide the styloid at its base and leave it attached to the ulnar collateral ligament (Fig. 6.46D).
- Reef and plicate the periosteal envelope and ligament to stabilize the end of the bone (Fig. 6.46E).

POSTOPERATIVE CARE No immobilization is necessary. Active exercises are allowed the day after surgery.

Partial distal ulnar resection arthroplasties are preferred for patients with distal radioulnar joint arthritis associated with distal radial malunions and often are done at the same time as distal radial osteotomies. Partial resection arthroplasties have the advantage of preserving the ulnocarpal ligaments and the triangular fibrocartilage complex. If there is positive ulnar variance, however, additional shortening procedures of the styloid or shaft must be done to avoid ulnocarpal impingement. Hemiresection procedures should be avoided in patients with an incompetent triangular fibrocartilage complex or global forearm axis instability (Essex-Lopresti injury). The Bowers arthroplasty is described in other chapter.

The Sauvé-Kapandji distal radioulnar arthrodesis with more proximal ulnar pseudarthrosis allows restoration of forearm rotation while reducing pain at the distal radioulnar joint. The ulnar carpal ligaments and ulnar bony support of the carpus are preserved. This technique is recommended for patients with fixed radioulnar joint subluxation and concomitant joint destruction associated with intraarticular fractures of the distal radius. The Sauvé-Kapandji procedure is described in other chapter.

In some patients, dorsal dislocation of the distal radioulnar joint is associated with a malunion of an ulnar styloid fracture. This type of malunion has been reported in association with Galeazzi, Colles, and Smith fractures of the distal

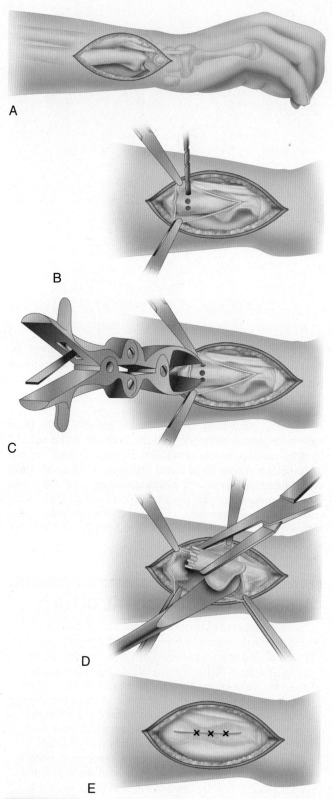

FIGURE 6.46 Darrach resection of distal ulna. Except for good reason, no more than 2.5 cm of bone should be resected (see text). **SEE TECHNIQUE 6.37.**

radius. The triangular fibrocartilage complex inserts on the proximal half of the ulnar styloid and is a major stabilizer of the distal radioulnar joint. Displaced fractures of the base of the ulnar styloid may result in dislocation of the joint. Patients present with ulnar-sided wrist pain, decreased forearm rotation, and decreased grip strength. CT scans show a dorsal dislocation of the distal radioulnar joint and palmar displacement of the ulnar styloid fragment. The ulnar styloid usually is displaced proximally as well. In such cases, Nakamura et al. recommended osteotomy of the ulnar styloid to allow reduction of the distal radioulnar joint. An ulnar incision is made, and an osteotomy is done at the base of the malunited ulnar styloid. The styloid fragment is translocated ulnarly and stabilized with a tension band and two 0.062-inch Kirschner wires. Ulnar shortening also is done if necessary to reduce the joint or correct positive ulnar variance. Postoperatively, a long arm cast is worn for 2 weeks and a short arm cast is worn for 6 weeks. In their series of four patients, the distal radioulnar joint was reduced in three but subluxation persisted in one; wrist function was improved in all four.

CARPUS

For malunited fractures of the carpal bones, surgery is not justified merely to restore alignment. There is usually either nonunion or dislocation. In some instances, fusion of the wrist or excision of one or more of the carpals may be indicated.

HAND

Malunited fractures of the hand are discussed in other chapter.

REFERENCES

FOOT

Aly T: Management of valgus extra-articular calcaneus fracture malunions with a lateral opening wedge osteotomy, *J Foot Ankle Surg* 50:703, 2011.

Banerjee R, Saltzman C, Anderson RB, Nickisch F: Management of calcaneal malunion, *J Am Acad Orthop Surg* 19:27, 2011.

Chiodo CP, Cicchinelli L, Kadakia AR, et al.: Malunion and nonunion in foot and ankle surgery, *J Trauma* 69:418, 2010.

Nery C, Raduan F, Baumfeld D: Joint-sparing correction in malunited Lisfranc joint injuries, *Foot Ankle Clin* 21(1):161, 2016.

Rammelt S, Zwipp H: Corrective arthrodeses and osteotomies for post-traumatic hindfoot malalignment: indications, techniques, and results, *Int Orthop* 37:1707, 2013.

Schneiders W, Rammelt S: Joint-sparing correction of malunited Chopart joint injuries, *Foot Ankle Clin* 21(1):147, 2016.

Shibuya N, Humphers JM, Fluhman BL, Jupiter DC: Factors associated with nonunion, delayed union, and malunion in foot and ankle surgery in diabetic patients, *J Foot Ankle Surg* 52:207, 2013.

Zwipp H, Rammelt S: Secondary reconstruction for malunions and nonunions of the talar body, *Foot Ankle Clin* 21(1):95, 2016.

ANKLE

Alonso-Rasgado T, Jimenez-Cruz D, Karski M: 3-D computer modelling of malunited posterior malleolar fractures: effect of fragment size and offset on ankle stability, contact pressure, and pattern, *J Foot Ankle Res* 10:13, 2017.

Bull PE, Berlet GC, Canini C, Hyer CF: Rate of malunion following bi-plane chevron medial malleolar osteotomy, *Foot Ankle Int* 37(6):620, 2016.

Egger A, Berkowitz MJ: Operative treatment of the malunited fibula fracture, *Foot Ankle Int* 39(10):1242, 2018.

Guo CJ, Li XC, Hu M, et al.: Realignment surgery for malunited ankle fracture, *Orthop Surg* 9(1):49, 2017.

Guo C, Liu Z, Xu Y, et al.: Supramalleolar osteotomy combined with an intra-articular osteotomy for the reconstruction of malunited medial impacted ankle fractures, *Foot Ankle Int*, 2018, 1071100728795309.

Hintermann B, Barg A, Knupp M: Corrective supramalleolar osteotomy for malunited pronation-external rotation fractures of the ankle, *J Bone Joint Surg* 93:1367, 2011.

Ohl X, Harisboure A, Hemery X, Dehoux E: Long-term follow-up after surgical treatment of talar fracture: twenty cases with an average follow-up of 7.5 years, *Int Orthop* 35:93, 2011.

Rammelt S: Secondary correction of talar fractures: asking for trouble? *Foot Ankle Int* 33:359, 2012.

Rammelt S: Zwipp H: intra-articular osteotomy for correction of malunions and nonunions of the tibia pilon, *Foot Ankle Clin* 21(1):63, 2016.

Van Wensen RJ, van den Bekerom MP, Marti RK, van Heerwaarden RJ: Reconstructive osteotomy of fibular malunion: review of the literature, *Strategies Trauma Limb Reconstr* 6(2):51, 2011.

Weber D, Weber M: Corrective osteotomies for malunited malleolar fractures, *Foot Ankle Clin* 21(1):37, 2016.

TIBIA

Buijze GA, Richardson S, Jupiter JB: Successful reconstruction for complex malunions and nonunions of the tibia and femur, *J Bone Joint Surg* 93A:485, 2011.

Kane JM, Raikin SM: Addressing hindfoot arthritis with concomitant tibial malunion or nonunion with retrograde tibiotalocalcaneal nailing: a novel treatment approach, *J Bone Joint Surg Am* 96:574, 2014.

Russell GV, Graves ML, Archdeacon MT, et al.: The clamshell osteotomy: a new technique to correct complex diaphyseal malunions: surgical technique, *J Bone Joint Surg* 92A((suppl 1) Pt 2):158, 2010.

Weinberg DS, Park JPJ, Liu RW: Association between tibial malunion deformity parameters and degenerative hip and knee disease, *J Orthop Trauma* 30:510, 2016.

KNEE

Fürnstahl P, Vlachopoulos L, Schweizer A, et al.: Complex osteotomies of tibial plateau malunions using computer-assisted planning and patient-specific surgical guides, *J Orthop Trauma* 29, 2015:e270.

Mastrokalos DS, Panagopoulos GN, Koulalis D, et al.: Reconstruction of a neglected tibial plateau fracture malunion with an open-book osteotomy, *JBJS Case Connect* 7:e21, 2017.

Pagkalos J, Molloy R, Snow M: Bi-planar intra-articular deformity following malunion of a Schatzker V tibial plateau fracture: correction with intra-articular osteotomy using patient-specific guides and arthroscopic resection of the tibial spine bone block, *Knee* 25:959, 2018.

Wang Y, Luo C, Hu C, et al.: An innovative intra-articular osteotomy in the treatment of posterolateral tibial plateau fracture malunion, *J Knee Surg* 30:329, 2017.

Wang H, Newman S, Wang J, et al.: Corrective osteotomies for complex intra-articular tibial plateau malunions using three-dimensional virtual planning and novel patient-specific guides, *J Knee Surg* 31:642, 2018.

Yang P, Du D, Zhou Z, et al.: 3D printing-assisted osteotomy treatment for the malunion of lateral tibial plateau fracture, *Injury* 47:2816, 2016.

FEMUR, HIP, AND PELVIS

Buijze GA, Richardson S, Jupiter JB: Successful reconstruction for complex malunions and nonunions of the tibia and femur, *J Bone Joint Surg* 93A:485, 2011.

Kendoff DO, Fragomen AT, Pearle AD, et al.: Computer navigation and fixator-assisted femoral osteotomy for correction of malunion after periprosthetic femur fracture, *J Arthroplasty* 25:333, 2010.

Lee KJ, Min BW, Oh GM, Lee SW: Surgical correction of pelvic malunion and nonunion, *Clin Orthop Surg* 7(3):396, 2015.

Phillips JR, Trezies AJ, Davis TR: Long-term follow-up of femoral shaft fracture: relevance of malunion and malalignment for the development of knee arthritis, *Injury* 42:156, 2011.

Pires RE, Gausden EB, Sanchez GT, et al.: Clamshell osteotomy for acute fractures in the malunion setting: a technical note, *J Orthop Trauma* 32(10):e415, 2018.

Saleeb H, Tosounidis T, Papakostidis C, Giannoudis PV: Incidence of deep infection, union and malunion for open diaphyseal femoral shaft fractures treated with IM nailing: a systematic review, *Surgeon*, 2018, [Epub ahead of print].

Sasidharan B, Shetty S, Philip S, Shetty S: Reconstructive osteotomy for a malunited medial Hoffa fracture – a feasible salvage option, *J Orthop* 13:132, 2016.

Wai T, Hamada M, Miyama T, Shino K: Intra-articular corrective osteotomy for malunited Hoffa fracture: a case report, *Sports Med Arthrosc Rehabil Ther Technol* 4:28, 2012.

SCAPULA

Cole PA, Talbot M, Schroder LK, Anavian J: Extra-articular malunions of the scapula: a comparison of functional outcome before and after reconstruction, *J Orthop Trauma* 25:649, 2011.

CLAVICLE

Bae DS, Shah AS, Kalish LA, et al.: Shoulder motion, strength, and functional outcomes in children with established malunion of the clavicle, *J Pediatr Orthop* 33:544, 2013.

Beirer M, Banke IJ, Harrasser N, et al.: Mid-term outcome following revision surgery of clavicular non-and malunion using anatomic locking compression plate and iliac crest bone graft, *BMC Musculoskelet Disord* 18(1):129, 2017.

Grewal S, Dobbe JGG, Kloen P: Corrective osteotomy in the symptomatic clavicular malunion using computer-assisted 3-D planning and patient-specific surgical guides, *J Orthop* 15(2):438, 2018.

Hillen RJ, Burger BJ, Pöll RG, et al.: Malunion after midshaft clavicle fractures in adults, *Acta Orthop* 81:273, 2010.

Jorgensen A, Troelsen A, Ban I: Predictors associated with nonunion and symptomatic malunion following nonoperative treatment of displaced midshaft clavicle fractures – a systematic review of the literature, *Int Orthop* 38:2543, 2014.

Kim D, Lee D, Jang Y, et al.: Effects of short malunion of the clavicle on in vivo scapular kinematics, *J Shoulder Elbow Surg* 26(9):e286, 2017.

Sidler-Maier CC, Dedy NJ, Schemitsch EH, McKee MD: Clavicle malunions: surgical treatment and outcome – a literature review, *HSS J* 14(1):88, 2018.

Smekal V, Deml C, Kamelger F, et al.: Corrective osteotomy in symptomatic midshaft clavicular malunion using elastic stable intramedullary nails, *Arch Orthop Trauma Surg* 130:681, 2010.

HUMERUS

Ballas R, Teissier P, Teissier J: Stemless shoulder prosthesis for treatment of proximal humeral malunion does not require tuberosity osteotomy, *Int Orthop* 40(7):1473, 2016.

Duparc F: Malunion of the proximal humerus, *Orthop Traumatol Surg Res* 99(1 Suppl):S1, 2013.

Giannicola G, Sacchetti FM, Postacchini R, Postacchini F: Hemilateral resurfacing arthroplasty in posttraumatic degenerative elbow resulting from humeral capitellum malunion, *J Shoulder Elbow Surg* 19:e12, 2010.

Jacobson JA, Duquin TR, Sanche-Sotelo J, et al: Anatomic shoulder arthroplasty for treatment of proximal humerus malunions, *J Shoulder Elbow Surg* 23:1232, 2014.

Martinez AA, Calvo A, Bejarano C, Carbonel I, Herrera: The use of the Lima reverse shoulder arthroplasty for the treatment of fracture sequelae of the proximal humerus, *J Orthop Sci* 17:141, 2012.

Martinez AA, Calvo A, Domingo J, et al.: Arthroscopic treatment for malunions of the proximal humeral greater tuberosity, *Int Orthop* 34:1207, 2010.

Pinkas D, Wanich TS, DePalma AA, Gruson KI: Management of malunion of the proximal humerus: current concepts, *J Am Acad Orthop Surg* 22:491, 2014.

Raiss P, Edwards TB, Collin P, et al.: Reverse shoulder arthroplasty for malunions of the proximal part of the humerus, (type-4 fracture sequelae), *J Bone Joint Surg* 98:893, 2016.

Ranalletta M, Bertona A, Rios JM, et al.: Corrective osteotomy for malunion of proximal humerus using a custom-made surgical guide based on three-dimensional computer planning: case report, *J Shoulder Elbow Surg* 26:e357, 2017.

Schweizer A, Mauler F, Vlachopoulos L, et al.: Computer-assisted 3-dimensional reconstructions of scaphoid fractures and nonunions with and without the use of patient-specific guides: early clinical outcomes and postoperative assessments of reconstruction accuracy, *J Hand Surg Am* 41:59, 2016.

Vlachopoulos L, Schweizer A, Graf M, et al.: Three dimensional postoperative accuracy of extra-articular forearm osteotomies using CT-scan based patient-specific surgical guides, *BMC Musculoskeletal Disord* 16:336, 2015.

Vlachopoulos L, Schweizer, Meyer DC, et al.: Three-dimensional corrective osteotomies of complex malunited humeral fractures using patient-specific guides, *J Shoulder Elbow Surg* 25:2040, 2016.

Wellmann M, Struck M, Pastor MF, et al.: Short and midterm results of reverse shoulder arthroplasty according to the preoperative etiology, *Arch Orthop Trauma Surg* 133(4):463, 2013.

Willis M, Min W, Brooks JP, et al.: Proximal humeral malunion treated with reverse shoulder arthroplasty, *J Shoulder Elbow Surg* 21(4):507, 2012.

FOREARM, ELBOW, AND WRIST

Abramo A, Geijer M, Kopylov P, Tägil M: Osteotomy of distal radius fracture malunion using a fast remodeling bone substitute consisting of calcium sulphate and calcium phosphate, *J Biomed Mater Res B Appl Biomater* 92:281, 2010.

Ali M, Brogren E, Wagner P, Atroshi I: Association between distal radial fracture malunion and patient-reported activity limitations: long-term follow-up, *J Bone Joint Surg Am* 100(8):633, 2018.

Barbaric K, Rujevcan G, Labas M, et al.: Ulnar shortening osteotomy after distal radius fracture malunion: review of literature, *Open Orthop J* 9:98, 2015.

Brogren E, Hofer M, Petranek M, et al.: Relationship between distal radius fracture malunion and arm-related disability: a prospective population-based cohort study with 1-year follow-up, *BMC Musculoskelet Disord* 12(9), 2011.

Brogen E, Wagner P, Petranek M, Atroshi I: Distal radius malunion increases risk of persistent disability 2 years after fracture: a prospective cohort study, *Clin Orthop Relat Res* 471:1691, 2013.

Bronstein A, Heaton D, Tencer AF, Trumble TE: Distal radius malunion and forearm rotation: a cadaveric study, *J Wrist Surg* 3(1):7, 2014.

Capo JT, Hashem J, Orillaza NS, et al.: Treatment of extra-articular distal radial malunions with intramedullary implant, *J Hand Surg* 35A:892, 2010.

Chia DS, Lim YJ, Chew WY: Corrective osteotomy in forearm fracture malunion improves functional outcome in adults, *J Hand Surg Eur* 36:102, 2011.

Coulet B, Id El Ouali M, et al.: Is distal ulna resection influential on outcomes of distal radius malunion corrective osteotomies? *Orthop Traumatol Surg Res* 97:479, 2011.

De Smet L, Verhaegen F, Degreef I: Carpal malalignment in malunion of the distal radius and the effect of corrective osteotomy, *J Wrist Surg* 3(3):166, 2014.

Disseldorp DJ, Poeze M, Hannemann PF, Brink PR: Is bone grafting necessary in the treatment of malunited distal radius fractures? *J Wrist Surg* 4(3):207, 2015.

Gong HS, Kim KH, Roh YH, et al.: Delayed-onset ulnar neuropathy at the wrist associated with distal radioulnar joint arthritis after radius malunion: report of two cases, *J Hand Surg* 35A:233, 2010.

Henry M: Immediate mobilization following corrective osteotomy of distal radius malunions with cancellous graft and volar fixed angle plates, *J Hand Surg Eur* 32:88, 2007.

Hollevoet N: Effect of patient age on malunion of operatively treated distal radius fractures, *Acta Orthop Belg* 76:743, 2010.

Hsieh MK, Chen AC, Cheng CY, et al.: Repositioning osteotomy for intra-articular malunion of distal radius with radiocarpal and/or distal radio-ulnar joint subluxation, *J Trauma* 69:418, 2010.

Hutchinson AJ, Dunn JC, Pirela-Cruz MA: Surgical correction of distal radius malunions using an anatomic radial locking plate, *Hand* 10(4):654, 2015.

Kilic A, Kabukcuoglu YS, Gül M, et al.: Fixed-angle volar plates in corrective osteotomies of malunions of dorsally angulated distal radius fractures, *Acta Orthop Traumatol Turc* 45:297, 2011.

Leong NL, Buijze GA, Fu EC, et al.: Computer-assisted versus noncomputer-assisted preoperative planning of corrective osteotomy for extra-articular distal radius malunions: a randomized controlled trial, *BMC Musculoskelet Disord* 11:282, 2010.

Lozano-Calderón SA, Brouwer KM, Doornberg JN, et al.: Long-term outcomes of corrective osteotomy for the treatment of distal radius malunion, *J Hand Surg Eur* 35:370, 2010.

Luo TD, Nunez FA, Newman EA, Nunez Sr FA: Early correction of distal radius partial articular malunion leads to good long-term functional recovery at mean follow-up of 4 years, *Hand*, 2018, [Epub ahead of print].

Mauler F, Langguth C, Schweizer A, et al.: Prediction of normal bone anatomy for the planning of corrective osteotomies of malunited forearm bones using a three-dimensional statistical shape model, *J Orthop Res* 35(12):2630, 2017.

Michielsen M, Van Haver A, Bertrand V, Vanhees M, Verstreken F: Corrective osteotomy of distal radius malunions using three-dimensional computer simulation and patient-specific guides to achieve anatomic reduction, *Eur J Orthop Surg Traumatol*, 2018, [Epub ahead of print].

Mulders MA, d'Ailly PN, Cleffken BI, Schep NW: Corrective osteotomy is an effective method of treating distal radius malunions with good long-term functional results, *Injury* 48(3):731, 2017.

Obert L, Lepage D, Sergent P, et al.: Post-traumatic malunion of the distal radius treated with autologous costal cartilage graft: a technical note on seven cases, *Orthop Traumatol Surg Res* 97:430, 2011.

Oka K, Kataoka T, Tanaka H, et al.: A comparison of corrective osteotomies using dorsal and volar fixation for malunited distal radius fractures, *Int Orthop*, 2018, [Epub ahead of print].

Opel S, Konan S, Sorene E: Corrective distal radius osteotomy following fracture malunion using a fixed-angle volar locking plate, *J Hand Surg Eur* 39(4):431, 2014.

Ozasa Y, Iba K, Oki G, et al.: Nonunion of the ulnar styloid associated with distal radius malunion, *J Hand Surg [Am]* 38(3):526, 2013.

Ozer K, Kilic A, Sabel A, Ipakthchi K: The role of bone allografts in the treatment of angular malunions of the distal radius, *J Hand Surg* 36A:1804, 2011.

Prommersberg KJ, Pillukat T, Mühldorfer M, van Schoonhoven J: Malunion of the distal radius, *Arch Orthop Trauma Surg* 132:693, 2012.

Roth KC, Walenkamp MM, van Geenen RC, et al.: Factors determining outcome of corrective osteotomy for malunited paediatric forearm fractures: systematic review and meta-analysis, *J Hand Surg Eur* 42(8):810, 2017.

Ruch DS, Wray 3rd WH, Papadonikolakis A, et al.: Corrective osteotomy for isolated malunion of the palmar lunate facet in distal radius fractures, *J Hand Surg* 35A:1779, 2010.

Slagel BE, Luenam S, Pichora DR: Management of post-traumatic malunion of fractures of the distal radius, *Hand Clin* 26:71, 2010.

Srinivasan RC, Jain D, Richard MJ, et al.: Isolated ulnar shortening osteotomy for the treatment of extra-articular distal radius malunion, *J Hand Surg [Am]* 38(6):1106, 2013.

Tarng YW, Yang SW, Hsu CJ: Palmar locking plates for corrective osteotomy of latent malunion of dorsally tilted distal radial fractures without structural bone grafting, *Orthopedics* 34:178, 2011.

Tiren D, Vos DI: Correction osteotomy of distal radius malunion stabilized with dorsal locking plates without grafting, *Strategies Trauma Limb Reconstr* 9(1):53, 2014.

Van der Slijs JA, Bron JL: Malunion of the distal radius in children: accurate prediction of the expected remodeling, *J Child Orthop* 10(3):235, 2016.

Wada T, Tatebe M, Ozasa Y, et al.: Clinical outcomes of corrective osteotomy for distal radial malunion: a review of opening and closing-wedge techniques, *J Bone Joint Surg* 93A:1619, 2011.

The complete list of references is available online at expertconsult.inkling.com.

CHAPTER 7

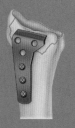

DELAYED UNION AND NONUNION OF FRACTURES

John C. Weinlein

DEFINITIONS	436	Electrical and electromagnetic		Lateral malleolus	459
Delayed union	436	stimulation	449	Fibular shaft	459
Nonunion	437	Extracorporeal shock-wave therapy	450	Patella	459
ETIOLOGY AND		**FACTORS COMPLICATING**		Femur	459
PATHOPHYSIOLOGY	438	**NONUNION**	450	Supracondylar area	459
GENERAL TREATMENT		Infection	450	Femoral shaft	460
OF NONUNIONS	439	Conventional treatment	450	Peritrochanteric and	
Preoperative workup	439	Active treatment	450	subtrochanteric region	460
Considerations before		Polymethyl methacrylate		Femoral neck	461
surgery	439	antibiotic Beads	451	Pelvis and acetabulum	464
Status of soft tissues and		Deformity, shortening, and		Clavicle	465
Neurovascular structures	439	segmental Bone loss	451	Humerus	466
Status of bones	439	Ilizarov method	451	Proximal third	466
Reduction and preparation of		Taylor spatial frame method	452	Humeral shaft	466
nonunions	442	Corticotomy	452	Distal humerus	467
Bone grafting	443	**NONUNION OF SPECIFIC**		Proximal third of the ulna with	
Ceramics	444	**BONES**	452	Dislocation of the radial head	467
Stabilization of fragments	445	Tibia	452	Forearm bones	467
Plating	445	Medial malleolus	453	Both radius and ulna	467
Intramedullary nailing	445	Tibial shaft	455	Radius or ulna alone	468
External fixation	445	Internal fixation	457	Proximal end of ulna	468
Arthroplasty	445	External fixation	459	Distal end of ulna	468
Amputation	448	Distal tibia	459		
Low-intensity ultrasound	449	Fibula	459		

Approximately 2 million long bone fractures are treated in the United States each year. Of this number, about 100,000 result in nonunion. Nonunions can be very problematic not only to the patient but also to society in general. Patients with nonunions have significant disability, and the associated cost of treatment is burdensome on the patient and society. Brinker reported significant physical (Fig. 7.1) and mental disability associated with tibial and femoral nonunions. Although patients undergoing successful treatment of nonunions can experience significant improvement, they often lag behind population-based norms for functional outcome scores. Antonova et al. found the median total cost of care for a tibial nonunion to be more than twice the cost associated with a tibial fracture that goes on to uneventful union. In addition, the duration of opioid use in patients who had a nonunion was twice that of those who did not have a nonunion (5.4 compared with 2.8 months).

Although orthopaedic surgeons may lead the charge in the treatment of nonunion, coordinated involvement of multiple personnel often is necessary, including an infectious disease physician, plastic surgeon, vascular surgeon, endocrinologist, internist, physical and occupational therapist, and psychiatrist or other mental health professional. Treatment of nonunions often is complex, but it also offers great reward because many of these patients have been significantly disabled for a prolonged period of time.

DEFINITIONS
DELAYED UNION

The definition of *delayed union* is arbitrary. *Delayed union* occurs when a fracture has not healed in the time frame that would be expected. The time frame for healing varies for different locations around the body and also is different based on the degree of associated soft-tissue injury. For example, the elapsed time frame for delayed union of a closed tibial shaft fracture would be different from that for delayed union of a type IIIB open tibial shaft fracture. Generally, the time frame for *delayed union* is between 3 and 6 months. *Delayed union* can be thought of as a precursor to nonunion. In appropriate circumstances, intervention for *delayed union* can prevent a nonunion. Intervention can include correction of metabolic or endocrine abnormalities; stabilization with a cast or brace; bone stimulation, with pulsed ultrasound, electrical (or electromagnetic) stimulation, or extracorporeal shock-wave therapy; or surgical intervention. The consequences to the patient of prolonged convalescence must always be considered when treating both delayed union and nonunion.

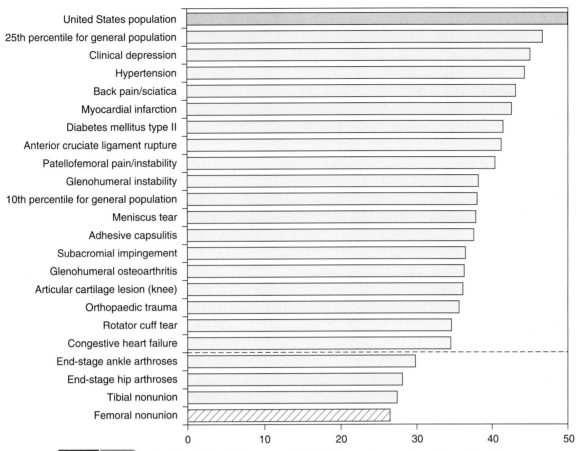

FIGURE 7.1 Significant disability associated with femoral nonunions. Mean Short Form (SF)-12 Physical Component Summary Scores according to diagnosis. *Striped bar,* femoral nonunions; *solid gray bar,* mean across noninstitutionalized U.S. population; medical conditions above dashed line associated with significantly ($P < 0.05$) better physical health than femoral nonunions. (From Brinker MR, Trivedi A, O'Connor DP: Debilitating effects of femoral nonunion on health-related quality of life, *J Orthop Trauma* 31:e37, 2017.)

Most surgeries performed on delayed unions correct issues associated with poor technique during the index procedure. An open reduction may be necessary to reduce widely displaced fracture fragments and remove interposed tissue. If surgery is in a location not prone to nonunion and the patient is a good host, then the surgeon can proceed with standard techniques for acute fracture fixation, and bone grafting may not be necessary. If surgery is in an area prone to nonunion or the patient is a poor host, then bone grafting should be at least considered. The method of stabilization also affects the surgeon's decision to bone graft. Bone grafting is also more likely to be used if delayed union is being treated with plate osteosynthesis than with an intramedullary nail or external fixator.

NONUNION

Similar to *delayed union,* the diagnosis of *nonunion* is also arbitrary. The U.S. Food and Drug Administration defines *nonunion* as "established when a minimum of 9 months has elapsed since injury and the fracture shows no visible progressive signs of healing for 3 months." This definition fails to include many fractures that have no chance of proceeding to union. The definition of *nonunion* from Brinker is probably more appropriate: "A fracture that, in the opinion of the treating physician, has no possibility of healing without further intervention." Generally speaking, the diagnosis of *nonunion* should not be made until clinical or radiographic evidence is noted that healing has ceased or that union is highly unlikely. The time frame for *nonunion* differs by location and by the degree of associated soft-tissue injury. A femoral neck fracture that has not united and displays implant failure at 3 months may appropriately be considered a nonunion, whereas a Gustilo and Anderson type 3B open tibial fracture that has received appropriate surgical treatment may not be considered a nonunion after this same 3-month time frame. However, waiting 9 months to intervene on many fractures that have not united may result in prolonged morbidity, inability to return to work, narcotic dependence, and emotional impairment.

TABLE 7.1	
Biologic Etiologies of Nonunion	
Local	Excessive soft-tissue stripping (from injury or surgeon)
	Bone loss
	Vascular injury
	Radiation
	Infection
Systemic	Age
	Chronic diseases
	Diabetes mellitus
	Chronic anemia
	Metabolic or endocrine abnormalities (vitamin D deficiency)
	Malnutrition
	Medications (steroids, NSAIDs, antiepileptics)
	Smoking

NSAIDs, Nonsteroidal antiinflammatory drugs.

TABLE 7.2	
Mechanical Etiologies of Nonunion	
Malreduction	Malposition
	Malalignment
	Distraction
Inappropriate stabilization	Too little or insufficient fixation
	Too much or too rigid fixation
	Inappropriate implant choice
	Inappropriate implant position
	Technical error(s)

ETIOLOGY AND PATHOPHYSIOLOGY

Without an understanding of normal fracture healing, the ability to successfully treat nonunions is compromised. Fractures treated nonoperatively and those treated with intramedullary nails, bridge plates, and many external fixators rely upon secondary bone healing. Relative stability is provided by these devices when attempting to obtain secondary bone healing. These fractures heal with callus formation and progress through stages: (1) inflammatory stage, (2) soft callus stage, (3) hard callus stage, and (4) remodeling phase. Interfragmentary motion is typically between 0.2 and 1 mm. Fractures fixed rigidly with plates rely on primary bone healing. Absolute stability is necessary; interfragmentary motion is less than 0.15 mm and the strain is less than 2%. Healing is similar to the remodeling phase of secondary bone healing, with osteoclasts converting woven bone to lamellar bone. In many cases of plate fixation, if fracture gaps are larger than 0.1 mm, primary bone healing does not occur. In this situation, gap healing may occur. With gap healing, the strain is still less than 2%; however, gaps up to 1 mm are tolerated.

There are many suspected etiologies for nonunions, and most nonunions likely have multiple etiologies. These etiologies are both biologic and mechanical. Biologic etiologies can be divided into local and systemic. Local biologic etiologies include excessive soft-tissue stripping, bone loss, vascular injury, irradiated bone, and infection. Excessive soft-tissue stripping can also be the result of surgery. Systemic biologic etiologies include age, chronic diseases (diabetes mellitus, chronic anemia), metabolic or endocrine abnormalities, malnutrition, medications (steroids, antiepileptic medications), and smoking (Table 7.1). The effects of anti-inflammatory medications, as well as alcohol and opioids, are controversial. Mechanical etiologies (Table 7.2) of nonunion include malreduction (malposition, malalignment, distraction) and inappropriate stabilization ("too little," or insufficient fixation; "too much" or "too rigid" fixation), inappropriate implant choice, inappropriate implant position, or technical error.

Brinker et al. specifically evaluated metabolic and endocrine abnormalities in a large series of nonunions that were not thought to have a mechanical etiology. Four percent of patients (37 of 883) were referred to an endocrinologist. Eighty-four percent (31 of 37) were diagnosed with a metabolic or endocrine abnormality. Sixty-eight percent (25 of 37) of patients were found to have a vitamin D deficiency. Other abnormalities included calcium imbalances, hypogonadism, and thyroid or parathyroid disorders. Other studies have reported similar prevalences of vitamin D deficiency in the general orthopaedic trauma population, and the effect of vitamin D deficiency and its treatment on nonunions is not clear. While many abnormalities have been associated with nonunion, assigning causation has still been elusive.

The use of tobacco has been implicated in the development of nonunions and delayed union. Pearson et al. recently reported just over twice the risk of delayed and/or nonunion in smokers. Smokers have decreased oxygen levels in the cutaneous and subcutaneous tissues, which leads to poor wound healing. Nicotine also has been associated with decreased vascularity at fracture sites. Although approximately 50% of smokers return to their habit, it is best for healing of bone and soft tissue if they can abstain while being treated for their nonunion. Nonsteroidal antiinflammatory drugs (NSAIDs) have been found to decrease fracture healing in multiple animal studies. The literature is still conflicting concerning the influence of NSAIDs on fracture healing in humans. Although numerous animal data suggest NSAIDs have a negative effect on fracture healing, the data in humans are more controversial. Several human studies have found delayed healing in subjects who were taking NSAIDs, whereas other studies refute the hypothesis that NSAIDs delay fracture healing. We use NSAIDs for acute pain management in fracture patients and believe treatment of short duration likely causes minimal negative consequences on fracture healing. We suggest that patients with a delayed union or nonunion abstain from using NSAIDs or steroids, if possible, during their nonunion treatment.

Opioids also may have an effect on fracture healing. Animal data have suggested a negative impact on fracture callus volume, maturation, and strength. Several retrospective human studies suggest an association with opioid use and nonunion; however, high-quality studies demonstrating causality between opioid use and nonunion are lacking.

TABLE 7.3	
Predicted Probability of Confirming Infection Using White Blood Cells, Erythrocyte Sedimentation Rate, and C-Reactive Protein	
NUMBER OF POSITIVE TESTS UNDER CONSIDERATION	**PREDICTED PROBABILITY OF INFECTION (%)**
0	19.6
1	18.8
2	56.0
3	100.0

From Stucken C, Olszewski DC, Creevy WR, et al: Preoperative diagnosis of infection in patients with nonunion, *J Bone Joint Surg* 95A:1409, 2013.

TABLE 7.4	
Predicted Probability of Excluding Infection Using White Blood Cells, Erythrocyte Sedimentation Rate, and C-Reactive Protein	
NUMBER OF NEGATIVE TESTS UNDER CONSIDERATION	**PREDICTED PROBABILITY OF NO INFECTION (%)**
0	0
1	48.0
2	76.4
3	81.6

From Stucken C, Olszewski DC, Creevy WR, et al: Preoperative diagnosis of infection in patients with nonunion, *J Bone Joint Surg* 95A:1409, 2013.

GENERAL TREATMENT OF NONUNIONS

PREOPERATIVE WORKUP

The workup for nonunion includes history, physical examination, radiographic examination, and laboratory evaluation. The history should include previous treatment, time frame of previous treatment, documented infection, signs and symptoms consistent with current or previous infection, and presence or absence of pain. The physical examination should include a detailed neurovascular examination and assessment for presence or absence of tenderness at the fracture site, deformity, malrotation, leg-length discrepancy, joint range of motion, compensatory contractures, erythema, and drainage. The radiographic examination begins with plain films. Oblique plain films can be useful in evaluating progression of long bones toward union, particularly around the distal tibia. CT scan may be indicated in certain situations. CT scan is highly sensitive for nonunion but does lack specificity. MRI and nuclear imaging may be useful in certain situations. The usefulness of nuclear imaging in diagnosing infection preoperatively, however, has been questioned. The goals of imaging include assessing union, monitoring progression toward union, determining etiology for delayed union or nonunion, evaluating integrity of implants, and checking for signs of infection.

The laboratory evaluation begins with a complete blood count (CBC) with differential, erythrocyte sedimentation rate (ESR), C-reactive protein (CRP), and 25-hydroxy vitamin D. Other laboratory values may be indicated in certain situations. When using CBC (white blood cells [WBCs]), ESR, and CRP to assess for infection, the positive predictive value when all three values are positive is 100% (Table 7.3). The negative predictive value when all three laboratory values are negative is 81.6% (Table 7.4). Wang et al. recently reported the use of preoperative serum D-dimer in the assessment of infected nonunions. The authors reported higher positive and negative predictive values when using D-dimer compared with isolated CRP or ESR. Further investigation may clarify the usefulness of this laboratory value in nonunion workup. A nonunion work sheet as suggested by Brinker can be helpful in organizing all of the important data necessary before treatment of a nonunion (Fig. 7.2).

CONSIDERATIONS BEFORE SURGERY

Metabolic and nutritional factors should be optimized. We continue to make attempts to optimize 25-hydroxy vitamin D levels before proceeding with nonunion surgery, but recognize that the data supporting this approach are lacking. Patients should be encouraged to discontinue tobacco and any other medications that may have an effect on fracture union.

■ STATUS OF SOFT TISSUES AND NEUROVASCULAR STRUCTURES

The condition of the soft tissues surrounding a nonunion must be considered in treatment planning. Significant soft-tissue scarring, especially on the concave side of a deformity, may result in skin necrosis requiring aggressive correction. Scarring also may limit some treatment options or require treatment of the nonunion with concomitant free-tissue transfer. Soft-tissue contractures must be considered if treatment of the nonunion would result in lengthening of the extremity.

In patients with histories of vascular injuries or patients with weak or absent peripheral pulses, an arteriogram may be indicated to evaluate vascular status. A significant vascular abnormality may limit treatment methods and fracture healing. Vascular abnormalities should be corrected, if possible.

Any nerve deficit should be carefully considered. In patients with long-standing significant deformity, Ilizarov or Taylor Spatial Frame (Smith & Nephew, Memphis, TN) treatment may be most appropriate for gradual deformity correction or lengthening of the nonunion. When the nerves are so damaged that sensation and motor function in a lower extremity are permanently lost, amputation usually is the more practical choice.

■ STATUS OF BONES

The status of the bones, especially at the nonunion, depends on the type and duration of the fracture and the method of any previous treatment. Nonunions are classified based on location, presence or absence of infection, and etiology:
- Epiphyseal, metaphyseal, or diaphyseal
- Septic or aseptic
- Hypertrophic, oligotrophic, or atrophic (Fig. 7.3)
- Pseudarthrosis

Septic nonunions are much more difficult to treat than aseptic nonunions. Hypertrophic nonunions (Fig. 7.4) have adequate vascularity, display abundant callus, and lack stability. Oligotrophic nonunions usually have adequate vascularity, display little or no callus, and often are associated with malreduction (distraction). Atrophic nonunions (Fig. 7.5) lack adequate vascularity and display no callus. Synovial pseudarthrosis (Fig. 7.6) involves sealed medullary canals with an

GENERAL INFORMATION

Patient Name: _____   Age: _____ Gender: _____

Referring Physician: _____   Height: _____ Weight: _____

Injury (description): _____

Date of Injury: _____   Pain (0 to 10 VAS):

Occupation: _____   Was injury Work Related?:   Y   N

PAST HISTORY

Initial Fracture Treatment (Date): _____

Total # of Surgeries for Nonunion: _____

     Surgery #1 (Date): _____

     Surgery #2 (Date): _____

     Surgery #3 (Date): _____

     Surgery #4 (Date): _____

     Surgery #5 (Date): _____

     Surgery #6 (Date): _____

     (Use backside of this sheet for other prior surgeries)

Use of Electromagnetic or Ultrasound Stimulation?

Cigarette Smoking   # of packs per day _____   # of years smoking _____

History of Infection? (include culture results) _____

History of Soft-Tissue Problems? _____

Medical Conditions: _____

Medications: _____

NSAID Use: _____

Narcotic Use: _____

Allergies: _____

PHYSICAL EXAMINATION

General: _____

Extremity:

     Nonunion: _____ Stiff   _____ Lax

     Adjacent Joints (RCM, compensatory deformities): _____

     Soft Tissues (defects, drainage): _____

     Neurovascular Exam: _____

RADIOLOGIC EXAMINATION

     Comments _____

OTHER PERTINENT INFORMATION _____

     _____

     _____

NONUNION TYPE

     _____ Hypertrophic

     _____ Oligotrophic

     _____ Atrophic

     _____ Infected

     _____ Synovial Pseudoarthrosis

FIGURE 7.2 Nonunion work sheet. (From Brinker MR: Nonunions: evaluation and treatment. In Browner BD, Jupiter JB, Levine AM, et al, editors: *Skeletal trauma: basic science, management, and reconstruction*, ed 4, Philadelphia, 2009, Saunders.)

associated pseudomembrane containing fluid. Radiographic appearance is variable, and technetium bone scan reveals a "cold cleft" between areas of increased activity. Classification of nonunions has historically guided treatment and is therefore important to understand.

Many options are available for treatment of nonunions, including invasive and noninvasive modalities. Noninvasive interventions include casting or bracing, low-intensity pulsed ultrasound (LIPUS), electric or electromagnetic stimulation, and extracorporeal shock-wave therapy. Invasive interventions include bone grafting (or bone grafting alternatives) and stabilization. Stabilization can take many forms but primarily involves plating, intramedullary nailing, or external fixation. To treat nonunions most effectively, a surgeon should have some experience with all forms of surgical stabilization.

Often a nonunion may be treated with several different interventions. The patient should be involved in the discussion because potential risks and benefits vary among treatments. When selecting treatment, thought should be given to future interventions that may be necessary if the fracture does not unite. Operations for nonunions are relatively invasive and should be undertaken only after nonunion has been proven clinically and radiographically or when union is extremely unlikely or impossible without a change in current treatment.

The requirements for successful nonunion treatment are biomechanical stability and a biologic vitality of the bone. These requirements can be obtained through reduction of fragments, bone grafting, and stabilization of the fragments. Many techniques or combinations of techniques meet these requirements, and some general guidelines apply to all techniques.

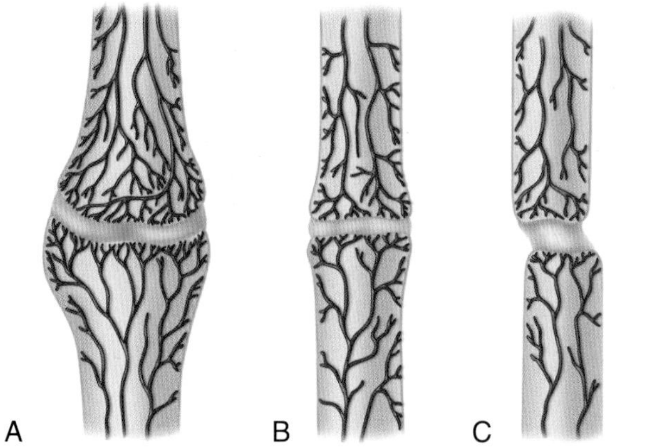

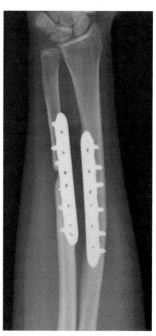

FIGURE 7.3 Types of nonunions. **A,** Hypertrophic. **B,** Oligotrophic. **C,** Atrophic.

FIGURE 7.5 Atrophic nonunion of ulna after treatment with internal fixation.

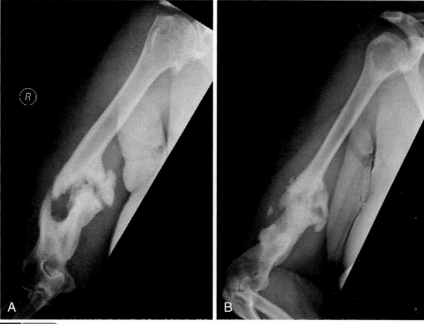

FIGURE 7.4 **A and B,** Hypertrophic humeral nonunion.

REDUCTION AND PREPARATION OF NONUNIONS

Malreduction (malposition, malalignment, distraction) of bone fragments (Fig. 7.7) can be responsible for nonunion. Malreduction can be particularly problematic in fractures that are rigidly fixed. The same reduction that would be considered satisfactory if stabilized by an intramedullary nail or circular fine wire external fixator may be unsatisfactory if stabilized rigidly with a plate. When malreduction is considered at least part of the etiology of the nonunion, reduction must be improved with the surgical intervention chosen. Depending on the mobility of the nonunion, the method of stabilization, and the decision regarding bone grafting, reduction may be performed open or closed. When an open reduction is performed to adequately reduce and stabilize fracture fragments, interposed fibrous tissue is removed by necessity. In contrast, when fracture fragments are satisfactorily aligned and without a gap, aggressive removal of intervening fibrous tissue may be undesirable. Minimizing further insult to periosteum, callus, and fibrous tissue around the major fragments may preserve vascularity and stability. A bridging cancellous graft placed after meticulous preparation of the proximal and distal fracture fragments (decorticating, petaling, fish scaling, or drilling) should lead to union of the fracture. When reduction is necessary to improve alignment, fragments are mobilized while preserving as much soft-tissue attachments as possible; medullary canals are debrided of fibrous tissue and reestablished to aid in medullary osteogenesis; rounded fracture ends are resected to maximize bone contact.

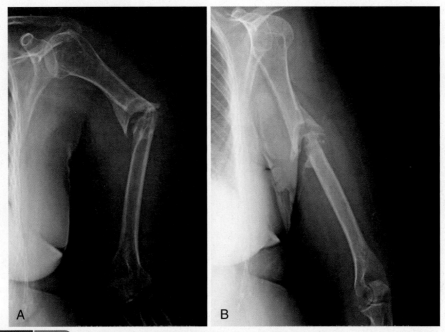

FIGURE 7.6   **A** and **B**, Synovial pseudoarthrosis of the humerus.

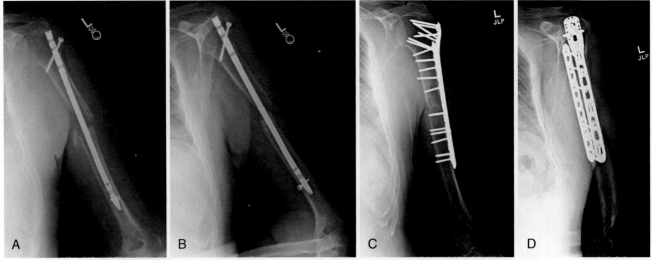

FIGURE 7.7   Treatment of humeral nonunion with plating. **A** and **B**, Radiographs of humeral nonunion after intramedullary nailing. **C** and **D**, After treatment of humeral nonunion with nail removal, plating, and bone grafting.

DECORTICATION

TECHNIQUE 7.1

- Incise the periosteum longitudinally approximately 4 cm proximal and distal to the nonunion site.
- Using a sharp osteotome, elevate "scales" of bone with care to keep them attached to overlying periosteum (Fig 7.8A). Homan retractors are useful to retract the osteoperiosteal layer as decortication continues.
- Decorticate over approximately two thirds of the bone circumference, but avoid decortication directly under the area of anticipated plate placement.

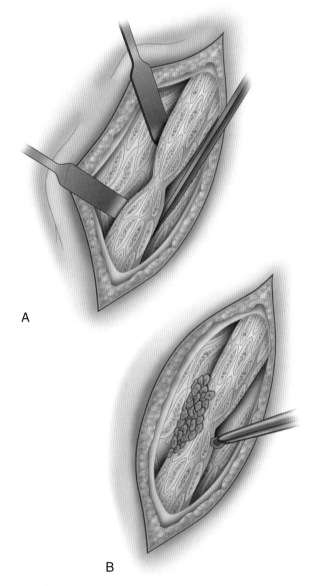

A

B

FIGURE 7.8 Decortication and grafting. **A,** Method of decortication. **B,** Insertion of autogenous cancellous graft (see text). **SEE TECHNIQUE 7.1.**

BONE GRAFTING

Bone grafting has been a staple of nonunion treatment for many years and is still used in most atrophic nonunions and many oligotrophic nonunions. Bone grafting is reserved for rare cases of hypertrophic nonunions because these usually do not need a biologic stimulus. Numerous techniques have been described throughout the years. Many, now mainly historical techniques, such as Boyd's dual onlay graft, Nicoll's cancellous insert graft, and Gill's massive sliding graft, have been illustrated in previous editions of this book.

Autogenous cancellous bone grafting remains a mainstay of nonunion treatment. Unfortunately, autogenous cancellous bone grafts are limited in quantity and can be associated with significant donor site morbidity. The osteoconductive, osteoinductive, and osteogenic properties of autogenous cancellous bone make it ideal for nonstructural grafting; it remains the standard against which other alternatives are compared. Autogenous cancellous grafts are obtained most frequently from the ilium (anterior or posterior iliac crest), proximal tibia, or distal femur. While mesenchymal stem cells derived from bone marrow do undergo negative age-related changes, a recent clinical study suggests no difference in the success of treatment of nonunions using iliac crest bone grafting in geriatric and nongeriatric patients. Allogenic bone for grafting can be used when the source of fresh autogenous bone is inadequate or inaccessible but usually serves as a graft extender. Clinical and experimental data show that the osteogenic properties of allogenic bone are inferior to the osteogenic properties of autogenous bone. When mixed with autogenous bone or perhaps even host bone marrow aspirate (BMA), cancellous allograft can be used in nonstructural applications with excellent results. Techniques of autogenous cancellous harvest are outlined in other chapter.

A more recent technique involves obtaining autogenous graft from the intramedullary canals of long bones (femur and tibia). The reamer-irrigator-aspirator (RIA, Synthes, Paoli, PA) has been found to obtain large quantities of graft that qualitatively compares favorably to iliac crest autograft. The advantages and risks of the RIA technique are described in chapter 1.

For structural applications, autologous cortical grafts, except from the fibula, are now rarely used because of donor site morbidity. Autologous tricortical iliac crest grafts can be used to fill defects in the forearm and clavicle. Autologous vascularized and nonvascularized (Fig. 7.9; Technique 7.2) fibular grafts are options for large defects in the upper extremity, particularly of the radius and ulna. Donor site morbidity is a consideration when obtaining an autogenous fibular graft. In adults, nonvascularized fibular grafts do not sufficiently hypertrophy, and vascularized fibular grafts do not hypertrophy quickly enough to be useful in lower extremity osseous defects. Distraction osteogenesis and the Masquelet technique are therefore better options for treating large lower extremity osseous defects. Frozen or freeze-dried cortical allografts provide structural strength, but their osteogenic properties are limited.

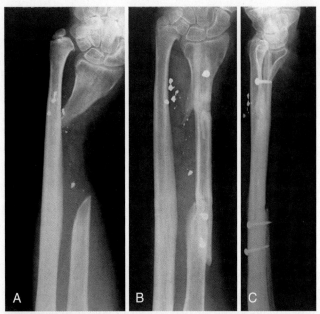

FIGURE 7.9 Avascular fibular autograft. Bridging of bone defect with whole fibular autograft or whole fibular transplant. **A,** Defect in radius was caused by shotgun wound. **B** and **C,** Ten months after defect was spanned by whole fibular autograft, patient had 25% range of motion in wrist, 50% pronation and supination, and 80% use of fingers. **SEE TECHNIQUE 7.2.**

FIBULAR AUTOGRAFT (NONVASCULARIZED)

TECHNIQUE 7.2

- Through an appropriate incision, expose the proximal and distal fragments of the nonunion, resect all sclerotic or nonviable bone, and square the ends with a rongeur.
- With a drill or a curet, ream out the medullary canals of both the fragments.
- Apply traction to the extremity and determine the maximal length that can be restored.
- Harvest a fibular autograft long enough to bridge the full defect and to overlap the fragments of the host bone far enough to permit stable fixation.
- Step-cut the transplant at both ends. Make its intact middle part the exact size of the defect to be bridged. Preserve the step-cut pieces from each end.
- With an osteotome, flatten the fragments of the nonunion to receive the step-cut ends of the fibular autograft.
- Fit the fibular autograft into the defect and fix it to both fragments with screws.
- Utilize remaining bone preserved from the step-cutting and place around the junctions of the fibular autograft and host bone; alternatively, cancellous autograft can be harvested and placed at the junctions (Fig. 7.8B).
- It may be impossible to apply one end of the fibula as a step-cut onlay because one host fragment is too short; the fibular autograft can then be inserted into the medullary canal at this end and applied as an onlay at the other.

- Consider protecting the fibular autograft by adding a small fragment plate to neutralize the construct while the graft incorporates.

POSTOPERATIVE CARE The postoperative care is similar to that after routine grafting, but more time is necessary for complete revascularization of the transplant. Although the ends of the fragments may be united with the transplant, strength is not restored until the entire graft has been revascularized. Consequently, support must be continued for an extended time to prevent a fracture of the fibula; preferably, a removable support or one with joints that allow active and passive motions is used.

INTRAMEDULLARY FIBULAR STRUT ALLOGRAFT (HUMERUS)

Intramedullary fibular strut allografts have been used successfully in the humerus (Fig. 7.10). Intramedullary strut allografts have the benefit of less soft-tissue dissection associated with insertion than extramedullary strut allografts.

TECHNIQUE 7.3

(WILLIS ET AL.)
- Choose an approach to the humerus that makes the most sense based on the location of fracture or previous intervention.
- Expose and mobilize the nonunion site.
- Debride devitalized bone and perform shortening as necessary to optimize bone contact.
- Open the medullary canal both proximally and distally using rongeurs, curets, and increasing diameter drill bits.
- Fashion a fibular allograft with a high-speed burr.
- The length of the allograft should be at least three to four times the diameter of the humerus at the nonunion site.
- Place the allograft within the canal of one fragment. The graft should be able to move freely and is placed initially almost entirely in this one fragment.
- Provisionally reduce the humerus. Using a bone clamp move the allograft across the nonunion site into the other fragment.
- Stabilize the nonunion beginning on one side with a large fragment plate: dynamic compression plate (DCP), limited contact dynamic compression plate (LC-DCP), or locking compression plate (LCP).
- Compress across the nonunion site using an articulating tensioning device, Verbrugge forceps, or other clamp as space allows.
- A minimum of one screw on each side of the nonunion should be placed through the allograft.
- Complete the construct by placing additional screws.

CERAMICS

Ceramics (hydroxyapatite, calcium phosphate, calcium sulfate, or some combination) have osteoconductive properties

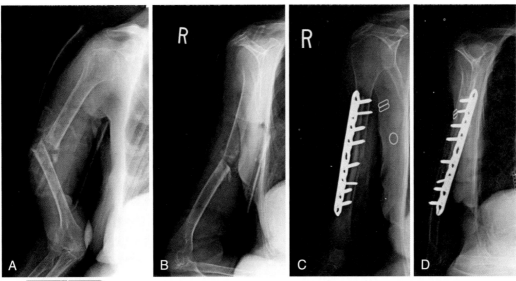

FIGURE 7.10 Intramedullary fibular strut allograft. **A** and **B,** Radiographs of humeral nonunion after conservative treatment. **C** and **D,** After treatment with fibular strut allograft and plating. **SEE TECHNIQUE 7.3.**

and avoid problems with donor site morbidity. Their role in treatment of nonunions is not completely defined, but they probably are best used as delivery devices (antibiotics) or bone graft extenders.

STABILIZATION OF FRAGMENTS

Satisfactory stabilization of fracture fragments is imperative to achieve successful results in the treatment of nonunions. One must carefully analyze the potential mechanical etiologies related to the nonunion and make sure that prior mistakes are not repeated. Adequate stabilization can be obtained with plating, intramedullary nails, or external fixation.

■ PLATING

Plating (Fig. 7.11) in the treatment of nonunions, as in acute fractures, should provide sufficient stability for fracture healing. The plating technique and choice of plate depend on the type of nonunion, the condition of the soft tissues and bone, the size and position of the bone fragments, and the size of the bony defect. Plating without bone grafting usually is adequate for hypertrophic nonunions if the bone is not osteoporotic and the fragments are large enough for secure screw fixation. Plating typically is performed with a compression technique, but it may be performed with a neutralization technique if lag screws were successfully placed across the nonunion. Bridge plating or wave plating also can be used.

■ INTRAMEDULLARY NAILING

Intramedullary nailing is very useful in nonunions of long bones, such as the tibia or femur (Fig. 7.12). However, intramedullary nailing, particularly exchange nailing, is not the best option for humeral nonunion. If alignment is acceptable or closed reduction can be obtained, the procedure can be performed without opening the fracture site. Bone grafting usually is not required. If necessary, long bone intramedullary reaming can generate a large amount of corticocancellous graft material that can be easily harvested with a RIA system with little increased morbidity. When an open

technique is required, usually only limited exposure and dissection are required. Early weight bearing is possible, and the effects of prolonged non–weight bearing may be minimized. A relative contraindication for intramedullary nailing is current infection; however, intramedullary nailing can be successful for infected nonunions once the infection has been eradicated.

A newer type of intramedullary nail, a magnetic compression nail (Precise, NuVasive, San Diego, CA), is being used with increasing frequency in the treatment of nonunions. This nail allows sustained compression at the nonunion site. Early results from this device have been positive in the treatment of humeral, tibial, and femoral nonunions. As with many new devices, comparative studies with standard treatments evaluating clinical results and cost implications have not yet been published.

■ EXTERNAL FIXATION

Circular fine wire fixation, such as the Ilizarov fixator, is a labor-intensive, but very effective, tool in the treatment of nonunions. It is especially useful in nonunions associated with infection, osseous defects, and deformity. The Taylor Spatial Frame is a more contemporary circular fine-wire fixator that relies on computer software to assist in deformity correction (Fig. 7.13). An advantage of external fixation is that it is relatively noninvasive and does not disturb soft tissues surrounding the nonunion. Other advantages are its ability to correct deformity and provide stable fixation. Similar to intramedullary nailing, early weight bearing is possible, and the effects of prolonged non–weight bearing may be minimized.

ARTHROPLASTY

Advances in arthroplasty techniques in the treatment of degenerative conditions have led to many of these techniques being used in some patients with a nonunion. Arthroplasty is an option for certain nonunions of the proximal (Fig. 7.14) and distal humerus and the proximal and distal femur that may not be best served with plating, intramedullary nailing, or external

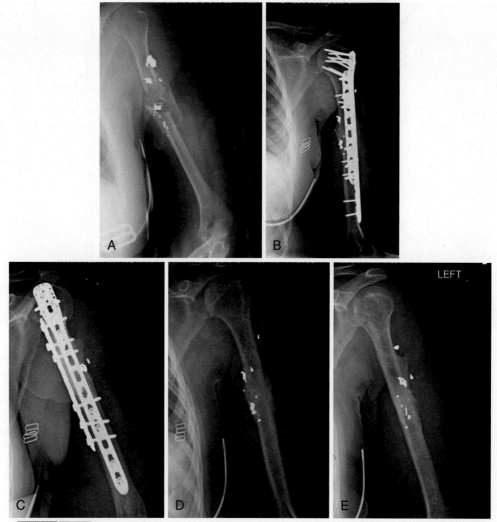

FIGURE 7.11 Plating in treatment of nonunion. **A,** Humeral nonunion after conservative treatment. **B** and **C,** Radiographs demonstrating union of humerus after plating and bone grafting. **D** and **E,** After implant removal.

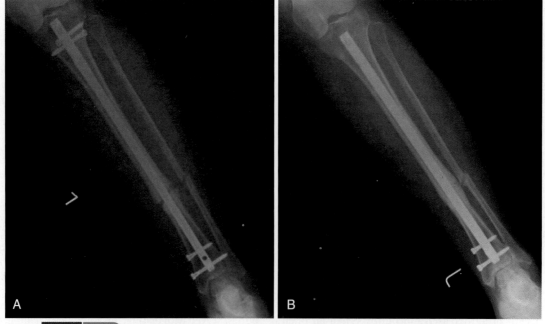

FIGURE 7.12 Intramedullary nailing in treatment of nonunion. **A,** Radiograph of tibial nonunion after intramedullary nailing. **B,** Union of tibia after exchange intramedullary nailing.

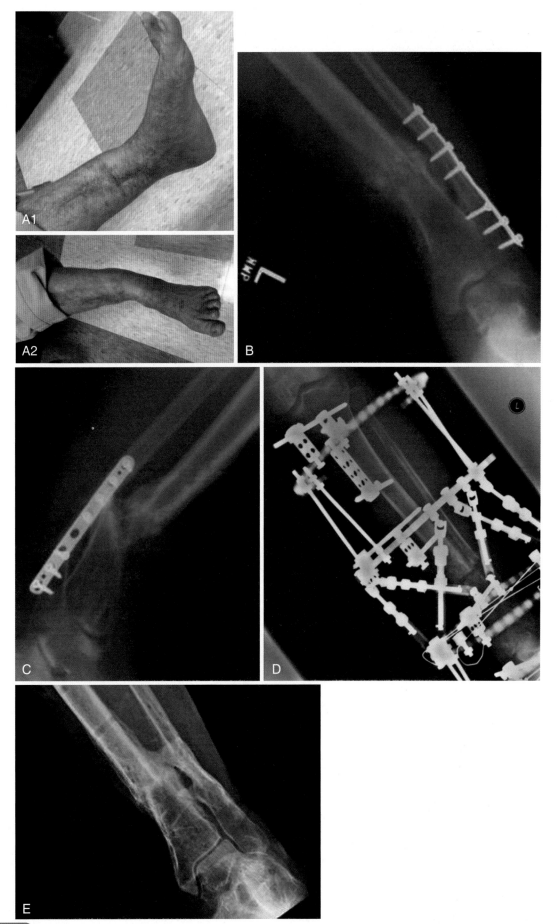

FIGURE 7.13 External fixation in treatment of nonunion. **A,** Clinical photos illustrating deformity and compromised soft tissues associated with tibial nonunion. **B and C,** Radiographs of tibial nonunion after initial fixation and subsequent tibial plate removal. **D,** After remaining implants removal and placement of circular fixator. **E,** Union after treatment with circular fixator.

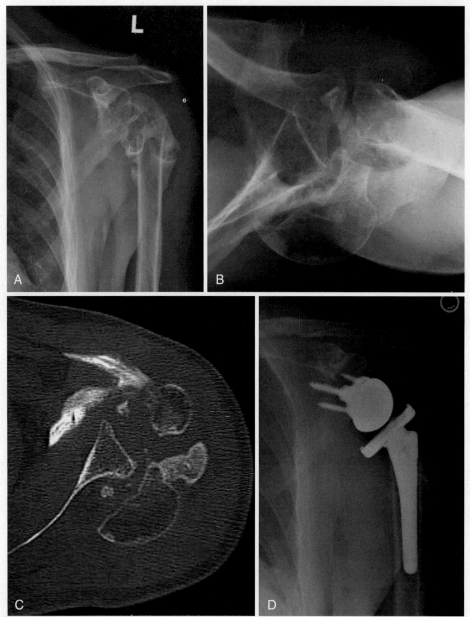

FIGURE 7.14   Arthroplasty in treatment of nonunion. **A** and **B**, Radiographs of proximal humeral nonunion. **C**, Computed tomography of proximal humeral nonunion. **D**, After treatment with reverse total shoulder arthroplasty.

fixation. Fixation in these areas may be limited by osteoporosis or short segments. Infection would obviously need to be eradicated before an attempt at arthroplasty is made. A benefit to arthroplasty is potential early weight bearing, which may help in the patient's overall functional recovery.

AMPUTATION

The function of a limb with a properly fitted prosthesis after amputation often is better than a painful extremity with limited usefulness. Amputation should not be viewed as a failure of treatment. An amputation should be considered a reconstructive procedure (Fig. 7.15). Amputation typically is the most reliable nonunion surgery. To proceed with amputation or further intervention in an attempt to obtain union is always a decision that involves the patient. The patient should

be encouraged to speak with as many individuals experienced in traumatic reconstruction as possible. Every alternative should be explored and explained to the patient for his or her final decision. The patient also must consider many factors not immediately surgical in nature, such as the length of hospitalization and the economic hardships involved in the alternatives.

The surgeon is likely to recommend amputation under the following circumstances:
1. When a reconstruction has failed
2. When a proposed plan of reconstruction would likely result in less satisfactory function than amputation and a properly fitted prosthesis
3. When the danger of major operations outweighs the anticipated benefit

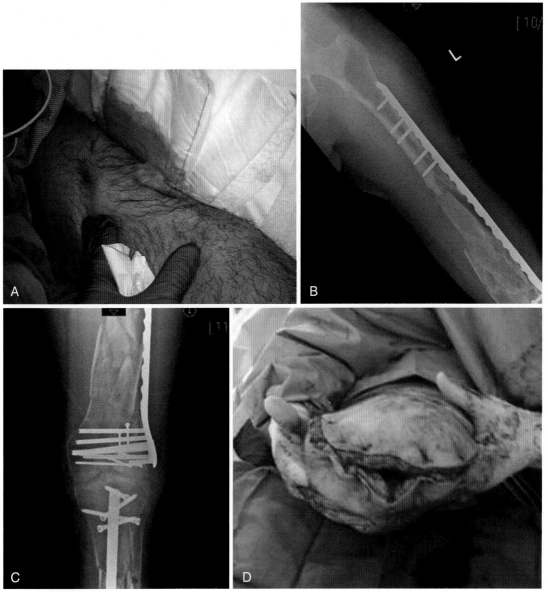

FIGURE 7.15 Amputation in treatment of nonunion. **A,** Clinical photo showing gross purulence associated with infected distal femoral nonunion. **B** and **C,** Radiographs of distal femoral nonunion. **D,** Clinical photo during above-knee amputation.

4. When the damaged part, such as a finger, cannot be well enough restored to prevent its interfering with the function of the extremity as a whole
5. When reconstruction is impossible

LOW-INTENSITY ULTRASOUND

Xavier and Duarte in Brazil first reported the successful use of low-intensity ultrasound to heal nonunions in humans in 1983. Before their report, several studies suggested that the stimulation of bone ends by ultrasound in animals would accelerate or enhance bone healing. Some studies showed increases in cellular activity at osteotomy sites and increases in mineralization of the bone and metabolic activity. It has been theorized that ultrasound stimulation promotes bone healing because it stimulates the genes involved in inflammation and bone regeneration. Another theory suggests that ultrasound increases blood flow through dilation of capillaries and enhancement of angiogenesis, increasing the flow of nutrients to the fracture site. Some studies have suggested that chondrocyte stimulation is enhanced by ultrasound, which leads to an increase in enchondral bone formation. A large meta-analysis reported a success rate of more than 80% with LIPUS for the treatment of nonunion. Interestingly, this study also suggested that LIPUS was twice as effective in hypertrophic nonunions compared with atrophic nonunions. LIPUS seems to be a reasonable, noninvasive treatment for fractures in which healing is delayed or at risk for nonunion. LIPUS also appears to be an option for nonunions in patients who are high risk for surgery.

ELECTRICAL AND ELECTROMAGNETIC STIMULATION

Improvements in electrical and electromagnetic bone growth stimulators continue to progress. External electrical stimulation is especially advantageous in infected nonunion management or when surgical intervention is contraindicated. Four electrical and electromagnetic methods are available for the treatment of nonunions (direct current, capacitive coupling, pulsed electromagnetic field, combined magnetic fields). These methods can be invasive (direct current), requiring the implantation of electrodes, and time-consuming. Use of capacitive coupling and pulsed electromagnetic field stimulation require 8 to 24 hours of use per day, and compliance may be an issue.

EXTRACORPOREAL SHOCK-WAVE THERAPY

Extracorporeal shock-wave therapy is another nonoperative option for nonunion treatment. Although there appear to be more contraindications with this method of fracture augmentation compared with ultrasound and electrical and electromagnetic stimulation, the efficacy in treatment of nonunions has been reported to be above 75% with just one treatment.

FACTORS COMPLICATING NONUNION

Nonunions may be complicated by infection, deformity, shortening, and segmental bone loss.

INFECTION

Considerable judgment is required to treat infected nonunions. Even when infection is not suspected based on the preoperative laboratory workup, intraoperative cultures should be obtained in every nonunion that has initially been managed with surgical treatment. Patients with "surprise positive cultures" (unexpected positive intraoperative cultures after negative preoperative workup) have a much lower incidence of successful nonunion treatment in terms of both union and recurrent infection. Classically, two entirely different approaches of treatment have been employed most often for this difficult problem. The first is the *conventional*, or *classic*, method used for many decades. The second is the *active* method. One or the other of these methods can be performed wholly or in part, depending on the circumstances in a given patient and the judgment of the surgeon. The two are described separately here, but the surgeon often uses parts of each in a single patient. The Ilizarov method is another method of treating infected nonunions that has similarities to the conventional and the active methods. The status of bone involvement (medullary, superficial, localized, and diffuse) and host competency help the surgeon decide on the potential healing of infected bone. The gold standard for diagnosis of infection has been multiple direct cultures of the fracture site (not the skin or sinus tract). A report, however, has questioned the sensitivity of cultures in the diagnosis of infection in nonunion treatment. The diagnosis of infection is discussed more in other chapter.

■ CONVENTIONAL TREATMENT

The objectives of the conventional method are to convert an infected and draining nonunion into one that has not drained for several months and to promote healing of the nonunion by bone grafting. This method of treatment often requires a prolonged period of time and many potential operations.

Debridement is performed with removal of all foreign, infected, or devitalized materials to provide a vascular bed. Providing some element of stabilization is considered at this point with appropriate coverage provided by the plastic surgery team. Infections can be controlled more easily when robust, highly vascular soft tissue is used to cover the fracture, especially with infected nonunions of the tibia. External fixation may initially be most appropriate. Antibiotics are used systemically and are based on intraoperative cultures. Bone grafting is deferred until the soft tissues have completely healed and become stabilized. In some patients, the fracture may unite and bone grafting becomes unnecessary.

When the clinical signs of infection have subsided, the soft tissues over the bone are good, and when nonunion persists, bone grafting is considered. There may never be a perfect time to graft the nonunion because whether an infection has been completely eradicated or is merely quiescent cannot be determined for sure, but a time must be selected or conventional treatment abandoned. The character and duration of the infection, the time of the last drainage, and the general condition of the extremity all must be considered.

When an infection has been active chiefly in the soft tissues or around sequestra, the risk of reactivating it by surgery is much less than when it has involved the cortex and medullary canal. When the infection has been prolonged and destructive, all the surrounding structures are presumed to have been deeply penetrated, and a dormant infection is likely. Bacteria can lie dormant for years, only to become active again after surgery or some other trauma. This danger is inherent in the treatment of infected nonunions and must be accepted. The use of antibiotics before and after surgery has reduced the danger because they can often control an infection within the limits of a vascular area, but they cannot be expected to sterilize an avascular area that they cannot penetrate. Reconstructive operations usually should be delayed until at least 6 months after all signs of infection have disappeared.

Controlling infection before attempting bone grafting always has been a sound clinical principle in the conventional treatment of nonunions. There are exceptions to this principle, however, especially in the tibia. Successful bone grafting in tibial nonunions, even in the presence of draining sinuses, has been reported. In sequestration or gross infection, the bone is saucerized through an anterior approach, the incision is closed or the wound is covered, and the infection is treated with antibiotics.

In treating the tibial nonunion itself, the anterior aspect of the tibia is avoided because the draining sinuses and poor skin usually are located here. The tibia is traditionally approached posterolaterally. The posterior aspect of the tibia (or the tibia and fibula) is decorticated proximal and distal to the nonunion. The entire area is grafted with autogenous cancellous iliac crest. The nonunion itself is not exposed; it is hoped that the grafted area will not communicate directly with the infected area.

■ ACTIVE TREATMENT

The objective of the active method is to obtain bony union early and shorten the period of convalescence and preserve motion in the adjacent joints. Judet and Patel and Weber and Cech described this method, and much of the following is taken from their reports.

The first step is restoration of bony continuity. This takes absolute priority over treatment of the infection. The nonunion is exposed through the old scar and sinuses. The ends of the fragments are decorticated subperiosteally, forming many small osteoperiosteal fragments; any grafts that become detached are discarded. Next, all devitalized and infected bone and soft tissues are removed. Then the fragments are aligned and stabilized, usually by an external fixation device. Compression is applied across the nonunion if possible. Autogenous cancellous bone grafts can be inserted. Internal fixation with a plate is used only when drainage has ceased, and then the approach is away from the area of old drainage, or when no other method of fixation is possible and the infection is mild. When the fracture already has been firmly fixed with a plate or intramedullary nail, the fixation is not disturbed, and the operation is done as described except decortication is omitted when an intramedullary nail has been used. The wound is then closed, and systemic antibiotics are administered based on intraoperative cultures.

If necessary for union, a second decortication with or without the addition of autogenous cancellous graft is performed. After the nonunion has healed, any residual sequestra are removed, and split-thickness skin grafts are applied to any remaining defect in the skin. Satisfactory results have been reported with this method of treatment with or without cancellous grafts, with success rates ranging from 83% to 98%.

■ POLYMETHYL METHACRYLATE ANTIBIOTIC BEADS

Antibiotic-impregnated polymethyl methacrylate (PMMA) beads can be used to treat infected nonunions. Thonse and Conway found that Palacos (Zimmer, Warsaw, IN) cement was superior in elution to Simplex (Stryker, Mahwah, NJ). Heat-stable antibiotics, such as tobramycin and gentamicin, can be mixed with PMMA and used locally to achieve 200 times the antibiotic concentration achieved with intravenous administration. The use of antibiotic-impregnated PMMA beads in conjunction with debridement in the management of infected nonunions was shown in one study to be more effective in treatment than systemic antibiotics. Placement of a PMMA spacer is another option that has the ability to provide some stability in an osseous defect situation. The body's reaction to PMMA beads or a spacer leaves a bioactive membrane, *Masquelet membrane* (Fig. 7.16). The use of cancellous bone graft to deliver antibiotics to infected nonunion sites has been described in a limited number of patients with satisfactory results; however, the optimal ratio of antibiotic to cancellous graft is not known.

DEFORMITY, SHORTENING, AND SEGMENTAL BONE LOSS
■ ILIZAROV METHOD

According to Ilizarov, to eliminate infection and obtain union, vascularity must be increased. Three basic modes of application exist for the Ilizarov frame: (1) monofocal, (2) bifocal, and (3) trifocal (Box 7.1). The Ilizarov frame allows multiple modes of treatment, including compression, distraction, lengthening, and bone transport. In the Ilizarov approach, vascularity is increased by corticotomy and application of a circular external fixator. Although infected

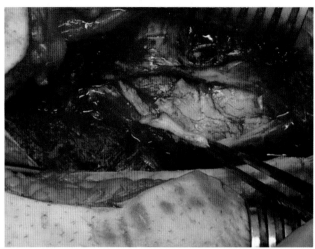

FIGURE 7.16 Masquelet technique. Clinical photo showing membrane formed around polymethyl methacrylate spacer.

BOX 7.1

Modes of Treatment With Circular External Fixation

Monofocal
- Compression
- Sequential distraction-compression
- Distraction
- Sequential compression-distraction

Bifocal
- Compression-distraction lengthening
- Distraction-compression transport (bone transport)

Trifocal
- Various combinations

---

nonunions frequently have been successfully treated without debridement, some authors recommend open debridement to remove necrotic and infected segments, followed by bone transport into the region and soft-tissue coverage. One study advocated segmental excision of the nonunion site followed by distraction osteogenesis. Catagni recommended compression for hypertrophic nonunions with minimal infection and no sequestered bone to increase formation of repair callus and vascularity. Monofocal compression also can be used for infected hypertrophic nonunions with deformity. For atrophic nonunions with diffuse infection or sequestered bone, open resection of the infected segment is performed and bifocal compression is used. If skin quality is poor, the bone is stabilized with the external fixator after resection of necrotic bone. When skin conditions improve and the infection has regressed, corticotomy is performed and bifocal compression (Fig. 7.17) is applied.

Combinations of several of the methods described for infection can be used for treatment of the separate components of a complex nonunion, but the Ilizarov method allows simultaneous treatment of all components, including

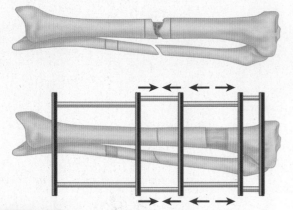

FIGURE 7.17 Bifocal treatment with Ilizarov fixator after debridement of necrotic bone and corticotomy.

angular, rotary, and translational deformities; shortening; and segmental bone loss. Although dramatic results can be obtained, this method is technically demanding and requires thorough training and experience. It is recommended that only surgeons knowledgeable in its biologic basis and the techniques required for its safe, effective application use this method.

Deformities of 10 or 15 degrees can be corrected immediately by frame application; larger deformities should be corrected gradually. Hypertrophic nonunions can be treated by gradual correction of the deformity, followed by compression. Atrophic nonunions with shortening can be treated by compression at the nonunion accompanied by a corticotomy in the metaphyseal region of the same bone and gradual lengthening through the corticotomy. Ilizarov showed marked hypervascularity of the limb and bone after corticotomy and gradual distraction. Conceivably, the corticotomy provides some of the same biologic benefits as a bone graft. Nonunions with segmental bone loss can be treated by corticotomy and gradual transport of a fragment. The leading edge of this transported fragment frequently requires bone grafting at the time of arrival to the principal fragment. Depending on the size of the defect and the anticipated time to docking, bone grafting can be performed at the time of frame application or just before docking if necessary.

The sequence of correction of complex deformities, including shortening, rotation, angulation, translation, or a combination of one or more, varies, but generally length must be reestablished before other deformities can be corrected. It sometimes is difficult to evaluate malrotation when major angulation and translation deformities are present, and its correction may be best left until last. If rotation is corrected last, the frame must be mounted carefully, with the bone centered within the frame; otherwise, translation of one bone fragment would occur during final rotation and would require an additional step of translation to reestablish full apposition. Some complex deformities can be resolved with a simple hinge, and some simple deformities can be best treated with more complex constructs. The maximal velocity of bone or soft-tissue elongation is approximately 1 mm every 24 hours. During the correction of a complex deformity, the structures being lengthened most may change during the treatment, and the structure at greatest risk during any phase of treatment must be appreciated and monitored.

The Ilizarov frame can be constructed to provide compression or distraction or both, and careful preoperative evaluation of deformities allows assembly of the proper frame before surgery. True anteroposterior and lateral views of the limb are necessary. The importance of these orthogonal views cannot be overemphasized because these films are used to characterize completely the plane and extent of angulation and translational deformities and, along with preoperative sizing of the limb, to determine correct ring diameter to allow frame construction before surgery. First, the plane and the extent of deformity in this plane are determined. Next, the type of hinge or linkage frame necessary to correct the deformity (e.g., opening wedge or distraction hinge) is determined. Finally, the exact locations of the hinges or linkages are determined.

■ TAYLOR SPATIAL FRAME METHOD

The more contemporary Taylor Spatial Frame fine-wire external fixator has simplified deformity correction through utilization of a computer program. The computer program and virtual hinge assists with determining the exact position of wires or pins, hinges, and linkages in the correction of complex deformities. Struts can be manipulated daily by patients until deformity is corrected. This fixator is especially useful in treating hypertrophic nonunions and nonunions associated with infection, soft-tissue compromise, bone loss, and leg-length discrepancy. Several authors have reported its successful use in infected and noninfected nonunions. Application of the spatial frame is described in chapter 2.

■ CORTICOTOMY

To lengthen a bone, a special type of percutaneous osteotomy, or corticotomy, is required (Fig. 7.18). Paley et al. described an effective method of corticotomy in which a 5 mm osteotome is used to cut the medial and lateral cortices, extending subperiosteally into the posteromedial and posterolateral corners. The osteotome is turned 90 degrees to wedge open the incomplete osteotomy and to crack the remaining posterior cortex. This maneuver is repeated with the osteotome in the posteromedial and posterolateral cortices. The fixator rings above and below can be rotated to complete the osteoclasis. The corticotomy preserves the soft tissue inside and outside the bone (the periosteal and endosteal circulation). On a radiograph, the corticotomy should appear as a nondisplaced osteotomy.

NONUNION OF SPECIFIC BONES
TIBIA

The tibia is the most common bone to proceed to nonunion. Nonunions are estimated to occur after 2% to 15% of all tibial fractures. The development of a tibial nonunion is closely related to the type and severity of the injury, but other factors may play a role, such as degree of fracture comminution, open fracture, degree of soft-tissue injury, medical comorbidities, and patient lifestyle (tobacco use, nutritional status, medications). Subsequent complications, such as infection or compartment syndrome, also may affect healing of the fracture. Infection rates as high as 24% have been reported in open tibial fractures. In a large recent study of open tibial fractures, deep infection was found to be an overwhelming predictor of fracture nonunion (OR = 12.75). Other predictors of nonunion

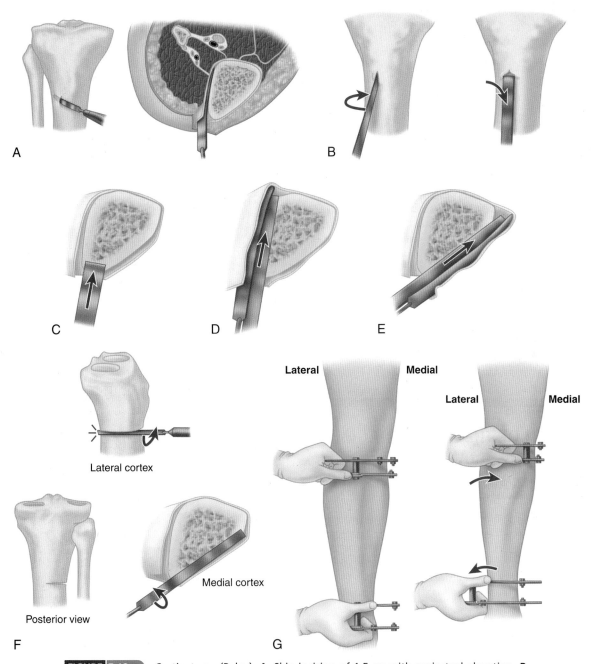

FIGURE 7.18 Corticotomy (Paley). **A,** Skin incision of 1.5 cm with periosteal elevation. **B,** Osteotome is twisted transversely to cut groove in anterior cortex only. **C,** Anterior groove is cut to, but not through, medullary cavity. **D,** Periosteum is elevated laterally, and lateral cortex is cut with 5-mm osteotome to and through posterolateral corner. **E,** Anteromedial periosteum is elevated, and medial cortex is cut. **F,** Osteotome is twisted 90 degrees in posteromedial cortex to crack it and is inserted in posterolateral cortex and twisted. **G,** Osteoclasis is completed by gentle controlled external rotation of fixator rings.

included soft-tissue wounds (Gustilo and Anderson type IIIA open fractures, OR = 2.49) and smoking (OR = 1.73). Investigators continue to try to identify patient, injury, and treatment factors that may predict subsequent nonunion.

■ MEDIAL MALLEOLUS

A fracture of the medial malleolus occasionally fails to unite, usually after closed treatment. Surgery may be indicated for the few nonunions in which other serious complications of

the fracture, such as posttraumatic arthrosis, are not seen on radiographs. The technique usually includes excision of the nonunion, application of autogenous bone grafts, and internal fixation of the malleolar fragment. When the nonunion is painful, it can be surgically managed in the following ways. When the bone adjacent to the nonunion is sclerotic or has been absorbed, and the proximal part of the malleolus is large enough to preserve the ankle mortise, resecting the ununited distal fragment is preferable to bone grafting (Fig. 7.19).

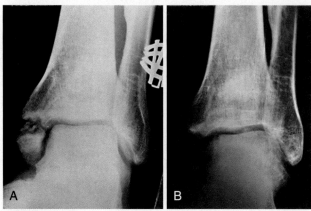

FIGURE 7.19 Resection of medial malleolus. **A,** Persistent nonunion of medial malleolus. **B,** Seven years after resection of medial malleolus. Ankle is stable, although mild arthritic changes are becoming evident. This is maximal amount of medial malleolus that can be removed if stability of ankle is to be preserved.

When the fragment is larger, bone grafting and stabilization usually are indicated. Bicortical lag screws probably are indicated; they have been shown to be more stable and less likely to be associated with nonunion.

RESECTION OF THE DISTAL FRAGMENT OF THE MEDIAL MALLEOLUS

TECHNIQUE 7.4

- Make a medial longitudinal incision 5 cm long over the malleolus and divide the periosteum and deltoid ligament in line with the skin incision.
- By sharp and blunt subperiosteal dissection, but without cutting the periosteum in a transverse direction or cutting the posterior tibial tendon, remove the distal fragment of the malleolus.
- Close the wound.

POSTOPERATIVE CARE Weight bearing in a three-dimensional boot or ankle corset can be started in 3 weeks.

SLIDING GRAFT

TECHNIQUE 7.5

- Expose the nonunion through an anteromedial curved incision 10 cm long.
- Reflect the periosteum anteriorly and posteriorly and remove the fibrous tissue from the nonunion; freshen the ends of the fragments, but remove no bone from their deeper edges; with a curet, carefully hollow out the distal fragment.

- Beginning at the nonunion and using a motor saw, remove a graft about 4 cm long and 1 cm wide from the proximal fragment.
- Displace the graft distally across the nonunion into the distal fragment; hold this fragment in its normal position, and transfix the fragments and the graft with a screw (Fig. 7.20).
- Check the position of the graft, the screw, and the fragments with radiographs.
- Place cancellous chips around the graft and close the wound.

POSTOPERATIVE CARE A short leg splint is initially applied. At 2 weeks, the sutures are removed and a walking cast is applied. Partial weight bearing is allowed during the next 2 weeks, and full weight bearing is allowed thereafter. The cast is discarded when radiographs show that the nonunion has healed, usually at 8 to 10 weeks.

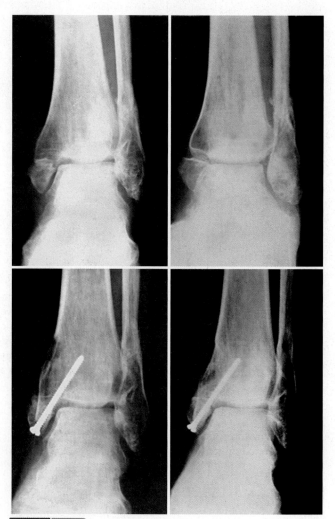

FIGURE 7.20 Nonunion of medial malleolus treated by sliding graft. **SEE TECHNIQUE 7.5.**

BONE GRAFT OF MEDIAL MALLEOLAR NONUNION

TECHNIQUE 7.6   *Figure 7.21*

(BANKS)

- Expose the nonunion through a medial longitudinal incision. The incision should be long enough to obtain graft. Prepare the nonunion site and place the hardware.
- Debride the nonunion surfaces by removing devitalized bone. A wedge-shaped defect with its apex at the articular surface of the ankle may be created; avoid damage to the articular surface.
- Restore the fragment to its anatomic position and provisionally stabilize.
- Make a window in the tibial metaphysis at the proximal end of the wound by removing a square piece of cortex. Alternatively, a round trephine can be used to access the tibial metaphysis.
- Fill the defect at the nonunion with cancellous bone obtained through the square or round window.
- Stabilize the medial malleolus with 3.5-mm cortical screws. Screws should be bicortical and can be placed in lag fashion if they are not used as position screws, if the defect is not excessively large, and when overcompression is not a concern.
- Replace the piece of cortex and close the wound.

POSTOPERATIVE CARE Postoperative care is the same as in Technique 7.5.

■ TIBIAL SHAFT

Many treatment methods have been highly successful in obtaining union of tibial shaft nonunions. Because the tibia is a weight-bearing bone and its length and alignment are important to function of the knee and ankle, simply obtaining union may not result in a satisfactorily functioning extremity. Plating, intramedullary nails, and external fixation can all be successful if chosen for the appropriate situation.

The technique selected depends on many variables, including whether the nonunion is hypervascular or avascular, and whether or not the alignment of the fragments is satisfactory. For nonunions with bony defects, infection, or deformity, an extensive procedure may be necessary. In hypertrophic nonunions, the bone ends have the capacity to unite. In this situation, fixation with a compression plate, intramedullary nail, or external fixator usually is all that is necessary. Bone grafting usually is not necessary for hypertrophic nonunions. Bone grafting is considered in hypertrophic nonunions if an open approach is being performed for reduction or stabilization (plating), a defect exists, or the patient is a poor host (has several risk factors for nonunion). In atrophic nonunions, fixation is supplemented by decortication of the bone ends and bone grafting. In recalcitrant cases of tibial nonunion, debate still exists on optimal treatment.

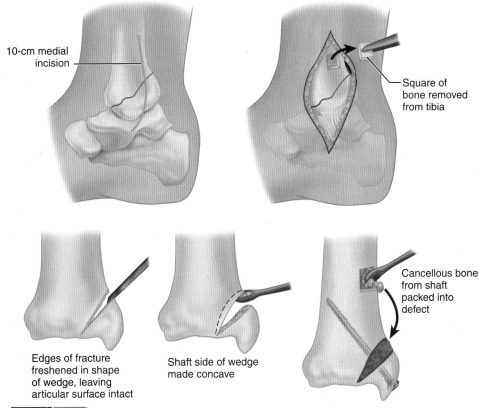

10-cm medial incision

Square of bone removed from tibia

Edges of fracture freshened in shape of wedge, leaving articular surface intact

Shaft side of wedge made concave

Cancellous bone from shaft packed into defect

FIGURE 7.21   Technique for grafting nonunion of medial malleolus. **SEE TECHNIQUE 7.6.**

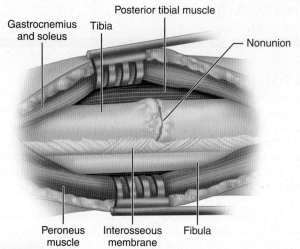

FIGURE 7.22 Posterolateral bone grafting. Tibia and fibula have been approached posterolaterally. Posterior aspect of tibia (or tibia and fibula) is decorticated and grafted with autogenous iliac bone (not shown). **SEE TECHNIQUE 7.7.**

▌ROLE OF THE FIBULA IN TIBIAL NONUNION TREATMENT

In all tibial nonunions, the fibula must be considered. When the fibula and the tibia are fractured, the fibula almost always heals first and may become a load-sharing structure that decreases axial loading across the tibia. When it is not fractured, the fibula may prevent close apposition of tibial fragments and prevent full axial loading of the tibia. Partial fibulectomy has been described in the past to promote union. We almost never perform fibulectomy in isolation, but it is important to evaluate the fibula, particularly in patients with tibial nonunions for which dynamization or exchange nailing is being considered.

The surgical technique is simple, and complications are rare. The full-thickness segment removed from the fibula should be approximately 2 to 2.5 cm long; removal of a smaller segment may allow healing of the fibula before the tibia unites.

POSTEROLATERAL BONE GRAFTING

Posterolateral bone grafting (Fig. 7.22) has most often been recommended for tibial fractures with infection or extensive bone loss. Reported rates of union after this procedure range from 80% to 97%, with an average time to union of 5 to 7 months. A more contemporary study reported a 74% union rate in the treatment of established tibial nonunions with posterolateral bone grafting using various combinations of bone graft. The main advantage of posterolateral grafting is that it is a single, nondestructive procedure with a high degree of success.

TECHNIQUE 7.7

- With the patient prone and a tourniquet inflated, make a longitudinal incision 1 to 2 cm posterior to the fibula and parallel to it. The length of the incision is determined by the amount of exposure required; expose 4 to 5 cm of bone above and below the nonunion.

- Divide the subcutaneous tissue and identify the deep fascial plane between the gastrocnemius-soleus muscle group and the peroneal muscles.
- Reflect the fibular origins of the flexor hallucis longus and soleus subperiosteally and reflect the origin of the posterior tibial muscle from the interosseous membrane.
- Expose the tibia by dissecting the remainder of the posterior tibial origin and the flexor hallucis longus from the fibula.
- Retract the posterior tibial artery and vein medially in the muscle mass, but do not expose them. Do not disturb the fibrous union or penetrate the interosseous membrane.
- With an osteotome, decorticate the tibia proximal and distal to the nonunion site.
- Next decorticate the medial side of the fibula.
- Obtain and place autogenous cancellous graft over the bone surfaces and interosseous membrane.
- Confirm graft placement with a radiograph made with the leg in 30 degrees of internal rotation.
- Loosely reapproximate the deep fascia over the muscle with a few interrupted sutures to hold the graft in place and close the skin in a routine manner. Apply a compression dressing.

POSTOPERATIVE CARE The dressing is removed when swelling subsides, usually within 3 days. Weight bearing depends on the stability of the nonunion and the fixation in place. For most patients, weight bearing is initially restricted and advanced with signs of consolidation.

ANTERIOR CENTRAL BONE GRAFTING

Ryzewicz et al. reported a retrospective review of 24 patients who had central bone grafting using the interval between the anterior compartment (extensor digitorum) and the lateral compartment (peroneals), creating a synostosis between the fibula and tibia. Fracture union occurred in 23 of 24 patients, and this approach was found to promote faster healing and require fewer operations than the posterolateral approach. Anterior central bone grafting (Fig. 7.23) may be a good alternative based on prior incisions and when soft tissues preclude a posterolateral approach.

TECHNIQUE 7.8

- Place the patient supine. Prepare the extremity and the ipsilateral iliac crest and apply a tourniquet.
- Make an incision just anterior to the fibula and develop the plane between the peroneal tendons and extensor digitorum. Take care to avoid the superficial peroneal nerve.
- Bluntly elevate the anterior compartment off the intermuscular septum.
- Elevate the periosteum of the tibia anteriorly as the tibia is decorticated proximally and distally to the nonunion site.

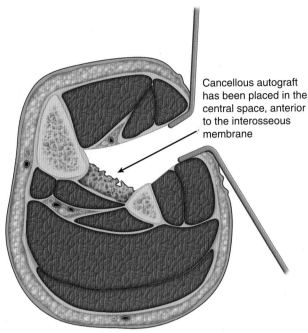

Cancellous autograft has been placed in the central space, anterior to the interosseous membrane

FIGURE 7.23 Central bone grafting. Cross-section through the mid-tibia, showing interval for approach and fibular decortication. Osteoperiosteal flap has been raised posteriorly off lateral aspect of the tibia, and the interosseous membrane is detached from the fibula, creating central space for graft placement. (Redrawn from Ryzewicz M, Morgan SJ, Lindford E, et al: Central bone graft for nonunion of fractures of the tibia. A retrospective series, *J Bone Joint Surg* 91B:522, 2009. Copyright British Editorial Society of Bone and Joint Surgery.)

- Continue the decortication posteriorly, detaching the interosseous membrane and elevating it as one layer with the periosteum from the tibia.
- Decorticate the medial aspect of the fibula.
- Leave the nonunion site undisturbed unless sequestrum or synovial pseudoarthrosis is present or alignment needs to be corrected.
- Place autogenous cancellous graft in this "central space."

POSTOPERATIVE CARE Postoperative care is the same as for posterolateral bone grafting.

PERCUTANEOUS BONE MARROW INJECTION

The use of bone marrow in treating a variety of diseases has led to its consideration in the treatment of nonunions. Percutaneous bone marrow injection is a simpler method of performing autologous bone grafting with less morbidity than standard techniques. It is not, however, a substitute for adequate stabilization of the fracture. Casting, bracing, plating, intramedullary nailing, or external fixation should be used if needed for stability. An 80% union rate has been reported using marrow injections. This technique has been shown to be the most effective in the treatment of delayed union to prevent the development of nonunion. Kettunen et al. found

percutaneous bone marrow grafting to be as effective as open techniques, with many advantages over open procedures, including decreased donor site morbidity and decreased cost.

Hernigou et al. reported that hematopoietic stem cells are pluripotent and are able to differentiate; however, the number of pluripotent cells is decreased in patients who use tobacco, alcohol, or steroids. Spinning down the donor sample will increase the number of pluripotent cells (located in the buffy coat). They have demonstrated that success is dependent on the number (concentration) of stem cells available for injection.

Brinker et al. reported a series evaluating unprocessed or nonconcentrated marrow (BMA) grafting in the treatment of distal tibial metadiaphyseal delayed unions or nonunions initially treated with plate fixation. Patients were treated with concentrated marrow grafting and nine of 11 healed. The role of concentrating the marrow (bone marrow aspirate concentrate, BMAC) is still not completely defined. Concentration certainly adds time and expense to the procedure. There are currently no large randomized trials evaluating the efficacy of BMA and BMAC.

TECHNIQUE 7.9

(CONNOLLY ET AL., BRINKER ET AL.)

- Aspiration and injection usually are performed with the patient under general anesthesia.
- Place the patient prone on the operating table (also may be performed supine with harvest from the anterior iliac crest).
- Make a small (2 to 3 mm) incision over the crest and insert a marrow aspiration needle (11 to 16 gauge) into multiple areas of the iliac crest.
- Obtain a minimum of 40 mL up to 150 mL of marrow. Marrow should be harvested in small (<5 mL) aliquots.
- To avoid clotting, use a heparinized syringe.
- Under image intensification, localize placement of an 18-gauge needle; first use a needle to create microtrauma at the nonunion site; then inject marrow into the site of nonunion or delayed union. The bone or muscle junction also can be injected as this area tends to be well vascularized.

■ INTERNAL FIXATION

The advantages of internal fixation are its ability to correct deformity and to promote healing of a nonunion. The use of internal fixation and the device used depend on the amount of deformity to be corrected, the size of the fracture gap, the presence of infection, and the vascularity of the fragments.

Closed reamed intramedullary nailing is the procedure of choice for tibial nonunions. Appropriate locking, static or dynamic or none, continues to be debated, as does the role of an associated fibular osteotomy or fibulectomy. If performed closed, the periosteal blood supply is increased, and reaming may add graft to the endosteal surface and stimulate union. Caution should be exercised if external fixation was initially used for a significant length of time. An increased risk of infection after the use of external fixation pins longer than 2 weeks has been reported with reamed intramedullary nailing. One also should consider other treatment options if the fracture was previously infected or use methods (antibiotic nail) to eradicate the infection before proceeding with intramedullary nailing. Closed intramedullary nailing is best reserved for treatment of closed fractures treated by casting and in which the medullary canals are still in close proximity. Otherwise, in the case of a bayonet alignment, open reduction of the fracture is necessary. Reamed nailing can be used in most diaphyseal nonunions with high union rates. The technique of reamed intramedullary nailing is covered in chapter 1. When using intramedullary nailing for nonunions, a pseudarthrosis chisel should be available.

Tibial fractures that do not unite after initial intramedullary nailing may be treated successfully with exchange intramedullary nailing. Swanson et al. reported a 98% union rate with exchange intramedullary nailing for aseptic tibial nonunions that had at least 50% cortical apposition. All types of aseptic nonunions were included: atrophic (four) and oligotrophic (25). A fibulectomy was performed in four patients when the fibula was thought to be preventing maximal axial compression at the tibial nonunion site (Fig. 7.24). Four patients underwent subsequent dynamization. Union for the entire cohort occurred at a mean of 4.8 months. Endocrine or metabolic abnormalities were sought and treated per the senior author's protocol.

TIBIAL EXCHANGE NAILING

TECHNIQUE 7.10

- Position the patient supine.
- Remove the current intramedullary nail.
- Perform fibulectomy if indicated (if fibula appears to be experiencing axial stress and "bowing" as seen on preoperative radiographs); remove approximately 2 to 2.5 cm of fibula.
- Correct any tibial deformity.
- Progressively ream the tibia in an attempt to place an intramedullary nail that is at least 2 mm larger than previous nail.

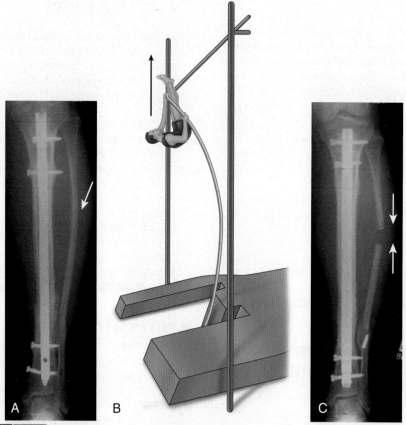

FIGURE 7.24 Fibulectomy with exchange intramedullary nailing. **A,** Anteroposterior radiograph of a nonunion 64 months after tibial fracture and 26 months after exchange nailing. Distal interlocking screws are broken, and fibula has significant bowing *(arrow)*. **B,** Axial loading was sufficient to break the screws. The bowed fibula may have provided a distraction force similar to force a bowed pole provides to lift a pole vaulter, which may have contributed to failure of the fracture to heal. **C,** Six months after exchange nailing and partial fibulectomy the patient had a solid bony union. Arrows indicate that partial fibulectomy removed the distraction force, allowing compression across the construct. (From Swanson EA, Garrard EC, O'Connor DP, Brinker MR: Results of a systematic approach to exchange nailing for the treatment of aseptic tibial nonunions, *J Orthop Trauma* 29:28, 2015.)

- Ream 1 mm larger than the intramedullary nail to be placed. (Consider placing a different manufacturer's intramedullary nail to get novel interlocking options.)
- Lock the nail distally first.
- Compress across the nonunion site by either "backslapping" a distally locked nail or using the nail's internal compression device.
- In proximal or distal fractures, add additional interlocking screws in the short segment as the nail allows. Also consider placing blocking screws around the nail to increase stability in the short proximal or distal segment.

POSTOPERATIVE CARE Ankle and knee motion are allowed immediately after surgery. Ambulation is allowed, and full weight bearing is encouraged.

▌PLATE FIXATION

Plate fixation, particularly applied to the tension (convex) side, may achieve healing through compression in tibial nonunions. Satisfactory reduction is achieved, and the fracture is sufficiently exposed so that a bone graft can be added. Care should be taken, however, not to devascularize the tibia any more than necessary. Interfragmentary lag screw technique should be used when possible. The plate should be contoured to the bone, rather than excessively debriding bone and callus to allow placement of a straight plate. Infection and implant failure remain the largest risks associated with this technique, and it probably should not be performed in patients who have had infections. Locking plates or blade plates can be useful when the distal fragment is very small or osteoporotic.

▪ EXTERNAL FIXATION

Because of the frequency of infection in tibial nonunions, external fixation is an attractive option. The application of an external fixator does not disturb the fracture site because it is applied percutaneously. External fixation allows correction of multiple deformities and bridging of large fracture gaps by bone transport techniques. Healing has been reported in 94% of nonunions with the use of dynamic axial external fixation, and high rates of union have been reported with the Ilizarov method, especially in complicated nonunions, and the Taylor Spatial Frame with bone grafting when necessary.

CT is helpful to determine if a tibial nonunion is present. It is imperative to distinguish a delayed union, which may proceed to union without surgical intervention, from a nonunion, which requires surgical intervention to achieve healing. CT allows excellent evaluation of fracture healing, even when implants are present; however, it does have a low specificity (62%). The orthopaedic surgeon must keep in mind that even if the CT scan shows a nonunion, the fracture may be united. Sometimes this cannot be confirmed except by surgical exploration. Data from the Study to Prospectively Evaluate Reamed Intramedullary Nails in Patients with Tibial Fractures (SPRINT) trial suggest that many tibial fractures proceed to union without intervention, if given enough time. Investigation continues into identifying factors that may predict nonunion and allow appropriate early treatment.

DISTAL TIBIA

Multiple techniques have been used for the treatment of distal tibial nonunions. Haller et al. reported union in seven of eight tibial pilon fractures treated with implant removal and intramedullary nailing. Bone grafting was not used. Arvesen et al. reported a 94% union rate using the Taylor Spatial Frame circular fine-wire fixator for treatment of distal tibial nonunions, many associated with preoperative bony defects, deformity, and infection. Compression followed by distraction was used, and 70% of cases did not require bone grafting.

FIBULA
▪ LATERAL MALLEOLUS

Nonunions of the lateral malleolus rarely require treatment. Nonunions without displacement usually are asymptomatic; some eventually heal spontaneously. Nonunion of the lateral malleolus in itself has not been found to cause traumatic arthritis or other abnormality and does not influence the final result in fractures of the ankle.

▪ FIBULAR SHAFT

Nonunion of the fibula in adults is rare. Asymptomatic or low-demand patients can be treated with observation. However, symptomatic nonunions can be treated with internal fixation and bone grafting or partial fibulectomy (2 to 5 cm) centered over the nonunion site. A diagnostic injection of bupivacaine (Marcaine) under fluoroscopic guidance can be helpful in determining which patients will benefit from further intervention for their nonunion.

PATELLA

Nonunions of the patella are rare. When a fresh fracture is comminuted, excision of the fragments eliminates the possibility of nonunion; when it is not comminuted, internal fixation usually results in union.

When the fragments of a nonunion are in good position, fibrous union may be compatible with satisfactory function; the severity of later arthritic changes is about proportional to the irregularity of the articular surface of the patella. When the fragments are separated, partial or complete excision of the patella, as for a fresh fracture, is indicated.

FEMUR

Femoral nonunions are much less common than in past years. Since the use of modern intramedullary nailing techniques, healing rates now approach 99% with closed shaft fractures. Since acute femoral fractures are almost exclusively treated operatively, nonunions of the femur invariably have some implant in place.

▪ SUPRACONDYLAR AREA

Although rates of union approach 99% with intramedullary nailing of closed femoral shaft fractures, nonunion does continue to be a problem with supracondylar femoral fractures. When a nonunion occurs in the supracondylar area, union can be difficult to obtain. A short supracondylar fragment can be treated by one of the following methods.

1. *Plating* (distal femoral locking plate or blade plate). A medial plate may be added through a subvastus approach if significant comminution is present. Bone grafting is used in atrophic or oligotrophic nonunions.

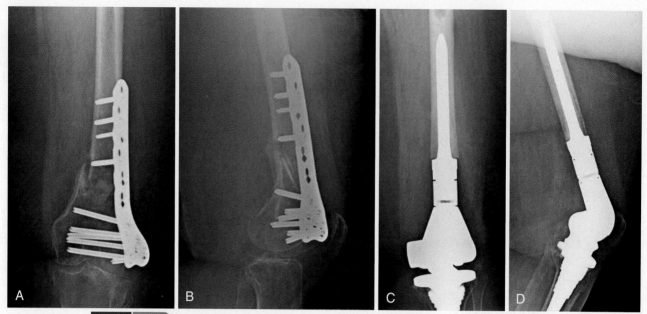

FIGURE 7.25 Treatment of distal femoral nonunion with arthroplasty. **A** and **B,** Radiographs of distal femoral nonunion. **C** and **D,** After treatment with arthroplasty using a tumor prosthesis.

2. *Intramedullary nailing.* Technology has increased our ability to obtain stable distal fixation with retrograde nails. Intramedullary nailing also can be used in combination with plating. Bone grafting is used in atrophic or oligotrophic nonunions. Attum et al. reported 100% union rate in a small series of 10 distal femoral nonunions treated with a combination of intramedullary nailing, plating, and bone grafting using the RIA system.

3. *Arthroplasty.* Alternatively, total knee replacement with a tumor prosthesis (Fig. 7.25) can be considered. A potential advantage of arthroplasty is immediate weight bearing.

External fixation has a limited role in the treatment of supracondylar femoral nonunions.

▪ FEMORAL SHAFT

Risk factors for femoral nonunion after intramedullary nailing are open fracture, delay in weight bearing, and tobacco use. The treatment of nonunion with a statically locked intramedullary nail in place is either bone grafting in situ, dynamization of the nail by locking screw removal, or exchange nailing. Swanson et al. recently reported a 100% union rate with exchange nailing (Fig. 7.26) of aseptic femoral nonunions. Seven of 50 fractures were atrophic. All exchange nails placed were at least 2 mm larger in diameter than the index nail. Six exchange nails were placed in the opposite direction (antegrade or retrograde) from the index procedure to increase stability in the smaller proximal or distal segment. Fourteen of 50 patients underwent dynamization, and endocrine or metabolic abnormalities were sought and treated per the senior author's protocol. The average time to union was 7 months. The technique for intramedullary nailing of femoral shaft fractures can be found in chapter 2. A recent systematic review compared dynamization to exchange intramedullary nailing for delayed unions and nonunions of the femur. Exchange intramedullary nailing was superior to dynamization for established nonunions (84.8% vs

66.4% success); however, dynamization was believed to have a role in delayed unions, with a success rate of 81.8%. No difference was found when comparing statically and dynamically locked exchange nailing.

Some authors have reported that exchange intramedullary nailing may not be as effective in metaphyseal regions of the femur. Another technique that may be useful in the distal femoral metaphysis or metadiaphysis is plating over an intramedullary nail (Fig. 7.27). This technique can be combined with bone grafting as appropriate. Lai et al. recently reported 92.3% success for plating around an intramedullary nail (compared with 60% with exchange nailing) in nonisthmic atrophic femoral nonunions. Decortication and bone grafting (ICBG) also were done in the plating group.

Historically, Judet and Patel reported excellent results of 195 nonunions of the femoral shaft treated with decortication and internal fixation with plates and screws or intramedullary nails. When possible, compression was applied across the nonunion. In only a few was the decortication unsatisfactory, and in these, iliac cancellous or tibial cortical grafts were added. Union failed after one operation in only nine patients (4.6%).

Defects of the femur can be treated by intramedullary nailing with autogenous bone grafting. Protected weight bearing is continued until the graft has incorporated sufficiently. Johnson and Urist reported excellent results with the use of a human bone morphogenetic protein and allograft for reconstruction of femoral nonunions. Large gaps also can be treated with the Ilizarov external fixator and internal bone transport. This technique may be most advantageous after thorough debridement when a septic nonunion is present.

▪ PERITROCHANTERIC AND SUBTROCHANTERIC REGION

Nonunions of the subtrochanteric region typically are treated by intramedullary nailing or blade plating. The technique for intramedullary nailing of subtrochanteric nonunions can be

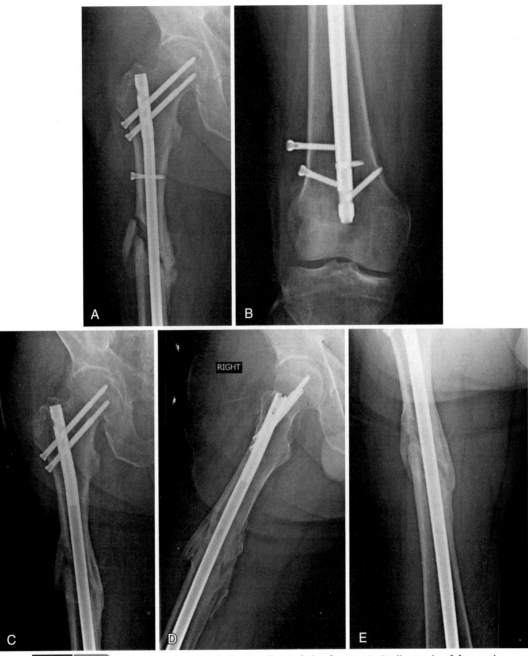

FIGURE 7.26 Exchange intramedullary nailing of the femur. **A,** Radiograph of femoral nonunion. **B,** Distal interlocking screw breakage. **C** to **E,** Treatment with exchange nailing.

found in chapter 2. Alignment should be corrected as necessary. Bone grafting should be performed based on the nature of the nonunion. A blade plate (Fig. 7.28) also can be successful when used in this area along with bone grafting when indicated.

■ FEMORAL NECK

Unfortunately, nonunions of the femoral neck still occur with an incidence of approximately 10% to 30%. Factors contributing to nonunions of the femoral neck include impaired vascularity, inaccurate reduction, and loss of fixation. CT with reconstructions can be helpful in the diagnosis of nonunion.

The appropriate treatment depends on several factors, including the physiologic age of the patient, the viability of the femoral head, the amount of resorption of the femoral neck, and the duration of the nonunion. Most patients with femoral nonunions are older than 60 years of age and may be poor surgical candidates, and extreme osteoporosis decreases the efficiency of any internal fixation. In long-standing nonunions, muscle contractures may prevent adequate lengthening, and the acetabular cartilage may be severely damaged.

Success has been reported with free vascularized fibular bone grafting in nonunions of femoral neck fractures in patients younger than 50 years old. Significant preoperative femoral neck shortening has been shown to compromise the success of this technique. Vascularized fibular grafting is highly demanding, however, and is done only at a few select centers throughout the United States.

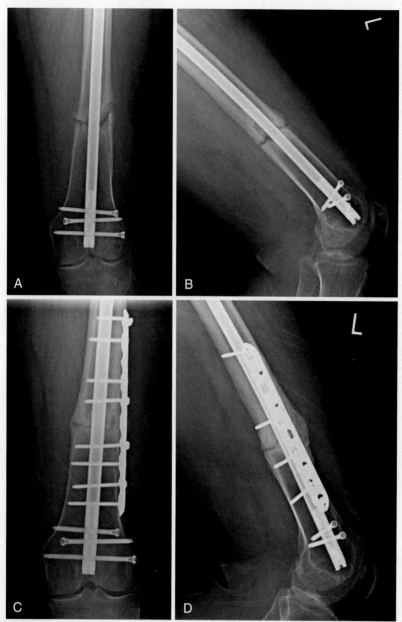

FIGURE 7.27 Treatment of femoral metadiaphyseal nonunion with combination of nailing and plating. **A** and **B,** Radiographs of femoral metadiaphyseal nonunion after retrograde intramedullary nailing. **C** and **D,** After treatment with combination of nailing, plating, and bone grafting.

In general, operations for nonunions of the femoral neck can be grouped into three general classes: (1) valgus intertrochanteric osteotomy, (2) prosthetic replacement (hemiarthroplasty or total hip arthroplasty), and (3) arthrodesis.

Some general guidelines are as follows:

1. In adults younger than 60 years old, nonunions in which the femoral head is viable can be treated by valgus intertrochanteric osteotomy (Fig. 7.29). This technique converts shear forces to compressive forces at the fracture site.
2. In children and in young adults, nonunions in which the femoral head is not viable may be treated with an arthrodesis. With increasing frequency, young adults are being treated with arthroplasty.
3. In adults, nonunions in which the femoral head is not viable can be treated with arthroplasty or arthrodesis, depending on the circumstances in the given patient and on the experience and preference of the surgeon. Arthrodesis, although being performed less and less frequently, still has some role in patients who are not candidates for arthroplasty. In patients older than 60 years, nonunions, regardless of the viability of the femoral head, usually are treated with a hemiarthroplasty or a total hip arthroplasty.

OSTEOTOMY

Valgus intertrochanteric osteotomy is an angulation osteotomy made through or just distal to the lesser trochanter. The mechanical advantage of an angulation osteotomy is that shear forces at the fracture are converted to compression forces, hopefully promoting an environment for union. A serious disadvantage is produced, however, if the femoral

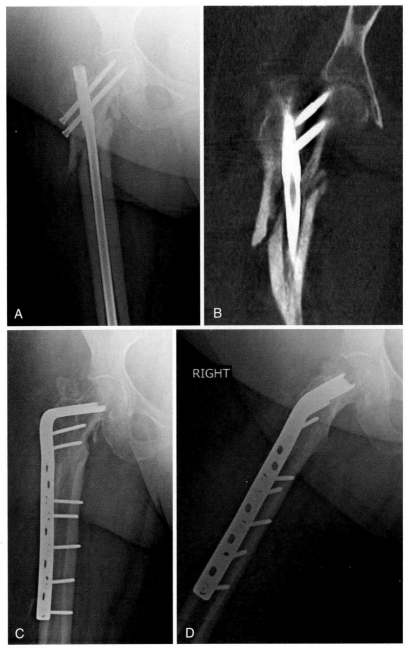

FIGURE 7.28 Treatment of reverse obliquity intertrochanteric femoral nonunion with blade plate. **A,** Radiograph of proximal femoral nonunion. **B,** Computed tomography of proximal femoral nonunion. **C** and **D,** Radiographs at union after valgus intertrochanteric osteotomy and fixation with blade plate.

neck and head are placed in an extreme valgus position. This position must be avoided if possible because it shortens the lever arm between the trochanter, on which the abductor muscles pull, and the head, which is the fulcrum. In 1935 Pauwels called attention to this mechanical problem. A valgus position must be used sometimes to obtain union of a non-united fracture of the femoral neck or to hasten healing of a comminuted trochanteric fracture; however, it predisposes to degenerative changes in a normal head and probably to osteo-necrosis when the neck has been fractured. Additionally, decreased functional results because of a persistent limp in patients treated with a valgus osteotomy have been reported.

Valgus intertrochanteric osteotomy is appropriate for nonunited fractures of the femoral neck in which the head is viable and the neck is fairly well preserved in children and in adults until approximately 60 years of age. The results of such an osteotomy are about proportional to the mechanical and physiologic status of the nonunion before surgery. When the head is viable and union occurs, function usually approaches normal, but the more abnormal the bony structure, the more unfavorable the result. Many excellent or good results at 1 year after surgery have been downgraded at 3 to 5 years because of progressive arthritic changes or osteonecrosis. Valgus intertrochanteric osteotomy is stabilized with a blade

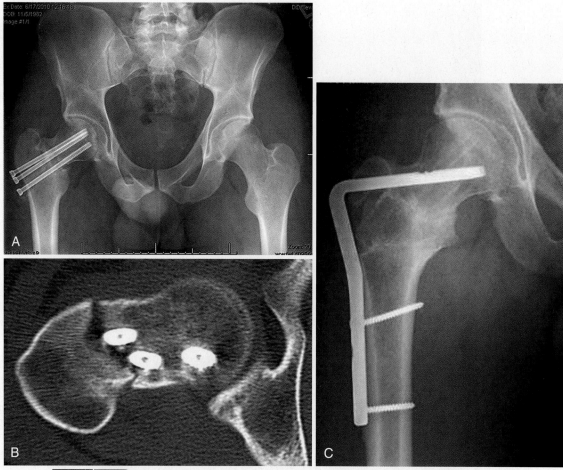

FIGURE **7.29** Nonunion of femoral neck fracture. Anteroposterior radiograph **(A)** and CT **(B)**. **C,** Union after fixation with a blade plate. (Courtesy of David Templeman, MD, Minneapolis, MN.)

plate or compression hip screw. Several reports have reported union rates of 86% to 97%. Yuan et al. reported excellent results with valgus intertrochanteric osteotomy in 32 patients with the goal of reducing Pauwels' angle to ≤50 degrees (generally, 20 degree osteotomy for preoperative Pauwels' angle less than 70 degrees; 30 degree osteotomy for Pauwels' angle of more than 70 degrees). Despite a more modest correction of Pauwels' angle (mean of 24 degrees), 97% of nonunions healed. Unfortunately, 22% of patients developed osteonecrosis, with three of seven proceeding to total hip arthroplasty. This more modest correction also may be of benefit to arthroplasty surgeons in patients who subsequently require total hip arthroplasty for degenerative changes or osteonecrosis.

PROSTHETIC REPLACEMENT

The indications for prosthetic replacement for femoral neck nonunions are still are not precisely defined. Usually a prosthesis should be reserved for older patients; rarely should it be used in patients younger than 50 years old and then only for good reason. A prosthesis is now indicated more frequently for acute fractures (see chapter 3) than for treatment of their complications. Prosthetic replacement can be used occasionally, however, in adults younger than 50 to 60 years old after fracture of the femoral neck, with or without union, in which the head is not viable, and an arthrodesis is undesirable. Hemiarthroplasty is not indicated in arthritis of the hip,

either traumatic or primary; rather, total hip arthroplasty or arthrodesis should be used.

Complication rates are higher after treatment of acute femoral neck fractures with arthroplasty. See other chapter for the management of complications after hemiarthroplasty or total hip arthroplasty for femoral neck and intertrochanteric fractures.

ARTHRODESIS

According to Gill, the advantages of an arthrodesis for nonunion of the femoral neck are freedom from pain, stability during weight bearing, and, consequently, a useful extremity. We sometimes recommend arthrodesis in children or adults younger than 50 years old whose work is heavy manual labor or who are not candidates for arthroplasty. Techniques of hip arthrodesis are described in other chapter.

PELVIS AND ACETABULUM

Nonunions and delayed unions of fractures of the pelvis do occur and require treatment (Fig. 7.30). Pennal and Massiah classified nonunions into three main groups according to the direction of the forces that caused them: anteroposterior compression, lateral compression, and vertical shear. The signs and symptoms included one or more of the following: pain, limp, instability, and clinical deformity. Deformity is assessed with anteroposterior pelvic, inlet, and outlet views.

CT of the pelvis can be helpful in diagnosing and planning surgery for a pelvic nonunion. In the sacroiliac area, Pennal and Massiah found that the fractures tended to be of the avascular type, and in the rami, the hypervascular type. Insufficient immobilization was thought to be the cause because the fragments were not adequately reduced or sufficiently stabilized. Twenty-four of their 42 patients were treated nonoperatively, and only five of these patients returned to the same job they had before their injury. Of the 16 patients who had bone grafting and stabilization of the unstable pelvis, all but one achieved solid bony union and returned to work, most returning to the job they had before injury.

Mears and Velyvis reported 79% excellent results and 21% satisfactory results in patients with nonunion treated with bone grafting and realignment procedures. Patients with nonunions, unstable malalignment, and heterotopic ossification had the poorest outcomes. We advocate open reduction and internal fixation with bone grafting for most pelvic nonunions.

Acetabular nonunions were thought to be rare, usually occurring in widely displaced and unreduced acetabular fractures. Of 569 acutely fixed acetabular fractures, Letournel and Judet reported only four nonunions. A nonunion of a displaced transverse pattern (transverse, transverse posterior wall, T-type) might make a subsequent reconstruction (total hip arthroplasty) extremely difficult. More recently, Sagi et al. reported nonunion of the posterior wall in patients undergoing acetabular surgery and being treated with indomethacin for heterotopic ossification prophylaxis. Patients treated with 6 weeks of indomethacin had a 62% incidence of radiographic nonunion (CT scan at 6 months) compared with 19% with placebo. The ramifications of radiographic nonunion of the posterior wall are not completely clear.

CLAVICLE

Nonunion of clavicular fractures has been shown to be much more common than historically thought. Despite the lateral clavicular fracture being the most likely to become a nonunion, it is the midshaft clavicular fracture that is the most common fracture site for nonunion because of its frequency.

Only patients who have sufficient symptoms should be considered for an operation. Symptomatic nonunions of the middle third of the clavicle are treated by plating with consideration given to bone grafting (Fig. 7.31). Often, sufficient local bone is present, and autogenous grafting from a distant donor site may not be necessary. Chen et al. recently reported a 100% union rate in 17 clavicular nonunions treated with

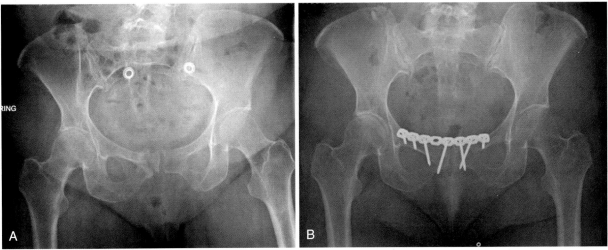

FIGURE 7.30 Treatment of pelvic nonunion (hypertrophic nonunion of parasymphyseal fracture) with plating. **A,** Radiograph of pelvic (parasymphyseal) nonunion. **B,** After treatment with plating.

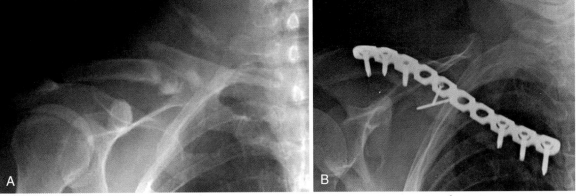

FIGURE 7.31 Treatment of clavicular nonunion with plating and bone grafting. **A,** Radiograph of clavicular nonunion. **B,** After treatment with plating and bone grafting.

plating without bone grafting. Up to 2 cm of shortening was done after resection or preparation of the nonunion site. Although defect size after resection did not correlate with functional outcomes in this small series, shortening may not be appropriate in every patient.

PLATE FIXATION AND BONE GRAFTING OF THE CLAVICLE
TECHNIQUE 7.11

- Make an incision parallel with and just distal to the clavicle. Incise the periosteum and decorticate the clavicle medial and lateral to the nonunion site.
- Plate placement may be superior or anteroinferior. Both approaches have advantages and disadvantages, and there are advocates of both approaches. Use a precontoured clavicular plate that allows at least six cortices of fixation on each side of fracture. Alternatively, a 3.5-mm dynamic compression can be used. Place local bone or autogenous cancellous bone graft around the nonunion and close the wound. Shortening can be considered if the defect after nonunion preparation is not large.

POSTOPERATIVE CARE A shoulder immobilizer or sling is worn for 1 to 2 weeks. Gentle active and pendulum exercises are begun to maintain shoulder mobility. Weight bearing is initiated as the fracture consolidates.

HUMERUS
■ PROXIMAL THIRD

Most often nonunions of the proximal humerus are two-part fractures at the surgical neck (Fig. 7.32). Locking plates sometimes with the use of intramedullary allograft (hypertrophic and oligotrophic nonunions) and autograft (atrophic nonunions),

especially in osteoporotic bone, have been useful. The locking plate is superior to traditional plates in that it is lower profile, demonstrates higher torsional strength and stiffness, and allows for multiple divergent proximal screw placements that provide better fixation in weak bone. Shoulder arthroplasty provides significant reduction in pain with improved motion but is less satisfying than when performed for primary arthritis. Reverse shoulder arthroplasty has also been used successfully in treatment of proximal humeral fracture nonunion in the low-demand elderly patient with a functional deltoid.

■ HUMERAL SHAFT

Nonunions occur in approximately 10% of patients with humeral shaft fractures regardless of the type of treatment. Nonunion is more common in the mid and proximal diaphysis, especially with a spiral or oblique fracture pattern. Gaps may result from distraction, overriding, soft-tissue interposition, or loss of bone. Comminuted fractures may have a disrupted blood supply. The type of nonunion and the age and comorbidities of the patient should be considered in treatment decisions. In most patients, operative treatment is indicated to correct deformity and regain function. However, in elderly patients with osteoporotic bone, diminished function because of a pseudoarthrosis may be preferable to the risks of open reduction and internal fixation. The use of a lightweight orthosis may allow enough function to avoid further treatment.

Most humeral nonunions can be treated by open reduction and compression plating with union rates well above 90%. The use of a fibular allograft in the medullary canal may improve stability and enhance union. Exchange intramedullary nailing of humeral nonunions has not been as successful as in other areas of the body. If the fracture site is opened, adding bone graft is considered. Recent studies have suggested that autogenous cancellous bone grafting may not be routinely necessary in the treatment of humeral nonunion. Lin et al. reported a 100% union rate in 31 atrophic nonunions treated with plating and bone grafting with allograft. Hierholzer et al. reported a 97% union rate with plating and bone grafting with demineralized bone matrix in 32 atrophic nonunions. Willis et al. reported a 95% union rate with plating over an intramedullary strut allograft in 20 patients with atrophic nonunions.

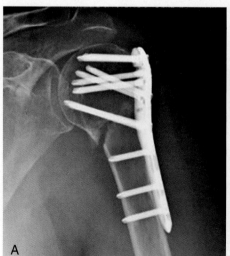
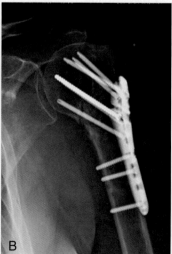
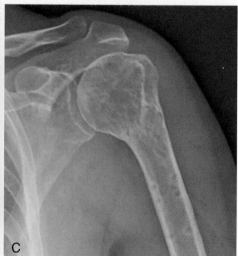

A　　　　　　　　　B　　　　　　　　　C

FIGURE 7.32　　**A,** Proximal humeral nonunion. **B,** After revision plating and bone grafting. **C,** After union and implant removal.

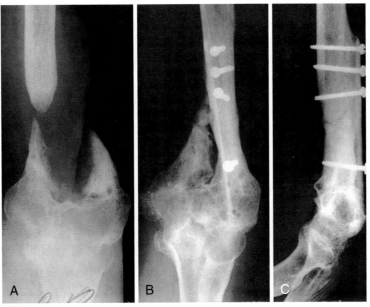

FIGURE 7.33 Treatment of humeral nonunion with avascular fibular autograft (whole fibular transplant). **A,** Large defect in distal metaphysis of humerus after open fracture. **B and C,** Twenty months after bridging of defect by avascular fibular autograft (whole fibular transplant). Cancellous bone was used to bridge expanded portion of metaphysis and shaft.

Treating a defect in the humeral shaft is easier than treating defects in the lower extremity. Shortening through the defect usually is well tolerated, even shortening up to 3 cm. Shortening combined with bone grafting and appropriate stabilization often yields successful results.

A longer defect can be bridged with a fibular transplant (Fig. 7.33); the distal end of the transplant is applied to the condyle that has the longest remaining metaphyseal part, preferably the lateral one. (This distal fragment should be large enough to engage two screws.) The normal metaphyseal expansion is restored with iliac bone. The Ilizarov method of internal bone transplant also can be used for humeral nonunions with bone loss and infection.

■ DISTAL HUMERUS

Poor initial fracture fixation is the major reason for nonunion in the supracondylar area. Many patients treated for distal humeral fracture nonunions can expect union; however, most will have residual morbidity. Those with nonunions extending into the trochlea fare worse than others despite eventual union of the fracture. Internal fixation, bone grafting, release of joint contractures, and ulnar nerve transposition or neurolysis, if ulnar nerve symptoms are present or motion about the elbow is expected to increase, are performed for most distal humeral nonunions. Bone healing takes precedence over motion when attempting to unite a nonunion. Restoration of motion can be treated after union has been achieved with physical therapy, dynamic splints, and capsular releases as needed. Mitsunagase, Bryan, and Linscheid obtained union in 25 of 32 patients treated by open reduction, internal fixation, and bone grafting of the nonunion. Six patients required secondary procedures for repeat bone grafting or revision of the fixation device, seven were treated by total elbow arthroplasty, and two required reoperation for loose humeral components. Union of the fractures resulted in relief of pain and good functional motion of the elbow. Total elbow arthroplasty was considered only as a salvage procedure. For distal humeral nonunions, Sanders and Sackett recommended rigid internal fixation with a plate and screws and a bone graft. Beredjiklian et al. used a free vascularized bone graft in patients with segmental bone loss in nonunions of the distal humerus when total elbow replacement would have a poor outcome, but they reserve this technique for younger patients with segmental bone loss for which conventional fixation and bone grafting are inappropriate. Infected nonunions in this region may be treated with removal of retained implants, debridement of devascularized tissue, capsulectomy, ulnar nerve transposition or neurolysis, bone grafting when appropriate, and application of a ring fixator. Total elbow replacement (linked) has the best outcome when the patient is older than 65 years, has previous arthritic changes, has compromised bone stock that cannot be internally fixed, has low demand on the arm, does not have infection, and has had only one previous operation. Limitations of arthroplasty include lifetime avoidance of repetitive lifting of 2 lb (0.9 kg) or more or one-time lifting of 10 lb (4.5 kg) or more.

PROXIMAL THIRD OF THE ULNA WITH DISLOCATION OF THE RADIAL HEAD

Long-standing nonunions of the proximal third of the ulna often are associated with dislocations of the radial head (Monteggia fracture). In these instances, no attempt is made to reduce the dislocation; instead, the radial head and as much of the neck as necessary are resected (see chapter 6). The nonunion is stabilized with a compression plate or wave plate, and the nonunion is typically bone grafted.

FOREARM BONES
■ BOTH RADIUS AND ULNA

Treatment of nonunions of forearm bones involves removing all sclerotic and devascularized tissue, recannulating the medullary canals with a drill, and, if using a bone graft, decorticating or "fish scaling" the cortices opposite the interosseous membrane. The nonunions can be treated by compression plating or wave plating and cancellous grafting, with care to preserve the interosseous space. The fragments must be carefully aligned and apposed in correct rotary relationship or pronation and supination will be limited. Recreation of the radial bow is essential for a good functional outcome. Limitation of rotation and pain in the distal radioulnar joint occurs if enough difference exists in the length of the two bones.

Defects in the radial head or neck or the distal 3.5 cm of the ulna can be treated by excising the fragment; these fragments are dispensable, and removing them is simpler than grafting. In some instances, prosthetic radial head replacement can be performed that can restore the function of the radial head, eliminate the nonunion, and provide resistance to proximal migration of the radius.

When bony defects are present in both bones, usually any sclerotic bone can be removed and the lengths of the bones can be equalized by resecting the ends of the fragments without too much shortening; plating with grafting is then sufficient. When this procedure would shorten the arm too much, each bone must be treated separately; sometimes the fragments of one bone can be freshened and apposed without too much shortening, and yet the other bone may require a graft to bridge a longer defect or the defect in both bones may be long enough to require bridging. Tricortical grafts can be used, however. Ring et al. reported good results with defects up to 6 cm (mean, 2.2 cm) using cancellous grafting and plating. When using bone graft, care must be taken to graft away from the other forearm bone to prevent iatrogenic synostosis. Good results also have been reported in segmental defects of the radius and ulna treated with free vascularized fibular grafts.

Infected nonunions of the forearm, particularly with bone defects, can be more difficult to treat. They may be managed with debridement of all devitalized tissue, placement of antibiotic beads or a spacer, and subsequent staged plating and bone grafting. Alternatively, bone transport may be considered. Zhang et al. reported a 100% union rate without recurrence of infection in 16 forearm nonunions with an average bone defect of 3.81 cm. The mean time to union was 6.19 months. In rare circumstances, such as an infected nonunion with significant bone loss, creation of a one-bone forearm is a salvage option that can offer satisfactory results.

■ RADIUS OR ULNA ALONE

After fractures of both bones of the forearm when one bone fails to unite and the other unites in an unsatisfactory position, enough bone is resected from the area of the malunion to equalize the length of the bones; the bones are grafted as just described.

When one bone unites in good alignment without shortening or was not fractured, and the other fails to unite, any defect cannot be closed because of splinting by the intact bone. Bridging such a defect is preferable to shortening the normal bone and risking the possibility of a second nonunion. Short defects can be bridged with a compression plate and the space between them filled with iliac bone.

▎ DISTAL END OF THE RADIUS

When the distal fragment of a nonunited distal radial fracture is fairly substantial, the technique for malunited Colles fracture (see chapter 6) can be used; usually, however, the distal

fragment is short and osteoporotic, and bone grafting and internal fixation with plating are indicated. Arthrodesis can be performed as a salvage procedure.

■ PROXIMAL END OF ULNA

Nonunions of the olecranon proximal to the middle of the trochlear notch are not difficult to treat. When there is strong fibrous union, the disability may be only slight, and in middle-aged or elderly patients, surgery may not be justified. If the ununited fragment is less than 50% of the olecranon surface, it can be simply excised, and the distal insertion of the triceps tendon is reattached to the ulna as for some fresh fractures (see chapter 5). For larger proximal fragments, precontoured plating with bone grafting provides appropriate stability for early elbow range of motion. Ring, Jupiter, and Gulotta generally reported excellent or good results in the proximal ulna after autogenous bone grafting and plate fixation

■ DISTAL END OF ULNA

Nonunions of the distal 3.5 cm of the ulna can be treated by resection or by fixation with a 2.7-mm or 3.5-mm compression plate with cancellous bone grafting. Occasionally, nonunion of the distal third of the ulna results in a disability insufficient to warrant surgery.

REFERENCES

INTRODUCTION AND DEFINITIONS

Antonova E, Le TK, Burge R, Mershon J: Tibia shaft fractures: costly burden of nonunions, *BMC Musculoskel Disord* 14:42, 2013.

Brinker MR, Hanus BD, Sen M, O'Connor DP: The devastating effects of tibial nonunion on health-related quality of life, *J Bone Joint Surg* 95A:2170, 2013.

Brinker MR, O'Connor DP: Nonunions: evaluation and treatment. In Browner BD, Jupiter JB, Krettek C, Anderson PA, editors: *Skeletal trauma*, ed 5, Philadelphia, 2015, Elsevier Saunders.

Hak DJ, Fitzpatrick D, Bishop JA, et al.: Delayed union and nonunions: epidemiology, clinical issues, and financial aspects, *Injury* 45S:S3, 2014.

Tay WH, de Steiger R, Richardson M, et al.: Health outcomes of delayed union and nonunion of femoral and tibial shaft fractures, *Injury Int J Care Injured* 45:1653, 2014.

Wichlas F, Tsitsilonis S, Disch AC, et al.: Long-term functional outcome and quality of life after successful surgical treatment of tibial nonunions, *Int Orthop* 39:521, 2015.

ETIOLOGY AND PATHOPHYSIOLOGY

Bottlang M, Doornink J, Lujuan TJ, et al.: Effects of construct stiffness on healing of fractures stabilized with locking plates, *J Bone Joint Surg* 92A(Suppl 2):12, 2010.

Chrastil J, Sampson C, Jones KB, et al.: Postoperative opioid administration inhibits bone healing in an animal model, *Clin Orthop Relat Res* 471:4076, 2013.

Donohue D, Sanders D, Serrano-Riera R, et al.: Ketorolac administered in the recovery room for acute pain management does not affect healing rates of femoral and tibial fractures, *J Orthop Trauma* 30:479, 2016.

Haines N, Kempton LB, Seymour RB, et al.: The effect of a single early high-dose vitamin D supplement on fracture union in patients with hypovitaminosis D: a prospective randomised trial, *Bone Joint Lett J* 99-B:1520, 2017.

Hood MA, Murtha YM, Della Rocca GJ, et al.: Prevalence of low vitamin D levels in patients with orthopedic trauma, *Am J Orthop (Belle Mead NJ)* 45:E522, 2016.

Jeffcoach DR, Sams VG, Lawson CM, et al.: Nonsteroidal anti-inflammatory drugs' impact on nonunion and infection rates in long-bone fractures, *J Trauma Acute Care Surg* 76:779, 2014.

McDonald E, Winters B, Nicholson K, et al.: Effect of postoperative ketorolac administration on bone healing in ankle fracture surgery, *Foot Ankle Int* 39:1135, 2018.

Nino S, Soin SP, Avilucea FR: Vitamin D and metabolic supplementation in orthopedic trauma, *Orthop Clin North Am* 50:171, 2019.

Pearson RG, Clement RG, Edwards KL, et al.: Do smokers have greater risk of delayed and non-union after fracture, osteotomy and arthrodesis? A systematic review with meta-analysis, *BMJ Open* 6:e010303, 2016.

Sprague S, Bhandari M, Devji T, et al.: Prescription of vitamin D to fracture patients: a lack of consensus and evidence, *J Orthop Trauma* 30:e64, 2016.

Weestgeest J, Weber D, Dulai SK, et al.: Factors associated with development of nonunion or delayed healing after an open long bone fracture: a prospective cohort study of 739 subjects, *J Orthop Trauma* 30:149, 2016.

GENERAL TREATMENT

Amorosa LF, Buirs LD, Bexkens R, et al.: A single-stage treatment protocol for presumptive aseptic diaphyseal nonunions: a review of outcomes, *J Orthop Trauma* 27:582, 2013.

Bhattacharyya T, Bouchard KA, Phadke A, et al.: The accuracy of computed tomography for the diagnosis of tibial nonunion, *J Bone Joint Surg* 96A:130, 2014.

Brinker MR, O'Connor DP: Nonunions: evaluation and treatment. In Browner BD, Jupiter JB, Krettek C, Anderson PA, editors: *Skeletal trauma*, ed 5, Philadelphia, 2015, Elsevier Saunders.

Conway J, Mansour J, Kotze K, et al.: Antibiotic cement-coated rods. An effective treatment for long bones and prosthetic joint nonunions, *Bone Joint Lett J* 96B:1349, 2014.

Fragomen AT, Wellman D, Rozbruch SR: The PRECECE magnetic IM compression nail for long bone nonunions: a preliminary report, *Arch Orthop Trauma Surg* 139:1551, 2019.

Lark RK, Lewis JS, Watters TS, Fitch RD: Radiographic outcomes of ring external fixation for malunion and nonunion, *J Surg Orthop Advances* 22:316, 2013.

Stucken C, Olszewski DC, Creevy WR, et al.: Preoperative diagnosis of infection in patients with nonunion, *J Bone Joint Surg* 95A:1409, 2013.

Yadav SS: The use of a free fibular strut as a "biologic intramedullary nail" for the treatment of complex nonunion of long bones, *JBJS Open Access* 3:e0050, 2018.

BONE GRAFTING

Braly Houston L, O'Connor DP, Brinker MR: Percutaneous autologous bone marrow injection in the treatment of distal meta-diaphyseal tibial nonunions and delayed unions, *J Orthop Trauma* 27:527, 2013.

Carlock KD, Hildebrandt KR, Konda SR, et al.: Autogenous iliac crest bone grafting for the treatment of fracture nonunion is equally effecting in elderly and nonelderly patients, *J Am Acad Orthop Surg* 27:696, 2019.

Conway JD: Autografts and nonunions: morbidity with intramedullary bone graft versus iliac crest bone graft, *Orthop Clin North Am* 41:75, 2010.

Dawson J, Kiner D, Gardner 2nd W, et al.: The reamer-irrigator-aspirator as a device for harvesting bone graft compared with iliac crest bone graft: union rates and complications, *J Orthop Trauma* 28:584, 2014.

Desai PP, Bell AJ, Suk M: Treatment of recalcitrant, multiply operated tibial nonunions with the RIA graft and rh-BMP2 using intramedullary nails, *Injury* 41:S69, 2010.

Flierl MA, Smith WR, Mauffrey C, et al.: Outcomes and complications rates of different bone grafting modalities in long bone fracture nonunions: a retrospective cohort study in 182 patients, *J Orthop Surg Res* 8:33, 2013.

Grimsrud C, Raven R, Fothergill AW, Kim HT: The in vitro elution characteristics of antifungal-loaded PMMA bone cement and calcium sulfate bone substitute, *Orthopedics* 34:390, 2011.

Marino JT, Ziran BH: Use of solid and cancellous autologous bone graft for fractures and non-union, *Orthop Clin North Am* 41:15, 2010.

Novotny AJ, Bauer M: Allograft safety: analysis of T106™ terminal sterilization system, Orlando, FL, TissueNet.

Rearick T, Charlton TP, Thordarson D: Effectiveness and complications associated with recombinant human bone morphogenetic protein-2 augmentation of foot and ankle fusions and fracture nonunions, *Foot Ankle Int* 35:783, 2014.

Ricci WM: Principles of nonunion and bone defect treatment. In Tornetta 3rd P, Ricci W, Court-Brown CM, et al.: *Rockwood and Green's fractures in adults*, ed 9, Philadelphia, 2020, Wolters Kluwer.

Sagi HC, Young ML, Gerstenfeld L, et al.: Qualitative and quantitative differences between bone graft obtained from the medullary canal (with a reamer/irrigator/aspirator) and the iliac crest of the same patients, *J Bone Joint Surg* 94A:2128, 2012.

Stafford PR, Norris BL: Reamer-irrigator-aspirator bone graft and bi Masquelet technique for segmental bone defect nonunions: a review of 25 cases, *Injury* 41(Suppl 2):S72, 2010.

Starman JS, Bosse MJ, Cates CA, Norton HJ: Recombinant human bone morphogenetic protein-2 use in the off-label treatment of nonunions and acute fractures: a retrospective review, *J Trauma* 72:676, 2012.

Takemoto R, Forman J, Taormina DP, Egol KA: No advantage to rhBMP-2 in addition to autogenous graft for fracture nonunion, *Orthopedics* 37:3525, 2014.

Willis MP, Brooks JP, Badman BL, et al.: Treatment of atrophic diaphyseal humeral nonunions with compressive locked plating and augmented with an intramedullary strut allograft, *J Orthop Trauma* 27:77, 2013.

Zhou S, Greenberger JS, Epperly MW, et al.: Age-related intrinsic changes in human bone-marrow-derived mesenchymal stem cells and their differentiation to osteoblasts, *Aging Cell* 7:335, 2008.

ULTRASOUND

Ebrahim S, Mollon B, Bance WS, et al.: Low-intensity pulsed ultrasonography versus electrical stimulation for fracture healing: a systematic review and network meta-analysis, *Can J Surg* 57:e105, 2014.

Higgins A, Glover M, Yang Y, et al.: EXOGEN ultrasound bone healing system for long bone fractures with non-union or delayed healing: a NICE medical technology guidance, *Appl Health Econ Health Policy* 12:477, 2014.

Mizra YH, Teoh KH, Golding D, et al.: Is there a role for low intensity pulsed ultrasound (LIPUS) in delayed or nonunion following arthrodesis in foot and ankle surgery?, *Foot Anklle Surg* 2018, [Epub ahead of print].

Nicholson JA, Tsang STJ, MacGillivray TJ, et al.: What is the role of ultrasound in fracture management? Diagnosis and therapeutic potential for fractures, delayed unions, and fracture-related infections, *Bone Joint Res* 8:304, 2019.

Watanabe Y, Ariai Y, Takenaka N, et al.: Three key factors affecting treatment results of low-intensity pulsed ultrasound for delayed unions and nonunions: instability, gap size, and atrophic nonunion, *J Orthop Sci* 18:803, 2013.

ELECTRICAL STIMULATION

Aleem IS, Aleem I, Evaniew N, et al.: Efficacy of electrical stimulators for bone healing: a meta-analysis of randomized sham-controlled trials, *Scii Rep* 6:31724, 2016.

Assiotis A, Sachinis NP, Chalidis BE: Pulsed electromagnetic fields for the treatment of tibial dealyed unions and nonunions. A prospective clinical study and review of the literature, *J Orthop Surg Res* 7:24, 2012.

Ryan Martin J, Vestermark G, Mullis B, et al.: A retrospective comparative analysis of the use of implantable bone stimulators in nonunions, *J Surg Orthop Adv* 26:128, 2017.

EXTRACORPOREAL SHOCK-WAVE THERAPY

Alkhawashki HM: Shock wave therapy of fracture nonunion, *Injury* 46:2248, 2015.

Ayeni OR, Busse JW, Bhandari M: Using extracorporeal shock-wave therapy for healing long-bone nonunions, *Clin J Sports Med* 21:74, 2011.

Elster EA, Stojadinovic A, Forsberg J, et al.: Extracorporeal shock wave therapy for non-union of the tibia, *J Orthop Trauma* 24:133, 2010.

Furia JP, Juliano PJ, Wade AM, et al.: Shock wave therapy compared with intramedullary screw fixation for non-union of proximal fifth metatarsal metaphyseal-diaphyseal fractures, *J Bone Joint Surg* 92A:846, 2010.

Kertzman P, Császár NBM, Furia JP, et al.: Radial extracorporeal shock wave therapy is efficient and safe in the treatment of fracture nonunions of superficial bones: a retrospective case series, *J Orthop Surg Res* 12:164, 2017.

Zelle BA, Gollwitzer H, Zlowodzki M, Bühren V: Extracorporeal shock wave therapy: current evidence, *J Orthop Trauma* 24:S66, 2010.

FACTORS COMPLICATING NONUNION (INFECTION)

Conway J, Mansour J, Kotze K, et al.: Antibiotic cement-coated rods. An effective treatment for long bones and prosthetic joint nonunions, *Bone Joint Lett J* 96B:1349, 2014.

Gaillard C, Dupond M, Brisou P, Gaillard T: Septic nonunions of lower limb long bones: don't neglect *Propionibacterium acnes!*, *Int J Lower Extr Wounds* 12:301, 2013.

McKee MD, Li-Bland EA, Wild LM, et al.: A prospective, randomized clinical trial comparing an antibiotic-impregnated bioabsorbable bone substitute with standard antibiotic-impregnated cement beads in the treatment of chronic osteomyelitis and infected nonunion, *J Orthop Trauma* 24:483, 2010.

Olszewski D, Streubel PN, Stucken C, et al.: Fate of patients with a "surprise" positive culture after nonunion surgery, *J Orthop Trauma* 30:e19, 2016.

Palmer MP, Altman DT, Altman GT, et al.: Can we trust intraoperative culture results in nonunions? *J Orthop Trauma* 28:384, 2014.

Selhi HS, Mahindra P, Yamin M, et al.: Outcome in patients with an infected nonunion of the long bones treated with a reinforced antibiotic bone cement rod, *J Orthop Trauma* 26:184, 2012.

Wang Z, Zheng C, Wen S, et al.: Usefulness of serum D-dimer for preoperative diagnosis of infection nonunion after open reduction and internal fixation, *Infect Drug Resist* 12:1827, 2019.

FACTORS COMPLICATING NONUNION (DEFORMITY, SHORTENING, AND SEGMENTAL BONE LOSS)

Blum ALL, Bongiovanni JC, Morgan SJ, et al.: Complications associated with distraction osteogenesis for infected non-union of the femoral shaft in the presence of a bone defect: a retrospective series, *J Bone Joint Surg* 92B:565, 2010.

NONUNION OF SPECIFIC BONES

TIBIA (MEDIAL MALLEOLUS AND TIBIAL SHAFT)

Antonova E, Le TK, Burge R, Mershon J: Tibia shaft fractures: costly burden of nonunions, *BMC Musculoskelet Disord* 14:42, 2013.

Arvesen JE, Tracy Watson J, Israel H: Effectiveness of treatment for distal tibial nonunions with associated complex deformities using a hexapod external fixation, *J Orthop Trauma* 31:e43, 2017.

Braly HL, O'Connor DP, Brinker MR: Percutaneous autologous bone marrow injection in the treatment of distal meta-diaphyseal tibial nonunions and delayed unions, *J Orthop Trauma* 27:527, 2013.

Brinker MR, Hanus BD, Sen M, O'Connor DP: The devastating effects of tibial nonunion on health-related quality of life, *J Bone Joint Surg* 95A:2170, 2013.

Brinker MR, O'Connor DP: Partial fibulectomy for symptomatic fibular nonunion, *Foot Ankle Int* 31:542, 2010.

Buijze GA, Richardson S, Jupiter JB: Successful reconstruction for complex malunions and nonunions of the tibia and femur, *J Bone Joint Surg* 93A:485, 2011.

Dailey HL, Wu KA, Wu PS, et al.: Tibial fracture nonunion and time to healing after reamed intramedullary nailing: risk factors based on a single-center review of 1003 patients, *J Orthop Trauma* 32:e263, 2018.

Ebraheim NA, Evans B, Liu X, et al.: Comparison of intramedullary nail, plate, and external fixation in the treatment of distal tibia nonunions, *Int Orthop* 41:1925, 2017.

Fong K, Truong V, Foote CJ, et al.: Predictors of nonunion and reoperation in patients with fractures of the tibia: an observational study, *BMC Musculoskel Disord* 14:103, 2013.

Foster MJ, O'Toole RV, Manson TT: Treatment of tibial nonunion with posterolateral bone grafting, *Injury* 48:2242, 2017.

Haller JM, Githens M, Dunbar R: Intramedullary nailing for pilon nonunions, *J Orthop Trauma* 31:e395, 2017.

Kan JM, Raikin SM: Addressing hindfoot arthritis with concomitant tibial malunion or nonunion with retrograde tibiotalocalcaneal nailing, *J Bone Joint Surg* 96A:574, 2014.

Khurana S, Karia R, Egol KA: Operative treatment of nonunion following distal fibula and medial malleolar ankle fractures, *Foot Ankle Int* 34:365, 2013.

Ko SB, Lee SW: Do fibula nonunions predict later tibia nonunions? *J Orthop Trauma* 27:150, 2013.

Litrenta J, Tornetta 3rd P, Mehta S, et al.: Determination of radiographic healing: an assessment of consistency using RUST and Modified RUST in metadiaphyseal fractures, *J Orthop Trauma* 29:516, 2015.

Ricci WM, Tornetta P, Borrelli Jr J: Lag screw fixation of medial malleolar fractures: a biomechanical, radiographic, and clinical comparison of unicortical partially threaded lag screws and bicortical fully threaded lag screws, *J Orthop Trauma* 26:602, 2012.

Ross KA, O'Halloran K, Castillo RC, et al.: Prediction of tibial nonunion at the 6-week time point, *Injury* 49:2075, 2018.

Sanders DW, Bhandari M, Guyatt G, et al.: Critical-sized defect in the tibia: is it critical? Results from the SPRINT trial, *J Orthop Trauma* 28:632, 2014.

Scaglione M, Fabbri L, Dell'Omo D, et al.: Long bone nonunions treated with autologous concentrated bone marrow-derived cells combined with dried bone allograft, *Musculoskelet Surg* 98:101, 2014.

Schemitsch EH, Bhandari M, Guyatt G, et al.: Prognostic factors for predicting outcomes after intramedullary nailing of the tibia, *J Bone Joint Surg* 94A:1786, 2012.

Schoenleber SJ, Hutson JJ: Treatment of hypertrophic distal tibia nonunion and early malunion with callus distraction, *Foot Ankle Int* 36:400, 2015.

Sugaya H, Mishima H, Aoto K, et al.: Percutaneous autologous concentrated bone marrow grafting in the treatment for nonunion, *Eur J Orthop Surg Traumatol* 24:671, 2014.

Swanson EA, Garrard EC, O'Connor DP, Brinker MR: Results of a systematic approach to exchange nailing for the treatment of aseptic tibial nonunions, *J Orthop Trauma* 29:28, 2015.

Tarkin IS, Siska PA, Zelle BA: Soft tissue and biomechanical challenges encountered with the management of distal tibia nonunions, *Orthop Clin North Am* 41:119, 2010.

Yang JS, Otero J, McAndrew CM, et al.: Can tibial nonunion be predicted at 3 months after intramedullary nailing? *J Orthop Trauma* 27:599, 2013.

FIBULA

Bhadra AK, Roberts CS, Giannoudis PV: Nonunion of fibula: a systematic review, *Int Orthop* 36:1757, 2012.

Brinker MR, O'Connor DP: Partial fibulectomy for symptomatic fibular nonunion, *Foot Ankle Int* 31:542, 2010.

PATELLA

Kadar A, Sherman H, Glazer Y, et al.: Predictors for nonunion, reoperation and infection after surgical fixation of patellar fracture, *J Orthop Sci* 20:168, 2015.

Nathan ST, Fisher BE, Roberts CS, Giannoudis PV: The management of nonunion and delayed union of patella fractures: a systematic review of the literature, *Int Orthop* 35:791, 2011.

Petrie J, Sassoon A, Langford J: Complications of patellar fracture repair: treatment and results, *J Knee Surg* 26:309, 2013.

PELVIS/ACETABULUM

Lee KJ, Min BW, Oh GM, et al.: Surgical correction of pelvic malunion and nonunion, *Clin Orthop Surg* 7:396, 2015.

Sagi HC, Jordan CJ, Barel DP, et al.: Indomethacin prophylaxis for heterotopic ossification after acetabular fracture surgery increases the risk for nonunion of the posterior wall, *J Orthop Trauma* 28:377, 2014.

FEMORAL SHAFT (SUPRACONDYLAR REGION, FEMORAL SHAFT, PERITROCHANTERIC AND SUBTROCHANTERIC REGION)

Amorosa LF, Jayaram PR, Wellman DS, et al.: The use of the 95-degree-angled blade plate in femoral nonunion surgery, *Eur J Orthop Surg Traumatol* 24:953, 2014.

Attum B, Douleh D, Whiting PS, et al.: Outcomes of distal femur nonunions treated with a combined nail/plate construct and autogenous bone grafting, *J Orthop Trauma* 31:e301, 2017.

Buijze GA, Richardson S, Jupiter JB: Successful reconstruction for complex malunions and nonunions of the tibia and femur, *J Bone Joint Surg* 93A:485, 2011.

Hierholzer C, Glowalla C, Herrier M, et al.: Reamed intramedullary exchange nailing: treatment of choice of aseptic femoral shaft nonunion, *J Orthop Surg Res* 9:88, 2014.

Lai PJ, Hsu YH, Chou YC, et al.: Augmentative antirotational plating provided a significantly higher union rate than exchanging reamed nailing in treatment for femoral shaft aseptic atrophic nonunion—retrospective cohort study, *BMC Musculoskelet Disord* 20:127, 2019.

Luo H, Su Y, Ding L, et al.: Exchange nailing versus augmentative plating in the treatment of femoral shaft nonunion after intramedullary nailing: a meta-analysis, *EFORT Open Rev* 4:513, 2019.

Metsemakers WJ, Roels N, Belmans A, et al.: Risk factors for nonunion after intramedullary nailing of femoral shaft fractures: remaining controversies, *Injury* 46:1601, 2015.

Monroy A, Urruela A, Singh P, et al.: Distal femur nonunion patients can expect good outcomes, *J Knee Surg* 27:83, 2014.

Papakostidis C, Psyllakis I, Vardakas D, et al.: Femoral-shaft fractures and nonunions treated with intramedullary nails: the role of dynamisation, *Injury Int J Care Injured* 42:1353, 2011.

Park J, Kim SG, Yoon HK, Yang KH: The treatment of nonisthmal femoral shaft nonunions with IM nail exchange versus augmentation plating, *J Orthop Trauma* 24:89, 2010.

Park J, Yang KH: Indications and outcomes of augmentation plating with decortication and autogenous bone grafting for femoral shaft nonunions, *Injury Int J Care Injured* 44:1820, 2013.

Rodriguez EK, Boulton C, Weaver MJ, et al.: Predictive factors of distal femoral fracture nonunion after lateral locked plating: a retrospective multicenter case-control study of 283 fractures, *Injury Int J Care Injured* 45:554, 2014.

Somford MP, van den Bekerom MPJ, Kloen P: Operative treatment for femoral shaft nonunions, a systematic review of the literature, *Strat Traum Limb Recon* 8:77, 2013.

Stella M, Santolini E, Autuori A, et al.: Masquetlet technique to treat a septic nonunion after nailing of a femoral open fracture, *Injury* 49(Suppl 4):S29, 2018.

Swanson EA, Garrard EC, Bernstein DT, et al.: Results of a systematic approach to exchange nailing for the treatment of aseptic femoral nonunions, *J Orthop Trauma* 29:21, 2015.

Vaughn JE, Shah RV, Samman T, et al.: Systematic review of dynamization vs exchange nailing for delayed/non-union femoral fractures, *World J Orthop* 9:92, 2018.

Wang Z, Liu C, Liu C, et al.: Effectiveness of exchange nailing and augmentation plating for femoral shaft nonunion after nailing, *Int Orthop* 38:2343, 2014.

Yang KH, Kim JR, Park J: Nonisthmal femoral shaft nonunion as a risk factor for exchange nailing failure, *J Trauma* 72:e60, 2012.

FEMORAL NECK

Banaszek D, Spence D, O'Brien P, et al.: Principles of valgus intertrochanteric osteotomy (VITO) after femoral neck nonunion, *Adv Orthop* 2018:5214273, 2018.

Deakin DE, Guy P, O'Brien PJ, et al.: Managing failed fixation: valgus osteotomy for femoral neck nonunion, *Injury Int J Care Injured* 46:492, 2015.

Magu NK, Singla R, Rohilla R, et al.: Modified Pauwels' intertrochanteric osteotomy in the management of nonunion of a femoral neck fracture following failed osteosynthesis, *Bone Joint Lett J* 96B:1198, 2014.

Medda S, Jinnah AH, Marquez-Lara A, et al.: Valgus intertrochanteric osteotomy for femoral neck nonunion, *J Orthop Trauma* 33(Suppl 1):S26, 2019.

Yang JJ, Lin LC, Chao KH, et al.: Risk factors for nonunion in patients with intracapsular femoral neck fractures treated with three cannulated screws placed in either a triangle or an inverted triangle configuration, *J Bone Joint Surg* 95A:61, 2013.

Yin J, Zhu H, Gao Y, et al.: Vascularized fibular grafting in treatment of femoral neck nonunion: a prognostic study based on long-term outcomes, *J Bone Joint Surg Am* 101:1294, 2019.

Yuan BJ, Shearer DW, Barel DP, et al.: Intertrochanteric osteotomy for femoral neck nonunion: does "undercorrection" result in an acceptable rate of femoral neck union? *J Orthop Trauma* 31:420, 2017.

CLAVICLE

Chen W, Tang K, Tao X, et al.: Clavicular non-union treated with fixation using locking compression plate without bone graft, *J Orthop Surg Res* 13:317, 2018.

Huang HK, Chiang CC, Ping Y, et al.: Role of autologous bone graft in the surgical treatment of atrophic nonunion of midshaft clavicular fractures, *Orthopedics* 35:e197, 2012.

Jorgensoen A, Troelsen A, Ban I: Predictors associated with nonunion and symptomatic malunion following nonoperative treatment of displaced midshaft clavicle fractures – a systematic review of the literature, *Int Orthop* 38:2543, 2014.

Murray IR, Foster CJ, Eros A, Robinson CM: Risk factors for nonunion after nonoperative treatment of displaced midshaft fractures of the clavicle, *J Bone Joint Surg* 95A:1153, 2013.

Riggenbach MD, Jones GL, Bishop JY: Open reduction and internal fixation of clavicular nonunions with allograft bone substitute, *Int J Shoulder Surg* 5:61, 2011.

HUMERUS (PROXIMAL HUMERUS, HUMERAL SHAFT, DISTAL HUMERUS)

Cadet ER, Yin B, Schulz B, et al.: Proximal humerus and humeral shaft nonunions, *J Am Acad Orthop Surg* 21:538, 2013.

De Domsure RB, Peter R, Hoffmeyer P: Uninfected nonunion of the humeral diaphysis: review of 21 patients treated with shingling, compression plate, and autologous bone graft, *Orthop Traumatol Surg Res* 96:139, 2010.

Ding L, He Z, Xiao H, et al.: Factors affecting the incidence of aseptic nonunion after surgical fixation of humeral diaphyseal fracture, *J Orthop Sci* 189:973, 2014.

DuQuin TR, Jacobson JA, Sanchez-Sotelo J, et al.: Unconstrained shoulder arthroplasty for treatment of proximal humeral nonunions, *J Bone Joint Surg* 94A:1610, 2012.

Kumar MN, Ravindranath P, Ravishankar MR: Outcome of locking compression plates in humeral shaft nonunions, *Indian J Orthop* 47:150, 2013.

Lin WP, Lin J: Allografting in locked nailing and interfragmentary wiring for humeral nonunions, *Clin Orthop Relat Res* 468:852, 2010.

Prasarn ML, Achor T, Paul O, et al.: Management of nonunions of the proximal humeral diaphysis, *Injury* 41:1244, 2010.

Raiss P, Edwards B, Ribeiro da Silva M, et al.: Reverse shoulder arthroplasty for the treatment of nonunions of the surgical neck of the proximal part of the humerus (type-3 fracture sequelae), *J Bone Joint Surg* 96A:2070, 2014.

Watson JT, Sanders RW: Controlled compression nailing for at risk humeral shaft fractures, *J Orthop Trauma* 31(Suppl 6):S25, 2017.

Willis MP, Brooks JP, Badman BL, et al.: Treatment of atrophic diaphyseal humeral nonunions with compressive locked plating and augmented with an intramedullary strut allograft, *J Orthop Trauma* 27:77, 2013.

Zafra M, Uceda P, Flores M, Carpintero P: Reverse total shoulder replacement for nonunion of a fracture of the proximal humerus, *Bone Joint Lett J* 96B:1239, 2014.

Zhang Q, Yin P, Hao M, et al.: Bone transport for the treatment of infected forearm nonunion, *Injury* 45:1880, 2014.

FOREARM

Devendra A, Velmurugesan PS, Dheenadhayalan J, et al.: One-bone forearm reconstruction: a salvage solution for the forearm with massive bone loss, *J Bone Joint Surg Am* 101:e74, 2019.

Kloen P, Buijze GA: Ring D: management of forearm nonunions: current concepts, *Strat Traum Limb Recon* 7:1, 2012.

Liu T, Liu Z, Ling L, Zhang X: Infected forearm nonunion treated by bone transport after debridement, *BMC Musculoskel Disord* 14:273, 2013.

The complete list of references is available online at ExpertConsult.com.

CHAPTER 8

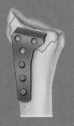

ACUTE DISLOCATIONS

Anthony A. Mascioli

INDICATIONS FOR OPEN REDUCTION	472	
ANKLE	472	
PATELLA	473	
Acute dislocations of the patella	473	
Intraarticular dislocations of the patella	475	
KNEE	475	
Proximal tibiofibular joint	477	
HIP	477	

Complications	480
Pubic symphysis and sacroiliac joints	481
STERNOCLAVICULAR JOINT	481
ACROMIOCLAVICULAR JOINT	482
Etiology and classification	482
Clinical findings	483
Treatment	483

SHOULDER	485
ELBOW	485
Dislocation of the radial head	486
Dislocation of radial head and fracture of proximal third of ulna (monteggia fracture)	486
Fracture-dislocation of elbow with severe damage of soft structures	487
DISTAL RADIOULNAR JOINT	487

Open techniques are occasionally necessary for acute dislocations. Closed reduction with intravenous analgesia or sedation with general anesthesia should be attempted first for most uncomplicated dislocations. If general anesthesia is necessary, operating room personnel should prepare for the possibility of an open surgical procedure if closed reduction is unsuccessful. Excessive force should not be used in closed reduction because soft tissue or bone sometimes becomes interposed between the articular surfaces, making closed reduction impossible. Forceful manipulation under these conditions can result in fractures or additional articular trauma. The use of image intensification may aid in reduction and help prevent these complications.

Acute dislocations should be reduced as soon as possible. If they are not reduced promptly, pathologic changes occur, especially around the hip. Immediate reduction of an acute dislocation does not guarantee a satisfactory result, however, and the patient should be informed of this at the time of the initial evaluation and treatment. Damage to the articular cartilage, joint capsule, ligaments, and vascularity of the bones can lead to posttraumatic arthritis. The patient also should be informed that heterotopic ossification, posttraumatic arthritis, and osteonecrosis might develop in any joint after open or closed reduction.

These complications are usually caused by the immense forces that caused the dislocation. Occasionally neurovascular structures are injured when a joint becomes dislocated, and complete physiologic block of the nerve or persistent neuritis results. Any nerve injury should be detected and carefully recorded on the patient's chart before closed or open reduction is performed. The nerve may be stretched, contused, or ruptured. Stretching occurs most often, and the nerve usually recovers spontaneously; no attempt should be made to explore it at the time of open reduction unless it is located in the immediate field of operation. If signs of recovery do not appear after a reasonable time, the nerve should be explored as described in other chapter. Arteriography and vascular studies are needed in any extremity with markedly diminished or absent pulses.

INDICATIONS FOR OPEN REDUCTION

Open reduction of an acute dislocation is usually indicated in the following circumstances:

1. If anatomic, concentric reduction cannot be achieved by gentle, closed techniques with the patient under general anesthesia. Interposed soft tissues or osteochondral fragments may contribute to the irreducibility.
2. If a stable reduction cannot be maintained. Articular fractures are often unstable and must be reduced and fixed to ensure stability of the reduction.
3. If careful evaluation before closed reduction reveals normal neurologic function and, after reduction, a definite, complete motor and sensory nerve deficit becomes evident.
4. If circulatory impairment distal to the injury is well documented before reduction and persists after reduction. Further assessment of the circulation is essential and should include vascular studies.
5. If ischemia is persistent. Surgical exploration with appropriate management of the vascular injury is indicated.

ANKLE

Dislocations of the ankle without fracture of either the medial or lateral malleolus or the anterior or posterior lip of the distal articular surface of the tibia are extremely rare. Usually, any dislocations that do occur are easily reduced by closed methods. Posterior dislocation of the

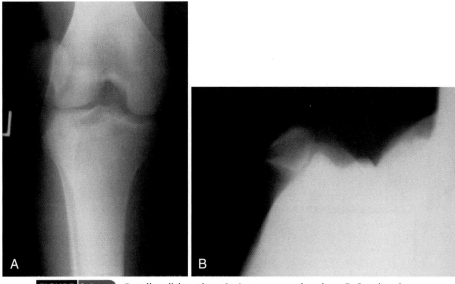

FIGURE 8.1 Patellar dislocation. **A,** Anteroposterior view. **B,** Sunrise view.

fibula behind the tibia may contribute to difficulty with closed reduction and at times may require open reduction. Ruptures of the deltoid ligament, the anterior tibiotalar ligament, and the anterior and posterior talofibular ligaments occur alone or in combination. Controversy exists over acute ligamentous repair without evidence of fracture. Good-to-excellent results are possible without acute ligamentous repair; however, syndesmosis and mortise widening should be treated operatively if present. (For discussion of acute fractures of the ankle, see chapter 2; of malunited fractures of the ankle, see chapter 6.)

PATELLA
ACUTE DISLOCATIONS OF THE PATELLA

Acute dislocations of the patella are usually managed by closed methods (Fig. 8.1). The patella is almost always dislocated laterally, and extension of the flexed knee with pressure applied to the lateral margin of the patella results in reduction. The limb is immobilized in a knee immobilizer until symptoms resolve, then motion and a Palumbo brace are encouraged for 3 to 6 weeks to promote the formation of strong collagen along the lines of stress. Radiographs should be evaluated carefully to ensure that no osteochondral fragments are displaced within the joint. If a hemarthrosis is present, MRI is warranted to detect any osteochondral fragments. One study demonstrated articular cartilage injury in 94% of patients; 72% had an osteochondral or chondral fracture, and 23% had patellar microfractures.

An MRI study by Balcarek et al. identified either a complete or partial tear of the medial patellofemoral ligament in most patients (98%) after an acute lateral patellar dislocation. The femoral origin was most frequently affected (50%), followed by the midsubstance (10%), and patellofemoral origin (10%). More than one site of injury was found in 22%. In their subgroup analysis, patellar height and trochlear facet asymmetry were significantly different on MRI in patients with patellar or femoral origin injury (or both) compared with patients in an age-matched control group, but no

significant differences were noted in patients with solely a midsubstance injury. In addition, the tibial tuberosity-trochlear groove distance in the patellar origin injury subgroup was significantly greater compared with the other subgroups (femoral origin, patellar and femoral origin, midsubstance, and control).

Because the sites of injury of the medial patellofemoral ligament may differ, treating the specific pathology is critical. Whereas a direct repair may be adequate for a lesion at the femoral or patellar origin, it may not be for a combined tear. Furthermore, direct repair is satisfactory only if the ligament is otherwise intact. If ligament quality is poor, or there is a combined tear, a reconstruction may be more appropriate.

Sufficient evidence does not exist to advocate surgical intervention for primary patellar dislocations. After a second dislocation there is a much higher dislocation rate (49%), and surgical intervention may be considered.

Good or excellent results have been reported in 75% of nonoperatively treated knees and 66% of operatively treated knees in one study. Recurrent dislocation occurred in 71% of nonoperatively treated knees and in 67% of operatively treated knees. Fifty-two percent of patients had their first redislocation within 2 years after the primary injury. The patient should be warned of the possibility of future episodes of recurrent patellar subluxation or dislocation.

In most patients, the long-term subjective and functional results after acute patellar dislocation are satisfactory. Initial operative repair of the medial structures combined with lateral release has not been shown to improve the long-term outcome, despite the very high rate of recurrent instability. Routine repair of the torn medial stabilizing soft tissues in acute patellar dislocation is not recommended in children or adolescents. However, one study found only a 31% success rate with nonoperative treatment in patients who were skeletally immature and had trochlear dysplasia.

Arthroscopic techniques for the repair of the medial patellar retinaculum after acute patellar dislocations have been described, but we prefer the open method at our institution if repair is indicated (Fig. 8.2).

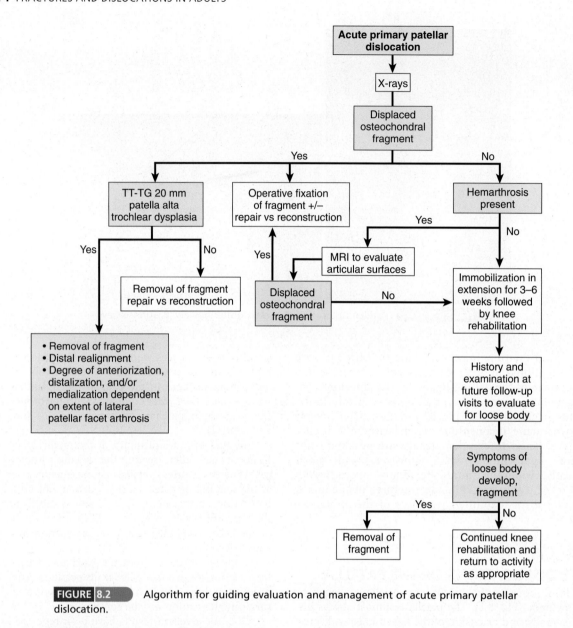

FIGURE 8.2 Algorithm for guiding evaluation and management of acute primary patellar dislocation.

OPEN REDUCTION AND REPAIR OF PATELLAR DISLOCATION

TECHNIQUE 8.1

- Through a medial parapatellar incision, explore the tear in the medial patellar retinaculum.
- Irrigate and explore the knee joint. Remove or fix any loose osteochondral fragments and make a thorough search for any further loose fragments or intraarticular damage to the joint.
- Repair any disruption in the vastus medialis muscle belly or in the medial patellar retinaculum.
- Pay careful attention to that portion of the vastus medialis that originates in the region of the femoral adductor tubercle. If this origin has been disrupted and has retracted

proximally, the angle of insertion of the vastus medialis muscle fibers into the patella is significantly changed. These fibers are vital to the prevention of recurrent lateral dislocation of the patella.
- A lateral release may be performed if indicated.
- Close the wound in layers and apply a knee immobilizer.

POSTOPERATIVE CARE The limb is immobilized in a knee immobilizer for 10 to 14 days. Early range of motion is begun to prevent arthrofibrosis and to promote the formation of strong collagen along the lines of stress. A Palumbo-type brace is added at 2 weeks. Crutches are discontinued when control of the limb is regained and limping is no longer a problem. Quadriceps strengthening is continued for 3 to 4 months, and strength can be documented objectively. We allow return to full activity (sports) when quadriceps strength reaches 90% of the uninvolved side. Walking on crutches with weight bearing to tolerance is begun during the first week. The crutches

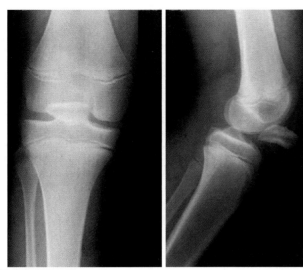

FIGURE 8.3 Intraarticular horizontal dislocation of patella. Quadriceps mechanism usually remains intact. (From Brady TA, Russell D: Interarticular horizontal dislocation of the patella: a case report, *J Bone Joint Surg* 47A:1393, 1965.)

are discontinued when full weight bearing can be tolerated. Appropriate rehabilitation of the musculature of the extremity is essential. Stiff-legged resistance exercises with weights, followed by short-arc knee extension exercises, are recommended. A full range of motion of the knee against resistance during early rehabilitation places excessive forces on the patellofemoral joint and should be avoided.

GRAFTING OF THE MEDIAL PATELLAR RETINACULUM

TECHNIQUE 8.2

- Prepare a semitendinosus autologous graft or allograft.
- Center the skin incision between the medial edge of the patella and adductor tubercle.
- Identify the extensor retinaculum.
- Make a small incision at the medial edge of the patella and just distal to the adductor tubercle.
- Using a hemostat, pass the graft through a tunnel between the capsule and retinaculum.
- Secure the graft to the femur using suture, interference screw, or a suture anchor. The attachment site for the medial patellofemoral ligament can be found radiographically just anterior to the intersection of the posterior femoral cortical line and Blumensaat's line on a lateral radiograph.
- Attach the graft through the midportion of the quadriceps tendon at its insertion to the superior pole of the patella as described by Fulkerson. Cycle the knee and stabilize with figure-of-eight sutures through the quadriceps tendon and the graft.
- Repair the retinaculum with figure-of-eight sutures.

- Close the wound in layers and apply a controlled-motion knee brace.

POSTOPERATIVE CARE The limb is immobilized in 30 degrees of flexion for the first 2 weeks. Motion is gradually increased under supervision, and the brace is locked in full extension for ambulation for 6 weeks. Otherwise, the rehabilitation protocol is the same as after repair.

INTRAARTICULAR DISLOCATIONS OF THE PATELLA

Intraarticular dislocations of the patella are rare and are of two types. The most common type is a horizontal intraarticular dislocation of the patella with detachment of the quadriceps tendon; the articular surface of the patella is directed toward the tibial articular surface (Fig. 8.3). In the other type, the patella also is dislocated horizontally, but its inferior pole is detached from the patellar tendon and the articular surface faces proximally. These dislocations are frequently difficult to reduce by closed methods, and open reduction generally is required, along with repair of the extensor mechanism.

OPEN REDUCTION AND REPAIR OF THE EXTENSOR MECHANISM

TECHNIQUE 8.3

- Through a medial parapatellar incision, expose the dislocated patella, usually found in the intercondylar notch.
- Replace the patella into its bed in the quadriceps or patellar tendon and reattach it there with sutures. Placing the sutures through holes drilled in the patella may help secure the repair.
- Inspect the knee and remove any loose osteochondral or cartilaginous fragments.
- Close the wound in layers.

POSTOPERATIVE CARE Postoperative care is the same as that for repair of acute lateral dislocation of the patella.

KNEE

Dislocation of the knee has been considered a rare injury, but it seems to have increased in frequency over the years. It has been noted that the incidence might be higher than recognized because many knee dislocations are reduced at the scene of the injury without subsequent accurate reporting of this diagnosis (Fig. 8.4).

Knee dislocations are designated as anterior, posterior, medial, lateral, or rotary, according to the displacement of the tibia in relation to the femur. Rotary dislocations are designated further as anteromedial, anterolateral, posteromedial, or posterolateral. Knee dislocations are true orthopaedic

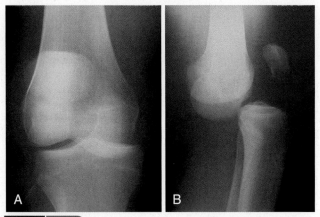

FIGURE 8.4 Knee dislocation. **A,** Lateral dislocation. **B,** Anterior dislocation.

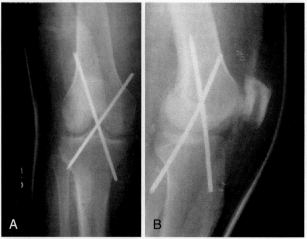

FIGURE 8.5 Radiograph showing transarticular pins. **A,** Anteroposterior view. **B,** Lateral view.

emergencies. Reported series have emphasized the extensive ligamentous damage and potential for vascular complications associated with these injuries. Prompt evaluation and early repair of any vascular damage in the injured extremity is universally recommended.

The incidence of vascular injuries in knee dislocations has been reported to range from 0% to 40%. Some centers use ankle-brachial indices to assess for vascular injury, but we recommend an arteriogram if the dislocation required reduction. When there is doubt concerning an injury to the popliteal artery, a thorough evaluation, including arteriography and early surgical exploration, is mandatory. Continued observation in anticipation of improvement often leads to disaster. The amputation rate is approximately 11% if vascular repair is done within 6 hours, and this increases to 86% if repair is delayed beyond this time period.

Nerve injuries occur in 16% to 43% of dislocations of the knee. The peroneal nerve is injured most often, and the prognosis for return of function after injury is guarded. If the nerve damage is complete, less than 40% of patients will regain dorsiflexion of foot. The majority of patients with incomplete palsy will regain full motor function.

Knee dislocations can usually be reduced satisfactorily by closed methods. After reduction and in the absence of additional complications, aspiration of the hemarthrosis using sterile technique and immobilizing the knee in full extension are satisfactory temporary treatments. The neurocirculatory status should be checked frequently for 5 to 7 days. A large transarticular pin can be placed through the intercondylar notch of the femur into the intercondylar eminence of the tibia to provide immediate stability for knees that redislocate in a splint or after vascular repair (Fig. 8.5). Transarticular pins have been associated with pin track infection and breakage and should be used with caution. We have found a transarticular pin to be useful when the posterior capsule is completely disrupted, preventing concentric reduction in full extension. The pin is left in place for 4 to 6 weeks, and range of motion is begun. A knee-spanning external fixator can be used in open knee dislocations with extensive soft-tissue injury or in unstable knees after vascular repair. When it is certain that the circulation is not impaired, treatment can be selected for repair of the injured ligaments, as discussed in other chapter. Closed reduction may be impossible, however, especially when the dislocation is posterolateral. Blocking of reduction by the interposition of the joint capsule and "buttonholing" of the femoral condyle medially through a tear in the capsule have been reported. A torn tibial collateral ligament or pes anserinus tendon also can block reduction. When an irreducible dislocation is encountered, open reduction through a medial approach often is necessary; however, the approach usually depends on the type of dislocation. The entrapping and torn structures are released and repaired, and the postoperative care is the same as for ligamentous injuries.

In complete knee dislocations, both cruciate ligaments usually are torn. In addition, the lateral or medial collateral ligament usually is completely disrupted. The decision to repair the ligaments surgically is affected by the presence of any other skeletal injuries, vascular deficits, or open wounds. If possible, the ligaments should be repaired or reconstructed early because early ligament repair has been shown to have more satisfactory long-term results than cast immobilization alone. If repair is impossible, however, such as in injuries requiring vascular repair or in injuries associated with large, open wounds, satisfactory results can be obtained by nonsurgical management. A long leg splint is applied and worn for approximately 2 weeks. Range of motion in a brace is then initiated. Patients who are not selected for surgical repair because of age, activity, or other coexistent pathology usually have stiffness rather than instability as a long-term problem.

Several authors have advocated early repair of all injured structures in order to obtain satisfactory outcomes. Only fair or poor results can be expected with nonoperative treatment. When open treatment is selected, the surgeon must be prepared to repair structures medially, laterally, anteriorly, and posteriorly as indicated. MRI can be a valuable tool in preoperative planning. Techniques for repair and reconstruction of the ligaments are found in other chapters.

Many dislocations result in avulsions, rather than midsubstance tears, of collateral or cruciate ligaments. This is particularly helpful in cruciate tears because primary repair of these structures is inferior to reconstruction, whereas replacement of avulsed bone and secure fixation can lead to acceptable results. Posterolateral corner injuries are particularly worrisome and should be treated early (2 to 3 weeks) to avoid having to perform less rewarding reconstructive procedures that become necessary thereafter.

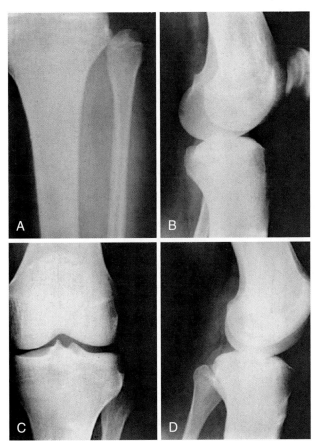

FIGURE 8.6 **A** and **B,** Acute dislocation of proximal tibiofibular joint. **C** and **D,** After closed reduction. Note change in position of fibular head in both views. (From Stewart MJ: Unusual athletic injuries, *Instr Course Lect* 17:377, 198.)

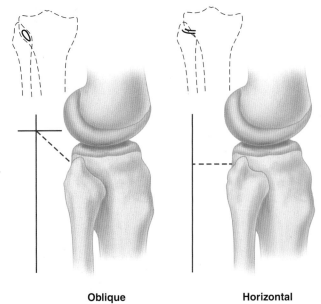

| Oblique | Horizontal |

FIGURE 8.7 Two basic types of proximal tibiofibular joints according to Ogden.

After stabilization of the patient and diligent neurovascular evaluation, we prefer to operate on these injuries within the first 3 weeks depending on which ligaments are involved, as discussed previously. Knees without posterolateral corner involvement can be treated when range of motion of 0 to 90 degrees is restored.

PROXIMAL TIBIOFIBULAR JOINT

Acute dislocation of the proximal tibiofibular joint is rare (Fig. 8.6). It is usually the result of a twisting trauma and may be seen in association with other injuries to the same extremity. Patients usually present with pain and a prominence in the lateral aspect of the knee. Injuries of the proximal tibiofibular joint frequently are overlooked. Patients with chronic dislocations or subluxation complain of popping and instability, which can be confused with a lateral meniscus injury. The proximal tibiofibular joint can be oblique or horizontal (Fig. 8.7). More motion is possible in horizontal joints, and the relative restriction of motion in oblique joints is presumably the reason why most injuries occur in them.

Ogden classified tibiofibular subluxations and dislocations into four types (Fig. 8.8): subluxation and anterolateral, posteromedial, and superior dislocations. Keogh et al. concluded after a cadaver study that the diagnosis of suspected dislocations of the proximal tibiofibular joint was best determined with an axial CT scan (Fig. 8.9).

Subluxation of the proximal tibiofibular joint is a recurring problem and is associated with pain and generalized joint hypermobility. Rarely, peroneal nerve deficits are present. If the symptoms fail to respond to cylinder cast immobilization, resection of the fibular head is recommended. Arthrodesis of the joint is discouraged because of its relationship to ankle motion and the potential for late, painful complaints referable to the ankle.

Anterolateral dislocations (see Fig. 8.6) were the most common proximal tibiofibular dislocations in Ogden's series. They usually were treated successfully by closed methods.

Posteromedial proximal tibiofibular dislocations are relatively uncommon. These are difficult to reduce and are usually associated with disruptions of the tibiofibular capsular ligaments and the lateral collateral ligament. When the dislocation is acute, open reduction is recommended with repair of the torn ligaments and lag screw fixation.

Superior dislocation of the proximal tibiofibular joint is also rare and is frequently associated with a fracture of the fibula or proximal dislocation of the lateral malleolus. If open reduction is necessary, the leg is immobilized in a long leg cast after surgery to prevent ankle motion and motion at the proximal joint. Immobilization of the knee in slight flexion should also relax the pull of the biceps femoris on the fibular head. Crutches are used until the long cast is removed at 3 weeks. A short leg walking cast is then applied.

HIP

The hip joint is inherently stable, and hip dislocations are generally produced by high-energy trauma. Often they are associated with multiple injuries to different organ systems. Motor vehicle accidents remain the most common mechanism of hip dislocation, followed by falls from a height, industrial accidents, and, more rarely, sports such as football or wrestling. Posterior dislocations occur much more frequently than anterior dislocations and result from a posteriorly directed force to the flexed knee with the hip also in a flexed position. Lesser degrees of hip flexion and increasing

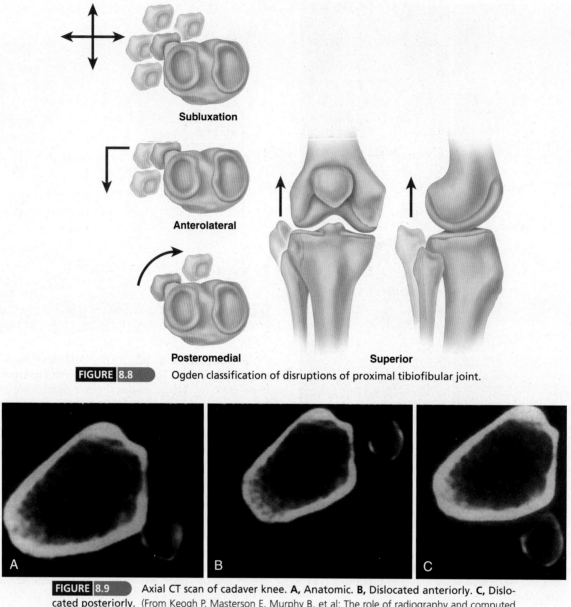

FIGURE 8.8 Ogden classification of disruptions of proximal tibiofibular joint.

FIGURE 8.9 Axial CT scan of cadaver knee. **A,** Anatomic. **B,** Dislocated anteriorly. **C,** Dislocated posteriorly. (From Keogh P, Masterson E, Murphy B, et al: The role of radiography and computed tomography in the diagnosis of acute dislocation of the proximal tibiofibular joint, *Br J Radiol* 66:108, 1993.)

amounts of hip abduction with similarly applied force often result in an acetabular fracture. Anterior dislocations are caused by an abduction and external rotation force to the affected limb.

Patients with an isolated posterior hip dislocation present with hip flexion, adduction, internal rotation, and a shortened extremity. Anterior dislocations cause the leg to be held in a position of abduction and external rotation. Although isolated hip dislocations are easily recognized, associated lower extremity injuries may distract the examining physician from an ipsilateral hip dislocation or may alter the classic position of the dislocated hip. As in any orthopaedic injury, careful physical examination is crucial, with particular attention paid to associated sciatic nerve or ipsilateral knee injuries.

Radiographic assessment of patients with a hip dislocation should include an anteroposterior view of the pelvis before reduction and is repeated after reduction, along with a 45-degree oblique Judet view of the pelvis. CT of the pelvis with 3-mm cuts and bone windows is also recommended after reduction

to rule out associated femoral head or acetabular fractures and incarcerated intraarticular fragments and to assess joint congruency. Patients with persistent pain or mechanical symptoms with negative plain radiographs or computed tomography may benefit from further workup; a 93% incidence of labral tears has been reported. Magnetic resonance imaging or arthrography has been shown to have an accuracy of 91% in one study; however, in that particular study, 15% of patients had loose bodies not detected on imaging. Arthroscopy is indicated as a diagnostic tool when imaging is equivocal.

Hip dislocations are classified according to the position of the femoral head in relation to the acetabulum and according to associated fractures of the acetabulum and proximal femur. Posterior dislocations have been classified by Thompson and Epstein into five types: type I, with or without a minor fracture; type II, with a large single fracture of the posterior acetabular rim; type III, with a comminuted fracture of the rim of the acetabulum, with or without a major fragment; type IV, with fracture of the acetabular rim and floor; and type V, with fracture of the femoral head. Types II through IV with significant associated acetabular fractures are discussed in chapter 4, and femoral head fractures are discussed in chapter 3.

Anterior dislocations have also been classified by Epstein as follows:

1. Pubic (superior)
   - With no fracture (simple)
   - With fracture of the head of the femur
   - With fracture of the acetabulum
2. Obturator (inferior) (Fig. 8.10)
   - With no fracture (simple)
   - With fracture of the head of the femur
   - With fracture of the acetabulum

The term *central dislocation* historically referred to a medial position of the femoral head after a fracture involving the medial wall of the acetabulum of varying types. This subtype is not very descriptive and may be more accurately discussed in terms of the underlying acetabular fracture.

A hip dislocation constitutes an orthopaedic emergency because delaying its reduction increases the risk of osteonecrosis of the femoral head. Hougaard and Thomsen recommended

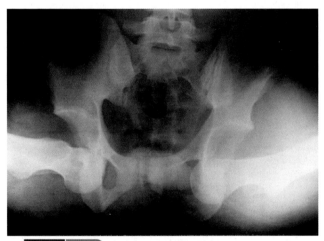

FIGURE 8.10 Bilateral obturator dislocations of hip.

reduction within 6 hours of the injury. They reported an osteonecrosis rate of 4.8% if reduction occurred within 6 hours of injury compared with 53% if reduction was delayed for more than 6 hours after injury. When the initial trauma survey has been made, and life-threatening injuries have been stabilized, the dislocated hip takes precedence over any other orthopaedic injury. Closed reduction of the hip should initially be attempted in the emergency department under intravenous sedation or general anesthesia, if readily available. If other injuries require emergency operative intervention, the initial hip reduction can be performed in the operating room.

The following guidelines for treatment refer to hip dislocations without significant associated femoral head or acetabular fractures (Thompson and Epstein type I). Several methods of closed reduction have been used successfully, all of which generally consist of recreating the injurious deforming force (for posterior dislocations—flexion, adduction, and internal rotation; for anterior dislocations—abduction and external rotation in extension). Traction in line with the affected femur and small amounts of rotation and abduction and adduction complete the reduction. The Allis maneuver is performed for posterior dislocations as previously described with the patient supine, whereas the Stimson maneuver is similarly performed with the patient prone (Fig. 8.11). Other reduction techniques involve levering the affected limb at the ankle over a fulcrum (Figs. 8.12 and 8.13). Regardless of the method chosen, only two or three attempts should be made at closed reduction. Multiple, increasingly forcible attempts at reduction could lead to an iatrogenic femoral head, neck, or shaft fracture or cartilaginous injury to the femoral head or acetabulum.

Failed closed reduction of the hip can be caused by "buttonholing" of the femoral head through the capsule, inversion of the labrum, or interposition of the piriformis into the acetabulum. Incarcerated bone fragments from the femoral head or acetabulum or displaced, unstable acetabular fractures that cannot completely contain the dislocated femoral head can cause hip incongruity. If closed reduction fails, anteroposterior and Judet views and a CT scan of the pelvis should be obtained quickly to assess the interposed structure. If the hip is reduced incongruently, skeletal traction with the femoral head slightly distracted is necessary to avoid further cartilaginous injury until surgery can be done. If the hip is irreducible by closed means, open reduction of the hip should be done immediately. Associated femoral head or acetabular fractures can wait a few days for definitive treatment.

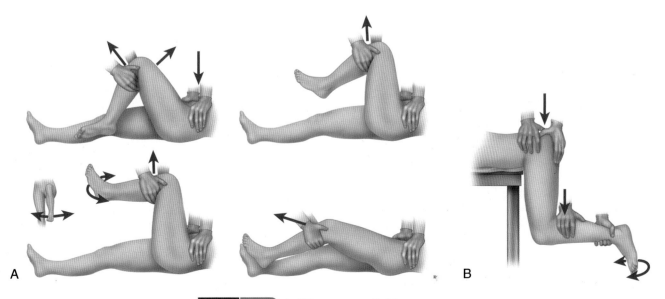

FIGURE 8.11 **A,** Allis maneuver. **B,** Stimson maneuver.

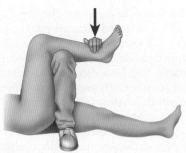

FIGURE 8.12 Lefkowitz maneuver using physician's knee as a fulcrum for affected limb. Left hand levers ipsilateral ankle and controls rotation.

The hip approach used is generally determined by the direction of the dislocation. Posterior dislocations are treated by the posterior Kocher-Langenbeck type of approach. Anterior dislocations can be reduced by the direct anterior approach of Smith-Petersen or by the anterolateral or direct lateral approaches of Watson-Jones and Hardinge. The anterolateral and direct lateral approaches offer better access to the posterior capsule, if necessary, whereas the anterior approach may offer a better view of femoral head fractures.

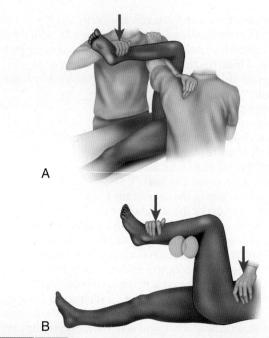

FIGURE 8.13 **A,** "East Baltimore lift" is shown with physician and assistant's arms as fulcrum and ankle as lever. **B,** Second assistant stabilizes pelvis.

OPEN REDUCTION OF HIP DISLOCATION

TECHNIQUE 8.4

- Regardless of the direction of the dislocation, when the approach has been made, assess the capsule first.
- If the femoral head is buttonholed, extend the traumatic capsulotomy in a T-shaped fashion along the acetabular rim, carefully preserving the labrum, if possible.
- Inspect the joint for intervening capsule, labrum, piriformis muscle, or bony fragments.
- If necessary, retract or distract the hip manually or with skeletal traction applied through a fracture table or femoral distractor for better assessment of the joint.
- When the joint has been cleared of debris, reduce the hip joint by releasing the traction.
- Repair the capsule along with the labrum.
- Close the wound routinely for the chosen approach.

POSTOPERATIVE CARE Gait training is begun when the patient regains control of the affected limb. Some authors have advocated postoperative traction and protected weight bearing to decrease the incidence of femoral head collapse from osteonecrosis. The benefits of these measures have not been proven. Patients are advised to avoid putting the hip in the position of the dislocation, and hip abductor and flexor strengthening and gentle range-of-motion exercises are initiated. An abduction pillow is useful in the postoperative period in sedated and noncompliant patients with previous posterior dislocation.

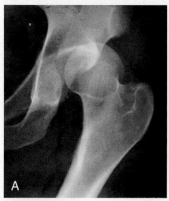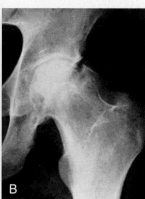

FIGURE 8.14 **A,** Posterior dislocation of hip. **B,** Osteonecrosis of femoral head 8 months after closed reduction. Note subchondral sclerosis, narrowed joint space, and femoral head collapse.

COMPLICATIONS

Osteonecrosis has been reported to occur in 4% to 22% of hip dislocations without associated femoral head or acetabular fracture (Fig. 8.14). Time to reduction plays a role in the development of this complication because multiple studies have shown a direct correlation between the time to reduction and the prevalence of osteonecrosis. In the best of circumstances, a percentage of patients develop avascular changes despite prompt reduction of a dislocated hip. Patients with posterior dislocations and multiple injuries are apparently at increased risk for the development of osteonecrosis. Most patients who develop osteonecrosis have symptoms within 2 years of injury, although late cases of osteonecrosis with radiographic changes delayed 5 years have been reported.

Osteoarthritis is the most common complication after hip dislocation. Although a percentage results from osteonecrosis, a significant number of patients develop osteoarthritic changes without radiographic signs of osteonecrosis. The radiographic distinction between these two entities can be difficult. Indentation fractures and transchondral fractures of the femoral head larger than 4 mm have been associated with increased risk of osteoarthritis.

Sciatic nerve palsy complicates simple posterior hip dislocation in 13% of patients. No neurologic sequelae have been reported after anterior hip dislocation. The peroneal portion of the sciatic nerve is more commonly affected than the tibial branch. The relationship of the peroneal distribution to the piriformis muscle, tethering of the nerve at the sciatic notch and fibular neck, and the overall morphology of the peroneal division are possible explanations for its relatively increased risk. At least partial recovery of nerve function can be expected in approximately two thirds of patients. Significant controversy exists regarding the merits and timing of surgical exploration of the sciatic nerve after hip dislocation if closed reduction has been successfully performed and nerve function does not improve. Tornetta and Mostafavi recommended nerve exploration only if sciatic function was normal before reduction and deteriorated after closed reduction of the hip.

Recurrent instability occurs extremely rarely after hip dislocation without fracture and is caused by capsular or labral defects or capsular laxity. Capsular repair, labral repair, and bone block augmentation have been advocated for the surgical treatment of recurrent hip instability. Soft-tissue repair seems warranted initially with the addition of bony augmentation if acceptable stability cannot be shown intraoperatively after capsular or labral pathology has been treated.

PUBIC SYMPHYSIS AND SACROILIAC JOINTS

Dislocations involving the symphysis pubis and sacroiliac joints occur only with high-energy trauma. Considerable force is required to overcome the complex ligamentous structures that provide stability to the adult pelvis. The relevant anatomy and appropriate diagnostic and treatment algorithms are included in chapter 4.

STERNOCLAVICULAR JOINT

Traumatic dislocation of the sternoclavicular joint usually results from an indirect force on the anterior shoulder with the arm abducted. The most frequent of these injuries is the anterior dislocation in which the medial end of the clavicle is displaced anteriorly. Posterior or retrosternal dislocations also occur. The sternoclavicular joint also can be dislocated congenitally and in developmental, degenerative, and inflammatory processes.

When traumatic dislocation is anterior, considerable pain and swelling and a prominent deformity over the dislocated joint occur. The anteriorly displaced clavicle may appear elevated in relation to the sternum or may remain depressed near the first rib, depending on the extent of ligamentous disruption. Acute anterior dislocations can usually be treated by nonoperative methods, but interposition of the joint capsule or the ligaments may cause the dislocation to be irreducible. If the joint remains dislocated, the medial end of the clavicle causes an unsightly prominence, but for sedentary patients, little disability is to be expected.

Posterior dislocation of the sternoclavicular joint, as already mentioned, is less common. It can be a much more serious injury than the anterior dislocation, however, because the trachea, esophagus, thoracic duct, or large vessels in the mediastinum may be damaged by the posteriorly displaced medial end of the clavicle. The posteriorly displaced medial end of the clavicle can produce respiratory distress, venous congestion or arterial insufficiency, brachial plexus compression, and myocardial conduction abnormalities. Occasionally, pressure on these structures makes the dislocation a true emergency. Whether the sternoclavicular joint subluxates or dislocates depends on the extent of the injury to the capsular ligaments, the articular disc, the interclavicular ligament, and the costoclavicular (rhomboid) ligament. Rockwood stressed the importance and the frequency of injuries to the physis of the medial end of the clavicle that may appear to be a sternoclavicular dislocation in patients younger than 25 years old. Groh et al. found that early recognition (<10 days) of posterior dislocations improves the probability of accomplishing a closed reduction. When a closed reduction fails, they recommend open reduction. Closed and open reduction both produced similar good or excellent results in 18 of 21 patients.

In addition to the physical examination and anteroposterior radiographs, CT scan can be helpful in making a diagnosis. An apical lordotic view of the upper thorax centered over the sternum is usually diagnostic. In this view, the medial end of the clavicle is anterior or posterior to that of the normal clavicle on the opposite side.

For acute anterior sternoclavicular dislocations, Heinig recommended closed reduction after infiltrating the hematoma with a local anesthetic. In this situation, a meticulous sterile technique must be used. With the patient supine and with a large sandbag between the scapulae, traction is applied to the affected extremity, and the arm is abducted and extended while pressure is applied downward over the dislocated end of the clavicle. When the dislocation is reduced, the joint may be unstable, and the decision must be made whether to accept a residual subluxation or perform an open reduction and an internal fixation. In anterior dislocations, the deformity generally is accepted. If later instability is painful, ligament reconstruction or resection of the medial end of the clavicle (see chapter 9) may be indicated.

If the sternoclavicular dislocation is posterior, the patient is placed supine with a large sandbag between the scapulae. Traction is applied to the affected extremity, and the arm is abducted and extended. The clavicle is grasped with the fingers or a sterile towel clip, and anterior traction is exerted to assist in reduction. If a towel clip is used, sterile preparation of the skin is carried out first. Buckerfield and Castle described a reduction maneuver consisting of traction on the affected arm with the shoulder in adduction while a posteriorly directed force is applied to the shoulder and distal clavicle. Most posterior dislocations are stable when reduced. After reduction, immobilization can be achieved with a figure-of-eight soft dressing, a commercially prepared clavicular strap, or a figure-of-eight plaster dressing for 4 weeks. Activities should be restricted for 6 weeks. If reduction of the posterior dislocation cannot be obtained by closed methods even with the patient under general anesthesia, open reduction is indicated because of the dangers of leaving the joint dislocated. Kennedy recommended open reduction and ligament reconstruction because of the significant injury to the joint capsule, articular disc, and extraarticular ligaments. If open reduction is necessary, a surgeon with thoracic surgery experience should be consulted.

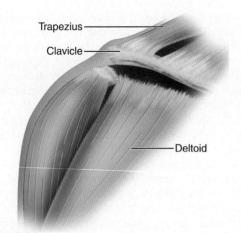

FIGURE 8.15 Dislocation of clavicle often causes tears in clavicular attachments of deltoid and trapezius muscles.

If open reduction is necessary, an attempt should be made to obtain stable fixation without the use of transarticular pins. Waters et al. advocated suture stabilization of costoclavicular and sternoclavicular ligaments for unstable reductions. Such considerations imply that surgical treatment should be reserved for irreducible posterior sternoclavicular dislocations and for significantly symptomatic, old, unreduced, or recurrent anterior sternoclavicular dislocations. If open reduction is required, the approach as described for old, unreduced (see chapter 9), and recurrent sternoclavicular dislocations can be modified.

ACROMIOCLAVICULAR JOINT
ETIOLOGY AND CLASSIFICATION

Injuries to the acromioclavicular joint are usually the result of a force applied downward on the acromion. The most common mechanism of injury is a fall directly onto the dome of the shoulder. The clavicle rests against the first rib, and the rib blocks further downward displacement of the clavicle. As a result, if the clavicle is not fractured, the acromioclavicular and coracoclavicular ligaments are ruptured. Injuries to the other structures in this area may include tears in the clavicular attachments of the deltoid and trapezius muscles (Fig. 8.15); fractures of the acromion, clavicle, and coracoid; disruption of the acromioclavicular fibrocartilage; and fractures of the articular cartilage of the acromioclavicular joint.

The severity of any superior or posterior displacement of the clavicle is determined by the severity of injury to the acromioclavicular and coracoclavicular ligaments, the acromioclavicular joint capsule, and the trapezius and deltoid muscles. In cadaver dissections, Rosenørn and Pedersen found that if the acromioclavicular ligament, the joint capsule, and these muscles were cut, proximal displacement of the clavicle ranged from 0.5 to 1.0 cm. More importantly, considerable anteroposterior instability was also present when the acromioclavicular ligament and joint capsule were sectioned. If, in addition to these structures, the coracoclavicular ligaments were also divided, the superior clavicular displacement ranged from 1.5 to 2.5 cm. Horn noted the clinical association of tears or avulsions of the deltoid and trapezius muscles with tears of the acromioclavicular and coracoclavicular ligaments.

Although many surgeons still use three grades of severity of separation, Rockwood and others subclassify these injuries

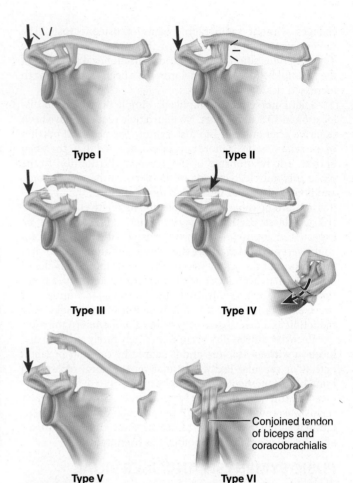

FIGURE 8.16 Rockwood classification of acromioclavicular injuries. *Type I:* neither acromioclavicular nor coracoclavicular ligaments are disrupted. *Type II:* acromioclavicular ligament is disrupted, and coracoclavicular ligament is intact. *Type III:* both ligaments are disrupted. *Type IV:* ligaments are disrupted, and distal end of clavicle is displaced posteriorly into or through trapezius muscle. *Type V:* ligaments and muscle attachments are disrupted, and clavicle and acromion are widely separated. *Type VI:* ligaments are disrupted, and distal clavicle is dislocated inferior to coracoid process and posterior to biceps and coracobrachialis tendons.

further into types I through VI (Fig. 8.16). Type I injuries result from minor strains of the acromioclavicular ligament and joint capsule. The acromioclavicular joint is stable, and pain is minimal. Although radiographs initially may be negative, periosteal calcification at the distal end of the clavicle may be apparent later. More significant forces cause type II, and the acromioclavicular ligament and the joint capsule are ruptured. The coracoclavicular ligaments remain intact. In this instance, the acromioclavicular joint is unstable. This instability, especially in the anteroposterior plane, causes deformity, and on radiographs, the lateral end of the clavicle may ride higher than the acromion, usually by less than the thickness of the clavicle even when stress is applied to the joint. Considerable pain and tenderness are present over the acromioclavicular joint, but stress radiographs are necessary to assess the degree of instability after these injuries. Injuries that result from a force sufficient to rupture the acromioclavicular and coracoclavicular ligaments have been considered grade III injuries.

CLINICAL FINDINGS

In addition to the physical findings of pain, swelling, and an unstable acromioclavicular joint with a mobile distal clavicle, radiographs are helpful in assessing the degree of injury. If the acromioclavicular ligament has been torn, and the coracoclavicular ligaments are intact, anteroposterior instability is the usual finding. Widening of the acromioclavicular joint is noted in the anteroposterior projection in these grade II injuries. Further instability in the acromioclavicular joint is detected by suspending 10 to 15 lb (4.5 to 6.8 kg) of weights to both of the patient's wrists. If possible, the weights should be tied to the wrists to avoid having the patient hold them; this allows the upper extremity muscles to relax completely. With the patient standing erect, anteroposterior radiographs are made of each acromioclavicular joint, and the two sides are compared. In significant subluxations, the lateral end of the clavicle is displaced superiorly, or the scapula and arm are displaced inferiorly, more than one half the thickness of the clavicle. In dislocations, the distal clavicle is displaced a distance that is equal to or more than its thickness (Fig. 8.17).

TREATMENT

Type I injuries are satisfactorily treated nonsurgically. This usually includes application of ice, use of mild analgesics, immobilization with a sling, early range-of-motion exercises, and reinstitution of activities when comfort permits. Most surgeons agree that type II injuries should be treated similarly unless significant instability is observed. If the distal clavicle is displaced no more than one half of its thickness, strapping, splinting, or immobilization with a sling for 2 to 3 weeks is usually successful. Six weeks usually must pass, however, before heavy lifting or contact sports can be resumed. Treatment of type III injuries has become less controversial in recent years. Isokinetic testing after nonsurgical treatment of acromioclavicular dislocation has revealed that strength and endurance are comparable on the affected and uninjured sides. Most patients have no difficulty with activities of daily living, but athletes occasionally report pain with contact sports and throwing. At this clinic, we generally treat all type III acromioclavicular joint separations nonoperatively initially with late reconstruction if necessary. In types IV, V, and VI injuries, most authors agree that the displacement of the acromioclavicular joint would be too great to accept and that open reduction and internal fixation are indicated.

It has been suggested that conservative treatment fails chiefly because of the interposition of the articular disc, frayed capsular ligaments, and fragments of articular cartilage between the acromion and the clavicle. The disadvantages of nonsurgical treatment by strapping, bracing, or splinting techniques include: (1) skin pressure and ulceration, (2) recurrence of deformity, (3) necessity of wearing the sling or brace for 8 weeks, (4) poor patient cooperation, (5) interference with activities of daily living, (6) loss of shoulder and elbow motion (in older patients), (7) soft-tissue calcification, (8) late acromioclavicular arthritis, and (9) late muscle atrophy, weakness, and fatigue. The avoidance of a surgical procedure is a major advantage of closed methods, and, when successful, closed techniques usually result in a stable joint and satisfactory function in the shoulder. To prevent possible complications, however, close observation on a regular basis is necessary and complete patient cooperation is essential.

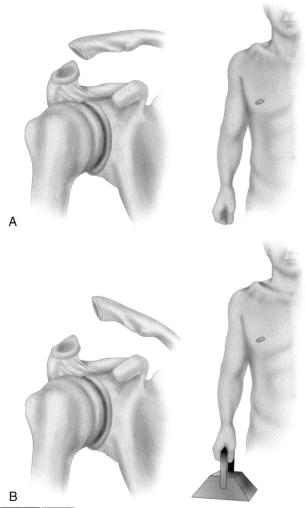

FIGURE 8.17 Stress views of acromioclavicular dislocation. **A,** Without weights. **B,** With weights.

Besides types I and II, Rockwood described types III, IV, V, and VI injuries. Type III injuries consist of disruption of the acromioclavicular and coracoclavicular ligaments and the distal clavicular attachment of the deltoid muscle. The distal clavicle is above the acromion by at least the thickness of the clavicle. Traditionally, this elevation of the clavicle has been attributed to the pull of the trapezius muscle; however, Rockwood suggested that the scapula, including the glenohumeral joint, is depressed, rather than the clavicle being elevated, creating the gap between the clavicle and the acromion. In type IV injuries, the same structures are disrupted as in grade III injuries. The distal clavicle is displaced posteriorly into or through the trapezius muscle. In type V injuries, the distal attachments of the deltoid and trapezius to the clavicle are detached from the distal half of the clavicle. The acromioclavicular joint is displaced 100% to 300%, and a gross separation between the clavicle and the acromion is present. Type VI injuries are rare and are caused by extreme abduction that tears the acromioclavicular and coracoclavicular ligaments. The distal clavicle is displaced under the coracoid and behind the conjoined tendons.

MRI may play a role in the treatment of this injury. In one series, 30% of patients had a concomitant injury that needed surgical treatment at the time of acromioclavicular joint repair or reconstruction.

The difficulties and problems associated with surgical methods include: (1) infection, (2) anesthetic risk, (3) hematoma formation, (4) scar formation, (5) recurrence of deformity, (6) metal breakage, migration, and loosening, (7) breakage or loosening of sutures, (8) erosion or fracture of the distal clavicle, (9) postoperative pain and limitation of motion, (10) second procedure required for removal of fixation, (11) late acromioclavicular arthritis, and (12) soft-tissue calcification (usually insignificant). Surgical treatment permits inspection of the injury to the joint and removal of any fracture fragments or other obstructions to reduction. It also permits an anatomic reduction and secure fixation that usually allows the resumption of shoulder motion earlier than is possible with closed techniques.

Many different procedures have been devised for the surgical treatment of dislocations of the acromioclavicular joint. They can be divided into five major categories: (1) acromioclavicular reduction and fixation; (2) acromioclavicular reduction, coracoclavicular ligament repair, and coracoclavicular fixation; (3) a combination of the first two categories; (4) distal clavicle excision; and (5) muscle transfers.

Acromioclavicular reduction and transarticular wire fixation, usually with smooth or threaded Kirschner wires, has been used. Acromioclavicular reduction with acromioclavicular repair or reconstruction and coracoclavicular fixation with coracoclavicular ligament repair or reconstruction also has been reported. Coracoclavicular fixation with heavy nonabsorbable suture and transfer of the coracoacromial ligament to the distal clavicle resulted in 89% satisfactory results in a study by Weinstein et al. These researchers also found that early repairs were more likely to have more satisfactory results than late reconstructions, and this was statistically significant. The superior acromioclavicular ligament can be repaired directly or can be reconstructed with the coracoacromial ligament or free tendon grafts. The coracoclavicular ligaments can also be repaired directly when they are not too frayed; they have been reconstructed using fascia lata, free tendon grafts, the coracoacromial ligament, and transfer of the tendon of the long head of the biceps.

Coracoclavicular fixation devices depend on an intact coracoid process and have included single and double wire loops, screws, nonabsorbable sutures, metallic and bioabsorbable suture anchors, and bone grafts. Coracoclavicular bone grafting creates an extraarticular acromioclavicular arthrodesis and reportedly results in no significant restriction of shoulder motion. We have had little experience with this procedure.

Resection of the lateral or distal end of the clavicle has been proposed for the treatment of acute and old acromioclavicular dislocations. If the coracoclavicular ligaments are disrupted, they must be repaired or reconstructed; internal fixation is required, either across the acromioclavicular defect or between the coracoid and the clavicle. Dewar and Barrington described transfer of the coracoid to the clavicle to hold the lateral end of the bone in position. This technique can be combined with resection of the lateral end of the clavicle (see chapter 9).

Our preferred method for treating acromioclavicular joint dislocations is a technique described by Mazzocca et al. It is an anatomic reconstruction of both the conoid and trapezoid ligaments. This procedure alleviates concerns over implant migration, inadequate acromioclavicular ligaments for repair, and nonanatomic positioning. Distal clavicular resection is performed routinely to correct altered acromioclavicular joint

biomechanics. Autologous semitendinosus graft is preferred, and the reconstruction is augmented preferably with suture tape. Biomechanical studies by Mazzocca et al. demonstrated superior fixation using this technique compared with pin fixation or repair. This technique also can be used for unstable distal clavicular fractures through appropriate drill holes in the clavicle.

Any surgical procedure for acromioclavicular dislocation should fulfill three requirements: (1) the acromioclavicular joint must be exposed and debrided; (2) the coracoclavicular and acromioclavicular ligaments must be repaired or reconstructed; and (3) stable reduction of the acromioclavicular joint must be obtained. Procedures that accomplish these three goals, no matter how the joint is fixed, should produce acceptable results.

Most of the procedures that reduce and fix the acromioclavicular joint should be reserved for patients younger than 45 years old. DePalma's anatomic dissections and studies suggest that early degenerative changes are developing in the acromioclavicular joint by the third decade and that significant changes are present by the fourth decade. Although procedures in which the distal clavicle is excised can be used satisfactorily in young patients, older patients with painful, disabling, old acromioclavicular dislocations with degenerative changes should especially be considered as candidates for such a procedure. Various arthroscopic techniques also have been described for acromioclavicular joint fixation, showing fair-to-good results at short-term follow-up. In one study the acromioclavicular joint was found to be unsatisfactory in 40% of patients as seen on postoperative radiographs. This technique should be performed only by an experienced arthroscopist. See other chapter for arthroscopic treatment of acromioclavicular joints. The treatment of old acromioclavicular dislocations is discussed in chapter 9.

ANATOMIC RECONSTRUCTION OF THE CONOID AND TRAPEZOID LIGAMENTS

TECHNIQUE 8.5

(MAZZOCCA ET AL.)

- Make a curvilinear incision 3.5 cm from the distal clavicle in the lines of Langer to the tip of the coracoid (Fig. 8.18A).
- Raise full-thickness flaps anteriorly and posteriorly on the clavicle, skeletonizing the clavicle.
- Resect the last 10 mm of the distal clavicle, beveling the inferior bone.
- Dissect the coracoid posterior to the deltoid. Once the coracoid is exposed, create a tunnel under the coracoid with a right-angle clamp to ensure easy graft passage.
- Drill the first tunnel 45 mm from the distal clavicle (35 mm if distal clavicular resection has already been performed) using an appropriate steel reamer. It should be positioned slightly posterior to re-create normal conoid position (Fig. 8.18A).
- Drill the second tunnel 15 mm lateral to the first tunnel slightly anteriorly to re-create trapezoid position (Fig. 8.18A).

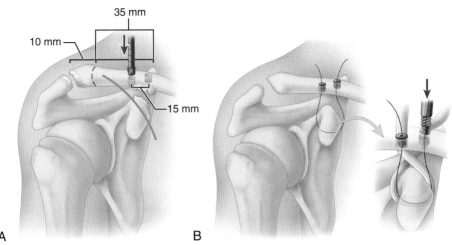

FIGURE 8.18 Mazzocca anatomic coracoclavicular reconstruction. **A,** Incision and tunnel placement. **B,** Graft passage. **SEE TECHNIQUE 8.5.**

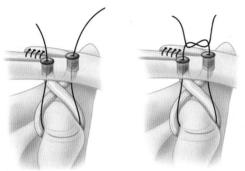

FIGURE 8.19 Mazzocca anatomic coracoclavicular reconstruction. Interference screw fixation of graft to clavicle. **SEE TECHNIQUE 8.5.**

- Pass the lateral limb of the graft with suture through the first (posterior) tunnel and cross it posteriorly so that it will ultimately be a figure-of-eight. Then feed the medial limb of the graft through the anterior tunnel. Do not cross the suture but pass it directly so that it will be a circle (Fig. 8.18B).
- Secure the graft with a soft-tissue interference screw in the posterior or anterior tunnel, bringing the suture up through the cannulated screw.
- With upper displacement of the scapulohumeral complex, slightly overreduce the acromioclavicular joint. After assessment of correct screw placement, place a second screw in the final bone tunnel.
- Confirm the reduction with C-arm Zanca view. Tie the suture (Fig. 8.19).
- Route the remaining lateral limb of the tendon graft and suture it to the acromion as in an acromioclavicular ligament reconstruction (Fig. 8.20).
- Close the deltotrapezial interval securely and close the skin with absorbable monofilament suture (Fig. 8.21).

POSTOPERATIVE CARE A brace is worn for 6 weeks, removed only for active-assisted and pendulum exercises. Strengthening begins at 12 weeks and return to sports is in 6 months.

SHOULDER

Uncomplicated dislocations of the shoulder rarely require open reduction. Some acute anterior dislocations of the shoulder are irreducible because of interposition of the long head of the biceps tendon, greater tuberosity, or fracture fragments of the glenoid. Fracture-dislocations of the shoulder are discussed in chapter 5. Rotator cuff tears that require repair have also been reported with shoulder dislocation. The biomechanics and pathoanatomy seen with recurrent dislocations are discussed in other chapter.

Recurrent instability in young patients has been reported in up to 90% of patients treated nonoperatively. Up to 12% recurrence has been reported in operatively treated shoulders. Arthroscopic stabilization has been recommended in active young patients with no history of subluxation or impingement who may otherwise have recurrent dislocations after acute traumatic dislocation. We currently favor initial nonoperative management for first-time dislocations but consider arthroscopic stabilization procedures an appropriate alternative in selected patients.

ELBOW

The elbow is the second most commonly dislocated joint in adults. Approximately 20% of dislocations are associated with fractures and up to 50% in children. Acute dislocation of the elbow is almost always reducible by closed methods, and most are stable after reduction. Open reduction may be required if fracture fragments in a fracture-dislocation block closed reduction. Late elbow instability and stiffness are rare after simple dislocations.

Treatment principles of simple dislocations include reduction of the joint and early motion. One study found that patients with unstable elbow joints treated nonoperatively had fewer symptoms than patients treated with ligament repair. Unprotected flexion and extension exercises within 2 weeks of dislocation have been recommended. Burra and Andrews recommended operative treatment when throwing movements are required by athletes.

DISLOCATION OF THE RADIAL HEAD

If dislocation of the radial head occurs without dislocation of the humeroulnar joint, the radial head is almost always displaced anteriorly and can be easily reduced manually. Because the annular ligament has been ruptured or displaced, the pull of the biceps muscle often causes the dislocation to recur, and unless the radial head remains reduced, it would limit flexion of the joint. Consequently, open reduction and repair or reconstruction of the annular ligament is indicated (1) when the dislocation recurs after closed reduction and immobilization of the elbow in more than 90 degrees of flexion; (2) when it has gone untreated for 2 to 4 weeks; or (3) when it is irreducible by closed means, usually because the radial head is trapped by interposed soft tissues. When the dislocation has gone untreated for more than 4 or 5 weeks in an adult, the radial head should be excised (see chapter 5).

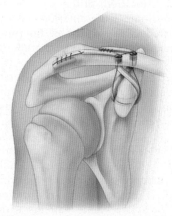

FIGURE 8.20 Mazzocca anatomic coracoclavicular reconstruction. Final placement of grafts. **SEE TECHNIQUE 8.5.**

OPEN REDUCTION OF RADIAL HEAD DISLOCATION

TECHNIQUE 8.6

- Make an incision over the posterior aspect of the radial head, expose the head and identify the annular ligament (Fig. 8.22).
- Reduce the dislocation and, if possible, repair the ligament and disrupted capsule with fine interrupted sutures.
- If repair is impossible, take a fascial graft 1.3 cm wide × 10 cm long from the outer aspect of the thigh (or from the deep fascia on the dorsal aspect of the forearm, as described in chapter 5).
- Expose the posterior surface of the ulna through a second incision 5.0 cm long and drill a hole transversely through the bone 1.3 cm distal to the level of the radial head.
- Pass the strip of fascia lata through this hole and around the radial neck and suture its ends together without tension, creating a new annular ligament.

POSTOPERATIVE CARE With the arm in a splint or a cast, the elbow is immobilized at 90 degrees of flexion with the forearm in neutral rotation for 2 to 3 weeks. Gentle active motion and especially rehabilitation of the muscles are begun. The elbow must not be manipulated, and motion must not be passively forced in any attempt to restore function. After motion and strength have been actively restored, the head may become slightly displaced, but, if so, it does not interfere significantly with function.

■ DISLOCATION OF RADIAL HEAD AND FRACTURE OF PROXIMAL THIRD OF ULNA (MONTEGGIA FRACTURE)

The treatment of a Monteggia fracture is described in chapter 5.

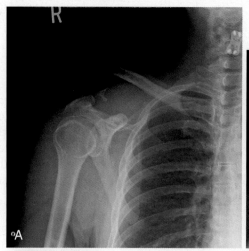

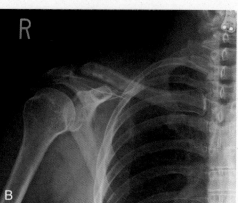

FIGURE 8.21 **A,** Grade V acromioclavicular dislocation. **B,** After Mazzocca anatomic reconstruction with Mumford procedure. **SEE TECHNIQUE 8.5.**

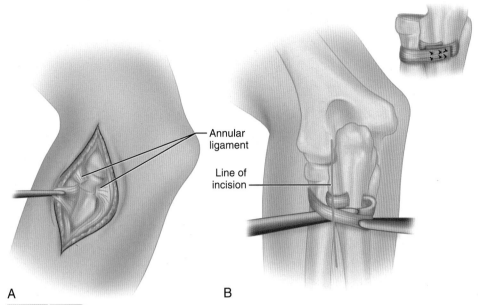

FIGURE 8.22 Dislocation of radial head. **A,** Annular ligament has been ruptured. Often, this ligament can be sutured satisfactorily. **B,** If necessary, annular ligament can be reconstructed with strip of fascia lata. *Inset,* Reconstruction has been completed. **SEE TECHNIQUE 8.6.**

▓ FRACTURE-DISLOCATION OF ELBOW WITH SEVERE DAMAGE OF SOFT STRUCTURES

Complex elbow dislocations with associated fractures may require surgical intervention to obtain joint stability. This typically includes ligament or fracture repair. A fracture-dislocation of the adult elbow in which the soft structures have been severely damaged should not be treated by closed methods but by debridement and repair. This operation is occasionally indicated if the radial head and the coronoid process of the ulna have been fractured and severe damage to the soft tissues is evident. Large periarticular fractures have been shown to affect functional results adversely. A fractured coronoid process strongly suggests that the elbow had become at least partially dislocated at the time of the injury. At surgery, the brachialis muscle may be found to be torn, the anterior part of the capsule of the elbow joint to be avulsed, and either one or both collateral ligaments to be ruptured. If the injuries of the soft structures are repaired at the same time as the injuries to the bone, the return of function can be hastened, the final range of motion can be improved, and the potential for myositis ossificans around the elbow can be reduced. This open reduction is only for fracture-dislocations of the elbow with severe damage (see chapter 5 for ligament repair techniques). In a severe fracture-dislocation of the elbow, it is important to assess the integrity of the distal radioulnar joint.

DISTAL RADIOULNAR JOINT

An injury to the distal radioulnar joint can occur in association with almost any fracture of the forearm or as an isolated injury. A dislocation of this joint may be simple or complex. Failure to recognize a simple dislocation of the distal radioulnar joint associated with a fracture of the forearm may result in inappropriate or inadequate immobilization of the joint after fixation of the fracture. Consequently, the injured triangular fibrocartilage complex may not heal, leading to recurrent postoperative instability. Failure to diagnose and treat a complex

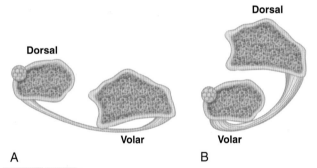

FIGURE 8.23 Distal radioulnar dislocation. **A,** Ulnar dorsal dislocation is maintained by pull of pronator quadratus muscle, which prevents overlapping of bones. **B,** In ulnar volar dislocation, pull of pronator quadratus muscle produces overlapping of distal radius and ulna.

distal radioulnar joint dislocation can lead to chronic persistent subluxation or dislocation and to symptomatic osteoarthrosis.

The chief function of the distal radioulnar joint is to stabilize the forearm during pronation and supination as the radius rotates on the distal end of the ulna. The distal ulna is completely covered by cartilage and articulates with the ulnar notch of the radius except on its ulnar side. The distal radioulnar joint is stabilized by the following structures: the ulnar collateral ligament, which is attached to the tip of the ulnar styloid and to the pisiform and triquetrum; the articular disc, which is attached to the base of the ulnar styloid and to the margin of the ulnar notch of the radius; the anterior and posterior radioulnar ligaments, which are parts of the joint capsule; and the pronator quadratus muscle, which spans the volar surface of the distal radius and ulna and the interosseous space. For the distal radioulnar joint to become dislocated, some or all of these structures must be injured.

A distal radioulnar dislocation can be dorsal or volar (Fig. 8.23). If the dislocation is with the ulna in the dorsal

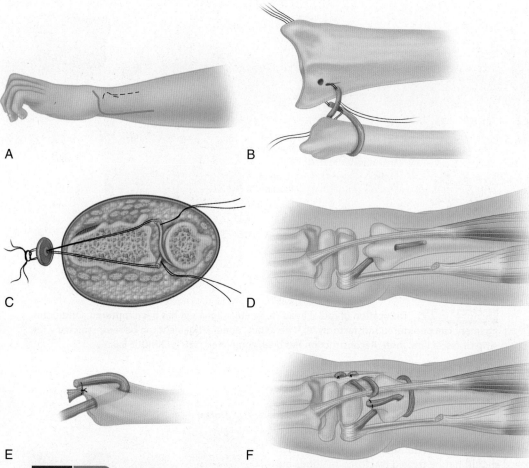

FIGURE 8.24 Bunnell technique to stabilize distal radioulnar joint. **A,** Skin incision. **B,** Annular ligament formed by looping small tendon graft around neck of ulna and attaching it to radius. **C,** Cross section of wrist showing method of attaching tendon graft to radius. **D,** Tenodesis of distal end of ulna, using split portion of flexor carpi ulnaris tendon. **E,** Detail of tenodesis. **F,** Final appearance after anchoring extensor carpi ulnaris tendon dorsally by separate tendon loop to prevent subluxation of tendon on flexion and pronation of wrist.

position, reduction is usually accomplished by supination of the forearm with pressure on the distal ulna. If the dislocation is with the ulna in the volar position, pronation of the forearm is usually successful in reducing the dislocation. An excellent result can usually be expected if it is reduced early and immobilized for 1 month in plaster. If the dislocation is less than 2 months old and cannot be reduced closed, open reduction with exposure and repair of the triangular fibrocartilage is advised. If the dislocation is reduced surgically after more than 2 months, consideration should be given to excision of the distal ulna and distal ligament reconstruction. According to Milch, rupture of the distal radioulnar ligaments usually causes diastasis of the distal radioulnar joint. He stated that this separation can be seen on radiographs and is a pathognomonic sign that the ligaments have been ruptured and should be repaired. Irreducible dislocations of the distal radioulnar joint have been described. In most patients, the extensor carpi ulnaris was entrapped in the joint and prevented closed reduction. A dorsal approach was used to free the extensor carpi ulnaris, and repair of the triangular fibrocartilage or transosseous pinning was used to stabilize the joint.

Rupture of the ligaments around the distal radioulnar joint without a fracture usually is considered to be only a sprain, and the joint seldom is properly immobilized. The ligaments may not heal well, and, if not, the damage is rarely discovered before 6 to 8 weeks after injury. By this time, degenerative changes in the articular surfaces of the joint may have become so severe that restoring the normal radioulnar relationship would be undesirable. In these instances, resection of the distal ulna (see chapter 6) is usually indicated; reconstruction of the ligaments is indicated only rarely. Operations to reconstruct permanently damaged ligaments of the distal radioulnar joint cannot be successful unless the component bones are undeformed.

Because operations to stabilize the distal radioulnar joint are so rarely indicated, the techniques for performing them are not described here. In Figures 8.24 and 8.25, two such operations are shown, and the reader is referred to the original works for details of the techniques. Acute dislocations of the wrist, the carpus, and the joints of the hand are discussed in other chapter.

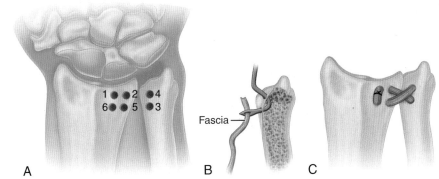

FIGURE 8.25 Liebolt technique to stabilize distal radioulnar joint. **A,** Location of holes drilled in radius and ulna. **B,** Method of passing tendon. **C,** Appearance after joint has been stabilized.

REFERENCES

Ahmad I, Mistry J: The management of acute and chronic elbow instability, *Orthop Clin North Am* 46(2):271, 2015.

Balcarek P, Ammon J, Frosch S, et al.: Magnetic resonance imaging characteristics of the medial patellofemoral ligament lesion in acute lateral patellar dislocations considering trochlear dysplasia, patella alta, and tibial tuberosity-trochlear groove distance, *Arthroscopy* 26:926, 2010.

Boyce RH, Singh K, Obremskey WT: Acute management of traumatic knee dislocations for the generalist, *J Am Acad Orthop Surg* 23(12):761, 2015.

Braun C, McRobert CJ: Conservative management following closed reduction of traumatic anterior dislocation of the shoulder, *Cochrane Database Syst Rev* 5:CD004962, 2019.

Chang N, Furey A, Kurdin A: Operative versus nonoperative management of acute high-grade acromioclavicular dislocations: a systematic review and meta-analysis, *J Orthop Trauma* 32(1):1, 2018.

Cunningham NJ, Farebrother N, Miles J: Review article: isolated proximal tibiofibular joint dislocation, *Emer Med Australas* 31(2):156, 2019.

De Carli A, Lanzetti RM, Ciompi A, et al.: Acromioclavicular third degree dislocation: surgical treatment in acute cases, *J Orthop Surg Res* 10:13, 2015.

Duryea DM, Payatakes AH, Mosher TJ: Subtle radiographic findings of acute, isolated distal radioulnar joint dislocation, *Skel Radiol* 45(9):1243, 2016.

Duthon VB: Acute traumatic patellar dislocation, *Orthop Traumatol Surg Res* 101(1 Suppl):S59, 2015.

Fuller JA, Hammil HL, Pronschinske KJ, Durall CJ: Operative versus nonoperative treatment after acute patellar dislocation: which is more effective at reducing recurrence in adolescents? *J Sport Rehabil* 27(6):601, 2018.

Gabl M, Arora R, Gassner EM, Schmidle G: Ulna rotation osteotomy in complete dislocation of the radioulnar joint, *J Wrist Surg* 6(1):74, 2017.

Gravesen KS, Kallemose T, Blond L, et al.: High incidence of acute and recurrent patellar dislocations: a retrospective nationwide epidemiological study involving 24,154 primary dislocations, *Knee Surg Sports Traumatol Arthrosc* 26(4):1204, 2018.

Groh GI, Wirth MA, Rockwood CA: Treatment of traumatic posterior sternoclavicular dislocations, *J Shoulder Elbow Surg* 20:107, 2011.

Heitmann M, Akoto R, Krause M, et al.: Management of acute knee dislocations: anatomic repair and ligament bracing as a new treatment option-results of a multicentre study, *Knee Surg Sports Traumatol Arthrosc* 27(8):2710, 2019.

Khakha RS, Day AC, Gibbs J, et al.: Acute surgical management of traumatic knee dislocations—average follow-up of 10 years, *Knee* 23(2):267, 2016.

Khanna V, Harris A, Farrokhyar F, et al.: Hip arthroscopy: prevalence of intra-articular pathologic findings after traumatic injury of the hip, *Arthroscopy* 30:299, 2014.

Kavaja L, Lähdeoja T, Malmivaara A, Paavola M: Treatment after traumatic shoulder dislocation: a systematic review with a network meta-analysis, *Br J Sports Med* 52(23):1498, 2018.

Kim HT, Can LV, Ahn TY, Kim IH: Analysis of radiographic parameters of the forearm in traumatic radial head dislocation, *Clin Orthop Surg* 9(4):521, 2017.

Lewallen LW, McIntosh AL, Dahm DL: Predictors of recurrent instability after acute patellofemoral dislocation in pediatric and adolescent patients, *Am J Sports Med* 41:575, 2013.

Mah J, Canadian Orthopaedic Trauma Society (COTS): General health status after nonoperative versus operative treatment for acute, complete acromioclavicular joint dislocation: results of a multicenter randomized clinical trial, *J Orthop Trauma* 31(9):485, 2017.

Metzler AV, Lattermann C, Johnson DL: Cartilage lesions of the patella: management after acute patellar dislocation, *Orthopedics* 38(5):310, 2015.

Mori D, Yamashita F, Kizaki K, et al.: Anatomic coracoclavicular ligament reconstruction for the treatment of acute acromioclavicular joint dislocation: minimum 10-year follow-up, *JBJS Open Access* 23(3):e0007, 2017.

Olds MK, Ellis R, Parmar P, Kersten P: Who will redislocate his/her shoulder? Predicting recurrent instability following a first traumatic anterior shoulder dislocation, *BMJ Open Sport Exerc Med* 5(1):e000447, 2019.

Park B: Acute management of shoulder dislocations, *J Am Acad Orthop Surg* 23(4):209, 2015.

Ranger P, Senay A, Gratton GR, et al.: LARS synthetic ligaments for the acute management of 111 acute knee dislocations: effective surgical treatment for most ligaments, *Knee Surg Sports Traumatol Arthrosc* 26(12):3673, 2018.

Shanchez-Sotelo J, Morrey M: Complex elbow instability: surgical management of elbow fracture dislocations, *EFORT Open Rev* 1(5):183, 2017.

Tauber M, Koller H, Hitzl W, Resch H: Dynamic radiologic evaluation of horizontal instability in acute acromioclavicular joint dislocations, *Am J Sports Med* 38:1188, 2010.

Watts AC: Primary ligament repair for acute elbow dislocation, *JBJS Essent Surg Techn* 9(1):e8, 2019.

Wight L, Owen D, Goldbloom D, Knupp M: Pure ankle dislocation: a systematic review of the literature and estimation of incidence, *Injury* 48(10):2027, 2017.

Woodmass J, Romatowski NP, Esposito JG, et al.: A systematic review of peroneal nerve palsy and recovery following traumatic knee dislocation, *Knee Surg Sports Traumatol Arthrosc* 23(10):2992, 2015.

Zheng X, Hu Y, Xie P, et al.: Surgical medial patellofemoral ligament reconstruction versus nonsurgical treatment of acute primary patellar dislocation: a prospective controlled trial, *Int Orthop* 43(6):1495, 2019.

The complete list of references is available online at ExpertConsult.com.

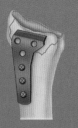
FOOT	490	**STERNOCLAVICULAR JOINT**	495	Posterior dislocations	506
ANKLE	490	Posterior dislocations	496	Hemiarthroplasty	508
PROXIMAL TIBIOFIBULAR JOINT	490	**ACROMIOCLAVICULAR JOINT**	497	Total shoulder arthroplasty	509
KNEE	491	**SHOULDER**	501	**ELBOW**	509
PATELLA	492	Treatment	503	Closed reduction	509
HIP	493	Closed reduction	503	Open reduction	509
Chronic anterior dislocations	493	Open reduction	504	Elbow arthroplasty	513
Chronic posterior dislocations	493	Anterior dislocations	505	Anterior dislocation of the radial head	513

Any dislocation should be reduced as soon as reasonably possible. While a joint is dislocated, the metabolism of its hyaline cartilage is disturbed and synovial fluid functions are impaired. Hyaline cartilage may begin to degenerate during this brief period, and irreversible changes rapidly occur. Consequently, when old unreduced dislocations are finally reduced, normal and painless joint motion and function should not be expected.

When old unreduced dislocations are encountered, especially in the elbow, hip, knee, or ankle, arthroplasty or arthrodesis may be necessary either at the time of reduction or shortly thereafter. The procedure selected depends on individual considerations, such as the joint affected, the condition of the articular cartilage, any associated injuries, and the patient's age and occupation. Treatment options include reduction alone, reduction with arthroplasty, or arthrodesis.

Reduction alone usually suffices for children and young adults. In older patients, reduction combined with arthroplasty or arthrodesis may be a better course. In patients in whom the dislocation is not restricting daily activities and is not excessively painful, reduction may not be indicated, especially in older patients.

Most old unreduced dislocations require open reduction. However, there is no arbitrary time limit beyond which a dislocation cannot be reduced by closed means. Skeletal traction sometimes will reduce a joint that has been dislocated for several weeks. If 2 to 3 weeks have passed since the injury, manipulation should be done cautiously and gently. Osteoporosis from disuse rapidly weakens the bones after a dislocation, and manipulative techniques may result in fractures. If open techniques are employed, similar care should be taken with use of instruments such as levers because articular surfaces may be further damaged. Excessive force thus should be avoided in both open and closed methods. The most common of old unreduced dislocations are discussed in this chapter.

FOOT

Fractures and dislocations around the foot are discussed in other chapter.

ANKLE

An old unreduced dislocation of the ankle without a fracture is extremely rare. The type and severity of the dislocation almost always depend on the type and treatment of any associated fractures. An anterior dislocation usually is complicated by a fracture of the anterior margin of the distal articular surface of the tibia. A posterior dislocation usually is complicated either by a fracture of the distal tibia, including its posterior margin and a part of the metaphysis, or by a trimalleolar-type fracture. A lateral dislocation is usually complicated by a lateral or bimalleolar fracture. Fractures of the lower extremity are discussed in chapter 2.

PROXIMAL TIBIOFIBULAR JOINT

Two types of proximal tibiofibular subluxations or dislocations have been described: idiopathic and posttraumatic. The idiopathic type occurs primarily in preadolescent or adolescent children and is more common in girls than in boys. It can also occur in patients in their late 40s and 50s with generalized laxity of ligaments. An idiopathic subluxation usually is treated nonoperatively. If the condition is symptomatic, initial treatment can be cast immobilization. Idiopathic subluxation in a young patient should probably not be treated surgically, because it appears to be a self-limited condition. Surgery may be indicated in older patients if subluxation becomes chronic and painful and does not respond to immobilization.

Posttraumatic, chronic subluxation of the proximal fibula occurs after injuries to the anterior and posterior capsular ligaments of the proximal tibiofibular joint and to the fibular collateral ligament of the knee, often initially not fully appreciated. The ligamentous and capsular structures around the proximal tibiofibular joint are shown in Fig. 9.1.

An old dislocation of the proximal fibula may not be symptomatic enough to require treatment. When symptoms do occur, it may be as lateral knee pain, instability, arthritis, or as ankle pain. Problems may be minimal with normal activities but experienced as clunking or giving way with certain more strenuous activities. Peroneal nerve dysfunction,

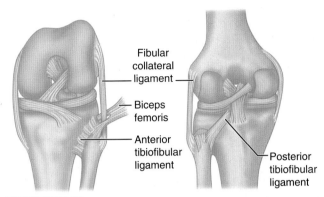

FIGURE 9.1 Anatomy of proximal tibiofibular joint. (Redrawn from Halbrecht JL, Jackson DW: Recurrent dislocation of the proximal tibiofibular joint, *Orthop Rev* 20:957–960, 1991.)

Labels on figure: Fibular collateral ligament, Biceps femoris, Anterior tibiofibular ligament, Posterior tibiofibular ligament

particularly decreased foot sensation, can also be troublesome. If symptoms demand, treatment is indicated.

Various treatment options exist. Because of the relative rarity of this problem, decisions on treatment may be hampered by lack of evidence from studies with large numbers or long-term follow-up. Closed reduction alone is not likely to be successful or helpful. Nonoperative treatment may be attempted using a supportive strap, an exercise program, and activity modification. However, when nonoperative treatment is inadequate, surgery may be indicated. Most authors have thought that resection of the proximal fibula is the best option, although some have expressed reservations about using this procedure in children, adolescents, and some athletes.

Arthrodesis has been performed but is problematic. It has been shown that during dorsiflexion of the ankle the proximal fibula rotates around its longitudinal axis. To accommodate lateral plane rotation of the talus and the ankle joint, the fibula must rotate externally.

Attempts at ligamentous reconstruction using biceps, and deep fascia or gracilis grafts have met with at least some early success, and temporary (3 to 6 months) screw fixation also has been described with good early results.

LIGAMENTOUS RECONSTRUCTION FOR OLD UNREDUCED DISLOCATION OF THE PROXIMAL TIBIOFIBULAR JOINT

TECHNIQUE 9.1

- See the technique for removal of a proximal fibular graft (see Technique 1.7).
- It is important when this technique is used that the lateral supporting structures of the knee joint be reconstructed. This is accomplished by preserving the proximal fibular styloid process with its attached ligaments for subsequent attachment to the tibia.
- The fibular dissection should be subperiosteal to prevent injury to the peroneal nerve.

POSTOPERATIVE CARE A long leg, bent-knee cast is applied and worn for 6 weeks. Treatment thereafter should be as described for acute injuries of the lateral knee ligaments in other chapter.

KNEE

Acute dislocation of the knee is usually a true emergency because of the possibility of vascular injury. Old unreduced dislocations of the knee are therefore rare. A useful range of motion is seldom restored after open reduction of such a dislocation. Even though at surgery the articular cartilage may look normal, adhesions usually develop between the articular surfaces (Fig. 9.2). Satisfactory results have been reported after open reduction as long as 4 months after dislocation, and there have been reports of successful gradual reduction of chronic dislocations using the Ilizarov device, the Taylor Spatial Frame, or similar circular and hinged external fixators. Some authors have followed this reduction with arthrodesis, whereas others have described arthroscopic ligamentous reconstruction after reduction as an alternative to an open procedure. In older patients with chronic dislocations, total knee arthroplasty (TKA) may be an option, but this has been reported in only a few patients. Because of recurrent dislocation after TKA with a nonconstrained implant, Chen and Chiu recommended a constraining implant in such situations.

OPEN REDUCTION FOR OLD UNREDUCED DISLOCATION OF THE KNEE

TECHNIQUE 9.2

- Use an anteromedial approach to expose the knee joint. If the patella has been displaced either medially or laterally, make the skin incision to correspond with the normal anatomic location of the medial borders of the quadriceps tendon, patella, and patellar tendon.
- If necessary, dissect the soft structures subperiosteally from the posterior aspect of the femur and tibia. Excise enough fibrous tissue to expose the articular surfaces completely.
- If the cartilage appears undamaged, reduce the dislocation. To maintain reduction, stabilize the joint for 6 weeks with one or two large Steinmann pins or a spanning external fixator. If the cartilage has been irreversibly damaged, proceed with arthrodesis of the knee if this is the indicated procedure.
- If arthroplasty is indicated, it is often better to reduce the joint, proceed with the rehabilitation of the extremity, allow the contractures to resolve, and then follow with arthroplasty at a later time. If this course is chosen, immobilize the extremity in a long leg cast or brace until knee motion has started.

POSTOPERATIVE CARE If arthroplasty is planned, postoperative care is the same as that for acute dislocation of

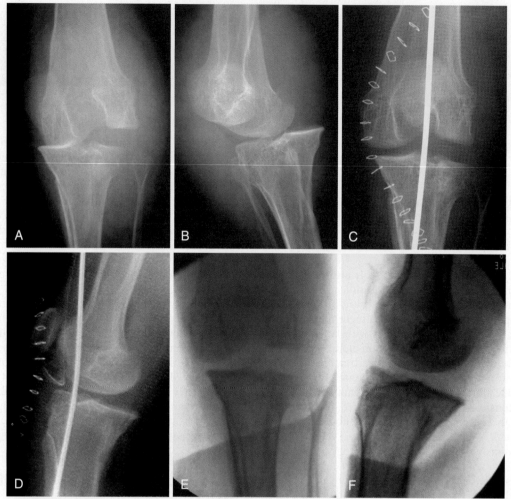

FIGURE 9.2 Seventeen-year-old girl with history of neurofibromatosis and 6-week history of acute knee dislocation and inability to walk. **A** and **B,** Anteroposterior and lateral radiographs of knee showing posteromedial (tibia) knee dislocation with medial dislocation of patella. **C** and **D,** Anteroposterior and lateral radiographs at time of open reduction and internal fixation with smooth Steinmann pin through quadriceps mechanism of femur and tibia. **E** and **F,** Postoperative anteroposterior and lateral radiographs showing mild persistent lateral subluxation but good reduction of knee and patellar dislocations.

the knee. If arthrodesis has been performed at the time of open reduction, postoperative care is the same as for arthrodesis.

If open reduction alone would require too much dissection or if this procedure would damage important structures, an arthroplasty or an arthrodesis is indicated.

PATELLA

Old unreduced dislocation of the patella after trauma is rare and should be distinguished clinically from congenital dislocation. Congenital dislocation often is not appreciated initially because the normal patellar ossification does not occur until 3 years of age. A high percentage of traumatic patellar dislocations (16%) are missed when associated knee dislocation is present. Therefore it is important to maintain a high index of suspicion of possible patellar dislocation when medial structures have been severely damaged.

The anatomic abnormalities found in posttraumatic dislocation differ from those found in the congenital type of dislocation. The congenital lesion is accompanied by a flexion contracture of the knee and incongruity of the patella and trochlea; these changes are part of the original pathologic process. In posttraumatic dislocation, an adaptive flattening of the patella occurs, and the knee contracture is a reactive change. Treatment of congenital dislocation of the patella is discussed in other chapter.

Old traumatic patellar dislocations may be treated by observation, patellar realignment, or patellectomy. Knee function can sometimes be satisfactory despite the old unreduced dislocation of the patella. Observation is then the treatment of choice. If the dislocation is not of long duration, if degenerative changes of the patella are minimal or absent, and if the tibiofemoral joint is essentially normal, then open reduction may be helpful. In dislocations of long duration, usually traumatic arthritis will have developed, motion in the joint will be limited, and pain and disability will have resulted. If the patellar degenerative changes appear significant, patellaplasty or patellectomy may be indicated. We have had no experience with patellar resurfacing or patellar prostheses for this condition. The long-term prognosis for useful function is guarded regardless of the procedure selected.

OPEN REDUCTION FOR OLD UNREDUCED DISLOCATION OF THE PATELLA

TECHNIQUE 9.3

- Make a 7.5-cm longitudinal midline incision.
- Dissect laterally deep to the subcutaneous tissue.
- Incise the capsule and synovium parallel with the lateral border of the quadriceps tendon.
- Free the deep surfaces of the quadriceps tendon and of the patella and place these structures in their normal positions.
- Excise the redundant part of the capsule from the medial side of the knee and close the capsule on this side.
- It is important that the general alignment of the extensor mechanism be normal at the completion of the procedure to prevent redislocation of the patella laterally. The fibers of the vastus medialis muscle should be appropriately oriented to the patella. This may require reattachment of a portion of the vastus medialis muscle to the adductor tubercle of the femur.
- Transfer the tibial tuberosity medially to realign the distal portion of the extensor mechanism if necessary.
- If the articular surface of the patella has degenerated, a patellectomy or a patellaplasty is necessary. Realignment of the extensor mechanism is just as important after patellectomy as it is after open reduction of the patella.

HIP

Old unreduced dislocations of the hip are relatively uncommon in adults. They are usually the result of a motor vehicle accident that also caused head injury, fracture of the ipsilateral femur, or dislocation or fracture of the opposite hip, which drew attention away from the dislocation.

In developing countries, unreduced traumatic dislocations are seen more frequently. The various treatment possibilities include closed reduction, open reduction, heavy traction and abduction, subtrochanteric osteotomy, Girdlestone procedure, arthrodesis, endoprosthetic replacement, and total hip replacement. Like acute dislocations, unreduced dislocations can be classified as anterior or posterior.

CHRONIC ANTERIOR DISLOCATIONS

Traumatic anterior dislocation of the hip is a comparatively rare injury, and little has been written about old unreduced anterior dislocations of the hip. Trochanteric osteotomy has

been reported to correct the deformity and improve body mechanics and balance. Although trochanteric osteotomy may give a stable hip, long-term results are not known. Subsequent salvage operations, such as total hip arthroplasty, may be more difficult if the proximal femoral anatomy is distorted.

INTERTROCHANTERIC OSTEOTOMY FOR CHRONIC ANTERIOR DISLOCATION OF THE HIP

TECHNIQUE 9.4

(AGGARWAL AND SINGH)
- The Gibson approach is used.
- Divide the femur along the line joining the greater and lesser trochanters. Then adduct, extend, and internally rotate the limb.

POSTOPERATIVE CARE The patient is kept in skin or skeletal traction for 6 weeks to prevent recurrence of the rotational deformity. The patient is allowed to walk with crutches 6 weeks after surgery, and full weight bearing is allowed in 3 to 4 months. Hamada recommended postoperative immobilization in a one and one half spica cast, which includes the normal leg down to the knee. With intertrochanteric osteotomy, early union usually is complete in 3 to 4 months.

A modified Girdlestone arthroplasty has been described for the treatment of unreduced anterior hip dislocations. The femoral neck is exposed through an anterior Smith-Petersen approach (see Technique 1.66) or a Watson-Jones anterolateral approach (see Technique 1.67). A subcapital osteotomy is performed, attempting to leave as much of the femoral neck as possible with the distal fragment. The femoral head is then removed. By manipulating the leg, the cut femoral neck is displaced upward into the acetabulum. Postoperative skeletal traction of 5 kg is maintained for 6 weeks. Gentle active hip flexion is started 10 days after surgery, and non–weight bearing with crutches is begun at 6 weeks. Gradual weight bearing is started at 3 months. Preservation of the femoral neck makes subsequent total hip arthroplasty easier, and this modified subcapital displacement osteotomy for neglected anterior dislocation of the hip treated 6 months or more after dislocation in young patients can serve as a temporizing procedure until definitive total hip arthroplasty is performed later.

CHRONIC POSTERIOR DISLOCATIONS

Unreduced posterior dislocations of the hip are much more common than the anterior type. Two factors that have been reported to contribute to poor results in old posterior dislocations are fracture of the femoral head or medial acetabular wall (Epstein types IV and V) and osteonecrosis, an unpredictable event that may not become apparent on plain radiographs for many months. Primary reconstructive procedures have been shown to give the best results. Although the viability of the femoral head in old unreduced posterior dislocations should determine treatment, use of bone scan or MRI to detect the vascularity of the femoral head before beginning treatment is not mentioned in the literature. In young patients, if the femoral head is thought to be viable, an effort should be made to save it.

For a type I posterior hip dislocation (no fracture or only a minor fracture of the acetabular rim less than 12 weeks from injury), with a viable femoral head, closed reduction under general anesthesia is recommended. After 12 weeks, the acetabulum may fill with fibrous tissue, making a concentric closed reduction impossible. If closed reduction fails, heavy traction and abduction should be considered. If the type I posterior hip dislocation with a viable femoral head has been present for more than 12 weeks, a concentric reduction most often cannot be obtained with closed reduction or heavy traction and abduction, and open reduction is indicated.

TRACTION AND ABDUCTION FOR CHRONIC POSTERIOR HIP DISLOCATION

TECHNIQUE 9.5

(GUPTA AND SHRAVAT)

- Place a tibial traction pin in the region of the tibial tubercle and place the patient in 18 kg of skeletal traction. The patient is kept in traction and under sedation and muscle relaxation during this time.
- Obtain radiographs on alternate days. Usually by the fifth day, the femoral head should be at or below the level of the acetabulum.
- Gradually abduct the limb and reduce the traction 3.6 kg every fourth day.

- Once the femoral head has been reduced into the acetabulum, maintain 7 kg of traction for the next 2 weeks.
- Remove the traction and begin non–weight bearing exercises for the next 4 weeks. Weight bearing is not allowed for 3 months (Fig. 9.3).

The success of the heavy traction technique depends on achieving a concentric reduction. If the reduction is not concentric, an open reduction to debride any interposed soft tissue or bone fragments is necessary.

For posterior hip dislocations with a viable femoral head that are type II (large uncomminuted fracture of the posterior acetabular rim) or type III (comminuted fracture of the posterior acetabular rim), open reduction and internal fixation should be considered if the injury is less than 3 months old. If the head of the femur is displaced superiorly, preoperative skeletal traction is necessary. With reduction thus accomplished, it is necessary to fix the bone fragments internally to restore stability.

Total hip arthroplasty is recommended for hips with posterior dislocations categorized as type IV (fracture of the acetabular rim and floor) or type V (fracture of the femoral head with or without other fractures) that have been dislocated for more than 3 months. Because of osteonecrosis, poor results have been noted in these types of fracture-dislocations even in some patients who had reduction within 24 hours after injury. If the femoral head is thought to be avascular on MRI or bone scan, a primary reconstructive procedure should be considered rather than open or closed reduction. In young patients, arthrodesis can be considered, although successful fusion may be difficult in the presence of osteonecrosis. As with any arthrodesis of the hip, the status of the ipsilateral knee, the contralateral hip, and the lumbar spine must be considered. Subtrochanteric osteotomy has also been used for old unreduced dislocations of the hip in areas of the world where arthroplasty or endoprosthetic

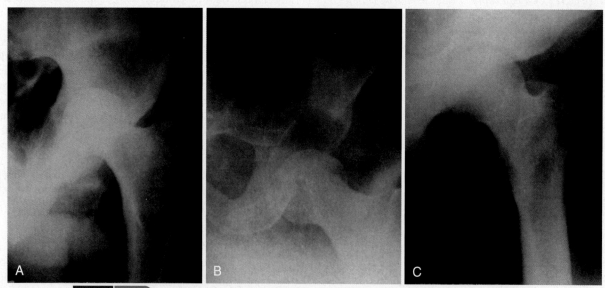

FIGURE 9.3 **A,** Anteroposterior radiograph of left hip in 27-year-old man demonstrating posterior dislocation with myositis ossificans 37 days after injury. **B,** Same hip on fifth day of traction. Head of femur is partially below acetabulum. **C,** Same hip on day 17 with reduced traction and extremity in abduction. (From Gupta RC, Shravat BP: Reduction of neglected traumatic dislocation of the hip by heavy traction, *J Bone Joint Surg* 59A:249–251, 1977.) **SEE TECHNIQUE 9.5.**

replacements are not readily available. This procedure may be indicated for patients who are relatively pain free and have a reasonable range of hip flexion but have joint contracture or limb-length inequality.

The best results have been reported after total hip arthroplasty. The main problem encountered with total hip arthroplasty in this situation is the creation of adequate acetabular stock when the posterior acetabular lip is fractured or displaced. This is accomplished by open reduction and internal fixation of the fracture fragment or by use of the femoral head as a bone graft. Ilyas and Rabbani reported successful one-stage total hip arthroplasty in 15 patients with chronic (over 6-month history) posterior dislocations; bulk femoral head autografts were used in 13 patients. Their short- to midterm results were quite satisfactory, especially considering the complex nature of these particular arthroplasties. All patients had decreased pain and increased range of hip motion after surgery.

In a patient who has had multiple procedures to stabilize a chronically dislocated hip, a total hip arthroplasty with a constrained acetabular component should be considered.

Young and Banza recommended osteotomy of the greater trochanter to improve access to the acetabulum for both anterior and posterior chronic dislocations.

STERNOCLAVICULAR JOINT

Most authors believe that old unreduced anterior dislocations of the sternoclavicular joint usually cause minimal if any disability, although reports of surgical intervention for this condition have indicated that untreated patients complain of weakness and fatigue of the arm during heavy use or athletic endeavors. Rarely, if ever, is surgical intervention required in this subset of patients. Surgery may, on occasion, be helpful in patients with underlying joint laxity.

Several basic surgical procedures have been described for individuals who may require surgery. The use of fascia lata around the clavicle and first rib was described by Speed, whereas others have used fascia lata between the clavicle and the sternum. The subclavius tendon also has been used to reconstruct the costoclavicular ligaments, and reconstructions using semitendinosus, palmaris longus, or gracilis tendons have had good clinical outcomes. Bak and Fogh reported successful reconstruction of the sternoclavicular joint in 27 patients with palmaris longus and gracilis tendon autografts. Quayle et al. described the use of an artificial ligament for reconstruction of the sternoclavicular joint and costoclavicular ligaments; all four of their young, active patients returned to full activity including competitive sports. Some authors have used a threaded Steinmann pin across the sternoclavicular joint, but migration of metallic fixation into the mediastinum can occur, often with disastrous consequences. Subperiosteal dissection of the sternal origin of the sternocleidomastoid muscle extending inferiorly with a strip of periosteum also has been described. This tendoperiosteal strip is threaded subperiosteally under the medial end of the first rib, up behind the rib, and up through a hole drilled from superior to inferior in the clavicle. It is then sutured back on itself.

Resection of the medial end of the clavicle has been recommended, although upper extremity weakness has been reported after this procedure. It has been emphasized that

if the medial end of the clavicle is to be removed because of degenerative changes, the surgeon should be careful not to damage the costoclavicular ligament.

Rockwood recommended a nonoperative "skillful neglect" treatment, although he stated that sternoclavicular arthroplasty with resection of the medial clavicle is occasionally necessary, especially in patients in whom attempts to reduce and to stabilize the joint with suture, fascia, and tendons have failed. He resected 1 inch of the medial clavicle, debrided the intraarticular disc ligament, and stabilized the remaining clavicle to the first rib with a 3-mm cotton Dacron tape or a strip of fascia. He recommended detachment of the clavicular head of the sternocleidomastoid to temporarily resist the upward pull of the clavicle by this muscle. We agree that surgery is rarely indicated primarily; however, if surgery is to be undertaken, we also recommend arthroplasty of the sternoclavicular joint.

RESECTION OR STABILIZATION OF THE MEDIAL END OF THE CLAVICLE FOR OLD ANTERIOR STERNOCLAVICULAR JOINT DISLOCATION

TECHNIQUE 9.6

- Expose the medial end of the clavicle subperiosteally through an incision approximately 6 cm long parallel to the bone.
- Free the medial end of the bone, grasp it with forceps, lift it anteriorly and superiorly, and clear it of soft-tissue attachments posteriorly. The costoclavicular ligaments are usually torn.
- If the ligaments are attached but stretched, remove only that part of the clavicle medial to these ligaments.
- If the ligaments are torn, resect about 2 cm of bone (Fig. 9.4).
- Bevel the anterosuperior corner of the remaining clavicle for cosmetic purposes.
- If instability is a problem, stabilize the clavicle to the first rib with a 3-mm cotton Dacron tape or a strip of fascia (Fig. 9.5). Detach the clavicular head of the sternocleidomastoid; plicate and close the periosteum.
- Alternatively, stabilize the joint as described by Kawaguchi et al. with a double figure-of-eight gracilis tendon autograft (Fig. 9.6). Harvest the autograft and reinforce it with Krakow-type nonresorbable suture.
- Stabilize the joint with a 2.0-mm Kirschner wire, pass the autograft in a double figure-of-eight through four drill holes, and secure with two 4.0-mm fully-threaded cancellous interference screws.
- Remove the Kirschner wire at 6 weeks.

POSTOPERATIVE CARE The shoulder girdle is immobilized in a Velpeau-type dressing or shoulder immobilizer for 3 weeks. A progressive active range-of-motion exercise program is then begun.

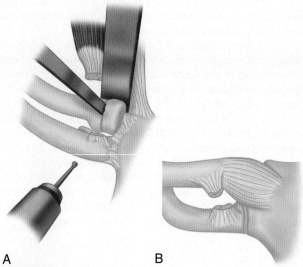

A   **B**

FIGURE 9.4   Technique for resecting medial end of clavicle. **A,** Site of osteotomy is outlined with drill, and 2.5 cm of bone is then resected with osteotome. **B,** Periosteum is plicated and closed around remaining medial end of clavicle. (**B** redrawn from Eskola A, Vainionpää S, Vastamäki M, et al: Operation for old sternoclavicular dislocation, *J Bone Joint Surg* 71B:63–65, 1989.) **SEE TECHNIQUE 9.6**.

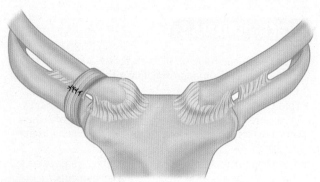

FIGURE 9.5   Stabilization of clavicle to first rib with fascial loops. **SEE TECHNIQUE 9.6**.

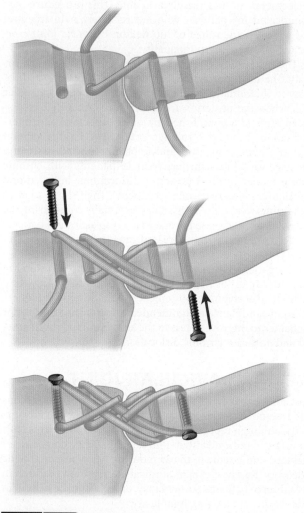

FIGURE 9.6   Reconstruction of chronic anterior sternoclavicular dislocation with a double figure-of-eight gracilis tendon autograft. (Redrawn from Kawaguchi K, Tanaka S, Yoshitoni H, et al: Double figure-of-eight reconstruction technique for chronic anterior sternoclavicular joint dislocation, *Knee Surg Sports Traumatol Arthrosc* 23:1559–1562, 2015.) **SEE TECHNIQUE 9.6**.

POSTERIOR DISLOCATIONS

Posterior dislocation of the sternoclavicular joint is an uncommon problem that is seen much less frequently than anterior dislocations. In a chronic state, posterior dislocation can be symptomatic and cause other significant complications involving the trachea, esophagus, or great vessels. Intrathoracic injury and thoracic outlet syndrome have also been reported. Most common symptoms include dysphagia, dyspnea, or cough. In view of the potential complications associated with this injury, especially subclavian artery compression, open reduction of the dislocation is recommended. Preoperative evaluation should include CT of the affected area and possibly arteriography to plan a surgical approach. Consultation with a thoracic surgeon should also be considered. If the reduction is unstable or cannot be achieved, the medial part of the clavicle can be resected. Except for some cosmetic defect, no functional disability has been noted from this procedure.

STABILIZATION OF OLD POSTERIOR STERNOCLAVICULAR JOINT DISLOCATION

TECHNIQUE 9.7

(WANG ET AL.)

- With the patient in the beach-chair position, prepare and drape the entire clavicle, shoulder, and upper extremity.
- Prepare and drape the ipsilateral lower leg and harvest a 16-cm portion of the gracilis tendon through a 2-cm vertical incision over the pes anserinus. Trim and whipstitch the graft to fit through 4.8-mm drill holes.
- Make a 10-cm transverse incision over the sternoclavicular joint and carefully debride the joint superiorly.

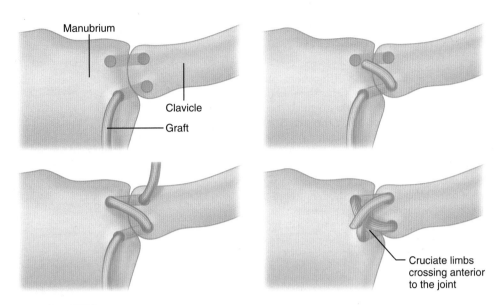

FIGURE 9.7   Steps for passing autograft for figure-of-eight left sternoclavicular joint reconstruction. (Redrawn from Wang D, Camp CL, Werner BC, et al: Figure-of-8 reconstruction technique for chronic posterior sternoclavicular joint dislocation, *Arthroscopic Tech* 6:e1749–e1753, 2018.) **SEE TECHNIQUE 9.7.**

- Elevate the medial end of the clavicle and drill two 4.8-mm parallel holes, one through the lateral manubrium and one through the distal clavicle (Fig. 9.7).
- Pass the graft in a figure-of-eight fashion with the cruciate limb crossing anterior to the joint.

ACROMIOCLAVICULAR JOINT

The same classification can be used for both old unreduced and acute dislocations of the acromioclavicular joint. Surgical treatment of acromioclavicular joint dislocations has been performed since 1861, and over 100 different surgical techniques have been described for acute and chronic dislocations.

Resection of the distal end of the clavicle (Mumford procedure) is indicated for symptomatic grade I or II unreduced dislocations in which the coracoclavicular ligaments are intact. With improvements in techniques and instrumentation, arthroscopic distal clavicular resection has become more widely used, with results equal to or better than those of open techniques. Reported advantages of arthroscopic resection include improved cosmetic results, easier postoperative rehabilitation, and faster return to function because of the preservation of the acromioclavicular joint ligaments and capsule and the deltotrapezial fascia. Most authors recommend resection of only 0.5 to 1 cm of the distal clavicle with the arthroscopic technique. Persistent symptoms after either open or arthroscopic distal clavicular resection may be caused by underresection, overresection leading to joint instability, stiffness, heterotopic ossification, untreated concomitant shoulder pathology, and infection; less common causes include distal clavicular fracture, reossification or fusion across the acromioclavicular joint, suprascapular neuropathy, and psychiatric disorders.

The Mumford procedure is not for acutely injured grade I or grade II acromioclavicular joints but rather for patients with chronic symptoms resulting from degenerative changes in the acromioclavicular joint. If this operation is performed in patients with more severe injuries in which the ligaments are torn, the clavicle will remain hypermobile and continue to irritate the soft tissues around the shoulder. Therefore in chronic dislocations of grades III, IV, and V, some type of reconstruction of the coracoclavicular ligaments is indicated.

RESECTION OF THE LATERAL END OF THE CLAVICLE FOR CHRONIC ACROMIOCLAVICULAR JOINT DISLOCATION

TECHNIQUE 9.8

(MUMFORD; GURD)
- Expose the lateral end of the clavicle through a short curved incision.
- By dissecting subperiosteally, free the lateral 2.5 cm of the clavicle of all soft-tissue attachments and with bone-cutting rongeurs resect about 2.5 cm of the bone.
- Smooth the superior border of the remaining lateral end of the bone with a file to eliminate any sharp bony ridge beneath the skin. It is unnecessary to disturb the cartilaginous surface of the acromion.
- Plicate and suture the periosteum and soft tissues over the raw end of the clavicle.

POSTOPERATIVE CARE The shoulder is immobilized in a Velpeau dressing for 1 week, and then active use is encouraged.

In chronic unreduced acromioclavicular dislocations of grades III, IV, and V, the coracoclavicular ligaments should be reconstructed. Neviaser described an operation in which the coracoacromial ligament is used to reconstruct the superior acromioclavicular ligament. This method does not reconstruct the coracoclavicular ligaments, however, and therefore can be followed by redislocation.

Neviaser used Kirschner wires for fixation of the acromioclavicular joint, but these wires have been thought to precipitate osteoarthritis and have been reported to cause severe complications from distant migration of the wire to the lung, spinal cord, or neck. The lateral end of the wire should be bent over on itself to prevent migration.

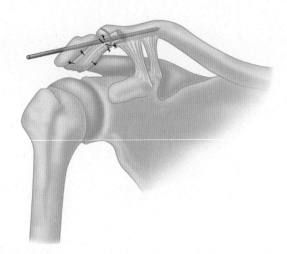

FIGURE 9.8 Neviaser technique for repairing dislocations of acromioclavicular joint (see text). (Redrawn from Neviaser JS: Acromioclavicular dislocation treated by transference of the coraco-acromial ligament: a long-term follow-up in a series of 112 cases, *Clin Orthop Relat Res* 58:57–68, 1968.) **SEE TECHNIQUE 9.9**.

RECONSTRUCTION OF THE SUPERIOR ACROMIOCLAVICULAR LIGAMENT FOR CHRONIC ACROMIOCLAVICULAR JOINT DISLOCATION

TECHNIQUE 9.9

(NEVIASER)
- Make a slightly curved incision that begins medially over the lateral half of the clavicle and ends laterally at the lateral border of the acromion.
- Strip the deltoid muscle from the lateral third of the clavicle.
- Expose the coracoacromial ligament and the dislocated acromioclavicular joint. Do not disturb the ruptured acromioclavicular and coracoclavicular ligaments or the articular disc.
- Reduce the acromioclavicular joint and fix it by inserting a Kirschner wire 1.6 mm in diameter through the skin and acromion into the clavicle (Fig. 9.8). This maneuver may be simplified by retrograde insertion of the wire, first through the center of the acromial articular surface and then out through the skin. To prevent the wire from working loose, embed its medial tip in the cortex of the clavicle near the apex of its lateral curve.
- Free the medial end of the coracoacromial ligament by resecting from the lateral border of the coracoid a small piece of bone that includes its attachment.
- Turn the coracoacromial ligament over the superior surface of the acromion and fix it there with three absorbable sutures passed through the soft tissues. Then bring the transferred ligament over the acromioclavicular joint to the superior surface of the clavicle and anchor it by roughening an area on the bone where the ligament is to be attached.
- Fix the ligament there with absorbable sutures passed through two holes drilled vertically into the bone.

- Pass a suture around the ligament and the clavicle and secure the small bone fragment and the new ligament in place.
- Suture the deltoid to the clavicle and close the wound.
- Cut off the Kirschner wire just beneath the skin and bend the end to prevent medial migration.
- Apply a modified Velpeau bandage.

POSTOPERATIVE CARE The wound is dressed, and the wire is inspected every week. Gentle passive motions of the shoulder are carried out weekly when the wound is dressed. At 5 weeks, the Kirschner wire is removed and normal activities are gradually resumed. Competitive sports should be avoided for a minimum of 8 weeks.

Another operation described for this injury is transfer of the end of the coracoid and its attached muscles to the clavicle to hold the lateral end of the bone in position. If the individual situation requires, it can be combined with resection of the lateral end of the clavicle. This technique provides a dynamic reduction force on the distal clavicle but not a static one.

In the classic Weaver and Dunn technique, the coracoacromial ligament is detached from the acromion and reattached to the remaining end of the distal clavicle. This procedure, usually combined with some kind of stabilizing fixation to protect the repair, has been an effective approach to reconstructing and repositioning the chronically dislocated distal clavicle. In the original report, however, the rate of incomplete reduction was 27%, and loss of reduction has been reported in other series, prompting a number of modifications to the original Weaver-Dunn technique, including those with autologous or allograft hamstring or semitendinosus tendon or synthetic ligament augmentation and the use of newer tendon fixation devices. Tauber et al. compared outcomes in 12 patients treated with a modified Weaver-Dunn procedure to those in 12 patients treated with semitendinosus tendon grafts and found that the tendon graft results in significantly superior clinical and radiographic outcomes.

Other reconstruction techniques (Figs. 9.9 through 9.12) include anatomic "double-bundle" reconstruction using the coracoacromial ligament and conjoined tendon or double suture buttons, a nonanatomic "docking" technique in which the coracoacromial ligament is passed into an intramedullary bone tunnel and tensioned before it is sutured in place through drill holes in the clavicle. Fauci et al. compared biologic grafts (semitendinosus) to synthetic ligaments in a prospective randomized comparative study of 40 chronic dislocations. Those with biologic grafts had significantly better scores than those with synthetic ligaments.

Rockwood described transfer of the coracoacromial ligament from the acromion to the clavicle while the clavicle is held reduced with a Bosworth screw.

TRANSFER OF THE CORACOACROMIAL LIGAMENT FOR CHRONIC ACROMIOCLAVICULAR JOINT DISLOCATION

TECHNIQUE 9.10

(ROCKWOOD)

- Make a skin incision over the distal clavicle along the lines of Langer around the shoulder (Fig. 9.13A).

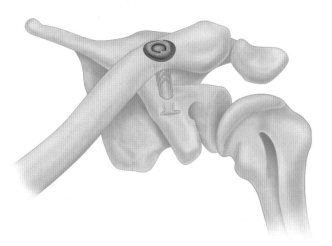

FIGURE 9.9   Single-bundle stabilization of the acromioclavicular joint. The oval subcoracoid button is connected to the supraclavicular round button by a FiberWire (Arthrex, Naples, FL), and the double-folded gracilis tendon is fixed within the clavicle by a tenodesis screw and held by a suture loop into the subcoracoid button. (From Tauber M, Valler D, Lichtenberg S, et al: Arthroscopic stabilization of chronic acromioclavicular joint dislocations: triple- versus single-bundle reconstruction, *Am J Sports Med* 44:482–489, 2015.)

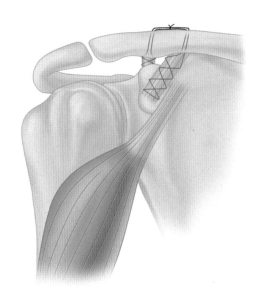

FIGURE 9.11   Anatomic double-bundle coracoclavicular reconstruction. The suture ends of the lateral half of the conjoined tendon have been passed through the conoid tubercle. (From Lee SK, Song DG, Choy WS: Anatomic double-bundle coracoclavicular reconstruction in chronic acromioclavicular dislocation, *Orthopedics* 38:e655–e662, 2015.)

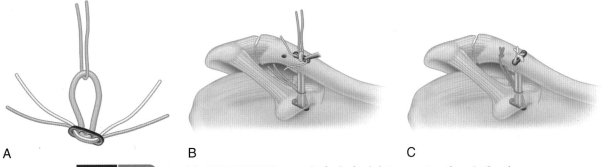

A   B   C

FIGURE 9.10   Double ENDOBUTTON acromioclavicular joint reconstruction. **A,** Continuous loop and suture limbs threaded through the ENDOBUTTON (Smith & Nephew, Memphis, TN) before deployment. **B,** ENDOBUTTON is passed through the continuous suture loop that has been pulled up through the prepared holes in the coracoid and clavicle. The free sutures will be passed through the peripheral holes in the button to secure it. **C,** Final appearance of the construct with an auxiliary stitch replicating the course to the trapezoid ligament. (From Struhl S, Wolfson TS: Continuous loop double EndoButton reconstruction for acromioclavicular joint dislocation, *Am J Sports Med* 43:2437–2444, 2015.)

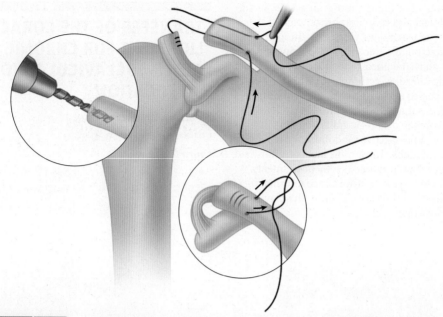

FIGURE 9.12 Acromioclavicular reconstruction with the docking technique. (From Millett PJ, Braun S, Gobezie R, et al: Acromioclavicular joint reconstruction with coracoacromial ligament transfer using the docking technique, *BMC Musculoskelet Dis* 10:6, 2009.)

- Expose the distal clavicle subperiosteally and resect about 2.5 cm of bone (Fig. 9.13B).
- Drill and curet the medullary canal of the distal clavicle to receive the transferred coracoacromial ligament.
- Use a knife to remove the acromial attachment of the coracoacromial ligament from the acromion, or, if desired, remove a sliver of bone from the undersurface of the acromion along with the coracoacromial ligament. This provides bone-to-bone fixation at the distal clavicle rather than ligament-to-bone fixation. This also might provide slightly more length to the coracoacromial ligament if it alone is too short. Further lengthening the coracoacromial ligament can be obtained, if necessary, by detaching the anterior fasciculus of the ligament off the waist of the coracoid process.
- Pass a heavy, nonabsorbable suture back and forth through the ligament so that the ends exit through the acromial end of the ligament (Fig. 9.13C).
- Drill two small holes into the superior cortex of the distal end of the clavicle, entering the medullary canal. Next, drill another hole through the distal clavicle directly above the base of the coracoid process. With the clavicle held in the corrected position, insert a drill bit through this hole and drill a hole through both cortices of the coracoid process.
- Pass the two ends of the suture in the coracoacromial ligament into the medullary canal of the clavicle and out through the holes in the superior cortex before inserting a lag screw. Then pass a lag screw (Bosworth screw) through the clavicle and into the coracoid and tighten it to hold the clavicle just above the coracoid.
- Tighten and tie the two ends of the suture in the coracoacromial ligament as the ligament is fed into the medullary canal of the clavicle (Fig. 9.13D).

POSTOPERATIVE CARE After surgery, the patient is allowed to use the arm for everyday living activities but not for any heavy lifting, pushing, or pulling. At 12 weeks postoperatively, the lag screw is removed under local anesthesia.

More recently, Boileau et al. reported similar reconstructions performed primarily arthroscopically with good short-term results.

ARTHROSCOPIC TRANSFER OF THE CORACOACROMIAL LIGAMENT FOR CHRONIC ACROMIOCLAVICULAR JOINT DISLOCATION

TECHNIQUE 9.11

(BOILEAU ET AL.)
- With the patient in the beach-chair or lateral decubitus position, define the landmarks and create arthroscopic portals sequentially as indicated (Fig. 9.14).
- Detach the distal end of the coracoacromial ligament, with a wafer of bone, using a high-speed burr.
- Reduce the distal clavicle remnant and fix with an Endo-Button (Smith & Nephew, Andover, MA).
- Transfer the coracoacromial ligament to the resected end of the clavicle and fix with sutures to the EndoButton (Smith & Nephew, Memphis, TN) (Fig. 9.15).

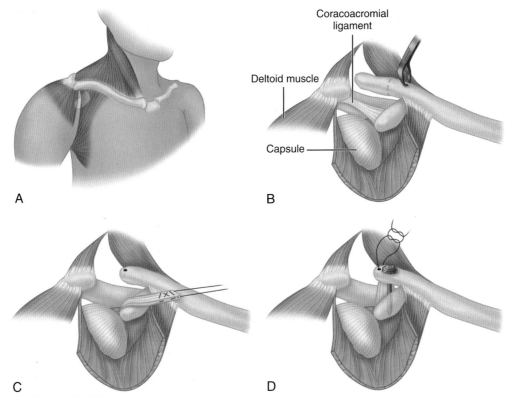

Coracoacromial ligament

Deltoid muscle

Capsule

A

B

C

D

FIGURE 9.13 **A-D,** Rockwood technique for reconstruction in type III acromioclavicular dislocation (see text) **SEE TECHNIQUE 9.10.**

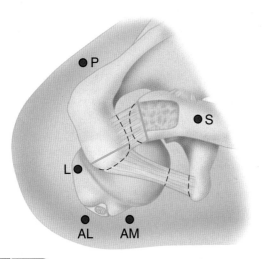

FIGURE 9.14 Five portals used for acromioclavicular joint reconstruction. *AL,* Anterolateral; *AM,* anteromedial; *L,* lateral; *P,* posterior; *S,* superior. (Modified from Boileau P, Old J, Gastaud O, et al: All-arthroscopic Weaver-Dunn-Chuinard procedure with double-button fixation for chronic acromioclavicular joint dislocation, *Arthroscopy* 26:149–160, 2010.) **SEE TECHNIQUE 9.11**.

POSTOPERATIVE CARE The arm is placed in a sling for 3 to 4 weeks postoperatively. During this period, normal use of the elbow, wrist, and hand is encouraged. The sling is removed for pendulum exercises and bathing. Strengthening exercises are begun at 2 months, and the patient can return to contact sports at 3 to 6 months postoperatively.

SHOULDER

Old unreduced dislocations of the shoulder usually occur in patients older than 50 years. The complaints are generally those of pain and limitation of motion. The pain usually is caused by attempts to move the shoulder beyond its restricted range. These old dislocations are most often traumatic but have frequently been produced by a trivial injury as a result of the patient's increasing age and weakness and degeneration of the soft tissue around the glenohumeral joint, such as the rotator cuff and subscapularis tendon. In younger patients, unreduced dislocations often occur in those with alcoholism, seizures, or multiple traumas. Many of these dislocations are complicated by fractures of the glenoid cavity, tuberosities, or other parts of the humerus. More than one third are complicated by neurologic deficits. Loss of motion is the chief clinical finding; abduction and internal rotation are restricted in old anterior dislocations, and abduction and external rotation are restricted in old posterior dislocations.

Complete radiographic evaluation should include anteroposterior and axillary views of the shoulder. CT and three-dimensional CT techniques are helpful in evaluating the bony injuries and the extent of damage to the articular surface of the humeral head. The degree of damage to the articular surface is a major determining factor in the procedure selected (Fig. 9.16).

These injuries produce pathologic conditions in both the soft tissue and the bone. After a few weeks, fibrous and capsular contractures occur across the base of the glenoid. The rotator cuff muscles also are contracted. The fibrosis can include other structures, such as the axillary artery and nerve. The natural anatomy is, therefore, often markedly distorted. Neviaser has described a capsular

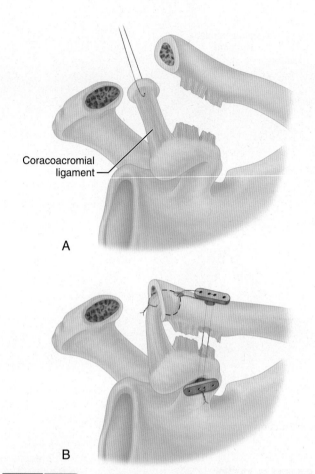

FIGURE 9.15 Weaver-Dunn-Chuinard procedure with double button fixation. **A,** Coracoacromial ligament is harvested with bone block from tip of acromion and is rerouted in distal end of clavicle. Arthritic distal clavicle has been resected and socket drilled in its medullary canal. **B,** Bone-ligament transfer is protected for time of bone healing by maintaining reduction with help of double-button (two titanium buttons connecting the clavicle and coracoid with four strands of suture). (Modified from Boileau P, Old J, Gastaud O, et al: All-arthroscopic Weaver-Dunn-Chuinard procedure with double-button fixation for chronic acromioclavicular joint dislocation, *Arthroscopy* 26:149–160, 2010.) **SEE TECHNIQUE 9.11**.

"bowstringing" phenomenon. The capsule itself becomes adherent in the glenoid fossa, preventing closed reduction (Fig. 9.17).

Bony pathologic change also is often seen. In chronic anterior dislocations, a compression fracture occurs in the posterolateral aspect of the humeral head, where it impinges against the anterior glenoid rim (Fig. 9.18). Because of the repeated efforts of the patient to achieve normal motion in the glenohumeral joint, this lesion often is larger than the usual Hill-Sachs lesion seen in recurring anterior dislocations of the shoulder. There are also compression fractures of the apposing glenoid rim or sometimes a pseudoarticulation with the scapula (Fig. 9.19). In chronic posterior dislocations, a bony lesion similar to the Hill-Sachs lesion of recurring anterior dislocations is found. This is a compression fracture caused by impingement of the posterior rim of the glenoid on the anteromedial aspect of the humeral head (Fig. 9.20). These lesions are also usually large because of the patient's continual attempts to increase the range of motion of the affected joint.

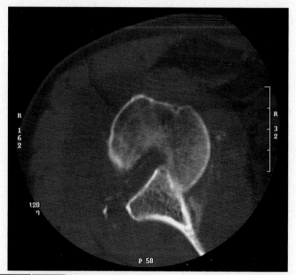

FIGURE 9.16 CT scan showing extent of damage to articular surface of glenoid head.

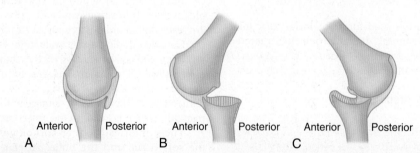

FIGURE 9.17 Relationships in unreduced dislocations of shoulder. **A,** Normal relationship of humeral head and glenoid cavity. **B,** In old anterior dislocation, adhesions of posterior capsule to glenoid surface develop. **C,** In old posterior dislocation, adhesions of anterior capsule to glenoid surface develop. (From Neviaser JS: *Arthrography of the shoulder: the diagnosis and management of the lesions visualized*, Springfield, 1975, Charles C. Thomas.)

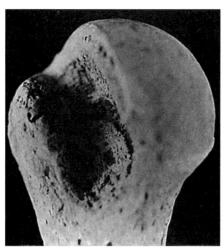

FIGURE 9.18 Large wedge-shaped defect in posterolateral aspect of humeral head in chronic anterior dislocation. (From Kirtland S, Resnick D, Sartoris D, et al: Chronic, unreduced dislocations of the glenohumeral joint: imaging strategy and pathologic correlation, *J Trauma* 28:1622–1631, 1988.)

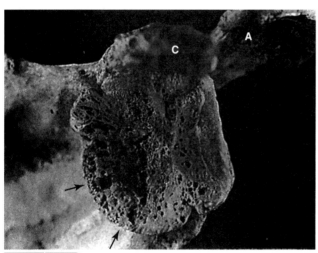

FIGURE 9.19 Pseudoarticulation *(arrows)* of humeral head with anterior aspect of glenoid cavity in chronic anterior dislocation of shoulder. *A,* Acromion; *C,* coracoid process. (From Kirtland S, Resnick D, Sartoris D, et al: Chronic, unreduced dislocations of the glenohumeral joint: imaging strategy and pathologic correlation, *J Trauma* 28:1622–1631, 1988.)

TREATMENT

The treatment options for an old unreduced dislocation of the shoulder are no treatment, closed reduction (arthroscopic-assisted), open reduction, hemiarthroplasty, and total shoulder replacement. Not all patients with old unreduced dislocations of the shoulder require treatment. In some patients, although motion is limited and slightly uncomfortable, the upper extremity remains functional. Also, if a patient is inactive and a poor risk for surgery, the option of nonoperative treatment should be considered. Patients with posterior dislocations who were not treated have been shown to have better results than those with untreated anterior dislocations. In unreduced posterior dislocations, the arm rests at the side in internal rotation, allowing the patient to reach the face, head, and rear of the body. The arm of a patient with an

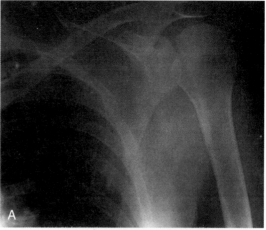

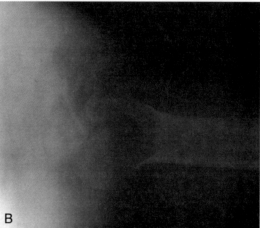

FIGURE 9.20 Posterior dislocation of shoulder. **A,** Anteroposterior radiograph shows only subtle changes. **B,** Axillary lateral radiograph shows posterior dislocation of humeral head with posterior rim of glenoid caught in humeral head defect.

unreduced anterior dislocation is held away from the body in external rotation, making it difficult to reach the face and impossible to reach the back.

■ CLOSED REDUCTION

As emphasized by many authors, manipulative reduction should not be undertaken before the patient's age, the degree of osteoporosis of the humerus, the vascular status, and the duration of the dislocation are all carefully considered. The size of the humeral depression defect also should be taken into account. A few cases of closed reduction of shoulders that have been dislocated for more than 6 to 8 weeks have been reported in the literature, but most agree that attempts at closed reduction should be considered carefully after 4 weeks. After this time, the soft-tissue contractures, the fibrous tissue within the glenoid cavity, and the retracted rotator cuff muscles usually make closed reduction impossible.

In general, it may be unwise to attempt closed reduction for a shoulder with an impression defect involving more than 20% of the articular surface of the humeral head or for a shoulder that has been dislocated for more than 3 to 4 weeks. If a closed reduction is attempted, it should be done with minimal traction, no leverage, and complete muscle relaxation under general anesthesia. In elderly patients

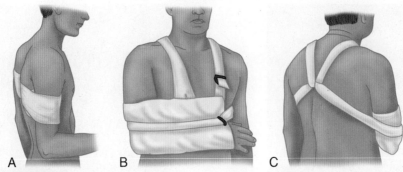

FIGURE 9.21 Rowe and Zarins method of immobilization after shoulder dislocations. **A,** After posterior dislocation, arm is prevented from moving anterior to coronal plane of body. **B** and **C,** After anterior dislocation, arm is prevented from moving posterior to coronal plane of body. (Redrawn from Rowe CR, Zarins B: Chronic unreduced dislocation of the shoulder, *J Bone Joint Surg* 64A:494–505, 1982.) **SEE TECHNIQUE 9.3.**

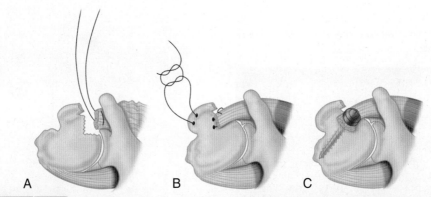

FIGURE 9.22 Technique for treatment of old unreduced posterior dislocation of shoulder. **A,** Two holes are drilled transversely through area of anterior defect. **B,** Mattress suture in freed subscapularis tendon is passed through holes and tied securely, fixing tendon in defect. **C,** Neer alternative in which subscapularis tendon is freed by osteotomy of lesser tuberosity and tuberosity is fixed in anterior defect with screw. **SEE TECHNIQUES 9.13 AND 9.14.**

with arterial vascular disease, rupture of the axillary artery is possible. If reduction is successful, the shoulder should be immobilized for 3 to 4 weeks. For posteriorly dislocated shoulders, we prefer to immobilize the arm posterior to the axis of the body. If the dislocation is anterior, the arm is immobilized anterior to the axis of the body (Fig. 9.21). Active and active-assisted range-of-motion and strengthening exercises should be initiated when the immobilization period is complete.

▮ OPEN REDUCTION

Two obstacles are generally encountered with open reduction. The first is difficulty in replacing the humeral head because of fibrosis, shortening of the muscle, contracture, bowstringing of the capsule across the glenoid cavity, defect of the articular surface in the humeral head at the point of impingement at the glenoid, and scar tissue in the glenoid fossa. The second obstacle is difficulty maintaining reduction because of instability.

When an open reduction is performed, it is often necessary to prevent recurrent dislocations caused by the humeral head defect. This problem is generally encountered more often in old unreduced posterior dislocations than in anterior

dislocations. Methods for treating this problem include filling the defect in the anterior part of the humeral head with the subscapularis tendon (Fig. 9.22A and B) and transplanting the subscapularis tendon with the lesser tuberosity attached (Fig. 9.22C). Elevation and bone grafting with an autograft or allograft also may be required. In general, these techniques can be used for defects of up to approximately 40% of the articular surface; for larger defects, the necessity of prosthetic replacement is more likely.

Rockwood recommended a posterior approach for old unreduced posterior dislocations of the shoulder if the anteromedial humeral head defect is less than 15%. If the head defect is greater than 15%, an anterior reconstruction through an anterior approach is recommended. Superior and anteromedial approaches for open reduction of these posterior dislocations also have been advocated.

El Shewy et al. treated chronic posterior dislocations (with head defects less than 25%) by reduction, and then posterior capsular shift (Fig. 9.23), with good pain relief and reasonable functional improvement.

A humeral rotational osteotomy has been described for patients who have locked posterior shoulder dislocations and meet the following criteria: (1) healthy articular cartilage, (2) humeral head defect involving less than 40% of the articular

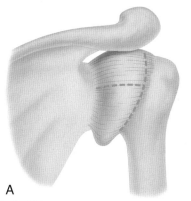 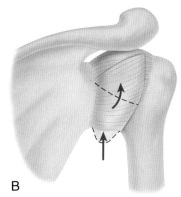

A   B

FIGURE 9.23 Open reduction and posterior capsular shift in old unreduced posterior shoulder dislocations. **A,** T-shaped incision of the posterior capsule. **B,** Upward shift of inferior flap with overlap by superior flap to reinforce the repair. (Modified from El Shewy MT, El Barbary HM, El Meligy YH, et al: Open reduction and posterior capsular shift for cases of neglected unreduced posterior shoulder dislocation, *Am J Sports Med* 36:133–136, 2008.)

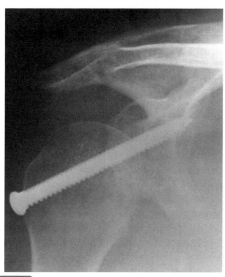

FIGURE 9.24 Use of Swiss screw to maintain reduction of shoulder in old unreduced dislocation. (From Neviaser TJ: Old unreduced dislocations of the shoulder, *Orthop Clin North Am* 11:287, 1980.)

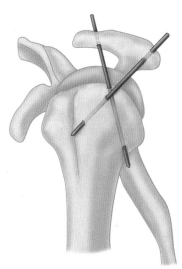

FIGURE 9.25 Wilson and McKeever method of stabilizing shoulder joint with two Kirschner wires after reduction of posterior dislocation. (From DePalma AF: *Surgery of the shoulder*, Philadelphia, 1950, JB Lippincott.)

surface, and (3) ability to participate in an active rehabilitation program.

Internal fixation may be a helpful (or necessary) adjunct to open reduction. A Swiss screw (Fig. 9.24) or crossed Kirschner wires through the acromion into the humeral head (Fig. 9.25) have been described. Kirschner wire fixation also has been used in anterior dislocations with transfer of the coracoid to the glenoid. Akinci et al. reported five excellent, four good, and one poor result with open reduction and Kirschner wire fixation of 10 old unreduced anterior shoulder dislocations. Some authors have found it unnecessary to transfix the shoulder joint at all and have recommended simply supporting the arm at the side in a position anterior to the coronal plane of the body for anterior dislocations and posterior to the coronal plane for posterior dislocations (Fig. 9.21).

ANTERIOR DISLOCATIONS

OPEN REDUCTION OF CHRONIC ANTERIOR SHOULDER DISLOCATION

TECHNIQUE 9.12

(ROWE AND ZARINS)

- An anterior approach to the shoulder through the deltopectoral interval is usually satisfactory. Make an incision extending from the lateral third of the clavicle inferiorly for 10 to 12.5 cm.

- Separate the deltoid and pectoralis major muscles and retract the short head of the biceps and the coracobrachialis. Inferior to the coracoid, the humeral head may be seen or felt with a blunt instrument.
- Before trying to reduce the dislocation, open the capsule and completely divide the coracohumeral ligament and free the glenoid cavity of fibrous tissue.
- Release of the subscapularis muscle will be necessary in performing this step. Replace the humeral head gently into the glenoid cavity. Avoid using too much mechanical force with tools to prevent fracturing of the osteoporotic bone of the humeral head or glenoid.
- Stretch the soft tissues gently, manipulating the shoulder until motion of the joint is almost normal.
- The capsule will be so contracted that it usually cannot be closed. Carefully repair the subscapularis muscle; remember that just inferior to this lies the axillary nerve (Fig. 9.26).
- If the anterior glenoid is deficient, osteotomize the coracoid process with attached conjoined tendon and transfer it to the anterior glenoid rim below the equator (see Bankart-Bristow-Latarjet technique, Technique 52.11).

POSTOPERATIVE CARE If internal fixation is used, support the arm in the desired position in an abduction splint or in a spica cast; the internal fixation is removed at 3 to 4 weeks. If the technique of Rowe and Zarins is used (Fig. 9.21), the arm supports are removed at about 3 weeks. At 3 to 4 weeks, gentle pendulum motion is begun. Active motion and passive motion of the shoulder are soon begun and are continued within the ranges of comfort. The shoulder should probably be supported in a splint at night for several months until fairly strong, active abduction has been regained.

Full function of the shoulder rarely is regained after this operation. Motion is often limited, especially in abduction and external rotation. The patient therefore should not expect full recovery, but some improvement in shoulder function should be expected.

POSTERIOR DISLOCATIONS

Posterior dislocation of the shoulder commonly is neglected because of presentation with the limb adducted and internally rotated. The mechanism of injury usually is a violent injury, a seizure, or an electric shock. A reverse Hill-Sachs lesion may be present in the anterior humeral head, which can be quite large if the dislocation is chronic, and the dislocation may be locked.

OPEN REDUCTION OF CHRONIC POSTERIOR SHOULDER DISLOCATION FROM A SUPERIOR APPROACH

TECHNIQUE 9.13

(ROWE AND ZARINS)
- The "utility" approach has been found to be superior for chronic posterior dislocations. Place the patient on the operating table on the contralateral side.

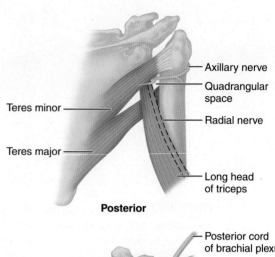

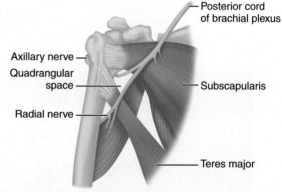

FIGURE 9.26 Relation of axillary nerve to subscapularis muscle, quadrangular space, and neck of humerus. With anterior dislocations, subscapularis is displaced forward, creating traction injury to axillary nerve. Nerve is entrapped and held above by brachial plexus and below where it wraps around behind neck of humerus. (Redrawn from Neer CS, Rockwood CA: Fractures and dislocations of the shoulder. In Rockwood CA, Green DP, editors: *Fractures in adults*, ed 2, Philadelphia, 1984, Lippincott.) **SEE TECHNIQUE 9.12.**

- Make the skin incision as shown in Fig. 9.27.
- Turn down the deltoid muscle together with a detached 5-mm-wide piece of the acromion at the middle third of the muscle. When the bony rim of acromion is reattached, the deltoid will heal in its anatomic position and not displace distally.
- Sharply separate from the clavicle and the spine of the scapula the anterior and posterior origins of the deltoid as far as necessary and then split the deltoid distally (as much as 5 cm) to allow complete anterior, posterior, and inferior exposure of the shoulder joint. Take care to avoid injury to the axillary nerve. The anatomic landmarks are easily obscured. The easiest landmark to locate is the long head of the biceps, which can be followed to the bicipital groove between the lesser and greater tuberosities.
- Incise and retract the rotator cuff and remove the fibrous tissue from the glenoid cavity. As an alternative, strip the capsule from the glenoid face first and then proceed to lyse adhesions of the rotator cuff from the anatomic neck of the humerus.

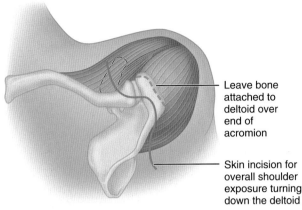

Leave bone attached to deltoid over end of acromion

Skin incision for overall shoulder exposure turning down the deltoid

FIGURE 9.27 Combined approach in which deltoid muscle is turned down to expose anterior and posterior aspects of shoulder. *Heavy dotted line* shows skin incision. *Light dotted line* shows skin osteotomy of acromion leaving 5 mm of bone attached to deltoid muscle. (Redrawn from Rowe CR, Zarins B: Chronic unreduced dislocation of the shoulder, *J Bone Joint Surg* 64A:494–505, 1982.) **SEE TECHNIQUE 9.13**.

- With the contractures released, carefully separate the humeral head from the posterior rim of the glenoid. If the dislocation is old, the humeral head may be soft and easily injured unless the exposure is adequate.
- Reduce the head of the humerus into the glenoid cavity.
- If the shoulder is unstable or a large anterior humeral head defect is present, dissect the subscapularis tendon sharply from its insertion and transfer it to fill the defect or resect the lesser tuberosity with the attached subscapularis tendon and transfer it (Fig. 9.22C).
- Internal fixation of the shoulder joint generally is not necessary if the arm is kept posterior to the coronal plane of the body with support after surgery (Fig. 9.21).
- Suture the rotator cuff tendons to the sites of their insertions.
- Reattach the rim of the acromion, which was removed by osteotomy, with sutures passed through three drill holes in the acromion.

POSTOPERATIVE CARE A support is applied to prevent motion of the arm anterior to the coronal plane of the body (Fig. 9.21). The elbow is left free for flexion and extension, and the shoulder can be moved posteriorly into extension. If the arm remains posterior to the coronal plane, the humeral head should not dislocate posteriorly. The support is removed at 3 weeks, and gentle pendulum motion is then begun together with guided isometric exercises and progressive use of the arm within the range of comfort.

OPEN REDUCTION OF CHRONIC POSTERIOR SHOULDER DISLOCATION THROUGH AN ANTEROMEDIAL APPROACH

TECHNIQUE 9.14

(MCLAUGHLIN)
- Expose the shoulder through an anteromedial approach (see Technique 1.92).
- Divide the subscapularis tendon transversely as close to its insertion as possible and retract it medially.
- Attempt to reduce the shoulder manually. If this attempt fails (and it usually does), insert a blunt periosteal elevator or bone skid between the humeral head and the rim of the glenoid cavity and gently lever them apart. As soon as the glenoid rim has become disengaged from the defect in the anterior part of the humeral head, reduction usually occurs.
- Thoroughly inspect the joint, including the humeral head and the defect.
- Curet the defect to bleeding bone and remove all debris and fibrous tissue, beginning on the lesser tuberosity and emerging in the defect in the humeral head (Fig. 9.22A).
- Drill two holes transversely through the bone and pass a mattress suture through these and the previously freed subscapularis tendon.
- Pull the tendon into the defect in the humeral head and tie the sutures securely (Fig. 9.22B).
- Alternatively, resect the lesser tuberosity and its attached subscapularis tendon and fix it in the defect with a bone screw. This allows bone-to-bone healing rather than tendon-to-bone healing. Do not disturb the posterior part of the joint unless the reduction is unstable (Fig. 9.22C).
- If the defect is too large for a less tuberosity transfer, add iliac crest autograft to the defect to correct the humeral head deformity, as described by Khira and Salama. Alternatively, use a femoral head osteochondral allograft, as described by Elmali et al.
- Close the wound and immobilize the arm in a Velpeau dressing.
- When the reduction is not stable enough after anchoring of the subscapularis tendon into the defect, a structural graft can be used posteriorly along the rim of the glenoid cavity and neck of the scapula as a block to dislocation. Such grafting is performed through a posterior approach (see Technique 1.99). The graft can be obtained from the posterior iliac crest or the posterior surface of the acromion. Use screws or threaded pins to fix the graft beneath the periosteum of the neck of the scapula posteriorly.

POSTOPERATIVE CARE A Velpeau dressing is applied and worn until the wound has healed. The sutures are removed in 2 weeks, and gentle, active, and pendulum range-of-motion exercises are begun. A shoulder immobilizer is worn at night for 6 weeks. Exercises are increased so that internal rotation and overhead exercises are underway by 4 to 6 weeks.

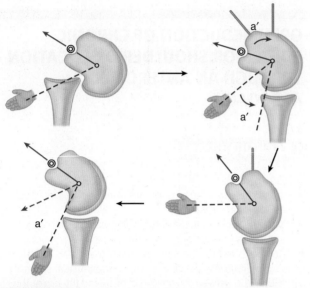

FIGURE 9.28 Diagrammatic representation of principle of rotational osteotomy in shoulder with locked posterior shoulder dislocation. (From Keppler P, Holz U, Thielemann FW, et al: Locked posterior dislocation of the shoulder: treatment using rotational osteotomy of the humerus, *J Orthop Trauma* 8:286–292, 1994.) **SEE TECHNIQUE 9.15**.

DELTOPECTORAL APPROACH FOR CHRONIC POSTERIOR SHOULDER DISLOCATION

TECHNIQUE 9.15

(KEPPLER ET AL.)
- Place the patient supine.
- Expose the shoulder joint through an anterior deltopectoral approach (Technique 1.92).
- Make a 10-cm incision in the deltopectoral groove.
- After minimal detachment of the deltoid muscle from the clavicle, make an L-shaped incision of the subscapularis tendon and the capsule.
- Reduction of the dislocation may be difficult and should be performed by unhooking the humeral head from the glenoid. Remove any fibrous and granulation tissue filling the glenoid fossa to maintain reduction of the humeral head.
- After reduction, determine the congruity of the joint and the range of motion necessary to prevent a redislocation. The shoulder usually will redislocate with internal rotation as the humeral head defect articulates with the glenoid. If insufficient internal rotation remains to allow activities of daily living, osteotomy is indicated.
- Perform a transverse osteotomy in the humeral surgical neck to allow internal rotation of the humeral shaft (Fig. 9.28).
- Fix the osteotomy with an angled blade plate. The stabilized osteotomy ensures that the humeral head defect is always anterior to the glenoid rim during normal motion (Fig. 9.29). After osteotomy fixation, the shoulder should have normal motion in all planes except external rotation.

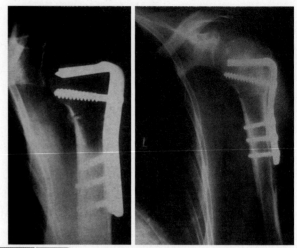

FIGURE 9.29 Internally fixed humerus after transverse osteotomy and internal rotation of humeral shaft. (From Keppler P, Holz U, Thielemann FW, et al: Locked posterior dislocation of the shoulder: treatment using rotational osteotomy of the humerus, *J Orthop Trauma* 8:286–292, 1994.) **SEE TECHNIQUE 9.15**.

- If the humeral head defect is large (greater than 40%), rotational osteotomy is unlikely to restore articular congruity and stability. Hemiarthroplasty or total shoulder arthroplasty should be considered.

POSTOPERATIVE CARE Postoperatively, the arm is held in a shoulder immobilizer. After removal of the suction drain on the second postoperative day, physical therapy is started with isometric exercises and gentle passive pendulum exercises. The patient should continue to wear the shoulder immobilizer at night. Guided passive exercises are begun 1 week after surgery, with a maximum of 90 degrees of flexion and abduction and with external rotation only to the neutral position. The shoulder immobilizer is discontinued as dictated by the patient's comfort. After 3 weeks, an active physical therapy program in all planes is initiated. External rotation is not allowed up to the sixth postoperative week. Six to 8 weeks after surgery, if good range of motion and strength have returned, activities such as swimming and throwing can be allowed. The angled plate is not routinely removed.

HEMIARTHROPLASTY

For very old (longer than 6 months) dislocations or for large head defects (larger than 45% to 50%), most authors suggest proceeding directly to arthroplasty, using hemiarthroplasty if the glenoid is normal and if the dislocation is more than 6 months old or the defect involves more than 45% of the articular surface as seen on the axillary radiograph or CT scan. Reducing the usual amount of retroversion of the humeral component decreases the tendency of the head to sublux posteriorly in posterior dislocations. For a posterior shoulder dislocation that has been present for more than 6 months, the humeral component is placed in approximately neutral version. For a posterior shoulder dislocation that has been present for less than 6 months, the component is placed in approximately

20 degrees of retroversion. The technique of hemiarthroplasty of the shoulder is further described in other chapter.

Occasionally, significant instability may persist even after arthroplasty requiring further soft-tissue reconstruction, such as posterior capsule augmentation using transplanted biceps tendon.

TOTAL SHOULDER ARTHROPLASTY

Total shoulder replacement is recommended if the glenoid has been destroyed and the dislocation is more than 6 months old or the defect involves more than 45% of the articular surface. A bone graft also may be necessary if extensive erosion of the posterior margin of the glenoid fossa has occurred. Appropriate radiographs and CT scans can determine whether such defects are present before surgery. The usual amount of retroversion of the humeral component must be reduced to lessen the tendency of the head to sublux posteriorly. The longer the dislocation has been present, the more retroversion must be reduced. Sahajpal and Zuckerman recommended decreasing the amount of retroversion by 10 to 15 degrees to provide a more stable construct. The correct amount of version can be determined by inserting trial components and testing the stability of the shoulder at the time of surgery, making adjustments if required. In addition, if necessary, the posterior part of the capsule can be plicated through the anterior approach after the humeral head has been osteotomized and before the components are inserted. Similarly, a large redundant posterior pouch can be corrected by plication of the capsule. For elderly patients with posterior dislocations and/or glenoid deficiency due to posterior instability, reverse total shoulder arthroplasty should be considered. The techniques of total shoulder arthroplasty, both anatomic and reverse, are described in other chapter.

ELBOW

Old unreduced dislocations of the elbow are rare and are more often seen in developing countries. Operative treatment for unreduced elbow dislocations has been reported mostly by surgeons practicing in the Middle East and Asia. Posterior dislocations are the most common; therefore, treatment for this alone is described. The arm generally is fixed in extension or in very slight flexion with minimal range of motion. Pronation and supination are limited. Pronation usually is more limited than supination because the biceps is under tension from angulation around the humeral condyles. The biceps then pulls the forearm into supination.

Pathologic findings with old unreduced dislocations of the elbow have been described, including extensive myositis ossificans around the joints, especially in the brachialis and the triceps brachii muscles; marked shortening of the triceps muscle and medial and collateral ligaments; tightening of the ulnar nerve with attempts at flexion; ossification or dense fibrous thickening of the joint capsule; and extensive dense, fibrous tissue filling the olecranon and coronoid fossae and the space between the distal end of the humerus and the proximal ends of the radius and ulna. A "radial humeral horn" (Fig. 9.30), seen in old unreduced dislocations, is the result of the ossification of the hematoma found near the periosteum adhering to the capsule near the head of the radius.

Treatment options for old unreduced posterior dislocations of the elbow include closed reduction, open reduction, excision arthroplasty, interposition or replacement arthroplasty, and arthrodesis.

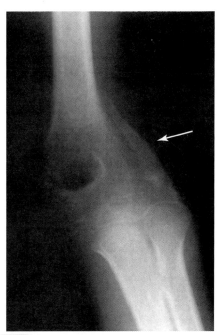

FIGURE 9.30 Anteroposterior radiograph showing lateral dislocation of the elbow and horn of ossification. (From Bruce C, Laing P, Dorgan J, et al: Unreduced dislocation of the elbow: case report and review of the literature, *J Trauma* 35:962–965, 1993.)

Although the results of open reduction of the elbow, if undertaken within 3 months, are acceptable, a normal functioning elbow should not be expected. In children, however, if the dislocation is not congenital, open reduction is worth an attempt no matter how long it has been since the dislocation occurred because children regain useful ranges of flexion and extension.

CLOSED REDUCTION

Most authors agree that closed reduction of the elbow is virtually impossible after 3 weeks. By that time, soft-tissue contracture and localized osteoporosis are sufficient to make closed reduction hazardous; the bone may fracture or the articular surfaces may be damaged at the time of reduction. Fracture can occur even during the early period, so the manipulation must be done carefully and gently with the patient under general anesthesia for complete muscle relaxation.

OPEN REDUCTION

Although some authors have reported that patients regain useful range of flexion-extension of the elbow after open reduction for old posterior dislocations regardless of the age of the patient and the duration of the unreduced dislocation, most report that the likelihood of restoring useful function by open reduction alone is inversely proportional to the length of time from injury to surgery.

In performing open reduction, the shortened triceps muscle must be lengthened and the shortened medial and lateral collateral ligaments must be released. The fibrous tissue between the distal humerus and the ulna should be removed. The radial humeral horn, if present, must be divided. It is wise to inspect and to decompress the ulnar nerve in all patients in whom open reduction of the elbow is required, and the nerve should be transposed if necessary. After reduction, the elbow is frequently unstable. For stability, some authors use Kirschner wires or Steinmann pins, transfixing the olecranon and the humerus or transfixing the capitellum and radial head. Others prefer a hinged fixator, which, although more complex, allows earlier motion, theoretically improving results. Others opt for ligament reconstruction with or without adjunctive fixation. Elbow arthroplasty may be the best choice for the most chronic or difficult cases. Good functional improvement has been reported in most patients with complete capsular and ligamentous release (including the collaterals) and a Speed "V-Y lengthening."

Anderson et al. reviewed 32 patients with chronic elbow dislocations without fractures that were treated with open reduction, complete soft-tissue release, intraarticular scar excision, and ulnar nerve transposition. The triceps tendon was left intact, although 25% required needle barbotage to incrementally lengthen the tendon. Ligament reconstruction, external fixation, or Steinmann pin fixation was not used. Using the Mayo Elbow Performance Index, 97% had good-to-excellent results at mean follow-up of almost 2 years.

Jupiter and Ring described a stable and mobile joint after open reduction and hinged external fixation in five patients at an average of 11 weeks after the initial injury. They reattached the lateral soft tissues, including the origin of the lateral collateral ligament complex to the lateral epicondyle in three patients, but they made no attempt to reconstruct the ligaments, tendons, or bone and performed no tendon lengthening or transfer and no deepening of the ulnar groove. To mobilize the elbow initially, a passive worm gear was incorporated into a hinged external fixation, and active mobilization was gradually introduced. The hinge was removed 5 weeks after the procedure.

Because of an approximately 30% recurrent dislocation rate after ligamentous repair alone, the use of a hinged fixator has been recommended to protect the repair, as well as to maintain joint reduction, permit motion, and enhance muscle-tendon stretching. The hinge usually is left in place for 8 weeks, during which time active and passive range of motion exercises are carried out (Figs. 9.31 and 9.32). Ivo et al. obtained good results in three patients with chronically unreduced complex elbow dislocations with a treatment protocol that included in situ neurolysis of the ulnar nerve, distraction and reduction of the joint with a unilateral hinged external fixator, and repair of the osseous stabilizers, without collateral ligament reconstruction. Pontini et al., however, warned that complications may be frequent with this technique: of their seven patients, four developed at least one complication, and three required additional procedures. The creation of an intraarticular "cruciate" ligament has been described to stabilize the joint and allow early flexion-extension exercises (Fig. 9.33). Most authors have found that lengthening of the triceps muscle is necessary to obtain reduction and use the V-Y technique described by Speed to lengthen the triceps muscle.

OPEN REDUCTION AND V-Y LENGTHENING OF TRICEPS MUSCLES FOR CHRONIC ELBOW DISLOCATION

TECHNIQUE 9.16

(SPEED)
- Make an incision over the posterolateral aspect of the elbow, beginning in the midline 10 cm proximal to the olecranon. Continue distally to just proximal to the tip of the olecranon, then slightly laterally over the lateral

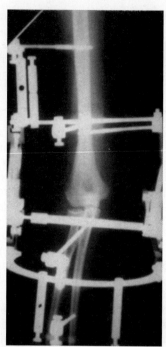

FIGURE 9.31 Late-discovered (6 weeks) medial elbow dislocation after open reduction with complete exposure of joint from medial side and hinged external fixation without ligament repair or reconstruction. (From Hotchkiss RN: Fractures and dislocations of the elbow. In Rockwood CA, Bucholz RW, Green DP, et al, editors: *Rockwood and Green's fractures in adults*, Philadelphia, 1996, Lippincott-Raven.)

humeral condyle and the radial head and continue farther distally for 5 cm on the forearm.
- Undermine and retract the edges of the wound and expose the tendinous insertion or aponeurosis of the triceps muscle on the posterior aspect of the elbow (Fig. 9.34A).
- Locate the ulnar nerve and dissect up from its bed along the groove in the medial humeral condyle and carefully retract it.
- Beginning proximally and using sharp dissection, reflect the aponeurosis of the triceps distally to form a flap of tissue attached to the olecranon.
- Beginning 7.5 cm proximal to the joint, make an incision in the midline of the arm through the fibers of the triceps muscle distally to the olecranon; then curve this deep incision around the lateral edge of the olecranon to the distal end of the skin incision.
- Subperiosteally, free all muscle attachments from the distal humerus, both anteriorly and posteriorly (Fig. 9.34B), and then release the attachments of the joint capsule and collateral ligaments around the condyles of the humerus. Some difficulty may be encountered in freeing the tissues around the medial condyle and along the anterior surface of the humerus just above the joint, but it is essential that they all be loosened and the lower end of the humerus be completely mobilized (Fig. 9.34C).
- There is often a great deal of callus on the posterior surface of the humerus and in the olecranon fossa as a result of the periosteum being elevated at the time of injury. Remove this callus along with any scar tissue.
- After completely freeing the distal humerus, expose the radial head and clear the trochlear notch of the ulna.

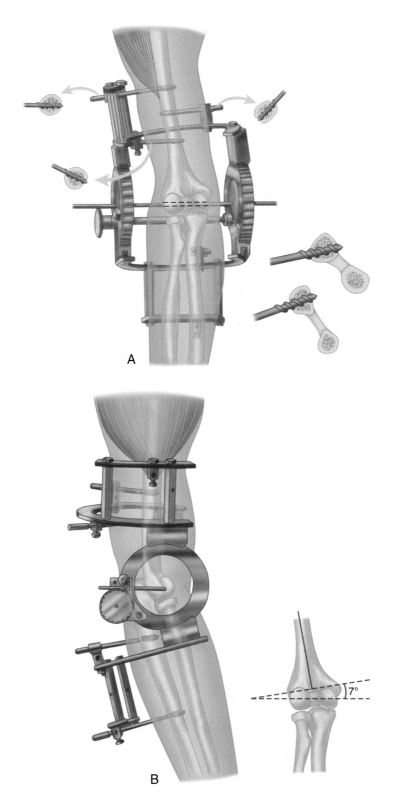

A

B

7°

FIGURE 9.32 Anterior **(A)** and lateral **(B)** views of representative pin placements for old elbow dislocation. Placements may need to be modified on basis of patient's needs. (Redrawn from Hotchkiss RN: *Compass elbow hinge surgical technique*, Memphis, 2004, Smith & Nephew.)

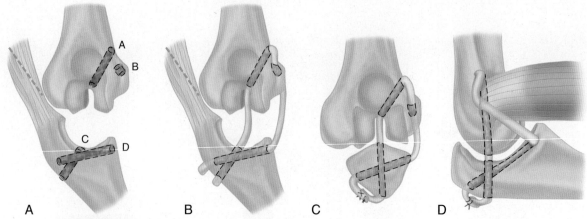

FIGURE 9.33   Reconstruction for old posterior dislocation of the elbow. **A** and **B,** Slot in trochlea and lines of drill holes *A* to *D* show course of tendon graft. **C** and **D,** Anteroposterior and lateral views of completed repair; note intact forearm flexor origin. (From Arafiles RP: Neglected posterior dislocation of the elbow: a reconstruction operation, *J Bone Joint Surg* 69B:199–202, 1987. © British Editorial Society of Bone and Joint Surgery.)

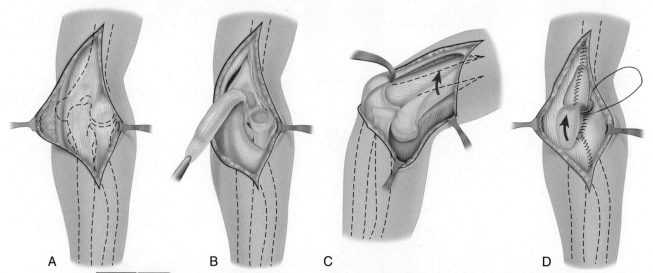

FIGURE 9.34   Speed technique of open reduction of old unreduced dislocation of elbow. **A,** Incision has been made, and ulnar nerve has been isolated. **B,** Triceps aponeurosis has been dissected free and reflected distally. Triceps muscle has been incised longitudinally, and it and other muscles have been stripped subperiosteally from distal humerus. **C,** Lateral view of elbow to show extent of mobilization occasionally necessary before reduction becomes possible. **D,** Closure (see text). **SEE TECHNIQUE 9.16.**

- Rotate the forearm and gently press on the anterior surface of the capitellum, bringing the radial head anteriorly into its normal position.
- If the radial head cannot be reduced easily, dissect the soft tissues more widely instead of applying force that may injure the articular surfaces.
- After the radial head has been reduced, slip the coronoid process distally and then anteriorly over the trochlea and repeat the reduction.
- Carry the joint through a full range of motion. If the elbow is unstable, as it usually is, transfix the olecranon to

the humerus with one or two small Steinmann pins or Kirschner wires with the elbow at 90 degrees.
- Cut the pins off and bend the proximal portion of the pin to prevent migration.
- Suture the periosteum and the triceps over the posterior surface of the humerus and the fascia over the radial head and then suture the tongue of the triceps aponeurosis into its normal position or, more generally, at a slightly more distal level (Fig. 9.34D).
- Decompress the wound with a suction drain.

POSTOPERATIVE CARE The arm is immobilized in a posterior splint at 90 degrees. The drain is removed after 24 hours. The pins are removed approximately 14 days after surgery. The splint is removed several times a day for gentle, active motion exercises. When a moderate range of strong active motion has been regained, the splint may be discarded during the day but should be worn at night for 2 or 3 more months. If a dislocation has been present for a long time, the best functional results can be obtained only by continuing exercises for a long time. Children usually regain motion more easily than adults do.

In an extensive review of the treatment of chronic elbow dislocation, Donohue and Mehlhoff stated that treatment is challenging and a stepwise approach to management is necessary. There are no large series of patients to guide treatment. The roles of primary ligament reconstruction and triceps lengthening remain controversial.

ELBOW ARTHROPLASTY

Most authors agree that an adult elbow that has remained unreduced for longer than 3 to 6 months may require some type of elbow arthroplasty or perhaps arthrodesis. Distraction interpositional arthroplasty has been well described by multiple authors. In cases of chronic dislocation with significant joint degeneration or incongruity in a patient too young for total elbow replacement (who declines arthrodesis), interpositional arthroplasty using fascia lata or a similar graft may be the best choice. The technique for fascial arthroplasty, the technique for total elbow replacement, and the technique for elbow arthrodesis are described in other chapters.

ANTERIOR DISLOCATION OF THE RADIAL HEAD

An old anterior dislocation of the radial head in an adult is sometimes compatible with useful function of the elbow, but flexion is hindered, and the limb is usually weak. If the disability is enough to justify surgery, the radial head probably should be excised. If the dislocation is not very old (e.g., 3 months), open reduction and temporary stabilization with a Kirschner wire can produce a good outcome. If the dislocation is associated with an ulnar shaft malunion, the malunion should be corrected, which should allow reduction of the radial head. If the radial head cannot be reduced, it should be excised or replaced with a radial head arthroplasty (see chapter 12). In a child, a dislocation may be congenital or may have occurred as an isolated injury or possibly in conjunction with a fracture of the ulnar shaft (Monteggia fracture). It may also sometimes be compatible with useful function, but as the child continues to grow, the carrying angle increases and the radial head becomes deformed. If the child is young and less than 1 year from dislocation, and it is not congenital, open reduction and reconstruction of the radial head and neck with or without an ulnar osteotomy can be performed.

Once growth is complete, if disability is severe enough, the radial head should be excised.

Old unreduced wrist and finger dislocations are discussed in other chapter.

REFERENCES

ANKLE

Shenoy R, Kubicek G, Pearse M: The Taylor Spatial Frame for correction of neglected fracture dislocation of the ankle, *J Foot Ankle Surg* 50:736, 2011.

Siddiqui RM, Parker S, Barry M, et al.: Consequences of a missed ankle dislocation in an adolescent, *Foot (Edinb)* 24:195, 2014.

Tellisi N, Deland JT, Rozbruch SR: Gradual reduction of chronic fracture dislocation of the ankle using Ilizarov/Taylor Spatial Frame, *HSS J* 7:85, 2011.

PROXIMAL TIBIOFIBULAR JOINT, KNEE, AND PATELLA

Angelini FI, Helito CP, Bonadio MB, et al.: External fixator for treatment of the sub-acute and chronic multi-ligament-injured knee, *Knee Surg Sports Traumatol Arthrosc* 23:3012, 2015.

Assaghir Y: Surgical realignment of knees with neglected congenital dislocations in a forty-three-year-old man, *J Bone Joint Surg* 92:443, 2010.

Banke IJ, Kohn LM, Meidinger G, et al.: Combined trochleoplasty and MPFL reconstruction for chronic patellofemoral instability: a prospective minimum 2-year follow-up study, *Knee Surg Sports Traumatol Arthrosc* 22:2591, 2014.

Belmoubarik A, Abouchane M, Gahsi M, et al.: Total knee arthroplasty for chronic neglected posterior knee dislocation: case report and literature review, *Open Access Lib J* 2:e1976, 2015.

Ferreira N, Marais LC: Chronic knee dislocation treated with a Taylor Spatial Frame, *SA Orthop J* 11:61, 2012.

Ilyas I, Rabbani SA: Total hip arthroplasty in chronic unreduced hip fracture-dislocation, *J Arthroplasty* 24:903, 2009.

Mani K, Raj D, Parimal A, et al.: Open reduction of neglected knee dislocation: case report of a rare injury, *Malays Orthop J* 10:56, 2016.

Moulton SG, Geeslin AG, LaPrade RF: A systematic review of the outcomes of posterolateral corner knee injuries, part 2: surgical treatment of chronic injuries, *Am J Sports Med* 44:1616, 2016.

Polyzois VD, Grivas TB, Stamatis E, et al.: Management of knee dislocation because of post-traumatic septic arthritis neglected for 40 years, *J Trauma* 64:E21, 2008.

Polyzois VD, Stathopoulos IP, Benetos JS, Pneumaticos SG: A two-stage procedure for the treatment of a neglected posterolateral knee dislocation: gradual reduction with an Ilizarov external fixator followed by arthroscopic anterior and posterior cruciate ligament reconstruction, *Knee* 23:181, 2016.

Van Seymortier P, Ryckaert A, Verdonk P, et al.: Traumatic proximal tibiofibular dislocation, *Am J Sports Med* 36:793, 2008.

Van Thiel GS, Baker III CL, Bush-Joseph C: A chronic posterolateral knee and patella dislocation: case report, *J Orthop Trauma* 23:541, 2009.

HIP

Alva A, Shetty M, Kumar V: Old unreduced traumatic anterior dislocation of the hip, *BMJ Case Rep* 2013, 2013.

Ilyas I, Rabbani SA: Total hip arthroplasty in chronic unreduced hip fracture-dislocation, *J Arthroplasty* 24:903, 2009.

Young S, Banza L: Neglected traumatic anterior dislocation of the hip. Open reduction using the Bernese trochanter flip approach—a case report, *Acta Orthop* 88:348, 2017.

CLAVICULAR JOINTS

Bak K, Fogh K: Reconstruction of the chronic anterior unstable sternoclavicular joint using a tendon autograft: medium-term to long-term follow-up results, *J Shoulder Elbow Surg* 23:245, 2014.

Boileau P, Old J, Gastaud O, et al.: All-arthroscopic Weaver-Dunn-Chuinard procedure with double-button fixation for chronic acromioclavicular joint dislocation, *Arthroscopy* 26:149, 2010.

Boutasta T, Nekhla A: Chronic posterior sternoclavicular dislocation with subclavian vein compression: a case report and review of literature, *Injury Extra* 44:46, 2013.

Broström Windhamre HA, von Heideken JP, Une-Larsson VE, Ekelund AL: Surgical treatment of chronic acromioclavicular dislocations: a comparative study of Weaver-Dunn augmented with PDS-braid or hook plate, *J Shoulder Elbow Surg* 19:1040, 2010.

Dearden PM, Ferran NA, Morris EW: Distal clavicle osteolysis following fixation with a synthetic ligament, *Int J Shoulder Surg* 5:101, 2011.

Elhassan B, Ozbaydar M, Diller D, et al.: Open versus arthroscopic acromioclavicular joint resection: a retrospective comparison study, *Arthroscopy* 25:1224, 2009.

Fauci F, Merolla G, Paladini P, et al.: Surgical treatment of chronic acromioclavicular dislocation with biologic graft vs synthetic ligament: a prospective randomized comparative study, *J Orthop Traumatol* 14:283, 2013.

Kawaguchi K, Tanaka S, Yoshitomi H, et al.: Double figure-of-eight reconstruction technique for chronic anterior sternoclavicular joint dislocation, *Knee Surg Sports Traumatol Arthrosc* 23:1559, 2015.

Lee SK, Song DG, Choy WS: Anatomical double-bundle coracoclavicular reconstruction in chronic acromioclavicular dislocation, *Orthopedics* 38:e655, 2015.

Millett PJ, Braun S, Gobezie R, Pacheco IH: Acromioclavicular joint reconstruction with coracoacromial ligament transfer using the docking technique, *BMC Musculoskel Dis* 10:6, 2009.

Pensak M, Grumet RC, Slabaugh MA, Bach Jr BR: Systematic review. Open versus arthroscopic distal clavicle resection, *Arthroscopy* 26:697, 2010.

Quayle JM, Arnander MW, Pennington RG, Rosell LP: Artificial ligament reconstruction of sternoclavicular joint instability: report of a novel surgical technique with early results, *Tech Hand Up Extrem Surg* 18:31, 2014.

Rushton PRP, Gray JM, Cresswell T: A simple and safe technique for reconstruction of the acromioclavicular joint, *Int J Shoulder Surg* 4:15, 2010.

Strauss EJ, Baker JU, McGill K, Verma NN: The evaluation and management of failed distal clavicle excision, *Sports Med Arthrosc Rev* 18:213, 2010.

Struhl S, Wolfson TS: Continuous loop double endobutton reconstruction for acromioclavicular joint dislocation, *Am J Sports Med* 43:2437, 2015.

Tauber M, Gordon K, Koller H, et al.: Semitendinosus tendon graft versus a modified Weaver-Dunn procedure for acromioclavicular joint reconstruction in chronic cases: a prospective comparative study, *Am J Sports Med* 37:181, 2009.

Tauber M, Valler D, Lichtenberg S, et al.: Arthroscopic stabilization of chronic acromioclavicular joint dislocations: triple-versus single-bundle reconstruction, *Am J Sports Med* 44:482, 2016.

Wang D: Camp Cl, Werner BC, et al: Figure-of-8 reconstruction technique for chronic posterior sternoclavicular joint dislocation, *Arthroscopy Tech* 6:e1749, 2017.

Wood TA, Rosell PA, Clasper JC: Preliminary results of the "Surgilig" synthetic ligament in the management of chronic acromioclavicular joint disruption, *J R Army Med Corps* 155:191, 2009.

SHOULDER

Akinci O, Kayali C, Akalin Y: Open reduction of old unreduced anterior shoulder dislocations: a case series including 10 patients, *Eur J Orthop Surg Traumatol* 20:123, 2010.

Aksekili MA, Ugurlu M, Isik C, et al.: Posterior bone block of chronic locked posterior shoulder dislocations with glenoid augmentation: a retrospective evaluation of ten shoulders, *Int Orthop* 40:813, 2016.

Babalola OR, Vrgoc G, Idowu O, et al.: Chronic unreduced shoulder dislocations: experience in a developing country trauma centre, *Injury* 46(Suppl 6):S100, 2015.

Elmali N, Tasdemir Z, Saglam F, et al.: One-stage surgical treatment of neglected simultaneous bilateral locked posterior dislocation of shoulder: a case report and literature review, *Eklem Hastalik Cerrahisi* 26:175, 2015.

El Shewy MT, El Barbary HM, El Meligy YH, Khaled SA: Open reduction and posterior capsular shift for cases of neglected unreduced posterior shoulder dislocation, *Am J Sports Med* 36:133, 2008.

Funk L: Treatment of glenohumeral instability in rugby players, *Knee Surg Sports Traumatol Arthrosc* 24:430, 2016.

Khira YM, Salama AM: Treatment of locked posterior shoulder dislocation with bone defect, *Orthopedics* 40:e501, 2017.

Kitayama S, Sugaya H, Takahashi N, et al.: Clinical outcome and glenoid morphology after arthroscopic repair of chronic osseous Bankart lesions. A five to eight-year follow-up study, *J Bone Joint Surg Am* 97:1833, 2015.

Kumar AJS, Oakley J, Wootton J: Dynamic posterior stabilization of shoulder hemiarthroplasty in long-standing neglected posterior dislocation of the glenohumeral joint, *Int J Shoulder Surg* 2:83, 2008.

Nordin JS, Aagaard KE, Lunsjö K: Chronic acromioclavicular joint dislocations treated by the GraftRope device, *Acta Orthop* 86:225, 2015.

Sahajpal DT, Zuckerman JD: Chronic glenohumeral dislocation, *J Am Acad Orthop Surg* 16:385, 2008.

Verhaegen F, Smets I, Bosquet M, et al.: Chronic anterior shoulder dislocation: aspects of current management and potential complications, *Acta Orthop Belg* 78:291, 2012.

ELBOW

Ahmed I, Mistry J: The management of acute and chronic elbow instability, *Orthop Clin North Am* 46:271, 2015.

Anderson DR, Haller JM, Anderson LA, et al.: Surgical treatment of chronic elbow dislocation allowing for early range of motion: operative technique and clinical results, *J Orthop Trauma* 32:196, 2018.

Bari MM, Shahidul J, Shetu NH, Mahfuzer RM: Treatment of neglected elbow dislocation using Ilizarov ring fixator, *MOJ Orthop Rheumatol* 3:000107, 2015.

Coulibaly NF, Tiemdjo H, Sane AD, et al.: Posterior approach for surgical treatment of neglected elbow dislocation, *Orthop Traumatol Surg Res* 98:552, 2012.

Damiani M, King GJ: Coronoid and radial head reconstruction in chronic posttraumatic elbow subluxation, *Instr Course Lect* 58:481, 2009.

Donohue KW, Mehlhoff TL: Chronic elbow dislocation: evaluation and management, *J Am Acad Orthop Surg* 24:413, 2016.

Duckworth AD, Ring D, Kulijdian A, McKee MD: Unstable elbow dislocations, *J Shoulder Elbow Surg* 17:281, 2008.

Elzohairy MM: Neglected posterior dislocation of the elbow, *Injury* 40:197, 2009.

Garg P, Paik S, Sahoo S, et al.: A new technique for surgical management of old unreduced elbow dislocations: results and analysis, *J Orthop Allied Sci* 2:45, 2014.

Ivo R, Mader K, Dargel J, Pennig D: Treatment of chronically unreduced complex dislocations of the elbow, *Strategies Trauma Limb Reconstr* 4:49, 2009.

Kamrani RS, Farhadi L, Zanjani LO: Old unreduced elbow fracture and fracture dislocation: treatment with open reduction and hinge external fixation, *Shafa Orthop J* 2:e1893, 2015.

Kanakaraddi S: Primary total elbow replacement in a patient with old unreduced complex posterior elbow dislocation, *Bull Hosp Jt Dis* 71:294, 2013.

Pontini VC, Ogunro S, Henry PD, et al.: Complications associated with hinged external fixation for chronic elbow dislocations, *J Hand Surg Am* 40:730, 2015.

The complete list of references is available online at ExpertConsult.com.

PART II

PERIPHERAL NERVE INJURIES OF THE UPPER AND LOWER EXTREMITIES

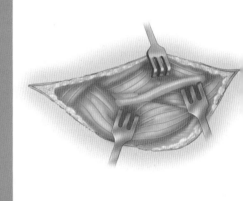

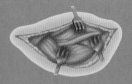

CHAPTER 10

PERIPHERAL NERVE INJURIES

Mark T. Jobe, Santos F. Martinez, William J. Weller

ANATOMY OF THE SPINAL NERVES 517
Components of mixed spinal nerves 517
  Motor 517
  Sensory 517
  Sympathetic 517
Gross anatomy 517
Microscopic anatomy 518

INTERNAL TOPOGRAPHY OF PERIPHERAL NERVES 519

NEURONAL DEGENERATION AND REGENERATION 519

CLASSIFICATION OF NERVE INJURIES 520

EFFECTS OF PERIPHERAL NERVE INJURIES 522
Motor 522
Sensory 522
Reflex 523
Autonomic 523
Complex regional pain syndrome (reflex sympathetic dystrophy) 524
  Clinical presentation 524
  Treatment 525

ETIOLOGY OF PERIPHERAL NERVE INJURIES 526

CLINICAL DIAGNOSIS OF NERVE INJURIES 526
Diagnostic tests 527
  Imaging 527
  Electrodiagnostic studies 527
  Tinel sign 528
  Sweat test 529
  Skin resistance test 529
  Electrical stimulation 529

GENERAL CONSIDERATIONS OF TREATMENT OF NERVE INJURIES 529

FACTORS THAT INFLUENCE REGENERATION AFTER NEURORRHAPHY 530
Age 530
Gap between nerve ends 530
Delay between time of injury and repair 530
Level of injury 530
Condition of nerve ends 531

GENERAL CONSIDERATIONS FOR SURGERY 531
Indications 531
Time of surgery 531
Instruments and equipment 531
Anesthesia 532
Preparation and draping 532

TECHNIQUE OF NERVE REPAIR 532
Endoneurolysis (internal neurolysis) 532
Partial neurorrhaphy 533
Neurorrhaphy and nerve grafting 533
  Methods of closing gaps between nerve ends 533
Techniques of neurorrhaphy 535
Results of operation 538

CERVICAL PLEXUS 538
Spinal accessory nerve 539
  Treatment 539
  Results of suture of the spinal accessory nerve 539

NERVE TRANSFERS 539

UPPER EXTREMITY NERVE INJURIES 544
Suprascapular nerve 544
  Examination 544
  Treatment 544
Long thoracic nerve 545
Axillary Nerve 545
  Examination 545
  Treatment 545
  Methods of closing gaps 546
  Results after axillary nerve injury 546
  Tendon and muscle transfers for paralysis of the deltoid 546
Musculocutaneous Nerve 546
  Examination 546
  Treatment 546
  Methods of closing gaps 546
  Results after injury to the musculocutaneous nerve 546
Radial Nerve 546
  Examination 546
  Treatment 547
  Methods of closing gaps 547
  Results of suture of the radial nerve 547

Critical limit of delay of suture 549
Ulnar Nerve 549
  Examination 550
  Treatment 550
  Methods of closing gaps 551
  Results of suture of the ulnar nerve 551
  Critical limit of delay of suture 552
  Nerve reconstruction 552
Median nerve 552
  Examination 553
  Treatment 553
  Methods of closing gaps 554
  Results of suture of the median nerve 555
  Critical limit of delay of suture 555

LUMBAR PLEXUS 555
Femoral nerve 556
  Examination 556
  Treatment 556
  Methods of closing gaps 557
  Results of suture of the femoral nerve 557

SACRAL PLEXUS 557
Sciatic nerve 557
  Examination 558
  Treatment 558
  Methods of closing gaps 559
  Results of suture of the sciatic nerve 560
  Critical limit of delay of suture 560
Common, superficial, and deep peroneal nerves 560
  Examination 560
  Treatment 560
  Methods of closing gaps 561
  Results of suture of the peroneal nerve 561
  Critical limit of delay of suture 561
  Tendon transfer for peroneal nerve paralysis 561
Tibial nerve 561
  Examination 562
  Treatment 562
  Methods of closing gaps 563
  Results of suture of the tibial nerve 563

Peripheral nerve injuries are common. Despite numerous advances in microsurgical technique and interfascicular nerve grafting, many treatment principles obtained from World War II experiences as set forth in the cumulative works of Seddon and Woodhall are still applicable today. Current research focusing on pharmacologic agents, immune system modulation, enhancing factors, and entubulation chambers, although promising, have had little clinical application so far, and the results of nerve repair remain modest with only 50% of patients regaining useful function.

In this chapter, the diagnosis and treatment of peripheral nerve injuries are described, with the details of surgical technique and postoperative care included in the discussion of each nerve. For details of embryology, microscopic anatomy, and physiology, the reader is referred to other works. The appropriate reconstructive operations are described in other sections of this book, and cross references are provided.

ANATOMY OF THE SPINAL NERVES

Each segmental spinal nerve is formed at or near its intervertebral foramen by the union of its dorsal, or sensory, root with its ventral, or motor, root. In most of the thoracic segments, these mixed spinal nerves retain their autonomy and supply one intercostal dermatomal and myotomal segment. In virtually all other segments of the spinal axis, the spinal nerves join with others to form a plexus that innervates a limb or a special body segment that no longer retains the primitive myomeric pattern. A total of 31 mixed spinal nerves leave their respective foramina on each side of the spine to innervate the homolateral trunk and extremities: eight cervical, 12 thoracic, five lumbar, five sacral, and one coccygeal.

COMPONENTS OF MIXED SPINAL NERVES

A typical mixed spinal nerve has three distinct components: motor, sensory, and sympathetic (Fig. 10.1).

■ MOTOR

Several rootlets leave the anterolateral sulcus of the spinal cord and unite to form each motor root. The fibers traversing

these roots arise from the anterior horn cells and innervate the skeletal muscles.

■ SENSORY

The sensory fibers arise from pain, thermal, tactile, and stretch receptors. Cell bodies for these fibers are located within the dorsal root ganglia with axons entering the posterolateral sulcus of the cord via several rootlets. The fibers conveying joint or position sensibility and some tactile fibers turn cephalad in the dorsal columns and do not synapse before reaching the gracile and cuneate nuclei at the cervicomedullary junction. Pain and temperature fibers synapse in the substantia gelatinosa and cross to ascend in the dorsal spinothalamic tract. Tactile fibers enter, synapse, and cross to ascend in the ventral spinothalamic tract.

■ SYMPATHETIC

The sympathetic component of all 31 mixed spinal nerves leaves the spinal cord along only 14 motor roots. The cells of origin are in the intermediolateral cell column that extends throughout the thoracic and upper lumbar cord segments. The fibers exit from the cord with the 12 thoracic and first two lumbar motor roots, enter the respective mixed spinal nerve, and promptly emerge from it as white rami. The white rami pass anteriorly to the corresponding sympathetic ganglion. Synapse may occur within the ganglion with which the ramus is associated, and postganglionic fibers pass back to the mixed spinal nerve as a gray ramus. More often, however, the fibers entering the ganglion via the white rami pass for variable distances up or down the paravertebral chain to synapse at higher or lower levels. The postganglionic fibers pass along gray rami to cervical, lower lumbar, or sacrococcygeal mixed spinal nerves having no white rami. Sweat glands, blood vessels, and erector pili are innervated also in a segmental pattern.

GROSS ANATOMY

Mixed spinal nerves, having left the intervertebral foramina, receive their sympathetic component and promptly branch into anterior and posterior primary rami. The posterior primary rami are directed posteriorly and supply the paraspinal musculature and the skin along the posterior aspect of the trunk, the neck, and the head. The upper three cervical posterior rami are larger than their corresponding anterior rami, supplying relatively large areas of the scalp posteriorly and the musculature around the craniocervical junction. With these exceptions, posterior primary rami are small, and the major part of each spinal nerve continues laterally in an anterior primary ramus to enter a plexus or to become an intercostal nerve.

Anterior primary rami of all the cervical, the first thoracic, and all the lumbosacral nerves join in the formation of plexuses. Alteration of the metameric pattern results from the migration of dermatomes and myotomes into the limb buds. The upper four cervical anterior rami form the cervical plexus, and the lower four cervical and first thoracic anterior rami form the brachial plexus. The first three and a part of the fourth lumbar anterior rami form the lumbar plexus. The sacral anterior rami along with the fifth lumbar and a part of the fourth join to form the lumbosacral plexus. The enlargement and prolongation of the limb bud markedly alter the myotomal pattern, resulting

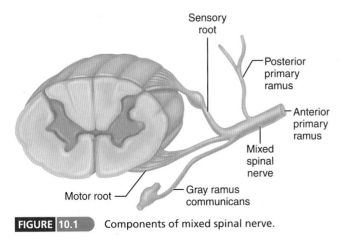

Sensory root

Posterior primary ramus

Anterior primary ramus

Mixed spinal nerve

Motor root

Gray ramus communicans

FIGURE 10.1 Components of mixed spinal nerve.

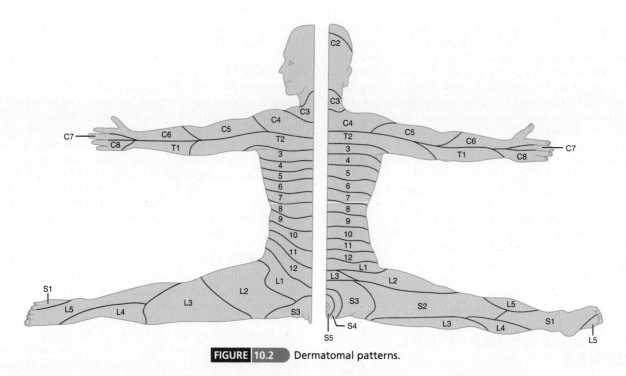

FIGURE 10.2 Dermatomal patterns.

in the union of some myotomes and the division or partial extended migration of others. The fibers of any one mixed spinal nerve may be distributed through several peripheral nerves. By the same token, any one peripheral nerve may contain fibers from several spinal nerves.

The area of skin supplied by the fibers of a single spinal root is called a dermatome. Segmental dermatomal patterns (Fig. 10.2) are well preserved in the thoracic region but not in the limbs. Migration of the limb buds accounts for the displacement of midcervical dermatomes along the lateral aspect of the arm and radial aspect of the forearm and of the lower cervical and upper thoracic dermatomes along the medial aspect of the arm and the ulnar aspect of the forearm. Lumbar and sacral dermatomal alignment along the various aspects of the lower extremity is similarly explained. The line separating the more rostral segmental dermatomes from the more caudal ones is called the axial line and may be followed into the spinal axis.

MICROSCOPIC ANATOMY

Each nerve fiber, or axon, is a direct extension of a dorsal root ganglion cell (sensory), an anterior horn cell (motor), or a postganglionic sympathetic nerve cell, and it is either myelinated or unmyelinated. Sensory and motor nerves contain unmyelinated and myelinated fibers in a ratio of 4:1 (Fig. 10.3). In the unmyelinated or sparsely myelinated fibers, several axons are wrapped by a single Schwann cell. In the more heavily myelinated fibers, the Schwann cell by rotation forms a multilaminated structure that encloses a myelin sheath around a single axon. The segment of myelinated nerve fiber enclosed by a single Schwann cell is referred to as an internode and varies in length from 0.1 to 1.8 mm, with the more heavily myelinated fibers having the longer internodes. The point at which one Schwann cell ends and the next begins is relatively sparse in myelin and is called the nodal gap, or node of Ranvier (Fig. 10.4). The axon with its

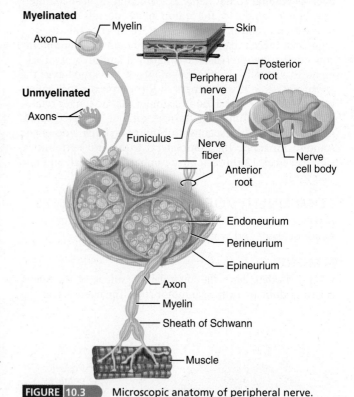

FIGURE 10.3 Microscopic anatomy of peripheral nerve.

Schwann cell and myelin sheath is surrounded by a veil of delicate fibrous tissue called the endoneurium. Seen longitudinally, the endoneurium forms a tube encircling individually the Schwann cell sheaths that cluster together to form a fascicle (or funicle as termed by Sunderland). Each fascicle or separate group of sheathed axons is surrounded by a denser layer of perineurium. The entire group of fascicles with their surrounding perineurium is encased as a mixed spinal or

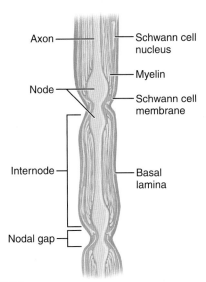

FIGURE 10.4 Basic anatomy of myelinated nerve fiber.

Labels: Axon, Schwann cell nucleus, Myelin, Node, Schwann cell membrane, Internode, Basal lamina, Nodal gap

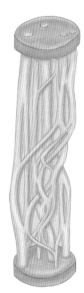

FIGURE 10.5 Internal topography of musculocutaneous nerve as depicted by Sunderland.

peripheral nerve in a denser epineurium. The blood supply to the peripheral nerve enters through the mesoneurium, which is loose connective tissue extending from the epineurium to the surrounding tissues. There is an extrinsic (segmental) and an intrinsic (longitudinal) blood supply to each nerve. The intrinsic blood supply that runs longitudinally within the epineurium, perineurium, and endoneurium is fairly extensive and allows surgical mobilization without complete devascularization over variable lengths of nerves.

INTERNAL TOPOGRAPHY OF PERIPHERAL NERVES

The internal topography or fascicular arrangement of the radial, median, and ulnar nerves was described by Sunderland in 1945 as a complex network of branching and intermingling fascicles that constantly change throughout the course of the nerve (Fig. 10.5). Studies have shown that although the fascicular arrangement is complex in the proximal aspect of a peripheral nerve, the distal fascicles can be dissected over long distances before merging occurs (Fig. 10.6). This characteristic is important to the surgeon when intraneural dissection is required for accurate neurorrhaphy.

NEURONAL DEGENERATION AND REGENERATION

Any part of a neuron detached from its nucleus degenerates and is destroyed by phagocytosis. This process of degeneration distal to a point of injury is called secondary, or *Wallerian degeneration* (Fig. 10.7). The reaction proximal to the point of detachment is called *primary, traumatic,* or *retrograde degeneration.* The time required for degeneration varies between sensory and motor segments and is related to the size and myelinization of the fiber.

During the first 3 days after injury, definite morphologic changes become apparent in the axon. Response to faradic stimulation can be obtained for periods of 18 to 72 hours.

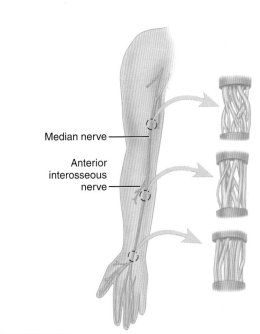

FIGURE 10.6 Complexity of internal topography diminishes in more distal portions of nerve.

Labels: Median nerve, Anterior interosseous nerve

After 2 or 3 days, the distal segment becomes fragmented, and with subsequent fluid loss the fragments begin to shrink and to assume a more oval or globular appearance. A concomitant fragmentation and shrinkage of the myelin sheath parallels the axonal degenerative change. By day 7, macrophages have reached the area in greater numbers, and clearing of the axonal debris is virtually complete after 15 to 30 days. Schwann cell division by mitosis is evident by day 7, the cells increasing in number to fill the area previously filled by the axon and myelin sheath.

The primary retrograde degeneration proceeds for at least an internode or more, depending on the degree of

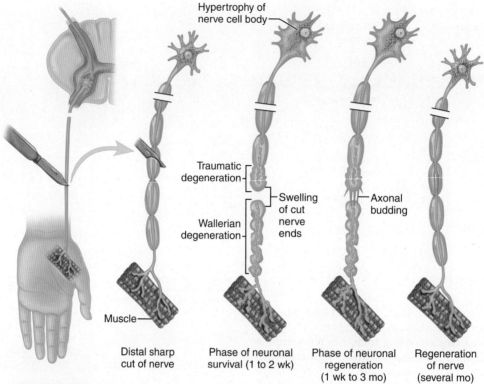

FIGURE 10.7 Physiologic changes in regeneration of peripheral motor nerve axon after division with sharp object.

proximal insult, and it is histologically identical to Wallerian degeneration. The changes in the parent cell body vary to some degree with the type of cell and the nearness of the injury to the cell body. The more proximal the site of injury, the more pronounced the changes. Chromatolysis with swelling of the cytoplasm and eccentric placement of the nucleus is commonly evident. This reaction within the cell body is evident by day 7, and death or evidence of beginning recovery is apparent after 4 to 6 weeks. With recovery, the edema begins to subside, the nucleus migrates toward the center of the cell, and Nissl substance begins to reaccumulate.

Distal to the point of injury or to the proximal extent of retrograde degeneration there is an endoneurial tube filled with Schwann cells to accept regenerating sprouts from the axonal stump. Axonal sprouting may occur within the first 24 hours after injury. All axonal sprouts initially are unmyelinated whether they arise from a myelinated or an unmyelinated fiber. If the endoneurial tube with its contained Schwann cells has been uninterrupted by the injury, the sprouts may pass readily along their former courses, and after regeneration the surviving cells innervate their previous end organs. If the injury has been severe enough to interrupt the endoneurial tube with its contained Schwann cells, however, sprouts that may number 100 from any one axonal stump may migrate aimlessly throughout the damaged area into the epineurial, perineurial, or adjacent regions to form a stump neuroma or neuroma in continuity. Other migrating axonal sprouts barred from their endoneurial tube by scar tissue might enter empty endoneurial tubes of other injured funiculi or, as shown by Cabaud et al., may regenerate through newly formed endoneurial tubes

only to terminate in myotomal or dermatomal areas other than their own. Axons regenerate as if they are influenced by certain neurotrophic substances contained within distal nerve tissue. Experimental work showed that in a primate model and through an inert silicone Y chamber, axons grow toward nerve tissue in preference to muscle or tendon. Some degree of end-organ specificity also exists in the experimental model, and there is a critical gap (2 mm) under which this neurotrophic effect does not exist.

Lesser injuries without disruption of the endoneurial and Schwann cell sheaths are associated with excellent or acceptable anatomic regeneration. Conversely, more extensive injuries with complete disruption of the entire nerve, with wide separation of the ends of the nerve, and with the regenerating fibers obstructed by extensive scar tissue result in little or no return of function.

CLASSIFICATION OF NERVE INJURIES

The classification of nerve injuries proposed by Seddon in 1943 was generally accepted but rarely used. He divided nerve injuries into three groups:

1. *Neurapraxia,* designating minor contusion or compression of a peripheral nerve with preservation of the axis-cylinder but with possibly minor edema or breakdown of a localized segment of myelin sheath. Transmission of impulses is physiologically interrupted for a time, but recovery is complete in a few days or weeks.

2. *Axonotmesis,* designating more significant injury with breakdown of the axon and distal Wallerian degeneration

TABLE 10.1

Classification of Nerve Injuries

DEGREE OF INJURY		HISTOPATHOLOGIC CHANGES					TINEL SIGN	
SUNDERLAND	SEDDON	MYELIN	AXON	ENDONEURIUM	PERINEURIUM	EPINEURIUM	PRESENT	PROGRESSES DISTALLY
I	Neurapraxia	±		–			–	–
II	Axonotmesis	+	+	–			+	+
III		+	+	+			+	+
IV		+	+	+	+		+	–
V	Neurotmesis	+	+	+	+	+	+	–

but with preservation of the Schwann cell and endoneurial tubes. Spontaneous regeneration with good functional recovery can be expected.

3. *Neurotmesis,* designating a more severe injury with complete anatomic severance of the nerve or extensive avulsing or crushing injury. The axon and the Schwann cell and endoneurial tubes are completely disrupted. The perineurium and epineurium also are disrupted to varying degrees. Segments of the latter two may bridge the gap if complete severance is not apparent. In this group, significant spontaneous recovery cannot be expected.

A more useful classification was described by Sunderland in 1951. This classification is more readily applicable clinically, with each degree of injury suggesting a greater anatomic disruption with its correspondingly altered prognosis. In this classification, peripheral nerve injuries are arranged in ascending order of severity from the first to the fifth degree. Anatomically, the various degrees represent injury to (1) myelin, (2) axon, (3) the endoneurial tube and its contents, (4) perineurium, and (5) the entire nerve trunk (Table 10.1).

In *first-degree injury,* conduction along the axon is physiologically interrupted at the site of injury but the axon is not disrupted. No Wallerian degeneration occurs, and recovery is spontaneous and usually complete within a few days or weeks. This injury coincides with the neurapraxia of Seddon. The loss of function varies. Usually, motor function is more profoundly affected than sensory function. Sensory modalities are affected in order of decreasing frequency as follows: proprioception, touch, temperature, and pain. Sympathetic fibers are the most resistant to this type of injury. If sensory modalities are markedly affected, paresthesias may be present for several days. If they are disturbed at all, sympathetic function often returns promptly; the modalities of pain and temperature also are commonly preserved or return promptly. Proprioception and motor function usually are the last to return. Electrical excitability of the nerve distal to the site of injury is preserved. A characteristic of this injury is the simultaneous return of motor function in the proximal and distal musculature; this would never occur in injuries with Wallerian degeneration in which the "motor march" is evident because of progressive regeneration or reinnervation of the more proximal motor units earlier in the course of recovery. Because there is neither axonal damage nor regeneration, no advancing Tinel sign is present. In most instances, the final result is complete restoration of function.

In *second-degree injury,* disruption of the axon is evident, with Wallerian degeneration distal to the point of injury and degeneration proximal for one or more nodal segments. The

integrity of the endoneurial tube (Schwann cell basal lamina) is maintained, providing a perfect anatomic course for regeneration. Any permanent deficit is related to the number of neural somas that die, such death being more common in injuries at the more proximal levels. Clinically, the neurologic deficit is complete with loss of motor, sensory, and sympathetic function. Motor reinnervation is accomplished in a progressive manner from proximal to distal in the order in which nerve branches leave the parent trunk. Commonly, an advancing Tinel sign can be followed along the course of the nerve usually at the rate of 1 inch per month, tracing the progression of regeneration. Usually, good functional return is achieved.

In *third-degree injury,* the axons and endoneurial tubes are disrupted but the perineurium is preserved. The result is disorganization resulting from disruption of the endoneurial tubes. Scar tissue within the endoneurium can obstruct certain tubes and divert sprouts to paths other than their own. Clinically, the neurologic loss is complete in most instances, and because of the additional time required for the regenerating axon tips to penetrate the fibrous barrier, the duration of loss is more prolonged than in second-degree injury. Returning motor function is evident from proximal to distal but with varying degrees of permanent motor or sensory deficit. As in a second-degree injury, an advancing Tinel sign usually is present; however, complete return of neural function does not occur, distinguishing this from a second-degree injury.

In *fourth-degree injury,* the axon and endoneurium are disrupted but some of the epineurium and possibly some of the perineurium are preserved, so complete severance of the entire trunk does not occur. Retrograde degeneration is more severe after this degree of injury, and the mortality among neuronal soma is higher, sometimes resulting in a significant reduction in the number of surviving axons. Essentially, nerve continuity is maintained only by scar tissue, preventing proximal axons from entering the distal endoneurial tubes. Axonal sprouts exit through defects in the perineurium and epineurium and wander about in the surrounding tissues. There is no advancing Tinel sign. Prognosis for significant return of useful function is uniformly poor without surgery.

In *fifth-degree injury,* the nerve is completely transected, resulting in a variable distance between the neural stumps. These injuries occur only in open wounds and usually are identified at the time of early surgical exploration. The likelihood of any significant bridging by axonal sprouts is remote, and the possibility of any significant return of function without appropriate surgery is equally remote.

Sixth-degree (Mackinnon) or *mixed injuries* occur in which a nerve trunk is partially severed, and the remaining part of the trunk sustains fourth-degree, third-degree, second-degree, or rarely even first-degree injury. A neuroma in continuity is present, and the recovery pattern is mixed depending on the degree of injury to each portion of the nerve. Surgical intervention to correct the fourth-degree and fifth-degree components may sacrifice the function of lesser injured fascicles.

EFFECTS OF PERIPHERAL NERVE INJURIES
MOTOR

When a peripheral nerve is severed at a given level, all motor function of the nerve distal to that level is abolished. All muscles supplied by branches of the nerve distal to that level are paralyzed and become atonic. Significant changes on electromyography (EMG) are not apparent for 8 to 14 days, at which time transient fibrillation potentials on needle insertion may become apparent. Spontaneous fibrillations may become evident after 2 to 4 weeks, coinciding with the onset of atrophic change within the muscle fibers. Atrophy of muscle bulk progresses rapidly to 50% to 70% at the end of about 2 months. Atrophy continues at a much slower rate, and the connective tissue component of the muscles increases. Striations and motor endplate configurations are retained for longer than 12 months, whereas the empty endoneurial tubes shrink to about one third their normal diameter. Complete disruption and replacement of muscle fibers may not become complete until after 3 years.

Several methods are used to evaluate motor return after peripheral nerve injuries. They involve assessment of muscle strength against gravity and against graded resistance. The use of pinch meters and grip meters and evaluation of endurance, speed of movement, and individual muscle function helps to document the progress of motor return. The British Medical Research Council established the following system for assessing the return of muscle function after peripheral nerve injuries: M0, no contraction has returned; M1, perceptible contraction in proximal muscles has returned; M2, perceptible contraction in proximal and distal muscles has returned; M3, all important muscles act against resistance; M4, all synergistic and independent movements are possible; M5, recovery is complete (Table 10.2).

SENSORY

Sensory loss usually follows a definite anatomic pattern, although the factor of overlap from adjacent nerves may confuse inexperienced surgeons. After severance of a peripheral nerve, only a small area of complete sensory loss is found. This area is supplied exclusively by the severed nerve and is called the *autonomous zone* or *isolated zone* of supply for that nerve. A larger area of tactile and thermal anesthesia is readily delineated and corresponds more closely to the gross anatomic distribution of the nerve (Fig. 10.8); this larger area is known as the *intermediate zone*. When a nerve is intact, and the adjacent nerves are blocked or sectioned, an area of sensibility exceeds the gross anatomic distribution of the nerve; this area is known as the *maximal zone*.

It has long been recognized that the autonomous zone becomes smaller during the first few days or weeks after injury, long before regeneration is possible. Livingston suggested that this is caused by ingrowth of adjacent nerves, but

TABLE 10.2	
Muscle Function Assessment After Peripheral Nerve Injuries	
MOTOR	**RECOVERY**
M0	No contraction
M1	Return of perceptible contraction in proximal muscles
M2	Return of perceptible contraction in proximal and distal muscles
M3	Return of function in proximal and distal muscles of such a degree that all important muscles are sufficiently powerful to act against resistance
M4	Return of function as in stage 3; in addition, all synergistic and independent movements are possible.
M5	Complete recovery

In the hand, proximal muscles are defined as extrinsic muscles and distal muscles are defined as intrinsic muscles.
From Leffert RD: Brachial plexus. In Green DP, editor: *Operative hand surgery*, ed 2, New York, 1988, Churchill Livingstone.

TABLE 10.3	
Sensibility Recovery Sequence	
I	Myelinated and unmyelinated fibers (restore perception of pain and temperature)
	Pseudomotor function
II	Touch perception
	Perception of 30 cycle per second (cps) of vibratory stimulus
	Perception of moving touch
	Perception of constant touch
	Perception of 256 cps vibratory stimulus

As outlined by Dellon AL, Curtis RM, Edgerton MT: Evaluating recovery of sensation in the hand following nerve injury, *Johns Hopkins Med J* 130:235, 1972.

resumption of or increase in function in anastomotic branches from adjacent nerves is a more plausible explanation. This decrease in the area of sensory loss might be interpreted by an inexperienced surgeon as evidence of regeneration or of incomplete injury and might be responsible for needless delay in exploration of the nerve.

In injury to the median and ulnar nerves, one study found that pinprick was the first perception to return, followed by 30 cycles/s vibratory stimulus, and then moving touch. The perception of constant touch and the perception of a 256 cycles/s vibratory stimulus were the last to return (Table 10.3). These investigators inferred that the early return of pain perception resulted from the faster regeneration of the small-diameter pain fibers. The larger-diameter touch fibers regenerated more slowly. The return of moving touch perception, mediated by quickly adapting fibers and Pacinian corpuscles, before the return of constant touch, mediated by slowly adapting fibers and the Merkel discs, was explained by differential maturation of the respective receptors, rather than by the diameter of the

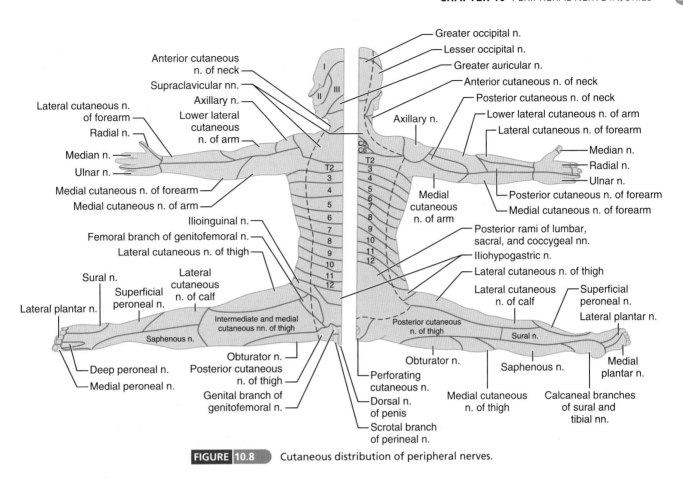

FIGURE 10.8 Cutaneous distribution of peripheral nerves.

fibers alone. The system of evaluating by moving touch, constant touch, vibratory stimulus, pinprick, and the Weber two-point discrimination was proposed as a method for screening patients to determine specific exercises for reeducation of constant-touch perception. The evaluation of sensory return after peripheral nerve injuries is important regardless of the site of the injury. This is especially true in the upper extremity, where sensibility in the hand is extremely important.

The clinical evaluation of sensory return also is done using other methods, such as pinprick appreciation and von Frey hairs. The British Medical Research Council established the following six-level grading scale for sensory return: S0, absence of sensibility in the autonomous area; S1, recovery of deep cutaneous pain within the autonomous area; S2, return of some superficial cutaneous pain and tactile sensibility within the autonomous area of the nerve; S3, return of superficial cutaneous pain and tactile sensibility throughout the autonomous area with disappearance of overreaction; S3+, some recovery of two-point discrimination within the autonomous area; S4, complete recovery (Table 10.4).

Two-point discrimination has been shown to directly correlate with return of hand function and object identification. The pick-up test (a timed test to measure fine and manual dexterity) and the triketohydrindene hydrate (ninhydrin) printing test also have been shown to be of use.

REFLEX

Complete severance of a peripheral nerve abolishes all reflex activity transmitted by that nerve. This is true in severance of the afferent or the efferent arc. Commonly, however, reflex

TABLE 10.4	
Sensation Assessment after Peripheral Nerve Injury	
SENSORY	**RECOVERY**
S0	Absence of sensibility in autonomous area
S1	Recovery of deep cutaneous pain sensibility within autonomous area of the nerve
S2	Return of some degree of superficial cutaneous pain and tactile sensibility within autonomous area of the nerve
S3	Return of superficial cutaneous pain and tactile sensibility throughout autonomous area, with disappearance of any previous overresponse
S3+	Return of sensibility as in stage 3; in addition, there is some recovery of two-point discrimination within autonomous area
S4	Complete recovery

From Leffert RD: Brachial plexus. In Green DP, editor: *Operative hand surgery*, ed 2, New York, Churchill Livingstone, 1988.

activity is abolished in partial nerve injuries when neither arc is completely interrupted and is not a reliable guide to the severity of injury.

AUTONOMIC

Interruption of a peripheral nerve is followed by loss of sweating and of pilomotor response and by vasomotor paralysis in the autonomous zone. The area of anhidrosis usually corresponds to, but may be slightly larger than, the sensory deficit. This area may be outlined easily by the starch-iodine test, by the ninhydrin printing test popularized by Aschan and Moberg, or by instruments for determining skin resistance (Richter dermometer). Another objective test described by O'Riain and by Leukens is the wrinkle test. When normal skin is immersed in water for a time, wrinkling occurs. Denervated skin does not wrinkle under these circumstances. As reinnervation occurs, wrinkling of the skin returns. If the injury is incomplete, and especially if it is associated with causalgia, sweating may be excessive and may involve areas beyond the intermediate zone of the nerve. Vasodilation occurs in complete lesions, and the area affected is at first warmer and pinker than the rest of the limb. After 2 to 3 weeks, however, the affected area becomes colder than the adjacent normal areas and the skin may be pale, cyanotic, or mottled in an area often extending beyond the maximal zone of the injured nerve. Trophic changes occur commonly and are most evident in the hands and feet. The skin becomes thin and glistening and, when subjected to trauma that ordinarily does little harm, breaks down to form ulcers that heal slowly. The fingernails become distorted, are often ridged or brittle, and may be lost entirely.

Osteoporosis often follows peripheral nerve injuries. It is more likely to be pronounced in incomplete lesions associated with pain. Incomplete lesions of the median nerve seem to be associated more often with osteoporosis, with changes occurring in the distal phalanges of the thumb and index and long fingers. Partial ankylosis from fibrosis of the periarticular structures also may develop. These changes are similar to atrophy of disuse but are much more severe.

COMPLEX REGIONAL PAIN SYNDROME (REFLEX SYMPATHETIC DYSTROPHY)

Complex regional pain syndrome (CRPS) represents autonomic and pain transmission dysregulation, resulting in peripheral sensitization with allodynia, dysesthesia, hyperpathia, and a reduced tolerance for pain when using the affected area for basic function. The condition occurs most commonly after a traumatic injury or iatrogenic insult. Classification of CRPS is based on the structures injured. The International Association for the Study of Pain delineated two main categories of the syndrome, replacing traditional terms, and through efforts by their Taxonomy Committee (iasp-pain.org), they continue to

update descriptions and terms. Although the attempt to simplify CRPS into types I and II is attractive, considerable overlap in pathology exists. CRPS I (formally *reflex sympathetic dystrophy*, RSD) theoretically represents patients who have had a musculoskeletal injury without a defined neural injury. CRPS II (causalgia) includes patients who fulfill the same criteria but who have evidence of a neural injury. In addition, there have been further efforts to define sympathetic-mediated and nonsympathetic-mediated varieties, with temporal transitions into "warm" and "cold" subtypes.

■ CLINICAL PRESENTATION

The most evident presentation in CRPS is avoidance behavior and an altered recovery pattern when the patient tries to use the area of the body that has been injured. CRPS may occur after a fracture, crush injury, routine surgical procedure, or a minor innocuous appearing injury. Chemical or electrical burns, metabolic neuropathies (e.g., diabetes mellitus), or infections, such as postherpetic neuralgia, all can contribute to this polymodal-mediated hyperpathia. A female predisposition has been noted, and upper extremity involvement is most frequently seen. CRPS also has been associated with smoking.

Early hallmark signs include a marked reduction in use or stimuli response of the affected area (e.g., an extremity) with sensitization and at times autonomic dysregulation. The condition may be self-limiting, but if not identified and treated aggressively, it can progress with a reduction in use and permanent impairment. Patients identified early (<6 months) have a better prognostic outcome than those with a delayed diagnosis (>1 year). This must be tempered, however, because a premature diagnosis in an impressionable patient who becomes invested in literature on the topic may actually lead to a self-fulfilling prophecy.

Harden et al. validated the Budapest criteria of CRPS to aid clinicians in identifying the signs and symptoms in four categories (Table 10.5). Although defined as types I and II, CRPS frequently exhibits with both musculoskeletal and neural injuries. Clinicians must be alert to disproportionate postoperative or posttraumatic clinical responses, such as allodynia, dysesthesia, hyperpathia, hyperalgesia, and hypoesthesia. The patient's exaggerated response to a relatively common injury may tempt the clinician to discount this as a psychologic issue. However, disproportionate symptoms

TABLE 10.5	
Budapest Diagnostic Criteria for Complex Regional Pain Syndrome	
1	Continued pain disproportionate to any inciting event
2	At least one symptom in three (clinical diagnostic criteria) or four (research diagnostic criteria) of the following: Sensory: hyperesthesia or allodynia Vasomotor: temperature asymmetry, skin color changes, or skin color asymmetry Sudomotor or edema: edema, changes or asymmetry in sweating Motor or trophic: decreased range of motion, motor dysfunction (weakness, tremor, or dystonia), or trophic changes (hair, nails, skin)
3	One sign at time of diagnosis in two or more categories: Sensory: hyperalgesia (to pinprick) or allodynia (to light touch), deep somatic pressure, or joint movement. Vasomotor: temperature asymmetry, skin color change or asymmetry Sudomotor or edema: edema, changes or asymmetry in sweating Motor or trophic: decreased range of motion or motor dysfunction (weakness, tremor, or dystonia), or trophic changes (hair, nails, or skin)
4	No other diagnosis better explains the signs and symptoms

TABLE 10.6

Bonica Stages of Reflex Sympathetic Dystrophy

STAGE	ONSET	SYMPTOMS	DURATION
Stage 1 dysfunction	1-3 months	Burning pain beyond dermatomes (follows thermatomes) Spasm and tendency for immobilization	2-8 weeks
Stage 2 dystrophy	3-7 months	Vasoconstriction Unilateral cold extremity Hair loss Tendency for weakness, tremor, and spasticity (flexed arm, extended legs)	2-4 months
Stage 3 atrophy	>7 months	Smooth glossy edematous skin Pale or cyanotic skin Lymphedema Atrophy of distal muscles Spasm, dystonia, tremor	>4 months
Stage 4	Several months to years	Loss of job and spouse in rare advanced severe cases Unnecessary surgery Orthostatic hypotension Hypertension Heart attack Neurodermatitis Angiectasis Depression, death caused by suicide	A few months

can be caused by an interruption of a nerve pathway, which results in abnormal firing of nociceptive mediators and dysfunction in neuromodulation within internuncial, ascending, and descending pathways in the spinal cord. There are differences in opinion as to whether certain psychologic traits predispose patients to CRPS or whether the psychologic factors are a sequela of the injury. In addition, secondary gain issues also must be considered and dealt with because, whether intentional or not, they inadvertently affect recovery.

Sympathetically mediated cases may result in homeostatic dysregulation of the autonomic nervous system, which clinically presents as edema, vasomotor effects, sudomotor dysfunction, temperature change, and color change (warm subtype), frequently occurring in the early phase. The affected area may be erythematous, swollen, and warm to touch with hyperhidrosis. Suspected metabolic and inflammatory mediators further enhance the vicious circle with progressive peripheral, and at times, central sensitization. Visual, emotional, and tactile stimuli may trigger impressive and disconcerting pain behavior. Even focal well-defined neural injuries may result in symptoms that are nondermatomal and nonsclerotomal (maladaptive neuroplasticity) in presentation, challenging one to consider the possibility of additional, more central cortical reprogramming, which is certainly concerning. This can progress to later phases with further alienation of the area and loss of volitional motion and trophic changes.

The extremity may appear pale and cool to touch (cold subtype), with altered skin texture and hair distribution, reduced nail growth, abnormal posturing, contracture, and reduction in bone mass. Although described under the former taxonomy of RSD, Bonica's description of sequential clinical stages still serves as a good reference for surgeons (Table 10.6).

Although certain features of CRPS can be quantified, no laboratory or biochemical testing is diagnostic. Patients exhibiting sympathetic dysregulation may have alterations delineated through autonomic testing, quantitative sudomotor axonal reflex testing, thermography, and asymmetric temperature measurements. The clinician's tactile temperature threshold difference may require upward of 5°F, although actual measurement is much more sensitive. Limb volume comparisons can be performed by submersion testing; however, such testing is frequently not readily available or practical. Reduced bone mass density may be suspected on standard radiographs with reduced bone density and periarticular reabsorption. The most sensitive radiographic study appears to be the triple phase bone scan. Changes seen on MRI have been described with noted muscle edema, interstitial edema, and hyperpermeability; however, it still is not very sensitive or specific.

■ TREATMENT

Although validation studies of treatment modalities for CRPS are still lacking despite the many thousands of patients treated, there is agreement that the best results are obtained with early diagnosis and an active function-oriented program that is multidisciplinary. Validation of a patient's symptoms is important, as is identification of possible secondary gain. Treatment strategies include pharmacologic, procedural, functional exercises, and psychologic evaluation. The treatment regimen is extremely time consuming and requires much patience and a coordination of efforts. Medication support generally includes antiinflammatory medication, analgesics (oral or topical), tricyclic antidepressants, calcitonin, bisphosphonates, selective serotonin reuptake inhibitors, anticonvulsants, and other antidepressants. The use of ketamine infusions in select patients has been proposed.

Interventional options include selective peripheral neural blocks/ablation techniques, trigger point injections, sympathetic blocks (single or indwelling), dorsal column stimulators, intrathecal infusions, and rarely sympathectomies (chemical or surgical). Descriptions of preventive anesthetic approaches for patients undergoing surgery have been limited. Favorable responses in pediatric patients with high-intensity physical therapy regimens alone have been reported. Therapy should be directed not only to all the joints of the involved extremity but also include more generalized movement patterns. Mirror-assisted movement patterns also may be incorporated. Some concern exists about overzealous therapy aggravating the condition; however, movement is paramount. For patients suspected of having sympathetic-mediated pain, a sympathetic blockade may be helpful for information and treatment. Kleinert et al. and Lankford reported favorable results with sequential stellate ganglion blocks combined with physical therapy in patients with CRPS involving the upper extremity. Pain relief and improved motion have been reported in 80% to 93% of patients with CRPS after sequential sympathetic blocks, although one study reported a 19% temporary response, and the patients required surgical sympathectomy. Poplawski, Wiley, and Murray reported 27 patients treated with intravenous regional blocks of lidocaine and corticosteroid followed by standard physical therapy. They found that the most important factor in predicting a favorable outcome was an interval between onset and treatment of less than 6 months.

ETIOLOGY OF PERIPHERAL NERVE INJURIES

Peripheral nerves can be injured by metabolic or collagen diseases; malignancies; endogenous or exogenous toxins; or thermal, chemical, or mechanical trauma. Only injuries caused by mechanical trauma are considered here. Every patient who has injured a limb or limb girdle should be evaluated for possible musculoskeletal, vascular, and peripheral nerve damage (Table 10.7).

Gunshot wounds often are complicated by peripheral nerve injury. Spontaneous recovery is expected in over 50%. The expected time to recovery after gunshot wounds is 3 to 9 months, with high-velocity injuries taking longer than low-velocity injuries to heal. Neurapraxia and axonotmesis occur with equal frequency in gunshot wounds.

TABLE 10.7

Frequency of Specific Nerve Involvement Associated with Long Bone Fractures Based on 300 Cases Reported by Spurling

EXTREMITY	BONE	NERVE	%
Upper, 74%	Humerus	Radial	70
		Median	8
		Ulnar	22
	Radius and/or ulna	Radial	35
		Median	24
		Ulnar	41
Lower, 20%	Femur	Complete sciatic	60
		Tibial component	20
		Peroneal component	20
	Tibia and/or fibula	Tibial	7
		Peroneal	70
		Both nerves	23

Bone or joint injury is often associated with peripheral nerve lesions. Primary injury of a peripheral nerve may result from the same trauma that injures a bone or joint; however, sometimes the neural injury is caused by displaced osseous fragments, by stretching, or by manipulation, rather than by the initial injuring force. Secondary injury results from involvement of the nerve by infection, scar, callus, or vascular complications. These complications include hematoma, arteriovenous fistula, ischemia, or aneurysm.

The radial nerve is most commonly injured. Of humeral shaft fractures, 14% are said to be complicated by injury of this nerve. Of radial nerve injuries, 33% are associated with fracture of the middle third of the humerus; 50%, with fracture of the distal third of the humerus; 7%, with supracondylar fracture of the humerus; and 7%, with dislocation of the radial head.

The ulnar nerve is injured in about 30% of patients with combined skeletal and neural injury involving the upper extremity. This injury is most commonly associated with fractures around the medial humeral epicondyle, but often it results from the formation of callus around the elbow.

The median nerve is injured in only about 15% of combined skeletal and neural injuries of the upper extremity. It is injured most commonly in dislocation of the elbow or secondarily in the carpal tunnel after injury of the wrist or distal forearm.

Axillary nerve stretch injuries occur in approximately 5% of shoulder dislocations. The peroneal nerve is injured most commonly at the fibular neck in fracture of the tibia and fibula or dislocation of the knee.

Branches of the lumbosacral plexus are injured in less than 3% of pelvic fractures; this plexus is reportedly injured in 10% to 13% of posterior dislocations of the hip. The tibial nerve may be injured in fractures of the proximal tibia and injuries around the ankle.

Peripheral nerve injuries should be carefully excluded in every patient with an acute extremity injury. Equal diligence should be applied in evaluation after surgery, manipulation, casting, and recovery from skeletal injury to detect secondary neural injury.

CLINICAL DIAGNOSIS OF NERVE INJURIES

Immediately after a severe injury to an extremity, recognition of a peripheral nerve injury is not always easy. Pain is often so severe that patient cooperation is limited at best. The preservation of life and limb is always the first objective. When possible, however, some simple tests should be conducted to detect injuries of major nerves of the extremity. In the upper extremity, loss of pain perception in the tip of the little finger indicates ulnar nerve injury. Loss of pain perception in the tip of the index finger indicates median nerve injury, and inability to extend the thumb in the hitchhiker's sign usually indicates radial nerve injury, although the extensor tendons may be severed and render this test invalid. Similarly, in the lower extremity, loss of pain perception in the sole of the foot usually indicates sciatic or tibial nerve injury, whereas inability to extend the great toe or the foot indicates peroneal or sciatic nerve injury. As with the radial nerve, injury to the tendons or muscle bellies may render these tests useless. They may be carried out quickly, however, and usually serve as effective screening procedures.

In evaluating peripheral nerve lesions, a precise knowledge of the course of the nerve, of the level of origin of its motor branches, and of the muscles that these branches supply is essential. Knowledge of common anatomic variations in nerve supply is extremely helpful. One must be familiar with the various zones of sensation and with the areas in which sweating may be diminished or absent and in which skin resistance may be increased. Evaluation of motor loss is crucial. This evaluation can be accurate only if one can palpate or see the tendon or muscle belly under consideration. If one relies on analysis of movement alone as an indication of intact nerve supply, errors can be made because of substitution and trick movement. Opposition of the thumb to the little finger can be accomplished by many patients even though the nerve supply to the opponens pollicis is completely severed and the muscle is paralyzed. In addition, the wrist can be partially extended, even when the muscles supplied by the radial nerve are completely paralyzed, by simple flexion of the fingers, and the elbow can be forcefully flexed, even when the musculocutaneous nerve is completely severed and the biceps paralyzed, by substitution of the brachioradialis. Palpation of the opponens pollicis, extensor tendons of the wrist, and biceps tendon or muscle prevents such deceptions. Some muscles cannot be tested by palpation or sight; these include the lumbricals, the short adductor of the thumb, and the interossei except for the first dorsal. There are enough muscles supplied by each nerve that can be so tested as to allow an accurate diagnosis in most instances. The muscles that can be examined accurately and easily are enumerated in the discussion of each nerve. A clinical assessment of the strength of the muscles is helpful. A scale recommended by Highet has been widely accepted. According to that scale, the following designations are assigned: 0 for total paralysis, 1 for muscle flicker, 2 for muscle contraction, 3 for muscle contraction against gravity, 4 for muscle contraction against gravity and resistance, and 5 for normal muscle contraction compared with the opposite side.

DIAGNOSTIC TESTS
■ IMAGING

Although a well-performed physical examination by an experienced examiner can usually provide sufficient information to accurately diagnose the presence or absence of a major nerve injury, further diagnostic studies are occasionally helpful, particularly in closed injuries in which the physical integrity of the nerve is in question. High-resolution ultrasound and MRI can accurately assess the physical integrity of the nerve immediately after injury and provide valuable information for surgical decision making. Intraneural and perineural injuries also can be identified with both of these techniques.

■ ELECTRODIAGNOSTIC STUDIES

The best and most accessible correlative electrophysiologic confirmations of a peripheral neural injury are nerve conduction and electromyographic mapping assessments. The surgeon must have specific objectives when ordering these tests to obtain the most useful information for clinical management. The timeline in ordering the studies is also important because the changes after injury and recovery follow a well-described pattern. The presence, location, severity, and possibly the prognosis of the neural insult can be determined from these studies, and information regarding the recovery pattern can be obtained when the study is done sequentially over

time. Alternative electrophysiologic uses include dynamic electromyographic assessment when considering optimal muscle transfer strategies, before tenotomy, or botulinum toxin injections in central and peripheral neuropathic conditions. Electrical stimulation can be used for optimal nerve localization when considering blocks or ablation procedures. Generally, both nerve conduction velocity studies and EMG are ordered for routine neural injury assessments because the information gained is complementary. Although full neuropathic changes are not observed in these studies for 2 or 3 weeks after injury, there may be instances in which early baseline studies should be done.

■ NERVE CONDUCTION VELOCITY

Standard nerve conduction techniques include orthodromic motor and antidromic-orthodromic sensory studies and retrograde studies (e.g., F wave study). F wave studies are especially useful for investigating peripheral nerve injuries that are more proximal and less accessible through other techniques. The suspected location of neural compromise is identified, and a protocol to electrically stimulate proximally, distally, and across the segment is formulated. Depending on whether it is an orthodromic or antidromic study, the evoked potential will be recorded at some defined point proximal and distal to the injury with a surface or needle electrode (Fig. 10.9, *Segment A*).

After a severe traumatic neural insult and Wallerian degeneration, there is a progressive structural degradation and neurotransmitter compromise expressed by alteration in nerve conduction and evoked motor and sensory configuration. Immediately after injury, conduction proximal and distal to the insult usually elicits a normal response, although stimulation across the injured segment may vary, depending on the presence of axonal or myelin injury. As Wallerian degeneration ensues (within 5 to 10 days), there is a progressive reduction in the amplitude and alteration in the configuration of the evoked potentials (Fig. 10.9, *Segment B*). If the insult produces only a temporary physiologic block (e.g., neurapraxia), conductivity distal to the lesion remains preserved even after 10 days and a more favorable prognosis can be expected. Evoked sensory amplitude assessments and comparisons also can assist in delineating further pathology.

With a more severe injury, not only is a conduction block across the segment present but a progressive decline in amplitude is noted in evoked potentials when stimulating distal to the injury; sometimes there is complete absence of a response (e.g., axonotmesis). Eventually, electromyographic changes evolve. Over a period of months, repeat studies may be performed to follow neural recovery patterns depending on the case.

■ ELECTROMYOGRAPHY

Manual muscle testing is routine with any musculoskeletal examination, but it is not sensitive for picking up more subtle neuropathic pathology. Myotomal sampling of the involved extremity with needle pick-up electrodes (e.g., monopolar, concentric, and single fiber) yields information regarding neuropathic injury and pathology. It can distinguish a recent injury from a chronic condition that predated the injury (e.g., workers' compensation or litigation). The basic monopolar needle electrode samples approximately eight muscle fibers, and by assessing different sites, fair representation of specifically innervated myotomal groups is possible. The muscle

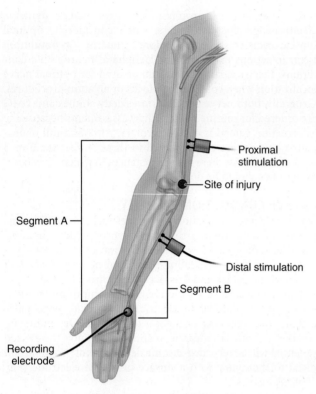

Injury pattern	Proximal stimulation (Segment A)	Immediately after injury distal stimulation (Segment B)	Ten days after injury distal stimulation (Segment B)
Neuropraxia	No response		
Axonotmesis or Neurotmesis	No response		No response

FIGURE 10.9 Neural injury pattern.

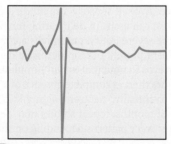

FIGURE 10.10 Diagram of electromyography tracing depicting normal insertion activity, which also may be present immediately after denervation.

initially is observed at rest (insertional activity, approximately 200 ms) and subsequently during volitional muscle recruitment. During the initial postinjury phase, needle sampling should be normal unless there has been a prior injury (Fig. 10.10). Recruitment at this point may vary depending on injury pattern and effort. At 10 to 14 days after neural injury, abnormal spontaneous rest potentials evolve (positive sharp waves) appearing in denervated myotomes where axonal

Positive sharp waves

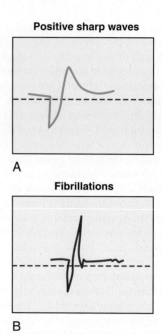

A

Fibrillations

B

FIGURE 10.11 **A,** Diagram of electromyography (EMG) tracing showing positive sharp wave consistent with denervation 10 to 14 days after injury. Rhythm is regular, amplitude is 100 to 400 μV, duration is 5 to 150 ms, and rate is 2 to 40 Hz. **B,** Diagram of EMG tracing showing spontaneous denervation fibrillation potentials present within 14 to 18 days after injury. Rhythm is regular, amplitude is 50 to 1000 μV, duration is 0.5 to 2 ms, and rate is 2 to 30 Hz.

injury has occurred (Fig. 10.11A). Between 14 and 18 days, fibrillations appear (Fig. 10.11B). Voluntary motor unit potentials, if present, may have attenuated amplitudes reflecting axonal compromise. Abnormal denervation patterns can be correlated with established intraneural topographic reference guides to assist in a clear anatomic mapping of the injury. Abnormal spontaneous rest potentials may last indefinitely until the muscle has become reinnervated or fibrotic.

At approximately 3 months after injury, some peripheral neural sprouting occurs and the motor unit potential amplitude progressively increases; this is preceded at times by polyphasic configuration potentials. Between 2 and 6 months after injury, larger than normal appearing potentials are established and remain so until the reinnervation is completed, at which time the motor unit potential configuration returns to a more normal-appearing pattern. Some surgeons monitor denervated myotomes over months (e.g., 3 months) before exploration, depending on the nature of injury and clinical presentation.

■ TINEL SIGN

The Tinel sign is elicited by gentle percussion by a finger or percussion hammer along the course of an injured nerve. A transient tingling sensation should be felt by the patient in the distribution of the injured nerve rather than at the area percussed, and the sensation should persist for several seconds after stimulation. It should be tested for in a distal-to-proximal direction. A positive Tinel sign is presumptive evidence that regenerating axonal sprouts that have not obtained complete myelinization are progressing along the endoneurial tube. With progressive regeneration, the positive response fades proximally, presumably because of progressive myelinization along the more proximal part of the regenerated segment. Distal progression of the response along the course of the nerve in question can be measured, and some have used the rate of this progression to establish prognosis or suggest the need for exploration. A distally advancing Tinel sign should occur in Sunderland types 2 and 3 nerve injuries. A Sunderland type 1 injury or neurapraxia should not show an advancing Tinel sign because Wallerian degeneration and axonal regeneration do not occur. A Sunderland type 4 or type 5 injury would not show an advancing Tinel sign unless repaired. The presence of such a sign alone with its progressive distal migration is encouraging. Electrodiagnostic techniques for the evaluation of nerve-evoked potentials and EMG in the office and operating room provide sophisticated means for evaluating the progress of nerve regeneration and for assessing neuromas in continuity. The work of Kline et al. in evaluating whole nerves and the reports of Terzis and of Williams and Terzis in assessing single fasciculi are recommended. A few regenerating sensory fibers can result in a positive Tinel sign; the presence of such a sign cannot be construed as absolute evidence that any motor fibers are regenerating or that significant sensory return is to be expected. Somatosensory evoked studies may be used as an adjunct including intraoperative monitoring for certain procedures (e.g., external fixation for limb lengthening).

■ SWEAT TEST

Sympathetic fibers within a peripheral nerve are resistant to mechanical trauma. The presence of sweating within the autonomous zone of an injured peripheral nerve reassures the examiner to a degree, suggesting that complete interruption of the nerve has not occurred. Preservation of sweating can be determined simply, as pointed out by Kahn, by observing beads of sweat through the +20 lens of an ophthalmoscope. The time-honored sweat test (iodine starch test) consists of dusting the extremity with quinizarin powder. Sweating is induced by various means. The powder remains dry and light gray throughout the denervated area and assumes a deep purple color throughout the area of normal sweating. The ninhydrin print test as recommended by Aschan and Moberg is another method of assessing sweat patterns in the hand.

■ SKIN RESISTANCE TEST

The skin resistance test is another method of evaluating autonomic interruption; in it a Richter dermometer is used. The autonomous zone with absence of sweating shows an increased resistance to the passage of electrical current. The adjacent innervated areas have a normal resistance, and further decreased resistance in these areas can be elicited by high external temperatures that do not affect the denervated area. The area outlined by the Richter dermometer roughly approximates the autonomous zone of the nerve in question.

■ ELECTRICAL STIMULATION

Electrical stimulation through the intact skin has been used in one form or another by many investigators and clinicians for a long time. Faradic stimulation is often of little value because normally innervated muscles may fail to respond to this current. Additionally, if response to faradic stimulation is still present after 3 weeks, the muscles in most instances are capable of voluntary contraction, and no additional information is obtained by the study. Galvanic stimulation is useful in determining chronaxy and the strength-duration curve. These determinations frequently give early evidence of denervation after nerve injury and are useful in following the evolution of reinnervation, which is less readily assessed by other methods.

GENERAL CONSIDERATIONS OF TREATMENT OF NERVE INJURIES

As in any other injury, initial management of a patient with peripheral nerve damage should begin with careful assessment of the vital functions. When indicated, appropriate actions to prevent cardiopulmonary failure and shock should be taken and systemic antibiotics and tetanus prophylaxis should be provided. When the extent of any injury to the major viscera has been determined, and appropriate resuscitative measures have been started, the injury to the peripheral nerve should be evaluated and the specific nerve deficit should be assessed carefully.

An open wound in which a peripheral nerve has been injured should be cleansed and debrided thoroughly of any foreign material and necrotic tissue, using local, regional, or general anesthesia. If the wound is clean and sharply incised, if the condition of the patient is satisfactory, and if a repair can be done in a quiet and unhurried setting with adequate personnel and equipment, immediate primary repair of the nerve is preferred. If the general medical condition of the patient does not permit adequate repair or if circumstances otherwise cause an undue delay, we prefer to perform the neurorrhaphy during the first 3 to 7 days after injury; in this instance, the wound is sutured, dressed sterilely, and observed for evidence of sepsis.

When open wounds are caused by blasting, abrading, or crushing agents, and when contamination with foreign material is severe, the wound is cleansed and debrided thoroughly, and a sterile dressing is applied. If the ends of the nerve can be identified, they are marked with sutures, such as Prolene or stainless steel, which can be easily identified later. In the absence of a significant nerve gap, loose end-to-end apposition prevents retraction of the nerve segments and makes later repair easier. In the presence of a segmental gap in the nerve, suturing the ends to the soft tissues prevents their retraction. Soft-tissue coverage of the wound consistent with the management of the injured part is carried out, and the nerve is repaired at a later date when the soft tissues have healed and the extent of neuroma formation is evident, usually 3 to 6 weeks after injury.

A closed injury in which a peripheral nerve has been damaged requires careful assessment of residual function and documentation of discrete deficits. After the initial pain has subsided and the wound has healed, early active motion of all joints of the involved extremity should be started. When necessary, gentle passive exercises that avoid disrupting nerves and tendons may be instituted. All joints of the extremity must be kept supple, and soft-tissue contractures must be avoided. Exercises help keep the soft tissues of the extremity in a better physiologic state so that when the nerve has regenerated, rehabilitation is easier. The specific effects of electrical stimulation of muscles are unclear. Regardless of the details of the treatment program, the patient must become actively involved in it to prevent contractures and to strengthen muscles with intact innervation. Similarly, an extremity with a peripheral nerve injury should not be immobilized indefinitely. Dynamic and static splinting to support joints and to prevent contractures should be used intermittently.

When closed fractures are complicated by peripheral nerve deficits, awaiting reinnervation seems reasonable, and early surgical exploration usually is avoided. Early ultrasound imaging of the involved nerve can determine the extent of injury. The progress of return of function in the injured extremity is evaluated with periodic EMG, nerve conduction velocity studies, and frequent clinical evaluation. Conversely, if the nerve deficit follows manipulation or casting of a closed fracture in the absence of a prior nerve deficit, early exploration of the nerve is favored.

FACTORS THAT INFLUENCE REGENERATION AFTER NEURORRHAPHY

Few worthwhile reports have been published on the results of neurorrhaphy and the factors that influence them, first, because few investigators have had access to a large enough group of patients to make evaluations statistically significant and, second, because reports have only rarely been based on sound criteria of regeneration. Valuable reports have been compiled from studies of such injuries incurred in World War II and later conflicts. As a result of these studies, the influence of many factors on regeneration after nerve suture is now better understood.

Rarely should a fracture interfere with nerve repair. In the usual situation, a nerve may be explored if the fracture requires open reduction. In many open injuries the nature of the wound may be such that early repair of the nerve cannot be done satisfactorily. Every effort should be made by repeated debridement of necrotic material to promote rapid healing of any open wounds without sepsis. Nerves may be repaired successfully during a second debridement, followed by closure and healing. Associated vascular injury can adversely affect nerve regeneration because of tissue ischemia.

Several important factors that seem to influence nerve regeneration are (1) the age of the patient, (2) the gap between the nerve ends, (3) the delay between the time of injury and repair, (4) the level of injury, (5) the condition of the nerve ends, and (6) the experience and techniques of the surgeon. The first five of these factors are discussed here.

AGE

Age undoubtedly influences the rate and degree of nerve regeneration. All other factors being equal, neurorrhaphies are more successful in children than in adults and are more likely to fail in elderly patients; why this is true has not been completely explained, but it may relate to the potential for central adaptation to the peripheral nerve injury. We do not know precisely what results can be expected in either of the extremes of age because practically all significant studies have dealt with military personnel whose average age was 18 to 30 years. A close correlation has been noted between age and two-point discrimination obtained after median and ulnar nerve repairs (30 mm at 20 to 40 years; 15 mm at 11 to 20 years; 10 mm at <10 years). After digital nerve repair, however, the final two-point discrimination was not as closely related to age. Another study found that a higher percentage of patients younger than 20 years at the time of repair had

two-point discrimination of less than 6 mm than did patients older than 20 years.

GAP BETWEEN NERVE ENDS

The nature of the injury is the most important factor in determining the defect remaining between the nerve ends after any neuromas and gliomas are resected. When a sharp instrument, such as a razor or knife, severs a nerve, damage is slight proximally and distally, and although the nerve ends inevitably do retract, the gap can usually be easily overcome. Conversely, when a high-velocity missile severs a nerve, proximal and distal nerve damage is extensive. Ultimately, both ends must be widely resected to expose normal funiculi, producing a larger gap. The gap is increased farther if part of the nerve is carried away by a missile, as in shrapnel injuries. Methods of closing troublesome gaps include (1) nerve mobilization, (2) nerve transposition, (3) joint flexion, (4) nerve grafts, and (5) bone shortening. The greater the defect, the more dissimilar the funicular pattern of the two ends because of the constantly changing arrangement of fibers within the nerve as it progresses distally. This is particularly important in the more proximal portion of peripheral nerves. Agreement is widespread that excessive tension on a neurorrhaphy harms nerve regeneration. Nerve grafting is advised if, after the nerve is mobilized, the gap cannot be closed by flexing the main joint of the limb 90 degrees. The observed upper limit of a gap beyond which results deteriorate is approximately 2.5 cm. The observations of Kirklin, Murphey, and Berkson in 1949 that recovery is slightly better when the gap is relatively small remain valid.

DELAY BETWEEN TIME OF INJURY AND REPAIR

Delay of neurorrhaphy affects motor recovery more profoundly than sensory recovery, most likely because of the survival time of denervated striated muscle. There is significant loss of motor endplates and increased muscle fibrosis by 18 months after denervation; therefore nerve repair needs to be performed early enough to allow reinnervation of muscle before this occurs. Experimental studies have shown better axonal survival with early nerve repair.

As a rule of thumb, Omer suggested that about 1% of recoverable nerve function is lost for each week of delay after 3 weeks postinjury. The influence of delay on sensory return is unclear; in the Veterans Administration study, little influence could be found and useful sensation returned in a few patients when suture was performed 2 years after injury. The critical limit of delay beyond which sensation does not return is unknown.

Our practice is to perform neurorrhaphies in clean, sharp wounds immediately or during the first 3 to 7 days. In the presence of extensive soft-tissue contusion, laceration, crushing, or contamination in which the proximal and distal extent of the nerve injury is impossible to delineate, a delay of 3 to 6 weeks is preferred.

LEVEL OF INJURY

The more proximal the injury, the more incomplete the overall return of motor and sensory function, especially in the more distal structures. Conditions are more favorable for recovery in the more proximal muscles because (1) the neurons that innervate the distal portions of the limb are more severely affected by retrograde changes after proximal injury,

(2) a greater proportion of the cross-sectional area of the nerve trunk is occupied by fibers to the proximal muscles, and (3) the potential for disorientation of regrowing axons and for axon loss during regeneration is greater for the distal muscles than for the muscles more proximally situated after a proximal injury. Except for parts of the brachial plexus, useful function at times returns regardless of the level of injury if the critical limit of delay has not passed.

CONDITION OF NERVE ENDS

The condition of the nerve ends at the time of neurorrhaphy is important. Meticulous handling of the nerve ends, asepsis, care with nerve mobilization, preservation of neural blood supply, avoidance of tension, and provision of a suitable bed with minimal scar all exert favorable influences on nerve regeneration. Distal stump shrinkage has been found to be maximal at about 4 months, leaving the distal fascicular cross-sectional area diminished to 30% to 40% of normal size. Intraneural plexus formation and fascicular dispersal make accurate fascicular alignment and appropriate axonal regeneration more difficult. A neurorrhaphy with a satisfactory external appearance is no guarantee of optimal internal fascicular alignment. Fascicular malalignment is a common finding. It is generally agreed that the nerve ends should be prepared in such a way that a satisfactory fascicular pattern is apparent in the proximal and distal stumps. No scar, foreign material, or necrotic tissue should be allowed to remain around the ends to interfere with axonal regeneration. Sometimes resection of the nerve ends so that satisfactory fasciculi are exposed leaves a gap that cannot be closed by end-to-end repair. As noted previously, clinical and experimental evidence indicates that excessive tension on the neurorrhaphy at the time of repair and when an acutely flexed limb is mobilized later causes excessive intraneural fibrosis. These findings and the promising results achieved after the interfascicular nerve grafting technique advocated by Millesi and by Millesi, Meissl, and Berger suggest that such a technique is preferable to repair of nerves under too much tension or with limbs in acutely flexed or awkward positions.

GENERAL CONSIDERATIONS FOR SURGERY

INDICATIONS

In the presence of a traumatic peripheral nerve deficit, exploration of the nerve is indicated as follows:

1. When a sharp injury has obviously divided a nerve, early exploration is indicated for diagnostic, therapeutic, and prognostic purposes. Neurorrhaphy can be done at the time of exploration or can be delayed.
2. When abrading, avulsing, or blasting wounds have rendered the condition of the nerve unknown, exploration is required for identification of the nerve injury and for marking the ends of the nerve with sutures for later repair.
3. When a nerve deficit follows blunt or closed trauma and no clinical or electrical evidence of regeneration has occurred after an appropriate time, exploration of the nerve is indicated. This also is true when a nerve deficit complicates a closed fracture. In this instance, it has been our practice to observe the patient for evidence of nerve regeneration for an appropriate time, depending on the nerve and its level of muscle innervation. Then if regeneration has not

occurred, we favor exploration. In situations in which a nerve has been intact before closed reduction and casting of a fracture, but a significant deficit is found immediately after, we explore the nerve as soon as feasible.
4. When a nerve deficit follows a penetrating wound, such as that caused by a low-velocity gunshot, the part is observed for evidence of nerve regeneration for an appropriate time. If there is no evidence of regeneration, exploration is indicated.

Conversely, delay in exploration of a nerve injury is indicated if progressive regeneration is evidenced by improvement in sensation, motor power, and electrodiagnostic tests and by progression of the Tinel sign.

TIME OF SURGERY

It has been the time-honored policy to advise primary suture when possible. This recommendation is logical when one considers what happens to the distal end of the nerve, motor endplates, sensory nerve ends, muscles, joints, and other tissues of the denervated extremity. The controversy concerning whether primary or secondary nerve repair is better is unresolved. Primary repair done in the first 6 to 8 hours or delayed primary repair done in the first 7 to 18 days is appropriate when the injury is caused by a sharp object, the wound is clean, and there are no other major complicating injuries. Ideally, such repairs should be performed by an experienced surgeon in an institution where adequate equipment and personnel are available. The development of magnification devices, new instruments, and new techniques and the modification of a variety of small instruments for use in nerve surgery have improved the technique of early repair. Primary repair should shorten the time of denervation of the end organs, and fascicular alignment should be improved because minimal excision of the nerve ends is required. Regarding war wounds, however, primary sutures have compared unfavorably with early secondary suture.

When the diagnosis of division of a peripheral nerve has been made, if conditions are suitable and repair is indicated, one should not delay repair in anticipation of spontaneous regeneration. Only if the patient's life or limb is seriously endangered should the operation be long postponed. A fracture is not a contraindication for operation. Operation before the fracture becomes united may be advantageous for two reasons: (1) if bone shortening is necessary, resection of an ununited or partially united fracture is a much less formidable procedure than resection of a fully united bone; and (2) restriction of joint motion is minimal if the nerve is repaired soon after the injury; later, motion would be more limited, perhaps so severely as to prevent flexing the joint enough to overcome a gap between the nerve ends.

INSTRUMENTS AND EQUIPMENT

A nerve stimulator should be available for all peripheral nerve procedures; many satisfactory permanent and disposable ones are available commercially. A stimulator is indispensable in investigating partially severed nerves and neuromas in continuity and in locating and preserving nerve branches given off proximal to or at the lesion that are still functioning but are encased in scar tissue. Intraoperative recording of somatosensory evoked potentials and nerve action potentials is useful in surgical planning and assessing nerve lesions. These techniques require sensitive and sophisticated recording and monitoring equipment and trained technicians. (For details of these monitoring techniques, the reader is referred to the references at the end of this chapter.)

Despite the technical difficulties involved in these methods, we have found intraoperative recording to be helpful when evaluating partial nerve lesions and neuromas in continuity. Instruments for handling and dissecting delicate tissues always are essential. Nerve surgery in the extremities also is made easier by the use of a pneumatic tourniquet, suction apparatus, and bipolar electrocautery. Gelfoam and thrombin are useful for controlling the bleeding from the cut ends of nerves. For suture material, we prefer 8-0, 9-0, and 10-0 monofilament nylon. The tensile strength, easy handling qualities, and minimal tissue reaction of nylon make it the most desirable suture material now available for neurorrhaphy. In our experience, most epineurial repairs are best done with 8-0 or 9-0 nylon. For perineurial or epiperineurial repair, 9-0 or 10-0 monofilament nylon is preferable.

ANESTHESIA

Peripheral nerve operations can be done with the patient under general, regional, or local anesthesia for the upper extremities or general, spinal, or local anesthesia for the lower extremities. Local anesthesia has the advantage of allowing evaluation of the passage of sensory impulses through the injured nerve. If evaluation is to be accurate, however, little if any anesthetic agent should be injected around the nerve, and, consequently, the procedure is painful. There is always the possibility that the agent would infiltrate the tissues around the nerve and interfere with motor response to stimulation. As a rule, we prefer general anesthesia for surgery in the upper extremities and neck and general or spinal anesthesia for surgery in the lower extremities.

PREPARATION AND DRAPING

Before preparing and draping, the correct side and site are identified and the site is marked with an indelible surgical marking pen. Because the exact length of an incision can rarely be predicted, it is mandatory that the entire extremity and its environs be prepared. For an operation on the upper extremity, the axilla, shoulder, neck, and chest should be included in the field of preparation; for an operation on the lower extremity, the buttock and the area up to the iliac crest posteriorly should be included. In operative procedures involving the distal portions of nerves only, such as below the elbow or knee, a well-padded pneumatic tourniquet placed above the elbow or knee is used, limiting the sterile field. A sterile tourniquet also can be helpful for more proximal lesions.

After preparation of the entire field, the proposed incision is marked on the extremity and is crosshatched with washable ink before any of the landmarks are covered. It is a good policy to mark the incision along the course of the nerve in the entire prepared area. The extremity is encased in a sterile stockinette so that it can be moved freely over the sterile drapes. If it is desirable to watch the movement of the muscles in the hand when the nerve is stimulated, the hand can be left exposed and bare.

TECHNIQUE OF NERVE REPAIR

In no type of surgery is the incision more important. Every incision should extend well proximal and distal to the lesion and when possible should follow the course of the nerve. An incision should never cross the flexor creases of the skin at a right angle. Short incisions are probably the cause of more futile nerve operations than any other factor except surgeon inexperience. One should never hesitate to extend an incision a great distance—even from the axilla to the wrist to overcome a large defect in the ulnar or median nerve.

It is essential that the injured nerve be exposed first proximal to and then distal to the lesion before approaching the site of injury. Dissection and exposure are made simpler, and there is less chance of damaging the nerve and any branches remaining in the scar. If one is confronted with a neuroma in continuity, the nerve should be stimulated proximal and distal to the lesion and the response recorded. When a nerve is dissected from scar tissue, it should be stimulated repeatedly to locate any branches that still might be functioning. Before the nerve is mobilized completely, sutures are placed in the epineurium proximal to and distal to the lesion for orientation so that if neurorrhaphy is necessary the ends can be joined without rotation. Also, inspection of the external surface of the nerve may allow alignment of the longitudinal epineurial vessels; this, too, can aid in appropriate rotation of the nerve ends.

Handling of the nerve during mobilization is made easier by the use of vessel loops. Any part of the nerve not being operated on at the moment should be covered with moist sponges.

If the nerve has not been completely severed, or if a neuroma in continuity is present, it can be difficult to decide whether neurolysis, partial neurorrhaphy, or complete neurorrhaphy would be best. The surgeon may need to call on all of the experience at his or her command to arrive at the wisest decision. Stimulation proximal to the injury for motor response distal to it is essential. If local anesthesia is used, stimulation distal to the lesion may give an idea of whether a significant number of sensory fibers have escaped injury or have regenerated, but sensory response is far less reliable than motor response. If a pneumatic tourniquet is used, it should be deflated to allow the muscles and nerves to recover from ischemia so that stimulation of the nerve to elicit motor response has more validity. Examination at the site of injury may assist in determining what course to pursue. The neuroma can be injected with saline solution, and if the solution passes up and down the nerve trunk with little difficulty, the neuroma probably should be left alone. This can be misleading, however, and unless both motor and sensory responses to stimulation are good, endoneurial exploration is advisable.

ENDONEUROLYSIS (INTERNAL NEUROLYSIS)

When an endoneurial exploration is undertaken, it should be borne in mind that neurolysis or partial or complete neurorrhaphy may be necessary, and one should preserve intact as much of the epineurium and normal nerve as possible. The epineurium is incised longitudinally proximal to the lesion, beginning not more than 0.5 cm from the level of gross changes in the nerve as determined by palpation. The incision is not extended more proximal to this point unless necessary because the epineurium may become frayed; and if neurorrhaphy becomes necessary, more of the nerve may have to be sacrificed. For the same reason, the distal end of the incision is limited. The flaps of epineurium on each side may be retracted laterally by nylon sutures and are undermined widely. The funiculi are separated if possible with a pointed or diamond-bladed knife, using sharp or blunt dissection as necessary. Spring-loaded microscissors also are helpful in this dissection. The surgeon constantly should be aware of the possibility of plexus formation between fascicles and protect these. Distinguishing between intraneural fibrosis and plexus formation is extremely difficult. If most of the fasciculi are intact and can be separated and traced through the neuroma, nothing further should be done. If stimulation fails to elicit a response, and few if any intact fasciculi can be found, resection of the neuroma and neurorrhaphy are probably indicated. Use of magnifying loupes or the operating microscope is essential when performing intraneural dissection to avoid injury to intact nerve tissue.

PARTIAL NEURORRHAPHY

Partial severance of the larger nerves, such as the sciatic nerve and the cords and trunks of the brachial plexus, is common. In such an injury, partial neurorrhaphy is best. It is occasionally necessary and justifiable in smaller nerves but is never quite as satisfactory technically as is complete neurorrhaphy. The decision to perform partial neurorrhaphy is likewise often difficult. The decision should be made only after the most careful investigation of the lesion. If one half of the nerve, especially a large one, is disrupted, partial neurorrhaphy is advisable. If the motor response to stimulation is good, however, it would be unwise in some nerves, such as the peroneal or ulnar, to risk injury of good motor funiculi in an attempt to restore sensation to a small area on the dorsum of the foot or to the little finger. If most of the fascicles in smaller nerves are severed, and if stimulation cannot show important function in the few that remain, complete neurorrhaphy probably is better. Suture of a few fascicles usually is impractical.

When the decision has been made to perform partial neurorrhaphy (Fig. 10.12), the incision is extended longitudinally

in the epineurium proximally and distally several centimeters, as necessary. The intact funiculi are dissected out for the same distance. The ends of the injured part of the nerve are resected to normal tissue. At the cut ends, an end-to-end neurorrhaphy is performed. If the epineurium is inadequate for placement of epineurial sutures, epiperineurial or perineurial (fascicular) sutures suffice. The proximal and distal dissection should be extensive enough to prevent kinking of the loop of intact nerve.

NEURORRHAPHY AND NERVE GRAFTING

When a nerve has been completely severed, and when conditions as already outlined are appropriate, neurorrhaphy after sufficient resection of the proximal and distal ends of the nerve is indicated. Sometimes a considerable gap or defect (actual loss of nerve tissue) remains after excision of any glioma and neuroma, and selecting a method for overcoming the gap is difficult. Extension of the incision proximally and distally can be helpful in permitting adequate dissection for closure of the gap. In general, direct neurorrhaphy may be possible with fairly large gaps in the median and ulnar nerves near the wrist and elbow after mobilization of proximal and distal segments, whereas gaps of 2 to 3 cm in the brachial plexus and radial, sciatic, and peroneal nerves and the median nerve at the midforearm level may require nerve grafting. Regardless of the technique used, there is general agreement that nerve repair under excessive tension is detrimental to satisfactory regeneration. It generally is recommended that if a single 8-0 nylon epineurial suture can maintain approximation of the nerve ends, excessive tension is not present.

▪ METHODS OF CLOSING GAPS BETWEEN NERVE ENDS

There are several methods of closing gaps between nerve ends without appreciable damage to the nerve itself. The methods most often used are mobilization of the nerve ends and positioning of the extremity. Other methods include nerve transplantation, bone resection, bulb suture, nerve grafting, and nerve crossing (pedicle grafting).

▌ MOBILIZATION

Most small gaps can be closed by mobilizing the nerve ends for a few centimeters proximal and distal to the point of injury. Mobilization of both nerve ends to some degree is required in all peripheral neurorrhaphies. The exact amount of mobilization a peripheral nerve can tolerate before its regenerating potential is compromised is unknown; however, extensive dissection of a nerve from its surrounding tissues does disrupt the segmental blood supply, causing subsequent ischemia and increased intraneural scarring. Mobilization has been shown to be more detrimental to the distal nerve segment. Nicholson and Seddon suggested that extensive mobilization adversely affects recovery after median nerve repairs in the forearm. Only 50% of patients had recovery to the M3 level or better if the gap was more than 2.6 cm and required extensive mobilization. Large gaps require extensive dissection of the nerve from its adjacent tissues for a relatively tension-free epineurial repair. Before subjecting a peripheral nerve to extensive dissection, the surgeon should have some idea of the maximal nerve gap over which mobilization may become a futile endeavor. The nerve gap is determined at the time of surgery with the extremity in the anatomic position

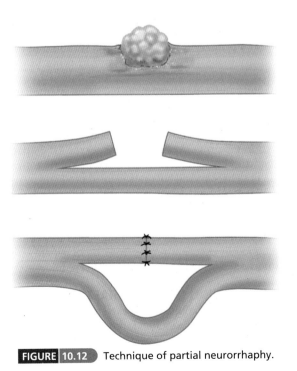

FIGURE 10.12 Technique of partial neurorrhaphy.

TABLE 10.8

Critical Nerve Gap Distances (Values of Grantham)

NERVE	LOCATION	DISTANCE (CM)
UPPER EXTREMITY		
Radial	Midarm	8
Median (not transposed)	Midforearm	4.5-6.5
Ulnar (not transposed)	Midforearm	3.2-5
Posterior interosseous	Forearm	1
LOWER EXTREMITY		
Sciatic	Midthigh	6-9
Tibial	Knee	4.5-9
Peroneal	Knee	6.4-8.1

From Spinner M: Current concepts of nerve suture, *Instr Course Lect* 33:487, 1984.

and after distal and proximal neuroma excision. Guidelines are extremely variable in the literature (2.5 to 9.0 cm, depending on the location; Table 10.8).

When mobilizing a peripheral nerve, care should be taken to avoid excessive stripping of the small vessels to the nerve. Motor and essential sensory branches should be carefully protected. Gaps distal to the motor branches of a peripheral nerve are closed more easily with mobilization. The branch of the radial nerve to the brachioradialis muscle commonly prevents closure of a gap proximal to the point where this branch emerges from the nerve, but if the biceps brachii is functioning, this branch can be sacrificed without much loss of function. Excessive tension must be avoided at all times.

▌POSITIONING OF EXTREMITY

Relaxing nerves by flexing various joints and occasionally by other maneuvers, such as abducting, adducting, rotating, and elevating the extremity, is as important as mobilization in closing large gaps in nerves. Through use of both methods, long gaps can be closed in nearly all of the peripheral nerves, and many unsatisfactory neurorrhaphies result from failure to make the most of their possibilities. When joints that are excessively flexed or awkwardly positioned are mobilized later, tension on the neurorrhaphy may be too great and may cause intraneural fibrosis that compromises axonal regeneration. Consequently, a joint should never be flexed forcibly to obtain end-to-end suture. It is a reasonable policy to flex the knee and elbow no more than 90 degrees. Also, flexion of the wrist more than 40 degrees is probably unwise. After the wound has healed sufficiently, the joint can be extended about 10 degrees per week until motion is regained. Flexing joints is most important in repairing gaps in the long nerves of the extremities. External rotation and abduction are helpful when repairing radial and axillary nerves, as in elevation of the shoulder girdle in brachial plexus injuries. Rarely, extension of a joint can be helpful, as in extension of the hip in sciatic injuries. Strong consideration should be given to nerve grafting in preference to drastic positioning of the extremity to produce a tension-free neurorrhaphy.

▌TRANSPOSITION

The anatomic course of some nerves can be changed to shorten the distance between severed ends. This is true especially of the ulnar nerve at the elbow. The median nerve also can be transposed anterior to the pronator teres if the lesion is distal to its branches to the long flexor muscles of the forearm, and the tibial nerve can be placed superficial to the soleus or gastrocnemius in the leg if the lesion is distal to its branches to the calf muscles. Most surgeons recommend transposition of the proximal end of the radial nerve anterior to the humerus and deep to the biceps to obtain needed length. Considerable length can be gained in most patients by the simpler maneuver of externally rotating the arm, provided that the mobilization has been carried into the axilla and that the branches of the radial nerve to the triceps muscle have been dissected well up the nerve.

▌BONE RESECTION

In civilian injuries, bone resection almost never should be necessary to accomplish neurorrhaphy. Even in war wounds, it was rarely employed, and when it was used, it was usually because the joints of the extremity had become so stiff from immobilization caused by fracture or injudicious use of casts that limited flexion. Intact long bones and most bones in children rarely should be shortened to aid in nerve repair. Bone resection is of particular value in the upper arm for closing large gaps in the ulnar, radial, or median nerves when the humerus already has been fractured. If early delayed suture is done in such patients before the fracture has healed, shortening the bone if necessary is not difficult. After the fracture has healed, however, osteotomy is more difficult. It rarely is worthwhile to shorten the femur in injuries of the sciatic nerve unless this bone already has been fractured; then shortening of the bone can be helpful. Both bones of the forearm or leg in the absence of a fracture should never be shortened.

▌NERVE GRAFTING

Interfascicular nerve grafting as described by Seddon and later by Millesi is indicated when primary nerve repair cannot be done without excessive tension. In general, a nerve gap that is caused simply by elastic retraction usually can be overcome with local nerve mobilization, limited joint positioning, and primary repair. If the defect is caused in part by loss of nerve tissue, however, nerve grafting is our procedure of choice. Autogenous sural nerve is the preferred source of graft. Good results have been reported using an interfascicular nerve autografting technique to close gaps without undue tension in injuries to the digital, medial, ulnar, and radial nerves. In the upper extremity especially, good results were achieved in repairing injuries to these nerves. Of 38 patients with median nerve grafts, 82% achieved useful motor recovery (M3 or better) and all but one regained protective sensibility. Of 39 patients with ulnar nerve grafts, all achieved useful motor recovery (M2+ or better) and 28% regained two-point discrimination. Of 13 patients with radial nerve grafts, 77% achieved an M4 or M5 level of function. Kallio and Vastamäki showed good or excellent results in 47 of 98 patients treated with interfascicular grafting for median nerve injuries.

▌NERVE CROSSING (PEDICLE GRAFTING)

Nerve-crossing operations in the extremities are rarely wise or possible. When a combined median and ulnar lesion is so great that the gap cannot be closed in either nerve in any other way, the ulnar nerve can be sectioned again in the upper arm, creating a segment long enough to bridge the gap between the two ends of the median nerve. The distal end of the median nerve is sutured to the distal end of the free segment of the ulnar nerve to form a U-shaped neurorrhaphy. The vasa nervorum should be left intact. The ulnar nerve is partially transected proximally to allow for sufficient graft length. At a second operation 6 weeks later, the ulnar nerve is completely transected and sutured into the distal segment of the median nerve. This procedure has been advised in situations such as nerve injury caused by massive ischemic necrosis of the forearm, but in light of current knowledge, other nerve grafting techniques seem more appropriate in these situations.

SOURCE OF NERVE FOR INTERFASCICULAR NERVE GRAFTING

Selecting a cutaneous nerve for nerve grafting should be done with great care. The sural nerve is the most commonly used, and in most situations it is recommended. From each leg, 40 cm of graft material can be obtained. The lateral antebrachial cutaneous nerve for digital nerve grafts can be used so that another limb would not be involved in the surgical procedure. Anatomic studies have shown no significant difference in fascicular area, area of the entire nerve bundle, and percentage of the nerve bundle occupied by the actual nerve fascicles. The lateral antebrachial cutaneous nerve is found most easily just lateral to the biceps tendon alongside the cephalic vein. Through a longitudinal incision, 20 cm of graft material can be obtained. The medial antebrachial cutaneous nerve, the terminal articular branch of the posterior interosseous nerve, and the dorsal sensory branch of the ulnar nerve also have been used for digital nerve grafting. The medial antebrachial cutaneous nerve is found adjacent to the basilic vein. The posterior interosseous nerve is located at the wrist just ulnar to the extensor pollicis longus tendon lying on the interosseous membrane. The superficial radial nerve is an excellent source of graft material when used in grafting a high radial nerve laceration because the neurologic deficit that otherwise would be created already exists. It is not recommended as a routine source because its sensory contribution to the hand is significant, especially when the median nerve is deficient.

NERVE ALLOGRAFTS

The use of fresh nerve allograft can potentially allow functional recovery equivalent to autograft; however, it requires systemic immunosuppression. Tacrolimus (Prograf) inhibits activation of T-cell proliferation and is administered starting 3 days preoperatively and continued for 18 months postoperatively. Grafts are selected from ABO blood type–compatible individuals (cadaveric or living related donors) and stored at 4°C in University of Wisconsin solution for 7 days before implantation. Rejection and increased vulnerability to opportunistic infection are potential complications. Acellularized nerve allografts are now available with the advantage of decreased host rejection. These grafts maintain the physical structure of the epineurium, perineurium, and endoneurial tubes, which are rapidly revascularized and repopulated with host cells. They are available in diameters of 1 to 5 mm and in lengths up to 5 cm. A multicenter retrospective study involving 56 patients and 71 nerve repairs demonstrated functional recovery in 86% of procedures, with sensory recovery ranging from S3 to S4 and motor recovery from M3 to M5. The majority of grafts were used in common digital and digital nerves (48 of 71); however, they were also used in median (10 of 71), ulnar (6 of 71), and radial nerves (2 of 71). The mean gap length was 23 ± 12 mm (range, 5 to 50 mm).

Evaluation of outcomes showed recovery in 89% of digital nerves, 75% of median nerves, and 67% of ulnar nerves. Although autograft is superior, acellularized nerve allograft has the advantages of shortened surgical time, avoidance of additional surgical site morbidity, and relatively unlimited supply.

SYNTHETIC NERVE CONDUITS

Synthetic conduits can be used to bridge neural gaps. Various conduit materials have been investigated including silicone, type I collagen, polyglactin, poly-L-lactic acid (PLLA), polyglycolic acid (PGA), and polyvinyl alcohol (PVA) hydrogel. We have had no experience with the use of synthetic conduits, but their use often is considered when there is the possibility of insufficient autogenous nerve graft. Currently, these are recommended for reconstruction of smaller-diameter sensory nerves with defects less than 3 cm.

TECHNIQUES OF NEURORRHAPHY

Fibrin clot, micropore tape, collagen tubulization techniques, adhesives, and many varieties of sutures and suture techniques have been proposed for neurorrhaphy. Neurorrhaphy by suture with nonreactive and nonabsorbable materials, such as stainless steel and monofilament nylon, has the widest application and acceptance. Magnification, appropriate small instruments, and meticulous technique are essential. Experimental evidence is conflicting concerning the relative merits of epineurial and perineurial (fascicular) neurorrhaphy techniques. Clinical evidence to support the use of one technique over the other is meager and inconclusive. The technique selected by the individual surgeon depends on training and experience. Proponents of repair supplementation with autologous fibrin glue, or other commercially available "nerve glues," cite less tendency for gapping at the repair site, fewer sutures required for the repair, and a possible barrier to invading scar tissue as advantages. None has been shown to increase the strength of the repair, and only one has been shown not to block axonal regeneration when interposed between nerve ends. Our preference is epiperineurial repair at the periphery of the nerve combined with perineurial (fascicular) neurorrhaphy for large fascicles within the nerve. Sunderland pointed out that funicular (fascicular) repair cannot be done accurately in every instance because (1) funicular patterns at nerve ends match exactly only after clean transection, (2) the numbers of funiculi at nerve ends may not correspond, and (3) any discrepancies in funiculi within the nerve would require excessive intraneural suture material. He suggested that funicular repair might be practical when (1) funicular groups are large enough to take sutures that maintain funicular apposition, (2) nerve ends show a funicular pattern that would predispose to wasteful regeneration of axons if epineurial repair were done, and (3) each funicular group is composed of nerve fibers to a particular branch occupying a constant position at the nerve ends. The last arrangement can be seen in the median and ulnar nerves at and above the wrist and the radial nerve at and just proximal to the elbow. Sunderland recommended suturing groups of funiculi in such situations.

EPINEURIAL NEURORRHAPHY

TECHNIQUE 10.1

- After exposing and dissecting the ends of the nerves, determine that any remaining gap can be closed by end-to-end repair without excessive tension.
- Resect the glioma and neuroma with a sharp razor blade or a diamond-bladed knife against a sterile wooden tongue depressor in a nerve miter box or with sharp nerve scissors.
- Make serial cuts about 1 mm apart in the end of the nerve until normal-appearing fasciculi are exposed; this is best determined by use of the operating microscope. If doubt remains concerning the amount of any remaining scar in the nerve end, frozen histologic sections of the nerve are helpful. Have permanent histologic sections made for later review to help in determining the prognosis.
- If the distal end contains glioma, or if more than one third of the proximal end consists of neuroma, carry out additional trimming as required.
- Control excessive bleeding with thrombin or Gelfoam.
- If positioning of the extremity is required to relieve tension, use an assistant at this point. Sometimes a traction or sling suture of 7-0 or 8-0 nylon passed through the nerve may be required. Our preference in such a situation is the gentle placement of a straight stainless steel Keith or Bunnell needle transversely through each of the nerve stumps with the nerve ends approximated, transfixing the nerve to the adjacent soft tissues.
- Determine appropriate rotational alignment by observing the orientation of surface vessels and the appearance and location of fasciculi within the nerve. Epineurial orientation sutures placed 1 cm from each cut edge also are helpful.
- Place a piece of plastic or rubber glove material beneath the nerve for visual contrast and less cumbersome handling of sutures. For this repair, 8-0 or 9-0 monofilament nylon usually is sufficient.
- Place the first suture in the posterior or deep surface of the nerve in the epineurium, and leave the suture long to make later rotation of the nerve easier. Place the next three sutures in the remaining three quadrants of the nerve, and leave them long, too.
- Determine as accurately as possible that no kinking or deviation of the fasciculi has occurred, and place sufficient interrupted sutures of 8-0 or 9-0 nylon to produce a satisfactory neurorrhaphy (Fig. 10.13).
- Rotate the nerve with the quadrant sutures to ensure satisfactory posterior surface repair. A 5-0 stainless steel suture can be placed 1 cm from each end of the repair in the epineurium to act as a radiographic marker to detect a rupture. (We rarely use this.)
- Before wound closure, remove the sling suture or steel needles from the nerve ends and place the extremity through a limited range of motion to assess positional tension at the repair site. This helps to determine the extent to which the extremity can be safely mobilized postoperatively.

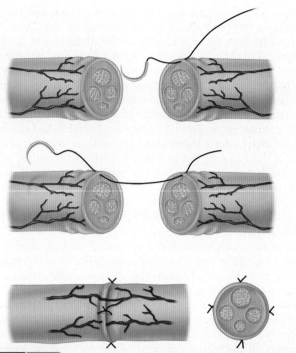

FIGURE 10.13 Epineurial neurorrhaphy (see text). **SEE TECHNIQUE 10.1.**

PERINEURIAL (FASCICULAR) NEURORRHAPHY

TECHNIQUE 10.2

- To perform perineurial (fascicular) neurorrhaphy, the surgeon must be proficient in the use of the operating microscope and must be able to handle the delicate 10-0 suture with ease and speed.
- Expose the nerve injury, and resect the ends of the nerve as described for epineurial neurorrhaphy (see Technique 10.1).
- Place the nerve ends in proper rotation.
- Using magnification, attempt to identify corresponding groups of fasciculi in the proximal and distal nerve stumps. It is helpful at this point to diagram the arrangement of the fascicular groups on sterile paper from glove or suture packages.
- Transfix the nerve ends to the soft tissues with stainless steel straight needles.
- Incise the epineurium longitudinally proximally and distally to expose the fasciculi; approximate them individually with interrupted 9-0 or 10-0 nylon sutures (Fig. 10.14). Where the nerve is composed of multiple small fasciculi, approximate several fasciculi as a group.
- After the fasciculi have been matched and approximated, close the epineurium with interrupted nylon sutures, or if the neurorrhaphy is secure and there is no tension on the repair, omit the epineurial closure to decrease the amount of fibrosis after surgery.

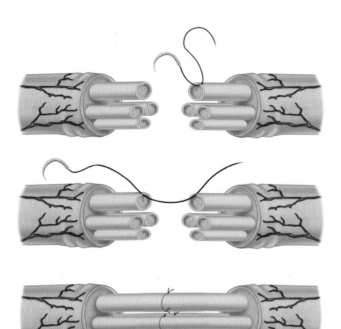

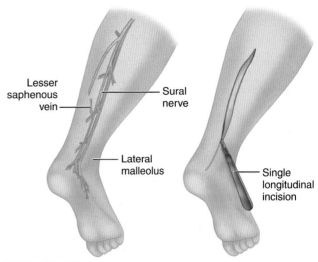

FIGURE 10.15 Sural nerve graft. If long nerve grafts are required, single longitudinal incision is used to minimize traction injury to nerve graft. **SEE TECHNIQUE 10.3.**

FIGURE 10.14 Perineurial (fascicular) neurorrhaphy (see text). **SEE TECHNIQUE 10.2.**

INTERFASCICULAR NERVE GRAFTING

TECHNIQUE 10.3

(MILLESI, MODIFIED)
- Keep the extremity in the extended position so that the graft is not under tension after surgery.
- Expose the nerve as for epineurial neurorrhaphy (see Technique 10.1).
- Beginning in normal-appearing tissue, dissect and expose the proximal and distal stumps.
- Incise the epineurium on the stumps in areas where the nerve appears normal.
- Excise a circumferential cuff of epineurium from each stump.
- Use the operating microscope to carry out intraneural dissection in the normal part of the nerve, working toward the neuroma and glioma in the proximal and distal ends. Attempt to identify large fasciculi and groups of smaller fasciculi.
- Ensure hemostasis by coagulating the smaller vascular branches with bipolar microcoagulating forceps.
- As intraneural fibrosis is encountered, transect each fasciculus or group of fasciculi individually at the level where the fibrosis begins. When this dissection has been completed, the fasciculi and groups should be transected at different levels depending on the extent of scarring. Four to six fasciculi or fascicular groups, all of different lengths, now should be present in each end of the stump.
- Deflate the tourniquet and compress the wound with saline-moistened packs.
- Draw a sketch of each nerve stump, and attempt to identify the corresponding fasciculi and groups of fasciculi in

each. The more proximal the lesion, the less well defined the fascicular groups. Use clinical judgment in matching the fasciculi and the fascicular groups in the ends of the stumps.
- By measuring the gaps remaining between the fasciculi and fascicular groups at each end of the nerve, estimate the length of nerve graft needed. Each major fasciculus or group requires a segment of graft; the graft should be 10% to 15% longer than the combined gaps to be filled.
- Nerves that can be used as donors are the sural, the saphenous, the lateral cutaneous of the thigh, the lateral and medial cutaneous of the forearm, the posterior cutaneous of the forearm, the superficial branch of the radial, the dorsal branch of the ulnar, and the intercostals (see Source of Nerve for Interfascicular Nerve Grafting). We prefer the sural nerve for most situations. A level for transection should be selected to allow the proximal end of the donor nerve to retract beneath fascia or muscles and avoid as much as possible the formation of a painful neuroma.
- If the sural nerve is to be used, expose it through a short transverse incision posterior to the lateral malleolus.
- Separate the nerve from the small saphenous vein that lies just anterior and superficial to it.
- Determine the course of the nerve in the calf by applying traction to the nerve.
- Along the course of the nerve, make additional transverse incisions to allow further dissection. If long segments of nerve are to be harvested, a single longitudinal incision is used (Fig. 10.15). This minimizes the potential harm caused by traction on the donor nerve during a difficult dissection. Although scissors or nerve strippers can be used during this part of the procedure, exercise care to avoid injuring the nerve graft.
- Transect the nerve so that its proximal end retracts beneath the fascia in the proximal calf.
- Close the incisions in the calf, and keep the graft moist with saline during the rest of the operation.

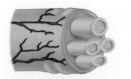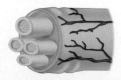

Nerve grafts placed between nerve ends

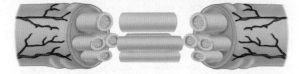

Nerve grafts sutured in place

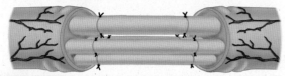

FIGURE 10.16 Interfascicular nerve grafting (see text). **SEE TECHNIQUE 10.3.**

- Dissect any excess fat from the ends of the graft, and section the graft so that shorter grafts of appropriate lengths can be placed between the ends of corresponding fasciculi or fascicular groups.
- Using the operating microscope, place each graft between the corresponding fasciculi and secure the epineurium of each end to the perineurium of the fasciculus or fascicular group with a single suture of 10-0 monofilament nylon (Fig. 10.16).
- If the extremity has been positioned in extension and if the grafts are placed without tension, the single sutures are sufficient. To reinforce the repair site and minimize the need for sutures, fibrin glue can be used as described by Narakas by mixing equal parts of thrombin and fibrinogen.
- Obtain meticulous hemostasis and close the wound. Avoid suction drainage tubes.
- The same technique can be used for a nerve lesion in continuity or for repair of an unsuccessful primary neurorrhaphy.

POSTOPERATIVE CARE After neurorrhaphy or nerve grafting, the extremity is immobilized in a plaster splint or cast. A posterior molded plaster splint usually is satisfactory for the arm, unless the shoulder girdle must be immobilized; a Velpeau dressing reinforced with plaster is then essential. After neurorrhaphy in the lower extremity, a spica cast may be needed. The use of a long leg cast alone frequently results in separation of the line of suture.

The wound should not be dressed until the 7th to 10th day. The sutures are then removed. In removing the splint or cast, extreme care is necessary to avoid tension on the line of suture.

Opinions differ widely as to when extension of the joints may be begun safely after end-to-end repairs. Our policy in the upper extremity is to retain the plaster splint for 4 weeks and then to replace it with a plastic splint that can be extended gradually over 2 to 3 weeks. In the lower extremity, especially when the peroneal or sciatic nerve has been

sutured, we keep the patient in the spica cast for at least 6 weeks; apply a long leg brace that controls extension of the knee; and allow 4 weeks or more, depending on the tension on the line of suture, for complete extension of the knee. Radiographs may be made monthly for the first 3 months to determine the integrity of the line of suture. Physical therapy is essential to recovery of function of the extremity.

After interfascicular grafting, the joints should be immobilized no longer than 10 days. Millesi recommended immobilization of the extremity in the exact position it was in at surgery. This maintains the graft in its elongated position and minimizes the potential for later disruption. The plaster cast or splint is removed, and active exercises of all joints are begun. The progress of regeneration is determined by the advance of the Tinel sign. As this sign progresses along the graft, it may stop at the distal repair temporarily; however, it usually resumes progress eventually. If the Tinel sign does not progress after 3 to 4 months, blockage at the distal line of suture is assumed and resection of this area followed by repair is indicated.

RESULTS OF OPERATION

The results of such procedures as neurolysis and partial neurorrhaphy cannot be determined accurately. We know, however, that neurorrhaphy is never followed by full return of motor and sensory function. Rarely, full return is approached after suture of the radial nerve and occasionally after suture of the median nerve in children. A useful degree of recovery often occurs when the factors that influence recovery are favorable (see "Factors that Influence Regeneration after Neurorrhaphy"). The degree of recovery varies from nerve to nerve and with the relative extent of damage to the motor and sensory components within each nerve. Recovery of function of the limb as a whole is not proportionate to neurologic recovery. A patient may recover fairly good neurologic function, but, because of other defects in the limb, overall functional recovery may be unsatisfactory. Because it is helpful to know what result can be expected after suture of any given nerve, a statement is made at the end of the discussion of each nerve when this information is available.

CERVICAL PLEXUS

The anterior primary rami of the first four cervical nerves unite to form the cervical plexus. Sensory fibers from the upper two or three segments course through the lesser occipital, greater auricular, and anterior cutaneous nerves of the neck. Sensory fibers from the lower two segments course through the supraclavicular nerves. Muscular branches join in the ansa hypoglossi to innervate the thyrohyoid, geniohyoid, omohyoid, sternothyroid, and sternohyoid muscles. Branches from C3, C4, and C5 unite to form the phrenic nerve. Fibers arising from the lateral aspect of the anterior horns of the upper five cervical segments unite to form the spinal accessory nerve, which ascends into the cranial cavity through the foramen magnum. At that point the nerve is joined by its cranial part, which consists primarily of rootlets destined to pass with the vagus nerve. These rootlets diverge from the spinal accessory nerve after its exit from the jugular foramen and thereafter course with the vagus fibers. The spinal accessory nerve descends in the neck beneath the posterior belly of the digastric muscle, receiving branches from the anterior primary rami of C2, C3, and C4 and branching to innervate the sternocleidomastoid. It then leaves the posterior aspect of this muscle and descends farther to innervate the superior third of the trapezius muscle.

SPINAL ACCESSORY NERVE

The spinal accessory nerve may be injured at any point along its course. Because of its superficial location in the posterior cervical triangle, it is especially susceptible to damage from penetrating injuries. It also may be injured during operations such as lymph node biopsy or radical neck dissection. Woodhall gave an accurate description of the symptoms and findings that follow surgical injury to this nerve: the patient reports generalized weakness in the affected shoulder girdle and arm, inability to abduct the shoulder more than 90 degrees, and a sensory disturbance that may vary from a pulling sensation in the region of the scar to aching in the shoulder and arm. The aching may radiate to the medial margin of the scapula and down the arm to the fingers and is sometimes incapacitating. The superior one third of the trapezius muscle on the affected side always atrophies, the shoulder sags, and power to elevate it is weak. The scapula rotates distally and laterally and flares slightly; its inferior angle is closer to the midline than is its superior angle. This position is accentuated when the arm is abducted; the flaring of the inferior angle disappears when the arm is raised anteriorly, in contrast to the usual deformity caused by paralysis of the serratus anterior.

◼ TREATMENT

If the nerve has been injured by a low-velocity missile, and if no vascular or visceral injuries require immediate surgical exploration, simple observation for 3 to 4 weeks may be best. If after that time electrodiagnostic examination reveals denervation of the trapezius, however, and if clinical evidence of return of function is absent, exploration of the nerve is indicated. When injury to the nerve is detected during an operation, and when circumstances permit, primary repair should be attempted. When the injury is not appreciated during an operation, however, or when removal of a segment of the nerve is necessary as part of an operation for malignancy, attempts to repair the nerve or any reconstructive procedure should be delayed 2 to 3 weeks to allow the initial wound to heal. When a segment of the nerve has been removed as part of an operation for malignancy, the condition of the patient or later treatment such as irradiation may preclude additional procedures. When the patient's condition permits, when symptoms warrant additional treatment, and when the gap created by segmental resection of the nerve is too great to close by end-to-end suture, interfascicular grafting (see Technique 10.3) or tendon transfer is the remaining alternative.

If the nerve is to be repaired, the approach described here allows satisfactory exposure for suture or nerve grafting. When the initial wound has healed well, the incision is made across the middle of the posterior triangle, following the skin folds of the neck. The terminal part of the spinal accessory nerve emerges at the junction of the proximal and middle thirds of the sternocleidomastoid muscle and courses diagonally distally and posteriorly to enter the lateral border of the trapezius muscle at the junction of its middle and distal thirds.

The incision should be long enough to permit exact identification of the distal and proximal parts of the nerve. Care must be taken not to confuse the lesser occipital and greater auricular nerves with the spinal accessory. The proximal part of the nerve should be stimulated. Contraction of the trapezius muscle indicates that the nerve has not been severed. The entire nerve is exposed in the posterior triangle. If scarring is extensive within or around the nerve, a neurolysis is performed. If the nerve has been divided, its ends should be mobilized and sectioned back to good funiculi. An end-to-end suture is performed under little or no tension. Awkward positioning of the head, neck, and shoulders in a cast to allow suturing of the nerve without tension should be avoided. Instead, interfascicular nerve grafting (Technique 10.3) may be a satisfactory alternative. If the line of suture is not under tension, the shoulder should be immobilized in a Velpeau bandage for 3 to 4 weeks. Gentle active exercises are started, and normal daily activities are resumed 6 to 8 weeks after surgery.

◼ RESULTS OF SUTURE OF THE SPINAL ACCESSORY NERVE

No statistically significant information on the results of suturing of the spinal accessory nerve is available. It has been suggested that neurolysis or repair when necessary may relieve symptoms and restore function. Good results may be expected because the spinal accessory nerve is purely a motor nerve.

NERVE TRANSFERS

Oberlin described the first neurotization procedure in 1994. It is indicated for musculocutaneous nerve injuries when elbow flexion power is lacking. This procedure was one of the first to describe the transfer of one nerve to another nerve for severe nerve injuries. This subsequently led to the development of other nerve transfers, such as the double fascicular transfer from the median and ulnar nerves to the musculocutaneous nerve, transfer of the branch of the radial nerve to the medial head of the triceps to the axillary nerve, and others described later.

TRANSFER OF THE ULNAR NERVE FASCICLES TO NERVE OF THE BICEPS MUSCLE

TECHNIQUE 10.4

(OBERLIN ET AL.)
- On the anterior aspect of the arm 4 cm distal to the humeral insertion of the pectoralis major tendon, outline on the skin the origin of the branch of the musculocutaneous nerve to the biceps muscle (Fig. 10.17A).
- Incise the skin longitudinally 8 to 10 cm, straddling this point. Incise the fascia over the biceps, and retract the muscle laterally (Fig. 10.17B).
- Identify the musculocutaneous nerve between the biceps and the coracobrachialis muscle. There are numerous variations of the origin and distribution of this nerve.
- Identify the ulnar nerve at the same level, using electrical stimulation to confirm identification.

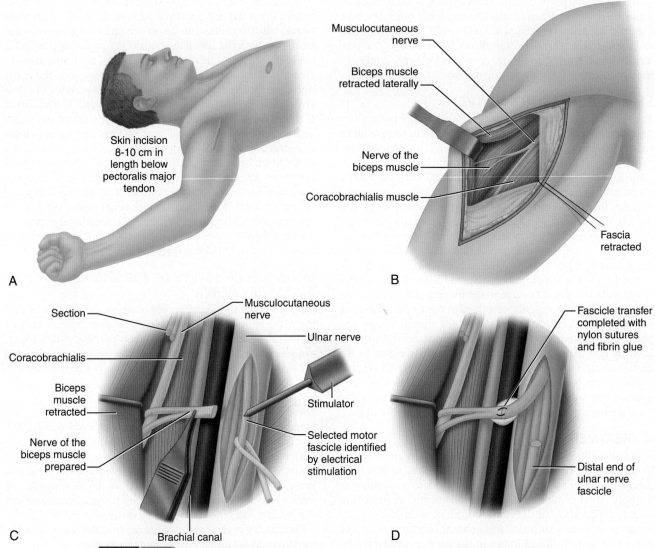

FIGURE 10.17 Transfer of ulnar nerve fascicles to nerve to biceps muscle. **A,** Skin incision. **B,** Approach to the musculocutaneous nerve. **C,** Microscopic dissection and nerve branching. Intraneural dissection and identification of motor fascicle by means of electrical stimulation. **D,** Repair completed. **SEE TECHNIQUE 10.4.**

- Under microscopic magnification, perform further dissection and identify branches to the biceps muscle. Usually, the vascular pedicle does not interfere with dissection of the nerve because it has a more transverse orientation.
- Split the branch(es) from the musculocutaneous nerve to the biceps muscle proximally 2 cm, and transect (Fig. 10.17C).
- Rotate the distal part medially toward the previously dissected ulnar nerve.
- Incise the epineurium of the ulnar nerve, and select one or two fascicle(s) with an adequate size. Use low-intensity electrical stimulation to distinguish precisely between sensory and motor fascicles. If a fascicle with the response in the extrinsic flexors is located, use this for transfer. (Often this fascicle is located anteriorly and medially within the ulnar nerve.)
- Separate the chosen fascicle from the rest of the ulnar nerve over 2 cm, and divide it distally.

- Turn the fascicle laterally and suture it to the nerve to the biceps (Fig. 10.17D) with 11-0 nylon without any tension at the repair site. Repair of the nerve is performed in front of the brachial vascular bundle. Add fibrin glue to the repair.

DOUBLE FASCICULAR TRANSFER FROM ULNAR AND MEDIAN NERVES TO NERVE OF THE BRACHIALIS BRANCHES

TECHNIQUE 10.5

(MACKINNON AND COLBERT)

- With the patient supine and the arm abducted, make a skin incision in the central portion of the bicipital groove, carrying the dissection down to the interval between the triceps and biceps muscles.

- Identify the ulnar nerve medial to the brachial artery, and identify the median nerve on the lateral surface of the artery.
- Identify the musculocutaneous nerve on the deep medial surface of the biceps muscle by palpation. Perform electrical stimulation of the brachialis and biceps branches to confirm lack of motor function.
- Dissect the biceps and brachialis branches at their points of proximal separation from the musculocutaneous nerve, and then drape them medially toward the ulnar and median nerves.
- Donor fascicle selection is based on the proximity to the recipient nerves. Usually, the biceps branch is closer to the median nerve and the brachialis to the ulnar nerve (Fig. 10.18), but not always. Plan the location of neurolysis to allow tension-free coaptation with the respective recipient nerves. As a rule-of-thumb, divide the donor nerve distally and the recipient nerve proximally. Use of a nerve stimulator can help identify redundant fascicles to the flexor carpi radialis and the flexor carpi ulnaris muscle. Alternative donors from the median nerve are redundant fascicles to the flexor digitorum sublimis and palmaris longus. The motor group fascicles of the median nerve are on the medial aspect of the nerve, and the motor groups of the ulnar nerve are in the lateral or central portion of the nerve.
- Take the elbow through range of motion to make sure the planned repair is tension free. After internal neurolysis, divide the isolated redundant fascicles at their distalmost points and repair them to their respective biceps and brachialis recipients with 9-0 nylon suture (Fig. 10.18).
- Place a drain and indwelling pain pump catheter as needed and place the patient's arm in a shoulder immobilizer, allowing gentle intermittent elbow and shoulder range of motion.

POSTOPERATIVE CARE The shoulder immobilizer is removed at approximately 7 days, and shoulder range-of-motion exercises are begun at 2 weeks. After return of the biceps and brachialis function, strengthening and reeducation are begun.

NEUROTIZATION OF THE SUPRASCAPULAR NERVE WITH THE SPINAL ACCESSORY NERVE

TECHNIQUE 10.6

(MACKINNON AND COLBERT)
- With the patient prone, identify the location of the distal accessory nerve and the suprascapular nerve at the suprascapular notch and mark the transverse incision (Fig. 10.19A).
- Make an incision and carry the dissection down to the trapezius muscle.

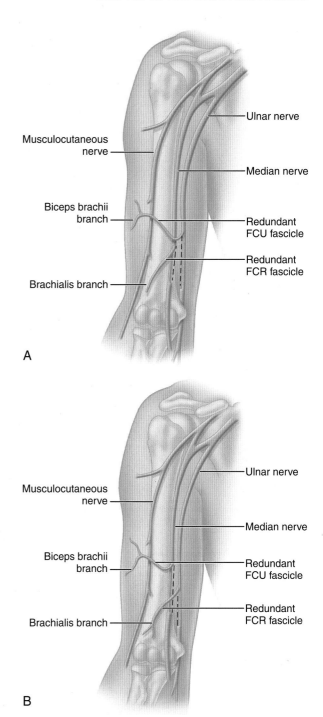

A

B

FIGURE 10.18 Double fascicular transfer for musculocutaneous nerve. **A,** Redundant flexor carpi ulnaris (FCU) fascicle from ulnar nerve is transferred to biceps branch. **B,** Redundant flexor carpi radialis (FCR) fascicle from the median nerve transferred to brachialis branch. **SEE TECHNIQUE 10.5.**

- Split the trapezius muscle along the transverse course of its fibers and identify the supraspinatus muscle below. Carry the dissection bluntly over the supraspinatus muscle to the superior border of the scapula.
- Identify the suprascapular notch by palpation. Expose the superior scapular ligament by blunt dissection with a "peanut" sponge, taking care not to injure the suprascapular

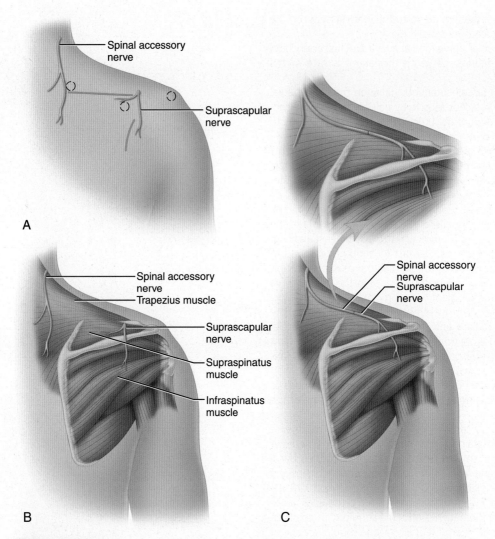

FIGURE 10.19   Spinal accessory nerve to suprascapular nerve transfer. **A,** Planned incision. **B,** Before nerve transfer. **C,** Nerve transfer for suprascapular nerve function. **SEE TECHNIQUE 10.6.**

artery, which courses superiorly over the ligament (Fig. 10.19B). Protect the artery while dividing the ligament under direct vision, revealing the suprascapular nerve.

- Stimulate the suprascapular nerve to confirm lack of function.
- Carry the dissection of the nerve as far proximally or anteriorly as possible to facilitate a tension-free repair. Carry the subtrapezius dissection medially toward the accessory nerve.
- Use blunt dissection and a nerve stimulator at a deep level to the trapezius muscle, working in a longitudinal direction to identify the nerve.
- Once the nerve is identified and confirmed intact by stimulation, dissect it as far distally or inferiorly as possible. Adequate dissection of both the suprascapular and accessory nerves allows transfer and tension-free repair without the need for a nerve graft.
- Divide the suprascapular nerve proximally and the accessory nerve distally.
- Suture the proximal end of the accessory nerve to the distal end of the suprascapular nerve with interrupted 9-0 nylon under an operating microscope (Fig. 10.19C).

POSTOPERATIVE CARE   The patient is placed in a shoulder immobilizer postoperatively to prevent abduction but care is taken to allow intermittent elbow range of motion to prevent stiffness and ulnar nerve irritation. Shoulder range of motion is begun at 2 weeks, and strengthening and reeducation exercises are begun after return of spinatus muscle function.

NEUROTIZATION OF THE AXILLARY NERVE WITH RADIAL NERVE

TECHNIQUE 10.7

(MACKINNON AND COLBERT)
- Place the patient prone.
- Make a longitudinal incision from a point overlying the quadrangular space at the posterior border of the deltoid

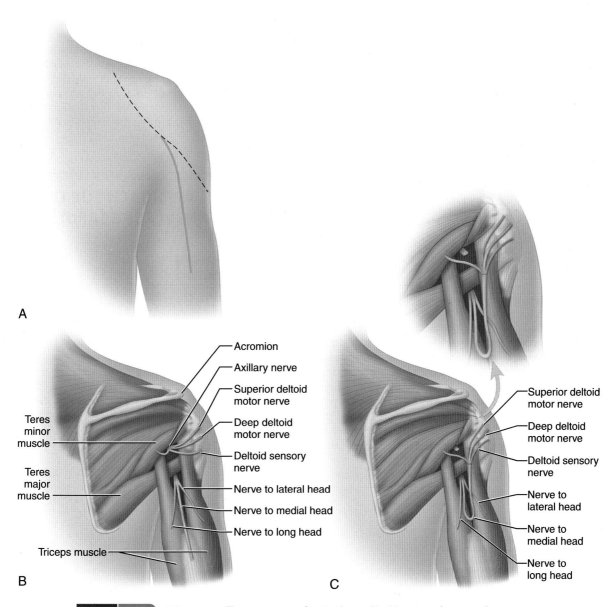

Teres
minor
muscle

Teres
major
muscle

Triceps muscle

Acromion

Axillary nerve

Superior deltoid
motor nerve

Deep deltoid
motor nerve

Deltoid sensory
nerve

Nerve to lateral head

Nerve to medial head

Nerve to long head

Superior deltoid
motor nerve

Deep deltoid
motor nerve

Deltoid sensory
nerve

Nerve to
lateral head

Nerve to
medial head

Nerve to
long head

A

B

C

FIGURE 10.20 Triceps to axillary nerve transfer. **A,** Planned incision. **B,** Before transfer. **C,** Nerve transfer for axillary nerve function. **SEE TECHNIQUE 10.7.**

muscle to the midposterior interval between the lateral and long heads of the triceps (Fig. 10.20A). Carry the dissection down to the level of the triceps and deltoid muscles.

- Open the triceps interval to expose the donor nerve running with the radial nerve on the posterior surface of the humerus and to facilitate identification of the quadrangular space, which transmits the axillary nerve (Fig. 10.20B).
- Retract the posterior border of the deltoid muscle superiorly. Often, the cutaneous branch of the axillary nerve courses deep to the deltoid muscle and dissection of the nerve proximally will help to identify the remainder of the axillary nerve. The transversely oriented tendinous portion of the teres major muscle, located deep to the long head of the triceps, is a key anatomic landmark.

- Locate the axillary nerve by blunt dissection superior to the teres major muscle and just superior to the posterior circumflex humeral vessels.
- Stimulate the axillary nerve to confirm lack of function.
- Identify the nerve branch to the medial head of the triceps, which is a distinct branch running adjacent to the radial nerve, by stimulation.
- Divide the branch at its most distal point and isolate it proximally to the inferior border of the teres major muscle.
- Sharply divide the proximal portion of the axillary nerve, including the component to the teres minor muscle.
- Repair the distal segment of the axillary nerve to the transferred proximal segment of the medial triceps nerve tension free under an operating microscope with interrupted 9-0 nylon suture (Fig. 10.20C).

POSTOPERATIVE CARE A shoulder immobilizer is placed postoperatively, allowing gentle intermittent elbow range of motion to prevent stiffness. Shoulder range-of-motion exercises are begun at 2 weeks, and strengthening and reeducation are begun after return of deltoid function.

UPPER EXTREMITY NERVE INJURIES

SUPRASCAPULAR NERVE

Arising from the upper trunk of the brachial plexus, the suprascapular nerve lies in the posterior triangle of the neck near the posterior belly of the omohyoid muscle. It courses across the posterior triangle, passing under the belly of the omohyoid muscle and the anterior border of the trapezius to the scapular notch. It traverses the scapular notch, passing below the superior transverse ligament (transverse scapular ligament), and enters the supraspinatus fossa, where it sends a motor branch to the supraspinatus muscle and an articular branch to the shoulder joint. It passes around the lateral border of the spine of the scapula (spinoglenoid notch) into the infraspinatus fossa, where it sends a muscular branch to the infraspinatus muscle with branches also to the shoulder joint and the scapula. The nerve may be injured by penetrating trauma in the posterior triangle of the neck; by cancer surgery in the same area; by blunt or penetrating trauma in the supraclavicular region; by fractures of the superolateral portion of the scapula, especially involving the region of the suprascapular notch; by anterior dislocations of the shoulder joint; by entrapment in the suprascapular notch; and by space-occupying lesions, such as a ganglion at the spinoglenoid notch.

■ EXAMINATION

Pain in the shoulder and weakness of the shoulder girdle are common complaints. Atrophy of the supraspinatus and infraspinatus muscles may be seen if the nerve is injured at or proximal to the suprascapular notch. Atrophy of only the infraspinatus muscle suggests entrapment distal to the supraspinatus fossa, as may occur at the spinoglenoid notch. Electrodiagnostic studies are helpful in confirming the diagnosis.

■ TREATMENT

POSTERIOR APPROACH FOR DIVISION OF THE TRANSVERSE SCAPULAR LIGAMENT

TECHNIQUE 10.8

(SWAFFORD AND LICHTMAN)
  Figure 10.21
- With the patient prone, make an incision parallel to and about 3 cm superior to the scapular spine.
- Elevate the trapezius subperiosteally, and expose the supraspinatus muscle.
- Identify the nerve by elevating the supraspinatus muscle and dissecting superior and inferior to the muscle.
- Identify the suprascapular notch, and release the transverse ligament.
- It may be necessary to enlarge the notch with a rongeur if it is narrow. Smooth the edges of the notch if it is enlarged.
- If no definite entrapment is identified in the notch, follow the nerve around the spinoglenoid notch to exclude

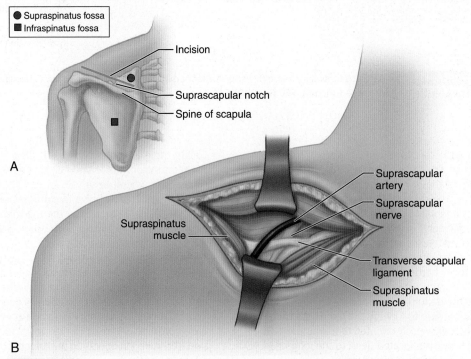

FIGURE 10.21 **A,** Posterior approach for division of transverse scapular ligament. **B,** Suprascapular artery is above and suprascapular nerve is beneath ligament. **SEE TECHNIQUE 10.8.**

- entrapment in that area, especially if only the infraspinatus muscle is involved.
- Return of function after release varies. Reports regarding results after suture of this nerve are inconclusive.

LONG THORACIC NERVE

The serratus anterior muscle alone is occasionally paralyzed by injury to the long thoracic nerve. Such injuries may result from either sharp or blunt trauma or from traction when the head is forced acutely away from the shoulder or when the shoulder is depressed, as when carrying heavy weights. Other causes include exposure to cold, viral infections, and placing patients in the Trendelenburg position with shoulder braces that compress the supraclavicular areas. When the serratus anterior is paralyzed, the patient cannot fully flex the arm above the level of the shoulder anteriorly; active abduction also may be restricted. When the patient attempts to exert forward pushing movements with the hands, "winging" of the scapula occurs and its vertebral border and inferior angle become unduly prominent.

When the nerve has been stretched rather than severed, it usually is enough to immobilize the shoulder girdle in extension with the arm against the chest. Contractures of the shoulder, elbow, and wrist should be avoided while awaiting recovery. According to Sunderland, the nerve may recover after 3 to 12 months. Early decompression of the long thoracic nerve has been recommended by Nath et al. Schippert et al. reported long thoracic nerve decompression through a supraclavicular approach for posttraumatic paralysis in six patients. All patients had decreased pain, disability, and scapular winging and improved shoulder range of motion. If paralysis persists, or if the nerve has been severed, the prognosis for recovery is poor and a reconstructive operation may be indicated (see also the discussion of muscle transfers and fascial transplants for paralysis of the scapular muscles in other chapter). There are no significant reports of results after suture of the long thoracic nerve. For reconstructive operations for paralysis of the long thoracic nerve, see other chapter.

AXILLARY NERVE

The axillary nerve, composed of fibers from C5 and C6, is a branch of the posterior cord of the brachial plexus emerging inferior to the subscapular and thoracodorsal nerves at the level of the humeral head; it winds around the neck of the humerus, passing through the quadrangular space to supply the deltoid and teres minor muscles. Ball et al. described the anatomy of the axillary nerve, emphasizing a posterior branch that innervates the teres minor and the posterior deltoid and supplies the cutaneous innervation through the superolateral brachial cutaneous nerve. The cutaneous portion traversed the fascia 6.3 to 10.9 cm below the posterolateral corner of the acromion along the medial border of the deltoid. The anterior branch continued in an anterolateral direction to supply most of the deltoid. In five of the 19 specimens, the posterior deltoid received its sole innervation from the anterior branch. This nerve commonly is injured by fractures or dislocations around the shoulder, penetrating wounds, and direct blows. It may be injured during a posterior approach to the shoulder and shoulder arthroscopy. The nerve most frequently is injured just proximal to the quadrilateral space. Rarely, compression of the axillary nerve or one of its major branches may occur in the quadrilateral space and cause chronic pain and paresthesia aggravated by forward flexion or abduction and external rotation of the humerus. This is referred to as the quadrilateral space syndrome.

■ EXAMINATION

Because a lesion of the axillary nerve sometimes does not cause anesthesia, the diagnosis must rest solely on the presence or absence of function in the deltoid muscle. Usually, deltoid paralysis is detected easily by the inability to abduct the arm actively. It is well documented, however, that full abduction of the arm is possible in the presence of deltoid paralysis because of the action of the supraspinatus and because of rotation of the scapula. It is essential to observe and palpate the deltoid muscle for contraction during the examination. Electrical stimulation of the nerve in situ is accomplished easily by inserting the needles along the posterior border of the deltoid. In quadrilateral space syndrome, there usually is no loss of sensation or strength and EMG may be normal. A subclavicular arteriogram may be indicated and is considered positive if posterior humeral circumflex artery occlusion occurs with less than 60 degrees of abduction.

■ TREATMENT

APPROACH TO THE AXILLARY NERVE

TECHNIQUE 10.9

- The patient should be placed in the lateral decubitus position to allow for anterior and posterior exposure and access to the sural nerve for grafting if necessary.
- If the wound is anterior, the axillary nerve is best exposed through the incision used for the more distal parts of the brachial plexus. Although occasionally it may be possible to expose the nerve in the axilla without detaching the pectoralis major tendon, dividing the insertion of this muscle greatly increases exposure.
- Externally rotate the arm so that the nerve can be followed into the quadrangular space.
- Release the coracobrachialis, short head of the biceps, and pectoralis minor off the coracoid.
- If the wound is posterior, the nerve can be exposed after it emerges from the quadrangular space through an incision beginning about 5 cm proximal to the posterior axillary fold, extending distally, parallel to the posterior border of the deltoid, and ending at a point posterior to the deltoid tuberosity of the humerus.
- Separate the posterior border of the deltoid muscle from the infraspinatus, teres minor and major, and triceps muscles.
- Locate the nerve as it emerges from the quadrangular space; the branch to the teres minor often arises proximal to this point. At varying distances, sometimes 2.5 cm, after emerging from the space, the axillary nerve divides into anterior and posterior branches as described.
- If the nerve is injured in the quadrangular space, or if a long gap must be closed, anterior and posterior incisions are necessary.

■ METHODS OF CLOSING GAPS

Interfascicular nerve grafting is the preferred method for bridging gaps; however, a gap of 4 to 5 cm can be closed by mobilizing the nerve and the posterior cord of the brachial plexus proximally to the clavicle and by stripping the nerve up the plexus for 3 to 4 cm. Rarely, other procedures used for mobilizing the brachial plexus, such as resecting part of the clavicle, may be indicated to gain more length. Positioning after surgery is the same as that for the brachial plexus.

Interfascicular nerve grafting to close gaps in the axillary nerve is preferable to extensive brachial plexus mobilization or clavicular osteotomy. Because minimal tension is placed on the nerve graft, early motion is allowed. As nerve transfers become more popular, transfer of a portion of the radial nerve into the axillary nerve may be considered to restore deltoid function.

■ RESULTS AFTER AXILLARY NERVE INJURY

If the injury is a closed one, signs of return of function may not be observed for 3 to 12 months; however, most patients progress to full recovery (approximately 90%).

■ TENDON AND MUSCLE TRANSFERS FOR PARALYSIS OF THE DELTOID

Tendon and muscle transfers for paralysis of the deltoid are discussed in other chapter.

MUSCULOCUTANEOUS NERVE

The musculocutaneous nerve, composed of fibers from C5 and C6, is a branch of the lateral cord of the brachial plexus. It most commonly is injured by penetrating injuries, but occasionally by anterior dislocation of the shoulder or fractures of the humeral neck. When this nerve is injured in the axilla, the injury often is in conjunction with injuries to other components of the brachial plexus. Complete division of the nerve may be overlooked because the sensory loss may be ill defined and flexion of the elbow by the brachioradialis may be strong enough to mask biceps paralysis. In these instances, it is essential to palpate the biceps while testing its function to identify specific muscle contractions.

■ EXAMINATION

The only muscle supplied by the musculocutaneous nerve that can be examined accurately is the biceps; the brachialis and the coracobrachialis are difficult to palpate. Sensory examination is of no great value because complete anesthesia is rare. Division of this nerve may cause less disability than that of any other major nerve in the body, and for this reason, especially in older patients, suture occasionally is not even indicated.

■ TREATMENT

APPROACH TO THE MUSCULOCUTANEOUS NERVE

TECHNIQUE 10.10

- The incision is the same as for exposing the more distal parts of the brachial plexus (see Fig. 10.17B). If it is certain

that no other nerves are involved, carry the incision in the proximal part of the arm about 2.5 cm anterior to that shown.
- Divide the tendon of the pectoralis major and identify the musculocutaneous nerve where it emerges from the lateral cord of the brachial plexus and before it pierces the coracobrachialis muscle.
- Follow the nerve through the coracobrachialis muscle, and, as it passes into the arm, locate it in the plane between the biceps and brachialis muscles.
- The muscular branches of the nerve to the biceps are given off just after the nerve emerges from the coracobrachialis muscle and those to the brachialis at or just proximal to the level of junction of the middle and distal thirds of the arm. Exposing the nerve distal to this point is unnecessary.

■ METHODS OF CLOSING GAPS

Gaps of 8 cm can be closed by mobilizing the lateral cord of the brachial plexus proximally into the neck and the musculocutaneous nerve distally to its muscular branches, by adducting the shoulder sharply, and by bringing the arm anteriorly across the chest as for relaxing the brachial plexus. Occasionally, the musculocutaneous nerve can be transposed so that it no longer pierces the coracobrachialis but runs across the axilla medial to this muscle between the biceps and brachialis muscles. As in repair of the brachial plexus, all sutures may be inserted in the nerve ends and the wound is closed except at the site of neurorrhaphy before the sutures are tied. Interfascicular grafting also can be done if the gap is too wide to close by mobilization and limb positioning.

■ RESULTS AFTER INJURY TO THE MUSCULOCUTANEOUS NERVE

Signs of recovery of the musculocutaneous nerve may appear at 4 to 9 months after injury. Excellent results have been reported after repair by secondary suture or grafting.

RADIAL NERVE

The radial nerve, a continuation of the posterior cord of the brachial plexus, consists of fibers from C6, C7, and C8 and sometimes T1. It is primarily a motor nerve that innervates the triceps; the supinators of the forearm; and the extensors of the wrist, fingers, and thumb. This nerve is injured most often by fractures of the humeral shaft. Gunshot wounds are the second most common cause of radial nerve injury. Other causes include lacerations of the arm and proximal forearm, injection injuries, and prolonged local pressure.

■ EXAMINATION

The following muscles supplied by the radial nerve can be tested accurately because their bellies or tendons or both can be palpated: the triceps brachii, brachioradialis, extensor carpi radialis, extensor digitorum communis, extensor carpi ulnaris, abductor pollicis longus, and extensor pollicis longus. Injury to this nerve results in inability to extend the elbow or supinate the forearm and in a typical wristdrop. An inexperienced examiner often may be misled by the patient's ability to extend the wrist merely by flexing the fingers. The examiner should be discriminating because analysis of movements often may result in error in evaluating the function of a nerve. The triceps is not seriously affected by injuries of the nerve at the level of the middle of the humerus or distally. In injuries of the nerve at its bifurcation into the deep and superficial branches, the brachioradialis and the extensor carpi radialis longus continue to function; the arm can be supinated, and the wrist can be extended. The nerve is especially susceptible to electrical stimulation in situ just proximal to the elbow; elsewhere this is difficult, and the results are uncertain.

Sensory examination is relatively unimportant, even when the nerve is divided in the axilla, because usually there is no autonomous zone. When present, the autonomous zone usually is over the first dorsal interosseous muscle, between the first and second metacarpals. It usually is too inconsistent to afford more than confirmatory evidence of complete interruption of the nerve proximal to its bifurcation at the elbow.

▤ TREATMENT

APPROACH TO THE RADIAL NERVE

TECHNIQUE 10.11

- Expose the radial nerve in the axilla and proximal third of the arm by the usual incision for the distal part of the brachial plexus, and carry this incision distally in the arm a little more posteriorly than is necessary for exposing the ulnar and median nerves.
- Incise the fascia over the neurovascular bundle, and expose the bundle between the triceps posteriorly and the biceps, brachialis, and coracobrachialis anteriorly.
- Expose and retract laterally the more superficial structures of the bundle—the ulnar nerve, the brachial artery and vein, and the median nerve—exposing the radial nerve and one or two of its branches, first to the long head and then to the medial head of the triceps.
- Trace the nerve to the point where it winds around the humerus.
- To expose the nerve on the posterior and lateral aspects of the humeral shaft, begin the incision along the posterior border of the distal third of the deltoid between the deltoid and the long head of the triceps. Curve it distalward along the lateral aspect of the arm, curving at first anteriorly along the medial aspect of the brachioradialis and then, if necessary, laterally at the elbow across the belly of this muscle and the extensor carpi radialis longus. Finally, if the deep radial nerve is to be explored, carry the incision distally on the dorsum of the forearm along the radial side of the extensor digitorum communis.
- In the incision proximal to the elbow it is wise to expose the nerve at its most superficial position by incising the fascia between the brachialis and brachioradialis and to identify the nerve at this point by retracting the brachioradialis laterally. The nerve can be exposed proximally by incising the fascia and retracting the lateral head of the triceps laterally to the point where the nerve winds around the humerus. This approach, with minor changes, is shown in Figure 10.22.
- The nerve can be carefully traced distally to the elbow; 5 or 6 cm proximal to the elbow it sends branches to the

brachioradialis and a little more distally to the extensor carpi radialis longus and brevis. At the elbow, the nerve divides into the superficial and deep radial (posterior interosseous) nerves.
- The superficial radial nerve is entirely sensory but should be protected to avoid painful neuromas. The deep radial nerve often is injured, and such an injury is quite disabling.
- Expose this nerve through the distal part of the incision just described, beginning 8 to 10 cm proximal to the elbow and continuing to the middle of the dorsum of the forearm (Fig. 10.23). Follow the nerve beneath the brachioradialis into the supinator muscle.
- If the injury is at this point or is more distal, expose the nerve distal to the supinator by incising the fascia between the extensor carpi radialis longus and brevis and the extensor digitorum communis and by developing this plane of cleavage.
- After exposing the nerve, follow it proximally to the distal border of the supinator where numerous branches are given off.
- After identifying these branches, incise the superficial part of the supinator at a right angle to the direction of its fibers to complete the exposure of the entire deep radial nerve.

▤ METHODS OF CLOSING GAPS

Interfascicular nerve grafting is the preferred method for bridging gaps, although extensive mobilization techniques have been described. In the axilla and in the proximal arm on the medial side proximal to the point of emergence of the branches to the triceps, closing a gap of more than 6 to 7 cm is difficult without sacrificing the branches to the triceps; this is hardly justifiable. Resecting the humerus rarely is feasible at this level.

In the middle third of the arm, defects of 10 to 12 cm can be closed by mobilizing the nerve from the elbow to the clavicle and widely stripping the branches of the nerve, by flexing the elbow, by externally rotating and strongly adducting the arm across the chest, and, if necessary, by sacrificing the branch to the brachioradialis (if the biceps is functioning). Transposing the nerve beneath the biceps anterior to the humerus, advocated by most authors on this subject, adds variable length and occasionally is worthwhile. In one patient, Gore reported mobilization of a proximal branch of the radial nerve to the triceps to suture to the distal end of the nerve with good results. In the presence of a nonunited fracture of the humerus, 3 to 4 cm of the bone can be resected, but if the procedures just mentioned are used, resecting part of a normal humerus almost never should be necessary to repair the radial nerve. Before such extreme dissection and awkward positioning are attempted, serious consideration should be given to interfascicular nerve grafting.

▤ RESULTS OF SUTURE OF THE RADIAL NERVE

Only motor recovery is important in suture of the radial nerve. Among patients with sutures of this nerve, 89% obtain recovery of proximal muscles, 63% regain useful function of all muscles supplied by the radial nerve, and 36% regain some fine control of the extensors of the fingers and thumb. When circumstances are most favorable, more than three fourths of these

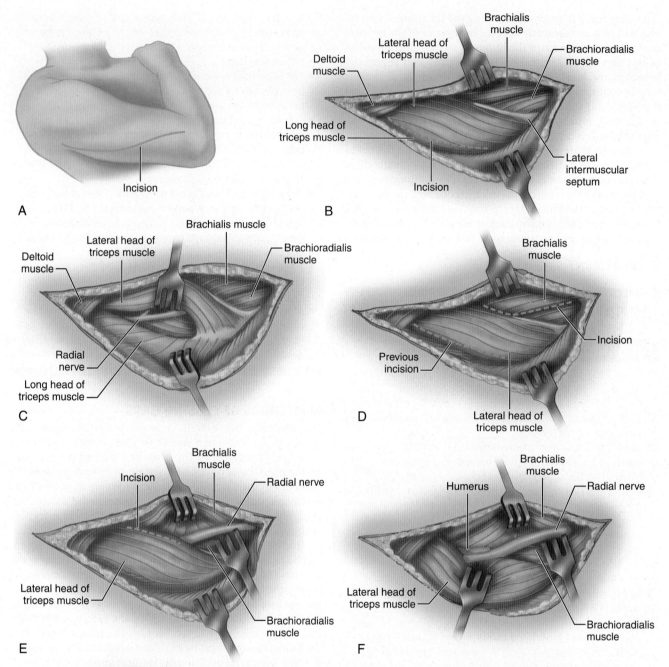

FIGURE 10.22 Exposure of radial nerve in middle and distal thirds of arm. **A,** Skin incision begins at posterior margin of deltoid muscle and extends distally in midline and laterally and anteriorly. It ends at interval between brachioradialis and brachialis. **B,** Posterior skin flap has been dissected and retracted; deep fascia is incised in line with skin incision. *Dotted line* indicates incision in triceps muscle between long and lateral heads. **C,** Radial nerve and accompanying vascular bundle have been exposed by retraction of these two heads of triceps muscle. Radial nerve has been dissected to point at which it passes beneath lateral head of triceps muscle. **D,** Arm is externally rotated a few degrees. Interval between proximal end of brachioradialis and brachialis is to be dissected, exposing radial nerve along anterolateral aspect of humerus. **E,** *Dotted line* indicates incision through which lateral head of triceps is mobilized from underlying bone, facilitating exposure of radial nerve deep to it. **F,** Exposure. **SEE TECHNIQUE 10.11.**

patients recover useful function of all the muscles supplied by this nerve. Lee et al. reported good-to-excellent motor recovery in six patients with high radial nerve palsy treated with 9 to 11 cm of interfascicular nerve grafting and recommended nerve reconstruction before resorting to tendon transfers. In their study of 244 patients with radial nerve injuries, Pan et al. found better outcomes of finger and thumb extension with injuries occurring distal to the lateral epicondyle. Wrist extension recovered in at least 80% of the patients, regardless of the level of injury in relation to the humerus. Primary repair of

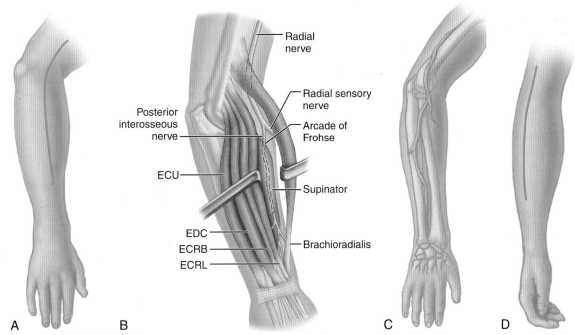

FIGURE 10.23 Exposure of posterior interosseous branch of radial nerve for repair or decompression in radial tunnel syndrome. **A,** Line of incision, forearm prone, elbow flexed. **B,** Nerve exposed. **C,** Diagram of course of nerve with arm in position A. **D,** Line of incision, elbow extended. **SEE TECHNIQUE 10.12.**

transected radial nerves associated with open humeral fractures is not recommended because of poor recovery.

■ CRITICAL LIMIT OF DELAY OF SUTURE

Return of motor function should not be expected when suture has been delayed for more than 15 months. Zachary found that return of function in muscles innervated by the posterior interosseous nerve is unlikely if the delay is more than 9 months.

ULNAR NERVE

The ulnar nerve is composed of fibers from C8 and T1 coming from the medial cord of the brachial plexus. It may be divided at any point along its course by missile wounds or lacerations. When it is injured in the upper arm, other nerves or the brachial artery because of their proximity also may be injured. In the middle of the arm the ulnar nerve is relatively protected, but in the distal arm and at the elbow it often is injured by dislocations of the elbow and supracondylar and condylar fractures. An ulnar nerve deficit complicating a fracture or dislocation may be caused by the initial trauma, by repeated manipulations of the osseous injury, or by scar formation developing sometime after injury. The nerve is injured most commonly in the distal forearm and wrist; in these locations it may be injured by gunshot wounds, lacerations, fractures, or dislocations. In civilian life, lacerations cause most of the injuries at the wrist.

Traction on the nerve, subluxation or dislocation of the nerve, and entrapment syndromes also can cause ulnar nerve deficits that may require surgical treatment. Tardy ulnar nerve palsy may develop after malunited fractures of the lateral humeral condyle in children, displaced fractures of the medial humeral epicondyle, dislocations of the elbow, and contusions of the nerve. In malunion of the lateral humeral

condyle, cubitus valgus develops; in this deformity, the ulnar nerve is gradually stretched and can become incompletely paralyzed. Tardy ulnar nerve palsy may also develop in patients who have a shallow ulnar groove on the posterior aspect of the medial humeral epicondyle, hypoplasia of the humeral trochlea, or an inadequate fibrous arch that normally keeps the nerve in the groove, resulting in recurrent subluxation or dislocation of the nerve. Recurrent subluxation or dislocation of the nerve has been found in 16.2% of 2000 elbows. Subluxation is more common than dislocation, and the ulnar nerve is more likely to be injured repeatedly in subluxations. In most patients, flexion of the elbow aggravated the symptoms of pain and paresthesias. Cubitus varus deformities also may be associated with tardy ulnar nerve palsy.

Entrapment or compression of the ulnar nerve may also occur at the supracondylar process of the humerus medially (also associated with median nerve compression), at the arcade of Struthers near the medial intermuscular septum, between the heads of origin of the flexor carpi ulnaris, and at the wrist in the Guyon canal. In 1958, Feindel and Stratford coined the term *cubital tunnel syndrome* to describe a compression neuropathy of the ulnar nerve around the elbow with no antecedent trauma. As the ulnar nerve enters the cubital tunnel it is first bordered by the medial epicondyle anteriorly, then by the elbow joint laterally, and finally by the two heads of the flexor carpi ulnaris medially. In other areas, the nerve may be compressed by tight fascia or ligaments, neoplasms, rheumatoid synovitis, aneurysms, vascular thromboses, or anomalous muscles.

Postoperative ulnar nerve palsy may result from direct pressure on the ulnar nerve at the elbow or prolonged flexion of the elbow during surgery. The ulnar nerve is especially vulnerable to compression when the forearm is allowed to rest in pronation. Some patients may have a preexisting subclinical cubital tunnel syndrome that may predispose them to this complication.

■ EXAMINATION

Interruption of the ulnar nerve proximal to the elbow is followed by paralysis of the flexor carpi ulnaris, the flexor profundus to the little and ring fingers, the lumbricals of the little and ring fingers, all of the interossei, the adductor of the thumb, and all of the short muscles of the little finger. Occasionally, when a nerve is completely divided at this level, the intrinsic muscles of the hand function normally because of anomalous innervation of these muscles by the median nerve. In these instances, the fibers that supply the intrinsic muscles may be incorporated in the median nerve down to the middle of the forearm where they leave the median nerve to join the ulnar nerve (Martin-Gruber anastomosis). Complete division of the ulnar nerve at the wrist usually causes paralysis of all ulnar-innervated intrinsic muscles, unless an anatomic variation connects the median and ulnar nerves in the palm (Riche-Cannieu anastomosis). Usually, when the nerve is divided at the wrist, only the opponens pollicis, the lateral or superficial head of the flexor pollicis brevis, and the lateral two lumbricals remain functional.

In practice, only three muscles—the flexor carpi ulnaris, the abductor digiti quinti, and the first dorsal interosseous—can be tested accurately. The bellies or tendons (or both) of these muscles may be easily palpated or seen. The surgeon may be tempted to test other muscles by their well-known functions but would be misled by the occasional patient who, by substituting other muscles, can perform perfectly the actions of paralyzed muscles.

Atrophy of the muscles supplied by the ulnar nerve and clawing of the little and ring fingers usually are confirmatory evidence of paralysis of the muscles supplied by this nerve. If the nerve has been injured proximal to the elbow, however, clawing of these two fingers may be absent because the flexor digitorum profundus to the ring and little fingers also is denervated. Electrical stimulation of the nerve in situ is easy at the elbow and wrist.

The sensory examination usually is straightforward, although anatomic variations may cause confusing sensory findings. The surgeon need examine only the middle and distal phalanges of the little finger, which compose the autonomous zone of the ulnar nerve (Fig. 10.24). Complete anesthesia to

pinpricks in this area strongly suggests total division of the nerve. If one is in doubt about the sensory examination, skin resistance studies or an iodine starch test is useful.

In patients suspected of having cubital tunnel syndrome, a positive percussion test over the ulnar nerve at the level of the medial epicondyle and a positive elbow flexion test strongly suggest a significant compressive neuropathy. With the elbow fully flexed, the patient complains of numbness and tingling in the small and ring fingers, often within 1 minute. A scratch collapse test also has been described by Mackinnon in which the examiner scratches the patient's skin lightly over the area of nerve compression while the patient performs resisted bilateral shoulder external rotation. A brief loss of muscle resistance will be elicited if the patient has allodynia from the compression neuropathy. Ochi et al. described an additional provocative test, the shoulder internal rotation test, that they found to be more sensitive than the elbow flexion test, with 80% of tested subjects having symptoms within 10 seconds of testing. To perform the test, the shoulder is held at 90 degrees of abduction and maximal internal rotation with the elbow at 90 degrees of flexion, the wrist at neutral, and the fingers fully extended. Nerve conduction studies are helpful and should show slowing in the ulnar nerve velocities across the elbow, although normal velocities may be maintained during early involvement. EMG may show fibrillations in the ulnar innervated intrinsic muscles.

■ TREATMENT

APPROACH TO THE ULNAR NERVE

TECHNIQUE 10.12

- In the axilla, the ulnar nerve is exposed through the usual more distal brachial plexus incision.
- To expose the nerve in the upper arm, begin the incision over the tendon of the pectoralis major and curve it into the natural folds of the axilla and distally along the medial aspect of the upper arm. At a point 6 to 8 cm proximal to the elbow, curve the incision posteriorly slightly behind the medial epicondyle (Fig. 10.25).
- To expose the nerve in the forearm, continue the incision distally along the ulnar side of the volar aspect of the forearm to the proximal flexor crease of the wrist.

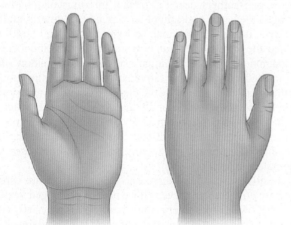

FIGURE 10.24 Autonomous sensory zone of ulnar nerve.

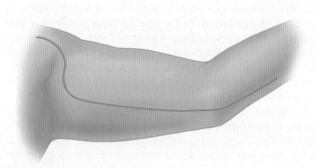

FIGURE 10.25 Skin incision for exploration of median and ulnar nerves in upper arm. **SEE TECHNIQUES 10.12 AND 10.14.**

- In the axilla and upper arm, the nerve lies just medial to the brachial artery, usually beneath the brachial vein. At about the middle of the upper arm, the nerve leaves the neurovascular bundle, gradually courses posteriorly through the intermuscular septum superficial to the medial head of the triceps muscle, and enters the ulnar groove behind the medial humeral epicondyle. The medial antebrachial cutaneous nerve may be confused with the ulnar nerve.
- In the region of the ulnar groove, the ulnar nerve gives off no important branches, although there are articular branches to the elbow joint and one or two branches to the flexor carpi ulnaris.
- Muscular branches to the medial half of the flexor digitorum profundus and additional branches to the flexor carpi ulnaris are given off distal to the groove.
- Trace the nerve into the forearm by freeing the flexor carpi ulnaris at its origin from the humeral epicondyle or by resecting the epicondyle.
- The nerve courses distally in the forearm on the flexor profundus on the radial side of the belly of the flexor carpi ulnaris. At the junction of the middle and proximal thirds of the forearm, the ulnar artery approaches the nerve from its lateral side and accompanies it into the hand. The dorsal cutaneous branch is given off 5 to 8 cm proximal to the pisiform and winds deep to the tendon of the flexor carpi ulnaris to reach the dorsum of the wrist and hand. The main trunk of the ulnar nerve courses distally lateral to the tendon of the flexor carpi ulnaris. At the distal forearm the motor branch is located in the dorsoulnar portion of the nerve as a single fascicular group making up about 30% of the nerve. At the distal aspect of the Guyon canal the ulnar nerve bifurcates into the superficial sensory and deep motor branches. The motor branch then passes deeply between the flexor and abductor digiti minimi muscles and continues radially innervating the intrinsics.

METHODS OF CLOSING GAPS

The ulnar nerve can be sutured at any point along its course. A gap in it probably can be closed more easily than in any other nerve, primarily because the nerve can be transposed to the antecubital fossa to gain length. If the lesion is distal to the muscular branches in the forearm, gaps of 12 to 15 cm can be closed by mobilization and transposition of the nerve, flexion of the wrist and elbow, intraneural dissection of the motor branches up the nerve, and sacrifice of the articular branches. Bunnell and Zachary reported that 13-cm gaps can be closed by elbow and wrist flexion and ulnar nerve transposition. Choudhry et al. compared subcutaneous, intramuscular, and submuscular transposition for gap reduction in a cadaver study and found that transposing the ulnar nerve reduced the repair gap required to cross the elbow regardless of transposition technique. When comparing individual techniques, however, they found that the greatest gap reduction was achieved by intramuscular transposition, followed by submuscular and subcutaneous transposition. A maximal gap reduction of 25 mm (average, 23 mm) was achieved using intramuscular transposition with the elbow in 90 degrees of flexion. Subcutaneous transposition actually increased the repair gap when the elbow was extended. Trumble and McCallister reported that a 2-cm gap in the forearm and a

4-cm gap at the elbow can be overcome by transposition. In a cadaver study, ulnar nerve transposition had no effect on closing nerve gaps in the distal forearm. In the proximal forearm, wrist and elbow flexion of more than 45 degrees is necessary to reduce a nerve gap of more than 11 mm after transposition.

The nerve should be transposed only after the most painstaking intraneural dissection of the branches to the flexor profundus and flexor carpi ulnaris. In our experience, satisfactory results have been achieved by placing the nerve on the fascia of the flexor-pronator group beneath the thick layer of fat in this region. The fat is sutured to the fascia medial to the nerve to keep the nerve from slipping back posterior to the epicondyle. Alternatively, the nerve can be transposed anteriorly deep to the flexor-pronator muscles by removing their origins from the medial epicondyle by dividing the flexor origin in its tendinous portion or by resecting and later reattaching the medial epicondyle; when this technique is used, the ulnar nerve is transposed anteriorly to a location near the median nerve. The medial intermuscular septum should be divided proximal to the elbow to allow flexion and extension of the joint without kinking or stretching the nerve. As an alternative to awkward positioning and extensive mobilization of the nerve, interfascicular nerve grafting should be considered and is our preferred technique.

If transposing the nerve and flexing the wrist and elbow have been necessary, a molded posterior plaster splint from the axilla to the metacarpophalangeal joints is necessary. If the lesion is in the forearm, and the gap is closed by flexing the wrist alone, the wrist is immobilized in a posterior molded plaster splint from just distal to the elbow to the metacarpophalangeal joints.

The sutures are removed at 7 to 10 days, and the splint is removed 4 weeks later. While wearing the splint, the patient should be encouraged to use the fingers and keep the metacarpophalangeal joints supple. After the splint is removed, the elbow and wrist, if flexed, are gradually extended during a period of 2 to 3 weeks, depending on the tension on the line of suture, by means of an adjustable hinged brace. After the elbow and wrist can be extended, physical therapy is started to help in regaining full motion in the joints. Splints are rarely used after the limb can be extended.

RESULTS OF SUTURE OF THE ULNAR NERVE

Motor recovery is more important than sensory recovery. After suture of the ulnar nerve, about half of these patients can be expected to show return of function in the long flexors of the fingers and wrist and some useful function in the interossei and hypothenar intrinsic muscles. Only 5% of the patients may recover independent function of the interossei; 78% may regain useful motor recovery under favorable circumstances, and 16% may show independent finger motion. About half of patients can be expected to regain useful sensation with return of sensitivity to touch and pain in the autonomous zone but with persistence of overresponse; 30% regain touch and pain sensation without overresponse; under favorable circumstances, this type of return may be obtained in half of these patients.

Good return of motor power (M3) has been reported in 50% to 90% of primary or secondary neurorrhaphies at the wrist. In a series of 26 ulnar nerve repairs performed within the Guyon canal, Kokkalis et al. reported restoration of good and excellent motor function in 25 (96%) with motor branch injury. Good and excellent sensory results were achieved in 15 (83%) of 18 with sensory branch injury. Outcomes were significantly better for those who had early repair (<4 weeks) than those who had repair 4 weeks after injury. There were no significant differences between outcomes after end-to-end repair or nerve grafting or between outcomes from repair of injuries in different zones. The authors concluded that early diagnosis and surgical treatment with careful dissection of the ulnar nerve branches within the canal are important for successful outcomes. Adequate exposure is required to repair the nerve in the Guyon canal. Nerve grafting at this level could give results similar to those of end-to-end repair.

The poorest motor return reported was after repair of the ulnar nerve in the axilla. The reported return of motor power of M3 or better has been reported in 79.5% after interfascicular grafting.

■ CRITICAL LIMIT OF DELAY OF SUTURE

Useful motor recovery of the ulnar nerve should not be expected if suture is delayed 9 months after injury in high lesions or 15 months in low lesions. Sensory recovery rarely occurs after 9 months in high lesions but has been reported to occur 31 months after injury in low lesions. Motor return cannot be expected after a delay of 29 months in lesions above the flexor carpi ulnaris and 18 months in lesions below the branches of the flexor digitorum profundus. Sensory return cannot be expected after a delay of 29 months in lesions above the flexor carpi ulnaris and 31 months below the flexor digitorum profundus.

■ NERVE RECONSTRUCTION

NERVE TRANSFER FOR ULNAR NERVE RECONSTRUCTION

In 1999, Mackinnon and Novak introduced a technique of transferring the distal portion of the anterior interosse-ous nerve into the motor branch of the ulnar nerve in an attempt to improve intrinsic return after ulnar nerve injuries. In 2002, Haase and Chung reported excellent return of intrinsic function in two patients using this technique.

TECHNIQUE 10.13

(MACKINNON AND NOVAK)
- Make an incision over the ulnar neurovascular bundle in the distal third of the forearm into the Guyon canal (Fig. 10.26A and B).
- Identify the motor branch of the ulnar nerve in the palm as it curves around the pisiform and carefully neurolyze it proximally to the level of the pronator quadratus (Fig. 10.26C).
- Dissect the motor nerve supplying the pronator quadratus along the undersurface of the muscle and transect it at its terminal branching.
- Transect the ulnar motor fascicles with enough length to perform a tension-free coaptation with the pronator nerve (Fig. 10.26D).
- Repair the nerve with 10-0 nylon suture using microscopic guidance.

POSTOPERATIVE CARE Postoperatively, no splinting is involved, allowing immediate range of motion and intrinsic stretching and strengthening exercises.

MEDIAN NERVE

The median nerve, formed by the junction of the lateral and medial cords of the brachial plexus in the axilla, is composed of fibers from C6, C7, C8, and T1 (Fig. 10.27). Median nerve injuries often result in painful neuromas and causalgia. From the sensory standpoint they are more disabling than injuries

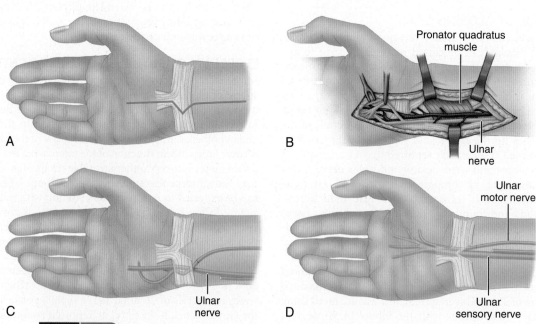

FIGURE 10.26 Terminal motor branch of anterior interosseous nerve to pronator quadratus can be transferred to deep motor branch of ulnar nerve. **A and B,** Incision and surgical exposure. **C and D,** Nerve transfer. **SEE TECHNIQUE 10.13.**

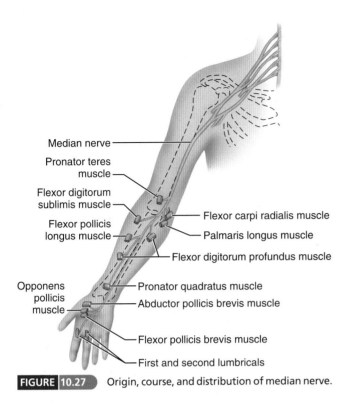

Median nerve

Pronator teres muscle

Flexor digitorum sublimis muscle

Flexor pollicis longus muscle

Flexor carpi radialis muscle

Palmaris longus muscle

Flexor digitorum profundus muscle

Opponens pollicis muscle

Pronator quadratus muscle

Abductor pollicis brevis muscle

Flexor pollicis brevis muscle

First and second lumbricals

FIGURE 10.27 Origin, course, and distribution of median nerve.

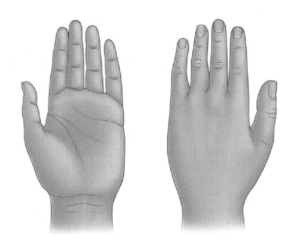

FIGURE 10.28 Autonomous zone of median nerve.

of the ulnar nerve because they involve the digits used in fine volitional activity.

Median nerve injuries often are caused by lacerations, usually in the forearm or wrist. Sunderland pointed out that in the upper arm the nerve can be injured by relatively superficial lacerations, excessively tight tourniquets, and humeral fractures, and when it is injured near the axilla, the ulnar and musculocutaneous nerves and the brachial artery also are commonly injured. In the arm, the median nerve may be compressed by the ligament of Struthers. At the elbow, the nerve may be injured in supracondylar fractures and posterior dislocations of the elbow.

■ EXAMINATION

Variations in the sensory supply of the median nerve also may be confusing, but usually the volar surface of the thumb, of the index and middle fingers, and of the radial half of the ring finger and the dorsal surfaces of the distal phalanges of the index and middle fingers are supplied by the median nerve. The smallest autonomous zone of the median nerve covers the dorsal and volar surfaces of the distal phalanges of the index and middle fingers (Fig. 10.28). The iodine starch test or ninhydrin print test may be helpful in diagnosis. Autonomic changes, such as anhidrosis, atrophy of the skin, and narrowing of the digits because of atrophy of the pulp, also are valuable signs of sensory deficit.

■ TREATMENT

Operative treatment may be indicated for most median nerve lesions. Surgical exploration and decompression of the median nerve for refractory pronator teres syndrome, as reported by Hartz et al. and by Johnson, Spinner, and Shrewsbury, have been successful in relieving symptoms in 80% to 92% of patients. Some persistence of symptoms has been reported in 66% of patients. In patients who have

symptoms of carpal tunnel syndrome and pronator teres syndrome, particular attention should be paid to the nerve conduction studies during preoperative planning. If the nerve conduction test is positive for carpal tunnel syndrome, we agree in recommending carpal tunnel release in anticipation that the proximal symptoms will resolve. If the nerve conduction test is negative for carpal tunnel syndrome, we recommend proximal median nerve exploration and proximal decompression as the initial procedure of choice. For the anterior interosseous syndrome, Spinner recommended the following plan. If the onset of paralysis has been spontaneous, the initial treatment is nonoperative. Surgical exploration is indicated in the absence of clinical or EMG improvement after 12 weeks. If an anterior interosseous nerve injury is caused by a penetrating wound, primary repair is recommended. In irreparable injury to the nerve, tendon transfers are indicated.

APPROACH TO THE MEDIAN NERVE

TECHNIQUE 10.14

- To expose the median nerve, use the same approach as that for the ulnar nerve in the arm and at the elbow and avoid crossing the folds of the antecubital fossa (see Fig. 10.25).
- To expose the median nerve in the forearm, continue the incision from the medial epicondyle onto the volar aspect of the forearm and distally over the course of the nerve. In approaching the wrist, curve it toward the radial side (or if exploration of the median and ulnar nerves is indicated, curve it toward the ulnar side). As the flexor creases of the wrist are reached, return the incision along one of them to the middle of the wrist. If the nerve is to be explored distal to the wrist, extend the incision down the thenar crease.
- Deepen the incision through the fascia along the course of the nerve. To accomplish this at the elbow, undermine the skin flap widely.
- In the arm, retract the brachial artery and vein medially to expose the nerve on the lateral aspect of the neurovascular bundle.

- At the junction of the middle and distal thirds of the arm, the nerve crosses to the medial side of the artery, usually coursing posteriorly, although occasionally anteriorly to it.
- The nerve enters the forearm beneath the lacertus fibrosus medial to the artery and then courses between the two heads of the pronator teres and continues distally in the forearm beneath the flexor sublimis, lying on the flexor profundus. Approaching the wrist, the nerve becomes more superficial, lies beneath the tendon of the flexor carpi radialis, and is easily found if approached between this tendon and that of the palmaris longus.
- At the elbow, expose the nerve by incising the fibers of the lacertus fibrosus at its attachment to the fascia over the pronator-flexor group.
- Dissect the fascia radially from this group of muscles, and incise it distally and radially along the proximal border of the pronator teres and then distally across this muscle and along the medial side of the flexor carpi radialis. The pronator teres may be widely mobilized and separated from the flexor carpi radialis, permitting easy exposure of the nerve and making closure easier later.
- Expose the nerve where it emerges from beneath the fibers of the flexor digitorum sublimis. Trace the nerve proximally by retracting the flexor carpi radialis laterally and the pronator proximally and by separating the fibers of the flexor digitorum sublimis. In this way, the nerve can be exposed over its entire course.
- As an alternative, cut the radial origin of the flexor digitorum sublimis in line with the nerve and sever the pronator teres by a Z-shaped incision near its insertion (Fig. 10.29).
- The median nerve gives off no branches in the upper arm.
- The branches to the pronator teres and flexor carpi radialis emerge as the nerve courses beneath the lacertus fibrosus. Usually, two branches go to the pronator: one to the superficial head and one to the deep head. Also, several branches go to the flexor carpi radialis and palmaris longus, one to the flexor sublimis, and one to the profundus.
- The anterior interosseous nerve emerges from the posteromedial side of the nerve after passing through the two heads of the pronator teres and supplies the flexor pollicis longus, the radial half of the flexor profundus, and the pronator quadratus. Farther distally, several more branches are given off to the flexor digitorum sublimis. No other significant branches are given off until the nerve enters the hand.
- When exposure of the anterior interosseous nerve deep to the pronator teres is required, or when anterior transposition of the median nerve is preferred, a method whereby the pronator teres insertion is released and is repaired by Z-plasty or a tongue-in-groove suture after the median nerve has been transposed is suitable.
- In decompressing the median nerve for pronator teres syndrome, explore and release all points of potential compression.
- If a ligament of Struthers is encountered, excise it from its origin on the supracondylar process to its insertion on the medial epicondyle.
- Divide the lacertus fibrosus, and trace the median nerve through the two heads of the pronator teres.
- Release any intermuscular tendinous bands within or under the pronator and fascial constricting bands between the superficial and deep heads of the muscle.
- If necessary, divide the deep head of the pronator teres.
- Alternatively, the superficial head of the pronator teres can be excised from its radial insertion, although this rarely is necessary in our experience.
- Retract the superficial head of the pronator teres anteriorly, distally, and ulnarward to allow exploration of the nerve into the flexor digitorum sublimis.
- Divide the aponeurotic arch, which commonly is encountered as the median nerve enters the sublimis muscle.
- If the Gantzer muscle is encountered, resect any proximal fibrous bands that may be compressing the median nerve.

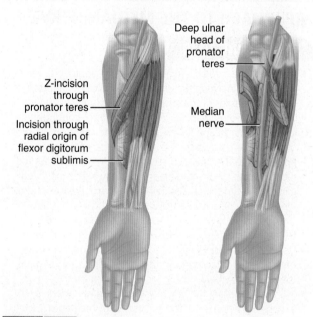

Z-incision through pronator teres

Incision through radial origin of flexor digitorum sublimis

Deep ulnar head of pronator teres

Median nerve

FIGURE 10.29 Alternative method of exposing median nerve throughout forearm (see text). **SEE TECHNIQUE 10.14.**

■ METHODS OF CLOSING GAPS

Interfascicular nerve grafting is the preferred method for closing gaps; however, the following techniques may be helpful at times. Extensively mobilizing the nerve, stripping back its branches in the main trunk, and flexing the wrist and elbow can allow closure of a gap of 8 to 10 cm proximal and of 12 to 15 cm distal to the elbow. Transposing the nerve anterior to the pronator teres gains more length if the lesion is distal to this muscle. The ease with which the nerve can be transposed anteriorly depends to some extent on the level at which the branches to the flexor-pronator group emerge. When they emerge distally, transposing the nerve is much more difficult than when they emerge more proximally. Transposition usually is necessary in large destructive wounds in the middle of the forearm. In these wounds, most of the branches to the flexor sublimis usually are destroyed and need not be considered.

Transposition is accomplished by stripping the branches to the pronator teres, the flexor carpi radialis, the palmaris longus, and the anterior interosseous nerve intraneurally from the main trunk well proximally in the upper forearm, then by mobilizing the distal end of the nerve all the way to the wrist and beneath the transverse carpal ligament, and then by flexing the wrist and the elbow and suturing the nerve anterior to the flexor-pronator group. By transposition, 2 or 3 cm may be gained in length, permitting neurorrhaphy, which could not be carried out otherwise. If too much tension is placed on the nerve, the fascia and lacertus fibrosus must be closed deep to it, and the nerve is left subcutaneous all the way to the wrist. Release of the deep head of the pronator teres and dissection and placement of the flexor carpi radialis deep to the median nerve may make mobilization and transposition of the nerve to the subcutaneous position easier.

Postoperative care is as described earlier for the ulnar nerve (see Technique 10.12).

■ RESULTS OF SUTURE OF THE MEDIAN NERVE

Motor recovery is crucial after median nerve repair; however, the hand without median nerve sensory supply is almost useless. Even with the best sensory recovery, the patient probably will have difficulty with stereognosis. Under favorable circumstances, about half of the patients with median nerve suture recover sensitivity to pain and touch and some degree of stereognosis. Under the same circumstances, about 90% of these patients recover a useful degree of motor function in the long flexors of the forearm. A much smaller number, perhaps one third, obtain useful recovery in the thenar muscles as well when the lesion is in the upper arm. In more distal lesions, about two thirds attain some useful motor recovery. Between 82% and 90% good and fair motor recovery has been reported and 97% sensory recovery after repair or interfascicular grafting.

■ CRITICAL LIMIT OF DELAY OF SUTURE

Motor recovery in the intrinsic muscles of the hand does not occur if suture is delayed 9 months in high lesions or 12 months in low ones. Useful sensory recovery only rarely occurs after 9 months in high lesions or 12 months in low ones, but it may occur when suture has been delayed 2 years. Zachary found that useful motor recovery cannot be expected after delays of 9 months in lesions above the pronator teres or 32 months in lesions below the flexor pollicis longus. For sensory return in adults, the critical period of delay seemed to be 12 months in lesions above the pronator teres and 9 months in lesions below the flexor pollicis longus. Sensory return in children is possible, however, after longer delays. Inasmuch as sensory recovery is so important, a second operation may be indicated if sensation does not return at the expected time because this is the only way that sensation can be regained.

LUMBAR PLEXUS

The lumbar plexus is formed by the junction of the anterior primary rami of L1, L2, L3, and L4. White rami leave L1 and L2, less often L3, and rarely L4. All nerves receive gray rami from the sympathetic chain. The L4 nerve makes a significant contribution to the formation of the sacral plexus, joining with the L5 anterior primary ramus to form the lumbosacral trunk (Fig. 10.30). The L4 nerve frequently is called the nervus furcalis because of its contribution to the lumbar and sacral plexuses.

The L1 anterior primary ramus extends laterally and divides into the iliohypogastric and ilioinguinal nerves. Its

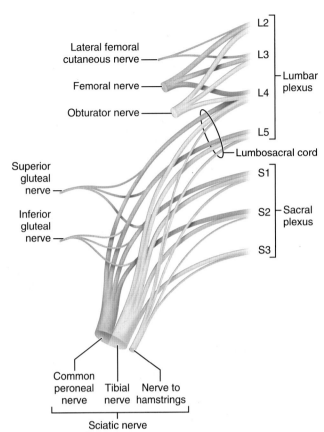

FIGURE 10.30 Simplified diagram of lumbosacral plexus. Contribution of L1 root is not shown. Lumbosacral trunk or cord is shown.

only branch leaves the nerve before this division and joins a fasciculus from the L2 nerve root to form the genitofemoral nerve. The L2, L3, and L4 roots divide into anterior and posterior divisions; the anterior divisions of all join to form the obturator nerve, and the posterior divisions of all join to form the femoral nerve. Smaller segments of the posterior divisions of L2 and L3 unite to form the lateral femoral cutaneous nerve. The lumbar nerve roots occasionally are injured by traction in fractures of the pelvis and dislocations of the sacroiliac joints. Myelography, EMG, and careful physical examination are helpful in evaluating these injuries. In contrast to cervical root avulsions, myelographic evidence of dural diverticula does not correlate well with avulsion of lumbar roots. Although repair of avulsed lumbar roots would seem futile, exploration may be helpful in prognosis. The plexus also may be injured by missile wounds.

The iliohypogastric nerve supplies a small area of skin over the superolateral gluteal region and an area just superior to the pubic bones on the anterior abdominal wall (See Fig. 10.8). The ilioinguinal nerve supplies a segmental strip of skin along the inguinal ligament overlying the symphysis pubis and the skin of the upper scrotum, the root and dorsal aspect of the penis, and the medial aspect of the thigh. The genitofemoral nerve traverses the inguinal canal and supplies the cremaster muscle and the skin of the scrotum and adjacent part of the thigh. From a surgical standpoint, these three nerves are significant because they may be injured in herniorrhaphy, resulting in persistent neuralgic discomfort that may require surgery.

The lateral femoral cutaneous nerve is formed from the roots of L2 and L3. It courses to the region of the anterior superior iliac spine to exit between the lateral attachments of the inguinal ligament and the anterior superior iliac spine and the sartorius muscle. The nerve becomes superficial, penetrating the fascia lata about 10 cm inferior to the inguinal ligament, and supplies the skin of the lateral aspect of the thigh. Compression of the nerve in the region of the anterior superior iliac spine by a tight-fitting brace or corset or injury to the nerve along its subcutaneous course often results in hypesthesias and dysesthesias in the area of its cutaneous distribution. This condition, known as meralgia paresthetica, may develop spontaneously. It often is associated with lumbar disc protrusion and impingement of the nerve, probably being the result of abnormal posture or persistent regional muscle spasm. In most instances, spontaneous recovery may be expected. Occasionally, symptoms are persistent, but rarely are they sufficiently severe to require decompression and neurolysis at the point of exit of the nerve beneath the inguinal ligament.

The obturator nerve is formed by union of the anterior divisions of the L2, L3, and L4 roots. It descends through the pelvis posterior to the common iliac vessels and exits through the obturator foramen to enter the thigh. Its cutaneous branches supply the medial thigh and occasionally the medial aspect of the knee. Its motor component is divided into anterior and posterior divisions. The anterior division supplies the adductor longus, the gracilis, the adductor brevis, the pectineus, and through articular branches the hip joint. The posterior division supplies the obturator externus, the adductor magnus, occasionally the adductor brevis, and through articular branches the knee joint. The obturator nerve may be compressed against the wall of the pelvis by a mass such as a tumor or a fetus. Because of its relationship to the pubis, it may be injured in pelvic fractures or in acutely flexed positions of the hip by being compressed against the pubis. Because of its nearness to the sacroiliac and hip joints, when these joints are diseased or injured, the obturator nerve may be involved, too. Obturator neurectomy sometimes is beneficial in relieving adductor spasm of the hip in spastic conditions that cause a scissoring of the lower extremities. In significant lesions of the obturator nerve, atrophy of the medial aspect of the thigh, sensory disturbances of the distal medial surface of the thigh and the medial surface of the knee, and weakness or paralysis of adduction of the hip are common findings.

FEMORAL NERVE

The femoral nerve is formed by union of the posterior divisions of the L2, L3, and L4 roots. It passes distally deep to the inguinal ligament, remaining lateral to the femoral artery as it enters the thigh. Just distal to the inguinal ligament, it divides into anterior and posterior branches. The anterior branch divides into the intermediate cutaneous and medial cutaneous nerves to supply the anteromedial aspect of the thigh. The motor branches of this part supply the pectineus and sartorius. The posterior branch of the femoral nerve gives off the saphenous nerve, which as the largest cutaneous branch continues distally with the femoral vessels in the subsartorial canal, pierces the fascia along the medial side of the knee to become subcutaneous, and supplies the skin on the anteromedial aspect of the leg distally to the medial malleolus and

arch of the foot. The muscular parts of the posterior branch supply the rectus femoris, the vastus lateralis, the vastus medialis, and the vastus intermedius.

The femoral nerve is often injured by penetrating wounds of the lower abdomen (the small intestine also may be injured at the same time). It also may be injured during an operation in this region. Because they are near each other, the iliac artery and femoral nerve may be injured together. Concern over the hemorrhage and the fact that active extension of the knee rarely is lost despite complete division of the femoral nerve cause injury to this nerve often to be overlooked, as is injury to the musculocutaneous nerve. Femoral neuropathies also may result from hematomas of the abdominal wall caused by hemophilia, anticoagulant therapy, or trauma. Branches of the femoral nerve may be contused or stretched in pelvic fractures. During operations in which the patient is prone, care must be taken to avoid excessive compression of the nerve.

■ EXAMINATION

Atrophy of the anterior thigh muscles is obvious. The patient usually is able to extend the knee slightly against gravity and can stand and walk, especially on level surfaces, because the gastrocnemius, the tensor fasciae latae, the gracilis, and the gluteus maximus aid in stabilizing the limb. The patient usually finds it difficult to go up a hill or stairs. The autonomous zone of supply usually consists of a small area just superior and medial to the patella; the anterior aspect of the thigh and the area supplied by the saphenous nerve show, at most, only varying degrees of hypesthesia. Electrical stimulation with needle electrodes inserted near the femoral nerve is valuable in assessing its function.

■ TREATMENT

APPROACH TO THE FEMORAL NERVE
TECHNIQUE 10.15

- Begin the incision 5 cm proximal to the anterior superior iliac spine, and direct it diagonally and distally to the point where the femoral nerve passes beneath the inguinal ligament. This point usually is 2.5 to 3.0 cm lateral to the femoral artery, which usually is palpable.
- Direct the incision medially for about 2.5 cm to avoid crossing the skin flexion creases at a right angle; continue it distally onto the anterior aspect of the thigh.
- Proximal to the inguinal ligament, deepen the incision through the fascia and the aponeurosis of the external oblique muscle.
- Open the transversalis fascia, and retract the peritoneum medially to expose the iliac fascia.
- The femoral nerve can be palpated beneath this thick fascia; split this fascia along the course of the nerve.
- The nerve can be exposed proximally to the point where it emerges from beneath the lateral edge of the psoas muscle and distally to the point where it passes beneath the inguinal ligament.
- If necessary, divide the inguinal ligament to expose the nerve as it enters the thigh and at once begins to divide into its motor and sensory branches.

■ METHODS OF CLOSING GAPS

Gaps of 8 to 10 cm can be closed without too much difficulty. The nerve is mobilized proximally to the point where it emerges from the lateral border of the psoas muscle and distally by freeing the branches of the nerve in the proximal thigh. The hip is flexed acutely, and the nerve is sutured. The inguinal ligament is reconstructed, and the wound is closed like any lower abdominal incision. A hip spica cast is applied, with the hip acutely flexed.

Postoperative care is as described for the sciatic nerve.

■ RESULTS OF SUTURE OF THE FEMORAL NERVE

No statistically significant information is available regarding grafting for defects in the femoral nerve.

SACRAL PLEXUS

The sacral plexus is formed by the anterior primary rami of L5, S1, S2, and S3 (Fig. 10.30). The anterior primary ramus of L4 contributes a large branch that joins with L5 to form the lumbosacral trunk. A segment of S4 joins a segment of S3 to form the pudendal nerve, which is considered by some to be a part of the sacral plexus, by others to be a separate or pudendal plexus, and by still others to be the superior part of the tiny coccygeal plexus. The anterior primary rami converge and split into anterior and posterior divisions. The trunk formed by the posterior divisions gives off the superior and inferior gluteal nerves and proceeds toward the sciatic notch as the common peroneal part of the sciatic nerve. The trunk formed by the anterior divisions becomes the tibial part of the sciatic nerve and proceeds toward the notch. Smaller branches that rarely are of concern surgically are given off within the pelvis to the quadratus femoris, obturator internus, superior gemellus, and piriformis. Smaller branches of S1, S2, and S3 unite to form the posterior femoral cutaneous nerve (posterior cutaneous nerve of the thigh). This is a relatively large nerve that leaves the sciatic notch medial to the sciatic trunk and lies just deep to the deep fascia as it courses distally in the middle of the thigh posteriorly, roughly overlying the sciatic trunk. It often is called the small sciatic nerve. It innervates the skin of the entire posterior aspect of the thigh and the popliteal fossa. The superior gluteal nerve leaves the sciatic notch proximal to the piriformis and supplies the gluteus medius and gluteus minimus, which function as abductors and internal rotators of the hip. The inferior gluteal nerve leaves the sciatic notch with the sciatic nerve and supplies the gluteus maximus, an important extensor of the hip. Paralysis of this muscle results in difficulty in rising from a squatting or sitting position and in ascending steps or a slope. The sacral plexus may be compressed by pelvic neoplasms or during labor and delivery, especially when forceps are used. Sacral fractures and sacroiliac dislocations also may be complicated by injuries of the sacral plexus.

The sciatic nerve is composed of fibers from L4, L5, S1, S2, and S3 (Fig. 10.31). It leaves the pelvis through the sciatic notch, and at this level the large trunk is easily separated into its common peroneal part laterally and its tibial part medially. Frequently, along the medial side of the trunk a smaller segment, the nerve to the hamstrings, is visible and can be dissected from it easily. Here the sciatic nerve is the largest one in the body, its transverse diameter being 2.0 to 2.5 cm.

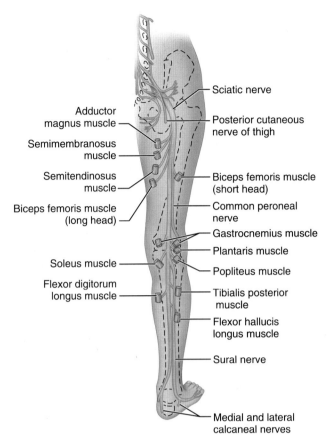

FIGURE 10.31   Origin, course, and distribution of sciatic nerve.

It supplies the muscles of the entire leg and foot and the posterior part of the thigh and carries most of the sensory fibers from these same parts. It descends deep to the gluteus maximus to the level of the inferior gluteal fold, where it lies in the depression between the ischial tuberosity and the greater trochanter. Distal to this level it follows a more superficial course to the distal third of the thigh, where it divides. While coursing through the posterior thigh, its upper part supplies articular branches to the hip joint. The nerve to the hamstrings, visible along the medial aspect of the trunk, sends branches medially to supply the adductor magnus, the semimembranosus, the semitendinosus, and the long head of the biceps femoris. A branch leaves the common peroneal part of the trunk laterally to supply the short head of the biceps femoris. Just proximal to the popliteal fossa, the sciatic nerve divides into its two large divisions: the common peroneal nerve, which deviates laterally, and the larger tibial nerve, which continues distally in the midline of the limb.

SCIATIC NERVE

The sciatic nerve is analogous in its importance in the lower extremity to the brachial plexus in the upper. Usually, it is injured by a gunshot wound to the thigh or buttock. Less often it is injured by posterior dislocation and fracture-dislocation of the hip, by intramuscular injection into the buttock, or during surgery around the hip joint. Sciatic nerve injury by wear debris from long-standing total hip replacements also has been described. When the nerve is injured in dislocations or fracture-dislocations of the hip, the peroneal half of the nerve is injured much more often than is the entire nerve.

Compression caused by anatomic variations in the relationship of the nerve to the gluteal and piriformis muscles and to the sciatic notch may cause sciatic pain. In the thigh, the nerve usually is injured by penetrating wounds and fractures of the femoral shaft. The semimembranosus and semitendinosus rarely are paralyzed by complete division of the proximal one third of the sciatic nerve as the result of a gunshot wound and rarely by a dislocation of the hip.

■ EXAMINATION

Of the muscles innervated by the sciatic nerve that can be tested accurately, those supplied by the tibial component include the hamstrings, the gastrocsoleus, the posterior tibial, and the long flexors of the toes; muscles supplied by the peroneal component include the anterior tibial and the long extensors of the toes (deep peroneal nerve) and the peroneus longus and the peroneus brevis (superficial peroneal nerve). Testing of the intrinsic muscles of the foot except the extensor digitorum brevis is impractical. An extremity in which the sciatic nerve has been divided may develop an equinus deformity of the foot, clawing of the toes, and atrophy of the muscles innervated by the nerve, depending on the level of the injury. Profound weakness of flexion of the knee, inability to dorsiflex the foot or extend the toes, inability to plantar-flex and evert the foot, and inability to flex the toes may be seen. When the peroneal part is involved, the sensory loss is primarily over the lateral aspect of the leg and dorsum of the foot. When the tibial nerve is involved, the sensory deficit is primarily over the plantar aspect of the foot. Anesthesia on the plantar surface may result in chronic ulceration. Autonomic disturbances and chronic pain may follow an injury to the sciatic or tibial nerve. The sciatic nerve is difficult to stimulate in situ because it is so deeply located. Stimulation is significant only when it causes contraction or pain. EMG is helpful in evaluating this nerve.

The autonomous zone of the sciatic nerve (Fig. 10.32) includes the area over the metatarsal heads and over the heel, the lateral and posterior aspects of the sole of the foot, the dorsum of the foot as far medially as the second metatarsal, and a narrow strip up the lateral aspect of the leg. The autonomous zones of the branches of the sciatic nerve—the tibial (branching into the lateral and medial plantar), the common peroneal (branching into the superficial and deep peroneal), and the sural—are smaller and are described later. As in other nerves, the skin resistance test or iodine starch test is helpful.

In multiple wounds, percussing along the course of the nerve to the point where tingling is most pronounced is a fairly accurate method of locating an injury. Exact knowledge of the point of emergence of the various nerve branches is helpful; however, if one attempts to locate an injury by this knowledge alone, one is more likely to err than when using percussion because a branch may be injured after it emerges from the nerve.

If an injury to a branch of the nerve has been caused by external compression, as occurs with a poorly fitted cast or with an unusual posture from crossing the legs, the cause should be corrected. If compression has been of long duration, exploration and neurolysis may be warranted, but the prognosis in these instances is extremely guarded. If a complete division of the sciatic nerve complicates a dislocation or fracture around the hip, exploration of the nerve assists in determining the extent of injury and whether repair is possible. If complete division of the nerve complicates a femoral shaft fracture or fracture-dislocation around the knee, exploration also is justified early when no signs of recovery are apparent. If a sciatic nerve lesion is caused by a penetrating injury, especially if the wound is proximal in the buttock, early exploration and repair may be worthwhile so that the distal structures are denervated for the shortest possible time.

■ TREATMENT

APPROACH TO THE SCIATIC NERVE

TECHNIQUE 10.16

- The sciatic nerve can be exposed easily from its emergence from the sciatic notch to the point of its division into the tibial and peroneal nerves in the popliteal fossa.
- For injuries near the sciatic notch, begin the incision at the posterior superior iliac spine and carry it diagonally distally and laterally in the direction of the fibers of the gluteus maximus to a point about 2.5 cm medial to the greater trochanter (Fig. 10.33). Curve the incision medially, distal to the gluteal fold, as far as the midpoint of the fold, and finally distalward along the posterior aspect of the thigh to a point 10 cm proximal to the skin creases of the popliteal fossa.

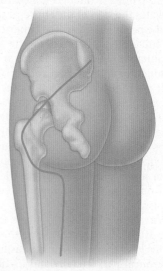

FIGURE 10.33 Skin incision for approach to proximal portion of sciatic nerve extends from posterior superior iliac spine to trochanter and is curved distally along posterior surface of thigh. **SEE TECHNIQUE 10.16.**

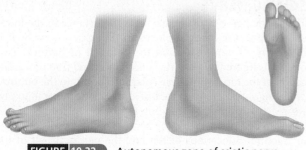

FIGURE 10.32 Autonomous zone of sciatic nerve.

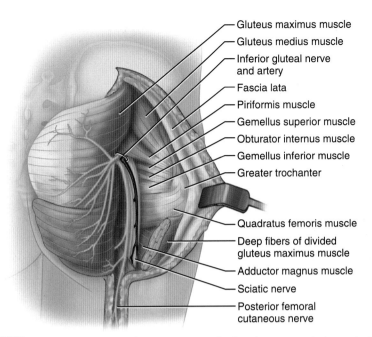

- Gluteus maximus muscle
- Gluteus medius muscle
- Inferior gluteal nerve and artery
- Fascia lata
- Piriformis muscle
- Gemellus superior muscle
- Obturator internus muscle
- Gemellus inferior muscle
- Greater trochanter
- Quadratus femoris muscle
- Deep fibers of divided gluteus maximus muscle
- Adductor magnus muscle
- Sciatic nerve
- Posterior femoral cutaneous nerve

FIGURE 10.34 Surgical anatomy of sciatic nerve and related structures in buttock. **SEE TECHNIQUE 10.16.**

- Deepen the proximal part of the incision through the gluteal fascia, and separate the fibers of the gluteus maximus muscle as far laterally as the greater trochanter.
- Incise the fascia of the thigh longitudinally to the gluteal fold and detach the insertion of the distal fibers of the gluteus maximus from the iliotibial band. The muscle with its nerve and blood supply can be reflected medially to expose the nerve as far proximally as the piriformis (Fig. 10.34).
- Sacrifice the piriformis to expose the nerve as it emerges from the sciatic notch.
- If better exposure of the nerve within the sciatic notch is necessary, remove with a rongeur a part of the sacrum.
- When the injury to the nerve is more distal to the sciatic notch, make the incision over the buttock likewise more distal.
- When the injury is in the thigh, begin the incision at the gluteal fold and continue it distally along the posterior aspect of the thigh, as just described, to a point 10 cm proximal to the knee.
- Open the fascia longitudinally in line with the skin incision.
- Protect the posterior femoral cutaneous nerve, which is just deep to the deep fascia. In the proximal thigh, identify the biceps femoris, retract it medially, and identify the sciatic nerve in the depths of the wound. Distally trace the nerve beneath the biceps to its point of bifurcation.
- For more exposure (Mayfield), curve the distal end of the incision to the lateral aspect of the knee when the peroneal nerve has been injured.
- Pass the incision distally along its course around the neck of the fibula. When the tibial nerve has been injured, pass the incision medially and then a few centimeters distally along the medial aspect of the leg. These incisions have two advantages. First, they do not cross the skin folds of the popliteal fossa; consequently, contractures and ulcerating scars are less likely. Second, closing the wound is easier with the knee flexed.

- When the lesion is located in the middle third of the thigh, a posterolateral approach may be preferable.

■ METHODS OF CLOSING GAPS

Mobilizing the nerve extensively including its two divisions, flexing the knee, and hyperextending the hip allow closure of a gap of 15 cm. When the femur has been fractured and the sciatic nerve divided, it is very important, even in the presence of draining sinuses, to operate on the nerve before the femur has united because, aside from the effect of time on the nerve ends and muscles, the knee may stiffen and it may be impossible to flex it enough to close large defects. Resecting a part of the femur may be necessary to help close the gap. When a fracture is present, such a resection may be justified and can be done with ease. In the absence of a femoral fracture, however, the bone should not be shortened. Instead, autogenous interfascicular nerve grafting may be a reasonable alternative, especially in young patients.

After any neurorrhaphy of the sciatic nerve, the limb should be immobilized in a double spica cast extending from the nipple line to the toes on the affected side and to above the knee on the opposite. On the affected side, the knee is flexed and the hip is extended if necessary. The cast is windowed to allow removal of the sutures after about 10 days. At 6 weeks, the cast is removed and a long leg brace with an adjustable knee hinge is applied so that the knee can be extended gradually during the next 6 weeks. Physical therapy and exercises are used to restore function to joints and soft parts. After extension of the knee is complete, an appropriate brace is applied to compensate for paralysis of the leg. When autogenous grafting has been used in repair of the sciatic nerve, the application of a spica cast after surgery is necessary but maintaining the hip and knee in awkward positions usually is unnecessary; in addition, the cast can be removed when the sutures are removed and motion of the joints can be started.

■ RESULTS OF SUTURE OF THE SCIATIC NERVE

According to Sunderland, the results of suture of the sciatic nerve are poor, especially in distally innervated muscles because of the extensive retrograde neuronal degeneration, intraneural intermixing of regenerating fibers with loss of fiber localization, and degenerative changes in the distal muscles that must remain denervated for a long time. Usually, significant recovery can be expected only in the proximally innervated muscles, especially the hamstring and calf muscles. If sensation returns, it usually is only of a protective nature. Delaria et al. reported 22 sciatic lesions treated surgically: 13 required neurolysis only, whereas nine were treated with nerve grafts. Of the lesions treated by neurolysis, five were excellent (complete recovery of muscles), seven were good, and one was poor. Of the lesions treated by grafting, four were excellent, four were good, and one was poor.

■ CRITICAL LIMIT OF DELAY OF SUTURE

Zachary found that useful motor and sensory recovery is to be anticipated if the sciatic nerve injured high in the thigh or in the buttock is sutured before 12 to 15 months.

COMMON, SUPERFICIAL, AND DEEP PERONEAL NERVES

The common peroneal nerve, a division of the sciatic nerve, is composed of fibers from L4, L5, S1, and S2. It is injured more often than the tibial nerve even where it is part of the sciatic nerve and is injured by trauma around the knee including ruptures of the fibular collateral ligament, by fractures and dislocations of the head of the fibula, by casts, and even by crossing the legs. Bony entrapment of the superficial peroneal nerve after fracture and entrapment by the margins of a deep fascial defect during exercise are other reported causes of injury. Release of compressing structures usually relieves the painful symptoms.

The common peroneal nerve is smaller than the tibial nerve after the two nerves separate near the proximal angle of the popliteal fossa. The former nerve deviates laterally in the popliteal fossa, arches around the posterior aspect of the fibular head, encircles the fibular neck, and divides into the superficial and deep peroneal nerves (Fig. 10.35). The common peroneal nerve itself is relatively short, having only two sensory branches and no motor branches. One sensory branch, the lateral sural cutaneous nerve, supplies the skin along the lateral aspect of the knee and the proximal third of the calf (see Fig. 10.8). The other sensory branch, the peroneal anastomotic branch, joins the tibial anastomotic branch to form the sural nerve, which supplies the skin over the posterolateral aspect of the calf and over the lateral malleolus, the lateral aspect of the foot, and the fourth and fifth toes. As already mentioned, at or just inferior to the fibular neck, the common peroneal nerve divides into its two branches, the superficial and deep peroneal nerves.

The superficial peroneal nerve continues distally in the leg between the peroneus longus and extensor digitorum longus muscles and the intermuscular septum. Along this route, it gives off two motor branches, one each to the peroneus longus and peroneus brevis. It divides into two cutaneous branches that pierce the deep fascia and course distally to supply the skin on the anterior and lateral aspects of the leg and the dorsum of the foot, with the exception of a small wedge-shaped area in the web between the great and second toes.

The deep peroneal nerve passes obliquely distally on the interosseous membrane beneath the extensor digitorum longus. Along this route, it gives off motor branches to the anterior

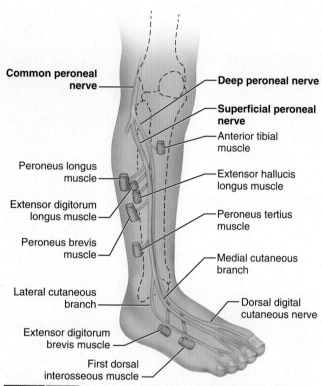

FIGURE 10.35 Common, superficial, and deep peroneal nerves.

Labels: Common peroneal nerve, Deep peroneal nerve, Superficial peroneal nerve, Anterior tibial muscle, Peroneus longus muscle, Extensor hallucis longus muscle, Extensor digitorum longus muscle, Peroneus tertius muscle, Peroneus brevis muscle, Medial cutaneous branch, Lateral cutaneous branch, Dorsal digital cutaneous nerve, Extensor digitorum brevis muscle, First dorsal interosseous muscle

tibial, the extensor digitorum longus, the extensor hallucis longus, the peroneus tertius, the extensor digitorum brevis, and the first dorsal interosseous. Its terminal branch divides into digital cutaneous nerves that supply the web between the great and second toe, the lateral aspect of the dorsum of the great toe, and the medial aspect of the dorsum of the second toe.

■ EXAMINATION

The muscles supplied by the common peroneal nerve that can be tested accurately have been listed previously (see Sciatic Nerve). Typically, injury of the peroneal nerve results in footdrop, which cannot be overcome or disguised by any supplementary or trick movement. The nerve may be stimulated easily in situ at the head of the fibula. The presence and extent of the autonomous zone of this nerve vary, but this zone may have value when present (Fig. 10.36).

■ TREATMENT

APPROACH TO THE COMMON, SUPERFICIAL, AND DEEP PERONEAL NERVES

TECHNIQUE 10.17

- The exposure of the peroneal nerve in the distal thigh and popliteal fossa has been described previously (see Technique 10.16).
- If the nerve is injured at the head of the fibula or distal to it, begin the incision at any point proximal to the injury as required; at the head of the fibula, curve it anteriorly over

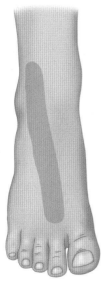

FIGURE 10.36 Autonomous zone of peroneal nerve.

the neck of the fibula and distally along the anterolateral aspect of the leg.
- Deepen it proximally through the fascia and identify the nerve on the medial side of the biceps tendon.
- Trace the nerve distally as it curves around the neck of the fibula between the origin of the peroneus longus and the bone; just distal to this point, it divides into the deep and superficial peroneal nerves. The superficial nerve continues distally in the leg between the peroneus longus and the extensor digitorum longus in the intermuscular septum. The deep nerve passes distally beneath the extensor digitorum longus, whose origin must be freed to expose completely this part of the nerve, from which numerous muscular branches arise; the nerve can be traced distally beneath the anterior tibial just lateral to the anterior tibial artery.

■ METHODS OF CLOSING GAPS

Autogenous interfascicular nerve grafting is the preferred technique for bridging gaps in the peroneal nerve, although mobilizing the nerve extensively and flexing the knee allows closure of a gap of 10 to 12 cm in the popliteal fossa. Distal to the neck of the fibula, length is hard to get. Even here, mobilizing the nerve in the thigh and the leg, stripping up branches in the leg, and flexing the knee allow closure of a considerable gap in either division of the common peroneal nerve. Wood noted that the ipsilateral sural nerve should be harvested for grafting only if sensory function is damaged and the sural nerve graft should be taken from the opposite leg if sensory function ipsilaterally is saved.

Although large gaps can be closed, lines of suture in the peroneal nerve are much more likely to separate than are those in other peripheral nerves, even when it is still a part of the sciatic nerve, presumably because it is especially vulnerable to stress between two bony points—the fibula and pelvis—between which no other soft-tissue structures effectively protect the nerve from tension. In most patients, immobilization in a hip spica cast for 6 weeks after surgery and gradual

extension of the knee during the next 6 weeks prevent such catastrophes. A long leg cast is not enough; the line of suture often separates unless a spica cast is used.

Postoperative care is as described for the sciatic nerve. If autogenous nerve grafting has been used, awkward positioning and prolonged use of casts and braces may not be required.

■ RESULTS OF SUTURE OF THE PERONEAL NERVE

Motor recovery is far more important than sensory recovery because the autonomous zone on the dorsum of the foot is so small. Motor recovery is useful only if it enables the patient to dorsiflex the foot against gravity. Under the most favorable circumstances, that is, after a low lesion with a small gap between the nerve ends and with early suture, 60% to 70% of patients reach this level of motor recovery. The percentage of success decreases as circumstances become less favorable but does not reach the point that suture is not worthwhile unless surgery is delayed too long. A second operation to resuture the nerve after initial failure to obtain motor recovery rarely is indicated. In a 2014 evidence-based structured review to assess the results of common peroneal nerve repair, George and Boyce concluded that common peroneal nerve repair was worthwhile in approximately half of all cases. They suggested that the results of common peroneal nerve repair will be suboptimal if surgery is performed more than 12 months after injury or if a graft of more than 12 cm is required.

■ CRITICAL LIMIT OF DELAY OF SUTURE

As mentioned earlier, useful motor function in the peroneal nerve is not to be expected when suture has been delayed 12 months after injury.

■ TENDON TRANSFER FOR PERONEAL NERVE PARALYSIS

Tendon transfer for peroneal nerve paralysis is discussed in other chapter.

TIBIAL NERVE

The tibial nerve, composed of fibers from L4, L5, S1, S2, and S3, is the larger and more important of the two divisions of the sciatic nerve. It begins in the distal third of the thigh just proximal to the popliteal fossa as the common peroneal nerve leaves the sciatic nerve to course laterally. It continues distally through the middle of the popliteal fossa and supplies branches to the plantaris, the soleus, the popliteus, and both heads of the gastrocnemius before passing beneath the arch of the soleus (Fig. 10.37). Also given off within the popliteal fossa is the tibial anastomotic branch, which joins the peroneal anastomotic branch to form the sural nerve already described. Deep to the soleus, the tibial nerve courses straight distally on the posterior tibial. It supplies motor branches to the posterior tibial, flexor hallucis longus, and flexor digitorum longus. In the distal calf, it gives off medial calcaneal branches to supply the skin on the medial aspect of the heel. The nerve passes beneath the laciniate ligament posterior and inferior to the medial malleolus and divides into the medial and lateral plantar nerves, which innervate the intrinsic muscles and the skin of the plantar surface of the foot much the same as the median and ulnar nerves innervate the hand. Injuries to the tibial nerve are severely disabling because of the large sensory deficit on the plantar surface of the foot.

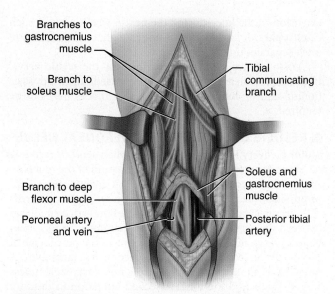

FIGURE 10.37 Anatomy of tibial nerve in popliteal space and proximal third of leg (see text for discussion of exposure).

Labels on figure:
- Branches to gastrocnemius muscle
- Branch to soleus muscle
- Branch to deep flexor muscle
- Peroneal artery and vein
- Tibial communicating branch
- Soleus and gastrocnemius muscle
- Posterior tibial artery

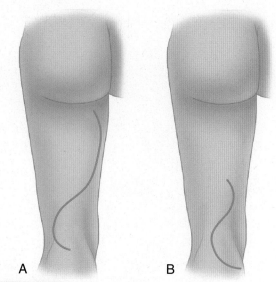

FIGURE 10.38 **A,** Mayfield incision for exposure of nerves in popliteal space. **B,** Ulceration and contracture are likely from incisions across skin folds.

Many such injuries are also associated with causalgia. The effect of a complete tibial nerve lesion on the function of the foot is comparable in importance to that of combined median and ulnar nerve lesions on function of the hand.

In the popliteal fossa, the tibial nerve, although protected by a muscular covering, may be injured in dislocations of the knee. In these instances, vascular injuries also may be present and careful evaluation is necessary. Deep to the soleus muscle, the tibial nerve most often is injured by penetrating wounds. Suture of the nerve distal to the muscular branches may result in disabling plantar hyperesthesia. It is worthwhile, however, to attempt such repair, especially in children and young adults, to prevent or minimize trophic ulceration on the plantar surface of the foot. Although division of the sural nerve may result in a troublesome neuroma, it rarely causes a severe clinical problem. Compression of this nerve at the lateral aspect of the ankle has been described, resulting in pain, paresthesias, dysesthesias, and hypesthesias. Relief was achieved by excision of a ganglion or release of a posttraumatic scar. On the medial side of the ankle, the tibial nerve may be compressed in the tarsal tunnel between the laciniate ligament and the medial surface of the talus distal to the medial malleolus.

■ EXAMINATION

The muscles supplied by this nerve that can be accurately examined were described in the discussion of the sciatic nerve. The autonomous zone of the tibial nerve (including the medial sural cutaneous branch) varies but generally includes the sole of the foot (except the medial border of the instep), the lateral surface of the heel, and the plantar surface of the toes. Because the nerve is deep in the popliteal fossa, stimulating the nerve in this area is not always dependable and, consequently, EMG is indicated. The posterior tibial, flexor digitorum longus, and flexor hallucis longus are supplied by branches of the tibial nerve after the nerve passes deep to the arch of the soleus muscle. The flexor digitorum longus and flexor hallucis longus can be difficult to test, but the tendon of the flexor hallucis longus can be palpated posterior to the medial malleolus as it

passes to cross the medial aspect of the plantar arch. Atrophy of the intrinsic muscles of the foot may allow palpation of the flexor digitorum longus tendons; otherwise, this muscle may not be palpable for testing. The autonomous zone of the tibial nerve as it passes deep to the soleus muscle is smaller than that of the nerve as it passes through the popliteal fossa because the sural nerve is excluded. Although EMG may be necessary for evaluating injury to the tibial nerve beneath the soleus, the nerve may be stimulated with relative ease at the posterior aspect of the medial malleolus.

■ TREATMENT
▌ APPROACH TO THE TIBIAL NERVE IN THE POPLITEAL FOSSA

The tibial nerve can be exposed in the popliteal fossa by the incision and the approach described for the sciatic nerve. As usual, crossing the skin folds in the popliteal fossa should be avoided, and if necessary the skin incision can be extended along the medial side of the hamstring tendons and distally on the leg just posterior to the medial border of the tibia (Fig. 10.38). Methods of closing gaps in this part of the nerve, immobilization, and care after surgery are the same as those described for the sciatic nerve.

APPROACH TO THE TIBIAL NERVE DEEP TO THE SOLEUS MUSCLE

TECHNIQUE 10.18

- Explore the tibial nerve deep to the soleus muscle or in the distal third of the leg through a longitudinal incision beginning posterior to the subcutaneous part of the tibia on the medial side of the leg and continuing parallel to the tibia distally to the ankle.
- Deepen the incision through the superficial fascia, and identify and retract laterally the Achilles tendon.

- Expose the deep fascia through which the nerve and artery can be easily palpated.
- Open this fascia longitudinally, and identify the nerve lateral to the artery. Distally this part of the nerve can be easily mobilized to the ankle, but proximally it is quite deep beneath the soleus muscle on the posterior tibial between the flexor hallucis longus laterally and the flexor digitorum longus medially.
- Proximal to the middle of the leg, the origin of the soleus from the tibia interferes with exposure and must be sectioned and reflected laterally to expose the tibial nerve as it comes under the arch of the soleus. Exposing and mobilizing the nerve require great care because of the many vessels with which it is intimately associated.
- Troublesome bleeding from these vessels can be minimized by using a pneumatic tourniquet and by wide exposure of the nerve in the distal two thirds of the leg.

■ METHODS OF CLOSING GAPS

Autogenous interfascicular grafting may prove to be a satisfactory alternative to awkward and sometimes disabling positioning when gaps are to be closed in the tibial nerve. Although the lesion itself can be fully exposed, a significant gap rarely can be closed by mobilizing this part of the nerve alone. Plantarflexing the foot to obtain length may lead to disabling equinus contracture of the ankle and is not recommended. Exposing and mobilizing the proximal part of the tibial nerve in the popliteal fossa or even farther proximally as already described are almost always necessary. By connecting the two incisions, the nerve can be exposed and mobilized from the thigh to the ankle. In addition, all muscular branches must be stripped back intraneurally for several centimeters by careful dissection. Flexing the knee to 90 degrees allows closure of a gap of 10 to 12 cm. Occasionally, more length can be obtained by transposing the nerve between the soleus and the gastrocnemius or superficial to both of these muscles. This is especially applicable when the distal muscular branches to the flexor hallucis and flexor digitorum longus have been destroyed, although it can be done with these branches intact if they are dissected proximally to the popliteal fossa. After one is certain that the defect can be closed, but before the nerve is sutured, especially if tension on the line of suture is likely, the incision in the popliteal fossa should be closed because closing the fascia may reduce slightly the length regained.

If the nerve has been transposed between the soleus and the gastrocnemius or superficial to both, the soleus also should be sutured to its origin before the nerve is sutured. If transposition has been unnecessary, the soleus is sutured after neurorrhaphy.

Postoperative care is as described for the sciatic nerve.

■ RESULTS OF SUTURE OF THE TIBIAL NERVE

Motor and sensory return is crucial. Even a slight return of pain sensation is valuable because an anesthetic foot tends to develop trophic lesions.

REFERENCES

GENERAL

Bergquist ER, Hammert WC: Timing and appropriate use of electrodiagnostic studies, *Hand Clin* 29:363, 2013.

Birch R, Eardley WGP, Ramasamy A, et al.: Nerve injuries sustained during warfare. Part I: Epidemiology, *J Bone Joint Surg* 94B:523, 2012.

Birch R, Eardley WGP, Ramasamy A, et al.: Nerve injuries sustained during warfare. Part II: Outcomes, *J Bone Joint Surg* 94B:529, 2012.

Boyd KU, Nimigan AS, Mackinnon SE: Nerve reconstruction in the hand and upper extremity, *Clin Plast Surg* 38:643, 2011.

Ducic I, Fu R, Iorio ML: Innovative treatment of peripheral nerve injuries. Combined reconstructive concepts, *Ann Plast Surg* 68:180, 2012.

Forli A, Bouyer M, Airbert M, et al.: Upper limb nerve transfers: a review, *Hand Surg Rehabil* 36:151, 2017.

Griffin JW, Hogan MV, Chhabra AB, Deal DN: Current concepts review. Peripheral nerve repair and reconstruction, *J Bone Joint Surg* 95A:2144, 2013.

Hoyng SA, Tannemaat MR, De Winter F, et al.: Nerve surgery and gene therapy: a neurobiological and clinical perspective, *J Hand Surg Eur* 36:735, 2011.

Isaacs J: Treatment of acute peripheral nerve injuries: current concepts, *J Hand Surg Am* 35A:491, 2010.

Issacs J: Major peripheral nerve injuries, *Hand Clin* 29:371, 2013.

Kaiser R, Ullas G, Havránek P, et al.: Current concepts in peripheral nerve injury repair, *Acta Chir Plast* 59:85, 2017.

Lee EY, Karjalainen TV, Sebastin SJ, et al.: The value of the tender muscle sign in detecting motor recovery after peripheral nerve reconstruction, *J Hand Surg Am* 40:433, 2015.

Lee EY, Sebastin SJ, Cheah A, et al.: Upper extremity innervation patterns and clinical implications for nerve and tendon transfer, *Plast Reconstr Surg* 140:1209, 2017.

Menorca RMG, Fussell TS, Elfar JC: Nerve physiology: mechanisms of injury and recovery, *Hand Clin* 29:317, 2013.

Missios S, Bekelis K, Spinner RJ: Traumatic peripheral nerve injuries in children: epidemiology and socioeconomics, *J Neurosurg Pediatr* 14:688, 2014.

Moore AM, Wagner IJ, Fox IK: Nerve repair in complex wounds of the upper extremity, *Semin Plast Surg* 29:40, 2015.

Novak CB, Anastakis DJ, Beaton DE, et al.: Relationships among pain disability, pain intensity, illness intrusiveness, and upper extremity disability in patients with traumatic peripheral nerve injury, *J Hand Surg Am* 35A:1633, 2010.

Novak CB, von der Heyde RL: Evidence and techniques in rehabilitation following nerve injuries, *Hand Clin* 29:383, 2013.

Ring D: Symptoms and disability after major peripheral nerve injury, *Hand Clin* 29:421, 2013.

Wang Y, Sunitha M, Chung KC: How to measure outcomes of peripheral nerve surgery, *Hand Clin* 29:349, 2013.

Zhu J, Liu F, Li D, et al.: Preliminary study of the types of traumatic peripheral injuries by ultrasound, *Eur Radiol* 21:1097, 2011.

Zuckerman SL, Kerr ZY, Pierpoint L, et al.: An 11-year analysis of peripheral nerve injuries in high school sports, *Phys Sportsmed* 1–7, 2018, [Epub ahead of print].

COMPLEX REGIONAL PAIN SYNDROME

Cappello ZJ, Kasdan ML, Louis DS: Meta-analysis of imaging techniques for the diagnosis of complex regional pain syndrome type I, *J Hand Surg Am* 37A:288, 2012.

Gierthmülen J, Maier C, Baron R, et al.: Sensory signs in complex regional pain syndrome and peripheral nerve injury, *Pain* 153:765, 2012.

Harden RN, Bruehl S, Perez RS, et al.: Validation of proposed diagnostic criteria (the "Budapest Criteria") for complex regional pain syndrome, *Pain* 150:268, 2010.

Marinus J, Moseley GL, Birklein F, et al.: Clinical features and pathophysiology of complex regional pain syndrome, *Lancet Neurol* 10:637, 2011.

Patterson RW, Li Z, Smith BP, et al.: Complex regional pain syndrome of the upper extremity, *J Hand Surg Am* 36A:1553, 2011.

Straube S, Derry S, Moore RA, Cole P: Cervico-thoracic or lumbar sympathectomy for neuropathic pain and complex regional pain syndrome, *Cochrane Database Syst Rev* 9:CD002918, 2013.

Xu J, Herndon C, Anderson S, et al.: Intravenous ketamine infusion for complex regional pain syndrome: survey, consensus, and a reference protocol, *Pain Med*, 2018, [Epub ahead of print].

Zyluk A, Mosiejczuk H: A comparison of the accuracy of two sets of diagnostic criteria in the early detection of complex regional pain syndrome following surgical treatment of distal radial fractures, *J Hand Surg Eur* 38:609, 2012.

Zyluk A, Puchalski P: Complex regional pain syndrome: observations on diagnosis, treatment and definition of a new subgroup, *J Hand Surg Eur* 38:599, 2012.

CLINICAL DIAGNOSIS OF NERVE INJURIES

Lee J, Bidwell T, Metcalfe R: Ultrasound in pediatric peripheral nerve injuries: can this affect our surgical decision making? A preliminary report, *J Pediatr Orthop* 33:152, 2013.

SURGICAL TECHNIQUE

Bassilios Habre S, Bone G, Jing XL, et al.: The surgical management of nerve gaps: present and future, *Ann Plast Surg* 80:252, 2018.

Chhabra A, Williams EH, Wang KC, et al.: MR neurography of neuromas related to nerve injury and entrapment with surgical correlation, *AJNR Am J Neuroradiol* 31:1362, 2010.

Cho MS, Rinker BD, Weber RV, et al.: Functional outcome following nerve repair in the upper extremity using processed nerve allograft, *J Hand Surg Am* 37:2340, 2012.

Gao W, Liu Q, Li S, et al.: End-to-side neurorrhaphy for nerve repair and function rehabilitation, *J Surg Res* 197:427, 2015.

George SC, Boyce DE: An evidence-based structured review to assess the results of common peroneal nerve repair, *Plast Reconstr Surg* 134:302e, 2014.

Koenig RW, Schmidt TE, Heinen CPG, et al.: Intraoperative high-resolution ultrasound: a new technique in the management of peripheral nerve disorders, *J Neurosurg* 114:514, 2011.

Kubiak CA, Kung TA, Brown DL, et al.: State-of-the-art techniques in treating peripheral nerve inujury, *Plast Reconstr Surg* 141:702, 2018.

Rinker B: Nerve transfers in the upper extremity: a practical user's guide, *Ann Plast Surg* 74(Suppl 4):S222, 2015.

Tung TH, Mackinnon SE: Nerve transfers: indications techniques and outcomes, *J Hand Surg Am* 35A:332, 2010.

Wali AR, Park CC, Brown JM, et al.: Analyzing cost-effectiveness of ulnar and median nerve transfers to regain forearm flexion, *Neurosurg Focus* 42:E11, 2017.

Wang E, Inaba K, Byerly S, et al.: Optimal timing for repair of peripheral nerve injuries, *J Trauma Acute Care Surg* 83:875, 2017.

Zhang SC, Ji F, Tong DK, Li M: Side-to-side neurorrhaphy for high-level peripheral nerve injuries, *Acta Neurochir (Wien)* 154:257, 2012.

NERVE REPAIR–TECHNIQUE

Ahmad I, Mir MA, Khan AH: An evaluation of different bridging techniques for short nerve gaps, *Ann Plast Surg* 79:482, 2017.

Braga Silva B, Marchese GM, Cauduro CG, et al.: Nerve conduits for treating peripheral nerve injuries: a systematic literature review, *Hand Surg Rehabil* 36:71, 2017.

Gesslbauer B, Furtmüller GJ, Schuhfried O, et al.: Nerve grafts bridging the thenar branch of the median nerve to the ulnar nerve to enhance nerve recovery: a report of three cases, *J Hand Surg Eur* 42:281, 2017.

Rbia N, Shin AY: The role of nerve graft substitutes in motor and mixed motor/sensory peripheral nerve injuries, *J Hand Surg Am* 42:367, 2017.

Rinker B, Zoldos J, Weber RV, et al.: Use of processed nerve allografts to repair nerve injuries greater than 25 mm in the hand, *Ann Plast Surg* 78(6S Suppl 5):S292, 2017.

CERVICAL PLEXUS (SPINAL ACCESSORY NERVE)

Bhandari PS, Deb P: Posterior approach for both spinal accessory nerve to suprascapular nerve and triceps branch to axillary nerve for upper plexus injuries, *J Hand Surg Am* 38:168, 2013.

Cambon-Binder A, Preure L, Dubert-Khalifa H, et al.: Spinal accessory nerve repair using a direct nerve transfer from the upper trunk results with 2 years follow-up, *J Hand Surg Eur* 43:589, 2018.

Camp SJ, Birch R: Injuries to the spinal accessory nerve: a lesson to surgeons, *J Bone Joint Surg Br* 93:62, 2011.

Göransson H, Leppänen OV, Vastamäki M: Patient outcome after surgical management of the spinal accessory nerve injury: a long-term follow-up study, *SAGE Open Med* 4: 2050312116645731, 2016.

Maldonado AA, Spinner RJ: Lateral pectoral nerve transfer for spinal accessory nerve injury, *J Neurosurg Spine* 26:112, 2017.

Restrepo CE, Tubbs RS, Spinner RJ: Expanding what is know of the anatomy of the spinal accessory nerve, *Clin Anat* 28:467, 2015.

SUPRASCAPULAR NERVE

Cabbad NC, Nuland KS, Pothula A: Intraoperative fluoroscopic imaging for suprascapular nerve localization during spinal accessory nerve to suprascapular nerve transfer, *J Hand Surg Am* 42:668.e1, 2017.

Yao K, Yew WP: Suprascapular nerve injury: a cause to consider in shoulder pain and dysfunction, *J Back Musculoskelet Rehabil*, 2016, [Epub ahead of print].

LONG THORACIC NERVE

Nath RK, Somasundaram C: Meta-analysis of long thoraqcic nerve decompression and neurolysis versus muscle and tendon transfer operative treatments of winging scapula, *Plast Reconstr Surg Glob Open* 5:e1481, 2017.

Schippert DW, Li A: Supraclavicular long thoracic nerve decompression for traumatic scapular winging, *J Surg Orthop Adv* 22:219, 2013.

AXILLARY NERVE

Dahlin LB, Cöster M, Björkman A, Backman C: Axillary nerve injury in young adults—an overlooked diagnosis? Early results of nerve reconstruction and nerve transfers, *J Plast Surg Hand Surg* 46:257, 2012.

Koshy JC, Agrawal NA, Seruya M: Nerve transfer versus interpositional nerve graft reconstruction for posttraumatic isolated axillary nerve injuries: a systematic review, *Plast Reconstr Surg* 140:953, 2017.

Wolfe SW, Johnsen PH, Lee SK, Feinberg JH: Long-nerve grafts and nerve transfers demonstrate comparable outcomes for axillary nerve injuries, *J Hand Surg Am* 39:1351, 2014.

MUSCULOCUTANEOUS NERVE

Leland HA, Aadgoli B, Gould DJ, et al.: Investigation into the optimal number of intercostal nerve transfers for musculocutaneous nerve reinnervation: a systematic review, *Hand (N Y)* 13:621, 2018.

O'Gorman CM, Kassardjian C, Sorenson EJ: Musculocutaneous neuropathy, *Muscle Nerve* 58:726, 2018.

RADIAL NERVE

Othman AM: Arthroscopic versus percutaneous release of common extensor origin for treatment of chronic tennis elbow, *Arch Orthop Trauma Surg* 131:383, 2011.

Pan CH, Chuang DC, Rodriguez-Lorenzo A: Outcomes of nerve reconstruction for radial nerve injuries based on the level of injury in 244 operative cases, *J Hand Surg Eur* 35:385, 2010.

Pet MA, Lipira AB, Ko JH: Nerve transfers for the restoration of wrist, finger, and thumb extension after high radial nerve injury, *Hand Clin* 32:191, 2016.

ULNAR NERVE

Choudhry IK, Bracey DN, Hutchinson ID, Li Z: Comparison of transposition techniques to reduce gap associated with high ulnar nerve lesions, *J Hand Surg Am* 39:2460, 2014.

Cobb TK: Endoscopic cubital tunnel release, *J Hand Surg Am* 35A:1690, 2010.

Dützmann S, Martin KD, Sobottka S, et al.: Open vs retractor-endoscopic in situ decompression of the ulnar nerve in cubital tunnel syndrome: a retrospective cohort study, *Neurosurgery* 72:604, 2013.

Kokkalis ZT, Efstathopoulos DG, Papanastassiou ID, et al.: Ulnar nerve injuries in Guyon Canal: a report of 32 cases, *Microsurgery* 32:296, 2012.

Ochi K, Horiuchi Y, Tanabe A, et al.: Comparison of shoulder internal rotation test with the elbow flexion test in the diagnosis of cubital tunnel syndrome, *J Hand Surg Am* 36:782, 2011.

Palmer BA, Hughes TB: Cubital tunnel syndrome, *J Hand Surg Am* 35:153, 2010.

Sallam AA, El-Deeb MS, Imam MA: Nerve transfer versus nerve graft for reconstruction of high ulnar nerve injuries, *J Hand Surg Am* 42:265, 2017.

MEDIAN NERVE

Andrea A, Gonzales JR, Iwanaga J, et al.: Median nerve palsies due to injections: a review, *Cureus* 9:e1287, 2017.

Bertelli JA, Soldado F, Lehn VL, et al.: Reappraisal of clinical deficits following high median nerve injuries, *J Hand Surg Am* 41:13, 2016.

Bertelli JA, Soldado F, Rodrigues-Baeza A, et al.: Transfer of the motor branch of the abductor digiti quinti for thenar muscle reinnervation in high medial nerve injuries, *J Hand Surg Am* 43:8, 2018.

Franco MJ, Nguyen DC, Phillips BZ, et al.: Intraneural medial nerve anatomy and implications for treating mixed median nerve injury in the hand, *Hand (N Y)* 11:416, 2016.

Gesslbauer B, Furtmüller GJ, Schuhfried O, et al.: Nerve grafts bridging the thenar branch of the median nerve to the ulnar nerve to enhance nerve recovery: a report of three cases, *J Hand Surg Eur* 42:281, 2017.

Pan TJ, White RJ, Zhang C, et al.: Baseline characteristics of the median nerve on ultrasound examination, *Hand (N Y)* 11:353, 2016.

Pederson WC: Median nerve injury and repair, *J Hand Surg Am* 39:1216, 2014.

Pulikkottil BJ, Schub M, Kadow TR, et al: Correlating median nerve cross-sectional area with nerve conduction studies, *J Hand Surg Am* 41:958, 2016.

Soldado F, Bertelli JA, Ghizoni MF: High median nerve injury: motor and sensory nerve transfers to restore function, *Hand Clin* 32:209, 2016.

LUMBAR PLEXUS (FEMORAL NERVE)

Fleischman AN, Rothman RH, Paravizi J: Femoral nerve palsy following total hip arthroplasty: incidence and course of recovery, *J Arthroplasty* 33:1194, 2019.

Patton RS, Runner RP, Lyons RJ, et al.: Clinical outcomes of patients with lateral femoral cutaneous nerve injury after direct anterior total hip arthroplasty, *J Arthroplasty* 33:2919, 2018.

Pritchett JW: Outcome of surgery for nerve injury following total hip arthroplasty, *Int Orthop* 42:2879, 2018.

SACRAL PLEXUS (SCIATIC NERVE, PERONEAL NERVES, TIBIAL NERVE)

Emamhadi M, Bakhshayesh B, Andalib S: Surgical outcome of foot drop caused by common peroneal nerve injuries: is the glass half full or half empty? *Acta Neurochir (Wein)* 158:1133, 2016.

Ferris S, Maciburko SJ: Partial tibial nerve transfer to tibialis anterior for traumatic peroneal nerve palsy, *Microsurgery* 37:596, 2017.

Immerman I, Price AE, Alfonso I, et al.: Lower extremity nerve trauma, *Bull Hosp Jt Dis* 72:43, 2013.

Ribak S, Fonesca JR, Tietzmann A, et al.: The anatomy and morphology of the superficial peroneal nerve, *J Recontr Microsurg* 32:271, 2016.

Ridley TJ, McCarthy MA, Bollier MJ, et al.: The incidence and clinical outcomes of peroneal nerve injuries associated with posterolatral corner injuries of the knee, *Knee Surg Sports Traumatol Arthrosc* 26:806, 2018.

Souter J, Swong K, McCoyd M, et al: Surgical results of common peroneal nerve neuroplasty at lateral fibular neck, *World Neurosurg* 112:e465, 20118.

The complete list of references is available online at Expert Consult.com.

PART **III**

AMPUTATIONS

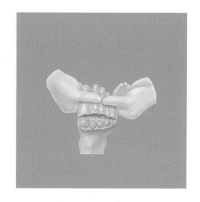

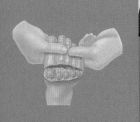

CHAPTER 11

GENERAL PRINCIPLES OF AMPUTATIONS

Patrick C. Toy

INCIDENCE AND INDICATIONS	568
Peripheral vascular disease	569
Trauma	569
Burns	571
Frostbite	571
Infection	572
Tumors	573

SURGICAL PRINCIPLES OF AMPUTATIONS	574
Determination of amputation level	574
Technical aspects	575
Skin and muscle flaps	575
Hemostasis	576
Nerves	576
Bone	576
Open amputations	576
Postoperative care	577

COMPLICATIONS	578
Hematoma	579
Infection	579
Wound necrosis	579
Contractures	579
Pain	579
Dermatologic problems	581
AMPUTATIONS IN CHILDREN	581

Amputation is the most ancient of surgical procedures. Advancements in surgical technique and prosthetic design historically were stimulated by the aftermath of war. Early surgical amputation was a crude procedure by which a limb was rapidly severed from an unanesthetized patient. The open stump was crushed or dipped in boiling oil to obtain hemostasis. The procedure was associated with high complication and mortality rates due to hemorrhage and infection. Surgeons during that time could rely only on their efficiency and technique to affect outcome and minimize pain. For patients who survived, the resulting stump was poorly suited for prosthetic fitting.

Hippocrates was the first to use ligatures; this technique was lost during the Dark Ages but was reintroduced in 1529 by Ambroise Paré, a French military surgeon. Paré also introduced the "artery forceps." He was able to reduce the mortality rate significantly while creating a more functional stump. He also designed relatively sophisticated prostheses. Further advances were made possible by Morel's introduction of the tourniquet in 1674 and Lister's introduction of antiseptic technique in 1867. Based on the microbial theory of infection, Lister instituted treating the patient's skin, the surgeon's hands, surgical instrumentation, and the surrounding operating theater air with phenol. As a result, the incidence of surgical sepsis and associated mortality fell dramatically. With the use of chloroform and ether for general anesthesia in the late 19th century, surgeons for the first time could fashion reasonably sturdy and functional stumps.

During the 1940s in the United States, veterans began to voice their concerns over the poor performance of their artificial limbs, which prompted the Surgeon General of the Army, Norman T. Kirk, to turn to the National Academy of Sciences. This led to the formation of the Advisory Committee on Artificial Limbs, later the Prosthetics Research Board, and finally the Committee on Prosthetics Research and Development.

Today, federally funded prosthetic research continues through university programs. With better understanding of biology and physiology, surgical technique and postoperative rehabilitation have improved. New information regarding biomechanics and materials has greatly improved prosthetic design. Patients with amputations now can enjoy higher levels of activity. Older patients, who previously would have been wheelchair dependent, are now more likely to regain ambulatory ability. Younger patients now have access to specialized prostheses that allow them to resume recreational activities such as running, golfing, skiing, hiking, swimming, and other competitive sports.

Now, more than ever, it is important that amputations be performed by surgeons who have a complete understanding of amputation surgical principles, postoperative rehabilitation, and prosthetic design. Improved prosthetic design does not compensate for a poorly performed surgical procedure. Amputation should not be viewed as a failure of treatment but rather as the first step toward a patient's return to a more comfortable and productive life. The operative procedure should be planned and performed with the same care and skill used in any other reconstructive procedure.

INCIDENCE AND INDICATIONS

The National Center for Health Statistics estimated that more than two million patients with amputations live in the United States. The number (~185,000) of amputations performed each year is increasing, mainly because of an aging population. More than 90% of amputations performed in the Western world are secondary to peripheral vascular disease. In younger patients, trauma is the leading cause, followed by malignancy.

The only absolute indication for amputation is irreversible ischemia in a diseased or traumatized limb. Amputation also may be necessary to preserve life in patients with uncontrollable infections and may be the best option in some patients with tumors, although advances in orthopaedic oncology now allow limb salvage in most cases. Injury not affecting circulation may result in a limb that it is not as functional as a prosthesis. Similarly, certain congenital anomalies of the lower extremity are best treated with amputation and prosthetic fitting. Each of these indications is discussed in further detail.

PERIPHERAL VASCULAR DISEASE

Peripheral vascular disease with or without diabetes, which most frequently occurs in individuals aged 50 to 75 years, is the most common indication for amputation. The treating physician should keep in mind that if vascular disease has progressed to the point of requiring amputation, it is not limited to the involved extremity. Most patients also have concomitant disease processes in the cerebral vasculature, coronary arteries, and kidneys. In addition to obtaining a vascular surgery consultation to evaluate the diseased limb, appropriate consultation is indicated to evaluate these other systems.

Approximately half of amputations for peripheral vascular disease are performed on patients with diabetes. The most significant predictor of amputation in diabetics is peripheral neuropathy, as measured by insensitivity to the Semmes-Weinstein 5.07 monofilament. Other documented risk factors include prior stroke, prior major amputation, decreased transcutaneous oxygen levels, and decreased ankle-brachial blood pressure index. Diabetics must be instructed on the importance of proper foot care and footwear and must examine their feet frequently. Ulcers should be treated aggressively with appropriate pressure relief, orthoses, total-contact casting, wound care, and antibiotics when indicated. Other risk factors, including smoking and poor glucose control, should be minimized.

Before performing an amputation for peripheral vascular disease, a vascular surgery consultation is almost always indicated. Improved techniques currently allow for revascularization of limbs that previously would have been unsalvageable. However, revascularization is not without risk. Although there is no conclusive evidence in the literature that peripheral bypass surgery compromises wound healing of a future transtibial amputation, our experience seems to indicate otherwise.

If amputation becomes necessary, all effort must be expended to optimize surgical conditions. All medical problems should be treated individually. Infection should be controlled as effectively as possible, and nutrition and immune status should be evaluated with simple screening tests. It has been shown that the risk for wound complications is greatly increased in patients whose serum albumin is less than 3.5 g/dL or whose total lymphocyte count is less than 1500 cells/mL. Perioperative mortality rates for amputation in peripheral vascular disease have been reported to be 30%, and 40% of patients die within 2 years. Critical ischemia develops in the remaining lower extremity in 30% of the remaining patients.

Determining the appropriate level of amputation is discussed later in this chapter. The energy required for walking is inversely proportional to the length of the remaining limb. In an elderly patient with multiple medical problems, energy reserves may not allow for ambulation if the amputation is at a proximal level. If a patient's cognitive function, balance, strength, and motivation level are sufficient for ambulatory rehabilitation to be a reasonable goal, amputation should be performed at the most distal level that offers a reasonable chance of healing to maximize function. Conversely, a nonambulatory patient with a knee flexion contracture should not undergo a transtibial amputation because a transfemoral amputation or knee disarticulation provides better function and less risk.

TRAUMA

Trauma is the leading indication for amputations in younger patients. Amputations caused by trauma are more common in men because of vocational and avocational hazards. These patients are often otherwise healthy and productive, and such injuries may have profound effects on their lives. The only absolute indication for primary amputation is an irreparable vascular injury in an ischemic limb. With improvements in prehospital care, acute resuscitation, microvascular techniques, and bone transport techniques, orthopaedic surgeons more often are faced with situations in which a severely traumatized limb can be preserved, although this involves substantial compromises.

Several studies have suggested guidelines to help decide which limbs are salvageable. Most of these studies have concentrated on severe injuries of the lower extremity. Most authors would agree that type III-C open tibial fractures, which include complete disruption of the tibial nerve, or a crush injury with warm ischemia time of more than 6 hours, are an absolute indication for amputation (Fig. 11.1). Relative indications for primary amputation include serious associated injuries, severe ipsilateral foot injuries, and anticipated protracted course to obtain soft-tissue coverage and tibial reconstruction. Although these relative indications are subject to various interpretations, they serve as reasonable guidelines.

Other authors have attempted to remove subjectivity from the decision-making process. To predict which limbs will be salvageable, available scoring systems include the predictive salvage index, the limb injury score, the limb salvage index, the mangled extremity syndrome index, and the mangled extremity severity score. Of these, we have found the mangled extremity severity score to be most useful (Table 11.1). This system, which is easy to apply, grades the injury based on the energy that caused the injury, limb ischemia, shock, and the

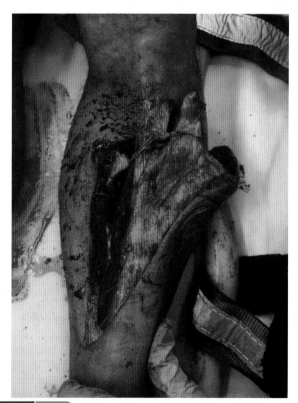

FIGURE 11.1   Lengthy warm ischemia time generally is an absolute indication for amputation.

TABLE 11.1			
Mangled Extremity Severity Score			
TYPE	**CHARACTERISTICS**	**INJURIES**	**POINTS**
1	Low energy	Stab wounds, simple closed fractures, small-caliber gunshot wounds	1
2	Medium energy	Open or multiple-level fractures, dislocations, moderate crush injuries	2
3	High energy	Shotgun blast (close range), high-velocity gunshot wounds	3
4	Massive crush	Logging, railroad, oil rig accidents	4
SHOCK GROUP			
1	Normotensive hemodynamics	Stable blood pressure in field and in operating room	0
2	Transiently hypotensive	Unstable blood pressure in field but responsive to intravenous fluids	1
3	Prolonged hypotension	Systolic blood pressure <90 mm Hg in field and responsive to intravenous fluid only in operating room	2
ISCHEMIA GROUP			
1	None	Pulsatile limb without signs of ischemia	0*
2	Mild	Diminished pulses without signs of ischemia	1*
3	Moderate	No pulse on Doppler imaging, sluggish capillary refill, paresthesia, diminished motor activity	2*
4	Advanced	Pulseless, cool, paralyzed, and numb without capillary refill	3*
AGE GROUP			
1	<30 years		0
2	>30 to <50 years		1
3	>50 years		2

*Points ×2 if ischemic time exceeds 6 hours.

From Helfet DL, Howey T, Sanders R, et al: Limb salvage versus amputation: preliminary results of the mangled extremity severity score, *Clin Orthop Relat Res* 256:80, 1990.

patient's age. The system was subjected to retrospective and prospective studies, with a score of 6 or less consistent with a salvageable limb. With a score of 7 or greater, amputation was the eventual result. Although we do not strictly follow these guidelines in all patients, we do calculate and document a mangled extremity severity score in the chart whenever we are considering primary amputation versus a complicated limb salvage.

No scoring system can replace experience and good clinical judgment. Amputation of an injured extremity might be necessary to preserve life. Attempts to salvage a severely injured limb may lead to metabolic overload and secondary organ failure. This is more common in patients with multiple injuries and in the elderly. It has been suggested that an injury severity score of greater than 50 is a contraindication to heroic attempts at limb salvage. Concomitant injuries and comorbid medical conditions must be considered before heading down a long road of multiple operations to save a limb.

After determining that a limb *can* be saved, the surgeon must decide whether it *should* be saved, and this decision must be made in concert with the patient. The surgeon must educate the patient regarding the tradeoffs involved with a protracted treatment course of limb salvage versus immediate amputation and prosthetic fitting. On entering the hospital, most patients are concerned only with saving the limb; they must be made to understand that this often comes at a great cost. They may have to face multiple operations to obtain bony union and soft-tissue coverage and multiple operations on other areas to obtain donor tissue. External fixation may be necessary for several years, and complications, including infection, nonunion,

or loss of a muscle flap, may occur. Chronic pain and drug addiction also are common problems of limb salvage because patients endure multiple hospital admissions and surgery, isolation from their family and friends, and unemployment. In the end, despite heroic efforts, the limb ultimately could require amputation, or a "successfully" salvaged limb may be chronically painful or functionless.

Patients also need to understand that the advances made in limb salvage surgery have been paralleled by advances made in the amputation surgery and prosthetic design. Early amputation and prosthetic fitting are associated with decreased morbidity, fewer operations, shorter hospital stay, decreased hospital costs, shorter rehabilitation, and earlier return to work. The treatment course and outcome are more predictable. Modern prosthetics often provide better function than many "successfully" salvaged limbs. A young, healthy patient with a transtibial prosthesis is often able to resume all previous activities with few restrictions. In long-term studies, patients who have undergone amputation and prosthetic fitting are more likely to remain working and are far less likely to consider themselves to be "severely disabled" than patients who have endured an extensive limb salvage.

Several comparisons of limb reconstruction and limb amputation have come to differing conclusions, with one large study of 545 patients projecting lifetime health care costs to be three times higher for patients with amputations than for those with reconstruction. A meta-analysis, on the other hand, concluded that length of rehabilitation and total costs are higher for patients who have undergone limb salvage procedures. Reports of functional results have been equally varied, with one study reporting a 64% return-to-work rate after limb salvage compared with 73% after amputation, and another study reporting that long-term functional outcomes were equivalent between limb salvage and primary amputation.

The worst-case scenario occurs when a limb must be amputated after the patient has endured multiple operations of an unsuccessful salvage or after years of pain following a "successful" salvage. After realizing the function that is possible with a prosthesis, many patients ask why the amputation was not performed initially. It is important to present all information from the very beginning so that the patient can make educated decisions regarding which course to follow. The physician cannot understand the importance each patient places on cosmesis, function, or body image without specifically asking these questions. Other important issues include the patient's ability to handle uncertainty, deal with prolonged immobilization, accept social isolation, and bear the financial burden. Without discussing all these issues, a physician would not be able to help patients make the "correct" decisions. The "correct" decisions are based on the patient as a whole, not solely on the extent of the limb injury.

When an amputation is performed in the setting of acute trauma, the surgeon must follow all the standard principles of wound management. Contaminated tissue must undergo debridement and irrigation followed by open wound management. Although all devitalized tissue must be removed, any questionable areas should be retained to preserve future reconstructive options and reevaluated at a repeat debridement in 24 to 48 hours. This time will not only allow the wound to further declare its course but also allow the patient to comprehend the severity of the problem. Functional stump length should be maintained whenever possible; this may require using nonstandard flaps or free muscle flaps for closure. Traction neurectomy for all named nerves and large cutaneous nerves should be performed proximal to the end of the residual limb to avoid sympathetic neuromas. Vascularized or nonvascularized tissue may be harvested from the amputated part to aid in this endeavor. If adequate length cannot be maintained acutely, the stump may be revised later using tissue expanders and the Ilizarov technique for bone lengthening. Negative pressure wound therapy is a useful adjuvant until the time of revision surgery. Controlled localized negative pressure promotes healing by promoting wound contraction, decreasing extracellular fluid, increasing tissue oxygenation, and stimulating formation of granulation tissue. A multidisciplinary approach involving other subspecialties (e.g., general surgery, vascular surgery) is recommended in the acute setting when patients are unable to be involved in the decision process secondary to their other injuries.

BURNS

Thermal or electrical injury to an extremity may necessitate amputation (Fig. 11.2). The full extent of tissue damage may not be apparent at initial presentation, especially with electrical injury. Treatment involves early debridement of devitalized tissue, fasciotomies when indicated, and aggressive wound care, including repeat debridements in the operating room. Compared with early amputation, delayed amputation of an unsalvageable limb has been associated with increased risk of local infection, systemic infection, myoglobin-induced renal failure, and death. In addition, length of hospital stay and cost are greatly increased with delayed amputation. Performing

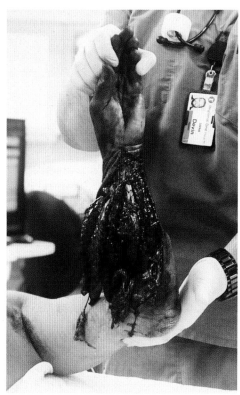

FIGURE 11.2 Electrical burn of the hand and forearm that necessitated an above-elbow amputation.

inadequate debridements with the unrealistic hope of saving a limb may put the patient in undue danger. Debridements must be aggressive and must include amputation when necessary.

FROSTBITE

Frostbite denotes the actual freezing of tissue in the extremities, with or without central hypothermia. Historically, frostbite was most prevalent in wartime; however, anyone exposed to subfreezing temperatures is at risk. This is a common problem for high-altitude climbers, skiers, and hunters. Also at risk are homeless, alcoholic, and schizophrenic individuals.

When heat loss exceeds the body's ability to maintain homeostasis, blood flow to the extremities is decreased to maintain central body temperature. The problem is exacerbated by exposure to wind or water. Actual tissue injury occurs through two mechanisms: (1) direct tissue injury through the formation of ice crystals in the extracellular fluid and (2) ischemic injury resulting from damage to vascular endothelium, clot formation, and increased sympathetic tone.

The first step in treatment is restoration of core body temperature. Treatment of the affected extremity begins with rapid rewarming in a water bath at 40°C to 44°C. This requires parenteral pain management and sedation. After initial rewarming, if digital blood flow is still not apparent, treatment with tissue plasminogen activator or regional sympathetic blockade may be indicated. Tetanus prophylaxis is mandatory; however, prophylactic systemic antibiotics are controversial. Blebs should be left intact. Closed blebs should be treated with aloe vera. Silver sulfadiazine (Silvadene) should be applied regularly to open blebs. Low doses of aspirin or ibuprofen also should be instituted. Oral antiinflammatory medication and topical aloe vera help stop progressive dermal ischemia mediated by

TABLE 11.2			
Differential Diagnosis of Infection With Gas-Forming Organisms			
FACTOR	**ANAEROBIC CELLULITIS**	**CLOSTRIDIAL MYONECROSIS**	**STREPTOCOCCAL MYONECROSIS**
Incubation	>3 days	<3 days	3–4 days
Onset	Gradual	Acute	Subacute
Toxemia	Slight	Severe	Severe (late)
Pain	Absent	Severe	Variable
Swelling	Slight	Severe	Severe
Skin	Little change	Tense, white	Tense, copper colored
Exudate	Slight	Serous hemorrhagic	Seropurulent
Gas	Abundant	Rarely abundant	Slight
Smell	Foul	Variable, "mousy"	Slight
Muscle involvement	No change	Severe	Moderate

From DeHaven KE, Evarts CM: The continuing problem of gas gangrene: a review and report of illustrative cases, *J Trauma* 11(12):983–991, 1971.

vasoconstricting metabolites of arachidonic acid in frostbite wounds. Physical therapy should be started early to maintain range of motion.

In stark contrast to traumatic, thermal, or electrical injury, amputation for frostbite routinely should be delayed 2 to 6 months. Clear demarcation of viable tissue may take this long. Even after demarcation appears to be complete on the surface, deep tissues still may be recovering. Despite the presence of mummified tissue, infection is rare if local wound management is maintained. Triple-phase technetium bone scan has helped delineate deep tissue viability. Performing surgery prematurely often results in greater tissue loss and increased risk of infection. An exception to this rule is the removal of a circumferentially constricting eschar.

INFECTION

Amputation may be necessary for acute or chronic infection that is unresponsive to antibiotics and surgical debridement. Open amputation is indicated in this setting and may be performed using one of two methods. A guillotine amputation may be performed with later revision to a more proximal level after the infection is under control. Alternatively, an open amputation may be performed at the definitive level by initially inverting the flaps and packing the wound open with secondary closure at 10 to 14 days.

Partial foot amputation with primary closure has been described for patients with active infection; the wound is closed loosely over a catheter through which an antibiotic irrigant is infused. The constant infusion is continued for 5 days. The wound must be closed loosely enough to allow the fluid to escape into the dressings. The dressings must be changed frequently until the catheter is removed on postoperative day 5. This method may allow for primary wound healing, while avoiding a protracted course of wound healing by secondary intention.

In the acute setting, the most worrisome infections are those produced by gas-forming organisms. Typically associated with battlefield injuries, gas-forming infections also may result from farm injuries, motor vehicle accidents, or civilian gunshot wounds. Any contaminated wound that is closed without appropriate debridement is at high risk for the development of gas gangrene.

Three distinct gas-forming infections must be differentiated (Table 11.2). The first is clostridial myonecrosis, which typically develops within 24 hours of closure of a deep contaminated wound. The patient has an acute onset of pain, swelling, and toxemia, often associated with a mental awareness of impending death. The wound develops a bronze discoloration with a serosanguineous exudate and a musty odor. Gram stain of the exudates shows gram-positive rods occasionally accompanied by other flora. Treatment consists of immediate radical debridement of involved tissue, high doses of intravenous penicillin (clindamycin may be used if the patient is allergic to penicillin), and hyperbaric oxygen. Emergency open amputation one joint above the affected compartments often is needed as a lifesaving measure but may be avoided if treatment is initiated early.

Streptococcal myonecrosis usually develops over 3 to 4 days. The onset is not as rapid, and patients do not appear as sick as patients with clostridial infections. Swelling may be severe, but the pain is typically not as severe as that experienced in clostridial myonecrosis. Abundant seropurulent discharge may be seen with only small amounts of gas formation. Debridement of involved muscle compartments, open wound management, and penicillin treatment usually allow for preservation of the limb.

The third entity that must be distinguished is anaerobic cellulitis or necrotizing fasciitis. Onset usually occurs several days after closure of a contaminated wound. Subcutaneous emphysema may spread rapidly, although pain, swelling, and toxemia usually remain minimal. Gas production may be abundant with a foul smell, but muscle compartments are not involved. Causative organisms include clostridia, anaerobic streptococci, *Bacteroides*, and gram-negative rods. Treatment includes debridement and broad-spectrum antibiotics. Amputation rarely is indicated.

Indications for amputation of a chronically infected limb must be defined on an individual basis. The systemic effects of a refractory infection may justify amputation. Disability from a nonhealing trophic ulcer, chronic osteomyelitis, or infected nonunion may reach a point at which the patient is better served by an amputation and prosthetic fitting. Rarely, a chronic draining sinus is the site of development of a squamous cell carcinoma, which necessitates amputation.

TUMORS

Advances in diagnostic imaging, chemotherapy, radiation therapy, and surgical techniques for reconstruction now make limb salvage a reasonable option for most patients with bone or soft-tissue sarcomas. Four issues must be considered when contemplating limb salvage instead of amputation:
1. Would survival be affected by the treatment choice?
2. How do short-term and long-term morbidity compare?
3. How would the function of a salvaged limb compare with that of a prosthesis?
4. Are there any psychosocial consequences?

Several studies have discussed the first question with regard to osteosarcoma. With the use of multimodal treatment, including surgery and chemotherapy, long-term survival for osteosarcoma patients has improved from 20% to 70% in most series. For osteosarcoma of the distal femur, the rate of local recurrence after wide resection and limb salvage is 5% to 10%, which is equivalent to the local recurrence rate after a transfemoral amputation for osteosarcoma. Although the rate of local recurrence of a tumor after hip disarticulation is extremely low, no study has shown a survival advantage for this technique. In general, provided that wide surgical margins are obtained, no study has proved a survival advantage of one technique over the other.

Amputation for malignancy may be technically demanding, often requiring nonstandard flaps, bone graft, or prosthetic augmentation to obtain a more functional residual limb (Fig. 11.3). Limb salvage is associated with greater perioperative morbidity, however, compared with amputation. Limb salvage involves a more extensive surgical procedure and is associated with greater risk of infection, wound dehiscence, flap necrosis, blood loss, and deep venous thrombosis. Long-term complications vary depending on the type of reconstruction. These include periprosthetic fractures, prosthetic loosening or dislocation, nonunion of the graft-host junction, allograft fracture, leg-length discrepancy, and late infection. A patient with a salvaged limb is more likely to need multiple subsequent operations for treatment of complications. After initial successful limb salvage surgery, one third of long-term survivors ultimately may require an amputation.

Regarding function, the location of the tumor is the most important factor. Resection of an upper extremity lesion with limb salvage, even with sacrifice of a major nerve, generally provides better function than amputation and subsequent prosthetic fitting. Similarly, resection of a proximal femoral or pelvic lesion with local reconstruction generally provides better function than hip disarticulation or hemipelvectomy. Sarcomas around the ankle and foot are frequently treated with amputation followed by prosthetic fitting. Treatment for sarcomas around the knee must be individualized.

Most patients with osteosarcoma around the knee are treated with one of three surgical procedures, which include either wide resection with prosthetic knee replacement, wide resection with allograft arthrodesis, or a transfemoral amputation. In one study of osteosarcoma patients, patients who had undergone resection and prosthetic knee replacement showed higher self-selected walking velocities and a more efficient gait with regard to oxygen consumption than patients with transfemoral amputations. Individuals with a transfemoral amputation functioned at more than 50% of their maximal aerobic capacity at free walking speeds, requiring anaerobic mechanisms to sustain muscle metabolism,

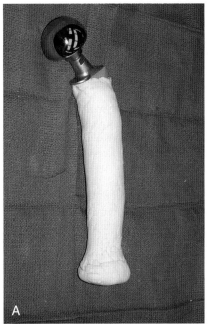

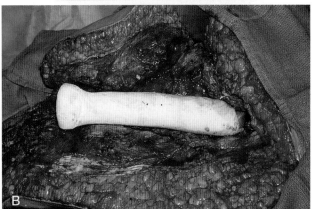

FIGURE 11.3 Hip disarticulation secondary to osteosarcoma. **A,** Proximal femoral replacement is constructed using hip hemiarthroplasty component and bone cement. **B,** Anterior and posterior flaps are repaired over prosthesis. Patient can function as transfemoral amputee.

which results in decreased endurance. The problem in many of these patients is compounded by decreased cardiac function from doxorubicin-induced cardiomyopathy.

In a comparison of the long-term function of amputation, arthrodesis, or arthroplasty for the treatment of tumors around the knee, patients with an amputation had difficulty walking on steep, rough, or slippery surfaces but were very active and were the least worried about damaging the affected limb. Patients with an arthrodesis performed the most demanding physical work and recreational activities, but they had difficulty with sitting, especially in the back seat of cars, theaters, or sports arenas. Patients who had arthroplasty generally led more sedentary lives and were more protective of the limb, but they had little difficulty with activities of daily living. These patients also were the least self-conscious about the limb.

No study has shown a significant difference between amputation and limb salvage with regard to psychologic outcome or quality of life in long-term sarcoma survivors.

The decision of limb salvage versus amputation involves more than the question of whether the lesion can be resected with wide margins. The patient ultimately must make the final decision based on long-term goals and lifestyle decisions.

Rarely, amputation may be indicated as a palliative measure for a patient with metastatic disease and pain that has been refractory to standard surgical treatment, radiation, chemotherapy, and narcotic pain management. Amputation may be indicated for treatment of a recurrent pathologic fracture in which stabilization is impossible. It also may be indicated if the malignancy has caused massive necrosis, fungation, infection, or vascular compromise (Fig. 11.4). Although cure is not the goal, amputation may dramatically improve the functional status and pain relief for the remaining months in some patients. The surgeon must remember, however, that survival is not always predictable. One such "palliative" hemipelvectomy was performed at this institution on a patient who subsequently lived comfortably for an additional 20 years.

SURGICAL PRINCIPLES OF AMPUTATIONS

DETERMINATION OF AMPUTATION LEVEL

Determining the appropriate level of amputation requires an understanding of the tradeoffs between increased function with a more distal level of amputation and a decreased complication rate with a more proximal level of amputation (Fig. 11.5). The patient's overall well-being, general medical condition, and rehabilitation all are important factors.

A vascular surgery consultation is almost always appropriate. Even if revascularization would not allow for salvage of the entire limb, it may allow for healing of a partial foot or ankle amputation instead of a transtibial amputation. As previously stated, however, peripheral bypass surgery may compromise wound healing of a future transtibial amputation.

Simple screening tests for nutritional status and immunocompetence should be performed. Use of tobacco products should be discouraged. Medical illness, infection, and major operations all induce a hypermetabolic state. Multiple studies have confirmed that malnourished or immunocompromised patients have markedly increased rates of perioperative complications.

Waters et al. studied the energy cost of walking for patients with amputations at the transfemoral, transtibial, and Syme levels secondary to trauma or chronic limb ischemia. Compared with controls without amputations, the self-selected walking velocity for vascular amputees was 66% at the Syme level, 59% at the transtibial level, and 44% at the transfemoral level. For traumatic amputees, generally younger patients, the rates were 87% at the transtibial level and 63% at the transfemoral level. At self-selected walking velocities, the slower rates for amputees seem to be a compensatory mechanism to conserve energy per unit time. Except for transfemoral amputations secondary to vascular insufficiency, all patients tended to ambulate at similar percentages of their maximal aerobic capacity compared with age-matched controls. Patients tended to decrease their velocities to keep their relative energy costs per minute within normal limits. Patients with transfemoral amputations secondary to vascular insufficiency were unable to accomplish this, however, often exceeding 50% of their maximal aerobic

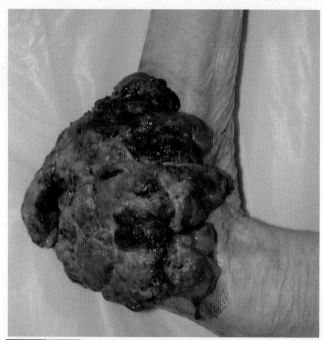

FIGURE 11.4 Fungating tumor required transhumeral amputation.

capacity even for minimal ambulation. In this state, as already mentioned, anaerobic mechanisms are summoned to sustain muscle function, and endurance is greatly compromised. As a result, fewer vascular transfemoral amputees regain functional ambulatory ability. It becomes apparent that amputation should be performed at the most distal level possible if ambulation is the chief concern.

If a patient has no ambulatory potential, wound healing with decreased perioperative morbidity should be the chief concern. A transtibial amputation in this setting is not a reasonable option because of the increased risk of wound problems and increased skin problems from knee flexion contractures. A knee disarticulation often provides the best function for these patients. Compared with transfemoral amputation, knee disarticulation provides a longer lever arm with balanced musculature to help with bed mobility and transfers. In addition, muscles are not divided and do not atrophy and contract over the femur as they often do after transfemoral amputation. Finally, better sitting stability and comfort are provided with a through-knee amputation.

Determining the most distal level for amputation with a reasonable chance of healing can be challenging. Preoperatively, clinical assessment of skin color, hair growth, and skin temperature provides valuable initial information. Preoperative arteriograms, although already obtained for vascular surgery consultation, are of little help in determining potential for wound healing. Segmental systolic blood pressures likewise offer little useful information because they are often falsely elevated owing to the noncompliant walls of arteriosclerotic vessels. Measurements of skin perfusion pressures may be of some benefit, however. Some authors have recommended thermography or laser Doppler flowmetry as methods to test skin flap perfusion. Others recommend determining the tissue uptake of intravenously injected fluorescein or the tissue clearance of intradermally injected xenon-133. We have found transcutaneous oxygen measurements to be most beneficial.

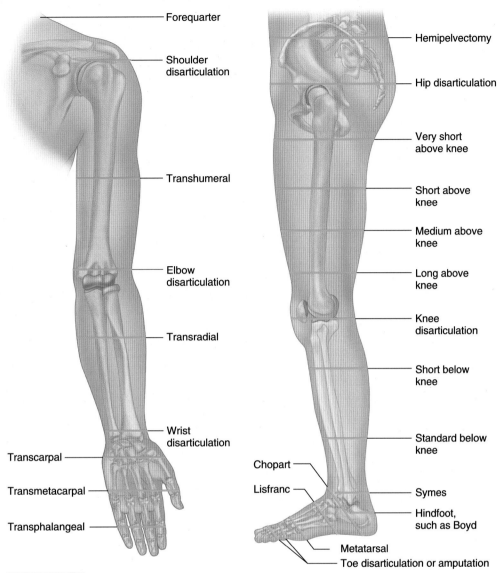

FIGURE 11.5 Levels of amputation: more distal levels are associated with increased function, more proximal levels are associated with a decreased complication rate.

Transcutaneous oxygen measurements can be determined at multiple sites along the limb. The test is performed by inserting a probe that is heated to 45°C for 10 minutes before oxygen tension is measured. This allows for a maximum vasodilatory response and a more accurate determination of perfusion potential. Various studies have recommended different cutoff levels, ranging from 20 to 40 mm Hg, for "good" healing potential. There is, however, no absolute cutoff because some studies have shown healing rates of 50% even when the transcutaneous oxygen level is less than 10 mm Hg. The measurement can be falsely decreased in circumstances that decrease the diffusion of oxygen, such as cellulitis or edema. The test can be improved by comparing the transcutaneous oxygen level before and after the inhalation of 100% oxygen. An increase of 10 mm Hg at a particular level is a good indicator for healing potential. Accuracy also can be improved by comparing supine and elevation of the extremity measurements in patients who fall into the 20 to 40 mm Hg gray zone. A decrease of greater than 15 mm Hg after 3 minutes of elevation of the involved limb is a poor prognostic indicator for healing. This information must be used in light of other patient variables, including age, concomitant medical problems, and ambulatory potential.

TECHNICAL ASPECTS

Meticulous attention to detail and gentle handling of soft tissues are important for creating a well-healed and highly functional amputation stump. The tissues often are poorly vascularized or traumatized, and the risk for complications is high.

■ SKIN AND MUSCLE FLAPS

Flaps should be kept thick. Unnecessary dissection should be avoided to prevent further devascularization of already compromised tissues. Covering the end of the stump with a sturdy soft-tissue envelope is crucial. Past studies have determined the best type of flaps for each level of amputation, but atypical flaps are always preferable to amputation at a more proximal level. With modern total-contact prosthetic sockets, the location of the scar is rarely important, but the scar should not be adherent to the underlying bone. An adherent scar makes prosthetic fitting extremely difficult, and this type of scar often breaks down after prolonged prosthetic use. Redundant soft tissues or large "dog ears" also create problems in prosthetic fitting and may prevent maximal function of an otherwise well-constructed stump (Fig. 11.6).

Muscles usually are divided at least 5 cm distal to the intended bone resection. They may be stabilized by *myodesis* (suturing muscle or tendon to bone) or by *myoplasty* (suturing muscle to the periosteum or the fascia of opposing musculature). Jaegers et al. showed that transected muscles atrophy 40% to 60% in 2 years if they are not securely fixed. If possible, myodesis should be performed to provide a stronger insertion, help maximize strength, and minimize atrophy (Fig. 11.7). Myodesed muscles continue to counterbalance their antagonists, preventing contractures and maximizing residual limb function. However, myodesis may be contraindicated in severe ischemia because of the increased risk of wound breakdown.

■ HEMOSTASIS

Except in severely ischemic limbs, the use of a tourniquet is highly desirable and makes the amputation easier. The limb may be exsanguinated by wrapping it with an Esmarch bandage before the tourniquet is inflated. However, in amputations for infections or malignancy, expressing blood from the limbs in this manner is inadvisable. In such instances, inflation of the tourniquet should be preceded by elevation of the limb for 5 minutes.

Major blood vessels should be isolated and individually ligated. Arteries and veins should be ligated separately, and larger vessels should be doubly ligated. The tourniquet should be deflated before closure, and meticulous hemostasis should be obtained. A drain should be used in most cases for 48 to 72 hours.

■ NERVES

A neuroma formation is inevitable after transection as the axons are unable to locate the distal nerve stump. A neuroma becomes painful if it forms in a position where it would be subjected to repeated trauma. Normal physiologic stimuli such as stretching, pressure, and vascular pulsations may be painful and, thus, limit prosthetic usage. Special techniques have been tried in the hopes of preventing the formation of painful neuromas. These include end-loop anastomosis, perineural closure, Silastic capping, sealing the epineurial tube with butyl-cyanoacrylate, ligation, cauterization, and methods to bury the nerve ends in bone or muscle. Most surgeons currently agree that nerves should be isolated, gently pulled distally into the wound, and divided cleanly with a sharp knife so that the cut end retracts well proximal to the level of bone resection. Strong tension on the nerve should be avoided during this maneuver; otherwise, the amputation stump may be painful even after the wound has healed. Crushing also should be avoided. Large nerves, such as the sciatic nerve, often contain relatively large arteries and should be ligated.

■ BONE

Excessive periosteal stripping is contraindicated and may result in the formation of ring sequestra or bony overgrowth.

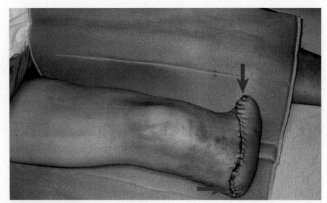

FIGURE 11.6 Redundant soft tissue or large "dog ears" can create problems in prosthetic fitting.

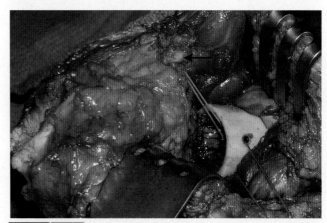

FIGURE 11.7 Myodesis in transfemoral amputation. Adductor magnus tendon *(arrow)* is pulled into cut end of distal femur and secured through drill hole in lateral cortex.

Bony prominences that would not be well padded by soft tissue always should be resected, and the remaining bone should be rasped to form a smooth contour. This is especially important in locations such as the anterior aspect of the tibia, lateral aspect of the femur, and radial styloid.

OPEN AMPUTATIONS

An open amputation is one in which the skin is not closed over the end of the stump. The operation is the first of at least two operations required to construct a satisfactory stump. It always must be followed by secondary closure, reamputation, revision, or plastic repair. The purpose of this type of amputation is to prevent or eliminate infection so that final closure of the stump may be done without breakdown of the wound. Open amputations are indicated in infections and in severe traumatic wounds with extensive destruction of tissue and gross contamination by foreign material. Appropriate antibiotics are given until the stump is finally healed (Fig. 11.8).

Previous editions of this book have described the techniques for open amputations with inverted skin flaps and circular open amputations with postoperative skin traction. More recently, in the setting of tissue contamination or severe trauma at the amputation site, we have employed the technique of vacuum-assisted closure. A wound vacuum-assisted closure is applied to the open stump immediately after the initial debridement. Subsequent debridements are scheduled at 48-hour intervals. The vacuum-assisted closure is reapplied

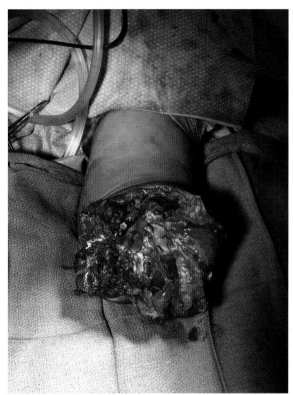

FIGURE 11.8 Open amputation. First stage, without skin closure, is aimed at preventing or eliminating infection before the second stage (closure, reamputation, revision, plastic repair).

after each debridement until the wound is ready for closure (Fig. 11.9).

POSTOPERATIVE CARE

Postoperative care of amputations often requires a multidisciplinary team approach. In addition to the surgeon, this team may include a physical medicine specialist, a physical therapist, an occupational therapist, a psychologist, and a social worker. An internist often is required to help manage postoperative medical problems. All the same precautions are followed as for any major orthopaedic surgery, including perioperative antibiotics, deep venous thrombosis prophylaxis, and pulmonary hygiene. Pain management includes the brief use of intravenous narcotics followed by oral pain medicine that is tapered as soon as can be tolerated. Several studies have noted decreased narcotic usage with improved pain management using an oral multimodal pain medication regimen (Table 11.3) and/or continuous postoperative perineural infusional anesthesia for several days.

Treatment of the stump from the time the amputation is completed until the definitive prosthesis is fitted is crucial if a strong and functional amputation stump capable of maximum prosthetic use is to be obtained. Since the mid-1970s, there has been a gradual shift from the use of "conventional" soft dressings to the use of rigid dressings, especially in centers that perform significant numbers of amputations. The rigid dressing consists of a plaster of Paris cast that is applied to the stump at the conclusion of surgery. Early weight bearing is not an essential part of the postoperative management program. If weight-bearing ambulation is not planned in the immediate postoperative

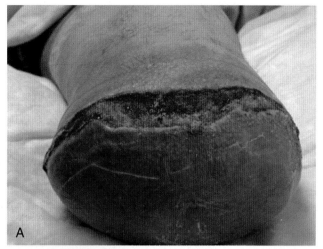

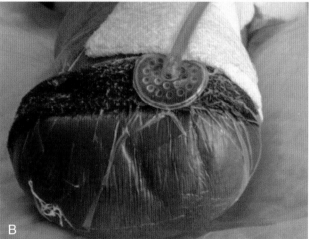

FIGURE 11.9 Postoperative below-knee amputation stump before **(A)** and after **(B)** negative-pressure wound therapy dressing. (From Sumpio B, Thakor P, Mahler D, Blume P: Negative pressure wound therapy as postoperative dressing in below knee amputation stump closure of patients with chronic venous insufficiency, *Wounds* 23[10]:301–308, 2011.)

period, the rigid dressing may be applied by the surgeon, observing standard cast application precautions, including appropriate padding of all bony prominences, avoiding proximal constriction of the limb, and use of dependable cast suspension methods. If weight-bearing ambulation in the immediate postoperative period is anticipated, a true prosthetic cast should be applied, preferably by a certified prosthetist, with appropriate use of stump socks, contoured felt padding over all bony prominences, and special suspension techniques. A metal pylon with a prosthetic foot is attached to the cast and properly aligned for ambulation. Specific details of such prosthetic cast applications for the major levels of amputation are provided after each discussion of surgical technique. Rigid stump dressings may be employed successfully and beneficially at essentially all levels of amputation in the lower and upper limbs and are applicable to all age groups.

Rigid dressings offer several advantages over soft dressings. Rigid dressings prevent edema at the surgical site, protect the wound from bed trauma, enhance wound healing and early maturation of the stump, and decrease postoperative

	TABLE 11.3	
Multimodal Analgesia: Pharmacologic Components		
	TYPE	**EXAMPLES**
Principal	Regional anesthesia	Central neuraxial or peripheral nerve block
		Single-shot or continuous catheter
		± Local infiltration analgesia
	Opioid analgesics	Oxycodone, morphine, fentanyl, hydromorphone
	Systemic nonopioid analgesics	Acetaminophen, nonsteroidal antiinflammatory drugs (NSAIDs)
Adjuvants	Gabapentinoids	Gabapentin, pregabalin
	N-methyl D-aspartate (NMDA) receptor antagonists	Ketamine, memantine, dextromethor phan, magnesium
	Alpha-2 adrenergic agents	Clonidine
	Glucocorticoids	Dexamethasone
	Other	Antidepressant, calcitonin, nicotine, capsaicin, cannabinoid, lidocaine

pain, allowing earlier mobilization from bed to chair and ambulation with support. For transtibial amputations, rigid dressings prevent the formation of knee flexion contractures. The physiologic benefits of upright posture to the respiratory, cardiovascular, urinary, and gastrointestinal systems are easily recognizable, but the psychologic benefits sometimes are more subtle. In most instances, the hospital stay can be decreased and the cost of care reduced accordingly. Finally, earlier definitive prosthetic fitting is possible and a higher percentage of patients are successfully rehabilitated.

Drains usually are removed at 48 hours. The patient is instructed on how to position the stump properly while in bed, while sitting, and while standing. The stump is elevated by raising the foot of the bed, which helps manage edema and postoperative pain. The patient is cautioned against leaving the stump in a dependent position. With transfemoral amputations, the patient is cautioned against placing a pillow between the thighs or beneath the stump or otherwise keeping the stump flexed or abducted. These precautions are necessary to help prevent flexion or abduction contractures. Exercises for the stump are started under the supervision of a physical therapist the day after surgery or as soon thereafter as tolerated. These should consist of muscle-setting exercises followed by exercises to mobilize the joints. Patients should be mobilized from bed to chair on the first postoperative day. Patients with lower extremity amputations should begin physical therapy within the first several days and begin ambulating using the parallel bars. This is followed shortly by ambulation with a walker or crutches when patients can control the limb and are comfortable enough.

The optimal time to begin prosthetic ambulation with protected weight bearing depends on many factors, including the age, strength, and agility of the patient as well as the patient's ability to protect the amputation stump from injury as a result of excessive weight bearing. The availability of a well-trained team of nurses, therapists, and prosthetists who can carry out a well-integrated prosthetic treatment program consistently and the desire and willingness of the surgeon to meticulously supervise such a treatment program are important factors.

The gradual application of functional mechanical stress in the appropriate distribution can enhance wound healing; however, shearing forces can lead to wound breakdown. Early unprotected weight bearing can result in sloughing of the skin or delayed wound healing. Any weight bearing before the stump has healed should be strictly supervised. Advancement of weight-bearing status should be individualized. A young patient with a traumatic amputation *above* the zone of injury probably could begin 25-lb partial weight bearing immediately postoperatively. A patient with a traumatic amputation *through* the zone of injury, or a patient with an amputation performed secondary to ischemia probably should wait until early wound healing is documented before gradually beginning partial weight bearing. Weight-bearing status should be reevaluated with each subsequent cast change. If the wound is progressing well, weight bearing can progress in 25-lb increments each week. Supervision is especially important in patients with peripheral neuropathy who may have difficulty judging how much weight they are placing on their stumps. Juvenile amputees also require close supervision because they are usually quite comfortable in a temporary prosthesis and often attempt to walk without support.

Regardless of when prosthetic ambulation is begun, the rigid dressing should be removed and the wound inspected in 7 to 10 days. Cast loosening, fever, excessive drainage, or systemic symptoms of wound infection are indications for earlier cast removal. If the wound is healing well, a new rigid dressing is applied, and ambulation with or without a pylon and prosthetic foot is continued. The cast should be changed weekly until the wound has healed. After the wound is well healed, the rigid dressing may be removed for bathing and stump hygiene, and, if desired, an elastic stump shrinker may be used at night in lieu of the rigid dressing. As stump shrinkage occurs, continued gentle compression of the stump is maintained by applying an additional stump sock before donning the plaster socket; this minimizes the need for repeated cast changes. Use of the rigid dressing is continued until the volume appears unchanged from the previous week. At that time, the prosthetist may apply the first prosthesis. One or more socket changes frequently are required over the first 18 months; therefore, many prosthetists prefer to make the initial prosthesis in a modular fashion.

COMPLICATIONS

In a review of 5732 patients with transmetatarsal, below-knee, or above-knee amputations, the overall complication rate was

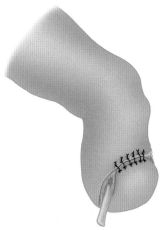

FIGURE 11.10   Partial closure of infected transtibial amputation.

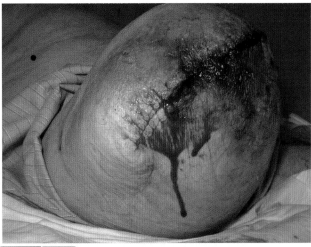

FIGURE 11.11   Tissue necrosis on stump wound.

43%, most of which consisted of wound-related complications. Independent predictors of readmission after amputation were chronic nursing-home residence, nonelective surgery, previous revascularization or amputation, preoperative congestive heart failure, and preoperative dialysis.

HEMATOMA

Meticulous hemostasis before closure, the use of a drain, and a rigid dressing should minimize the frequency of hematoma formation. A hematoma can delay wound healing and serve as a culture medium for bacterial infection. If a hematoma does form, it should be treated with a compressive dressing. If the hematoma is associated with delayed wound healing with or without infection, it should be evacuated in the operating room.

INFECTION

Infection is considerably more common in amputations for peripheral vascular disease, especially in diabetic patients, than in amputations secondary to trauma or tumor. Any deep wound infection should be treated with immediate debridement and irrigation in the operating room and open wound management. Antibiotics should be tailored according to the results of intraoperative cultures. Delayed closure may be difficult because of edema and retraction of the flaps. Smith and Burgess described a method whereby the central one third of the wound is closed and the remainder of the wound is packed open (Fig. 11.10). This method allows for continued open wound management while maintaining adequate flaps for distal bone coverage.

WOUND NECROSIS

The first step in evaluating significant wound necrosis is to reevaluate the preoperative selection of the amputation level. If transcutaneous oxygen studies were not obtained preoperatively, they should be obtained at this point to evaluate wound healing potential. A serum albumin level and a total lymphocyte count should be obtained. Many authors have reported significantly more problems with wound healing in patients with serum albumin levels less than 3.5 g/dL or total lymphocyte counts less than 1500 cells/mL. Nutritional supplementation has been shown to promote wound healing in this setting. Patients who smoke tobacco should quit immediately because smoking severely compromises cutaneous blood

flow, lowering tissue oxygen pressure. In a study by Lind et al., the risk of infection and reamputation was 2.5 times higher in smokers than in nonsmokers.

Necrosis of the skin edges less than 1 cm can be treated conservatively with open wound management (Fig. 11.11). There are several alternatives for management of more severe wound necrosis. The wound can be treated conservatively with local debridements combined with nutritional supplementation. In patients who are better rehabilitation candidates, some authors recommend total-contact casting with continued progression of weight bearing and rehabilitation. These authors state that weight bearing in a properly fitted total-contact cast stimulates wound healing and stump maturation. We prefer to postpone prosthetic use until the wound has healed. We have made extensive use of vacuum-assisted closure in this setting.

In cases of severe necrosis with poor coverage of the bone end, wedge resection may be indicated. The basic principle of wedge resection is to regard the end of the amputation stump as a hemisphere. Although local resection increases local tension on already compromised tissues, resection of a wedge incorporating the full diameter of the stump would allow for reformation of the hemisphere while minimizing local pressures (Fig. 11.12). Finally, hyperbaric oxygen therapy and transcutaneous electrical nerve stimulation have been shown in some studies to promote wound healing.

CONTRACTURES

Mild or moderate contractures of the joints of an amputation stump should be prevented by proper positioning of the stump, gentle passive stretching, and having the patient engage in exercises to strengthen the muscles controlling the joint. At the knee, increased ambulation tends to reduce a contracture. In some patients, prosthetic modification may be necessary to adapt to the contracture. Rarely, severe fixed contractures may require treatment by wedging casts or by surgical release of the contracted structures.

PAIN

Because pain is complex and mediated by multiple pathways, Kehlet and Dahl introduced the concept of multimodal analgesia for the management of acute postoperative pain. This

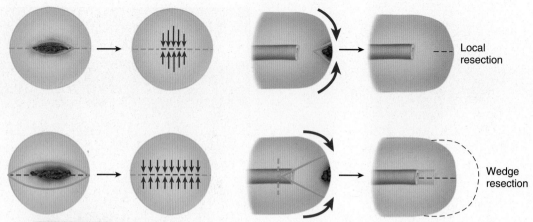

FIGURE 11.12 Diagrams of end-on and side views of amputation stumps. Local resection produces uneven tension; this is reduced and evenly distributed after wedge resection.

algorithm has proven to be valuable at our institution, and examples are shown in Table 11.3. Effectively treating postoperative pain will promote function, enhance psychologic well-being, and potentially minimize the risk of developing chronic pain.

After the immediate postoperative pain has been resolved, some patients continue to feel chronic pain as a result of various causes. The first step in management is to diagnose the cause accurately. Phantom limb pain must be differentiated from residual limb pain, and both must be distinguished from pain arising from a distant site, such as from a herniated lumbar disc.

Mechanical lower back pain has been shown to be more prevalent in amputees than in the general population. In a study of 92 patients with amputations, back pain was rated more bothersome than phantom limb pain or residual limb pain. In addition to other accepted treatments for back pain, patients must be instructed on proper prosthetic ambulation to minimize abnormal stresses on the lumbar spine.

Residual limb pain is often caused by a poorly fitting prosthesis. Pressure is placed on tissues of the remaining leg or arm that were not designed to be pressure bearing. An intimate fit is required to provide maximal function and avoid focal pressure points that can often be uncomfortable or painful.

The stump should be evaluated for areas of abnormal pressure, especially over bony prominences. Distal stump edema, often called "choking," may result if the end is not completely seated in the prosthesis, and ulceration or gangrene could result. These problems can be avoided with socket modifications.

A neuroma always forms after division of a nerve. A painful neuroma occurs when the nerve end is subjected to pressure or repeated irritation. A painful neuroma usually can be prevented by gentle traction on the nerve followed by sharp proximal division, allowing the nerve end to retract deep into the soft tissue. A painful neuroma usually is easily palpable and often has a positive Tinel sign. Treatment initially consists of socket modification. If this fails to relieve symptoms, simple neuroma excision or a more proximal neurectomy may be required. Some authors recommend neuroma excision combined with centrocentral anastomosis of the proximal stump or a procedure to seal the epineurial sleeve. Rarely, it may be difficult to distinguish a neuroma from a possible recurrent tumor. Provost et al. have provided some helpful descriptions of the ultrasound features of a neuroma.

Other possible causes of residual limb pain may be unrelated to the amputation stump. Osteoarthritis of the hip in a patient with an amputation should be treated the same way as with any other patient. If conservative measures fail to relieve symptoms, total hip arthroplasty should be offered as a reasonable option. Pain from osteoarthritis of the knee in a patient with a transtibial amputation, although rare, may be partially relieved by adding a knee joint and thigh corset to the prosthesis to allow load sharing with the thigh.

Phantom limb sensations are common after an amputation and they should be considered normal. Most patients do not find these to be bothersome. The most important part of management is simply to educate the patient regarding these sensations so that they are not surprised by their presence. During the first year after amputation, many patients experience a phenomenon referred to as "telescoping," whereby the phantom limb gradually shortens to the end of the residual limb.

Phantom limb pain is far less common. The exact incidence is difficult to determine because many authors fail to differentiate between phantom limb pain and phantom limb sensations. Other authors fail to distinguish between the mere presence of phantom limb pain versus the presence of severe phantom limb pain, which has a significant effect on the patient. Subsequently, some reports state that phantom limb pain is present in 80% of amputees. Most authors would agree that truly bothersome phantom limb pain is much less common and is probably present in less than 10% of amputees. In our experience, phantom limb pain is more often present with proximal amputations, such as forequarter and hindquarter amputations. Phantom pain also appears to be more common in patients who felt pain in the limb before amputation. Subsequently, some investigators claim that phantom limb pain can be prevented with the use of epidural anesthesia beginning the day before surgery. Other investigators have failed to substantiate these claims. When significant pain is established, however, it can be extremely difficult to treat. Although no one specific method is universally beneficial, some patients may benefit from such diverse measures as massage, ice, heat, increased prosthetic use, relaxation training, biofeedback, sympathetic blockade, oral medications, local nerve blocks, epidural blocks, ultrasound, transcutaneous electrical nerve stimulation, and placement of a dorsal column stimulator. Other general treatment guidelines have been suggested to be helpful. These include controlling stump edema, decreasing anxiety and stress, establishing good sleep hygiene patterns, decreasing depression, and encouraging smoking cessation. Treatment algorithms have been developed for both residual limb pain and phantom limb pain (Figs. 11.13 and 11.14).

DERMATOLOGIC PROBLEMS

Patients should be instructed to wash their stumps with a mild antimicrobial soap at least once a day. The stump should be thoroughly rinsed and dried before donning the prosthesis. Likewise, the prosthesis should be kept clean and should be thoroughly dried before donning.

Contact dermatitis is common and may be confused with infection. Skin inflammation is associated with intense itching and burning when wearing the socket. The most common cause is failure to rinse detergents from stump socks thoroughly. Other sensitizers include nickel, chromates used in leathers, skin creams, antioxidants in rubber, topical antibiotics, and topical anesthetics. Treatment consists of removal of the irritant, soaks, steroid cream, and compression.

Bacterial folliculitis may occur in areas of hairy, oily skin. The problem may be exacerbated by shaving and by poor hygiene. Treatment initially consists of improved hygiene and possibly socket modifications to relieve areas of abnormal pressure. Occasionally, cellulitis develops that requires antibiotic treatment or an abscess forms that requires incision and drainage.

Epidermoid cysts may develop at the socket brim. These frequently occur late and are best treated with socket modification. Excision may be required.

Verrucous hyperplasia refers to a wart-like overgrowth of the skin at the end of the stump. It is caused by proximal constriction that prevents the stump from fully seating in the prosthesis. This "choking," as previously mentioned, causes distal stump edema followed by thickening of the skin, fissuring, ulceration, and possibly subsequent infection. Treatment initially is directed toward treating the infection. The skin should be treated with soaks and salicylic acid to soften the keratin. Socket modification is mandatory because pressure on the distal skin is essential to treat the problem and to prevent recurrences.

AMPUTATIONS IN CHILDREN

Amputations in children may be divided into two general categories: congenital and acquired. Surveys of specialized child amputee clinics have shown that approximately 60% of childhood amputations are secondary to congenital limb deficiencies and 40% are secondary to acquired conditions. Acquired amputations most often are secondary to trauma, followed by neoplasm and infection. Motor vehicle accidents, gunshot wounds, and power tool injuries are the most common causes of limb loss from injury in older children; in young children, accidents with power tools, such as lawnmowers, and other household accidents are the most common causes. Dysvascular amputations in children are rare, but when they do occur, they usually are secondary to thrombotic or embolic events caused by another underlying problem. Congenital amputations are discussed in other chapter; only acquired amputations in children are considered here.

Most of the techniques of amputation described for adults also are useful for children, but in pediatric patients, general body growth and stump growth are significant factors. Krajbich summarized the general principles of childhood amputation surgery as follows: (1) preserve length, (2) preserve important growth plates, (3) perform disarticulation rather than transosseous amputation whenever possible, (4) preserve the knee joint whenever possible, (5) stabilize and normalize the proximal portion of the limb, and (6) be prepared to deal with issues in addition to limb deficiency in children with other clinically important conditions.

Preserving length is crucial. Seventy-five percent of the growth of the femur occurs at the distal growth plate. Consequently, any transfemoral amputation performed in a young child would result in a very short stump as an adult. Conversely, even a very short transtibial stump in a young child may result in a functional stump as an adult if the growth plate is preserved.

Disarticulation can provide a child with a well-balanced, sturdy stump capable of end weight bearing. Length and physes are preserved without the risks of terminal overgrowth. Additionally, prosthetic suspension is improved with a disarticulation secondary to preservation of the metaphyseal flares. This is important because of the high mechanical demands that children often place on their prostheses.

Terminal bone overgrowth is a significant problem in a child amputee with a transosseous amputation. The problem does not occur after disarticulation. The overgrowth is caused by appositional new bone formation and is unrelated to the growth of the physis. The resulting bone is elongated and often pencil shaped. It may cause swelling, edema, pain, and bursa formation, and in severe cases may penetrate the skin. Overgrowth is more common after traumatic amputations than after amputations performed for other indications. It is also more common in younger children than in older children and occurs most often in the humerus and fibula and less often in the tibia, femur, radius, and ulna, in that order. The exact incidence is difficult to determine because of variables in the definition of *significant* overgrowth and variations in the age cutoff of different studies. In one study, 27% of child amputees experienced overgrowth severe enough to require revision surgery.

Terminal overgrowth is treated effectively with surgical resection of the excess bone. Epiphysiodesis has been unsuccessful and is contraindicated. Capping the bone with a synthetic device has had only limited success and has been complicated by infection or fracture of the implant or bone. Improved results have been obtained by capping the bone with an epiphyseal graft harvested from the amputated limb at the index procedure (Fig. 11.15) or by capping with tricortical iliac crest graft at a revision operation.

Because of growth issues and increased body metabolism, children often can tolerate procedures on amputation stumps that are not tolerated by adults, including more forceful skin traction, the application of extensive skin grafts, and the closure of skin flaps under moderate tension. In addition, complications after surgery tend to be less severe in children. Painful phantom sensations do not develop, and neuromas rarely are troublesome enough to require surgery. Even extensive scars usually are tolerated well. One or more spurs usually develop on the end of the bone, but, in contrast to terminal overgrowth, almost never require resection. Psychologic problems after amputation are rare in children until they reach adolescence, at which time they may become severe enough to require treatment.

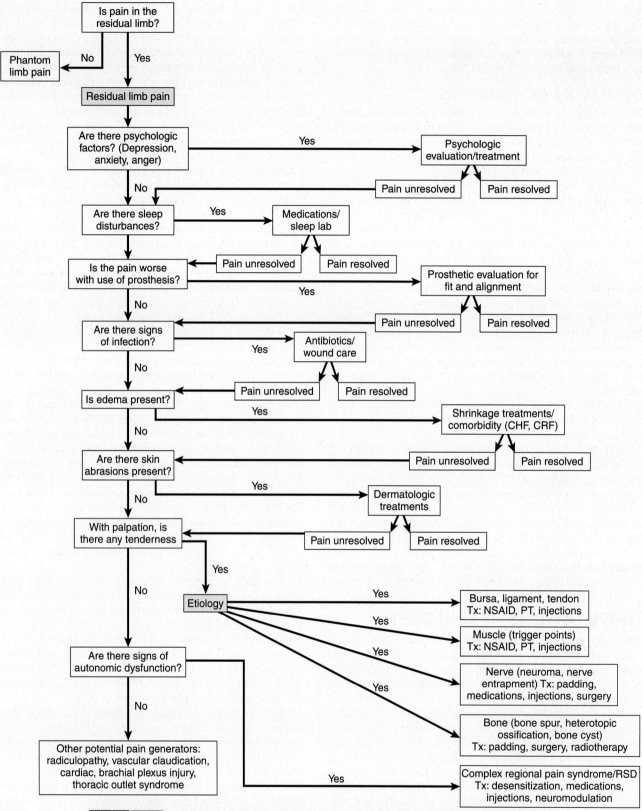

FIGURE 11.13 Residual limb pain algorithm. *CHF,* Chronic heart failure; *CRF,* chronic renal failure; *NSAID,* nonsteroidal antiinflammatory drugs; *PT,* physical therapy; *RSD,* reflex sympathetic dystrophy. (From Hompland S: Pain management for upper extremity amputation. In: Meier RH, Atkins DJ, editors: *Functional restoration of adults and children with upper extremity amputation,* New York, Demos, 2004.)

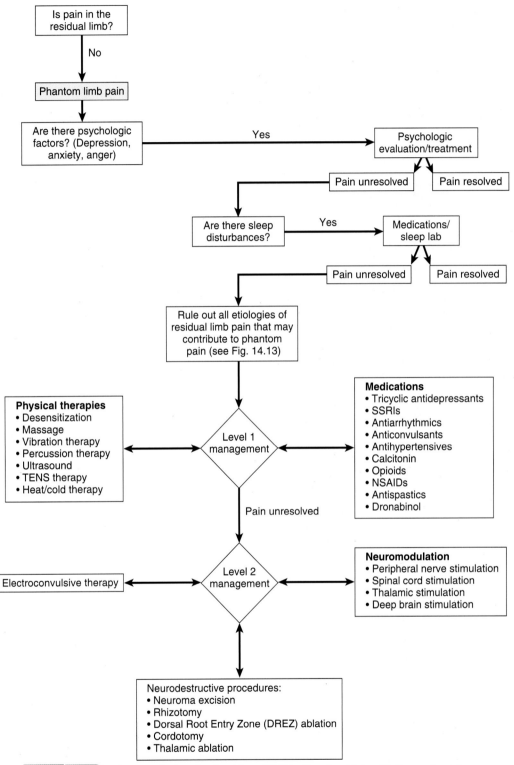

FIGURE 11.14 Phantom limb pain algorithm. *NSAIDs,* Nonsteroidal antiinflammatory drugs; *SSRIs,* selective serotonin reuptake inhibitors; *TENS,* transcutaneous electrical nerve stimulation. (From Hompland S: Pain management for upper extremity amputation. In: Meier RH, Atkins DJ, editors: *Functional restoration of adults and children with upper extremity amputation*, New York, Demos, 2004.)

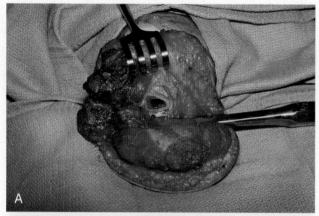

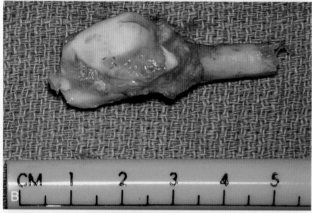

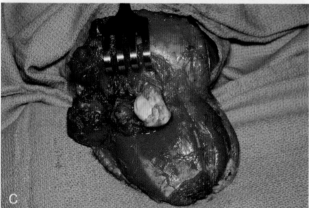

FIGURE 11.15 Stump capping procedure. **A,** Transtibial amputation in a 2-year-old child. **B,** Distal fibula from amputated leg is fashioned to fit into cut end of tibia. **C,** Fibula is press-fit into tibia.

activities. Because of their activity level and growth, children with amputations must be observed closely for prosthetic repair, for frequent changes in the socket, and for fitting with new prostheses.

Children use prostheses extremely well, and their proficiency increases as they age and mature. In general, a progressive prosthetic program should be designed that parallels normal motor development. At a young age, children function well with simple prostheses. As they grow, modifications may be made, such as the addition of a knee joint, a mobile elbow joint, or a mechanical hand. By the time children reach adolescence, they may begin to take advantage of the most sophisticated prostheses, including those for specialized

REFERENCES

Alothman S, Alenazi A, Waitman LR, et al.: Neuropathy and other risk factors for lower extremity amputation in people with diabetes using a clinical data repository system, *J Allied Health* 47:217, 2018.

Ayling OG, Montbriand J, Jiang J, et al.: Continuous regional anesthesia provides effective pain management and reduces opioid requirement following major lower limb amputation, *Eur J Vasc Endovasc Surg* 48:559, 2014.

Borghi B, D'Addabbo M, Borghi R: Can neural blocks prevent phantom limb pain? *Pain Manag* 4:261, 2014.

Chang CP, Hsiao CT, Lin CN, et al.: Risk factors for mortality in the late amputation of necrotizing fasciitis: a retrospective study, *World J Emerg Surg* 13:45, 2018.

Chopra A, Azarbal AF, Jung E, et al.: Ambulation and functional outcome after major lower extremity amputation, *J Vasc Surg* 67:1521, 2018.

Churilov I, Churilov L, Murphy D: Do rigid dressings reduce the time from amputation to prosthetic fitting? A systematic review and meta-analysis, *Ann Vasc Surg* 28:1801, 2014.

Ciufo DJ, Thirukumaran CP, Marchese R, et al: Risk factors for reoperation, readmission, an early complications after below knee amputation, Injury Oct 30, doi: 10.1016/j.injury.2018. [Epub ahead of print].

Collins KL, Russell HG, Schumacher PJ, et al.: A review of current theories and treatments for phantom limb pain, *J Clin Invest* 128:2168, 2018.

Coulston JE, Tuff V, Twine CP, et al.: Surgical factors in the prevention of infection following major lower limb amputation, *Eur J Vasc Endovasc Surg* 43:556, 2012.

Curran T, Zhang JQ, Lo RC, et al.: Risk factors and indications for readmission after lower extremity amputation in the American College of Surgeons National Surgical Quality Improvement Program, *J Vasc Surg* 60:1315, 2014.

Ebrahimzadeh MH, Moradi A, Khorasani MR, et al.: Long-term clinical outcomes of war-related bilateral lower extremities amputation, *Injury* 46:275, 2015.

Fisher TFm Kusnezov NA, Bader JA, et al.: Predictors of acute complications following traumatic upper extremity amputation, *J Surg Orthop Adv* 27:113, 2018.

Lim S, Javorski MJ, Halandras PM, et al.: Through-knee amputation is a feasible alternative to above-knee amputation, *J Vasc Surg* 68:197, 2019.

Markatos K, Karamanou M, Saranteas T, et al.: Hallmarks of amputation surgery, *Int Orthop*, 43(2):493, 2019.

Penna A, Konstantatos AH, Cranwell W, et al.: Incidence and associations of painful neuroma in a contemporary cohort of lower-limb amputees, *ANZ J Surg* 88:491, 2018.

Phair J, DeCarlo C, Scher L, et al.: Risk factors for unplanned readmission and stump complications after major lower extremity amputation, *J Vasc Aurg* 67:848, 2018.

Pisansky AJB, Brovman EY, Kuo C, et al.: Perioperative outcomes after regional versus general anesthesia for above the knee amputations, *Ann Vasc Surg* 48(53), 2018.

Polfer EM, Hoyt BW, Senchak LT, et al.: Fluid collections in amputations are not indicative or predictive of infection, *Clin Orthop Relat Res* 472:2978, 2014.

Reichmann JP, Stevens PM, Rheinstein J, et al.: Removable rigid dressings for postoperative management of transtibial amputations: a review of published evidence, *PM R* 10:516, 2018.

Shah SK, Bena JF, Allemang MT, et al.: Lower extremity amputations: factors associated with mortality or contralateral amputation, *Vasc Endovascular Surg* 47:608, 2013.

Shawen SB, Keeling JJ, Branstetter J, et al.: The mangled foot and leg: salvage versus amputation, *Foot Ankle Clin* 15:63, 2010.

Shin JY, Roh SG, Sharaf B, et al.: Risk of major limb amputation in diabetic foot ulcer and accompanying disease: A meta-analysis, *J Plast Reconstr Aesthet Surg* 70:1681, 2017.

Srivastava D: Chronic post-amputation pain: peri-operative management – review, *Br J Pain* 11:192, 2017.

Sumpio B, Thakor P, Mahler D, Blume P: Negative pressure wound therapy as postoperative dressing in below knee amputation stump closure of patients with chronic venous insufficiency, *Wounds* 23:301, 2011.

Uustal H, Meier III RH: Pain issues and treatment of the person with an amputation, *Phys Med Rehabil Clin N Am* 25:45, 2014.

von Plato H, Kontinen V, Hamunen K: Efficacy and safety of epidural, continuous perineural infusion and adjuvant analgesics for acute postoperative pain after major limb amputation – a systematic review, *Scan J Pain* 18:3, 2018.

Wang X, Yi Y, Tang D, et al.: Gabapentin as an adjuvant therapy for prevention of acute phantom-limb pain in pediatric patients undergoing amputation for malignant bone tumors: a prospective double-blind randomized controlled trial, *J Pain Symptom Manage* 55:721, 2017.

Wied C, Tengberg PT, Holm G, et al.: Tourniquets do not increase the total blood loss or re-amputation risk in transtibial amputations, *World J Orthop* 8:62, 2017.

The complete list of references is available online at Expert Consult.com

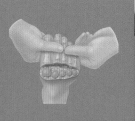

CHAPTER 12

AMPUTATIONS OF THE FOOT

David R. Richardson

TOE AMPUTATIONS   587   **MIDFOOT AMPUTATIONS**   595   **HINDFOOT AND ANKLE AMPUTATIONS**   600

As a percent of amputations involving the lower extremity, those around the foot and ankle are becoming increasingly common (Fig. 12.1). With advances in vascular and perfusion assessment and improvements in foot prostheses and footwear, success with ankle and partial foot amputations, as measured by functional, independent living, seems to be improving. When it is determined that limb salvage is not in a patient's best interest, ablation by amputation or disarticulation should be viewed as a reconstructive procedure rather than a treatment failure.

Indications for distal lower extremity amputation include trauma, peripheral vascular disease, neuropathy, infection, and tumor. Surgeons must be aware of advances in knowledge, technique, and technology that may influence the decision for or against amputation. Over the past few years, more literature has emerged to better define indications for amputation. The Lower Extremity Assessment Project (LEAP) study suggests that injury severity scoring systems, including the Limb Salvage Index, Predictive Salvage Index, and Mangled Extremity Severity Score, are insensitive in indicating those patients who ultimately benefit from amputation. The LEAP study did, however, find the Mangled Extremity Severity Score highly specific in ruling out patients who do not require amputation.

Presently, diabetic patients comprise over 70% of amputations because of ischemia, and over 30% of diabetic patients with a partial foot amputation will ultimately progress to a more proximal level of limb loss. Research indicates patients with diabetes fear major amputation more than death. Therefore, compassion and education are critical components of treatment.

Current guidelines for diabetic foot infections recommend histological analysis and culture for a diagnosis of osteomyelitis. However, bone biopsy may not be as reliable as once thought.

Severe postoperative infections have been found to be significantly more frequent in patients with complicated diabetes (defined as the presence of neuropathy, history of ulcers, Charcot neuroarthropathy, or vascular disease) than in those with uncomplicated diabetes or patients without diabetes. Despite the definitive nature of an amputation, diabetic patients with severe neuroarthropathy or ulceration perceive their quality of life as equal to that of those with lower extremity amputation. The roles of the certified pedorthist, orthotist, and prosthetist should not be undervalued in maximizing function and minimizing complications after amputations of the lower extremity.

Nutritional status and limb perfusion must be evaluated before surgery. With over one third of foot and ankle amputations in diabetic patients progressing to a higher level, it is important to optimize healing potential preoperatively. Critical values have been established to predict wound healing after amputation in the lower extremity. Indications of adequate perfusion include an ultrasound Doppler ankle-brachial index of more than 0.5, although this may be falsely elevated in patients with noncompressible vessels (Monckeberg sclerosis) and transcutaneous oxygen perfusion pressure on room air of more than 40 mm Hg. Toe pressures may be the most reliable noninvasive vascular measure, with 45 mm Hg or greater predictive of healing. The nutritional status of a patient also is crucial in wound healing after ablation procedures around the foot and ankle. A serum albumin value less than 3.5 g/dL and a total lymphocyte count less than 1500/mL have been shown to correlate with poor healing. A healing rate of 82% can be obtained with a total lymphocyte count of more than 1500/mL and an albumin level of at least 3.5 g/dL. Patients with poor nutritional status should be evaluated for dietary supplementation before surgery to maximize healing. Alternatively, a higher-level amputation may be chosen if delaying amputation carries an unacceptable risk to the patient. Gangrene upon admission and insulin-dependent diabetes are significant risk factors for reamputation.

Meticulous surgical technique, including avoidance of excessive pressure on the skin edges with forceps and use of thick skin flaps, may decrease wound complications. Refraining from tourniquet use, controlling hemostasis, and avoiding hematoma formation may be beneficial.

Expanding coverage options and advances in wound management have allowed greater success in more distal amputations. Advancement, rotation, transposition, and pedicle flaps are possible for limited coverage requirements around the foot and ankle; however, vascularized free flaps often are necessary for more extensive coverage. Consulting a plastic and reconstructive specialist early in treatment often is beneficial. There

Syme — Chopart — Transmetatarsal — Metatarsal phalangeal disarticulation

Lisfranc

Toe amputation or disarticulation

FIGURE 12.1   Levels of partial foot amputation.

are many types of dressings, including hydrocolloid, hydrogel, alginate, and debriding agents, and other types of biological dressings, such as Allomatrix and Graftjacket regenerative tissue matrix (Wright Medical, Memphis, TN). Platelet-rich plasma gel application has shown promise for treating diabetic, dysvascular wounds, as have growth factor and biologic wound products. Negative-pressure wound (vacuum-assisted closure) dressings also may be beneficial in larger wounds of the midfoot, hindfoot, and ankle. The vacuum-assisted closure system has been shown to heal diabetic foot wounds proximal to the transmetatarsal level faster and more predictably than moist gauze dressing changes. Vacuum-assisted closure dressings may be of less benefit in small forefoot wounds and wounds with severe peripheral vascular disease. It has been suggested that gauze-dressing changes may be more efficacious for patients with peripheral vascular disease. Larger, condition-specific studies are needed to better determine the role of each of these treatment options. What is evident is the benefit of treatment by a multidisciplinary team willing to collaborate to help the patient.

TOE AMPUTATIONS

Amputation of a single toe, with few exceptions, causes little disturbance in stance or gait. Amputation of the great toe does not functionally affect standing or walking at a normal pace. However, if the patient walks rapidly or runs, a limp appears because of the loss of push-off normally provided by the great toe. Amputation of the second toe frequently is followed by severe hallux valgus because the great toe tends to drift toward the third to fill the gap left by amputation. Smith recommended a second ray amputation and narrowing the foot. Screw fixation is used in this technique (Fig. 12.2) to prevent a severe valgus deformity from occurring. Amputation of any of the other toes causes little disturbance. Toe amputations are the most common partial foot amputation and, of these, the fifth toe is most commonly amputated, the usual indication being overriding on the fourth toe. Here amputation often is preferred to reconstructive procedures because it is simple and definitive

(Fig. 12.3). Toe amputation is a significant predictor of future limb loss. Amputation of all toes causes little disturbance in ordinary slow walking but is disabling during a more rapid gait and when spring and resilience of the foot are required. It interferes with squatting and tiptoeing. Usually, amputation of all toes requires no prosthesis, other than a shoe filler (Fig. 12.4). Amputation of more than two rays often is more disabling than a transmetatarsal amputation.

Amputation through the metatarsals is disabling in proportion to the level of amputation—the more proximal the level, the greater the disability. The loss of push-off in the absence of a positive fulcrum in the ball of the foot is chiefly responsible for impairment of gait. No prosthesis is required other than a shoe filler.

Foot amputations proximal to the transmetatarsal level result in considerable gait disturbance because of the loss of support and push-off. Such procedures occasionally are indicated, however, after severe trauma and in diabetic patients. Better preoperative tests for tissue perfusion have

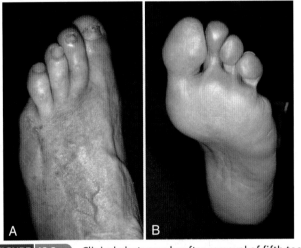

FIGURE 12.3 Clinical photographs after removal of fifth toe.

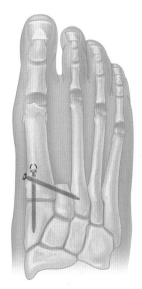

FIGURE 12.2 Second ray amputation with screw fixation to narrow the foot.

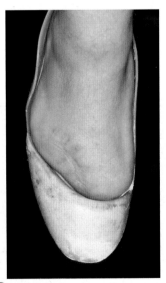

FIGURE 12.4 Custom shoe insert for transmetatarsal amputation.

made it possible to predict with reasonable accuracy the patients in whom toe, ray, and partial foot amputations will heal. In addition to using the ankle-brachial index, toe pressures of greater than 45 mm Hg and transcutaneous partial pressure of oxygen of more than 37 mm Hg correlate with healing of wounds. A transcutaneous partial pressure of oxygen of less than 20 mm Hg indicates that healing is unlikely at that level.

Good healing and functional results may be expected in diabetic patients after open Lisfranc or Chopart amputations with secondary closure. However, amputation at either level often results in an equinus deformity, because of loss of the foot dorsiflexor attachments (Fig. 12.5) and may require an ankle arthrodesis or revision to a higher level because such deformities prevent ambulation. Heel cord tenotomy or tenectomy can prevent early equinus deformities from becoming fixed, which can decrease the number of patients requiring revision to a higher level. Lisfranc (Fig. 12.6) and Chopart amputations done for severe foot trauma have a higher failure rate. Patients who heal function well with simple prosthetic devices, and good results can be achieved with amputation levels that have been unsatisfactory in the past.

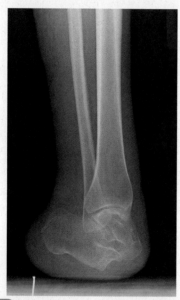

FIGURE 12.5 Severe equinus deformity after amputation through Chopart joints.

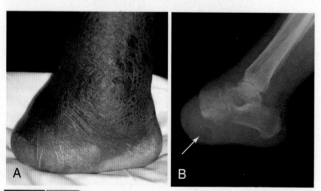

FIGURE 12.6 Amputation through Lisfranc joint. Note recurrent seroma on lateral radiograph.

TERMINAL SYME AMPUTATION

This amputation shares the name of the Syme amputation through the ankle because of the similar reconstruction of the plantar flap used for coverage. Indications include hallux terminal ulcerations, chronic ingrown nails with paronychia or nail deformity, hallux tuft osteomyelitis, or traumatic injury to the tip of the hallux involving the nail bed. Care must be taken to remove the entire matrix while attempting to maintain the insertion of the extensor and flexor hallucis longus.

TECHNIQUE 12.1

- Palpate the hallux interphalangeal joint and mark the dorsal incision just distal to this level in a transverse fashion. A digital tourniquet can be used but is usually not needed.
- Extend the incision on both sides of the hallux nail bed to include the paronychia. Distally extend the incision to include the terminal aspect of the hallux (Fig. 12.7A).
- Remove the nail plate, nail bed, contiguous soft tissue and distal aspect of the distal phalanx (retaining the extensor hallucis longus and flexor hallucis longus insertion) (Fig. 12.7B).
- Close the skin in a single everted layer (Fig. 12.7C). Do not attempt to contour the skin tags because they will remodel over time (Fig. 12.7D) and removing them can lead to wound problems.
- Dress the wound in a mildly compressive forefoot dressing.

POSTOPERATIVE CARE A sterile dressing is kept in place for 2 weeks. The sutures are removed at 12 to 16 days. Weight bearing is allowed in a stiff-soled shoe until the wound is healed. Then the patient may transition to a shoe with a wide toe box.

AMPUTATION AT THE BASE OF THE PROXIMAL PHALANX

Maintaining the base of the proximal phalanx often is preferable to metatarsophalangeal joint disarticulations. This allows for retention of some weight-bearing properties, especially in the hallux, where 1 cm of proximal phalanx allows for contribution by the flexor hallucis brevis and the plantar fascia. It also may slow the deviation of adjacent toes when one of the lesser digits is amputated (Fig. 12.8).

TECHNIQUE 12.2

- The skin incision varies with the toe involved. For the great toe, make a long medial incision and then circumscribe the digit. Begin the incision over the first metatarsal head in the midline medially and curve it distally over the lateral and posterior aspects for a distance slightly greater than the anteroposterior diameter of the digit and slightly longer plantarly than dorsally (Fig. 12.9A).

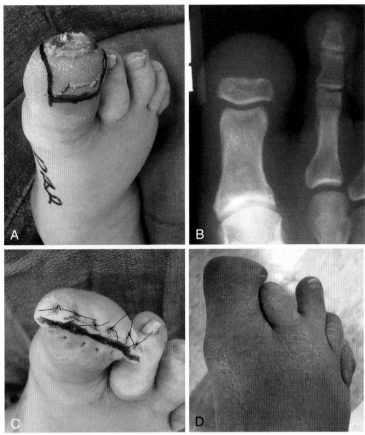

FIGURE 12.7   Terminal Syme amputation. **A,** Incision. **B,** Removal of distal aspect of phalanx along with nail plate and nail bed. **C,** Skin closure. **D,** Final appearance of toe. **SEE TECHNIQUE 12.1.**

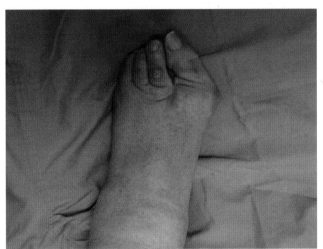

FIGURE 12.8   Hallux valgus deformity after second metatarsophalangeal joint disarticulation.

- With an oscillating saw, osteotomize the base of the first proximal phalanx 1 cm from the base. Ensure that the attachments of the flexor and extensor hallucis brevis are preserved (Fig. 12.9B).
- In the second, third, and fourth toes, amputation is done through a short dorsal racquet-shaped incision (Fig. 12.9C). Begin the incision 1 cm proximal to the metatarsophalangeal joint and extend it distally to the base of

the proximal phalanx, then curve it to pass around the toe across the plantar surface at the level of the flexor crease.
- With an oscillating saw, osteotomize the proximal phalanx 1 cm from the base, ensuring the integrity of the flexor and extensor digitorum brevis.
- In the fifth toe, fashion a lateral incision and extend it circumferentially around the medial aspect of the toe distally to the level of the proximal interphalangeal joint. Again leave 1 cm of bone at the base of the proximal phalanx.
- Draw the extrinsic tendons distally, divide them, and allow them to retract.
- Identify the digital nerves and divide them proximal to the end of the bone and divide and ligate the digital vessels.
- In either the great toe or fifth toe, copiously irrigate the wound, obtain hemostasis, and close the wound by approximating the skin edges (Fig. 12.9D).
- In amputation of the second, third, or fourth toe, close the skin edges with interrupted nonabsorbable sutures, as shown in Fig. 12.9E.

POSTOPERATIVE CARE   Protect the amputation site with a sterile dressing for 12 to 16 days. Remove the sutures in dysvascular patients at 21 to 23 days, unless the wound has obviously healed sooner. Protected weight bearing usually is not needed. A shoe with the toe box cut out or a wooden-soled postoperative shoe is worn until the sutures are removed. When the edema has subsided, ambulation in a supportive, soft-soled, accommodating shoe is allowed.

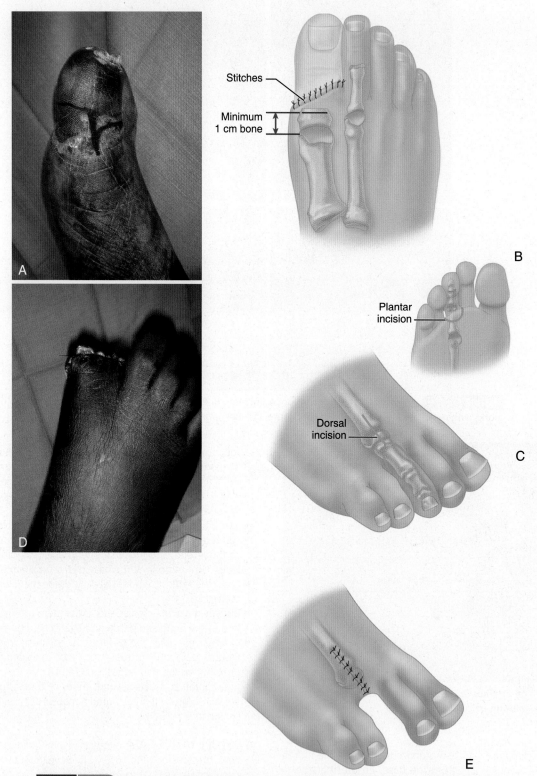

FIGURE 12.9 Amputation at base of phalanx. **A,** Incision. **B,** Osteotomy of first proximal phalanx 1 cm from base. **C,** Racquet-shaped incision. Osteotomy of lesser toes also is made 1 cm from the base of the proximal phalanx. **D** and **E,** Wound closure. **SEE TECHNIQUES 12.2 AND 12.4.**

METATARSOPHALANGEAL JOINT DISARTICULATION

In the diabetic foot, ischemia or osteomyelitis or both are the most compelling indications for amputation at the metatarsophalangeal joint.

TECHNIQUE 12.3

- Fashion a long plantar and a short dorsal skin flap. Begin the incision at the level of intended bone section at the midpoint on the medial side of the toe and curve it over the dorsal aspect to end at a similar point on the lateral side. Fashion a similar plantar flap but make it slightly longer than the dorsoplantar diameter of the toe at the level of bone section.
- Dissect the skin flaps proximally to the level of bone section.
- Divide the flexor and extensor tendons and let them retract just proximal to the end of the bone.
- Isolate and divide the digital nerves and ligate and divide the digital vessels.
- Section the bone at the selected level and smooth its end with a rasp.
- Close the flaps with interrupted nonabsorbable sutures.

TECHNIQUE 12.4

- Disarticulation of the metatarsophalangeal joint is carried out in the same manner as amputation through the base of the proximal phalanx, differing only in the level and manner of amputation of bone. The skin flaps may vary.
- Continue the incision distally to the level of the metatarsophalangeal joint and extend it distally and circumferentially while proceeding plantarward (Fig. 12.9C).
- Identify the capsule of the metatarsophalangeal joint and, with the toe in acute flexion, incise its dorsal side first; straighten the toe and expose and incise the remainder of the capsule after dividing the flexor tendons and neurovascular bundles, cauterizing the latter. Divide the neurovascular bundle distal to the bifurcation so as not to jeopardize the adjacent digits.
- For the first and fifth digit, fashion the incision in the same manner as described in Technique 12.2. If the skin allows, a longer plantar flap is probably indicated (Fig. 12.10).
- When performing a metatarsophalangeal disarticulation of the hallux, removing the sesamoids in the insensate foot is recommended. Stay close to the periosteum over the sesamoids (Fig. 12.11).

POSTOPERATIVE CARE Postoperative care is the same as after Technique 12.2.

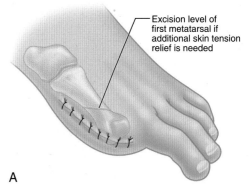

Excision level of first metatarsal if additional skin tension relief is needed

A

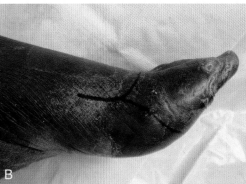

B

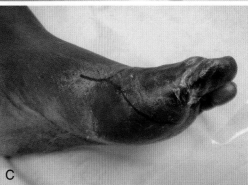

C

FIGURE 12.10 **A,** Disarticulation at metatarsophalangeal joint of great toe. **B** and **C,** Severe ischemia of hallux to level of metatarsophalangeal joint. **SEE TECHNIQUES 12.4 AND 12.5.**

FIRST OR FIFTH RAY AMPUTATION (BORDER RAY AMPUTATION)

TECHNIQUE 12.5

- For amputations at the first or fifth ray (border digit), the following incision is used. Base the incision medially (first digit) (see Fig. 12.10A) or dorsolaterally (fifth digit) (Fig. 12.12A), extending from the midline of the medial eminence (or lateral eminence of the fifth metatarsal) dorsally and plantarward to about the level of the middle of the metatarsal. If the ray is being amputated because of acute or chronic deep infection, such as in a diabetic foot with osteomyelitis, press the incision to bone because the tissue planes are obscured, and this flap may not survive if left thin.

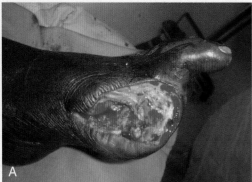
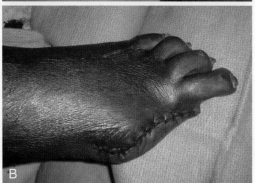

FIGURE 12.11 **A,** Sesamoids removed after first ray amputation in diabetic patient. **B,** Closure. Note longer plantar flap. **SEE TECHNIQUE 12.4.**

- When the dorsal full-thickness flap has been raised to the metatarsal, complete the plantar flap in the same manner.
- Open the capsule dorsal to the plantar flap and, retracting both flaps proximally, complete the disarticulation.
- Cauterize the neurovascular bundles.
- For the hallux, removing the sesamoids usually is not indicated unless the metatarsal head is retained.
- By extending the racquet-shaped incision proximally along the metatarsal shaft, part or all the first (or fifth) metatarsal may be removed. Take the incision to bone, raise the flaps at bone level, and section the first metatarsal from proximal plantar and medial to distal dorsal and lateral. Section the fifth metatarsal from proximal plantar and lateral to distal dorsal and medial (Fig. 12.12B, C).
- After lifting the bone, section the soft tissues to remove the intended segment. This is made easier by first disarticulating the digit at the metatarsophalangeal joint.
- If a disarticulation of the first metatarsal at the medial cuneiform is done, try to preserve the penetrating branch of the dorsalis pedis artery, coursing plantarward about 1 cm distal to the joint. Cautery or suture ligature often is necessary if it is sectioned. Also, consider reattaching the tibialis anterior if this has been detached. This tendon has a broad attachment to the base of the first metatarsal and the first cuneiform (Fig. 12.12D). Careful dissection may allow the tibialis anterior to remain attached to the first cuneiform, obviating the need for reattachment. Reattachment of the peroneus longus is not necessary.
- In fifth ray amputations, preserve the base of the fifth metatarsal to maintain the attachment of the peroneus

brevis. If the entire metatarsal is removed, reattach the brevis locally or tenodese to the peroneus longus.
- Close in a single layer of nonabsorbable suture (Fig. 12.12E).

POSTOPERATIVE CARE Postoperative care is the same as after Technique 12.2.

MULTIPLE RAY AMPUTATION

Usually, if more than two rays need to be removed, especially medially, a transmetatarsal amputation would be more functional. However, there is literature to suggest preservation of the medial two rays, even if a free flap is required, may result in significant improvement in maximally achieved ambulatory function.

After a first ray resection, the second ray also can be removed through the same incision (Fig. 12.13). If skin for coverage is limited, a fillet flap can be based laterally. If the form of the amputation is dictated by trauma rather than infection or arteriosclerosis, preservation of as much bony architecture as possible is reasonable. This may require a free vascularized flap, particularly in a younger patient (Fig. 12.14).

Partial foot amputations are especially desirable in a diabetic patient whose opposite foot is at significant risk. Amputation of the medial two or lateral two or even three rays often provides a functional weight-bearing foot (Fig. 12.15).

CENTRAL RAY AMPUTATION

Occasionally, because of infection with or without ischemia, particularly in a diabetic foot, and after trauma, partial or complete removal of one or more of the central rays is indicated. If the third and fourth rays require removal, it is particularly difficult to secure closure because of immobility of the recessed second ray. An osteotomy of the base of the fifth metatarsal may facilitate the closure (Fig. 12.16).

TECHNIQUE 12.6

- Begin a dorsal longitudinal incision over the metatarsal shaft of the ray to be resected; place the incision between the metatarsals if two are to be removed. Leaving a small remnant of the base of the metatarsal, if not contraindicated because of infection, expedites the excision.
- Disarticulation at the cuneiform level is tedious because of the limited exposure, the strength of the supporting capsuloligamentous structures, and the angles of planes at the tarsometatarsal joints. Disarticulating the toe at the metatarsophalangeal joint before excising the metatarsal also facilitates excision. The extensor tendons can be retracted or removed to enhance exposure.
- By sharp and blunt dissection, remove the intrinsic muscles on either side, transect the bone transversely, and,

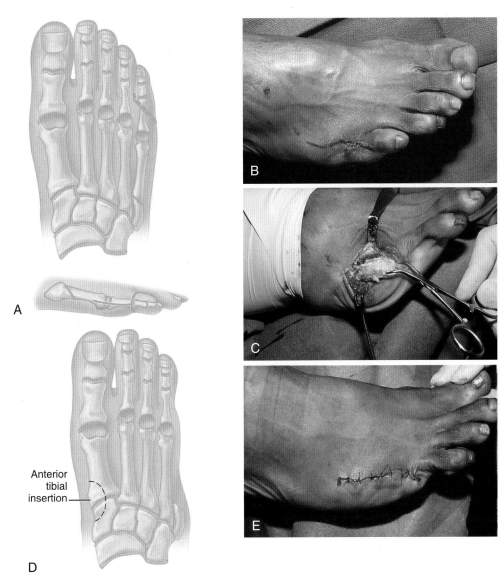

FIGURE 12.12 Fifth ray amputation. **A** to **C,** Incision and removal of sectioned metatarsal. **D,** Final resection of fifth metatarsal. **E,** Wound closure. **SEE TECHNIQUE 12.5.**

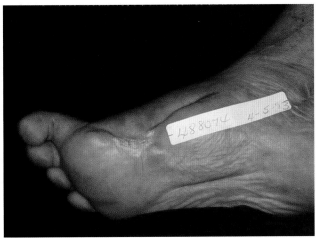

FIGURE 12.13 Complete amputation of first ray through medial incision.

lifting proximal to distal, clear the undersurface (plantar surface) of the metatarsal.

- After skeletonizing the bone to the level of the osteotomy, section the bone from dorsal distal to plantar proximal to avoid excess pressure with weight bearing (see Fig. 12.16).
- Disarticulation at the cuneiform or cuboid is an alternative technique.
- Unless the wound has been rendered surgically clean, leave it open and inspect it in 48 to 96 hours.
- Close primarily or with a skin graft when the wound allows. Consider placement of a drain (Fig. 12.17).

POSTOPERATIVE CARE Protected weight bearing for 3 to 4 weeks is recommended. When the edema has subsided, which may take several weeks, a noncustom-designed soft shoe is worn.

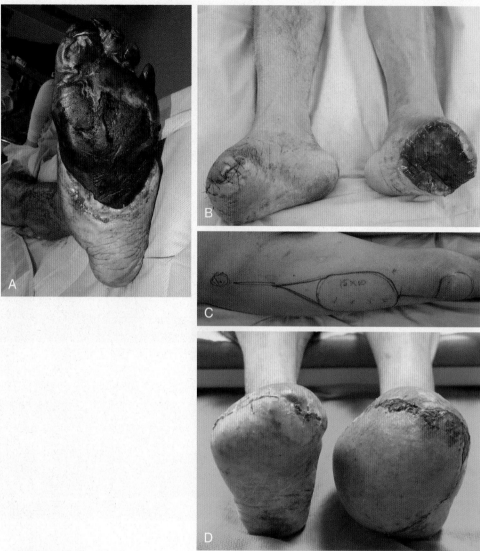

FIGURE 12.14 **A,** Vasopressor-induced necrosis in bilateral feet. Due to contralateral transmetatarsal amputation, every effort was made to preserve bony architecture. **B,** After transmetatarsal amputation and temporary coverage. **C** and **D,** Anterolateral thigh vascularized free flap was used. Debulking was required to allow for reasonable shoe wear. This amputation and graft are indicated when preservation of bony architecture is paramount, and caution is required when deep infection or arteriosclerosis is present.

A deep central space abscess with necrosis of the intrinsic muscles of the foot may be managed by external debridement and excision of one or more central rays with lateral border metatarsal osteotomy to close the gap. A few large retention sutures (when vascularity of the remaining part of the foot is not in question) approximating the medial and lateral borders of the foot provide a loose closure and allow drainage; the remainder of the wound heals by secondary intention. In this extenuating circumstance, where salvage of any functional part of the foot is the goal, angulation of the metatarsal osteotomy is not of prime importance or consequence.

TRANSMETATARSAL AMPUTATION

Transmetatarsal amputation allows patients to ambulate with a shoe filler and steel shank with rocker soles but without a prosthesis. Limb length is preserved, and gait is maintained fairly well. It is important to recognize the high morbidity and mortality rate of those undergoing nontraumatic amputations. Although transmetatarsal amputations heal less predictably than transtibial amputations, if the patient's vascularity allows, the benefits often outweigh the risk of needing a second surgery for revision. Despite

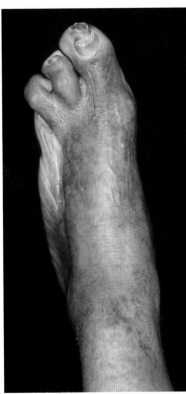

FIGURE 12.15   Lateral two rays amputated in elderly diabetic patient with ischemia and infection of lateral border of foot, including osteomyelitis.

preserving the dorsiflexion strength of the anterior tibial tendon, an Achilles tendon lengthening or gastrocnemius recession is almost always warranted because of the tendency to develop a plantarflexion contracture as a result of the shortened lever arm of the foot limiting dorsiflexion. A lengthening procedure also decreases the pressure on the terminal aspect of the amputation during walking. The Achilles tendon lengthening should be done first to prevent contamination and to allow for a long-lever arm to help with dorsiflexion correction.

Indications for transmetatarsal amputation include infection or gangrene involving multiple digits and possibly some of the dorsal skin proximal to the metatarsophalangeal joints. Essentially all the plantar skin proximal to the metatarsophalangeal joints must be preserved. Because of the inconsistency of wound healing, poor vascularity is a relative contraindication depending on severity and the patient's willingness and ability to undergo revision surgery if needed.

TECHNIQUE 12.7

- To fashion long plantar and short dorsal full-thickness flaps (Fig. 12.18A), begin the dorsal incision at the level of intended bone section on the anteromedial aspect of the foot and curve it slightly distal to the level of bone section to reach the midpoint of the lateral side of the foot (Fig. 12.18B). Begin the plantar incision at the same point as the dorsal, carry it distally beyond the metatarsal heads, and curve it proximally to end at the midpoint of the lateral side of the foot (Fig. 12.18C). Because of the

greater cross-sectional diameter to be covered with skin medially, the incision is slightly longer on the medial than on the lateral side. Fashion the plantar flap to include the subcutaneous fat and a layer of plantar muscles.
- Remove the toes at the metatarsophalangeal joints and section the metatarsals in a beveled fashion dorsal-distal to plantar-proximal at the junction of the middle and distal thirds (Fig. 12.18D). The metatarsals should be removed in a cascading fashion with the second metatarsal osteotomy only a few millimeters shorter than the first metatarsal, while each successive cut is 2 to 3 mm shorter than the previous medial metatarsal (Fig. 12.18E, F). The fifth metatarsal should be even shorter (4 to 5 mm shorter than the fourth). Always use a power saw to resect the metatarsal to try to prevent subsequent bony overgrowth. Use a rongeur and rasp to smooth any bony prominences. If infection is present distally, try not to violate any abscess, leaving the metatarsophalangeal joint intact.
- Identify the nerves and divide them well proximally so that their cut ends fall proximal to the end of the bones.
- Divide the tendons under tension so that they retract into the foot. As an alternative, suture the flexor and extensor tendons to each other to form a myoplasty. A drain may be used as necessary.
- Bring the long plantar flap over the ends of the bones and suture it to the dorsal flap with interrupted nonabsorbable sutures (Fig. 12.18G–I). Be careful about "contouring" skin tags at the medial and lateral edges because this may jeopardize the blood supply to the flap. This excessive tissue disappears with time.
- Apply a light compressive dressing and place the foot in a carefully padded posterior splint with the ankle in neutral to slight dorsiflexion.

POSTOPERATIVE CARE Except for the need for a shoe filler, the postoperative care is the same as after Technique 12.2.

MIDFOOT AMPUTATIONS

Amputations through the middle of the foot include Lisfranc amputation at the tarsometatarsal joints and Chopart amputation at the transverse tarsal joints (see Fig. 12.1), both of which may lead to severe equinovarus deformity (see Fig. 12.5), and Pirogoff amputation, in which the calcaneus is rotated forward to be fused to the tibia after vertical section through its middle. Equinovarus deformity after a Lisfranc amputation can be mitigated with meticulous surgical technique to preserve the insertion of the tibialis anterior and peroneus longus at the medial cuneiform and the peroneus brevis at the base of the fifth metatarsal. The base of the second metatarsal should be spared to preserve the proximal transverse arch. In a Chopart amputation, one or more dorsiflexors of the ankle must be transferred. Lessening the plantarflexion strength of the Achilles tendon is also necessary. Tenectomy of the Achilles tendon (removing 2 to 3 cm of the tendon) is recommended, rather than a simple lengthening. The patient should be placed in a slight dorsiflexion rigid dressing for 6 weeks to prevent equinus deformity and allow for

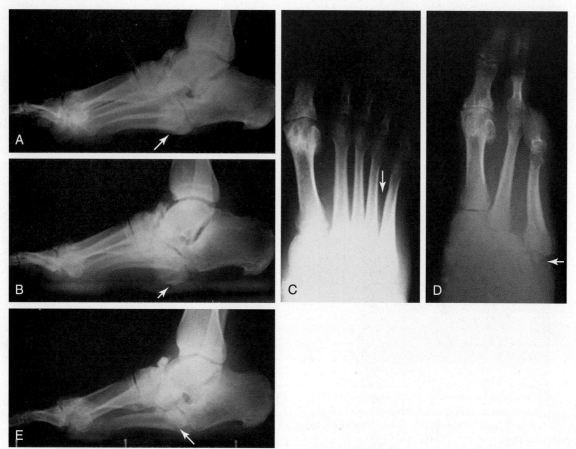

FIGURE 12.16 **A** and **B,** Progressive collapse of midfoot and hindfoot with loss of bony architecture in elderly patient with diabetes mellitus and Charcot arthropathy. **C,** Deep plantar space abscess and osteomyelitis or neuropathic periostitis followed by collapse deformity with ulceration. **D** and **E,** By osteotomizing border metatarsal or incising capsule at articulation with tarsus, the gap created by multiple central ray amputations can be closed and occasionally managed without skin graft or flap coverage. **SEE TECHNIQUE 12.6.**

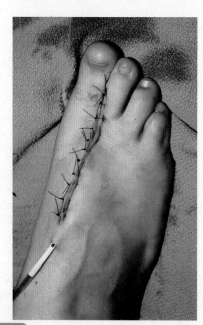

FIGURE 12.17 Central ray amputation; approximation of medial and lateral borders of the foot provides a loose closure and allows drainage. **SEE TECHNIQUE 12.6.**

incorporation of the transferred ankle dorsiflexors. To salvage tarsometatarsal and midtarsal amputations in which fixed equinus deformity has developed, both Burgess and Lieberman et al. recommend division of the Achilles tendon and placement in a rigid dressing in slight dorsiflexion for 6 weeks. By this means, the equinus is corrected, and weight is borne, as it should be, on the plantar skin of the heel and remaining part of the foot. Alternatively, an ankle or tibiotalocalcaneal arthrodesis may be added immediately or in a delayed fashion to prevent or treat equinovarus deformity. In general, the basic requirements for a successful midfoot amputation include palpable posterior tibial pulse, distal infections not extending proximally to the midfoot level, transcutaneous oxygen pressure (TcPO$_2$) greater than 37 mm Hg, hemoglobin level of more than 10 g/dL, and serum albumin level of more than 30 g/L.

Calcaneal deformity may develop but often causes no difficulty either in fitting the shoe or as a source of pain. Although push-off is compromised, the stump before lengthening of the Achilles tendon is not capable of much push-off in the presence of a fixed equinus deformity. By this simple method, skin problems, pressure irritation, and pain associated with excessive weight on the end of the stump are largely eliminated.

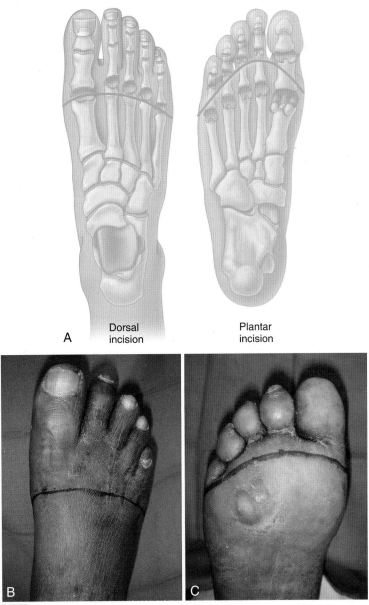

FIGURE 12.18 **A,** Dorsal and plantar incisions for transmetatarsal amputation and disarticulation at the metatarsophalangeal joints. **B,** Dorsal incision. **C,** Plantar incision.

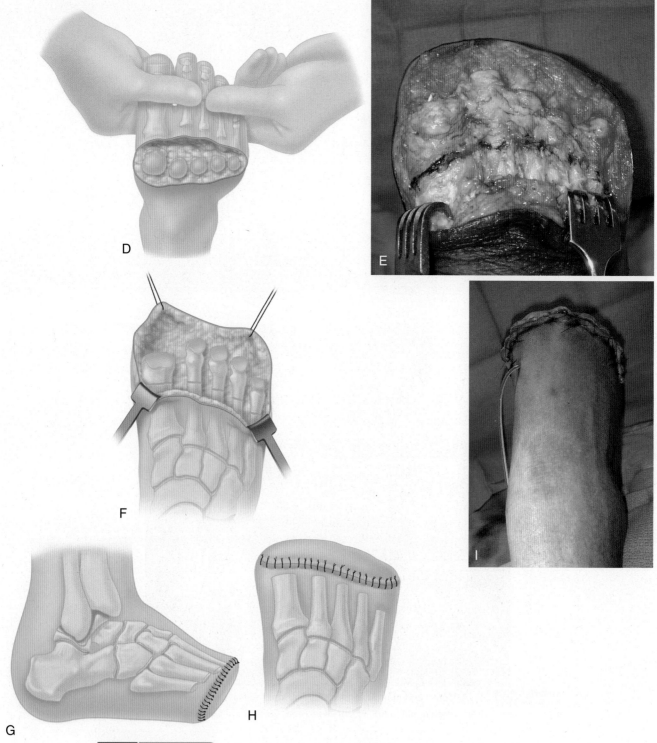

FIGURE 12.18, Cont'd **D to F,** Level of bone transection in transmetatarsal amputation. **G** and **H,** Osteotomy locations are gently curved with flap brought over the ends of bones. **I,** One-layer closure using monofilament nonabsorbable suture. **SEE TECHNIQUE 12.7.**

CHOPART AMPUTATION

TECHNIQUE 12.8

- To avoid contamination, begin by making a posteromedial incision and then perform a tenotomy of the Achilles tendon. Excise 2 cm of tendon and attempt to preserve the sheath of the Achilles tendon. Handle the soft tissue with care.
- Mark the skin incision preoperatively, creating a "fishmouth" flap on the plantar surface. Begin the incision at the transtarsal joints medially and laterally. Extend the flaps in a dorsal and plantar direction, creating adequate skin flaps for coverage (Fig. 12.19A–C). Carry the incision through the skin and subcutaneous tissue.
- Locate and pull the superficial sensory nerves distally, then transect them and allow them to retract.
- Identify the anterior tibial and extensor hallucis longus tendons (Fig. 12.19D), resect them distally, and prepare them for transfer.
- Identify the transverse tarsal (calcaneocuboid and talonavicular) joints and disarticulate them by releasing the dorsal and plantar ligaments (Fig. 12.19E, F).
- Transfer the anterior tibial tendon to the lateral aspect of the neck of the talus, using a bone tunnel with a biotenodesis screw or by creating a trough in the talus and using a suture anchor or staple to secure fixation (Fig. 12.19G, H). Several authors have suggested that a single tendon transfer is inadequate to balance the foot in this setting, so in addition to transferring the anterior tibial tendon to the neck of the talus we also transfer the peroneus brevis or extensor hallucis longus to the anterior process of the calcaneus. Also, the anterior tibial and the extensor hallucis longus tendons can be tenodesed and transferred to the neck of the talus, and the extensor digitorum longus can be transferred to the anterior aspect of the calcaneus.
- Close the wound by approximating the fascial layers plantarly and dorsally and then the skin in a tension-free manner. Place a drain as needed after hemostasis has been obtained and the wound copiously irrigated (Fig. 12.19I, J).
- Apply a well-padded dorsiflexion rigid dressing.

POSTOPERATIVE CARE The dorsiflexion rigid dressing is changed intermittently to check the wound. Sutures are kept in place for 4 to 6 weeks to allow for adequate healing. The splint must be worn for 6 to 8 weeks to prevent equinus contracture of the hindfoot. The patient will need an ankle-foot orthosis in a rocker-sole shoe (e.g., running shoe) for ambulation (Fig. 12.19K).

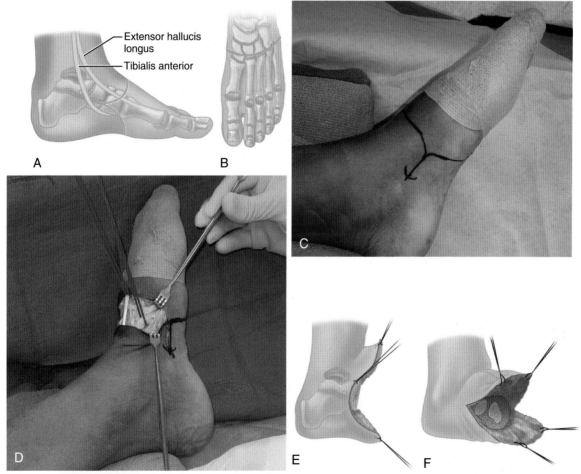

Extensor hallucis longus

Tibialis anterior

A   B

C

D   E   F

FIGURE 12.19 Chopart amputation. **A,** Incisions: lateral view of dorsal and plantar flaps. **B,** Dorsal view of incision. **C,** Dorsal flaps outlined. **D,** Anterior tibial and extensor hallucis longus tendons (marked by vessel loops) will be transferred to the neck of talus to help counter equinus deformity. **E** and **F,** Flaps retracted after resection of distal foot.

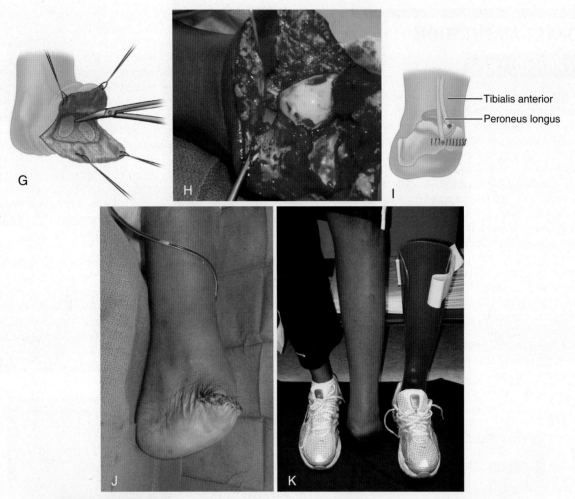

FIGURE 12.19, Cont'd **G,** Transfer of anterior tibial tendon through tunnel in neck of talus. **H,** Trough created in talus for transfer of anterior tibial tendon. **I** and **J,** After closure of incisions. **K,** Ankle-foot orthosis used for ambulation. **SEE TECHNIQUE 12.8.**

HINDFOOT AND ANKLE AMPUTATIONS

Amputations around the ankle joint not only must fulfill the requirements of an end-bearing stump but also must leave enough space between the end of the stump and the ground for the construction of some type of ankle joint mechanism for the artificial foot. In 1843, Syme described an amputation that meets these requirements better than any other in this region. The Syme amputation consists of a bone section at the distal tibia and fibula 0.6 cm proximal to the periphery of the ankle joint and passing through the dome of the ankle centrally. The tough, durable skin of the heel flap provides normal weight-bearing skin. There is apparently no middle ground for this amputation: when good, it is the most satisfactory functional level in the lower extremity, but when bad, it is valueless, and the extremity must be amputated at a more proximal level. The most common causes of an unsatisfactory Syme stump are posterior migration of the heel pad and skin slough resulting from overly vigorous trimming of "dog ears" or a compromised posterior tibial artery. These can be minimized by attention to preoperative planning and surgical technique.

The chief objection to this amputation is cosmetic. The prosthesis used must accommodate the flare of the distal tibial metaphysis that is covered with heavy plantar skin and is large and bulky. The prosthesis used for a classic Syme amputation consists of a molded plastic socket, with a removable medial window to allow passage of the bulbous end of the stump through its narrow shank, and a solid-ankle, cushioned-heel foot prosthesis (Fig. 12.20).

Sarmiento described a modification of the Syme technique that produces a less bulbous stump and allows the use of a more cosmetic prosthesis. He advised transection of the tibia and fibula approximately 1.3 cm proximal to the ankle joint and excision of the medial and lateral malleoli. This produces a stump that is only slightly larger in circumference than the diaphyseal portion of the leg and allows fitting with a prosthesis that incorporates an expandable socket, rather than a removable window.

In the past, most surgeons did not use the Syme amputation for ischemic limbs because the failure rate of wound healing was unacceptably high. More recently, preoperative determination of local tissue perfusion and oxygenation by such techniques as Doppler ultrasound measurement of segmental blood pressures, radioactive xenon clearance tests, and transcutaneous oxygen measurements have significantly increased the success rate of the Syme amputation in these limbs. A two-stage technique of the Syme amputation has been described for use in diabetic patients with an infected or gangrenous foot lesion and has achieved marked success in properly selected patients. Several authors have reported, however, that both stages can be safely combined

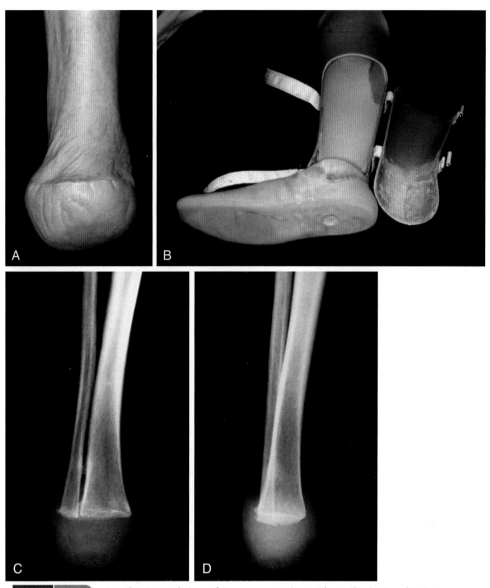

FIGURE 12.20   **A** and **B,** Frontal view of Syme amputation and prosthesis. **C** and **D,** Anteroposterior and lateral radiographs of Syme amputation. Note absence of malleoli.

when infection is not adjacent to the heel pad. A systematic review reveals children have better outcomes than adults, with almost 70% participating in sports. However, the results in adults are promising as well, despite higher rates of reamputation and complications. Those achieving a successful Syme amputation demonstrate improved levels of functional independence compared to those undergoing a transtibial amputation.

The Boyd amputation also produces an excellent end-bearing stump around the ankle and eliminates the problem of posterior migration of the heel pad that sometimes occurs after a Syme amputation. It involves talectomy, forward shift of the calcaneus, and calcaneotibial arthrodesis. The arthrodesis makes the procedure technically more difficult than the Syme amputation and produces a more bulbous stump. A satisfactory prosthesis that is cosmetically acceptable has been designed for use after this amputation, however.

The Pirogoff amputation involves arthrodesis between the tibia and part of the calcaneus; the calcaneus is sectioned vertically, its anterior part is removed, and its remaining posterior part and the heel flap are rotated forward and upward 90 degrees until the raw surface of the calcaneus meets the denuded distal end of the tibia. This amputation has no advantage over that of Boyd and technically is more difficult.

SYME AMPUTATION

TECHNIQUE 12.9

- A single long posterior heel flap is used. Begin the incision at the distal tip of the lateral malleolus and pass it across the anterior aspect of the ankle joint at the level of the distal end of the tibia to a point one fingerbreadth inferior to the tip of the medial malleolus; extend it directly plantarward and across the sole of the foot to the lateral aspect, and end it at the starting point (Fig. 12.21A).

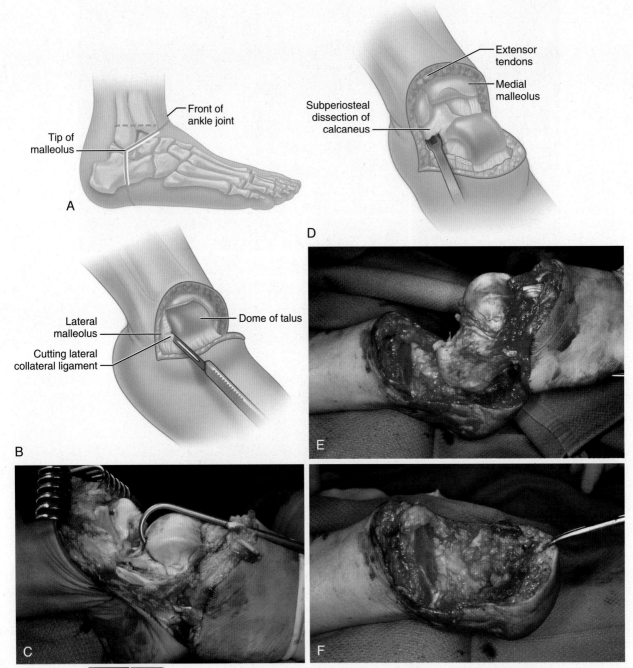

FIGURE 12.21 Syme amputation. **A,** Incision and bone level. **B,** Exposure of ankle and division of ligaments. **C,** Bone hook pulling talus distally, exposing distal articular surface of tibia and fibula. **D,** Dissection of soft tissues from calcaneus. **E** and **F,** Subperiosteal removal of calcaneus, leaving heel pad intact.

- Divide all structures to the bone.
- For excision of the tarsus, place the foot in marked equinus and divide the anterior capsule of the ankle joint.
- Insert a knife into the joint space between the medial malleolus and the talus and draw it inferiorly to section the deltoid ligament, protecting the posterior tibial artery; repeat this maneuver on the lateral side to section the calcaneofibular ligament (Fig. 12.21B).
- Place a bone hook in the posterior aspect of the talus to provide further equinus and proceed with dissection pos-

teriorly, dividing the posterior capsule of the ankle joint (Fig. 12.21C).
- Continue the dissection posteriorly, close to the superior surface of the calcaneus.
- Identify and expose the Achilles tendon and divide it at its insertion on the calcaneus, taking care not to damage the overlying skin because this may lead to necrosis of the entire flap.
- With a periosteal elevator, dissect the soft tissues from the lateral and medial surfaces of the calcaneus and pull

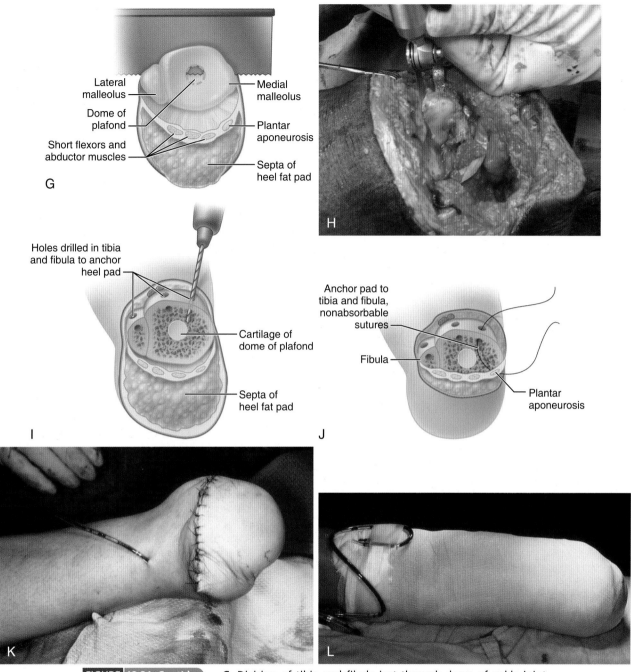

FIGURE 12.21, Cont'd **G,** Division of tibia and fibula just through dome of ankle joint centrally. **H,** Plane of transection to keep cut surfaces of tibia and fibula parallel to ground with patient standing. **I,** Holes drilled in anterior edge of tibia and fibula to anchor heel pad. **J,** Edge of deep fascia lining heel pad is anchored to tibia and fibula. **K and L,** Skin closure over drain, and application of above-knee cast. **SEE TECHNIQUE 12.9.**

the bone into even more equinus (Fig. 12.21D). Continue subperiosteal dissection on the inferior surface of the calcaneus until the distal end of the plantar skin flap is reached (Fig. 12.21E, F).

- Remove the entire foot except the heel flap. Retract the flap posteriorly and dissect the soft tissue from the tibia and malleoli.
- Incise the periosteum circumferentially 0.6 cm proximal to the joint line and divide the tibia and fibula at this level so

that the line of transection passes just through the dome of the ankle joint centrally (Fig. 12.21G, H). The plane of the transection should be such that the cut surfaces of the tibia and fibula are parallel to the ground when the patient is standing. Round and smooth all sharp corners of bone.

- Dissect the medial and lateral plantar nerves and divide them proximal to the end of the bone.
- Pull inferiorly and section all visible tendons to retract proximally into the leg.

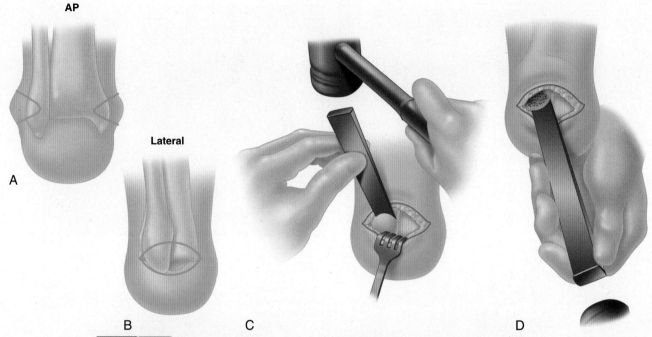

AP

Lateral

A

B   C   D

FIGURE 12.22 Second stage of Wagner-Syme amputation. **A** and **B**, Removal of "dog ears" over each malleolus. **C** and **D**, Resection of metaphyseal flare parallel with shaft of fibula; same procedure is carried out at distal tibia. **SEE TECHNIQUE 12.10.**

- Isolate the posterior tibial artery and vein and ligate them just proximal to the cut distal edge of the heel flap. Ligate the anterior tibial artery as it lies in the anterior flap.
- Perform minimal debridement of any soft-tissue tags of plantar muscle and fascia lining the inner surface of the heel flap and preserve intact the subcutaneous fat and its septa because this is specialized pressure-tolerant tissue.
- Several techniques have been used to prevent migration of the heel pad on the end of the stump, such as taping the heel flap to the leg with adhesive strips, skewering the heel flap to the bone with a Kirschner wire, or leaving a small sliver of calcaneus attached to the heel flap, which fuses to the end of the tibia. The technique of Wagner is simple and has been effective in his hands.
- Drill several holes through the anterior edge of the tibia and fibula and suture the deep fascia lining the heel flap to the bones through these holes (Fig. 12.21I and J).
- Under no tension, approximate the skin edge of the heel flap to the skin edge of the anterior flap with interrupted nonabsorbable sutures (Fig. 12.21K). Large protruding tags of skin, or "dog ears," are found at each end of the suture line; these should never be removed because they carry a large share of the blood supply to the heel flap and disappear later under bandaging.
- Apply a cast extending above the knee over a drain and remove the drain 24 to 48 h after surgery (Fig. 12.21L).

POSTOPERATIVE CARE A soft dressing can be applied and treatment continued as discussed in chapter 11. A preferable approach is to apply a properly padded rigid dressing in the operating room at the conclusion of surgery. If ambulation is to be delayed until wound healing is ensured, a simple well-padded cast is adequate. If early ambulation is preferred, or when subsequent prosthetic ambulation is to be instituted in the postoperative period, a true prosthetic cast should be applied as follows. Apply a light sterile dressing to the wound and apply a sterile stump sock. Sterile felt pads are appropriately fashioned and skived by the prosthetist to relieve pressure over the tibial crest and the edges of the transected bones; the prosthetist glues these pads to the stump sock with medical adhesive and applies the plaster cast. Use elastic plaster of Paris in the initial wrap to provide good control of tension; reinforce this with conventional plaster. Gentle compression should be maximal over the end of the stump and gradually decrease proximally. The cast need not extend above the knee because the shape of the stump and the intimate fit between the stump and the rigid dressing provide adequate suspension. The end of the rigid dressing is flattened for weight bearing by pressing a board against the wet plaster. The proximal part of the dressing is molded to create a patellar bar and a popliteal bulge, as in a patellar tendon-bearing prosthesis, to allow partial weight bearing by the patellar tendon and tibial condyles. A filler block is added if needed to correct leg-length discrepancy, and a Syme prosthetic foot or a rubber walking heel is attached to the cast. A waist belt and suspension straps are used for additional suspension. Gait training and further postoperative care proceed as discussed in the section on below-knee amputations in chapter 13.

TWO-STAGE SYME AMPUTATION

The two-stage Syme amputation procedure was developed to increase the success rate of amputations performed at the Syme level in patients with gross infection of the forefoot. It has proved to be extremely beneficial in diabetic patients, especially when coupled with the use of sophisticated techniques for preoperatively determining segmental limb viability. Several authors have reported that both stages can be safely combined when infection is not adjacent to the heel pad.

The procedure consists of performing an ankle disarticulation as the first stage, preserving the tibial articular cartilage and the malleoli, and performing a Syme-type closure over a suction-irrigation system that allows installation of an antibiotic solution into the wound. Irrigation is continued until local and systemic signs of infection have resolved. After 6 weeks, if the stump is healed, a second procedure is performed to remove the malleoli and narrow the stump for good prosthetic fitting.

TECHNIQUE 12.10

(WYSS ET AL.; MALONE ET AL.; WAGNER)

FIRST STAGE

- To allow slightly longer skin flaps to cover the malleoli, start the incision 1 cm distal and 1 cm anterior to the tip of each malleolus. Carry the inferior incision directly across the sole of the foot to connect these two points, cutting all layers down to the bone. Carry the superior incision obliquely across the ankle joint, connecting the two points and cutting all layers down to the bone.
- Pull the tendons on the dorsum of the foot distally into the wound and transect them so that they retract well proximal to the skin edge.
- Identify and ligate the dorsalis pedis artery. Incise the anterior capsule of the ankle joint, plantarflex the foot, and transect the medial and lateral collateral ankle ligaments, preserving the posterior tibial artery.
- Use a bone hook in the body of the talus to pull the foot into even greater plantarflexion and begin subperiosteal dissection on the superolateral surface of the calcaneus. Continue this dissection posteriorly and medially, transect the Achilles tendon near its insertion on the calcaneus, and protect the posterior tibial artery medially.
- Separate the foot from the leg by transection of the plantar aponeurosis.
- Ligate the posterior tibial artery near the margin of the heel flap and transect the tibial nerve so that its cut end retracts well proximal to the skin edge.
- Insert suction-irrigation tubes into the wound.
- Trim the distal edge of the heel flap to allow accurate closure with no tension, but do not attempt to trim the "dog ears" from the sides of the wound.
- Occasionally, it is necessary to divide fascial bands in the heel pad to prevent medial or lateral shifting of the pad. Similarly, it may be necessary to make small incisions into the fat pad to make a nest for each malleolus. These maneuvers usually allow secure seating of the heel pad on the end of the bones.
- Suture the deep fascia of the anterior flap to the deep fascia of the posterior flap with interrupted absorbable sutures and approximate the skin edges with interrupted nonabsorbable sutures.
- Cover the wound with a soft compression dressing.

- After surgery, the wound is irrigated with an antibiotic solution for 48 to 72 h or until local and systemic signs of infection have subsided.
- After the drains are removed, apply a well-padded plaster cast to the stump, using contoured felt pads to protect the "dog ears."
- Ambulation with or without weight bearing can be started at this point under strict supervision. Healing usually is secure enough at 6 weeks to perform the second stage or definitive amputation.

SECOND STAGE

- Make an elliptical incision over each malleolus to remove the "dog ears." The volume of tissue removed should be equal to that of the malleolus (Fig. 12.22A, B).
- Expose the malleoli by subperiosteal dissection, protecting the posterior tibial artery medially.
- Resect each malleolus flush with the joint surface and remove the adjacent metaphyseal flares parallel with the shafts of the tibia and fibula (Fig. 12.22C, D). This narrows and flattens the stump medially and laterally but still leaves anterior and posterior flares for prosthetic suspension.
- Tailor the soft tissues to allow secure positioning of the heel pad over the ends of the bones.
- Suture the deep fascia of the sole through holes drilled in the bone and close the wound with interrupted sutures.

POSTOPERATIVE CARE Apply a soft compression dressing until wound healing is apparent. Apply a walking cast and begin weight bearing 10 to 12 days after surgery. The cast should be changed at 2-week intervals or more often if it becomes loose or uncomfortable. Definitive prosthetic fitting usually is possible about 8 weeks after surgery.

BOYD AMPUTATION

TECHNIQUE 12.11   *Figure. 12.23*

- Fashion a long plantar flap and a short dorsal flap. Begin the incision at the tip of the lateral malleolus and pass it over the dorsum of the foot at the level of the talonavicular joint to a point one fingerbreadth inferior to the medial malleolus; curve it inferiorly and distally across the sole of the foot at the level of the metatarsal bases; and carry it superiorly and proximally to the tip of the lateral malleolus.
- Elevate the skin flaps and amputate the forefoot through the midtarsal joints.
- Divide the ligaments between the calcaneus and tibia by sharp dissection close to the bone and then remove the talus.
- Excise the anterior part of the calcaneus by transverse osteotomy just distal to the peroneal tubercle.
- Remove the cartilage from the appropriate surfaces of the tibia, fibula, and calcaneus to prepare them for arthrodesis.
- Draw distally any tendons present in the wound and section them proximally and allow them to retract.

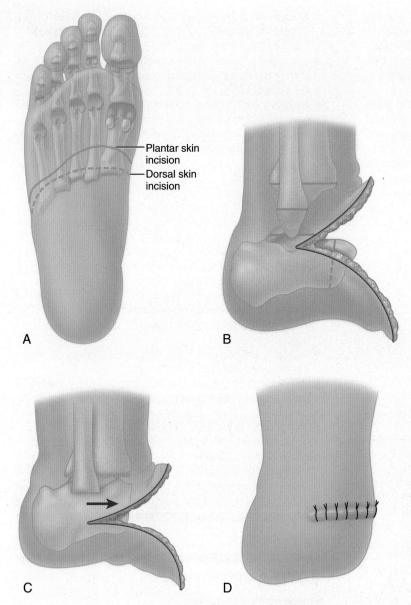

A

Plantar skin incision
Dorsal skin incision

B

C

D

FIGURE 12.23 Boyd amputation with calcaneo-tibial fusion. **A,** Full-thickness flaps with longer plantar extension in midtarsal amputation. These flaps extend distal to the metatarsophalangeal joints so that wound can be closed without skin tension. **B,** Midtarsal joint disarticulation, talectomy, and partial fibulectomy. **C,** Talus has been excised. Calcaneus and tibial platform prepared for arthrodesis. **D,** Single-layer closure with 2-0 monofilament nonabsorbable suture (over a drain). **SEE TECHNIQUE 12.11.**

- Section the medial and lateral plantar nerves to prevent them from being subject to pressure.
- Shift the calcaneus forward in its relationship to the ankle joint and mortise it into position for arthrodesis, its undersurface being parallel with the ground.
- If desired, pass a Steinmann pin or cannulated screw superiorly through the heel to fix the calcaneus to the tibia in proper position.
- Approximate the skin flaps with interrupted sutures and insert a drain, which is removed at 48 to 72 h.

POSTOPERATIVE CARE The sutures are removed after 2 weeks, and any Steinmann pin is removed after 4 weeks. Weight bearing on the stump is prohibited until 8 weeks. A walking cast is then applied and left in place until arthrodesis is complete.

REFERENCES

Adams BE, Edlinger JP, Ritterman Weintraub ML, Pollard JD: Three-year morbidity and mortality rates after nontraumatic transmetatarsal amputation, *J Foot Ankle Surg* 57(5):967, 2018.

Andrews KL, Dib MY, Shives TC, et al.: Noninvasive arterial studies including transcutaneous oxygen pressure measurements with the limbs elevated or dependent to predict healing after partial foot amputation, *Am J Phys Med Rehabil* 92:385, 2013.

Attinger CE, Meyr AJ, Fitzgerald S, Steinberg JS: Preoperative Doppler assessment for transmetatarsal amputation, *J Foot Ankle Surg* 49:101, 2010.

Aydin K, Isildak M, Karakaya J, Gürlek A: Change in amputation predictors in diabetic foot disease: effect of multidisciplinary approach, *Endocrine* 38:87, 2010.

Brown ML, Tang W, Patel A, Baumhauer JF: Partial foot amputation in patients with diabetic foot ulcers, *Foot Ankle Int* 33:707, 2012.

Chiu YC, Chung TC, Wu CH, et al.: Chopart amputation with tibiotalocalcaneal arthrodesis and free flap reconstruction for severe foot crush injury, *Bone Joint J* 100-B(10):1359, 2018.

Faglia E, Clerici G, Caminiti M, et al.: Influence of osteomyelitis location in the foot of diabetic patients with transtibial amputation, *Foot Ankle Int* 34:222, 2013.

Fergason J, Keeling JJ, Bluman EM: Recent advances in lower extremity amputations and prosthetics for the combat injured patient, *Foot Ankle Clin North Am* 15:151, 2010.

Finkler ES, Marchwiany DA, Schiff AP, Pinzur MS: Long-term outcomes following Syme's amputation, *Foot Ankle Int* 38(7):732, 2017.

Gessmann J, Citak M, Fehmer T, et al.: Ilizarov external frame technique for Pirogoff amputations with ankle disarticulation and tibiocalcaneal fusion, *Foot Ankle Int* 34:856, 2013.

Griffin KJ, Rashid TS, Bailey MA, et al.: Toe amputation: a predictor of future limb loss? *J Diabetes Complications* 26:251, 2012.

Janisse DJ, Janisse EJ: Shoes, orthoses, and prostheses for partial foot amputation and diabetic foot infection, *Foot Ankle Clin* 15:509, 2010.

Jeans KA, Browne RH, Karol LA: Effect of amputation level on energy expenditure during overground walking by children with an amputation, *J Bone Joint Surg* 93A:49, 2011.

Kim SW, Jeon SB, Hwang KT, Kim YH: Coverage of amputation stumps using a latissimus dorsi flap with a serratus anterior muscle flap: a comparative study, *Ann Plast Surg* 2014. [Epub ahead of print].

Kono Y, Muder RR: Identifying the incidence of risk factors for reamputation among patients who underwent foot amputation, *Ann Vasc Surg* 26(8):1120, 2012.

Krause FG, Pfander G, Henning J, et al.: Ankle dorsiflexion arthrodesis to salvage Chopart's amputation with anterior skin insufficiency, *Foot Ankle Int* 34:1560, 2013.

Kuehn BM: Prompt response, multidisciplinary care key to reducing diabetic foot amputation, *JAMA* 308:19, 2012.

Langeveld ARJ, Oostenbroek RJ, Wijffels MPJM, Hoedt MTC: The Pirogoff amputation for necrosis of the forefoot: a case report, *J Bone Joint Surg* 92A:968, 2010.

Mijuskovic B, Kuehl R, Widmer AF, et al.: Culture of bone biopsy specimens overestimates rate of residual osteomyelitis after toe or forefoot amputation, *J Bone Joint Surg Am* 100(17):1448, 2018.

Nather A, Song KL, Lim AS, et al.: The modified Pirogoff's amputation in treating diabetic foot infections: surgical technique and case series, *Diabet Foot Ankle* 5, 2014, https://doi.org/10.3402/dfa.v5.23354.

Ng VY, Berlet GC: Evolving techniques in foot and ankle amputation, *J Am Acad Orthop Surg* 18:223, 2010.

Pinzur MS: Syme's ankle disarticulation, *Foot Ankle Clin* 15:487, 2010.

Pinzur MS, Gottschalk F, Pinto MA, Smith DG: Controversies in lower extremity amputation, *Instr Course Lect* 57:663, 2008.

Sangeorzan BJ: Residual infection after forefoot amputation in diabetic foot infection: is new information helpful even when negative? *J Bone Joint Surg* 100(17):1447, 2018.

Serra R, Buffone G, Dominijanni A, et al: Application of platelet-rich gel to enhance healing of transmetatarsal amputations in diabetic dysvascular patients, *Int Wound J* 20:612, 2013.

Shaikh N, Vaughan P, Varty K, et al.: Outcome of limited forefoot amputation with primary closure in patients with diabetes, *Bone Joint J* 95B(8):1083, 2013.

Singla S, Garg R, Kumar A, Gill C: Efficacy of topical application of beta urogastrone (recombinant human epidermal growth factor) in Wagner's Grade 1 and 2 diabetic foot ulcers: comparative analysis of 50 patients, *J Nat Sci Biol Med* 5:273, 2014.

Sohn MW, Stuck RM, Pinzur M, et al.: Lower-extremity amputation risk after Charcot arthropathy and diabetic foot ulcer, *Diabetes Care* 33:98, 2010.

Suh YC, Kushida-Contreras BH, Suk H, et al.: Does reconstruction preserving the first or first two rays benefit over full transmetatarsal amputation in diabetic foot?, *Plast Reconstr Surg* 2018. [Epub ahead of print].

Tosun B, Buluc L, Gok U, Unal C: Boyd amputation in adults, *Foot Ankle Int* 32:1063, 2011.

Wukich DK, Raspovic KM, Suder NC: Patients with diabetic foot disease fear major lower-extremity amputation more than death, *Foot Ankle Spec* 11(1):17, 2018.

The complete list of references is available online at Expert Consult.com.

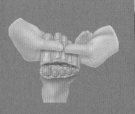

CHAPTER 13

AMPUTATIONS OF THE LOWER EXTREMITY

Marcus C. Ford

FOOT AND ANKLE
 AMPUTATIONS 608
TRANSTIBIAL (BELOW-KNEE)
 AMPUTATIONS 609
Nonischemic limbs 609

Rehabilitation in
 nonischemic limbs 611
Ischemic limbs 611
Rehabilitation in
 ischemic limbs 613

DISARTICULATION OF
 THE KNEE 614
TRANSFEMORAL (ABOVE-
 KNEE) AMPUTATIONS 617
REHABILITATION AFTER
 TRANSFEMORAL
 AMPUTATION 619

Lower limb amputations are the most common of all amputations. Despite advances in revascularization techniques, the most common indication for lower extremity amputation remains a dysvascular limb, including that caused by diabetes mellitus and peripheral vascular disease. Peripheral vascular disease from all causes affects over 8 million Americans. The rate of lower extremity amputation in this population is around 4 per 1000. Amputation of the contralateral limb is necessary within 5 years in 30% to 50% of patients who have an amputation of a dysvascular lower limb. Twenty percent of below-knee amputations are converted to above-knee amputations. Over 50% of nontraumatic amputations occur from diabetes-related pathology. In the diabetic population, first-year mortality rates after amputation are reported to be as high as 40%, while overall mortality rates range from 60% to 70%.

The number of amputations for causes other than diabetes and vascular disease, such as tumors and infection, has decreased in the United States because of surgical and medical advances. In war-torn countries, improvised explosive devices and land mines continue to be frequent causes of traumatic amputations. Also, a high rate of combat-related lower extremity amputations remains in the military population. Current level I and II studies are underway to investigate optimal lower extremity amputation techniques in this highly active population.

We advocate a multidisciplinary approach to the medical management of lower extremity amputations. Diabetic patients and those with vascular insufficiency who have had lower extremity amputation demonstrate high rates of 30-day mortality, stump complications, and hospital readmissions. Associated coronary artery disease and end-stage renal disease are predictors for perioperative medical complications and hospital readmissions.

The level of amputation is always a difficult decision and has a major effect on a patient's quality of life. Morbidity is more frequent after transfemoral amputations than after transtibial amputations. Energy expenditure is an important consideration in choosing the level of amputation. The increased energy consumption of bipedal locomotion for transtibial amputees ranges from 40% to 50%, compared with 90% to 100% in transfemoral amputees. Patients with transfemoral amputations are less likely to use a prosthesis successfully and consistently than are patients with more distal amputations. Higher-level amputations, even in children, are associated with a decline in physical function and quality of life.

Younger patients with traumatic amputations or amputations required for tumor treatment are more successful with prosthetic use than are patients with amputations of dysvascular limbs; dialysis patients are even less successful with prostheses. In dysvascular limbs, the level of amputation is critical because of poor wound healing. The most distal level should be chosen where the wound will have the best chance of healing. This decision process can be augmented using clinical tools such as transcutaneous oxygen tension, determining the nutritional status of patients (albumin level of >3 g/dL, lymphocyte count of >1500/mL) and preoperative medical frailty.

Amputation should not be viewed as a failed limb salvage or reconstruction. The amputation must be viewed as an opportunity to reestablish or enhance a patient's functional level and facilitate a return to near-normal locomotion. Transtibial amputation after failed attempted limb preservation can still be successful in improving pain, decreasing narcotic use, and improving function. This is especially true in the young, highly active trauma population. Meticulous surgical attention is necessary to provide an optimal base of support because the residual limb functions as a "sensorimotor end organ" with tolerance requirements at the stump-prosthesis interface to meet the dynamic weight-bearing challenges of ambulation. Anesthesia pain specialty teams often are helpful in the management of postoperative pain.

Developments in the prosthetic field range from early-stage fitting techniques (computer-assisted stump contour scanning) to the use of advanced prosthetic components (lighter materials, silicone gel liners, computer-assisted knee units, suspension device alternatives, and ankle-foot accommodative and energy storage systems). Osseointegrated prosthetic components have been investigated over the past several decades in transfemoral and transtibial amputees. Potential advantages include improved quality of life and body image, increased proximal joint range of motion, greater prosthetic comfort, better osseoperception, and improved walking ability. Minor complications include frequent superficial infections and stump irritation, and rare major complications include deep infection, osteomyelitis, peri-implant fracture, and failure of osseointegration. Tillander et al. reported a 20% cumulative risk of developing osteomyelitis.

FOOT AND ANKLE AMPUTATIONS

Amputations around the foot and ankle are discussed in chapter 12.

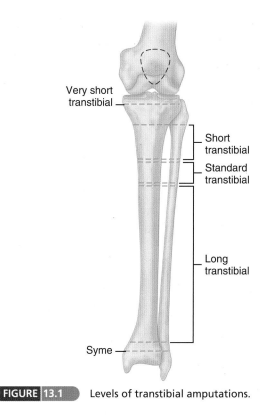

Very short
transtibial —

Short
transtibial

Standard
transtibial

Long
transtibial

Syme —

FIGURE 13.1   Levels of transtibial amputations.

TRANSTIBIAL (BELOW-KNEE) AMPUTATIONS

Transtibial amputation is the most common lower extremity amputation. The importance of preserving the patient's own knee joint in the successful rehabilitation of a patient with a lower extremity amputation cannot be overemphasized. Transtibial amputations can be divided into three levels (Fig. 13.1). The appropriate level must be determined for each individual patient. Although many variations in technique exist, all procedures may be divided into those for nonischemic limbs and those for ischemic limbs. General techniques vary primarily in the construction of skin flaps, muscle stabilization, and osseous stabilization techniques. In nonischemic limbs, skin flaps of various design and muscle stabilization techniques, such as tension myodesis and myoplasty, frequently are used. These techniques are employed to prepare a stump more suited for weight bearing and to protect from wound breakdown. In tension myodesis, transected muscle groups are sutured to bone under physiologic tension; in myoplasty, muscle is sutured to soft tissue, such as opposing muscle groups or fascia. In most instances, myoplastic closures are performed, but some authors have advocated the use of the firmer stabilization provided by myodesis in young, active individuals. In addition, some surgeons advocate creating a bone bridge between the distal tibia and fibula (Technique 13.2). Advocates of the Ertl technique claim that a bone bridge creates a more stable end-bearing construct and decreases the incidence of proximal tibiofibular joint instability. In addition, closure of the intramedullary canal in osteomyoplastic transtibial amputation has been shown to increase blood flow to the residual limb. In ischemic limbs, tension myodesis is relatively contraindicated because it may compromise further an already marginal blood supply. Also, a

long posterior myocutaneous flap and a short or even absent anterior flap are recommended for ischemic limbs because anteriorly the blood supply is less abundant than elsewhere in the leg.

In combat injuries that result from blasts or fragmentation wounds, the use of standard flaps may be impossible. Often flaps have to be fashioned from viable remaining tissue. Skin grafts may be used to cover soft-tissue defects, but skin grafts are not ideal for a stump-prosthesis interface.

NONISCHEMIC LIMBS

Rehabilitation after transtibial amputations in nonischemic limbs generally is quite successful, partly because of a younger, healthier population with fewer comorbidities. The optimal level of amputation in this population traditionally has been chosen to provide a stump length that allows a controlling lever arm for the prosthesis with sufficient "circulation" for healing and soft tissue for protective end weight bearing. The amputation level also is governed by the cause (e.g., clean end margins for tumor, level of trauma, and congenital abnormalities). A longer residual limb would have a more normal gait appearance, but stumps extending to the distal third of the leg have been considered suboptimal because there is less soft tissue available for weight bearing and less room to accommodate some energy storage systems. The distal third of the leg also has been considered relatively avascular and slower to heal than more proximal levels. Contemporary liners and ankle-foot storage systems now allow more options for accommodating a longer residual limb, but the long-term risk of skin breakdown in older patients with these newer prosthetic components is unknown. Our recent war experiences have shown that early posttraumatic amputations decrease the risk of chronic residual limb infection. If only one posttraumatic debridement procedure and 5 days or fewer pass before definitive amputation, the risk of infection is limited.

In adults, the ideal bone length for a below-knee amputation stump is 12.5 to 17.5 cm, depending on body height. A reasonably satisfactory rule of thumb for selecting the level of bone section is to allow 2.5 cm of bone length for each 30 cm of body height. Usually the most satisfactory level is about 15 cm distal to the medial tibial articular surface. A stump less than 12.5 cm long is less efficient. Stumps lacking quadriceps function are not useful. In a short stump of 8.8 cm or less, it has been recommended that the entire fibula together with some of the muscle bulk be removed so that the stump may fit more easily into the prosthetic socket. Many prosthetists find, however, that retention of the fibular head is desirable because the modern total-contact socket can obtain a better purchase on the short stump. Transecting the hamstring tendons to allow a short stump to fall deeper into the socket also may be considered. Although the procedure has the disadvantage of weakening flexion of the knee, this has not been a serious problem, and genu recurvatum has not been reported.

Amputations in nonischemic limbs result from tumor, trauma, infection, or congenital anomaly. In each, the underlying lesion dictates the level of amputation and choice of skin flaps. Microvascular techniques have made preservation of transtibial stumps possible with the use of distant free flaps and "spare part" flaps from the amputated limb. A description of the classic transtibial amputation using equal anterior and posterior flaps follows.

TRANSTIBIAL AMPUTATION

TECHNIQUE 13.1

- Place the patient supine on the operating table and use a pneumatic tourniquet for hemostasis.
- Beginning proximally at the anteromedial joint line, measure distally the desired length of bone and mark that level over the tibial crest with a skin-marking pen.
- Outline equal anterior and posterior skin flaps, with the length of each flap being equal to one half the anteroposterior diameter of the leg at the anticipated level of bone section.
- Begin the anterior incision medially or laterally at the intended level of bone section and swing it convexly distalward to the previously determined level and proximally to end at a similar position on the opposite side of the leg (Fig. 13.2A).
- When crossing the tibial crest, deepen the incision and mark the periosteum with a cut to establish a point for future measurement.
- Begin the posterior incision at the same point as the anterior and carry it first convexly distalward and then proximally as in the anterior incision (see Fig 13.2A).
- Deepen the posterior incision down through the deep fascia, but do not separate the skin or deep fascia from the underlying muscle.
- Reflect as a single layer with the anterior flap the deep fascia and periosteum over the anteromedial surface of the tibia.
- Continue this dissection proximally to the level of intended bone section.

- Because it contracts, the anterior flap cannot be used to measure the level of intended bone section. Instead, use the mark already made in the tibial periosteum to measure the original length of the flap and reestablish the level of bone section. With a saw, mark the bone at this point.
- Insert a curved hemostat in the natural cleavage plane at the lateral aspect of the tibia so that its tip follows along the interosseous membrane and passes over the anterior aspect of the fibula to emerge just anterior to the peroneus brevis muscle.
- Identify and isolate the superficial peroneal nerve in the interval between the extensor digitorum longus and peroneus brevis, gently draw it distally, and divide it high so that it retracts well proximal to the end of the stump.
- Divide the muscles in the anterior compartment of the leg at a point 0.6 cm distal to the level of bone section so that they retract flush with the end of the bone. As these muscles are sectioned, take special care to identify and protect the anterior tibial vessels and deep peroneal nerve.
- Isolate these structures and ligate and divide the vessels at a level just proximal to the level of intended bone section.
- Exert gentle traction on the nerve and divide it proximally so that it retracts well proximal to the end of the stump.
- Before sectioning the tibia, bevel its crest with a saw: begin 1.9 cm proximal to the level of the bone section and cut obliquely distalward to cross this level 0.5 cm anterior to the medullary cavity.
- Section the tibia transversely and section the fibula 1.2 cm proximally.
- Grasp their distal segments with a bone-holding forceps so that they can be pulled anteriorly and distally to expose the posterior muscle mass.

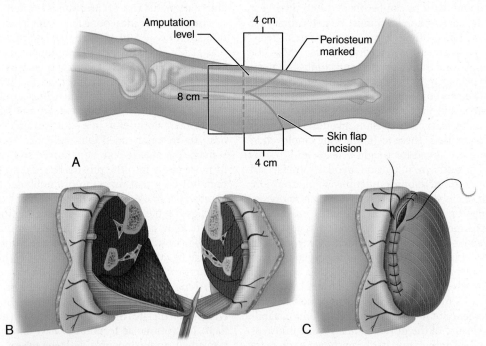

FIGURE 13.2 Amputation through middle third of leg for nonischemic limbs. **A,** Fashioning of equal anterior and posterior skin flaps, each one half anteroposterior diameter of leg at level of bone section. **B,** Fashioning of posterior myofascial flap. **C,** Suture of myofascial flap to periosteum anteriorly. **SEE TECHNIQUE 13.1.**

- Divide the muscles in the deep posterior compartment 0.6 cm distal to the level of bone section so that they retract flush with the end of the bone. This exposes the posterior tibial and peroneal vessels and the tibial nerve lying on the gastrocnemius-soleus muscle group. Doubly ligate and divide the vessels and section the nerve so that its cut end retracts well proximal to the end of the bone.
- With a large amputation knife, bevel the gastrocnemius-soleus muscle mass so that it forms a myofascial flap long enough to reach across the end of the tibia to the anterior fascia (Fig. 13.2B).
- Smoothly round the ends of the tibia and fibula with a rasp and irrigate the wound to remove all bone dust.
- Release the tourniquet and clamp and ligate or electrocoagulate all bleeding points.
- Bring the gastrocnemius-soleus muscle flap over the ends of the bones and suture it to the deep fascia and the periosteum anteriorly (Fig. 13.2C).
- Place a plastic suction drainage tube deep to the muscle flap and fascia and bring it out laterally through the skin 10 to 12 cm proximal to the end of the stump.
- Fashion the skin flaps as necessary for smooth closure without tension and suture them together with interrupted nonabsorbable sutures.

TECHNIQUE 13.2

(MODIFIED ERTL; TAYLOR AND POKA)
- Place the patient supine on a radiolucent bed; a tourniquet is used for hemostasis.
- Make an anterior incision at the level of the intended tibial resection and a posterior flap incision. The posterior flap should measure 1 cm more than the diameter of the leg at the level of bone division (Fig. 13.3A).
- Sharply incise the anterior compartment fascia, transect the musculature of the anterior compartment, and ligate the anterior neurovascular bundle.
- Identify the saphenous nerve, transect it proximally under tension, and allow it to retract.
- Identify the tibial resection site and elevate an osteoperiosteal sleeve proximal to the intended transection level both anteriorly and posteriorly before making the tibial cut (Fig. 13.3B).
- Measure the medial-to-lateral distance between the tibia and fibula at the area of transection and transect the peroneal muscle and fibula at this distance distal to the transected tibia.
- Transect the peroneal musculature and ligate the lateral neurovascular bundle.
- Transect the deep posterior compartment at the level of the tibial transection and sharply bevel the superficial posterior compartment to fashion a future flap.
- Identify the posterior compartment neurovascular bundle, ligate and transect it, allowing for retraction.
- Identify the sural nerve and transect it in the posterior subcutaneous flap.
- Remove the amputated limb from the operative field, saving bone for possible grafting.

- Osteotomize the remaining fibula at the level of the resected tibia; with a burr, create notches in the fibula and tibia for placement of the cut fibular autograft strut (Fig. 13.3C,D).
- Drill holes to accommodate heavy suture passage: two in the medial tibia, two in the medial fibular autograft, two in the lateral fibular autograft, and two in the distal fibula (screw fixation may alternatively be used; Fig. 13.3E).
- Secure the autograft strut with heavy suture and sew the tibial periosteal sleeve around the strut distally. Autogenous bone graft may augment the distal bone bridge if necessary.
- Release the tourniquet and achieve hemostasis.
- Mobilize the peroneal musculature distally to cover the end of the bone bridge and suture it to the medial aspect of the tibia.
- Suture the posterior musculature to the anterior tibial periosteum and close the subcutaneous tissues. Use nonabsorbable stitches in a mattress fashion to close the skin.

REHABILITATION IN NONISCHEMIC LIMBS

Rehabilitation after transtibial amputation in a nonischemic limb is fairly aggressive unless the patient is immunocompromised, there are skin graft issues, or there are concomitant injuries or medical conditions that preclude early initiation of physical therapy. An immediate postoperative rigid dressing helps control edema, limits knee flexion contracture, and protects the limb from external trauma.

A prosthetist can be helpful with such casting and can apply a jig that allows attachment and alignment for early pylon use. Weight bearing is limited initially, with bilateral upper extremity support from parallel bars, a walker, or crutches. The dressing is changed every 5 to 7 days for skin care. Within 3 to 4 weeks, the rigid dressing can be changed to a removable temporary prosthesis if there are no skin complications. The patient is shown the proper use of elastic wrapping or a stump shrinker to control edema and help contour the residual limb when not wearing the prosthesis. The physiatrist and therapist can assist in monitoring progress through the various transitions of temporary prosthetics to the permanent design, which may take several months. Endoskeletal designs have been more frequently used because modifications are simpler. Formal inpatient rehabilitation is brief, with most prosthetic training done on an outpatient basis. A program geared toward returning the patient to his or her previous occupation, hobbies, and educational pursuits can be structured with the help of a social worker, occupational therapist, and vocational counselor.

ISCHEMIC LIMBS

The frequent comorbidities in patients with ischemic limbs demand precautionary measures and interaction with a vascular surgical team. Because the skin's blood supply is much better on the posterior and medial aspects of the leg than on the anterior or anterolateral sides, transtibial amputation techniques for the ischemic limb are characterized by skin flaps that favor the posterior and medial side of the leg. The long posterior flap technique popularized by Burgess is most commonly used, but medial and lateral flaps of equal length

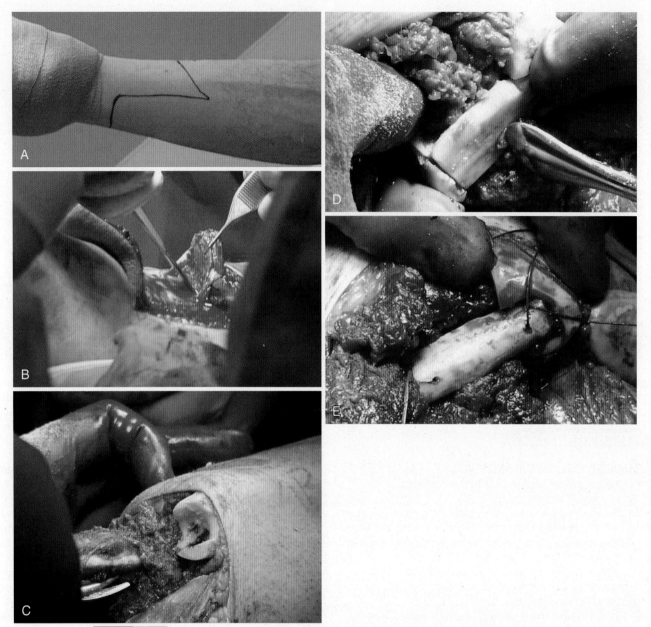

FIGURE 13.3   Modified Ertl technique. **A,** Skin incision marked to create long posterior flap. **B,** Elevation of osteoperiosteal flap from the tibia. **C,** Provisional notch created in distal tibia and fibula for fibular strut. **D,** Fibular strut placed into the tibial and fibular notches. **E,** Fibular strut secured via sutures through bone tunnels.   (A, B, and E, From: Taylor BC, Poka A: Osteomyoplastic transtibial amputation: the Ertl technique, *J Am Acad Orthop Surg* 24:259, 2013. C and D, From Taylor BC, Poka A: Osteomyoplastic transtibial amputation: technique and tips, *J Orthop Surg Res* 6:13, 2011.) **SEE TECHNIQUE 13.2.**

as described by Persson, skew flaps, and long medial flaps are being used. All techniques stress the need for preserving intact the vascular connections between skin and muscle by avoiding dissection along tissue planes and by constructing myocutaneous flaps. Also, amputations performed in ischemic limbs are customarily at a higher level (e.g., 10 to 12.5 cm distal to the joint line) than amputations in nonischemic limbs. Tension myodesis and osteomyoplasty, which may be of value in young, vigorous patients, historically have been contraindicated in patients with ischemic limbs due

to concerns of blood flow restriction. However, recent data demonstrate that the Ertl procedure may be safe in these high-risk patients.

Traditionally, tourniquets have not been used in the amputation of dysvascular limbs to avoid damage to more proximal diseased arteries. However, recent studies (including randomized controlled trials) demonstrate decreased blood loss, decreased postoperative transfusion rates, and no increased risk of vascular or wound complications with the use of a tourniquet.

TRANSTIBIAL AMPUTATION USING LONG POSTERIOR SKIN FLAP

TECHNIQUE 13.3

(BURGESS)

- Position the patient supine on the operating table; do not apply a tourniquet. Prepare and drape the limb so that an above-knee amputation can be performed if bleeding and tissue viability are insufficient to permit a successful transtibial amputation. For ischemic limbs, Burgess recommended amputation 8.8 to 12.5 cm distal to the line of the knee joint.
- Outline a long posterior flap and a short anterior one. The posterior flap should measure 1 cm more than the diameter of the leg at the level of bone division.
- Fashion the anterior flap at about the level of anticipated section of the tibia (Fig. 13.4A).
- Reflect as a single layer with the anterior flap the deep fascia and periosteum over the anteromedial surface of the tibia.
- Divide the anterolateral muscles down to the intermuscular septum, ligating and dividing the anterior tibial vessels and peroneal nerves as encountered.

- Section the tibia, and at a level no more than 0.9 to 1.3 cm higher, section the fibula. Dissect the soft tissues from the posterior aspect of the tibia and fibula distally to the level of the posterior transverse skin division and separate and remove the leg, ligating and dividing the nerves and vessels (Fig. 13.4B).
- Carefully round the tibia and form a short bevel on its anterior and medial aspects. Tension myodesis is not recommended in this instance.
- Bevel and tailor the posterior muscle mass to form a flap (see Fig. 13.4B) and carry it anteriorly, suturing it to the deep fascia and periosteum (Fig. 13.4C).
- Obtain meticulous hemostasis.
- Place a plastic suction drainage tube deep to the muscle flap and fascia and bring it out laterally through the skin 10 to 12.5 cm proximal to the end of the stump; if preferred, a through-and-through Penrose drain may be used, but it is more difficult to remove.
- Fashion the skin flaps as necessary to obtain smooth closure without too much tension. Trim any "dog ears" sparingly; otherwise, the circulation in the skin may be disturbed.
- Close the skin with interrupted nonabsorbable sutures.

■ REHABILITATION IN ISCHEMIC LIMBS

Rehabilitation in patients with ischemic limbs must proceed cautiously because of potential skin healing compromise

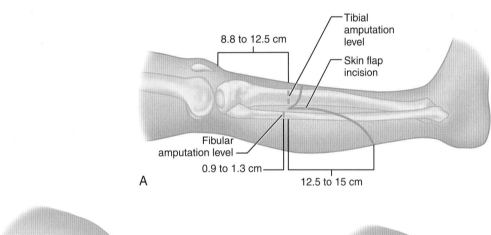

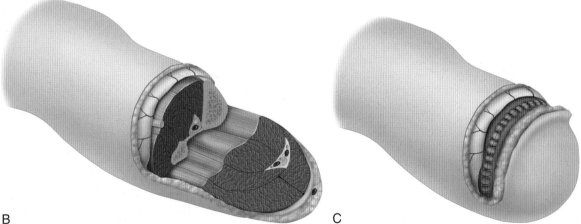

FIGURE 13.4 Transtibial amputation in ischemic limbs. **A,** Fashioning of short anterior and long posterior skin flaps. **B,** Separation and removal of distal leg. Muscle mass is tailored to form flaps. **C,** Suture of flap to deep fascia and periosteum anteriorly. (Redrawn from Burgess EM, Zettl JH: Amputations below the knee, *Artif Limbs* 13:1, 1969.) **SEE TECHNIQUE 13.3.**

and accompanying medical conditions. Initial postoperative efforts are centered on skin healing. After transtibial amputation, a soft dressing can be applied but a rigid dressing is preferred and can be used regardless of whether early ambulation is prescribed. If immediate or prompt prosthetic ambulation is not to be pursued, the stump can be dressed in a simple, well-padded cast that extends proximally to midthigh and is applied in such a manner as to avoid proximal constriction of the limb. Good suspension of the cast is essential to prevent it from slipping distally and impairing stump circulation. This may require compressive contouring of the cast in the supracondylar area and a waist band, suspension strap, or both. The cast should be removed in 5 to 7 days; and if wound healing is satisfactory, a new rigid dressing or prosthetic cast is applied. If immediate or prompt prosthetic ambulation is pursued, a properly constructed prosthetic cast is best applied by a qualified prosthetist. Success of rehabilitation depends on multiple variables, including cognitive status, premorbid functional level, condition of the upper extremities and contralateral lower limb, and coexisting medical and neurologic conditions. Early rehabilitation efforts may be geared toward independence in a wheelchair, stump care education, skin care techniques to avoid decubitus ulcers, care of the contralateral intact lower limb, and preprosthetic general conditioning. Weight bearing on the residual limb is usually delayed until skin healing has progressed. If a more aggressive approach is taken toward prosthetic training, more frequent rigid dressing changes are recommended and possibly the use of clear sockets to allow monitoring of the skin. Some patients may require further medical evaluation and clearance (e.g., chemically induced cardiac stress test or echocardiogram or vascular studies of the contralateral limb) to evaluate tolerance for prosthetic training. A pain management specialist may be needed to help treat postoperative phantom limb pain. Many patients receive inpatient rehabilitation training with subsequent therapy on an outpatient basis or in an extended-care facility or home health setting. Proposed rehabilitation goals also dictate which prosthetic components would be approved by insurance carriers.

DISARTICULATION OF THE KNEE

Disarticulation of the knee results in a functional end-bearing stump. Newer socket designs and prosthetic knee mechanisms that provide swing phase control have improved function in patients with knee disarticulation. Although the benefit of its use in children and young adults has been proven, its use in the elderly and especially in patients with ischemia has been limited in the United States. Knee disarticulations are more commonly used in cases of trauma. Based on published data, it remains unclear if knee disarticulation provides additional functional benefit and improved complication rates compared to transfemoral amputation.

Potential advantages of knee disarticulation include (1) preservation of the large end-bearing surfaces of the distal femur covered by skin and other soft tissues that are naturally suited for weight bearing, (2) creation of a long lever arm controlled by strong muscles, and (3) stability of the prosthesis. Techniques have been described for reducing the bulk of bone at the end of the stump to allow more cosmetic prosthetic fitting while still retaining the weight-bearing, suspension, and rotational control features of the stump. Modified

skin incisions allow greater use of this amputation level in patients with ischemia. In nonambulatory patients, additional extremity length provides adequate sitting support and balance. Knee flexion contractures and associated distal ulcers common with transtibial amputations also are avoided.

KNEE DISARTICULATION

TECHNIQUE 13.4

(BATCH, SPITTLER, AND MCFADDIN)

- Measuring from the inferior pole of the patella, fashion a long, broad anterior flap about equal in length to the diameter of the knee (Fig. 13.5A).
- Measuring from the level of the popliteal crease, fashion a short posterior flap equal in length to one half of the diameter of the knee. Place the lateral ends of the flaps at the level of the tibial condyles.
- Deepen the anterior incision through the deep fascia to the bone and dissect the anterior flap from the tibia and adjacent muscle. Include in the flap the insertion of the patellar tendon and the pes anserinus (Fig. 13.5B).
- Expose the knee joint by dissecting the capsule from the anterior and lateral margins of the tibia; divide the cruciate ligaments, and dissect the posterior capsule from the tibia (Fig. 13.5C).
- Identify the tibial nerve, gently pull it distally, and divide it proximally so that it retracts well proximal to the level of amputation (Fig. 13.5D).
- Identify, doubly ligate, and divide the popliteal vessels.
- Free the biceps tendon from the fibula, complete the amputation posteriorly, and remove the leg.
- Do not excise the patella or attempt to fuse it to the femoral condyles. Do not disturb the articular cartilage of the femoral condyles and patella. Perform a synovectomy only if specifically indicated.
- Suture the patellar tendon to the cruciate ligaments and the remnants of the gastrocnemius muscle to tissue in the intercondylar notch (Fig. 13.5E).
- Place a through-and-through Penrose drain in the wound.
- Close the deep fascia and subcutaneous tissues with absorbable sutures and the skin edges with interrupted nonabsorbable sutures.
- If sufficient skin for a loose closure is unavailable, resect the posterior part of the femoral condyles rather than risk loss of the skin flaps. The wound usually heals quickly, however, and a permanent prosthesis usually can be fitted in 6 to 8 weeks because shrinkage of the stump is not a factor. If the wound fails to heal primarily, there is no reason for apprehension or reamputation because it usually granulates and heals satisfactorily without additional surgery.

KNEE DISARTICULATION

Mazet and Hennessy recommended a method that features resection of the protruding medial, lateral, and posterior surfaces of the femoral condyles for creating a knee disarticulation stump for which a more cosmeti-

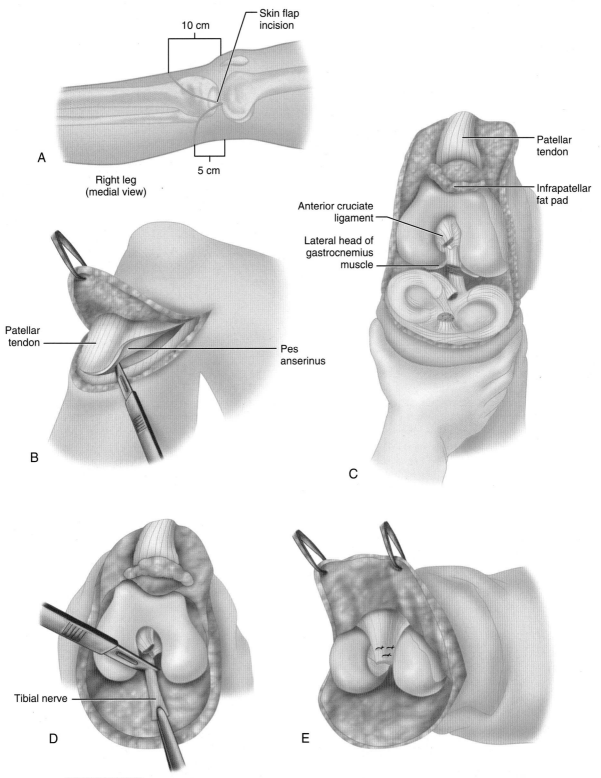

FIGURE 13.5 Disarticulation of knee joint. **A,** Skin incision. **B,** Anterior flap elevated, including insertion of patellar tendon and pes anserinus. **C,** Cruciate ligaments and posterior capsule divided. **D,** Tibial nerve divided high. **E,** Patellar tendon sutured to cruciate ligaments. **SEE TECHNIQUE 13.4.**

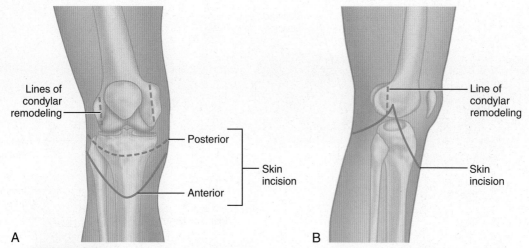

Lines of
condylar
remodeling

Posterior

Skin
incision

Anterior

A

Line of
condylar
remodeling

Skin
incision

B

FIGURE 13.6 Mazet and Hennessy disarticulation of knee. **A,** Anterior view. **B,** Lateral view. **SEE TECHNIQUE 13.5.** (Redrawn from Mazet R Jr, Hennessy CA: Knee disarticulation: a new technique and a new knee-joint mechanism, *J Bone Joint Surg* 48A:126, 1966.)

cally acceptable prosthesis can be constructed. With this technique, tolerances within the socket are greater, more adduction of the stump is permitted in the alignment of the prosthesis, and the decreased bulk of the stump permits greater ease in the application and removal of the prosthesis. The debulked stump requires smaller skin flaps, which may be beneficial for wound healing in dysvascular limbs. These patients may use a suction type prosthesis, which is less cumbersome to apply than a traditional above-knee amputation prosthesis and does not require removal for toileting needs.

TECHNIQUE 13.5

(MAZET AND HENNESSY)

- Fashion the usual fish-mouth skin incision, making the anterior flap longer and extending 10 cm distal to the level of the knee joint and making the posterior flap shorter and extending only about 2.5 cm distal to the same level (Fig. 13.6).
- Reflect the skin and deep fascia well proximal to the femoral condyles.
- Divide the patellar tendon midway between the patella and the tibial tuberosity.
- Flex the knee and section the collateral and cruciate ligaments.
- Increase flexion of the knee to 90 degrees, identify and ligate the popliteal vessels, and isolate and divide the tibial nerve.
- Detach the hamstring muscles from their insertions and remove the leg.
- Dissect the patella from its tendon and discard it.
- Remodel the femoral condyles in the following manner. Drive a wide osteotome vertically in a proximal direction through the medial femoral condyle to emerge at the level of the adductor tubercle. Start this cut along a line that extends from the medial articular margin anteriorly

to the midpoint of the distal articular surface posteriorly (the condyle is wider posteriorly). Discard the medial half of the condyle.

- Resect the lateral part of the lateral femoral condyle in a similar manner, starting at the junction of the medial two thirds and lateral one third of the distal articular surface.
- Direct attention to the posterior aspect of both condyles. Resect the posterior projecting bone by a vertical osteotomy in the frontal plane, starting at the point where the condyles begin to curve sharply superiorly and posteriorly.
- Smoothly round all bony prominences with a rasp, but do not disturb the remaining articular cartilage. At this point, each condyle has a fairly broad weight-bearing area, whereas the projecting side and posterior aspect of each have been removed and the remaining bone has been smoothly rounded.
- Suture the patellar tendon to the hamstrings in the intercondylar notch under slight tension. Insert drains at each end of the wound, and close the deep fascia and the skin in separate layers.

KNEE DISARTICULATION

TECHNIQUE 13.6

(KJØBLE)

- With the patient prone on the operating table, outline a lateral flap that is one half the anteroposterior diameter of the knee in length and a medial flap that is 2 to 3 cm longer to allow adequate coverage of the large medial femoral condyle (Fig. 13.7). By constructing shorter medial and lateral flaps,

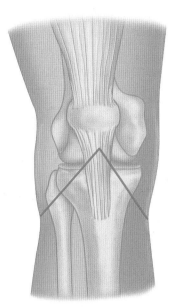

FIGURE 13.7　Kjøble disarticulation of knee with medial and lateral skin flaps. **SEE TECHNIQUE 13.6.**

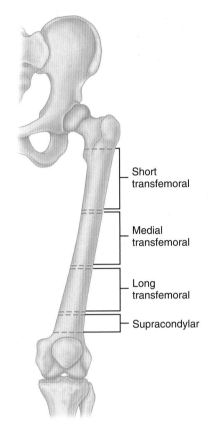

Short transfemoral

Medial transfemoral

Long transfemoral

Supracondylar

FIGURE 13.8　Levels of transfemoral amputations.

this technique provides more frequent healing in ischemic limbs than techniques using long anterior and posterior flaps.

- Begin the incision just distal to the lower pole of the patella and extend it distally to the tibial tuberosity, curving medially from this point for the medial flap and laterally from this point for the lateral flap.
- Carry both incisions posteriorly to meet in the midline of the limb at a point 2.5 cm proximal to the joint line.
- Deepen the incisions through the subcutaneous tissue and fascia down to bone.
- Divide the patellar tendon at its insertion, and release the medial and lateral hamstring tendons at their insertions.
- Divide the collateral ligaments and the cruciate ligaments.
- Divide the posterior joint capsule and expose, doubly ligate, and divide the popliteal vessels. Identify and sharply transect the peroneal and tibial nerves so that their cut ends retract well proximal to the end of the stump.
- Release the gastrocnemius origins from the distal femur and divide any remaining soft tissues.
- Suture the patellar tendon and the hamstring tendons to each other and to the cruciate ligaments in the intercondylar notch.
- Approximate the skin edges with interrupted nonabsorbable sutures.

POSTOPERATIVE CARE　If desired, a soft dressing may be applied, and conventional aftercare instituted as previously described (see chapter 11). Preferable treatment is to apply a rigid dressing or prosthetic cast with or without immediate or early weight-bearing ambulation. If non–weight bearing is desired, the rigid dressing need consist only of a properly padded cast extending to the groin and securely suspended by compressive contouring of the cast in the supracondylar area or by a waist belt, suspension strap, or both. If weight-bearing ambulation is pursued, the prosthetic cast should be applied by a qualified prosthetist. Postoperative care is similar to that outlined after transfemoral amputation (see section on transfemoral amputations).

TRANSFEMORAL (ABOVE-KNEE) AMPUTATIONS

Amputation levels above the knee can be classified as short transfemoral, medial transfemoral, long transfemoral, and supracondylar (Fig. 13.8). Amputation through the thigh is second in frequency only to transtibial amputation. In this procedure the patient's knee joint is lost, so it is extremely important for the stump to be as long as possible to provide a strong lever arm for control of the prosthesis. The conventional, constant friction knee joint used in conventional above-knee prostheses extends 9 to 10 cm distal to the end of the prosthetic socket, and the bone must be amputated this far proximal to the knee to allow room for the joint. Modern computer-assisted knee prostheses using variable friction for knee stiffness allow for shorter distal femoral segments. These prostheses that have highly sensitive sensors use hydraulic or magnetic units to allow for more natural knee motion, especially deceleration during the swing phase of gait. This also allows for longer femoral length without uneven levels of knee joint function. Amputation stumps in which the level of bone section is less than 5 cm distal to the lesser trochanter function as and are prosthetically fitted as hip disarticulations.

Muscle stabilization by myodesis or myoplasty is important when constructing a strong and sturdy amputation stump. Gottschalk pointed out that in the absence of myodesis of the adductor magnus, most transfemoral amputations result in at least 70% loss of adduction power.

TRANSFEMORAL (ABOVE-KNEE) AMPUTATION OF NONISCHEMIC LIMBS

TECHNIQUE 13.7

- Position the patient supine on the operating table and perform the surgery using tourniquet hemostasis.
- Beginning proximally at the anticipated level of bone section, outline equal anterior and posterior skin flaps. The length of each flap should be at least one half the anteroposterior diameter of the thigh at this level. Atypical flaps always are preferred to amputation at a higher level.
- Fashion the anterior flap with an incision that starts at the midpoint on the medial aspect of the thigh at the level of anticipated bone section. The incision passes in a gentle curve distally and laterally, crosses the anterior aspect of the thigh at the level determined as noted earlier, and curves proximally to end on the lateral aspect of the thigh opposite the starting point (Fig. 13.9A).
- Fashion the posterior flap in a similar manner.
- Deepen the skin incisions through the subcutaneous tissue and deep fascia and reflect the flaps proximally to the level of bone section.

- Divide the quadriceps muscle and its overlying fascia along the line of the anterior incision and reflect it proximally to the level of intended bone section as a myofascial flap.
- Identify, individually ligate, and transect the femoral artery and vein in the femoral canal on the medial side of the thigh at the level of bone section. Incise the periosteum of the femur circumferentially and divide the bone with a saw immediately distal to the periosteal incision.
- With a sharp rasp, smooth the edges of the bone and flatten the anterolateral aspect of the femur to decrease the unit pressures between the bone and the overlying soft tissues.
- Identify the sciatic nerve just beneath the hamstring muscles, ligate it well proximal to the end of the bone, and divide it just distal to the ligature.
- Divide the posterior muscles transversely so that their ends retract to the level of bone section and remove the leg (Fig. 13.9B).
- Isolate and section all cutaneous nerves so that their cut ends retract well proximal to the end of the stump. Irrigate the wound with saline to remove all bone dust.
- Through several small holes drilled just proximal to the end of the femur, attach the adductor and hamstring muscles to the bone with nonabsorbable or absorbable sutures (Fig. 13.9C). The muscles should be attached under slight tension (alternatively, suture anchors with heavy nonabsorbable suture or suture tape may be used instead of bone tunnels).

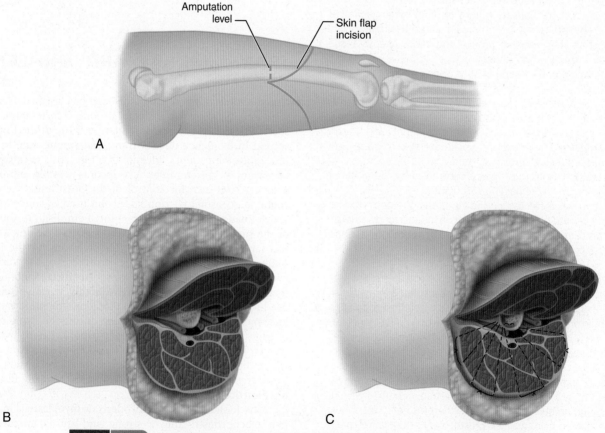

FIGURE 13.9   Amputation through middle third of thigh. **A,** Incision and bone level. **B,** Myofascial flap fashioned from quadriceps muscle and fascia. **C,** Adductor and hamstring muscles attached to end of femur through holes drilled in bone. **SEE TECHNIQUE 13.7.**

- Divide the femur 12 cm above the knee joint.
- Drill holes in the lateral, anterior, and posterior aspects of the femur, 1.5 cm from its end.
- Hold the femur in maximal adduction and suture the adductor magnus to its lateral aspect using previously drilled holes (Fig. 13.10). Also, place anterior and posterior sutures to prevent its sliding backward or forward.
- Suture the quadriceps to the posterior femur by drawing it over the adductor magnus while holding the hip in extension.
- Suture the remaining posterior muscles to the posterior aspect of the adductor magnus. Close the investing fascia and skin and apply a soft dressing.

REHABILITATION AFTER TRANSFEMORAL AMPUTATION

A soft dressing is adequate initially for elderly dysvascular patients, whereas immediate postoperative rigid dressings and earlier weight bearing with a locked-knee pylon are appropriate in younger patients. Patients seem more comfortable if weight bearing is delayed until sutures or staples are removed. Subsequently, ambulation can be progressed with an unlocked knee and less upper extremity support. For the definitive prosthesis, a variety of prosthetic knee units are available that are lighter and accommodate constant or variable gait cadences and provide good stability during weight bearing.

Many concepts and strategies relevant to these patients were discussed earlier under postoperative care of transtibial amputations. The emphasis is on the recognition that patients with ischemic limbs generally are less healthy than patients with nonischemic limbs; the rehabilitative program generally progresses much more slowly and more cautiously. A major obstacle to rehabilitation after transfemoral amputation is the loss of the knee joint, which exponentially increases the energy expenditure for locomotion with a prosthesis. This has consequences for cardiac patients and patients with ischemic contralateral limbs. The patient and family must be aware of the risks involved with a physically demanding rehabilitation program. Many transfemoral amputees with vascular disease never use a prosthesis consistently. Patients with bilateral transfemoral amputations frequently elect to use a wheelchair because it is faster, and oxygen consumption is four to seven times more using bilateral transfemoral prostheses. Younger patients can experience progress more rapidly, as discussed under transtibial postoperative care.

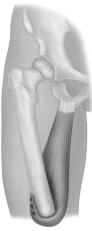

FIGURE 13.10 Attachment of adductor magnus to lateral femur. *(Redrawn from Gottschalk F: Transfemoral amputations. In: Bowker JH, Michael JW, editors: Atlas of limb prosthetics: surgical, prosthetic, and rehabilitation principles, ed 2, St. Louis: Mosby, 1992.)* **SEE TECHNIQUE 13.8.**

- At this point, release the tourniquet and attain meticulous hemostasis.
- Bring the "quadriceps apron" over the end of the bone and suture its fascial layer to the posterior fascia of the thigh, trimming any excess muscle or fascia to permit a neat, snug approximation.
- Insert plastic suction drainage tubes beneath the muscle flap and deep fascia, and bring them out through the lateral aspect of the thigh 10 to 12.5 cm proximal to the end of the stump.
- Approximate the skin edges with interrupted sutures of nonabsorbable material.

TRANSFEMORAL (ABOVE-KNEE) AMPUTATION OF NONISCHEMIC LIMBS

TECHNIQUE 13.8

(GOTTSCHALK)
- Place the patient supine with a roll under the buttock of the affected side.
- Develop skin flaps using a long medial flap in the sagittal plane when possible.
- Detach the quadriceps just proximal to the patella, retaining part of its tendon.
- Reflect the vastus medialis off the intermuscular septum.
- Detach the adductor magnus from the adductor tubercle and reflect it medially to expose the femur. Identify and ligate the femoral vessels at Hunter's canal.
- Divide the gracilis, sartorius, semimembranosus, and semitendinosus 2.5 to 5 cm below the intended bone section.

REFERENCES

Al Muderis M, Khemka A, Lord SJ, et al.: Safety of osseointegrated implants for transfemoral amputees: a two-center prospective cohort study, *J Bone Joint Surg Am* 98(11):900, 2016.

Albino FP, Seidel R, Brown BJ, et al.: Through knee amputation: technique modifications and surgical outcomes, *Arch Plast Surg* 41:562, 2014.

Baril DT, Ghosh K, Rosen AB: Trends in the incidence, treatment, and outcomes of acute lower extremity ischaemia in the United States Medicare population, *J Vasc Surg* 60:669, 2014.

Bell JC, Wolf EJ, Schnall BL, et al.: Transfemoral amputations: is there an effect of residual limb length and orientation on energy expenditure? *Clin Orthop Relat Res* 472:3055, 2014.

Bosse MJ, Morshed S, Reider L, et al.: Transtibial amputation outcomes study (TAOS): comparing transtibial amputation with and without a tibiofibular synostosis (Ertl) procedure, *J Orthop Trauma* 31(Suppl 1):S63, 2017.

Brown BJ, Iorio ML, Klement M, et al.: Outcomes after 294 transtibial amputations in the posterior myocutaneous flap, *Int J Low Extrem Wounds* 13:33, 2014.

Czerniecki JM, Thompson ML, Littman A, et al.: Predicting reamputation risk in patients undergoing lower extremity amputation due to the complications of peripheral artery disease and/or diabetes, *Br J Surg* 106(8):1026, 2019.

Easterlin MC, Chang DC, Wilson SE: A practical index to predict 30-day mortality after major amputation, *Ann Vasc Surg* 27:909, 2013.

Fang ZB, Hu FY, Arya S, et al.: Preoperative frailty is predictive of complications after major lower extremity amputation, *J Vasc Surg* 65(3):804, 2017.

Fergason J, Keeling JJ, Bluman EM: Recent advances in lower extremity amputation and prosthetics for the combat injured patient, *Foot Ankle Clin* 15:151, 2010.

Fleming ME, O'Daniel A, Bharmal H, Valerio I: Application of the orthoplastic reconstructive ladder to preserve lower extremity amputation length, *Ann Plast Surg* 73:183, 2014.

Goodney PP, Holman K, Henke PK, et al.: Regional intensity of vascular care and lower extremity amputation rates, *J Vasc Surg* 57:1471, 2013.

Hasanadka R, McLafferty RB, Moore CJ, et al.: Predictors of wound complications following major amputation for critical limb ischemia, *J Vasc Surg* 54:1374, 2011.

Hsu AR: Transfemoral amputation adductor myodesis using FiberTape and knotless anchors, *Foot Ankle Int* 39(7):874, 2018.

Jain A, Glass GE, Ahmadi H, et al.: Delayed amputation following trauma increases residual lower limb infection, *J Plast Reconstr Aesthet Surg* 66:531, 2013.

Jones WS, Patel MR, Dai D, et al.: High mortality risks after major lower extremity amputation in Medicare patients with peripheral artery disease, *Am Heart J* 165:809, 2013.

Kahle JT, Highsmith MJ, Kenney J, et al.: The effectiveness of the bone bridge transtibial amputation technique: a systematic review of high-quality evidence, *Prosthet Orthot Int* 41(3):219, 2017.

Karam J, Shepard A, Rubinfeld I: Predictors of operative mortality following major lower extremity amputations using the National Surgical Quality Improvement Program public use data, *J Vasc Surg* 58:1276, 2013.

Kwah LK, Webb MT, Goh L, Harvey LA: Rigid dressings versus soft dressings for transtibial amputations, *Cochrane Database Syst Rev* 6:CD012427, 2019.

Leijendekkers RA, van Hinte G, Frölke JP, et al.: Functional performance and safety of bone-anchored prostheses in persons with a transfemoral or transtibial amputation: a prospective one-year follow-up cohort study, *Clin Rehabil* 33(3):450, 2019.

Lowenberg DW, Buntic RF, Buncke GM, Parrett BM: Long-term results and costs of muscle flap coverage with Ilizarov bone transport in lower limb salvage, *J Orthop Trauma* 27:576, 2013.

Mangan KI, Kingsbury TD, Mazzone BN, et al.: Limb salvage with intrepid dynamic exoskeletal orthosis versus transtibial amputation: a comparison of functional gait outcomes, *J Orthop Trauma* 30(12):e390, 2016.

Nelson MT, Greenblatt DY, Soma G, et al.: Preoperative factors predict mortality after major lower-extremity amputation, *Surgery* 152:685, 2012.

O'Brien PJ, Cox MW, Shortell CK, Scarborough JE: Risk factors for early failure of surgical amputations: an analysis of 8,878 isolated lower extremity amputation procedures, *J Am Coll Surg* 216:836, 2013.

Penn-Barwell JG: Outcomes in lower limb amputation following trauma: a systematic review and meta-analysis, *Injury* 42:1474, 2011.

Phair J, DeCarlo C, Scher L, et al.: Risk factors for unplanned readmission and stump complications after major lower extremity amputation, *J Vasc Surg* 67(3):848, 2018.

Plucknette BF, Krueger CA, Rivera JC, Wenke JC: Combat-related bridge synostosis versus traditional transtibial amputation: comparison of military-specific outcomes, *Strategies Trauma Limb Reconstr* 11(1):5, 2016.

Polfer EM, Hoyt BW, Bevevino AJ, et al.: Knee disarticulations versus transfemoral amputations: functional outcomes, *J Orthop Trauma* 33(6):308, 2019.

Prinsen E, Nederhand MJ, Olsman J, Rietman JS: Influence of a user-adaptive prosthetic knee on quality of life, balance confidence, and measures of mobility: a randomised cross-over trial, *Clin Rehabil* 29:581, 2015.

Reichmann JP, Stevens PM, Rheinstein J, Kreulen CD: Removal rigid dressings for postoperative management of transtibial amputations: a review of published evidence, *PM R* 10(5):516, 2018.

Rosen N, Gigi R, Haim A, et al.: Mortality and reoperations following lower limb amputations, *Isr Med Assoc J* 16:83, 2014.

Ryan SP, DiLallo M, Klement MR, et al.: Transfemoral amputation following total knee arthroplasty: mortality and functional outcomes, *Bone Joint J* 101-B(2):221, 2019.

Schuett DJ, Wyatt MP, Kingsbury T, et al.: Are gait parameters for through-knee amputees different from matched transfemoral amputees? *Clin Orthop Relat Res* 477(4):821, 2019.

Seker A, Kara A, Camur S, et al.: Comparison of mortality rates and functional results after transtibial and transfemoral amputations due to diabetes in elderly patients – a retrospective study, *Int J Surg* 33:78, 2016.

Shah SK, Bena JF, Allemang MT, et al.: Lower extremity amputations: factors associated with mortality or contralateral amputation, *Vasc Endovascular Surg* 47:608, 2013.

Singleton JA, Walker NM, Gibb IE, et al: Case suitability for definitive through knee amputation following lower extremity blast trauma: analysis of 146 combat casualties, 2008-2010, *J R Army Med Corps* 160(187):2014.

Spahn K, Wyatt MP, Stewart JM, et al.: Do Gait and functional parameters change after transtibial amputation following attempted limb preservation in a military population? *Clin Orthop Relat Res* 477(4):829, 2019.

Sumpio B, Shine SR, Mahler D, Sumpio BE: A comparison of immediate postoperative rigid and soft dressings for below-knee amputations, *Ann Vasc Surg* 27:774, 2013.

Swaminathan A, Vemulapalli S, Patel MR, Jones WS: Lower extremity amputation in peripheral artery disease: improving patient outcomes, *Vasc Health Risk Manag* 10:417, 2014.

Taylor BC, Poka A: Osteomyoplastic transtibial amputation: technique and tips, *J Orthop Surg Res* 6:13, 2011.

Taylor BC, Poka A: Osteomyoplastic transtibial amputation: the Ertl technique, *J Am Acad Orthop Surg* 24(4):259, 2016.

Theeven PJ, Hemmen B, Geers RP, et al.: Influence of advanced prosthetic knee joints on perceived performance and everyday life activity level of low-functional persons with a transfemoral amputation or knee disarticulation, *J Rehabil Med* 44:454, 2012.

Tillander J, Hagberg K, Berlin Ö, et al.: Osteomyelitis risk in patients with transfemoral amputations treated with osseointegration prostheses, *Clin Orthop Relat Res* 475(12):3100, 2017.

Tintle SM, Keeling JJ, Shawen SB, et al.: Traumatic and trauma-related amputations: part I: general principles and lower-extremity amputations, *J Bone Joint Surg* 92A:2852, 2010.

Tintle SM, Shawen SB, Forsberg JA, et al.: Reoperation after combat-related major lower extremity amputations, *J Orthop Trauma* 28:232, 2014.

Tsai CY, Chu SY, Wen YW, et al.: The value of Doppler waveform analysis in predicting major lower extremity amputation among dialysis patients treated for diabetic foot ulcers, *Diabetes Res Clin Pract* 100:181, 2013.

Tseng CL, Rajan M, Miller DR, et al.: Trends in initial lower extremity amputation rates among Veterans Health Administration health care system users from 2000 to 2004, *Diabetes Care* 34:1157, 2011.

Vallier HA, Fitzgerald SJ, Beddow ME, et al.: Osteocutaneous pedicle flap transfer for salvage of transtibial amputation after severe lower-extremity injury, *J Bone Joint Surg* 94A:447, 2012.

Wied C, Tengberg PT, Holm G, et al.: Tourniquets do not increase the total blood loss or re-amputation rise in transtibial amputations, *World J Orthop* 8(1):62, 2017.

Whitehead A, Wolf EJ, Scoville CR, Wilken JM: Does a microprocessor-controlled prosthetic knee affect stair ascent strategies in persons with transfemoral amputation? *Clin Orthop Relat Res* 472:3093, 2014.

Zayad M, Bech F, Hernandez-Boussard T: National review of factors influencing disparities and types of major lower extremity amputations, *Ann Vasc Surg* 28:1157, 2014.

The complete list of references is available online at ExpertConsult.com.

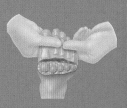

CHAPTER 14

AMPUTATIONS OF THE HIP AND PELVIS

Kevin B. Cleveland

| DISARTICULATION OF THE HIP | 621 | EXTERNAL HEMIPELVECTOMY (HINDQUARTER AMPUTATION) | 623 |

Hip disarticulation and the various forms of hemipelvectomy most often are performed for the treatment of primary bone tumors and rarely for metastases, infection, or trauma. Improved treatments with chemotherapy, radiation, and biologics are increasing survival of patients with malignancies, which has increased the indications for aggressive treatment of these tumors. The dimensions of the amputation vary with oncologic requirements, and nonstandard flaps often are necessary. For patients with such high-level amputations, the energy requirements to use a prosthesis have been estimated to be 250% of normal ambulation. Wheelchair and crutch locomotion are 50% faster and require less energy expenditure; however, especially in younger patients, providing prosthetic walking ability for even short distances may be beneficial to physical and mental health. With new advances in prosthetics, such as polycentric hip joints and microprocessor knees, more patients are increasing their independence and functional mobility. These newer advances provide greater ability to negotiate environmental obstacles such as stairs or inclines and allow variable cadence as well as minimize the need for ambulatory aides. Lighter-weight prostheses also have resulted in less oxygen consumption and more compliance with prosthetic use. The main goals of a prosthesis are to improve function and provide an improved self-body image. Only 43% of patients use a prosthetic device, however, and wear them on average for 5.8 hours per day. Although the only significant metric for unsuccessful prosthetic wear is coronary artery disease, the most common reason that patients do not use a prosthesis is that they were never offered one. We have found that consultation with a prosthetist is most valuable. A multidisciplinary team should be involved in the care of these patients, and thorough preoperative planning is imperative.

DISARTICULATION OF THE HIP

Hip disarticulation occasionally is indicated after massive trauma, for arterial insufficiency, for severe infections, for massive decubitus ulcers, or for certain congenital limb deficiencies. Most frequently, however, hip disarticulation is necessary for treatment of bone or soft-tissue sarcomas of the femur or thigh that cannot be resected adequately by limb-sparing methods. Hip disarticulation accounts for 0.5% of lower extremity amputations. Mortality rates vary in studies from 0% to 44%. The inguinal or iliac lymph nodes are not routinely removed with hip disarticulation. The anatomic method of Boyd and the posterior flap method of Slocum are described here. However, modifications frequently are required based on the location of the pathology.

ANATOMIC HIP DISARTICULATION

TECHNIQUE 14.1

(BOYD)

- With the patient in the lateral decubitus position, make an anterior racquet-shaped incision (Fig. 14.1A), beginning the incision at the anterior superior iliac spine and curving it distally and medially almost parallel with the inguinal ligament to a point on the medial aspect of the thigh 5 cm distal to the origin of the adductor muscles. Isolate and ligate the femoral artery and vein, and divide the femoral nerve; continue the incision around the posterior aspect of the thigh about 5 cm distal to the ischial tuberosity and along the lateral aspect of the thigh about 8 cm distal to the base of the greater trochanter. From this point, curve the incision proximally to join the beginning of the incision just inferior to the anterior superior iliac spine.
- Detach the sartorius muscle from the anterior superior iliac spine and the rectus femoris from the anterior inferior iliac spine. Reflect them both distally.
- Divide the pectineus about 0.6 cm from the pubis.
- Rotate the thigh externally to bring the lesser trochanter and the iliopsoas tendon into view; divide the latter at its insertion and reflect it proximally.
- Detach the adductor and gracilis muscles from the pubis and divide at its origin that part of the adductor magnus that arises from the ischium.
- Develop the muscle plane between the pectineus and obturator externus and short external rotators of the hip to expose the branches of the obturator artery. Clamp, ligate, and divide the branches at this point. Later in the operation the obturator externus muscle is divided at its insertion on the femur instead of at its origin on the pelvis because otherwise the obturator artery may be severed and might retract into the pelvis, leading to hemorrhage that could be difficult to control.
- Rotate the thigh internally and detach the gluteus medius and minimus muscles from their insertions on the greater trochanter and retract them proximally.
- Divide the fascia lata and the most distal fibers of the gluteus maximus muscle distal to the insertion of the tensor fasciae latae muscle in the line of the skin incision, and separate the tendon of the gluteus maximus from its insertion on the linea aspera. Reflect this muscle mass proximally.

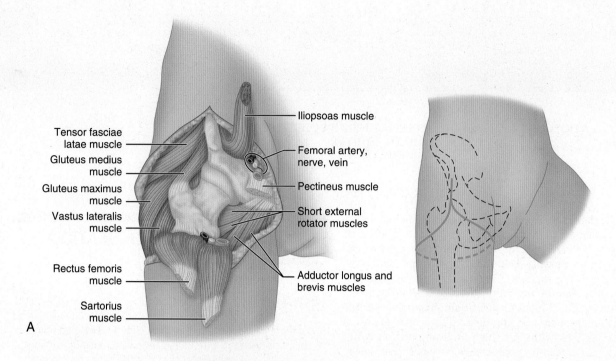

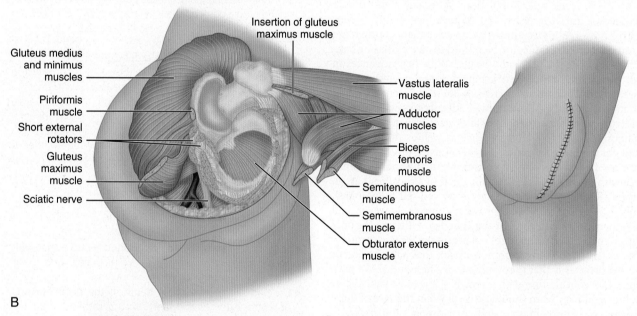

FIGURE 14.1 Boyd disarticulation of hip. **A,** Femoral vessels and nerve have been ligated, and sartorius, rectus femoris, pectineus, and iliopsoas muscles have been detached. *Inset,* Line of skin incision. **B,** Gluteal muscles have been separated from insertions, sciatic nerve and short external rotators have been divided, and hamstring muscles have been detached from ischial tuberosity. Inset, Final closure of stump. **SEE TECHNIQUE 14.1.** (Redrawn from Boyd HB: Anatomic disarticulation of the hip, *Surg Gynecol Obstet* 84:346, 1947.)

- Identify, ligate, and divide the sciatic nerve.
- Divide the short external rotators of the hip (i.e., the piriformis, gemelli, obturator internus, obturator externus, and quadratus femoris) at their insertions on the femur and sever the hamstring muscles from the ischial tuberosity.
- Incise the hip joint capsule and the ligamentum teres to complete the disarticulation (Fig. 14.1B).

- Bring the gluteal flap anteriorly and suture the distal part of the gluteal muscles to the origin of the pectineus and adductor muscles.
- Place a drain in the inferior part of the incision and approximate the skin edges with interrupted nonabsorbable sutures.

POSTERIOR FLAP

TECHNIQUE 14.2

(SLOCUM)
- Begin the incision at the level of the inguinal ligament, carry it distally over the femoral artery for 10 cm, curve it along the medial aspect of the thigh, continue it laterally and proximally over the greater trochanter, and swing it anteriorly to the starting point. A posteromedial flap long enough to cover the end of the stump is formed.
- Isolate, ligate, and divide the femoral vessels, and section the femoral nerve to fall well proximal to the inguinal ligament.
- Abduct the thigh widely and divide the adductor muscles at their pubic origins.
- Section the two branches of the obturator nerve so that they retract away from pressure areas.
- Free the origins of the sartorius and rectus femoris muscles from the anterior superior and anterior inferior iliac spines. Moderately adduct and internally rotate the thigh and divide the tensor fasciae latae muscle at the level of the proximal end of the greater trochanter; at the same level, divide close to bone the muscles attached to the trochanter. Next, abduct the thigh markedly and divide the gluteus maximus at the distal end of the posterior skin flap.
- Identify, ligate, and divide the sciatic nerve.
- Divide the joint capsule and complete the disarticulation.
- Swing the long posteromedial flap containing the gluteus maximus anteriorly and suture it to the anterior margins of the incision.

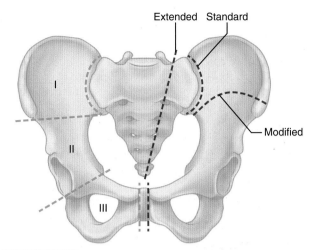

FIGURE 14.2 Modified hemipelvectomy. Bony section divides ilium above acetabulum *(red dotted line)*, preserving iliac crest. (Redrawn from: Bibbo C, Newman AS, Lackman RD, Levin LS, Kovach SJ: A simplified approach to reconstruction of hemipelvectomy defects with lower extremity free fillet flaps to minimize ischemia time, *J Plast Reconstr Aesth Surg* 68:1750, 2015)

EXTERNAL HEMIPELVECTOMY (HINDQUARTER AMPUTATION)

Hemipelvectomy most often is performed for tumors that cannot be adequately resected by limb-sparing techniques or hip disarticulation. Other indications for hemipelvectomy include life-threatening infection such as necrotizing fasciitis and arterial insufficiency. Chan et al. reported hemipelvectomy for decubitus ulcers in patients with spinal cord injury. In contrast to hip disarticulation, all types of hemipelvectomy remove the inguinal and iliac lymph nodes.

The standard hemipelvectomy employs a posterior or gluteal flap and disarticulates the symphysis pubis and sacroiliac joint and the ipsilateral limb. An extended hemipelvectomy includes resection of adjacent musculoskeletal structures, such as the sacrum or parts of the lumbar spine. In a modified hemipelvectomy, the bony section divides the ilium above the acetabulum, preserving the crest of the ilium (Fig. 14.2). Sherman, O'Connor, and Sim base their decision on when to perform a hemipelvectomy or a pelvic resection on three parameters: the sciatic nerve, the femoral neurovascular bundle, and the hip joint, including the periacetabular region. If two of the three are involved, they recommend hemipelvectomy over pelvic resections to obtain proper margins. Internal hemipelvectomy is a limb-sparing resection, often achieving proximal and medial margins equal to the corresponding amputation. This is currently the preferred method but should not be performed at the expense of quality margins. This procedure is discussed in other chapter.

All types of hemipelvectomy are extremely invasive and mutilating procedures. Gordon-Taylor called hindquarter amputations "one of the most colossal mutilations practiced on the human frame." These operations require optimizing the patient's nutritional status, preparing for blood replacement, and adequate monitoring during surgery. Early reports of mortality from hemipelvectomy was greater than 50%, but with more recent advances including radiation, chemotherapy, and patient optimization, mortality is less than 10%. Complications, however, are common and have been reported in up to 80% of patients. Many patients have significant phantom pain in the early postoperative course. Residual limb spasm has been reported to occur more commonly than phantom pain and may present weeks or even months after the procedure; it is most common after traumatic hemipelvectomy. Flap necrosis and wound sloughs are common complications. In their review of 160 external hemipelvectomies, Senchenkov et al. reported a morbidity rate of 54%, including intraoperative genitourinary (18%) and gastrointestinal injuries (3%). Wound complications were the most common postoperative complications, including infection and flap necrosis. Patients with a posterior flap, who had ligation of the common iliac vessels, were 2.7 times more likely to have flap necrosis than those patients who had ligation of the external iliac vessels alone. Apffelstaedt et al. found no statistical difference between flap failure and ligation of the common iliac artery compared to ligation of the external iliac artery only. We still recommend preservation of the common iliac artery when feasible. Increased operative time and complexity of the resection also lead to an increase in flap necrosis and infection. Up to 80% of flaps have been reported to have complications. The best option (86% success rate) for reconstructive flaps is use of the amputated tissue (free fillet flaps). Utilization of the fillet flap preserves the original soft tissue that can be used if the fillet flap should fail. To reduce ischemic time, it is recommended that the fillet flap be harvested before the hemipelvectomy is undertaken. Custom implants and trabecular metal can also be used to improve outcomes. The surgical techniques continue to evolve as advances in prosthetics continue to progress. New advances in 3D printed models and the use of intraoperative navigation systems improve the surgeon's understanding of the tumor as well as the resection required. Appropriate emotional and psychologic support is an important part of rehabilitation. Techniques for the standard, anterior flap and conservative hemipelvectomy are described.

STANDARD HEMIPELVECTOMY

TECHNIQUE 14.3

- Insert a Foley catheter. Place the patient in a lateral decubitus position with the involved side up. Support the patient so that the table can be tilted to facilitate anterior and posterior dissection.
- Perform the anterior dissection first, making an incision extending from 5 cm above the anterior superior iliac spine to the pubic tubercle (Fig. 14.3A). Deepen the incision through the tensor fascia, external oblique aponeurosis, and internal oblique and transversalis muscles.
- Retract the spermatic cord medially.
- Expose the iliac fossa by blunt dissection.
- Elevate the parietal peritoneum off of the iliac vessels and permit it to fall inferiorly with the viscera.
- Ligate the inferior epigastric vessels.
- Release the rectus muscle and sheath from the pubis.
- Identify the iliac vessels, retract the ureter medially, and ligate and divide the common iliac artery and vein. Put lateral traction on the iliac artery and vein and ligate and divide their branches to the sacrum, rectum, and bladder, separating the rectum and bladder from the pelvic side wall and exposing the sacral nerve roots (Fig. 14.3B, C). If necessary for exposure, divide the symphysis pubis and sacroiliac joint before this dissection.
- Pack the anterior wound with warm, moist gauze packs.
- Make a posterior skin incision, extending from 5 cm above the anterior superior iliac spine, coursing over the anterior aspect of the greater trochanter, paralleling the gluteal crease posteriorly around the thigh, and connecting with the inferior end of the anterior incision (see Fig. 14.3A).
- Raise the posterior flap by dissecting the gluteal fascia directly off the gluteus maximus. Include the fascia with the flap. If possible, include the medial portion of the gluteus maximus with the flap. Superiorly elevate the flap off the iliac crest.
- Divide the external oblique, sacrospinalis, latissimus dorsi, and quadratus lumborum from the crest of the ilium.
- Reflect the gluteus maximus from the sacrotuberous ligament, coccyx, and sacrum (Fig. 14.3D).
- Divide the iliopsoas muscle; genitofemoral, obturator, and femoral nerves; and lumbosacral nerve trunk at the level of the iliac crest.
- Abduct the hip, placing tension on the soft tissues around the symphysis pubis. Pass a long right-angle

clamp around the symphysis, and divide it with a scalpel (Fig. 14.3E).
- Divide the sacral nerve roots, preserving the nervi erigentes if possible. Reflect the iliacus muscle laterally, exposing the anterior aspect of the sacroiliac joint.
- Divide the joint anteriorly with a scalpel or osteotome and divide the iliolumbar ligament.
- Place considerable traction on the extremity, separating the pelvic side wall from the viscera. Proceeding from anterior to posterior, divide the following from the pelvic side wall: urogenital diaphragm, pubococcygeus, ischiococcygeus, iliococcygeus, piriformis, sacrotuberous ligament, and sacrospinous ligaments (Fig. 14.3F). All of these structures must be divided under tension. Move the extremity anteriorly and divide the posterior aspect of the sacroiliac joint to complete the dissection.
- Place suction drains in the wound and suture the gluteal fascia to the fascia of the abdominal wall. Close the skin.

POSTOPERATIVE CARE The drains and Foley catheter should be left in place for several days. Pressure should be kept off the posterior flap for several days.

ANTERIOR FLAP HEMIPELVECTOMY

Anterior flap hemipelvectomy is indicated for lesions of the buttock or posterior proximal thigh that cannot be adequately treated by limb-sparing methods. The larger posterior defect is covered by a quadriceps myocutaneous flap maintained by the superficial femoral vessels and may include part of the sartorius muscle.

TECHNIQUE 14.4

- Insert a Foley catheter. Place the patient in the lateral decubitus position with the operated side up and secure the patient to the table so that it can be tilted to facilitate the anterior and posterior dissections. Prepare the skin from toes to rib cages and drape the extremity free. Mark out the skin incision such that the length and width of the anterior flap adequately covers the posterior defect that is to be created (Fig. 14.4A).
- Make an incision superiorly across the iliac crest to the midlateral point, around the buttock just lateral to the anus, and to the midmedial point of the thigh. Carry the incision down the thigh a distance adequate to cover the posterior defect, across the front of the thigh to the midlateral point, and superiorly to join the superior incision.
- Perform the posterior dissection first. Preserve a skin margin of 3 cm from the anus. Detach the gluteus maximus and sacrospinalis from the sacrum. Detach the external oblique, sacrospinalis, latissimus dorsi, and quadratus lumborum muscles from the iliac crest.
- Flex the hip and place the tissues in the region of the gluteal crease under tension. Detach the remaining origins of the gluteus maximus from the coccyx and sacrotuberous ligament (Fig. 14.4B). Bluntly dissect lateral to the rectum into the ischiorectal fossa.

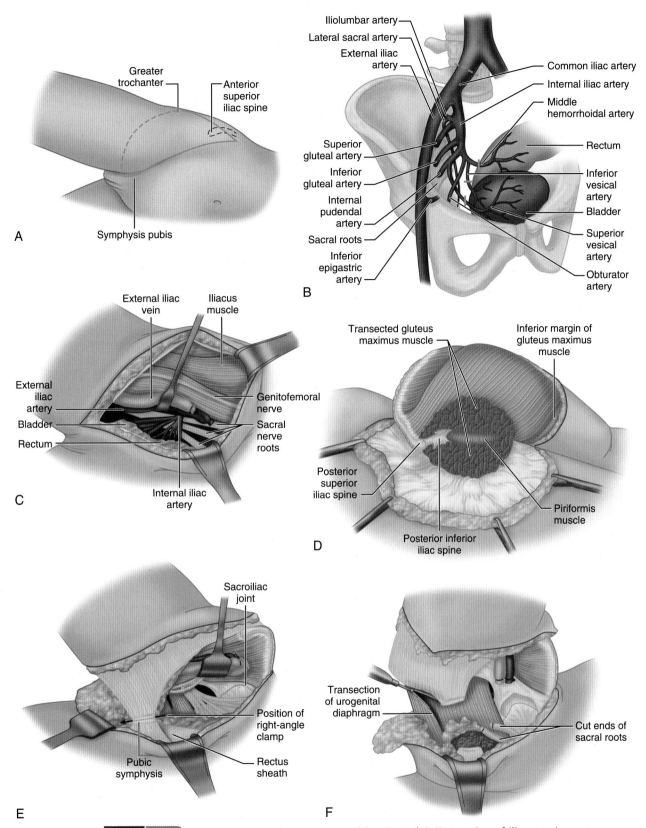

FIGURE 14.3 Standard hemipelvectomy. **A,** Incision. **B,** and **C,** Transection of iliac arteries and division of internal iliac vessels. **D,** Release of iliac crest and gluteus maximus. **E,** Division of symphysis pubis. **F,** Division of muscles from pelvis. **SEE TECHNIQUE 14.3.**

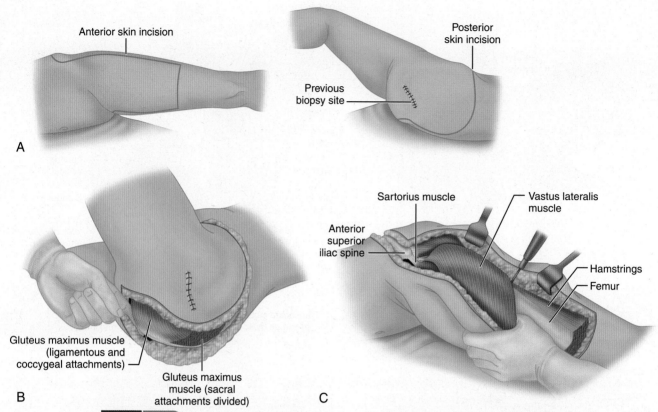

Anterior skin incision

Posterior skin incision

Previous biopsy site

A

Sartorius muscle

Vastus lateralis muscle

Anterior superior iliac spine

Hamstrings

Femur

Gluteus maximus muscle (ligamentous and coccygeal attachments)

Gluteus maximus muscle (sacral attachments divided)

B

C

FIGURE 14.4 Anterior flap hemipelvectomy. **A,** Anterior and posterior incision. **B,** Detachment of gluteus maximus origins from coccyx and sacrotuberous ligament. **C,** Severing vastus lateralis from femur and separating tensor fascia femoris from fascia.

- Move to the front of the patient and deepen the anterior incision at the junction of the middle and distal thirds of the thigh through the quadriceps to the femur. Continue the dissection laterally from this point in a cephalad direction to the anterior superior spine severing the vastus lateralis from the femur and separating the tensor fascia femoris from its fascia such that it is included with the specimen (Fig. 14.4C).
- Start the medial dissection at Hunter's canal and ligate and divide the superficial femoral vessels. Trace the vessels superiorly to the inguinal ligament, dividing and ligating multiple small branches to the adductor muscles.
- Place upward traction on the myocutaneous flap and detach the vastus medialis muscle and intermedius from the femur.
- Ligate and divide the profunda femoris vessels at their origin from the common femoral artery and vein.
- Separate the myocutaneous flap from the pelvis by releasing the abdominal muscles from the iliac crest, the sartorius from the anterior superior spine, the rectus femoris from the anterior inferior spine, and the rectus abdominis from the pubis (Fig. 14.4D).
- Retract the flap medially and dissect along the femoral nerve into the pelvis to expose the iliac vessels.

- Divide the symphysis pubis while protecting the bladder and urethra.
- Ligate and divide the internal iliac vessels at their origin from the common iliacs. While placing medial traction on the bladder and rectus, divide the visceral branches of the internal iliac vessels. Divide the psoas muscle as it joins the iliacus muscle and divide the underlying obturator nerve, but protect the femoral nerve going into the flap. Divide the lumbosacral nerve and the sacral nerve roots (Fig. 14.4E).
- Put traction on the pelvic diaphragm by elevating the extremity and divide the urogenital diaphragm, levator ani, and piriformis near the pelvis.
- Divide the sacroiliac joint and the iliolumbar ligament and remove the specimen.
- Turn the quadriceps flap onto the posterior defect and close the wound over suction drains by suturing the quadriceps to the abdominal wall, sacrospinalis, sacrum, and pelvic diaphragm.

POSTOPERATIVE CARE The patient may ambulate when comfort and stability permit. The drains and Foley catheter should be left in place for several days. Skin slough is much less common than with the classic posterior flap.

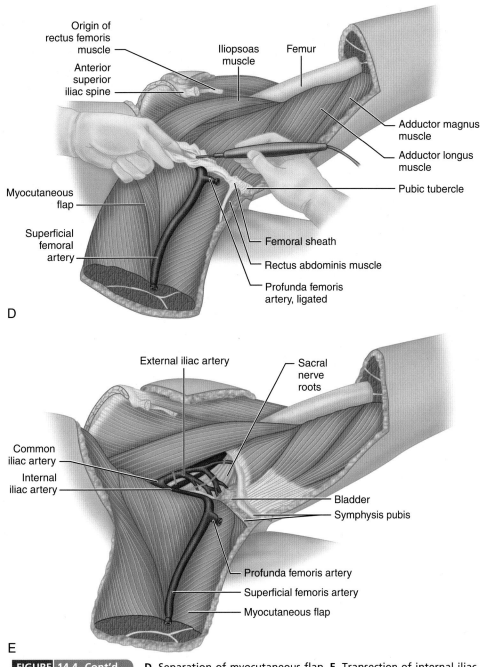

FIGURE 14.4, Cont'd **D,** Separation of myocutaneous flap. **E,** Transection of internal iliac vessels and branches. **SEE TECHNIQUE 14.4.**

CONSERVATIVE HEMIPELVECTOMY

Conservative hemipelvectomy is indicated for tumors around the proximal thigh and hip that cannot be resected adequately by limb-sparing techniques and do not require sacroiliac disarticulation for satisfactory proximal margins. The operation is a supraacetabular amputation that divides the ilium through the greater sciatic notch.

TECHNIQUE 14.5

- Insert a Foley catheter. Place the patient in a lateral decubitus position with the operated side up and secure the patient to the table so that it can be tilted to either side.
- Start the incision 1 to 2 cm above the anterior superior iliac spine and continue it posteriorly and laterally across the greater trochanter to the gluteal crease. Follow the crease to the medial thigh posteriorly. Begin a second inci-

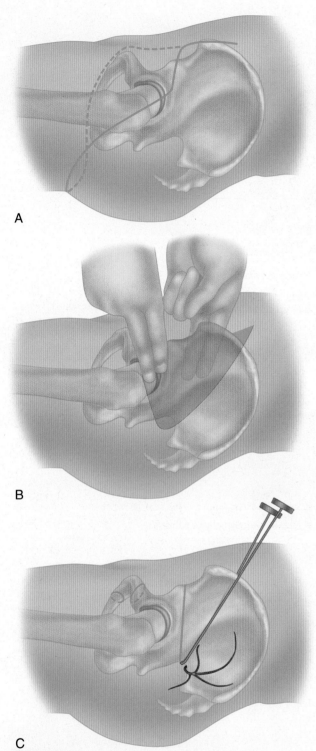

A

B

C

FIGURE **14.5** Conservative hemipelvectomy. **A,** Racquet type of incision. **B,** Separation of muscles from ilium. **C,** Division of ilium by Gigli saw. **SEE TECHNIQUE 14.5.** (Redrawn from Sherman CD Jr, Duthie RB: Modified hemipelvectomy, *Cancer* 13:51, 1960.)

sion from the first incision 5 cm below its starting point and continue it to just above and parallel to the inguinal ligament to the pubic tubercle. Carry the incision posteriorly across the medial thigh to join the first incision (Fig. 14.5A).
- Perform the anterior dissection first. Divide the abdominal wall muscles, exposing the peritoneum (Fig. 14.5B).

- Bluntly dissect the retroperitoneal space exposing the iliac vessels. Ligate and divide the external iliac vessels just distal to the internal iliacs.
- Divide the symphysis pubis, protecting the bladder and urethra.
- Divide the ilium through the greater sciatic notch as follows: bluntly dissect the iliopsoas muscle from the medial wall of the ilium by passing a finger from the anterior superior spine to the greater sciatic notch. Similarly dissect the gluteal muscles from the lateral aspect of the ilium. Pass a Gigli saw through the greater sciatic notch below the origin of the gluteus minimus and divide the ilium (Fig. 14.5C).
- Now the extremity can be positioned to place the various muscle groups under tension so that they can be divided at appropriate levels along with the femoral, obturator, and sciatic nerves. Care should be taken to divide the urogenital and pelvic diaphragms at their pelvic attachments, protecting the bladder and rectum.
- Close the wound over suction drains.

POSTOPERATIVE CARE The drains and Foley catheter are left in place for several days. Pressure should be kept off the posterior flap for several days after surgery.

REFERENCES

Akiyama T, Clark JC, Miki Y, Choong PF: The non-vascularized fibular graft: a simple and successful method of reconstruction of the pelvic ring after internal hemipelvectomy, *J Bone Joint Surg Br* 92:999, 2010.

Angelini A, Calabro T, Pala E, et al.: Resection and reconstruction of pelvic bone tumors, *Orthopedics* 38(2):87, 2015.

Bibbo C, Newman AS, Lackman RD, Levin LS, Kovach SJ: A simplified approach to reconstruction of hemipelvectomy defects with lower extremity free fillet flaps to minimize ischemia time, *J Plast Recon Aesthe Surg* 68:1750, 2015.

Brown TS, Salib CG, Rose PS, et al.: Reconstruction of the hip after resection of periacetabular oncological lesions, *Bone Joint J* 100-B(1 Suppl A):22, 2018.

Chao AH, Neimanis SA, Chang DW, et al.: Reconstruction after internal hemipelvectomy: outcomes and reconstructive algorithm, *Ann Plast Surg* 74:342, 2015.

Clarke MJ, Adnik PL, Groves ML, et al.: En bloc hemisacrectomy and internal hemipelvectomy via the posterior approach, *J Neurosurg Spine* 21:458, 2014.

D'Alleyrand JC, Fleming M, Gordon WT, et al.: Combat-related hemipelvectomy, *J Surg Orthop Adv* 21:38, 2012.

Ebrahimzadeh MH, Kachooei AR, Soroush MR, et al.: Long-term clinical outcomes of war-related hip disarticulation and transpelvic amputation, *J Bone Joint Surg Am* 95:e114, 2013.

Griesser MJ, Gillette B, Crist M, et al.: Internal and external hemipelvectomy or flail hip in patients with sarcomas. Quality-of-life and functional outcomes, *Am J Phys Med Rehabil* 91:24, 2012.

Grimer RJ, Chandrasekar CR, Carter SR, et al.: Hindquarter amputation: is it still needed and what are the outcomes? *Bone Joint J* 95:127, 2013.

Guo Y, Fu J, Palmer JL, et al.: Comparison of postoperative rehabilitation in cancer patients undergoing internal and external hemipelvectomy, *Arch Phys Med Rehabil* 92:620, 2011.

Guzik G: Oncological, surgical and functional results of the treatment of patients after hemipelvectomy due to metastases, *BMC Musculoskeletal Disorders* 19:63, 2019.

Henrichs MP, Singh G, Gosheger G, et al.: Stump lengthening procedure with modular endoprostheses—the better alternative to disarticulartions of the hip joint? *J Arthroplasty* 30:681, 2015.

Houdek MT, Andrews K, Kralovec ME, et al.: Functional outcome measures of patients following hemipelvectomy, *Prosthet Orthot Int*, 40(5):566, 2016.

Houdek MT, Kralovec ME, Andrews KL: Hemipelvectomy: high-level amputation surgery and prosthetic rehabilitation, *Am J Phys Med Rehabil* 93:600, 2014.

Kalson NS, Gikas PD, Aston W, et al.: Custom-made endoprostheses for the femoral amputation stump. An alternative to hip disarticulation in tumour surgery, *J Bone Joint Surg Br* 92:1134, 2010.

Kralovec ME, Houdek MT, Andrews KL, et al.: Prosthetic rehabilitation after hip disarticulation or hemipelvectomy, *Am J Phys Med Rehabil* 94(12):1035, 2015.

Liang H, Ji T, Zhang Y, Wang Y, Guo W: Reconstruction with 3D-printed pelvic endoprostheses after resection of a pelvic tumour, *J Bone Joint Surg* 99-B:267, 2017.

Mat Saad AZ, Halim AS, Faisham WI, et al.: Soft tissue reconstruction following hemipelvectomy: eight-year experience and literature review, *Sci World J* 2012:702904, 2012.

Mavrogenis AF, Soultanis K, Patapis P, et al.: Pelvic resections, *Orthopedics* 35:e232, 2012.

Mayerson JL, Wooldridge AN, Scharschmidt TJ: Pelvic resection: current concepts, *J Am Acad Orthop Surg* 22:214, 2014.

Ogura K, Sakuraba M, Miyamoto S, et al.: Pelvic ring reconstruction with a double-barreled free vascularized fibula graft after resection of malignant pelvic bone tumor, *Arch Orthop Trauma Surg* 135:619, 2015.

Robertson L, Roche A: Primary prophylaxis for venous thromboembolism in people undergoing major amputation of the lower extremity, *Cochrane Database Syst Rev* 12:CD010525, 2013.

Roulet S, Le Nail L-R, Va G, et al.: Free fillet lower leg flap for coverage after hemipelvectomy or hip disarticulation, *Orthop Traumatol*, 105:47, 2019.

Salunke AA, Shah J, Warikoo V, et al.: Surgical management of pelvic bone sarcoma with internal hemipelvectomy: oncologic and functional outcomes, *J Clin Orthop Trauma* 8:249, 2017.

Senchenkov A, Moran SL, Petty PM, et al.: Predictors of complications and outcomes of external hemipelvectomy wounds: account of 160 consecutive cases, *Ann Surg Oncol* 15:355, 2008.

Sherman CE, O'Connor MI, Sim FH: Survival, local recurrence, and function after pelvic limb salvage at 23 to 38 years of followup, *Clin Orthop Relat Res* 470:712, 2012.

Stihsen C, Panotopoulos J, Puchner SE, et al.: The outcome of the surgical treatment of pelvic chondrosarcomas. A competing risk analysis of 58 tumours from a single centre, *Bone Joint J* 99B:686, 2017.

Stranix JT, Vranis NM, Lam G, Rapp T, Saadeh PB: Posterior "open book" approach for type I internal hemipelvectomy, *Hip Int* 29(3):336, 2019.

Sun W, Li J, Li Q, et al.: Clinical effectiveness of hemipelvic reconstruction using computer-aided custom-made prostheses after resection of malignant pelvic tumors, *J Arthroplasty* 26:1508, 2011.

Van Houdt WJ, Griffin AM, Wunder JS, Ferguson PC: Oncologic outcome and quality of life after hindquarter amputation for sarcoma: is it worth it? *Ann Surg Oncol* 25:378, 2018.

Ver Halen JP, Yu P, Skoracki RM, Chang DW: Reconstruction of massive oncologic defects using free fillet flaps, *Plast Reconstr Surg* 125:913, 2010.

Wang B, Xie X, Yin J, et al.: Reconstruction with modular hemipelvic endoprosthesis after pelvic tumor resection: a report of 50 consecutive cases, *PloS ONE* 10(5):e0127263, 2015.

Wang G, Zhou D, Shen WJ, et al.: Management of partial traumatic hemipelvectomy, *Orthopedics* 36:e1340, 2013.

Wilson RJ, Free TH, Halpern JL, Schwartz HS, Holt GE: Surgical outcomes after limb-sparing resection and reconstruction for pelvic sarcoma, *JBJS Reviews* 6(4):e10, 2018.

Zhang Y, Wen L, Zhang J, et al.: Three-dimensional printing and computer navigation assisted hemipelvectomy for en block resection of osteosarcoma. A case report, *Medicine* 96(12), 2017.

The complete list of references is available online at Expert Consult.com

CHAPTER 15

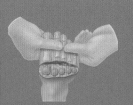

MAJOR AMPUTATIONS OF THE UPPER EXTREMITY

Kevin B. Cleveland

HAND AMPUTATIONS 630

WRIST AMPUTATIONS 630

FOREARM AMPUTATIONS (TRANSRADIAL) 631

ELBOW DISARTICULATION 633

ARM AMPUTATIONS (TRANSHUMERAL) 634

SHOULDER AMPUTATIONS 636

FOREQUARTER AMPUTATIONS 638

TARGETED MUSCLE REINNERVATION (TMR) AFTER SHOULDER OR TRANSHUMERAL AMPUTATION 641

Many orthopaedic surgeons consider amputation as a failure to restore function to an individual; however, an amputation should be considered the start of rehabilitation. Major amputations of the upper extremity are classified as being from the wrist distally to the axilla proximally. Major amputations of the upper extremity account for 8% of all amputations and are approximately 20 times less common than amputations of the lower extremity. Over 100,000 people in the United States are living with major upper extremity amputations today. Trauma is the most common reason for upper extremity amputations, with male predominance much greater than female. Shoulder disarticulation and forequarter amputations are performed more commonly for malignant tumors.

Most traumatic amputees benefit more from completion of the amputation and early prosthetic fitting than from heroic attempts at salvage procedures. However, most patients prefer reimplantation if possible over amputation because prostheses currently confer little in the way of sensation and psychological wellbeing. Approximately 13% of patients develop major complications after amputation.

Generally, all possible length should be preserved in upper extremity amputations. Length preservation can be maintained by careful evaluation and lengthening of a short stump by distraction osteogenesis (the method of Ilizarov) and microvascular anastomosis. Distal-free flaps and spare-part flaps (fillet flaps) from the amputated limb also should be used to preserve length. A shortening osteotomy may be required on occasion. However, prosthetists are able to fit even small stumps with prostheses to improve function. Often a small stump distal to the elbow can functionally be better than a long above-elbow amputation. A prosthetic limb cannot adequately replace the sensibility of the hand, and the function of a prosthetic limb decreases with higher levels of amputation. Few patients with amputations around the shoulder are regular prosthetic users. The use of a rigid dressing and subsequent early temporary prosthetic fitting (within 30 days) in patients with transhumeral or more distal amputations encourages the resumption of bimanual activities, softens the psychologic blow of limb loss, and decreases the prosthetic rejection rate. After 4 to 6 weeks postoperatively, the soft tissues have healed significantly, and the edema should be controlled enough to proceed with a definitive socket for the patient. A myoelectrical prosthesis may be an option for patients with a below-elbow amputation. These prostheses continue to evolve rapidly. The first-generation myoelectric prostheses used electromyographic (EMG) signals and allowed motion in only one plane (flexion and extension). EMG with the addition of targeted muscle reinnervation (TMR) allows more motion and more intuitive use of the prosthesis. Currently the addition of pattern recognition with TMR actually predicts the motion that is about to occur. However, with these advances the algorithms are limited to sequentially controlling the degrees of freedom to only two at a time. This is the limiting factor that keeps these advances from mimicking a natural limb. In manual workers, a more traditional device may be more effective. Some institutions use hybrid systems consisting of a locking shoulder joint with a body-powered elbow and externally powered wrist and terminal devices. These systems are most useful in amputations of the dominant extremity. Recipients use the prosthesis for approximately 14 hours a day. Some reports indicate that 50% of patients discontinue the use of the prosthesis after 5 years. Prosthetic rejection rates can be decreased with better patient education, more distal amputation levels, and prosthetic fitting within 30 days. Various terminal devices are available and are easily interchanged (Fig. 15.1). Phantom pain has been reported in over 50% of patients; however, it rarely causes impaired prosthetic use or unemployment. Myodesis, myoplasty, and myofascial closures should all be performed when possible.

New techniques of upper extremity amputations are evolving rapidly with the use of TMR, EMG pattern recognition, and to a lesser degree composite tissue allotransplantation. A multi-disciplinary team approach, including an experienced upper extremity surgeon, a skilled prosthetist or orthotist, a pain management physician, and a skilled physical therapist, should be employed. To obtain this most patients benefit from transfer to a level I hospital. Regardless, experienced prosthetists are invaluable in ensuring that patients have proper functional devices, and they should be consulted, when available, for each patient preferably before surgery.

HAND AMPUTATIONS

Hand amputations are discussed in chapter 16.

WRIST AMPUTATIONS

Whenever feasible, transcarpal amputation or disarticulation of the wrist is preferable to amputation through the forearm because, provided that the distal radioulnar joint remains normal, pronation and supination are preserved. Although only 50% of any pronation and supination is transmitted to

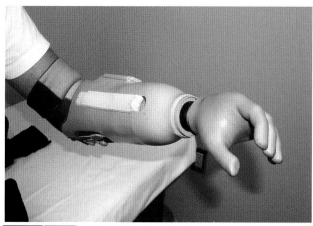

FIGURE 15.1 Myoelectrical prosthesis for forearm amputation with interchangeable terminal devices.

- At convenient points in line with their normal insertions, anchor the tendons of the wrist flexors and extensors to the remaining carpal bones so that active wrist motion is preserved.
- With interrupted nonabsorbable sutures, close the subcutaneous tissue and skin at the end of the stump, and insert a rubber tissue drain or a plastic tube for suction drainage.

the prosthesis, these motions are extremely valuable to the patient, and every effort should be made to preserve them. In transcarpal amputations, flexion and extension of the radiocarpal joint also should be preserved so that these motions, too, can be used prosthetically. Although difficult, prosthetic fitting of transcarpal amputation stumps can be achieved by a skilled prosthetist. Excellent wrist disarticulation prostheses are now available, and thin prosthetic wrist units can be used that, to a considerable extent, eliminate the previous objection of the artificial hand or prosthetic hook extending below the level of the opposite hand. Compared with more proximal amputations, the long lever arm afforded by amputation at the wrist increases the ease and power with which the prosthesis can be used.

AMPUTATION AT THE WRIST

TECHNIQUE 15.1

- Fashion a long palmar and a short dorsal skin flap in a ratio of 2:1. Use the thick palmar skin when available. Dissect the flaps proximally to the level of proposed bone section and expose the underlying soft structures.
- Draw the tendons of the finger flexors and extensors distally, divide them, and allow them to retract into the forearm.
- Identify the tendons of the wrist flexors and extensors, free their insertions, and reflect them proximal to the level of bone section. Identify the median and ulnar nerves and the fine filaments of the radial nerve. Draw the nerves distally and section them well proximal to the level of amputation so that their ends retract well above the end of the stump to help avoid a residual painful neuroma.
- Just proximal to the level of intended bone section, clamp, ligate, and divide the radial and ulnar arteries, and divide the remaining soft tissues down to bone.
- Transect the bones with a saw and rasp all rough edges to form a smooth, rounded contour.

DISARTICULATION OF THE WRIST

TECHNIQUE 15.2

- Fashion a long palmar and a short dorsal skin flap (Fig. 15.2A). Begin the incision 1.3 cm distal to the radial styloid process, carry it distally and across the palm, and curve it proximally to end 1.3 cm distal to the ulnar styloid process.
- Form a short dorsal skin flap by connecting the two ends of the palmar incision over the dorsum of the hand; atypical flaps may be fashioned, if necessary, to avoid amputation at a higher level. Reflect the skin flaps together with the subcutaneous tissue and fascia proximally to the radiocarpal joint.
- Just proximal to the joint, identify, ligate, and divide the radial and ulnar arteries.
- Identify the median, ulnar, and radial nerves and gently draw them distally into the wound. Section them so that they retract well proximal to the level of the amputation. Also identify the superficial radial nerve, the palmar cutaneous branch, and the dorsal ulnar cutaneous nerve. Preserve the cutaneous nerves that supply sensation to the residual skin stump.
- At a proximal level, divide all tendons and perform a tenodesis of the flexors and extensor tendons.
- Incise the wrist joint capsule circumferentially, completing the disarticulation (Fig. 15.2B, C).
- Retain if possible or resect (if they prevent tensionless closure) the radial and ulnar styloid processes and rasp the raw ends of the bones to form a smoothly rounded contour. Take care to avoid damaging the distal radioulnar joint, including the triangular ligament, so that normal pronation and supination of the forearm are preserved and pain in the joint is prevented (Fig. 15.2D).
- With interrupted nonabsorbable sutures, close the skin flaps over the ends of the bones (Fig. 15.2E) and insert a rubber tissue drain or a plastic tube for suction drainage.

FOREARM AMPUTATIONS (TRANSRADIAL)

Transradial amputations represent 40% of all major upper extremity amputations. As elsewhere, preserving as much length as possible is desirable. We recommend preserving a

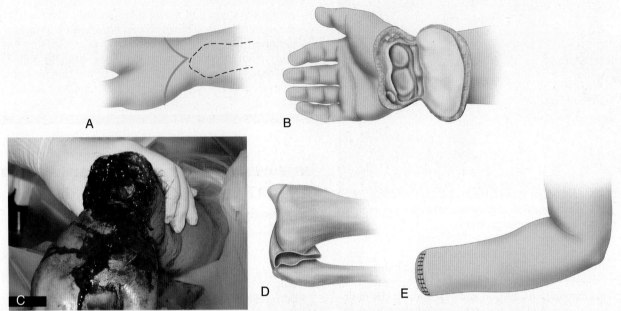

FIGURE 15.2
Disarticulation of the wrist. **A,** Skin incision. **B** and **C,** Reflection of the palmar flap and section of wrist joint capsule. **D,** Resection of tips of radial and ulnar styloids with preservation of the triangular ligament and underlying joint space. **E,** Completed amputation. **SEE TECHNIQUE 15.2.**

minimum of two thirds of the forearm length when possible. When circulation in the upper extremity is severely impaired, however, amputations through the distal third of the forearm are less likely to heal satisfactorily than those at a more proximal level because distally the skin is often thin and the subcutaneous tissue is scant. The underlying soft tissues distally consist primarily of relatively avascular structures, such as fascia and tendons. In these exceptional circumstances, an amputation at the junction of the middle and distal thirds of the forearm is preferable. In amputations through the proximal third of the forearm, even a short below-elbow stump 5 cm long is preferable to an amputation through or above the elbow because it preserves elbow function at this level and allows for prosthetic suspension. From a functional standpoint, preserving the patient's own elbow joint is crucial (5 cm of ulna). By using improved prosthetic fitting techniques, a skilled prosthetist can provide an excellent prosthetic device for even a short below-elbow stump. The benefits of TMR to transradial amputees can be substantial.

DISTAL FOREARM (DISTAL TRANSRADIAL) AMPUTATION

TECHNIQUE 15.3

- Beginning proximally at the intended level of bone section, fashion equal anterior and posterior skin flaps (Fig. 15.3A); make the length of each about equal to one half of the diameter of the forearm at the level of amputation. Together with the skin flaps, reflect the subcutaneous tissue and deep fascia proximally to the level of bone section.

- Clamp, doubly ligate, and divide the radial and ulnar arteries just proximal to this level.
- Identify the radial, ulnar, and median nerves; draw them gently distally; and transect them high so that they retract well proximal to the end of the stump.
- Cut across the muscle bellies transversely distal to the level of bone section and interpose the muscle tissue between the radius and the ulna. Distally, use the pronator quadratus and more proximally use one flexor tendon and one extensor tendon. Tenodese these muscles to the bone to help prevent painful convergence and instability.
- Divide the radius and ulna transversely and rasp all sharp edges from their ends (Fig. 15.3B).
- Close the deep fascia with fine absorbable sutures and the skin flaps with interrupted nonabsorbable sutures (Fig. 15.3C) and insert deep to the fascia a rubber tissue drain or, if preferable, a plastic tube for suction drainage.
- A myoplastic closure should be done in this amputation as follows. After raising appropriate flaps of skin and fascia, fashion an anterior flap of flexor digitorum sublimis muscle long enough so that its end can be carried around the end of the bones to the deep fascia dorsally.
- Divide the remaining soft tissues transversely at the level of bone section.
- After dividing the bones and contouring their ends, carry the muscle flap dorsally and suture its end to the deep fascia over the dorsal musculature. To prevent excessive bulk, the entire anterior muscle mass should never be used in this manner.
- Close the stump as already described.

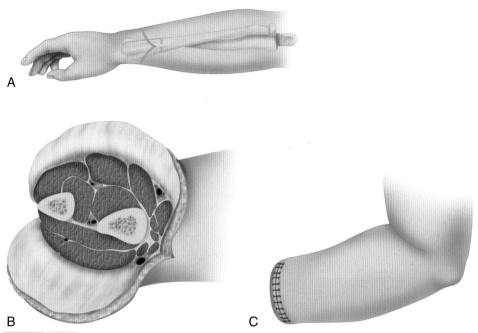

FIGURE 15.3 **Amputation through distal forearm. A,** Skin incision and bone level. **B,** Flaps are reflected, and bones and soft structures are divided. **C,** Completed amputation. **SEE TECHNIQUE 15.3.**

PROXIMAL THIRD OF FOREARM (PROXIMAL TRANSRADIAL) AMPUTATION

TECHNIQUE 15.4

- When good skin is available, fashion anterior and posterior skin flaps of equal length; if good skin is unavailable, fashion atypical flaps as necessary rather than amputate at a more proximal level. Reflect proximally the deep fascia together with the skin flaps to the level of intended bone section.
- Just proximal to this level, identify, doubly ligate, and divide the major vessels.
- Identify the median, ulnar, and radial nerves; gently pull them distally; and section them proximally so that their ends retract well proximal to the end of the stump.
- Divide the muscle bellies transversely distal to the level of bone section so that their proximal ends retract to that level. Carefully trim away all excess muscle.
- Divide the radius and ulna transversely and smooth their cut edges. Attempt to maintain at least 5 cm of the ulna proximally. If a more proximal osteotomy is required, tenodesis of the biceps tendon to the proximal portion of the residual ulna is needed. This lengthens the stump functionally and enhances prosthetic fitting. Even without biceps function, the elbow can be flexed satisfactorily by the brachialis muscle.
- With interrupted absorbable sutures, close the deep fascia; with interrupted nonabsorbable sutures, close the skin edges. Insert deep to the fascia a rubber tissue drain or a plastic tube for suction drainage.

ELBOW DISARTICULATION

The elbow joint is an excellent level for amputation because the broad flare of the humeral condyles can be grasped firmly by the prosthetic socket and humeral rotation can be transmitted to the prosthesis. In more proximal amputations, humeral rotation cannot be thus transmitted, so a prosthetic elbow turntable is necessary. The difficulties previously experienced in prosthetic fitting at this level have been overcome by modern prosthetic techniques, and most surgeons now believe that disarticulation of the elbow is usually preferable to a more proximal amputation.

Additionally, a humeral shortening osteotomy can be done to preserve the elbow.

DISARTICULATION OF THE ELBOW

TECHNIQUE 15.5

- Fashion equal anterior and posterior skin flaps as follows. Beginning proximally at the level of the humeral epicondyles, extend the posterior flap distally to a point about 2.5 cm distal to the tip of the olecranon and the anterior flap distally to a point just distal to the insertion of the biceps tendon. If necessary, fashion atypical flaps. Next, reflect the flaps proximally to the level of the humeral epicondyles and, on the medial aspect of the elbow, begin dissection of the deep structures.
- Identify and divide the lacertus fibrosus, free the origin of the flexor musculature from the medial humeral epicondyle, and reflect the muscle mass distally to expose the

neurovascular bundle that lies against the medial aspect of the biceps tendon.

- Proximal to the joint level, isolate, doubly ligate, and divide the brachial artery.
- Gently draw the median nerve distally and with a sharp knife divide it proximally so that it retracts at least 2.5 cm proximal to the joint line. Identify the ulnar nerve in its groove posterior to the medial epicondyle and treat it in a similar manner. Alternatively, they can be inserted into local muscle by TMR techniques (see Technique 15.12).
- Free the insertion of the biceps tendon from the radius and the insertion of the brachialis tendon from the coronoid process of the ulna.
- Identify the radial nerve in the groove between the brachialis and brachioradialis; isolate it, draw it distally, and section it far proximally.
- About 6.3 cm distal to the joint line, divide transversely the extensor musculature that arises from the lateral humeral epicondyle and reflect the proximal end of the muscle mass proximally.
- Divide the posterior fascia along with the triceps tendon near the tip of the olecranon.
- Divide the anterior capsule of the joint to complete the disarticulation and remove the forearm.
- Leave intact the articular surface of the humerus. Bring the triceps tendon anteriorly and suture it first to the humerus and then perform a myoplasty to the tendons of the brachialis and biceps muscles.
- Fashion a thin flap from the extensor muscle mass left attached to the lateral humeral epicondyle, carry it medially, and suture it to the remnants of the flexor muscles at the medial epicondyle. Cover all bony prominences and exposed tendons at the end of the humerus by passing additional sutures through the periosteum and the muscle flap.
- Trim the skin flaps for a snug closure without tension and approximate their edges with interrupted sutures of nonabsorbable material. Insert deep to the fascia a rubber tissue drain or a plastic tube for suction drainage.

ARM AMPUTATIONS (TRANSHUMERAL)

Amputation through the arm, or transhumeral amputation, is defined as amputation at any level from the supracondylar region of the humerus distally to the level of the axillary fold proximally. More distal amputations, such as the transcondylar, are fitted prosthetically and function as elbow disarticulations; amputations proximal to the level of the axillary fold function as shoulder disarticulations. As in all other amputations, as much length as possible should be preserved. If the humeral condyles cannot be preserved, a transhumeral osteotomy should be done approximately 3 to 5 cm proximal to the elbow joint. The prosthesis with which a patient having a transhumeral amputation is fitted must include an inside elbow-lock mechanism and an elbow turntable. The elbow-lock mechanism is required to stabilize the joint in full extension, full flexion, or a position in between. The turntable mechanism substitutes for humeral rotation.

The elbow-lock mechanism extends about 3.8 cm distally from the end of the prosthetic socket and to be cosmetically pleasing should lie at the level of the opposite elbow. Therefore, when performing transhumeral amputations, the level of the bone section should be at least 3.8 cm proximal to the elbow joint to allow room for this mechanism. During a transhumeral amputation, consideration must be given to an angulation osteotomy. The angulation ostectomy may avoid the need for a shoulder harness for suspension of a myoelectric arm and will markedly improve rotational control (Fig. 15.4). An angled osteotomy requires a minimum of 6 cm of residual bone length cut at an angle of 70 degrees with a posterior fixation plate. Although an amputation at the level of the axillary fold or more proximally must be fitted prosthetically as a shoulder disarticulation, preserving the most proximal part of the humerus, including the head, is valuable; the normal contour of the shoulder is retained, which is cosmetically desirable, and the disarticulation prosthesis is more stable on a shoulder in which some humerus remains that may be grasped by its socket. Every attempt should be made to preserve 5 to 7 cm of the proximal humerus. Osseointegration for transhumeral amputations is a technique used in Europe for over 2 decades. It involves placement of a suspension metallic intramedullary component that exits the skin, providing a bone implant interface that avoids the pitfalls of socket fixation such as poor fit, skin irritation, and excessive sweat. Despite the skin implant interface, deep infection is relatively low; however, superficial skin infections occur in up to 50% of patients requiring oral antibiotic treatment. Research to improve the skin-implant interface is underway.

In children younger than 12 years, osseous overgrowth of diaphyseal amputations has been reported with the humerus and fibula being most common. In general, disarticulation at the elbow is recommended; however, if disarticulation is not feasible, a capping graft of the humeral bone end should be done. Several authors have suggested using fascia, metal, or iliac crest grafts. We have used the amputated part of the distal humerus as a capping graft at the time of primary amputation with good results. Close clinical follow up is mandatory, and revisions are sometimes necessary.

SUPRACONDYLAR AREA

TECHNIQUE 15.6

- Beginning proximally at the level of intended bone section, fashion equal anterior and posterior skin flaps, each being in length one half of the diameter of the arm at that level (Fig. 15.5A).
- Doubly ligate and divide the brachial artery just proximal to the level of bone section and transect the median, ulnar, and radial nerves at a higher level so that their proximal ends retract well proximal to the end of the stump. Or consider a TMR procedure.
- Divide the muscles in the anterior compartment of the arm 1.3 cm distal to the level of intended bone section so that they retract to this level.

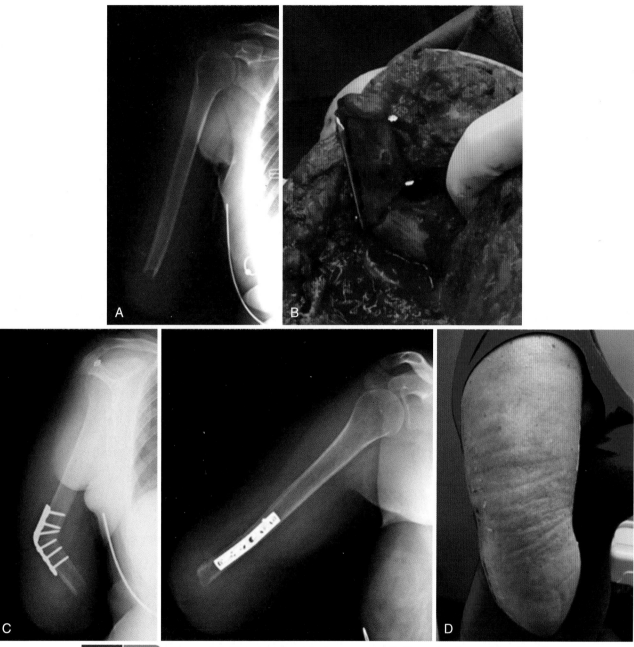

FIGURE 15.4 Humeral flexion osteotomy to improve prosthetic suspension and functional upper-extremity motion. **A,** Long transhumeral amputation. **B,** Humeral osteotomy performed through a posterior approach in same setting as targeted muscle reinnervation. **C,** Postoperatively after humeral osteotomy. **D,** Residual limb. (From: Pierrie SN, Gaston RG, Loeffler BJ: Current concepts in upper-extremity amputation, *J Hand Surg Am* 43:657, 2018.)

- Free the insertion of the triceps tendon from the olecranon, preserving the triceps fascia and muscle as a long flap. Reflect this flap proximally and incise the periosteum of the humerus circumferentially at a level at least 3.8 cm proximal to the elbow joint to allow room for the elbow mechanism of the prosthesis.
- Divide the bone at this level and with a rasp smoothly round its end (Fig. 15.5B).

- Trim the triceps tendon to form a long flap, carry it across the end of the bone, and tenodese it to the humerus, followed by myoplasty to the fascia over the anterior muscles.
- Insert deep to this flap a Penrose drain or a plastic tube for suction drainage. Close the fascia with fine absorbable sutures and the skin flaps with interrupted nonabsorbable sutures (Fig. 15.5C).

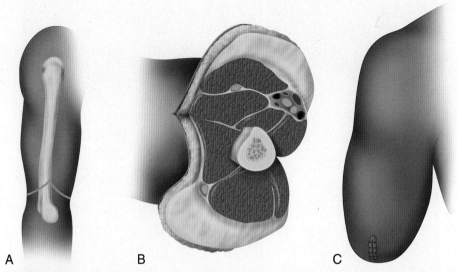

FIGURE 15.5   **Amputation through arm at supracondylar level. A,** Skin incision and bone level. **B,** Anterior muscles are divided transversely, triceps and fascial flap is constructed, and bone is sectioned. **C,** Completed amputation. **SEE TECHNIQUE 15.6.**

AMPUTATION PROXIMAL TO THE SUPRACONDYLAR AREA

TECHNIQUE 15.7

- Beginning proximally at the level of intended bone section, fashion equal anterior and posterior skin flaps, the length of each being slightly greater than one half of the diameter of the arm at that level.
- Just proximal to the level of intended bone section, identify, doubly ligate, and divide the brachial artery and vein.
- Identify, gently pull distally, and divide at a more proximal level the major nerves so that their proximal ends retract well proximal to the end of the stump. If the patient is a candidate, perform a TMR (see Technique 15.12).
- Section the muscles of the anterior compartment of the arm 1.3 cm distal to the level of bone section so that their cut ends retract to this level.
- Divide the triceps muscle 3.8-5 cm distal to the level of bone section and retract its proximal end proximally.
- Incise the periosteum circumferentially and divide the humerus. Using a rasp, smoothly round the end of the bone.
- Bevel the triceps muscle to form a thin flap, carry it over the end of the bone, and suture it to the humerus and the anterior muscle fascia.
- Deep to the flap, insert a rubber tissue drain or a plastic tube for suction drainage; then close the fascia with interrupted absorbable sutures. Approximate the skin edges with interrupted nonabsorbable sutures.

SHOULDER AMPUTATIONS

Most amputations in the shoulder area are performed for the treatment of malignant bone or soft-tissue tumors that cannot be treated by limb-sparing methods. Less commonly, amputation in this area is indicated for arterial insufficiency and rarely for trauma or infection. The extent of the amputation and design of the skin flaps must be modified often. Phantom pain is common and probably is best treated by proximal nerve blocks performed by a skillful anesthesiologist. Few patients regularly use a prosthesis, but a cosmetic shoulder cap is useful after forequarter amputation. TMR should be considered if the patient is a candidate for a myoelectric prosthesis (see Technique 15.12).

AMPUTATION THROUGH THE SURGICAL NECK OF THE HUMERUS

TECHNIQUE 15.8

- Place the patient supine with a sandbag well beneath the affected shoulder so that the back is at a 45-degree angle to the operating table.
- Begin the skin incision anteriorly at the level of the coracoid process and carry it distally along the anterior border of the deltoid muscle to the insertion of the muscle and along the posterior border of the muscle to the posterior axillary fold. Connect the two limbs of the incision by a second incision that passes through the axilla (Fig. 15.6A).
- Identify, ligate, and divide the cephalic vein in the deltopectoral groove.
- Separate the deltoid and pectoralis major and retract the deltoid muscle laterally. Next, divide the pectoralis major muscle at its insertion and reflect it medially.
- Develop the interval between the pectoralis minor and coracobrachialis muscles to expose the neurovascular bundle. Isolate, doubly ligate, and divide the axillary artery and vein immediately inferior to the pectoralis minor.

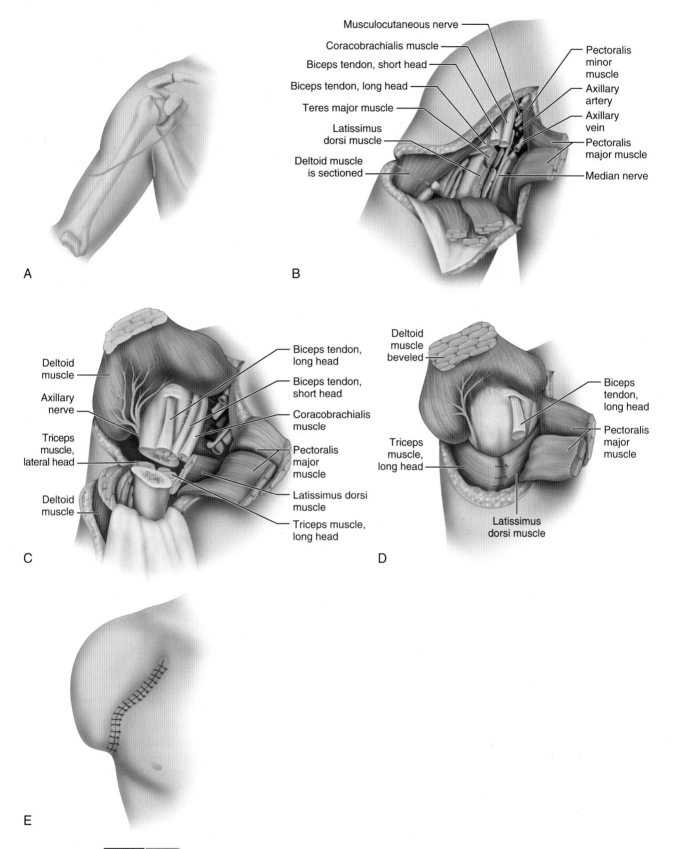

FIGURE 15.6 **Amputation through surgical neck of humerus. A,** Skin incision. **B,** Section of anterior muscles. **C,** Bone level and completed muscle section. **D,** Closure of muscle flap. **E,** Completed amputation. **SEE TECHNIQUE 15.8.**

- Isolate the median, ulnar, radial, and musculocutaneous nerves; gently draw them distally into the wound, and divide them so that their proximal ends retract well proximal to the pectoralis minor (Fig. 15.6B) if the patient is not a candidate for myoelectric prosthesis. Otherwise, perform a TMR procedure.
- Divide the deltoid muscle at its insertion and reflect it superiorly together with the attached lateral skin flap.
- Near their insertions at the bicipital groove, divide the teres major and latissimus dorsi muscles. At a point proximally 2 cm distal to the level of intended bone section, sever the long and short heads of the biceps, the triceps, and the coracobrachialis.
- Section the humerus at the level of its neck and smooth the cut end with a rasp (Fig. 15.6C).
- Suture the long head of the triceps, both heads of the biceps, and the coracobrachialis over the end of the humerus; swing the pectoralis major muscle laterally, and suture it to the end of the bone (Fig. 15.6D).
- Tailor the lateral skin flap and underlying deltoid muscle to allow accurate apposition of the skin edges and suture the edges with interrupted nonabsorbable material (Fig. 15.6E). Deep to the muscles and at the end of the bone, insert Penrose drains or plastic tubes for suction drainage.

DISARTICULATION OF THE SHOULDER

TECHNIQUE 15.9

- Position the patient supine with a sandbag under the affected shoulder so that the back is at a 45-degree angle to the operating table.
- Begin the skin incision anteriorly at the coracoid process and continue it distally along the anterior border of the deltoid muscle to its insertion and then superiorly along the posterior border of the muscle to end at the posterior axillary fold. Join the two limbs of this incision with a second incision passing through the axilla (Fig. 15.7A).
- Identify, ligate, and divide the cephalic vein in the deltopectoral groove.
- Separate the deltoid and the pectoralis major and retract the deltoid laterally.
- Divide the pectoralis major muscle at its insertion and reflect it medially. Develop the interval between the coracobrachialis and short head of the biceps to expose the neurovascular bundle. Isolate, doubly ligate, and divide the axillary artery and vein; identify the thoracoacromial artery, and treat it in a similar manner (Fig. 15.7B). Allow the vessel to retract superiorly beneath the pectoralis minor muscle.
- Identify and isolate the median, ulnar, musculocutaneous, and radial nerves; gently draw them inferiorly into the wound, and divide them far proximally so that they also

retract beneath the pectoralis minor or transfer the nerves to the shoulder girdle muscles if the patient is a candidate for a myoelectric prosthesis.
- Divide the coracobrachialis and short head of the biceps near their insertions on the coracoid process. Free the deltoid muscle from its insertion on the humerus and reflect it superiorly to expose the capsule of the shoulder joint. Near their insertions, divide the teres major and latissimus dorsi muscles.
- Place the arm in internal rotation to expose the short external rotator muscles and the posterior aspect of the shoulder joint capsule and divide all of these structures (Fig. 15.7C).
- Place the arm in extreme external rotation and divide the anterior aspect of the joint capsule and the subscapularis muscle (Fig. 15.7D). Section the triceps muscle near its insertion and divide the inferior capsule of the shoulder to sever the limb completely from the trunk.
- Reflect the cut ends of all muscles into the glenoid cavity and suture them there to help fill the hollow left by removing the humeral head (Fig. 15.7E).
- Carry the deltoid muscle flap inferiorly and suture it just inferior to the glenoid.
- Deep to the deltoid flap, insert Penrose drains or plastic tubes.
- Partially excise any unduly prominent acromion process to give the shoulder a more smoothly rounded contour.
- Trim the skin flaps for accurate fitting and close their edges with interrupted nonabsorbable sutures (Fig. 15.7F).

FOREQUARTER AMPUTATIONS

Forequarter amputation removes the entire upper extremity in the interval between the scapula and the chest wall. Usually it is indicated for malignant tumors that cannot be adequately removed by limb-sparing resections, such as the Tikhoff-Linberg procedure. Most tumors can be evaluated for limb-sparing procedures in place of amputation by magnetic resonance angiography or arteriography, which will show compression of the artery, limb edema, and neurologic deficits that necessitate amputation. However, careful inspection at the time of surgery will determine the appropriate procedure. Extension of the operation to include resection of the chest wall is occasionally required. Provisions for adequate blood replacement and monitoring of the patient are needed.

The anterior approach of Berger and our preferred posterior approach of Littlewood are described. The operation is performed more rapidly and easily using the Littlewood technique. Ferrario et al. described a combined anterior and posterior approach. This technique is useful for patients in whom the normal tissue planes have been obliterated because of radiation to the axilla. Excellent exposure is obtained and ligation of the subclavian vessels occurs at the thoracic inlet instead of where the vessels cross the third rib (Fig. 15.8). Kumar et al. described a single incision anterior approach that can be used with the patient supine.

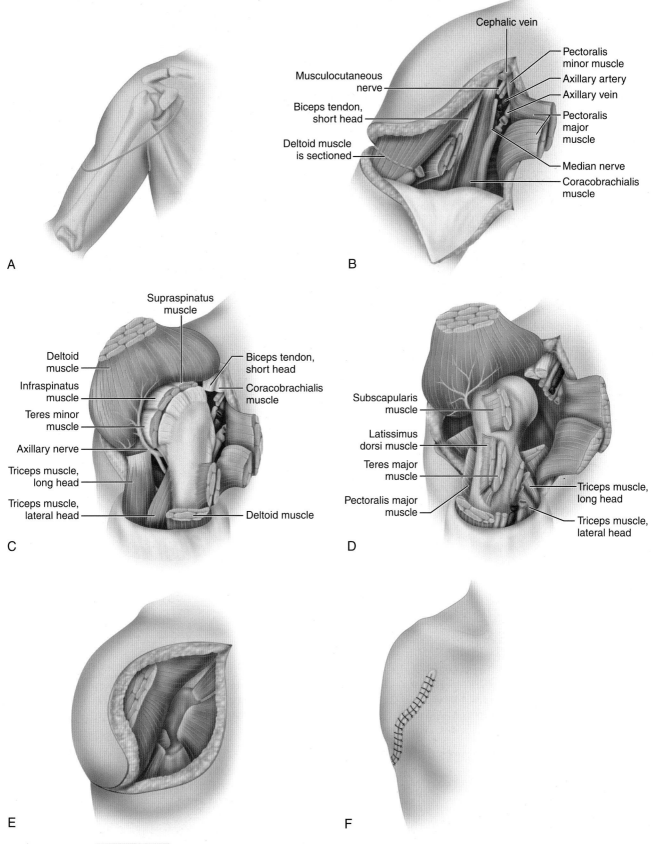

FIGURE 15.7 **Disarticulation of shoulder. A,** Incision. **B,** Exposure and sectioning of neurovascular bundle. **C,** Reflection of deltoid; arm is placed in internal rotation; sectioning of supraspinatus, infraspinatus, and teres minor muscles and of posterior capsule; sectioning of coracobrachialis and biceps at coracoid. **D,** Arm is placed in external rotation; subscapularis and anterior capsule are sectioned. **E,** Suture of muscles in glenoid cavity. **F,** Completed amputation. **SEE TECHNIQUE 15.9.**

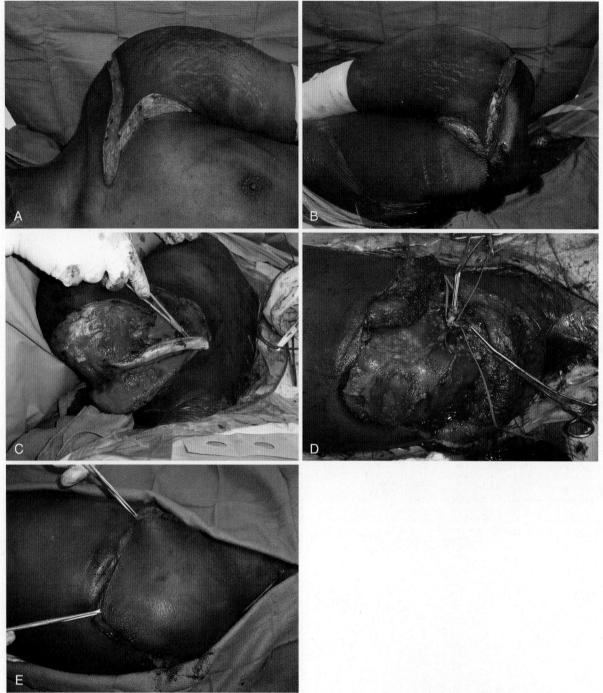

FIGURE 15.8 Forequarter amputation through combined anterior and posterior approach. **A,** Anterior flap. **B,** Posterior flap. **C,** Osteotomy performed through clavicle medially. **D,** Dissection deep to the scapula. **E,** Vessels ligated and forequarter removed; flap closed.

ANTERIOR APPROACH

TECHNIQUE 15.10

(BERGER)

■ Begin the upper limb of the incision at the lateral border of the sternocleidomastoid muscle and extend it laterally along the anterior aspect of the clavicle, across the acromioclavicular joint, over the superior aspect of the

shoulder to the spine of the scapula, and across the body of the scapula to the scapular angle. Begin the lower limb of the incision at the middle third of the clavicle and extend it inferiorly in the groove between the deltoid and pectoral muscles and across the axilla to join the upper limb of the incision at the angle of the scapula (Fig. 15.9A).

■ Deepen the clavicular part of the incision to bone and release and reflect distally the clavicular origin of the pectoralis major muscle.

■ Divide the deep fascia over the superior border of the clavicle close to bone and, by dissection with a finger and a blunt curved dissector, free the deep aspect of the clavicle. Retract the external jugular vein from the field or, if it is in the way, section it after ligating it.

- Divide the clavicle at the lateral border of the sternocleido-mastoid with a Gigli saw, lift the bone superiorly, and remove it by dividing the acromioclavicular joint (Fig. 15.9B).
- To complete the exposure of the neurovascular bundle, release the insertion of the pectoralis major from the humerus and the origin of the pectoralis minor from the coracoid process (Fig. 15.9C). Isolate, doubly ligate, and divide the subclavian artery and vein.
- Dissect the brachial plexus and by gentle traction inferiorly bring it well into the operating field; section the nerves in sequence and allow them to retract superiorly (Fig. 15.9D).
- Release the latissimus dorsi and remaining soft tissues that bind the shoulder girdle to the anterior chest wall and allow the limb to fall posteriorly.
- While holding the arm across the chest and exerting gentle downward traction, divide from superiorly to inferiorly the remaining muscles that fix the shoulder to the scapula.
- Divide the muscles that hold the scapula to the thorax, starting with the trapezius and continuing through the omohyoids, levator scapulae, rhomboids major and minor, and serratus anterior (Fig. 15.9E). The limb falls free and can be removed.
- To form additional padding, suture the pectoralis major, trapezius, and any other remaining muscular structures over the lateral chest wall. Bring the skin flaps together and trim them to form a smooth closure. Insert Penrose drains or plastic tubes for suction drainage and close the skin edges with interrupted nonabsorbable sutures (Fig. 15.9F).

POSTERIOR APPROACH

TECHNIQUE 15.11

(LITTLEWOOD)
- Insert a Foley catheter. Place the patient in a lateral decubitus position with the operated side up. Secure the patient to the operating table so that it may be tilted anteriorly and posteriorly.
- Two incisions are required: one posterior (cervicoscapular) and one anterior (pectoroaxillary) (Fig. 15.10A). Make the posterior incision first, beginning at the medial end of the clavicle and extending it laterally for the entire length of the bone. Carry the incision over the acromion process to the posterior axillary fold and continue it along the axillary border of the scapula to a point inferior to the scapular angle. Finally, curve it medially to end 5 cm from the midline of the back. Elevate a flap of skin and subcutaneous tissue medial to the vertebral border of the scapula, extending it from the inferior angle of the scapula to the clavicle (Fig. 15.10B).
- Identify the trapezius and latissimus dorsi muscles and divide them near the scapula.

- Draw the scapula away from the chest wall with a hook or retractor and divide the levator scapulae and the rhomboids minor and major (Fig. 15.10C).
- Ligate branches of the superficial cervical and descending scapular vessels.
- Divide the superior digitation of the serratus anterior close to the superior angle of the scapula and the remaining insertion of the serratus anterior along the vertebral border of the scapula.
- Divide the clavicle and subclavius muscle at the medial end of the bone. This allows the extremity to fall anteriorly, placing the neurovascular bundle under tension. The latter is found in the fibrofatty tissue near the superior digitation of the serratus anterior. Divide the cords of the brachial plexus close to the spine and doubly ligate and divide the subclavian artery and vein (Fig. 15.10D, E). Take care to avoid injury to the pleural dome.
- Divide the omohyoid muscle and ligate and divide the suprascapular vessels and external jugular vein.
- Make the anterior incision, starting it at the middle of the clavicle and curving it inferiorly just lateral to but parallel with the deltopectoral groove. Extend it across the anterior axillary fold and carry it inferiorly and posteriorly to join the posterior incision at the lower third of the axillary border of the scapula.
- Divide the pectoralis major and minor muscles and remove the limb.
- Close the flaps over suction drains without excessive tension. Occasionally, it is necessary to attach a flap to the chest wall and complete the closure with a skin graft.

POSTOPERATIVE CARE Phantom pain in the early postoperative period is common. Nerve blocks by an experienced anesthesiologist may be helpful. Although few patients find a prosthesis useful, a cosmetic shoulder cap is desirable.

TARGETED MUSCLE REINNERVATION (TMR) AFTER SHOULDER OR TRANSHUMERAL AMPUTATION

To improve function of upper extremity prostheses, Kuiken et al. developed a biologic neural-machine interface called *targeted reinnervation*. The goal of TMR is to take a nerve that formerly directed hand function and transfer it to a muscle segment that otherwise has no function because of the amputation. The reinnervated muscle segment amplifies the nerve signals to a myoelectric prosthesis, allowing movement of multiple prosthetic joints. According to Kuiken et al., this technique has several advantages: it is relatively simple to implement, no hardware is implanted into the body that could break and require additional surgery, and it can be used with existing myoelectric prosthetic technology. In addition to accelerating maximal control and function of myoelectric prostheses and avoiding secondary procedures, TMR has been shown to decrease the risk of painful neuromas. Approximately 25% of patients with major upper extremity amputations have painful neuromas. TMR provides an end organ for the damaged nerve to reinnervate. Studies have shown that TMR provides the neuroma a way to return to a more normal nerve structure.

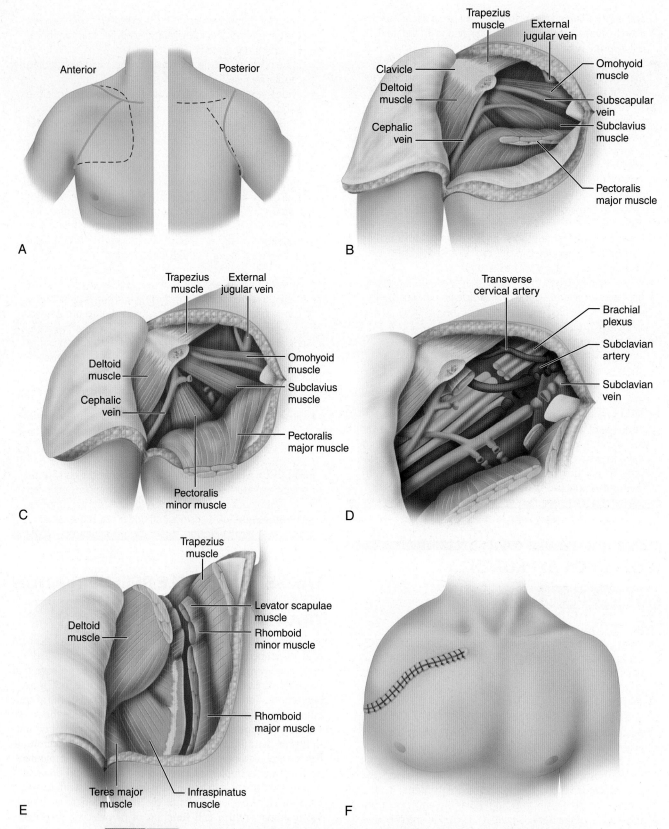

FIGURE 15.9 **Forequarter amputation through anterior approach. A,** Incision. **B,** Resection of clavicle. **C,** Lifting pectoral lid. **D,** Sectioning of vessels and nerves after incision through axillary fascia and insertion of pectoralis minor, costocoracoid membrane, and subclavius. **E,** Sectioning of supporting muscles of scapula. **F,** Completed amputation. **SEE TECHNIQUE 15.10.**

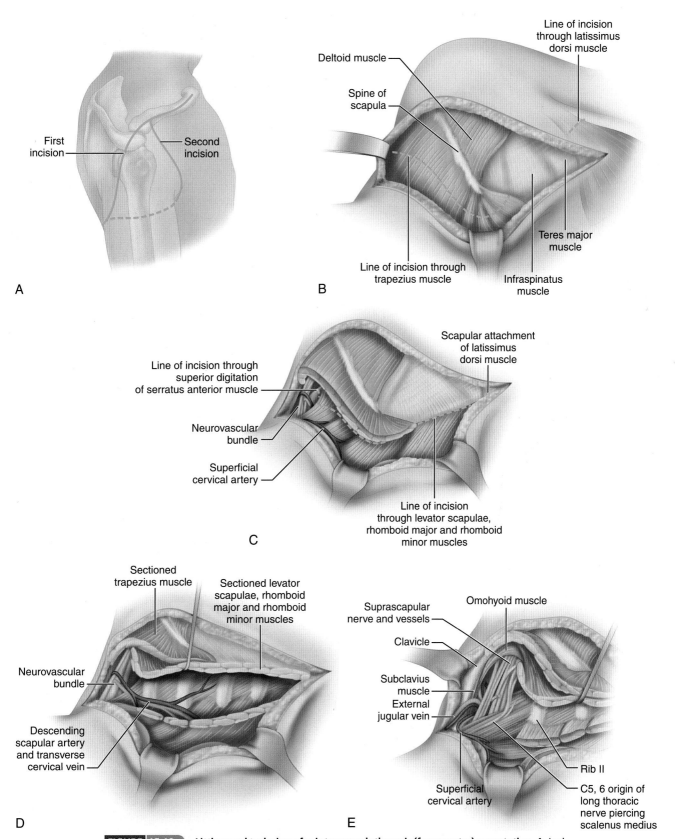

FIGURE 15.10   **Littlewood technique for interscapulothoracic (forequarter) amputation. A,** Incision. **B,** Skin flaps undermined from clavicle. **C,** Scapula drawn away from chest wall with hook or retractor; levator scapulae and rhomboids minor and major divided. **D,** Exposure of neurovascular structures. **E,** More detailed view of neurovascular structures. **SEE TECHNIQUE 15.11.**

In general, TMR begins with identifying the functional nerve, mobilizing it, and preserving its length. Excising the end neuromas and trimming of the fascicles to the level of axoplasmic sprouting should be performed. The targeted muscle and its native nerve are then identified. The native nerve must be trimmed back approximately 1 cm to the neuromuscular junction and the residual nerve buried away from the original muscle to avoid dual innervation (cross talk). The donor nerve is then coapted to the target muscle with end-to-end tension-free repair. Augmentation with epineurium to epimysium is beneficial. If the native nerve stump in the targeted muscle is not available, then the donor nerve can be directly sutured into the muscle. The subcutaneous adipose tissue should be debulked to decrease the distance between skin and the targeted muscle to improve the strength of the EMG.

The success of TMR has spawned interest into targeted sensory reinnervation (TSR). The ultimate prosthesis would provide motor as well as sensory functions. The sensory nerves are used to reinnervate more proximal, intact cutaneous nerves that provide varying degrees of light touch, pain, temperature, and proprioception. Multiple studies have shown that cortical remapping occurs, and a long-term effect can be established. The goal is to provide amputees with a more intuitive prosthesis by combining new technology that reinnervates residual muscle.

In patients with transhumeral amputation, the median nerve is transferred to the medial head of the biceps (hand-closing) and the distal radial nerve is transferred to the motor nerve of the brachialis muscle (hand-opening). In patients with a long residual humerus, the ulnar nerve is transferred to the motor nerve of the brachialis muscle. The intact lateral head of the biceps is still used for prosthetic elbow flexion and the triceps muscle for extension. In patients with more proximal amputations at the shoulder level, nerves that originally innervated the amputated limb are rerouted to muscles on the chest wall, creating an interface for a myoelectric prosthesis that is controlled by the same nerves that previously controlled the amputated limb.

Contraindications to TMR include ipsilateral brachial plexopathy, major comorbidities, or anticipated patient noncompliance with prosthetic wear. The pattern of nerve transfers is dictated by the availability of donor nerves and muscle. The mechanism of injury, residual nerve length, presence of healthy muscle, and a Tinel's sign are important preoperative predictors of successful TMR. It is critical to denervate the targeted muscle before TMR to avoid dual innervation, which can cause "cross talk" between the two nerves and compromise successful TMR. Placing adipofascial tissue into the repair site also can reduce the chance of cross-talk.

TARGETED MUSCLE REINNERVATION AFTER TRANSHUMERAL AMPUTATION

TECHNIQUE 15.12

(O'SHAUGHNESSY ET AL., 2008)

MEDIAN NERVE TRANSFER

- With the patient under general anesthesia and without muscle relaxation (so that motor nerves can be stimulated), make an anterior incision directly over the muscle bellies of the biceps muscle, beginning just inferior to the lower edge of the deltoid muscle.
- Inject the soft tissue liberally with dilute epinephrine solution (1:500,000) to open tissue planes, increase visual contrast between tissues, and improve hemostasis. Use electrocautery for coagulation.
- Open the fascia overlying the muscle bellies and develop the interspace between the heads of the biceps. Dissect the area immediately inferior to the deltoid muscle between the biceps heads to expose the musculocutaneous nerve, the motor branches to the medial and lateral biceps heads, and the motor nerve to the brachialis muscle (Fig. 15.11A).
- While paying close attention to the vascular supply of the medial head of the biceps muscle, mobilize the muscle segment away from the humerus to expose the median nerve that runs parallel and inferior to the biceps.
- Separate the muscle bellies from each other to expose the brachial artery and the median nerve (Fig. 15.11B). Leave the proximal and distal ends of the muscle bellies undisturbed so that the muscles remain long and in the proper position to permit later detection of electromyographic signals. With this approach, the median nerve is superficial to the ulnar nerve.
- To facilitate the nerve transfers, dissect the musculocutaneous nerve in such a way as to preserve the motor nerve innervating the lateral head of the biceps and to divide the motor nerve innervating the medial head of the biceps at a point 5 mm from its entry into the muscle substance.
- Mobilize the proximal part of the motor nerve and bury it into the lateral head of the biceps to prevent reinnervation of the medial head.
- Divide the continuation of the musculocutaneous nerve, which innervates the brachialis muscle, just after the intact takeoff of the nerve to the lateral head.
- Cut the median nerve back to healthy fascicles and sew it to the motor branch of the medial head of the biceps with 5-0 polypropylene suture. Incorporate some epimysium of the muscle belly itself in the suturing process to protect the small motor nerve from tearing. Median nerve fibers are now abutted to transected medial biceps nerve fibers to reinnervate the muscle.

RADIAL NERVE TRANSFER

- Make a second lateral incision over the distal and lateral aspect of the residual limb and develop the interspace between the triceps and brachialis to locate the septum between these muscles.
- Continue dissection superiorly at a level just superficial to the periosteum of the humerus to identify the distal radial nerve where it lies in the humeral groove.
- Follow the radial nerve from this location out distally toward the end of the amputation to gain additional length and cut the nerve back to healthy appearing fascicles.
- Identify and divide any aberrant innervation between the radial nerve and brachialis muscle to ensure that the target muscle regions are completely denervated.
- The motor nerve to the brachialis muscle is the continuation of the musculocutaneous nerve after the branches to the biceps muscle; it was prepared during the median nerve transfer.

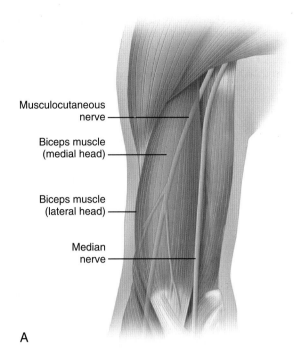

Musculocutaneous nerve

Biceps muscle (medial head)

Biceps muscle (lateral head)

Median nerve

A

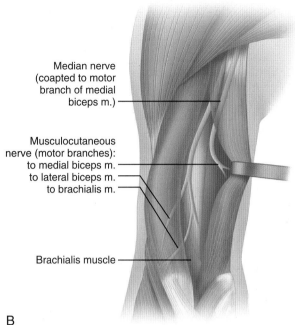

Median nerve (coapted to motor branch of medial biceps m.)

Musculocutaneous nerve (motor branches): to medial biceps m. to lateral biceps m. to brachialis m.

Brachialis muscle

B

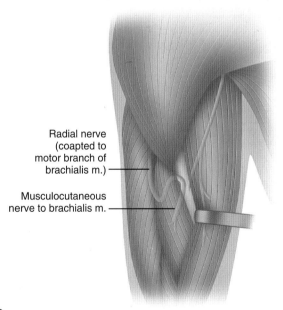

Radial nerve (coapted to motor branch of brachialis m.)

Musculocutaneous nerve to brachialis m.

C

FIGURE 15.11 Targeted reinnervation to improve prosthesis control after upper extremity amputation. **A,** Musculature of the right arm from the anterior position. **B,** Biceps-splitting approach to the musculocutaneous nerve. **C,** Anterolateral view of the right arm showing nerve transfer of the distal portion of the radial nerve to the motor nerve of the brachialis muscle. (Redrawn from O'Shaughnessy KD, Dumanian GA, Lipschutz RD, et al: Target reinnervation to improve prosthesis control in transhumeral amputees. A report of three cases, *J Bone Joint Surg Am* 90:393, 2008.) **SEE TECHNIQUE 15.12**.

- Mobilize the motor nerve to the brachialis muscle and the radial nerve to reach each other at the lateral border of the brachialis muscle and sew them together in an end-to-end fashion with 5-0 polypropylene suture (Fig. 15.11C).

COMPLETION OF PROCEDURE

- Thin a 4- to 5-cm area of subcutaneous fat over all four muscle regions to decrease the separation between the epidermis and the muscle; this maximizes the electromyo-

graphic amplitude over each muscle region of interest and minimizes electromyographic cross-talk between muscle regions.
- Resect the lateral and distal aspect of the lateral head of the biceps to better expose the brachialis muscle.
- A vascularized fascial flap can be interposed between the two heads of the biceps muscle to provide space between the muscle bellies and improve separation of electromyographic signals from the medial and lateral biceps heads.

- Tenodese the medial head of the biceps to the end of the amputation soft tissues to prevent lateral and proximal migration of the muscle belly.

POSTOPERATIVE CARE Patients are admitted to the hospital overnight for observation and pain management. Subcutaneous drains are removed on the day after surgery, and lightly compressive dressing is applied. Muscle twitches may be apparent around 4 months after surgery, and strong independent contractions at about 6 months. Generally, approximately 20 hours of training is required for efficient use of the myoelectric prosthesis.

Dumanian et al. described modifications to the original targeted innervation procedure, primarily handling of the radial nerve and the initial raising of a proximally based, U-shaped adipofascial flap to improve exposure for identification of the muscle raphes. Placement of the flaps between the muscle bellies decreases the chances for aberrant reinnervation and improves electromyographic signal detection. The radial nerve is exposed through a straight posterior approach between the long and lateral heads of the triceps. A motor branch to the lateral head, selected for its size and distal entry into the muscle, is followed proximally and transected off the radial nerve. The radial nerve proper is identified and followed distally toward the amputation stump, transected, cut back to healthy fascicles, and coapted to the motor nerve to the lateral head of the triceps. This requires less mobilization of the nerve to reach the motor nerve of the lateral triceps.

REFERENCES

Carlsen BT, Prigge P, Peterson J: Upper extremity limb loss: functional restoration from prosthesis and targeted reinnervation to transplantation, *J Hand Ther* 27:106, 2014.

Cheesborough JE, Smith LH, Kuiken TA, Dumanian GA: Targeted muscle reinnervation and advanced prosthetic arms, *Semin Plast Surg* 29:62, 2015.

Cheesborough JE, Souza JM, Dumanian GA, et al.: Targeted muscle reinnervation in the initial management of traumatic upper extremity injury, *Hand* 9:253, 2014.

Fisher TF, Kusnezov NA, Bader JA, Blair JA: Predictors of acute complications following traumatic upper extremity amputation, *J Surg Orthop Adv* 27(2):113, 2018.

Fitzgibbons P, Medvedev G: Functional and clinical outcomes of upper extremity amputation, *J Am Acad Orthop Surg* 23:751, 2015.

Freeland AE, Psonak R: Traumatic below-elbow amputations. , Available online at www.orthosupersite.com/print.aspx?rid=20414. Accessed 27 September 2010.

Garg MS, Souza JM, Dumanian GA: Targeted muscle reinnervation in the upper extremity amputee: a technical roadmap, *J Hand Surg Am* 40(9):1877, 2015.

Hebert JS, Olson JL, Morhart MJ, et al.: Novel targeted sensory reinnervation technique to restore functional hand sensation after transhumeral amputation, *IEEE Trans Neural Syst Rehabil Eng* 22:765, 2014.

Inkellis E, Low EE, Langhammer C, Morshed S: *Incidence and characterization of major upper-extremity amputations in the National Trauma Data Bank*, JBJS Open Access, 2018, p 30038.

Kuiken TA, Barlow AK, Hargrove LJ, Dumanian GA: Targeted muscle reinnervation for the upper and lower extremity, *Tech Orthop* 32:109, 2017.

Kumar A, Narange S, Gupta H, et al.: A single incision surgical new anterior technique for forequarter amputation, *Arch Orthop Trauma Surg* 131:955, 2011.

Littlewood H: Amputations at the shoulder and at the hip, BMJ 1:381, 1922..

Mioton LM, Dumanian GA: Targeted muscle reinnervation and prosthetic rehabilitation after limb loss, *J Surg Oncol* 118:807, 2018.

Misra S, Wilkens SC, Chen NC, Eberlin KR: Patients transferred for upper extremity amputation: participation of regional trauma centers, *J Hand Surg Am* 42(12):987, 2017.

Morgan EN, Potter BK, Souza JM, Tingle SM, Nanos GP: Targeted muscle reinnervation for transradial amputation: description of operative technique, *Tech Hand Surg* 20:166, 2016.

Morris CD, Potter BK, Athanasian EA, Lewis VO: Extremity amputations: principles, techniques, and recent advances, *Instr Course Lect* 64:105, 2015.

Otto IA, Kon M, Schuurman AH, van Minnen LP: Replantation versus prosthetic fitting in traumatic arm amputations: a systematic review, *PloS ONE* 10(9):e0137729, 2015.

Ovadia SA, Askari M: Upper extremity amputations and prosthetics, *Semin Plast Surg* 29:55, 2015.

Pet MA, Ko JH, Friedly JL, et al.: Does targeted nerve implantation reduce neuroma pain in amputees? *Clin Orthop Relat Res* 472:2991, 2014.

Pet MA, Morrison SD, Mack JS, et al.: Comparison of patient-reported outcomes after traumatic upper extremity amputation: replantation versus prosthetic rehabilitation, injury, *Int J Care Injured* 47:2783, 2016.

Pierrie SN, Gaston RG, Loeffler BJ: Current concepts in upper-extremity amputation, *J Hand Surg Am* 43(7):657, 2018.

Pierrie SN, Gaston RG, Loeffler BJ: Targeted muscle reinnervation for prosthesis optimization and neuroma management in the setting of transradial amputation, *J Hand Surg Am* Feb 4. pii:S0363-5023(18)30502-1, 2019.

Renninger CH, Rocchi VJ, Kroonen LT: Targeted muscle reinnervation of the brachium: an anatomic study of musculocutaneous and radial nerve motor points relative to proximal landmarks, *J Hand Surg Am* 40(11):2223, 2015.

Resnik L, Klinger S, Etter K: The DEKA arm: its features, functionality, and evolution during the Veterans Affairs Study to optimize the DEKA arm, *Prosthet Orthot Int* 38:492, 2014.

Serino A, Akselrod M, Salomon R, et al.: Upper limb cortical maps in amputees with targeted muscle and sensory reinnervation, *BRAIN* 140:2993, 2017.

Solarz MK, Thoder JJ, Rehman S: Management of major traumatic upper extremity amputations, *Orthop Clin N Am* 47:127, 2016.

Tennent DJ, Wenke JC, Rivera JC, Krueger CA: Characterisation and outcomes of upper extremity amputations, *Injury* 45:965, 2014.

Tintle SM, LeBrun C, Ficke JR, Potter BK: What is new in trauma-related amputations, *J Orthop Trauma* 30(10):S16, 2016.

Tsikandylakis G, Berlin Ö, Branemark R: Implant survival, adverse events, and bone remodeling of osseointegrated percutaneous implants for transhumeral amputees, *Clin Orthop Relat Res* 472:2947, 2014.

Vadala G, Di Pino G, Ambrosio L, Diaz Balzani L, Denaro V: Targeted muscle reinnervation for improved control of myoelectric upper limb prostheses, *J Biol Regul Homeost Agents* 31 4(S1):183, 2017.

Yao J, Chen A, Kuiken T, Carmona C, Dewald J: Sensory cortical re-mapping following upper-limb amputation and subsequent targeted reinnervation: a case report, *NeuroImage* 8:329, 2015.

The complete list of references is available online at ExpertConsult.com.

CHAPTER 16

AMPUTATIONS OF THE HAND

James H. Calandruccio, Benjamin M. Mauck

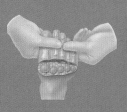

CONSIDERATIONS FOR
    AMPUTATION   647
PRINCIPLES OF FINGER
    AMPUTATIONS   647
FINGERTIP AMPUTATIONS   648
Free skin graft   651
Flaps for fingertip coverage   652
AMPUTATIONS OF SINGLE
    FINGERS   659
Index finger   659

Middle or ring finger ray
    amputations   660
    Ring avulsion injuries   662
Little finger
    amputations   664
THUMB AMPUTATIONS   664
AMPUTATIONS OF
    MULTIPLE DIGITS   665
PAINFUL AMPUTATION
    STUMP   666

RECONSTRUCTIONS AFTER
    AMPUTATION   666
Reconstruction after amputation of the
    hand   666
Reconstruction after amputation of
    multiple digits   668
Reconstruction of the thumb   668
    Pollicization   672

Acute fingertip and thumb injuries are common and require prompt and meticulous composite soft-tissue repair in incomplete amputations. Complete amputations proximal to the eponychial fold in the thumb or multiple digits may be salvaged by microvascular techniques; however, more distal devascularizing injuries rarely can be salvaged by such means and usually require special composite soft-tissue coverage techniques or complete amputation.

In general, every effort should be made to maintain or provide good skin sensation, joint mobility, and digital length with well-padded bony elements. Prolonged efforts to preserve severely damaged structures, especially those that are insensate, can delay healing, increase disability, and lead to a painful series of surgical procedures that may not enhance the final outcome. Thus primary amputation may be the procedure of choice in many patients. Achieving supple soft-tissue coverage of the ends of the thumb and fingers is essential. In amputations of several digits, pinch and grasp are the chief functions to be preserved. Revision amputation through the fingers or metacarpals is a reconstructive procedure to preserve as much function as possible in injured and uninjured parts of the hand.

CONSIDERATIONS FOR AMPUTATION

Amputations may be considered for a variety of conditions in which function is limited by pain, stiffness, insensibility, and cosmetic issues. A request for amputation of an injured part by a patient is usually the culmination of a critical thought process and is usually justified. More often, other factors must be considered in deciding whether amputation is advisable. The ultimate function of the part should be good enough to warrant salvage.

An analysis of the five tissue areas—skin, tendon, nerve, bone, and joint—is sometimes helpful in making the decision

to amputate. If three or more of these five areas require special procedures, such as grafting of skin, suture of tendon or nerve, bony fixation, or closure of the joint, amputation should be considered because the function of the remaining fingers may be compromised by survival of a mutilated finger. In children, amputation rarely is indicated unless the part is nonviable and cannot be made viable by microvascular techniques. Principles of replantation are discussed in other chapter.

Even if amputation is indicated, it may be wise to delay it if parts of the finger may be useful later in a reconstructive procedure. Skin from an otherwise useless digit can be used as a free graft. Skin and deeper soft structures can be useful as a filleted graft; if desired, the bone can be removed primarily and the remaining flap suitably fashioned during a second procedure. Skin well supported by one or more neurovascular bundles but not by bone can be saved and used as a vascular or neurovascular island graft. Segments of nerves can be useful as autogenous grafts. A musculotendinous unit, especially a flexor digitorum sublimis or an extensor indicis proprius, can be saved for transfer to improve function in a surviving digit (e.g., to improve adductor power of the thumb when the third metacarpal shaft has been destroyed or to improve abduction when the recurrent branch of the median nerve is nonfunctional). Tendons of the flexor digitorum sublimis of the fifth finger, the extensor digiti quinti, and the extensor indicis proprius can be useful as free grafts. Bones can be used as peg grafts or for filling osseous defects. Under certain circumstances, even joints can be useful. Every effort should be made to salvage the thumb (Fig. 16.1).

PRINCIPLES OF FINGER AMPUTATIONS

Whether an amputation is done primarily or secondarily, certain principles must be observed to obtain a painless and

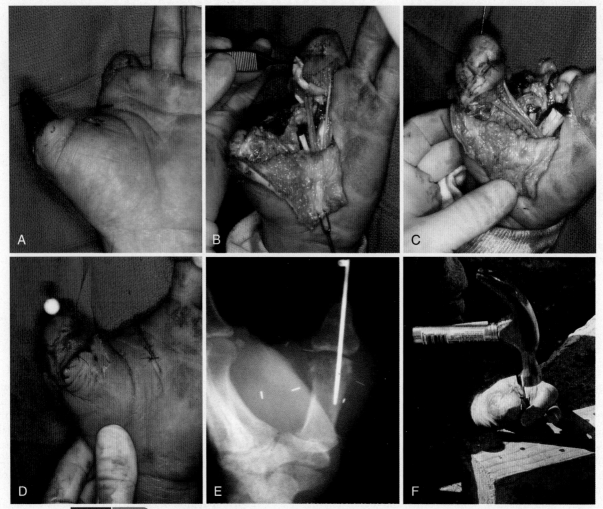

FIGURE 16.1 Thumb reconstruction. **A,** Failed thumb replantation after saw injury with concomitant primary ray amputation of index finger and partial amputation through middle finger. **B–D,** Metacarpophalangeal joint level thumb disarticulation and neurovascular island transfer of proximal phalanx segment of middle finger for thumb reconstruction. **E,** Radiographic appearance of transfer of middle finger proximal phalanx to thumb complex tissue. **F,** Example of functional hand use restored after sensory innervated composite thumb reconstruction.

useful stump. The volar skin flap should be long enough to cover the volar surface and tip of the osseous structures and preferably to join the dorsal flap without tension. The ends of the digital nerves should be dissected carefully from the volar flap, gently placed under tension so as not to rupture more proximal axons, and resected at least 6 mm proximal to the end of the soft-tissue flap. Neuromas are inevitable, but they should be allowed to develop only in padded areas where they are less likely to be painful. When scarring or a skin defect makes the fashioning of a classic flap impossible, a flap of a different shape can be improvised, but the end of the bone must be padded well. Flexor and extensor tendons should be drawn distally, divided, and allowed to retract proximally. When an amputation is through a joint, the flares of the osseous condyles should be contoured to avoid clubbing of the stump. Before the wound is closed, the tourniquet should be released and vessels cauterized to control bleeding.

FINGERTIP AMPUTATIONS

Fingertip amputations vary markedly depending on the amount and configuration of skin lost, the depth of the soft-tissue defect, and whether the phalanx has been exposed or even partially amputated (Fig. 16.2). In the United States, replantation is not performed for most fingertip amputations. Proper treatment is determined by the injury type and whether other digits also have been injured.

Injuries with loss of skin alone can heal by secondary intention or can be covered by a skin graft (Fig. 16.3). Despite continuous descriptions of new finger flaps, healing by secondary intention can in most cases provide equivalent preservation of sensation and function. In general, revision amputation or conservative measures, such as healing by secondary intention, may have improved restoration of static two-point discrimination when compared to other coverage methods. Some studies also suggest improved overall total arc of motion with

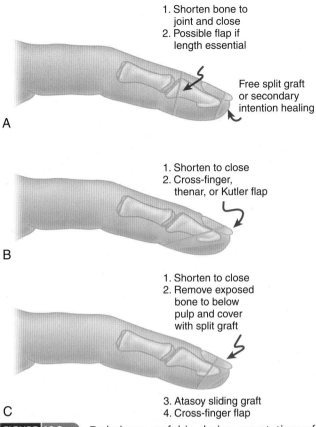

1. Shorten bone to joint and close
2. Possible flap if length essential

Free split graft or secondary intention healing

A

1. Shorten to close
2. Cross-finger, thenar, or Kutler flap

B

1. Shorten to close
2. Remove exposed bone to below pulp and cover with split graft

3. Atasoy sliding graft
4. Cross-finger flap

C

FIGURE 16.2 Techniques useful in closing amputations of fingertip. **A,** For amputations at more distal levels, a free split graft is applied; at more proximal levels, bone is shortened to permit closure, or if length is essential, dorsal flaps can be used. **B,** For amputations through green area, bone can be shortened to permit closure or cross-finger or thenar flap can be used. **C,** For amputations through green area, bone can be shortened to permit closure, exposed bone can be resected, and a split-thickness graft can be applied; Kutler advancement flaps can be used, or a cross-finger flap can be applied. In small children, fingertips commonly heal without grafts.

conservative methods; however, a higher incidence of cold intolerance should be taken into consideration. When tendon, nerve, or bone is exposed, soft-tissue coverage may be achieved in numerous ways. If half of the nail is unsupported by the remaining distal phalanx, a nail bed ablation usually is indicated; otherwise, a hook nail may develop. Reamputation of the finger at a more proximal level can provide ample skin and other soft tissues for closure but requires shortening the finger. If other parts of the hand are severely injured or if the entire hand would be endangered by keeping a finger in one position for a long time, amputation may be indicated. This is especially true for patients with arthritis or for patients with a less physically demanding lifestyle. A free skin graft can be used for coverage, but normal sensibility is rarely restored. A split-thickness graft is often sufficient if the bone is only slightly exposed and its end is nibbled off beneath the fat. Such a graft contracts during healing and eventually becomes about half its original size. Sometimes a full-thickness graft is available from other injured parts of the hand, but the fat should be removed from its deep surface. Occasionally, the amputated part of the fingertip is recovered and replaced as a free graft or

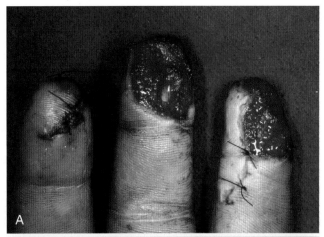

A

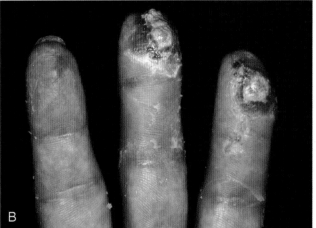

B

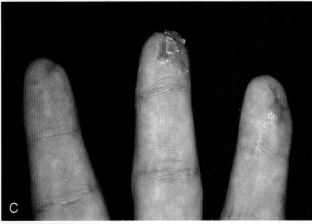

C

FIGURE 16.3 Abrasion injury to left hand treated by secondary-intention healing. **A,** Volar view soon after injury with 2 × 2 cm full-thickness pulp skin loss of middle and ring fingers. **B,** Same fingers with local wound care at 4 weeks. **C,** Result at 8 weeks with no operative intervention.

cap technique (Fig. 16.4). This procedure requires removing bone debris and partially defatting the distal part before reattachment. The cap procedure is quite successful in both children and adults. These free composite grafts should be secured by a stent dressing tied over the end of the finger.

The medial aspect of the arm just distal to the axilla, elbow flexion crease, volar forearm and wrist, and hypothenar

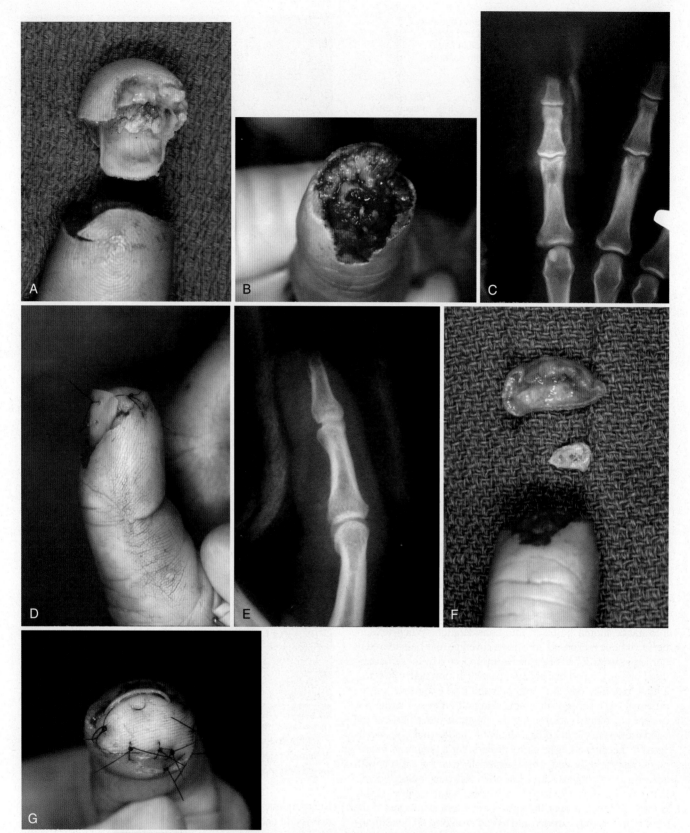

FIGURE 16.4 Cap technique. **A** and **B,** Composite soft-tissue loss from left index finger sustained while changing a tire. **C** and **D,** Biplanar views of finger, indicating inadequate soft-tissue coverage. **E,** Deboned and defatted distal part with good quality skin and sterile matrix. **F** and **G,** Composite tissue reattached with the old nail used as a nail matrix frame.

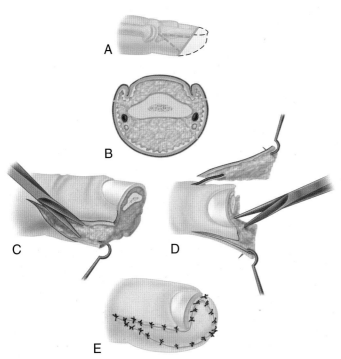

FIGURE 16.5 Kutler V-Y advancement flaps. **A,** Advancement flaps over neurovascular pedicles carried down to bone. **B–D,** Fibrous septa are defined **(B)** and divided **(C)**, permitting free mobilization on neurovascular pedicles alone **(D)**. **E,** Flaps advance readily to midline. **SEE TECHNIQUE 16.1.**

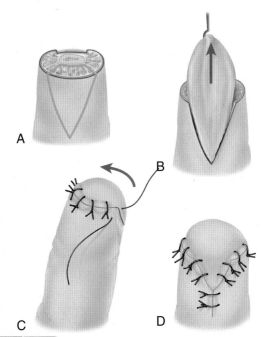

FIGURE 16.6 Atasoy V-Y technique. **A,** Skin incision and mobilization of triangular flap. **B,** Advancement of triangular flap. **C,** Suturing of base of triangular flap to nail bed. **D,** Closure of defect, V-Y technique. **SEE TECHNIQUE 16.2.**

eminence are convenient areas from which skin grafts can be obtained.

If deeper tissues and skin must be replaced to cover exposed tendon and bone, various flaps or grafts can be used. Frequently used distal advancement flaps include the Kutler double lateral V-Y and Atasoy volar V-Y advancement flaps (Figs. 16.5 to 16.7). These flaps involve tissue advancement from the injured finger and provide limited coverage. The dorsal pedicle flap is useful when a finger has been amputated proximal to the nail bed (Fig. 16.8). If further shortening is unacceptable, however, this type of flap can be raised from the dorsum of the injured finger and carried distally without involving another digit. Dorsal defects may be managed by adipofascial turnover flaps in which the proximal subdermal adipofascial tissues are flipped distally over a vascularized zone of the same tissue (Fig. 16.9). Advantages of same-digit coverage techniques include no need for a second operation for flap division (as with a cross-finger flap), prevention of adjacent finger stiffness that occurs with adjacent finger coverage techniques (especially in patients with underlying arthritic conditions), and the opportunity for coverage in patients in whom adjacent fingers are injured. The cross-finger flap provides excellent coverage but may be followed by stiffness not only of the involved finger but also of the donor finger. This type of coverage requires operation in two stages and a split-thickness graft to cover the donor site. The thenar flap also requires operation in two stages. It usually does not cover as large a defect as a cross-finger flap and sometimes is followed by tenderness of the donor site. It does have the advantage, however, of involving only one finger

directly. Thenar flaps also have been shown to be a safe and reliable option in the pediatric population. An alternative to this method is the palmar pocket method in which the distal fingertip (except that of the thumb) can be buried in the ipsilateral palm. The finger is removed from the pocket 16 to 20 days after surgery. Results were successful in 13 of 16 patients according to Arata et al. In children, we have observed that merely resuturing the defatted fingertips back in place usually results in a satisfactory result.

A local neurovascular island pedicle flap can be advanced distally and provides a good pad with normal sensibility. Flaps of 2×1.5 cm^2 and advancement of 18 mm have been reported (Fig. 16.10). Retrograde island pedicle flaps require tedious dissection but offer excellent distal coverage and utility for dorsal and volar defects (Fig. 16.11). Donor site morbidity may be reduced in retrograde island pedicle flaps that use the subdermal elements only (Fig. 16.12). Comparative studies have shown no significant differences between the two flaps at 12 months.

Composite soft-tissue transfer to the small finger may be accomplished by use of an ulnar hypothenar flap. This retrograde flow flap is based on the ulnar digital artery and may be used to supply sensation when the dorsal sensory branch of the ulnar nerve is included in the skin flap (Fig. 16.13). Eponychial flaps have historically been used to improve overall functional and cosmetic outcomes of distal amputations (Fig. 16.14).

Despite the variability of coverage options, patient-reported outcomes demonstrate satisfactory or good-to-excellent results independent of treatment type, with minimal influence on ability to perform activities of daily living or in quality of life.

FREE SKIN GRAFT

The techniques for applying free skin grafts are described in other chapter.

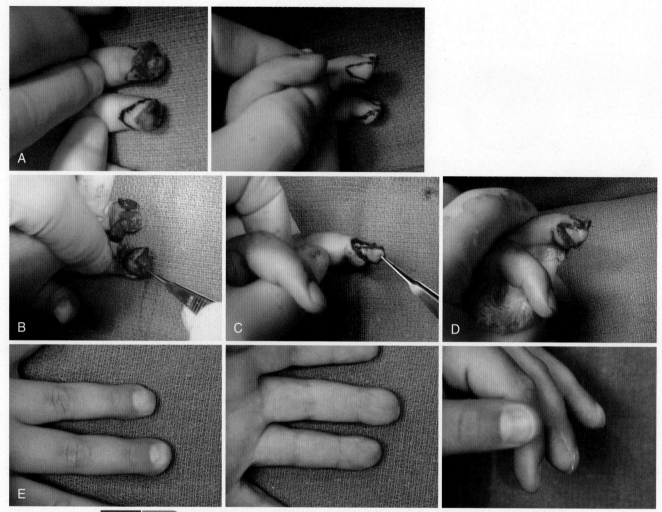

FIGURE 16.7   Distal fingertip amputation suitable for a V-Y advancement flap. **A,** Ample pulp skin with outline of intended skin incision. **B** and **C,** Flap raised with sequential dissection from the distal phalangeal periosteum and flexor digitorum profundus tendon centrodorsally, and dorsoradial and dorsoulnar margins by dissection down to the distal phalangeal bone laterally, and septal release volarly. Note that the neurovascular bundles must be carefully kept with the pulp skin, and direct inspection of them is not always possible. **D,** Flap sutured into position with proximal open area left open to heal by secondary intention. **E,** Clinical result at 6 weeks postoperatively. **SEE TECHNIQUE 16.1.**

FLAPS FOR FINGERTIP COVERAGE

KUTLER V-Y OR ATASOY TRIANGULAR ADVANCEMENT FLAPS

Kutler double lateral V-Y or Atasoy volar V-Y advancement flap fingertip coverage is appealing because it involves just the injured finger. It provides only limited coverage, however, and does not result consistently in normal sensibility. The injury pattern determines which flap to use. When more of the pulp skin remains, then the Atasoy flap is useful. When the pulp is compromised and the lateral hyponychial skin is uninjured, the Kutler flap can be used.

TECHNIQUE 16.1

(KUTLER; FISHER)
- Local anesthesia is preferred in adults; children may require general anesthesia. Anesthetize the finger by digital block at the proximal phalanx and apply a digital tourniquet.
- Debride the tip of the finger of uneven edges of soft tissue and any protruding bone (Fig. 16.5).
- Develop two triangular flaps, one on each side of the finger with the apex of each directed proximally and centered in the midlateral line of the digit. Avoid making the flaps too large; their sides should each measure about 6 mm, and their bases should measure about the same or slightly less.

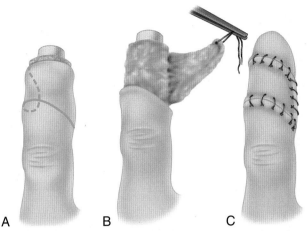

FIGURE 16.8 Dorsal pedicle flap useful for amputations proximal to the nail when preserving length is essential. It may have two pedicles or, as illustrated here, only one. **A,** Flap has been outlined. **B,** Flap has been elevated, leaving only a single pedicle. **C,** Flap has been sutured in place over end of stump, and remaining defect on dorsum of finger has been covered by split-thickness skin graft. **SEE TECHNIQUE 16.3.**

- Develop the flaps farther by incising deeper toward the nail bed and volar pulp. Take care not to pinch the flaps with thumb forceps or hemostats. Rather, insert a skin hook near the base of each and apply slight traction in a distal direction. With a pair of small scissors and at each apex, divide the pulp just enough (usually not more than half its thickness) to allow the flaps to be mobilized toward the tip of the finger. Avoid dividing any pulp distally.
- Round off the sharp corners of the remaining part of the distal phalanx and reshape its end to conform with the normal tuft.
- Approximate the bases of the flaps and stitch them together with small interrupted nonabsorbable sutures; stitch the dorsal sides of the flaps to the remaining nail or nail bed.
- Frequently, closure of the proximal and lateral defects is impossible without placing significant tension on the flaps. In such instances, the sides of the triangular flaps should be left without sutures and heal satisfactorily by secondary intention (Fig. 16.7D). Apply Xeroform gauze and a protective dressing.

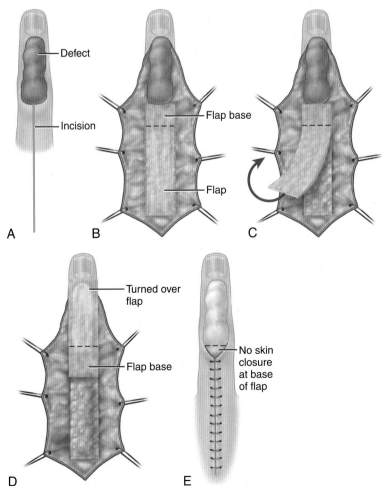

FIGURE 16.9 Turnover adipofascial flap. **A,** Complex defect. **B,** Design of adipofascial flap. Flap base is immediately proximal to the defect, and flap width is slightly wider than the defect. **C,** Development of a distally based flap by separating it from the underlying paratenon of the extensor tendon. (Intact paratenon ensures tendon gliding after surgery.) **D,** Flap is turned over on itself to cover the defect and the flap base. **E,** Flap covered with thin skin graft. Skin closure is not performed at base of flap to avoid tension. **SEE TECHNIQUE 16.4.**

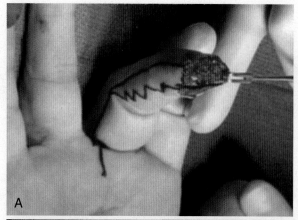

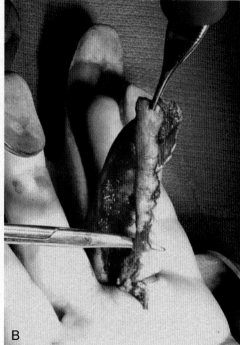

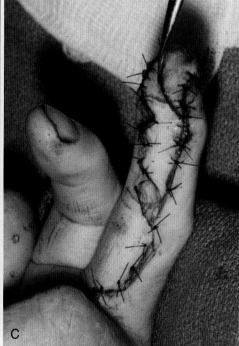

FIGURE 16.10   Homodigital antegrade-flow neurovascular pedicle flap. **A,** Flap pattern on middle finger outlined with dorsal border on midaxial line with progressively narrower sawtooth pattern volarly converging just proximal to the proximal interphalangeal joint. **B,** Flap raised with intact neurovascular bundle. **C,** Distally advanced and inset flap, with area proximally requiring ulnar-palm free skin graft.   (From Henry M, Stutz C: Homodigital antegrade-flow neurovascular pedicle flaps for sensate reconstruction of fingertip amputation injuries, *J Hand Surg* 31[7]:1220–1225, 2006.)

ATASOY TRIANGULAR ADVANCEMENT FLAPS

TECHNIQUE 16.2

(ATASOY ET AL.)

- Under tourniquet control and using an appropriate anesthetic, cut a distally based triangle through the pulp skin only, with the base of the triangle equal in width to the cut edge of the nail (Fig. 16.6).
- Develop a full-thickness flap with nerves and blood supply preserved. Carefully separate the fibrofatty subcutaneous tissue from the periosteum and flexor tendon sheath using sharp dissection.
- Selectively cut the vertical septa that hold the flap in place and advance the flap distally.
- Suture the skin flap to the sterile matrix or nail. The volar defect from the advancement can be left open and left to heal by secondary intention if closure compromises vascularity. A few millimeters of the phalanx can be removed to the level of the sterile matrix. The base of the flap may be difficult to suture to the sterile matrix or nail, and a 22-gauge needle can be used as an intramedullary pin in the distal phalanx to keep the flap in position.

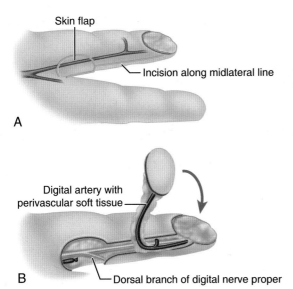

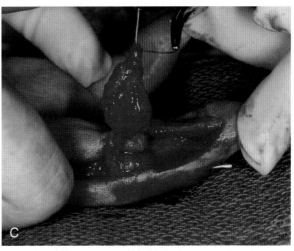

FIGURE 16.11 Reverse digital artery island flap. **A,** Flap design. **B** and **C,** Digital artery is ligated proximally. Skin flap is elevated along with artery and perivascular soft tissue. Dorsal branch of digital nerve can be incorporated and microanastomosed with transected contralateral digital nerve to facilitate innervation of flap. **SEE TECHNIQUE 16.8.**

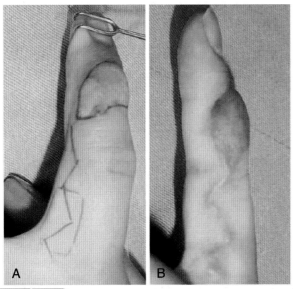

FIGURE 16.12 Reverse adipofascial flap. **A,** Skin incision outlining flap and defect. **B,** Postoperative result with free skin graft over defect site. (From Chang KP, Wang WH, Lai CS, et al: Refinement of reverse digital arterial flap for finger defects: surgical technique, *J Hand Surg Am* 30[3]:558–561, 2005.)

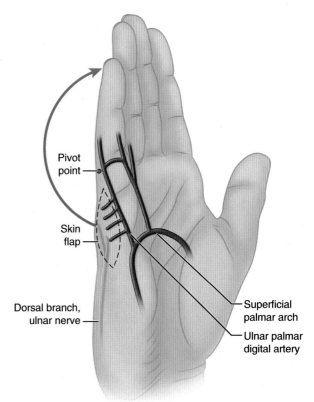

FIGURE 16.13 Reverse ulnar hypothenar flap design. **SEE TECHNIQUE 16.9.**

BIPEDICLE DORSAL FLAPS

A bipedicle dorsal flap is useful when a finger has been amputated proximal to its nail bed and when preserving all its remaining length is essential, but attaching it to another finger is undesirable. When this flap can be made wide enough in relation to its length, one of its pedicles can be divided, leaving it attached only at one side (Fig. 16.8).

TECHNIQUE 16.3

- Beginning distally at the raw margin of the skin and proceeding proximally, elevate the skin and subcutaneous tissue from the dorsum of the finger.

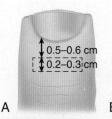 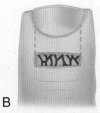 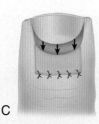

0.5–0.6 cm
0.2–0.3 cm

A B C

FIGURE 16.14 Eponychial flap for fingertip amputation. **A,** Dorsal fold advancement flap design to increase nail exposure. **B,** Proximal de-epithelialization of bed for flap advancement. **C,** After dorsal fold flap advancement into area of de-epithelialization. (Redrawn from Peterson SL, Peterson EL, Wheatley MJ: Management of fingertip amputations, *J Hand Surg Am* 39[10]:2093–2101, 2014.)

- At a more proximal level, make a transverse dorsal incision to create a bipedicle flap long enough, when drawn distally, to cover the bone and other tissues on the end of the stump.
- Suture the flap in place and cover the defect created on the dorsum of the finger by a split-thickness skin graft. The flap can be made more mobile by freeing one of its pedicles, but this decreases its vascularity.

ADIPOFASCIAL TURNOVER FLAP

The adipofascial turnover flap is a de-epithelialized flap that may be used to cover distal dorsal defects 3 cm in length.

TECHNIQUE 16.4

- Under tourniquet control, repair the traumatic defects as indicated, such as extensor tendon repair and fracture fixation.
- Outline the planned flap with a skin pen. Make the width 2 to 4 mm wider than the traumatic defect. The base-to-length ratio should be 1:1.5 to 1:3. The flap base should be 0.5 to 1 cm in length and is made just proximal to the defect. The flap length should be at least this much longer than the defect (Fig. 16.9B).
- Develop the adipofascial flap superficial to the extensor tendon paratenon from proximal to distal (Fig. 16.9C).
- After the flap is detached proximally and along its sides to the flap base, flip it over and suture it distally (Fig. 16.9D).
- Do not place sutures at the turnover site to avoid tension on the vascular pedicle (Fig. 16.9E).
- Use a split-thickness graft to cover the defect at the flap site.
- Immobilize the digit in a protective splint.

POSTOPERATIVE CARE The first dressing change is 3 weeks after surgery, and digital motion is begun as wound healing and other concomitant injuries allow.

CROSS-FINGER FLAPS FOR RECONSTRUCTION OF FINGERTIP AMPUTATIONS

The technique of applying cross-finger flaps is described in other chapter.

THENAR FLAP

Middle and ring finger coverage can be accomplished by the use of the thenar flap. Donor site tenderness and proximal interphalangeal joint flexion contractures can occur, and the flaps should not be left in place for more than 3 weeks.

TECHNIQUE 16.5

- With the thumb held in abduction, flex the injured finger so that its tip touches the middle of the thenar eminence. Outline on the thenar eminence a flap that when raised is large enough to cover the defect and is properly positioned; pressing the bloody stump of the injured finger against the thenar skin outlines by bloodstain the size of the defect to be covered (Fig. 16.15A,B).
- With its base proximal, raise the thenar flap to include most of the underlying fat; handle the flap with skin hooks to avoid crushing it even with small forceps. Make the flap sufficiently wide so that when sutured to the convex fingertip it is not under tension. Make its length no more than twice its width. By gentle undermining of the skin border at the donor site, the defect can be closed directly without resorting to a graft.
- Attach the distal end of the flap to the trimmed edge of the nail by sutures passed through the nail. The lateral edges of the flap should fit the margins of the defect, but to avoid impairing circulation in the flap, suture only their most distal parts, if any, to the finger. Prevent the flap from folding back on itself and strangulating its vessels (Fig. 16.15C and D).
- Control all bleeding, check the positions of the flap and finger, and apply wet cotton gently compressed to follow the contours of the graft and the fingertip.
- Hold the finger in the proper position by gauze and adhesive tape and splint the wrist.

POSTOPERATIVE CARE At 4 days, the graft is dressed again and then kept as dry as possible by dressing it every 1 or 2 days and by leaving it partially exposed. At 2 weeks, the base of the flap is detached and the free skin edges are sutured in place. The contours of the fingertip and the thenar eminence improve with time.

LOCAL NEUROVASCULAR ISLAND FLAP

An antegrade neurovascular island graft can provide satisfactory padding and normal sensibility to the most important working surface of the digit.

on the bundles. Should tension compromise the circulation in the graft, dissect the bundles more proximally or flex the distal interphalangeal joint, or both.
- Suture the graft in place with interrupted small nonabsorbable sutures.
- Cover the defect created on the volar surface of the finger with a free full-thickness graft.
- Carefully place contoured sterile dressings such as glycerin-soaked cotton balls over the grafts to lessen the likelihood of excess pressure on the neurovascular bundles.
- Apply a compression dressing until suture removal at 10 to 14 days.

POSTOPERATIVE CARE Begin digital motion therapy as soon as the wounds permit.

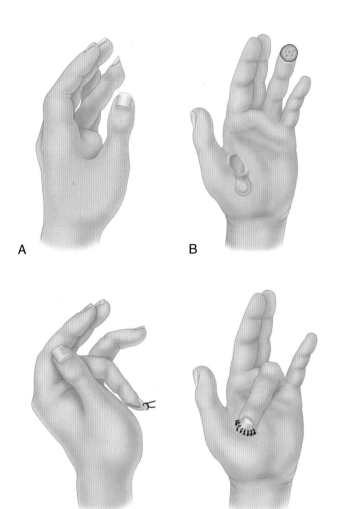

A

B

C

D

FIGURE 16.15 Thenar flap for amputation of fingertip. **A,** Tip of ring finger has been amputated. **B,** Finger has been flexed so that its tip touches middle of thenar eminence, and thenar flap has been outlined. **C,** Split-thickness graft is to be sutured to donor area before flap is attached to finger. **D,** End of flap has been attached to finger by sutures passed through nail and through tissue on each side of it. **SEE TECHNIQUE 16.5.**

TECHNIQUE 16.6

- Make a midlateral incision on each side of the finger (or thumb) beginning distally at the defect and extending proximally to the level of the proximal interphalangeal joint or thumb interphalangeal joint.
- On each side and beginning proximally, carefully dissect the neurovascular bundle distally to the level selected for the proximal margin of the graft (Fig. 16.16A). Here make a transverse volar incision through the skin and subcutaneous tissues, but carefully protect the neurovascular bundles (Fig. 16.16B).
- If necessary, make another transverse incision at the margin of the defect, freeing a rectangular island of the skin and underlying fat to which the two neurovascular bundles are attached.
- Carefully draw this island or graft distally and place it over the defect (Fig. 16.16C). Avoid placing too much tension

ISLAND PEDICLE FLAP

The axial-pattern island pedicle flap may be used to provide sensation or merely composite soft tissue to adjacent fingers or thumb. The skin paddle size can vary to suit the defect.

TECHNIQUE 16.7

- This procedure is performed as outpatient surgery, and general anesthesia is preferred.
- Inflate the arm tourniquet after using a skin pen to outline clearly the intended flap design.
- Measure the defect size after appropriate debridement and draw a slightly larger flap onto the donor digit.
- Use a midaxial or a volar zigzag incision to expose the neurovascular bundle of the area of the superficial arch, the usual pivot point of the flap.
- If a neurovascular island flap is desired to provide sensation to a given area, it is imperative that the ulnar border of the small finger and radial border of the index finger not be used as donors because maintaining or achieving sensation in these areas is desirable. The skin paddle is ideally centered over the neurovascular bundle.
- Under tourniquet control, locate the neurovascular bundle proximally and carefully dissect this to its superficial arch origin. Leave a cuff of soft tissue around the neurovascular bundle because discrete veins are not readily visible but exist in the periarterial tissues. Dissect the bundle deeply and use bipolar cautery well away from the proper digital artery to control perforating vessels entering the flexor sheath.
- Elevate the skin paddle, taking care to ensure the vascular bundle is reasonably centered under the flap, and divide the artery distally.
- Use a simple 5-0 nylon suture to secure the distal vascular bundle to the distal edge of the skin flap.
- Place the paddle over the recipient site to determine the best path for the pedicle because the pedicle should not be under any tension. The skin between the pivot point

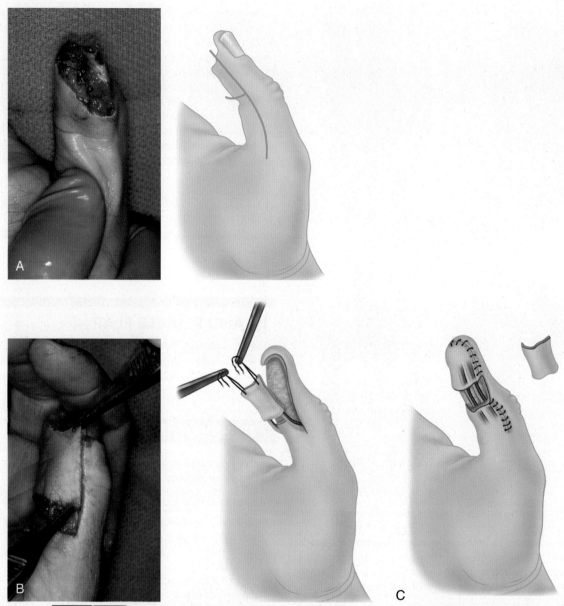

FIGURE 16.16   A–C, Local neurovascular island graft (see text). **SEE TECHNIQUE 16.6.**

can be undermined and enlarged by gently yet liberally spreading a hemostat in the intended pedicle path. The tunnel must allow easy passage of the flap. Frequently, a 2 to 3 cm skin bridge can be left between the proximal donor and recipient incisions. However, if any doubt remains in regard to the pedicle tension or impingement, these incisions should be connected.

- Deflate the tourniquet and control bleeding.
- Draw the 5-0 nylon suture gently through the skin bridge, taking care not to place shear stress between the pedicle and flap.
- Suture the flap loosely into position and close the remaining wounds. Ensure the flap remains well vascularized before placing a loose dressing and protective splint.
- *Note: When this procedure is performed as a vascular island pedicle flap, the proper digital nerve should be carefully preserved and protected to prevent problematic*

neuromas. Transient dysesthesias that commonly occur with this technique usually resolve in 6 to 8 weeks.

POSTOPERATIVE CARE The patient is seen in 5 to 7 days, and motion therapy is begun as soon as the wounds permit, usually 2 to 3 weeks postoperatively.

RETROGRADE ISLAND PEDICLE FLAP

This retrograde homodigital island flap is well suited to cover dorsal and volar defects distally. The procedure relies on retrograde flow through the proper digital artery, supplying the proximal composite tissue (Fig. 16.11). This flap can be performed with skin or adipofascial tissue.

TECHNIQUE 16.8

- After preparing the recipient site appropriately, determine the donor defect size.
- Expose the vascular pedicle using a linear or zigzag incision over the digit, the length of which is 1 to 1.5 cm larger than the distance between the proximal defect edge and distal donor edge.
- Dissect from proximal to distal under tourniquet control.
- Separate the proper digital artery proximal to the donor flap from the underlying digital nerve. Ligate and divide the artery and raise the flap carefully with its pedicle. Leave a 1-cm section of undamaged vascular bundle undisturbed distally to nourish the flap and act as the pivot point for the flap.
- Deflate the tourniquet and control bleeding with bipolar cautery.
- Suture without tension on the recipient site and close the remaining wound loosely so as not to compromise the pedicle.
- Donor defects typically require a split-thickness skin graft and a soft nonadherent conforming dressing, such as Xeroform gauze and glycerin-soaked cotton balls.
- *Note: This flap can be used as a de-epithelialized retrograde homodigital island to lessen the morbidity associated with the skin paddle. In such a modification, the skin graft is applied over the composite graft at the recipient site.*

POSTOPERATIVE CARE The dressing is removed 7 to 10 days postoperatively, and motion therapy is begun depending on wound healing.

ULNAR HYPOTHENAR FLAP

The ulnar hypothenar flap is a retrograde vascular pedicle flap that relies on the distal half of the hypothenar skin's vascular supply from the small finger ulnar digital artery. The flap can be used to cover defects as large as 5 × 2 cm. Based on the proper digital artery to the small finger, this flap may provide sensation by suturing the ulnar digital nerve to a cutaneous nerve sensory branch that is harvested with the flap.

TECHNIQUE 16.9

- Outline the flap on the distal half of the hypothenar eminence to correspond to the recipient defect.
- Under tourniquet control and general anesthesia, dissect in the subfascial plane, beginning on the dorsal side of the hand. Include the multiple vascular perforators with the flap before dividing the ulnar palmar digital artery proximally.
- Take the distal dissection of the pedicle to the pivot point of the proximal interphalangeal joint (Fig. 16.13).
- Close the wounds loosely after bleeding is controlled and apply a bulky soft dressing.

POSTOPERATIVE CARE The bulky soft dressing is removed within 1 week after surgery, and metacarpophalangeal and proximal interphalangeal joint motion therapy is begun.

AMPUTATIONS OF SINGLE FINGERS
INDEX FINGER

When the index finger is amputated at or more proximal to its proximal interphalangeal joint level, the remaining stump is useless and can hinder pinch between the thumb and middle finger. In most instances, when a primary amputation must be at such a proximal level, any secondary amputation should be through the base of the second metacarpal. This index ray amputation is especially desirable in women for cosmetic reasons. Because it is a more extensive operation than amputation through the finger, however, it can cause stiffness of the other fingers and may be contraindicated in arthritic hands. The middle finger radial digital nerve should be carefully isolated and dissected free from the second web space common digital nerve. Improper technique can result in a sunken scar on the dorsum of the hand or in anchoring the first dorsal interosseous to the extensor mechanism, rather than to the base of the proximal phalanx, causing intrinsic overpull.

INDEX RAY AMPUTATION

TECHNIQUE 16.10

- With a marking pen, outline the planned incisions (Fig. 16.17A). Begin the palmar line in the second web space at the radial base of the middle finger and continue this line proximally to the midpalmar area, being careful not to cross the palmar flexion creases at 90 degrees. Begin a second palmar line approximately 1 cm distal to the palmar digital flexion crease of the index finger radial base and extend this line proximally to meet the first incision in the midpalmar area. Zigzag incisions in the palmar skin may lessen the incidence of longitudinal skin scar contractures.
- Outline the dorsal part of the incision that extends from the palmar lines to converge at a point on the index carpometacarpal joint dorsally.
- Now make the incisions as just outlined.
- Ligate and divide the dorsal veins, and at a more proximal level divide the branches of the superficial radial nerve to the index finger.
- Retract the index extensor digitorum communis and the extensor indicis proprius tendons distally, sever them, and allow them to retract proximally.
- Detach the tendinous insertion of the first dorsal interosseous and dissect the muscle proximally from the second metacarpal shaft (Fig. 16.17B). Detach the volar interosseous from the same shaft and divide the transverse metacarpal ligament that connects the second and third metacarpal

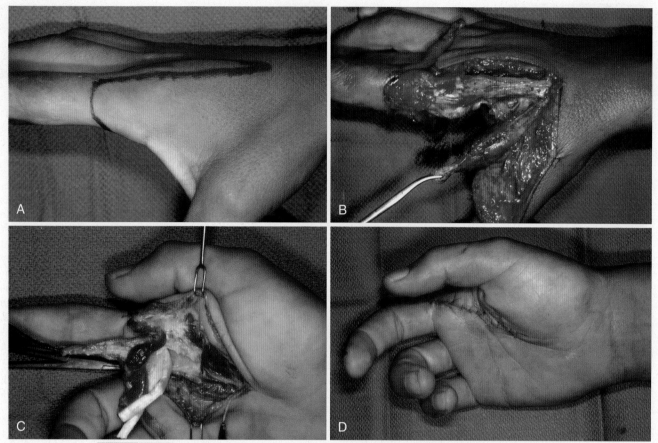

FIGURE 16.17 Technique for index ray amputation. **A,** Dorsal skin incisions planned with marking pen. Palmar skin incision can be outlined in matching *zigzag* fashion to reduce skin suture line contracture. **B,** Flexor digitorum superficialis and flexor digitorum profundus tendons severed proximal to lumbrical origin after isolation and division of appropriate neurovascular structures. **C,** First dorsal interosseous retained for insertion into radial base of middle finger proximal phalanx. **D,** Appearance after index ray amputation. **SEE TECHNIQUE 16.10.**

heads. Take care not to damage the radial digital nerve of the middle finger.

- Carefully divide the second metacarpal obliquely from dorsoradial proximally to volar-ulnar distally about 2 cm distal to its base. Do not disarticulate the bone at its proximal end. Smooth any rough edges on the remaining part of the metacarpal.
- Divide both flexor tendons of the index finger and allow them to retract (Fig. 16.17C).
- Ligate and divide digital arteries to the index finger.
- Carefully identify and divide both digital nerves leaving sufficient length so that their ends can be buried in the interossei.
- Anchor the tendinous insertion of the first dorsal interosseous to the base of the proximal phalanx of the middle finger. Do not anchor it to the extensor tendon or its hood because this might cause intrinsic overpull.
- With a running suture, approximate the muscle bellies in the area previously occupied by the second metacarpal shaft.
- Ligate or cauterize all obvious bleeders.

- Approximate the skin edges over a drain and remove the tourniquet (Fig. 16.17D).
- Apply a well-molded wet dressing that conforms to the wide new web between the middle finger and the thumb and support the wrist by a large bulky dressing or a plaster splint.

POSTOPERATIVE CARE The hand is elevated immediately after surgery for 48 hours. At 24 hours, the drain is removed. Digital motion therapy is initiated at 5 to 7 days postoperatively.

MIDDLE OR RING FINGER RAY AMPUTATIONS

In contrast to the proximal phalanx of the index finger, the proximal phalanx of either the middle or the ring finger is important functionally. Its absence in either finger makes a hole through which small objects can pass when the hand is used as a cup or in a scooping maneuver; its absence makes the remaining fingers tend to deviate toward the midline of

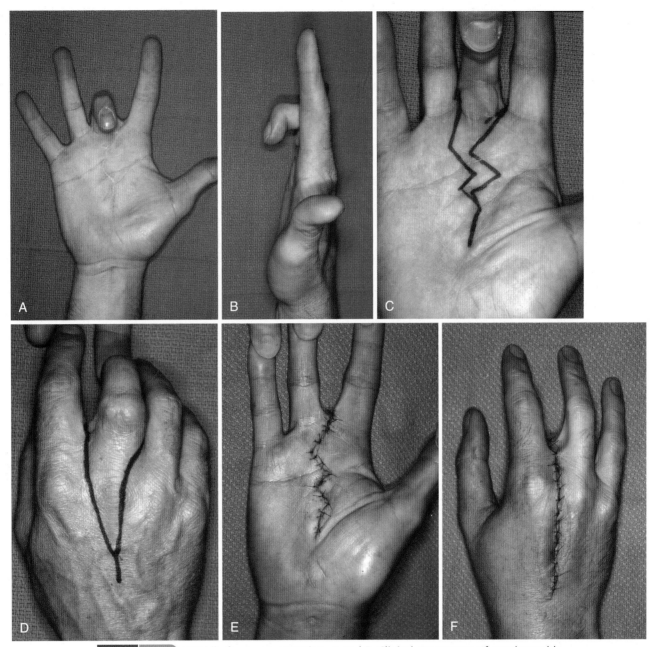

FIGURE 16.18 Middle finger ray resection. **A** and **B,** Clinical appearance of unsalvageable contracted and stiff middle finger after gunshot wound to hand. **C** and **D,** Planned palmar and dorsal incisions for ray resection. **E** and **F,** Cosmetic appearance after partial middle finger metacarpal amputation.

the hand. In multiple amputations, the length of either the middle or the ring finger becomes even more important. The third and fourth metacarpal heads are also important because they help stabilize the metacarpal arch by providing attachments for the transverse metacarpal ligament.

In a child or woman, when the middle finger has been amputated proximal to the proximal interphalangeal joint, and especially when it has been amputated proximal to the metacarpal head, transposing the index ray ulnarward to replace the third ray may be indicated. This operation results in more natural symmetry, removes any conspicuous stump, and makes the presence of only three fingers less obvious.

Transposition of the index metacarpal after partial middle finger metacarpal amputation is technically challenging and has significant complications. If this more cosmetic procedure is chosen, great care should be taken to achieve proper rotation and solid bone fixation. Union of midshaft metacarpal osteotomies is more difficult, and we recommend metaphyseal fixation in such instances.

Excising the third metacarpal shaft removes the origin of the adductor pollicis and weakens pinch. The index ray should not be transposed unless this adductor can be reattached elsewhere. The operation is contraindicated if the hand is needed for heavy manual labor (Fig. 16.18).

Similarly, when the ring finger has been amputated, transposing the fifth ray radialward to replace the fourth rarely is indicated. Resection of the fourth metacarpal at its base or at the carpometacarpal joint and closure of the skin to create a common web permits a "folding-in" of the fifth digit to close the gap without transposing the fifth metacarpal. Disarticulation of the ring finger at the carpometacarpal joint allows the small finger metacarpal base to shift radially over the hamate facet, essentially eliminating radial deviation of the ray (Fig. 16.19).

TRANSPOSING THE INDEX RAY

TECHNIQUE 16.11

(PEACOCK)
- Plan the incision so that a wedge of skin is removed from the dorsal and volar surfaces of the hand (Fig. 16.20).
- In the region of the transverse metacarpal arch, plot the exact points that must be brought together to form a smooth arch across the dorsum of the hand when the second and fourth metacarpal heads are approximated.
- Curve the proximal end of the dorsal incision slightly toward the second metacarpal base so that the base can be exposed easily.
- Fashion the distal end of the incision so that a small triangle of skin is excised from the ring finger to receive a similar triangle of skin from the stump or the area between the fingers; transferring this triangle is important to prevent the suture line from passing through the depths of the reconstructed web.
- After the dorsal and volar wedges of skin have been removed and the flaps have been elevated, expose the third metacarpal through a longitudinal incision in its periosteum.
- The index ray is the right length when its metacarpal is moved directly to the third metacarpal base. With an oscillating saw, transversely divide the third metacarpal as close to its base as possible. Excise the third metacarpal shaft and the interosseous muscles to the middle finger. Take care not to damage the interosseous muscles of the remaining fingers.
- Identify the neurovascular bundles of the middle finger; individually ligate the arteries and veins and divide the digital nerves.
- While the wrist is held flexed, draw the flexor tendons distally as far as possible and divide them.
- Retract the extensor tendons of the index finger, expose the second metacarpal at its base, and divide the bone at the same level as the third metacarpal.
- From the radial side of the second metacarpal, gently dissect the intrinsic muscles just enough to allow this metacarpal to be placed on the base of the third metacarpal without placing undue tension on the muscles. Obliquely bevel the second metacarpal base to produce a smooth contour on the side of the hand.
- From the excised third metacarpal, fashion a key graft to extend from one fragment of the reconstructed metacarpal to the other.

- Insert a Kirschner wire longitudinally through the metacarpophalangeal joint of the transposed ray and bring it out on the dorsum of the flexed wrist; draw it proximally through the metacarpal until its distal end is just proximal to the metacarpophalangeal joint.
- With the wrist flexed, cut off the proximal part of the wire and allow the remaining end to disappear beneath the skin.
- Flex all the fingers simultaneously to ensure correct rotation of the transposed ray and insert a Kirschner wire transversely through the necks of the fourth and the transposed metacarpals. Bony fixation with a small plate and screws can also be used. This requires precise technique and should be applied only after correct rotational alignment has been determined. Attaching the plate to the distal fragment first and flexing the metacarpophalangeal joints fully before proximal plate fixation is secured reduces the chance for malrotation.
- Close the skin and insert a rubber drain.
- Apply a soft pressure dressing; no additional external support is needed.

POSTOPERATIVE CARE At 2 days the rubber drain is removed, and at 8 to 10 days the entire dressing and the sutures are removed. A light volar plaster splint is applied to keep the wrist in the neutral position and support the transposed ray; however, the splint is removed daily for cleaning the hand and exercising the small joints. At about 5 weeks, when the metacarpal fragments have united, the Kirschner wires are removed with the use of local anesthesia.

■ RING AVULSION INJURIES

The soft tissue most commonly of the ring finger usually is forcefully avulsed at its base when a metal ring worn on that finger catches on a nail or hook. The force usually is sufficient to cause separation of the skin and nearly always damages the vascular supply to the distal tissue. The modification of the Urbaniak classification by Kay et al. (Box 16.1) is useful to quantify injury and prognosis. Fractures and ligamentous damage also can occur, but the tendons seem to be the last to separate. Attempts at salvage routinely fail unless

BOX 16.1

Classification of Ring Avulsion Injuries

I   Circulation adequate, with or without skeletal injury
II Circulation inadequate (arterial and venous), no skeletal injury
III Circulation inadequate (arterial and venous), fracture or joint injury present
    A. Arterial circulation only inadequate
    B. Venous circulation only inadequate
IV Complete amputation

From Kay S, Werntz J, Wolff TW: Ring avulsion injuries: classification and prognosis, *J Hand Surg Am* 14(2 Pt 1):204–213, 1989.

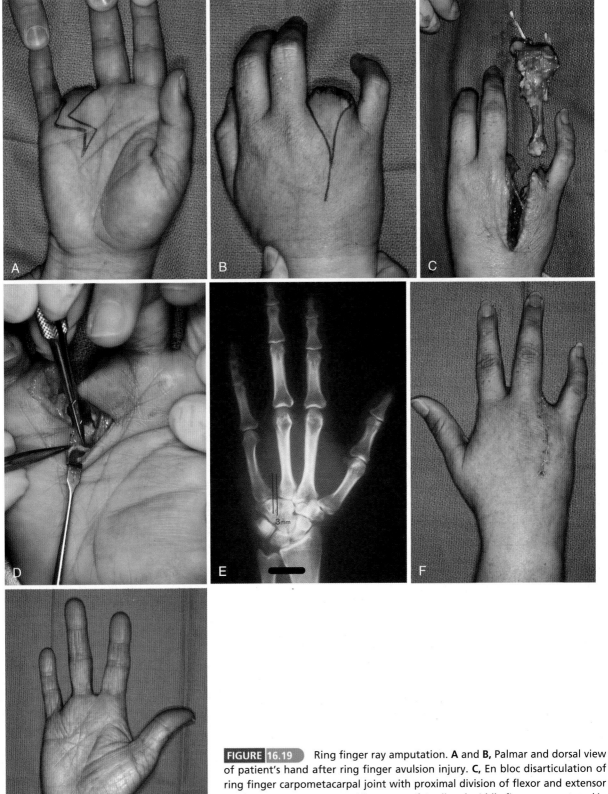

FIGURE 16.19 Ring finger ray amputation. **A** and **B,** Palmar and dorsal view of patient's hand after ring finger avulsion injury. **C,** En bloc disarticulation of ring finger carpometacarpal joint with proximal division of flexor and extensor tendons. **D,** Intermetacarpal ligaments of small and middle fingers are sutured in overlapped position to prevent splaying of small finger. **E,** Radiograph of hand indicating radialization of the small finger metacarpal base on hamate facet. **F** and **G,** Clinical appearance after ring finger ray resection.

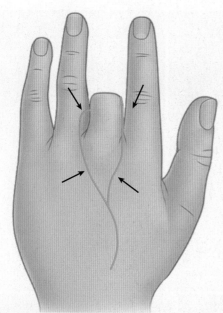

FIGURE 16.20 Peacock technique of transposing index ray. Dorsal incision is shown; *arrows* indicate points along skin edges that will be brought together. Similar palmar incision is made (see text). **SEE TECHNIQUE 16.11.**

the vascular supply can be reestablished. Recent advances in microvascular techniques have improved outcomes, making replantation a viable option for the skilled microvascular surgeon. Even with successful microvascular repair, stiffness and abnormal sensation are unavoidable. Amputation of the fourth ray with closure of the web is the procedure of choice in a child or woman. Simple metacarpal amputation rather than resection may be indicated in a heavy laborer. A report comparing metacarpal amputation with ray resection suggested that despite the poor cosmesis and palmar incompetence, metacarpal amputation preserved greater strength. By resecting the fourth ray at its base or at the carpometacarpal joint, the fifth ray closes without having to be surgically transposed. Simple amputation of the finger itself should be done in the presence of necrosis and infection; and, if indicated, the ray amputation is done later as an elective procedure.

LITTLE FINGER AMPUTATIONS

As much of the little finger as possible should be saved, provided that all the requirements for a painless stump are satisfied. Often this finger survives when all others have been destroyed, and it becomes important in forming a pinch with the thumb. When the little finger alone is amputated, and when the appearance of the hand is important or the amputation is at the metacarpophalangeal joint, the fifth metacarpal shaft is divided obliquely at its middle third. The insertion of the abductor digiti quinti is transferred to the proximal phalanx of the ring finger just as the first dorsal interosseous is transferred to the middle finger in the index ray amputation already described. This smooths the ulnar border of the hand and is used most often as an elective procedure for a contracted or painful little finger.

THUMB AMPUTATIONS

In partial amputation of the thumb, in contrast to amputation of a single finger, reamputation at a more proximal level to obtain closure should not be considered because the thumb rarely should be shortened. The wound should be closed primarily by a free graft, an advancement pedicle flap (described later), or a local or distant flap.

If a flap is necessary, taking it from the dorsum of the hand or the index or middle finger is preferable. A flap from one of these areas provides a touch pad that is stable but that does not regain normal sensibility.

Covering the volar surface of the thumb with an abdominal flap is contraindicated; even when the flap is thin, abdominal skin and fat provide a poor surface for pinch because they lack fibrous septa and roll or shift under pressure. Skin of the abdomen is dissimilar in appearance to that of the hand and its digits. When the skin and pulp, including all neural elements, have been lost from a significant area of the thumb, a neurovascular island graft may be indicated. The defect should be closed primarily by a split-thickness graft; the neurovascular island graft or, if feasible, a local neurovascular island graft or advancement flap as described for fingertip amputations (see Technique 16.1) is applied secondarily.

If the thumb has been amputated so that a useful segment of the proximal phalanx remains, the only surgery necessary, if any, except for primary closure of the wound is deepening the thumb web by Z-plasty. When amputation has been at the metacarpophalangeal joint or at a more proximal level, reconstruction of the thumb may be indicated (see Technique 16.15) if replantation cannot be accomplished.

ADVANCEMENT PEDICLE FLAP FOR THUMB INJURIES

Advancement flaps for fingertip injuries usually survive if the volar flap incisions are not brought proximal to the proximal interphalangeal joint. In the thumb, the venous drainage is not as dependent on the volar flap, however, and this technique is safer, and the flap can be longer (Fig. 16.21).

TECHNIQUE 16.12

- Using tourniquet control and appropriate anesthesia, make a midlateral incision on each side of the thumb from the tip to the metacarpophalangeal joint (Fig. 16.22A).
- Elevate the flap that contains both neurovascular bundles without disturbing the flexor tendon sheath (Fig. 16.22B).
- Flex the joints to allow the flap to be advanced and carefully sutured over the defect with interrupted sutures (Fig. 16.22C).

POSTOPERATIVE CARE The joints should be maintained in flexion postoperatively for 3 weeks. This large flap is used only when a large area of thumb pulp is lost.

AMPUTATIONS OF MULTIPLE DIGITS

In nonreplantable partial amputations of all fingers, preserving the remaining length of the digits is much more important than in a single finger amputation. Because of the natural hinge action between the first and fifth metacarpals, any remaining stump of the little finger must play an important role in prehension with the intact thumb, and

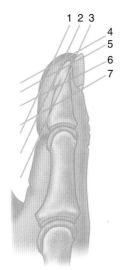

Thumb tip amputation levels. Acceptable procedures by level are *1*, split-thickness graft; *2*, cross-finger flap or advancement flap; *3*, advancement flap, cross-finger flap, or shorten thumb and close; *4*, split-thickness skin graft; *5*, shorten bone and split-thickness skin graft, advancement flap, or cross-finger flap; *6*, advancement flap or cross-finger flap; and *7*, advancement flap and removal of nail bed remnant. **SEE TECHNIQUE 16.12.**

this hinge action can be increased about 50% by dividing the transverse metacarpal ligament between the fourth and fifth rays. In partial amputation of all fingers and the thumb, function can be improved by lengthening the digits relatively and by increasing their mobility. Function of the thumb can be improved by deepening its web by Z-plasty and by osteotomizing the first and fifth metacarpals and rotating their distal fragments toward each other (Fig. 16.23) while, if helpful, tilting the fifth metacarpal toward the thumb. If the first carpometacarpal joint is functional but the first metacarpal is quite short, the second metacarpal can be transposed to the first to lengthen it and to widen and deepen the first web.

In complete amputation of all fingers, if the intact thumb cannot easily reach the fifth metacarpal head, phalangization of the fifth metacarpal is helpful. In this operation, the fourth metacarpal is resected and the fifth is osteotomized, rotated, and separated from the rest of the palm. Lengthening of the fifth metacarpal is also helpful. In complete amputation of all fingers and the thumb in which the amputation has been transverse through the metacarpal necks, phalangization of selected metacarpals can improve function. The fourth metacarpal is resected to increase the range of motion of the fifth, and function of the fifth metacarpal is improved further by osteotomy of the metacarpal in which the distal fragment is rotated radialward and flexed. The second metacarpal is resected at its base, but to preserve the origin of the adductor pollicis, the third metacarpal is not resected. The thumb should not be lengthened by osteoplastic reconstruction unless sensibility can be added to its volar surface. When the amputation has been through the middle of the metacarpal shafts, prehension probably cannot be restored, but hook can be accomplished by flexing the stump at the wrist. This motion at the wrist can be made even more useful by fitting an artificial platform to which the palmar surface of the stump can be actively opposed.

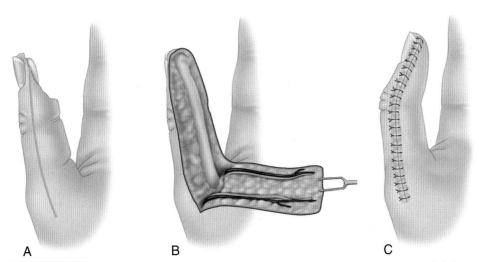

Advancement pedicle flap for thumb injuries. **A,** Deep thumb pad defects exposing bone can be covered with advancement pedicle flap. **B,** Advancement of neurovascular pedicle. **C,** Flexion of distal joint of thumb is necessary to permit placement of flap (see text). **SEE TECHNIQUE 16.12.**

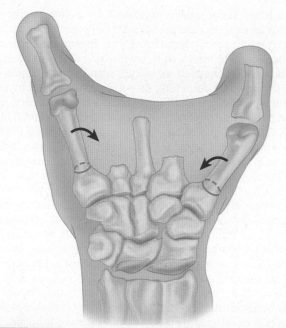

FIGURE 16.23 In multiple amputations including thumb, function can be improved by osteotomizing first and fifth metacarpals and rotating their distal fragments toward each other (see text).

PHALANGIZATION OF FIFTH METACARPAL

TECHNIQUE 16.13

- Over the fourth metacarpal, make dorsal and volar longitudinal incisions that join distally.
- Expose and resect the transverse metacarpal ligament on each side of the fourth metacarpal head.
- Divide proximally the digital nerves to the ring finger and ligate and divide the corresponding vessels.
- Resect the fourth metacarpal shaft just distal to its carpometacarpal joint. Through the same incision, osteotomize the fifth metacarpal near its base.
- Slightly abduct and flex the distal fragment and rotate it toward the thumb. Fix the fragments with a Kirschner wire.
- Cover the raw surfaces between the third and fifth metacarpals with split-thickness grafts, creating a web at the junction of the proximal and middle thirds of the bones. Ensure that the padding over the fifth metacarpal head is good and, if possible, that sensation is normal at its point of maximal contact with the thumb.

PAINFUL AMPUTATION STUMP

Revision surgery is a frequent elective procedure for the management of painful amputation stumps, especially those resulting from traumatic injuries. Revision rates can be influenced by finger involvement, mechanism of injury, or workman's compensation status of the patient. A neuroma located in an unpadded area near the end of the stump is the usual cause of pain. Symptomatic neuromas occur in approximately 7% of traumatic amputations and are most common in the index finger and avulsion type injuries. A well-localized area of extreme tenderness associated with a small mass, usually in line with a digital nerve, is diagnostic. Some painful neuromas can be treated by padding and desensitization, although surgical excision frequently is required. The neuroma is dissected free from scar, and the nerve is divided at a more proximal level. Another neuroma will develop but should be painless when located in a padded area. Suturing the radial and ulnar digital nerves end to end (compared with proximal resection as mentioned previously) has not been shown to reduce resting pain, cold intolerance, or perceived tenderness. Reduction in tenderness is achieved by this end-to-end nerve union, but at the expense of touch sensibility.

Pain in an amputation stump can also be caused by bony prominences covered only by thin skin, such as a split-thickness graft, or by skin made tight by scarring. In these instances, excising the thin skin or scar, shortening the bone, and applying a sufficiently padded graft may be indicated. Amputation stumps that are painful because of thin skin coverage at the pulp and nail junction can be improved by using a limited advancement flap as described in the section on thumb amputations. In the finger, proximal dissection to develop these flaps should not extend proximal to the proximal interphalangeal joint.

Finally, painful cramping sensations in the hand and forearm can be caused by flexion contracture of a stump resulting from overstretching of extensor tendons or adherence of flexor tendons; release of any adherent tendons is helpful.

RECONSTRUCTIONS AFTER AMPUTATION

RECONSTRUCTION AFTER AMPUTATION OF THE HAND

Hand amputation is an extremely disabling injury. In most patients, when replantation is not possible, prosthetic use is required. The field of prosthetics and orthotics is ever advancing. With new developments in 3D printing, myoelectric prosthetics, and groundbreaking operations, such as targeted muscle reinnervation or the starfish procedure, patients have shown significant improvements in use and function. For patients with bilateral hand amputations, advances in transplantation are continually being made. However, transplantation is not yet commonplace except at a few centers in the United States, and prosthetic use still remains the standard of care.

In selected patients, the Krukenberg operation is helpful. It converts the forearm to forceps in which the radial ray acts against the ulnar ray. Swanson compared function of the reconstructed limb with the use of chopsticks. Normal sensibility between the tips of the rays is ensured by proper shifting of skin during closure of the wound. The operation is especially helpful in blind patients with bilateral amputations because it provides not only prehension but also sensibility at the terminal parts of the limb. It is also helpful in other patients with similar amputations, especially in surroundings where modern prosthetic services are unavailable. According to Swanson, children with bilateral congenital amputation find the reconstructed limb much more useful than a mechanical prosthesis; they transfer dominance to this limb when a prosthesis is used on the opposite one. In children, the appearance of the limb after surgery has not been distressing, and the operation does not prevent the wearing of an ordinary prosthesis if desired.

KRUKENBERG RECONSTRUCTION

TECHNIQUE 16.14

(KRUKENBERG; SWANSON)
- Make a longitudinal incision on the flexor surface of the forearm slightly toward the radial side (Fig. 16.24A). Make

a similar incision on the dorsal surface slightly toward the ulnar side, but on this surface elevate a V-shaped flap to form a web at the junction of the rays (Fig. 16.24B).
- Separate the forearm muscles into two groups (Fig. 16.24C, D): The radial side comprises the radial wrist flexors and extensors, the radial half of the flexor digitorum sublimis, the radial half of the extensor digitorum communis, the brachioradialis, the palmaris longus, and the pronator teres; the ulnar side comprises the ulnar wrist flexors and extensors, the ulnar half of the flexor digitorum sublimis, and the ulnar half of the extensor digitorum communis. If the stump is made too bulky or the wound hard to close, resect as necessary the pronator quadratus, the flexor digitorum profundus, the flexor pollicis longus,

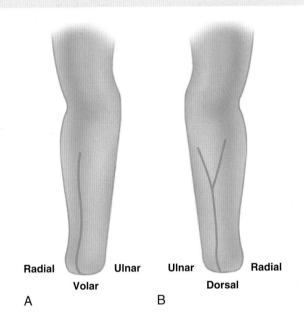

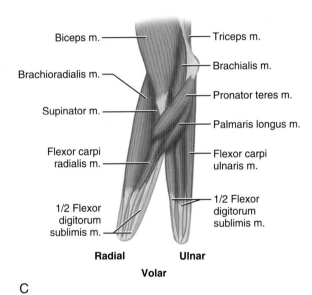

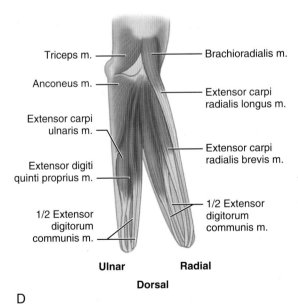

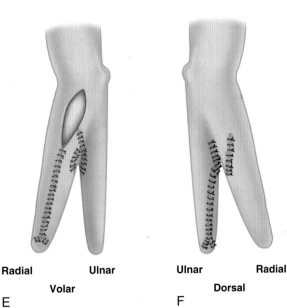

FIGURE 16.24 Krukenberg operation. A, Incision on flexor surface of forearm. B, Incision on dorsal surface (see text). C and D, Forearm muscles have been separated into two groups (see text). E, Closure of skin on flexor surface of forearm; the area yet to be closed indicates location of any needed split-thickness skin graft. F, Closure of skin on dorsal surface (see text). SEE TECHNIQUE 16.14.

the abductor pollicis longus, and the extensor pollicis brevis. Take care not to disturb the pronator teres.

■ Incise the interosseous membrane throughout its length along its ulnar attachment, taking care not to damage the interosseous vessel and nerve.

■ The radial and ulnar rays can be separated 6 to 12 cm at their tips depending on the size of the forearm; motion at their proximal ends occurs at the radiohumeral and proximal radioulnar joints. The opposing ends of the rays should touch; if not, osteotomize the radius or ulna as necessary. Now the adductors of the radial ray are the pronator teres, the supinator, the flexor carpi radialis, the radial half of the flexor digitorum sublimis, and the palmaris longus; the abductors of the radial ray are the brachioradialis, the extensor carpi radialis longus, the extensor carpi radialis brevis, the radial half of the extensor digitorum communis, and the biceps. The adductors of the ulnar ray are the flexor carpi ulnaris, the ulnar half of the flexor digitorum sublimis, the brachialis, and the anconeus; the abductors of the ulnar ray are the extensor carpi ulnaris, the ulnar half of the extensor digitorum communis, and the triceps.

■ Remove the tourniquet, obtain hemostasis, and observe the circulation in the flaps.

■ Excise any excess fat, rotate the skin around each ray, and close the skin over each so that the suture line is not on the opposing surface of either (Fig. 16.24E, F).

■ Excise any scarred skin at the ends of the rays and, if necessary to permit closure, shorten the bones; in children, the skin usually is sufficient for closure, and the bones must not be shortened because growth at the distal epiphyses would still be incomplete.

■ Preserve any remaining rudimentary digit. Next, suture the flap in place at the junction of the rays and apply any needed split-thickness graft.

■ Insert small rubber drains and, with the tips of the rays separated 6 cm or more, apply a compression dressing.

POSTOPERATIVE CARE The limb is continuously elevated for 3 to 4 days. The sutures are removed at the usual time. After 2 to 3 weeks, rehabilitation is begun to develop abduction and adduction of the rays.

RECONSTRUCTION AFTER AMPUTATION OF MULTIPLE DIGITS

Several reconstructive operations are useful after amputation of multiple digits at various levels. After soft-tissue stabilization is achieved, digital lengthening by callotasis is an option. Thumb pollicization may be required when transposition of remaining digits permits. Restoration of opposition by sensate opposable digits often necessitates a protracted reconstructive course that challenges the creativity of the surgeon and patience of the patient.

RECONSTRUCTION OF THE THUMB

Traumatic or congenital absence of the thumb causes a severe deficiency in hand function; such an absence usually is considered to constitute a 40% disability of the hand as a whole. When the thumb is partially or totally absent, reconstructive surgery is appealing. Before any decision for surgery is made,

however, several factors must be considered, including the length of any remaining part of the thumb, the condition of the rest of the hand, the occupational requirements and age of the patient, and the knowledge and experience of the surgeon. If the opposite thumb is normal, some surgeons question the need for reconstructing even a totally absent thumb. Function of the hand can be improved, however, by a carefully planned and skillfully executed operation, especially in a young patient.

Usually the thumb should be reconstructed only when amputation has been at the metacarpophalangeal joint or at a more proximal level. When this joint and a useful segment of the proximal phalanx remain, the only surgery necessary, if any, is deepening of the thumb web by Z-plasty. When amputation has been through the interphalangeal joint, the distal phalanx, or the pulp of the thumb, only appropriate coverage by skin is necessary, unless sensibility in the area of pinch is grossly impaired. In this latter instance, a more elaborate coverage, such as by a neurovascular island transfer, may be indicated.

A reconstructed thumb must meet five requirements. First and most important, sensibility, although not necessarily normal, should be painless and sufficient for recognition of objects held in the position of pinch. Second, the thumb should have sufficient stability so that pinch pressure does not cause the thumb joints to deviate or collapse or cause the skin pad to shift. Third, there should be sufficient mobility to enable the hand to flatten and the thumb to oppose for pinch. Fourth, the thumb should be of sufficient length to enable the opposing digital tips to touch it. Sometimes amputation or stiffness of the remaining digits may require greater than normal length of the thumb to accomplish prehension. Fifth, the thumb should be cosmetically acceptable because if it is not it may remain hidden and not be used.

Several reconstructive procedures are possible, and the choice depends on the length of the stump remaining and the sensibility of the remaining thumb pad (Figs. 16.25 and 16.26). The thumb can be lengthened by a short bone graft or distraction osteoplasty. In the face of an adjacent mangled finger, an "on-top plasty" can be considered. Sensibility can be restored by skin rotation flaps, with the nonopposing surface skin grafted as in the Gillies-Millard "cocked hat" procedure. Another possibility is pollicizing a digit. A promising possibility is microvascular free transfer of a toe to the hand.

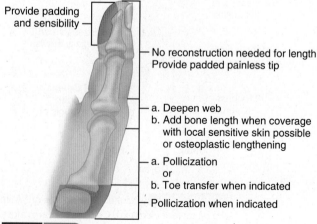

Provide padding and sensibility

No reconstruction needed for length
Provide padded painless tip

a. Deepen web
b. Add bone length when coverage with local sensitive skin possible or osteoplastic lengthening

a. Pollicization
or
b. Toe transfer when indicated

Pollicization when indicated

FIGURE 16.25 Thumb reconstruction at various levels. Basic needs are sensibility, stability, mobility, and length.

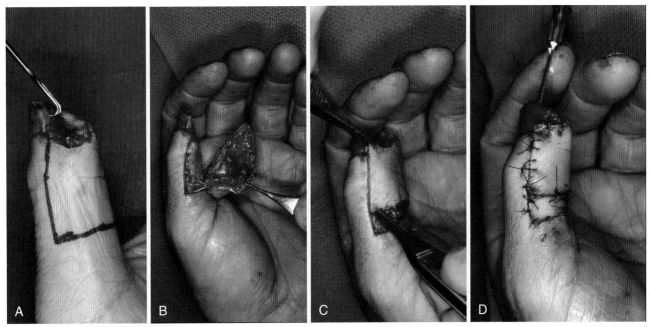

FIGURE 16.26 Moberg advancement flap. **A,** Thumb pulp defect with flap outlined. **B,** Flap raised on bilateral neurovascular pedicles. **C,** Flap advanced 1.5 cm. **D,** Flap sutured into position with hypothenar free full-thickness skin flap at flap base.

TABLE 16.1

Lister Classification

GROUPS	AMPUTATION	RECONSTRUCTION OPTIONS
Group 1	Acceptable length and poor soft-tissue coverage	*Glabrous:* Moberg advancement; V-Y advancement; NV island; free flap, free toe pulp transfer *Nonglabrous:* FDMA flap; distal free flap (PIA; RFF; groin flap)
Group 2	Subtotal amputation with questionable length	First web deepening; rotational flaps; ectopic banking or ectopic replantation, rigid or free flaps; distraction osteogenesis
Group 3	Total amputation with preservation of basal joint	Toe transfer; metacarpal lengthening (distraction osteogenesis); osteoplastic reconstruction; pollicization
Group 4	Total amputation with absence of basal joint	Toe transfer; pollicization

FDMA, First dorsal metacarpal artery; *PIA,* posterior interosseous flap; *RFF,* radial forearm flap.

In this procedure, sensory restoration is never normal. The osteoplastic technique with a bone graft and tube pedicle skin graft supplemented by a neurovascular pedicle is now rarely recommended. Lister's classification is useful in selecting appropriate treatment (Table 16.1).

Pollicization also is a viable option for thumb reconstruction (Techniques 16.17 to 16.19).

LENGTHENING OF THE METACARPAL AND TRANSFER OF LOCAL FLAP

When amputation of the thumb has been at the metacarpophalangeal joint or within the condylar area of the first metacarpal, the thenar muscles are able to stabilize the digit. In these instances, lengthening of the metacarpal by bone grafting and transfer of a local skin flap may be indicated. The technique as described by Gillies and Millard can be completed in one stage, and the time required for surgery and convalescence is less than in some other reconstructions. Disadvantages of this procedure include bone graft resorption and ray shortening and skin perforation after flap contraction. This procedure requires that there be minimal scarring of the amputated stump.

TECHNIQUE 16.15

(GILLIES AND MILLARD, MODIFIED)

- Make a curved incision around the dorsal, radial, and volar aspects of the base of the thumb (Fig. 16.27A).
- Undermine the skin distally, but stay superficial to the main veins to prevent congestion of the flap. Continue the undermining until a hollow flap has been elevated and slipped off the end of the stump; the blood supply to the flap is from a source around the base of the index finger in the thumb web. (If desired, complete elevation of the flap can be delayed.)

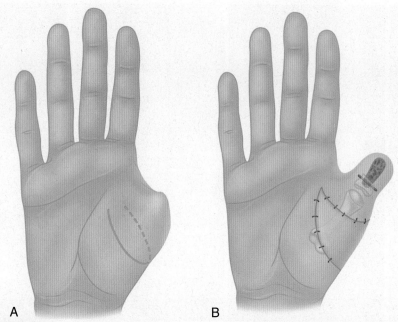

FIGURE 16.27 Reconstruction of thumb by technique of Gillies and Millard, modified. **A,** Outline of curved incision around dorsal, radial, and volar aspects of base of thumb. **B,** Hollow flap has been undermined and elevated, iliac bone graft has been fixed (this time to base of proximal phalanx), and raw area at base of thumb has been covered by split-thickness skin graft. **SEE TECHNIQUE 16.15.**

- Attach an iliac bone graft or a phalanx excised from a toe to the distal end of the metacarpal by tapering the graft and fitting it into a hole in the end of the metacarpal.
- Fix the graft to the bone by a Kirschner wire and place iliac chips around its base. Ensure that the graft is small enough that the flap can be placed easily over it.
- Cover the raw area at the base of the thumb by a split-thickness skin graft (Fig. 16.27B).

POSTOPERATIVE CARE The newly constructed thumb is immobilized by a supportive dressing, and a volar plaster splint is applied to the palm and forearm. The Kirschner wire is removed when the graft has united with the metacarpal. Minor Z-plasties may be necessary later to relieve the volar and dorsal web formed by advancing the flap.

OSTEOPLASTIC RECONSTRUCTION AND TRANSFER OF NEUROVASCULAR ISLAND GRAFT

Verdan recommended osteoplastic reconstruction, especially when the first carpometacarpal joint has been spared and is functional. It is a useful method when the remaining part of the first metacarpal is short. As in the technique of Gillies and Millard, no finger is endangered, and all are spared to function against the reconstructed thumb. Transfer of a neurovascular island graft supplies discrete sensibility to the new thumb, but precise sensory reorientation is always lacking (Fig. 16.28).

TECHNIQUE 16.16

(VERDAN)
- Raise the subpectoral region, or some other appropriate area a tubed pedicle graft that contains only moderate subcutaneous fat, from the abdomen.
- Excise the skin and subcutaneous tissue over the distal end of the first metacarpal; make this area for implantation of the tubed graft a long oval and as large as possible so that the graft can include many vessels and nerves and will not constrict later.
- Insert into the end of the first metacarpal an iliac bone graft shaped like a palette to imitate the normal thumb. Do not place the graft in line with the first metacarpal, but rather place it at an obtuse angle in the direction of opposition. Ensure that the graft is not too long. Place the end of the tubed pedicle over the bone graft and suture it to its prepared bed on the thumb.
- Immobilize the hand and tubed pedicle to allow normal motion of the fingers and some motion of the shoulder and elbow.
- After 3 to 4 weeks, free the tubed pedicle.
- Close the skin over the distal end of the newly constructed thumb, or transfer a neurovascular island graft from an appropriate area to the volar aspect of the thumb to assist in closure and to improve sensation and circulation in the digit.

POSTOPERATIVE CARE A supportive dressing and a volar plaster splint are applied. The newly constructed thumb is protected for about 8 weeks to prevent or decrease

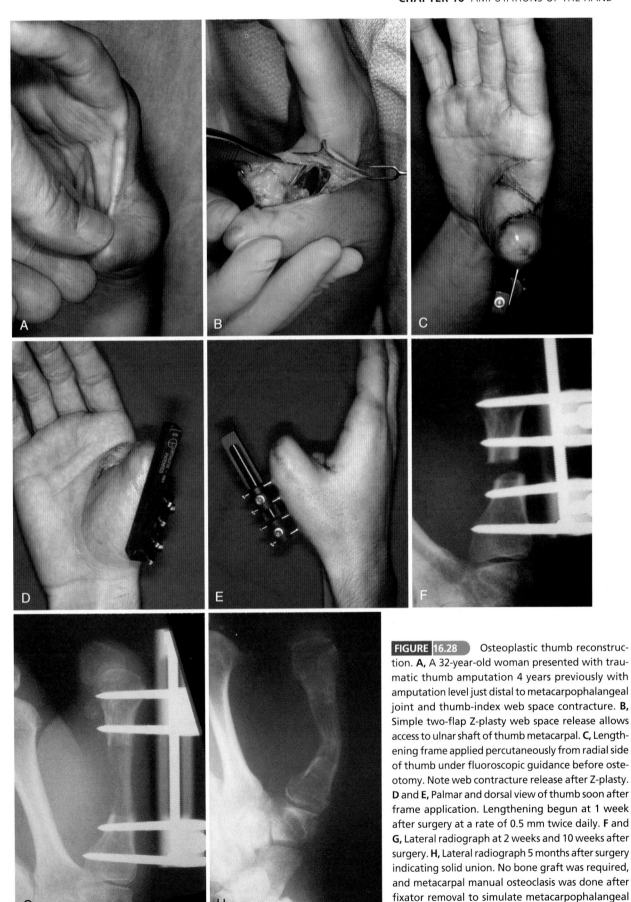

FIGURE 16.28 Osteoplastic thumb reconstruction. **A,** A 32-year-old woman presented with traumatic thumb amputation 4 years previously with amputation level just distal to metacarpophalangeal joint and thumb-index web space contracture. **B,** Simple two-flap Z-plasty web space release allows access to ulnar shaft of thumb metacarpal. **C,** Lengthening frame applied percutaneously from radial side of thumb under fluoroscopic guidance before osteotomy. Note web contracture release after Z-plasty. **D and E,** Palmar and dorsal view of thumb soon after frame application. Lengthening begun at 1 week after surgery at a rate of 0.5 mm twice daily. **F and G,** Lateral radiograph at 2 weeks and 10 weeks after surgery. **H,** Lateral radiograph 5 months after surgery indicating solid union. No bone graft was required, and metacarpal manual osteoclasis was done after fixator removal to simulate metacarpophalangeal joint fusion. **SEE TECHNIQUE 16.16.**

resorption of the bone graft. If a neurovascular island graft was not included in the reconstruction, this transfer must be done later.

■ POLLICIZATION

Pollicization (transposition of a finger to replace an absent thumb) may endanger the transposed finger; therefore, some surgeons recommend transposition only of an already shortened or otherwise damaged finger. When amputation has been traumatic, extensive scarring may require resurfacing by a pedicle skin graft before pollicization. In such instances, full function of the new thumb hardly can be expected; indeed full function cannot be expected even after successful transposition of a normal finger. However, in amputations near the carpometacarpal joint, especially in patients with significant bilateral thumb-level amputations, pollicization may be of benefit.

In the hands of an experienced surgeon, pollicization is worthwhile, especially in *pouce flottant* (floating thumb) and congenital absence of a thumb, assuming that the digit to be pollicized is relatively normal. Pollicization is performed when the child is 9 to 12 months of age; however, when the thumb is congenitally absent, the age of pollicization is not as important as a cerebral cortex awareness of a radial opposition post.

RIORDAN POLLICIZATION

In the Riordan technique, the index ray is shortened by resection of its metacarpal shaft. To simulate the trapezium, the second metacarpal head is positioned palmar to the normal plane of the metacarpal bases, and the metacarpophalangeal joint acts as the carpometacarpal joint of the new thumb. The first dorsal interosseous is converted to an abductor pollicis brevis, and the first volar interosseous is converted to an adductor pollicis. The technique as described is for an immature hand with congenital absence of the thumb, including the greater multangular, but it can be modified appropriately for other hands.

TECHNIQUE 16.17

(RIORDAN)
- Beginning on the proximal phalanx of the index finger, make a circumferential oval incision (Fig. 16.29A, B) on the dorsal surface.
- Place the incision level with the middle of the phalanx and on the palmar surface level with the base of the phalanx. From the radiopalmar aspect of this oval, extend the incision proximally, radially, and dorsally to the radial side of the second metacarpal head, then palmarward and ulnarward to the radial side of the third metacarpal base in the middle of the palm, and finally again radially to end at the radial margin of the base of the palm.

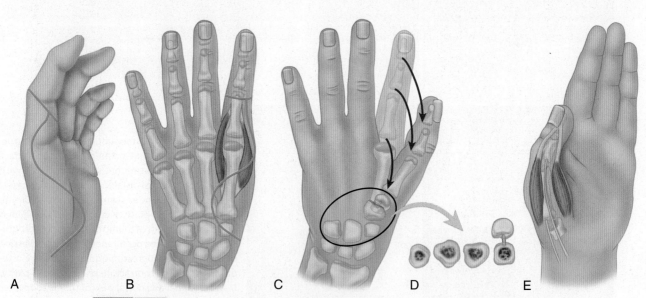

FIGURE 16.29 Riordan pollicization for congenital absence of thumb, including greater trapezium, in an immature hand. **A** and **B**, Incision (see text). Skin of proximal phalanx (*pink area* in **A**) is elevated as full-thickness skin flap. **C** and **D**, Second metacarpal has been resected by dividing base proximally and by cutting through epiphysis distally, and finger has been relocated proximally and radially. Second metacarpal head has been anchored palmar to second metacarpal base and simulates greater trapezium (see text). **E**, Insertion of first dorsal interosseous has been anchored to radial lateral band of extensor mechanism of new thumb and origin to soft tissues at base of digit; insertion of first volar interosseous has been anchored to opposite lateral band and origin to soft tissues. **SEE TECHNIQUE 16.17.**

- Dissect the skin from the proximal phalanx of the index finger, leaving the fat attached to the digit and creating a full-thickness skin flap.
- Isolate and free the insertion of the first dorsal interosseous and strip from the radial side of the second metacarpal shaft the origin of the muscle.
- Isolate and free the insertion of the first volar interosseous and strip from the ulnar side of the metacarpal shaft the origin of this muscle. Take care to preserve the nerve and blood supplies to the muscle in each instance.
- Separate the second metacarpal head from the metacarpal shaft by cutting through its epiphysis with a knife; preserve all of its soft-tissue attachments.
- Divide the second metacarpal at its base, leaving intact the insertions of the extensor carpi radialis longus and flexor carpi radialis; discard the metacarpal shaft.
- Carry the index finger proximally and radially and relocate the second metacarpal head palmar to the second metacarpal base so that it simulates a trapezium (Fig. 16.29C); take care to rotate and angulate it so that the new thumb is properly positioned.
- Anchor it in this position with a wire suture (Fig. 16.29D). Anchor the insertion of the first dorsal interosseous to the radial lateral band of the extensor mechanism of the new thumb and its origin to the soft tissues at the base of the digit; this muscle now functions as an abductor pollicis brevis (Fig. 16.29E).
- Anchor the insertion of the first volar interosseous to the opposite lateral band and its origin to the soft tissues; this muscle now functions as an adductor pollicis.
- Shorten the extensor indicis proprius by resecting a segment of its tendon; this muscle now functions as an extensor pollicis brevis. Also, shorten the extensor digitorum communis by resecting a segment of its tendon.
- Anchor the proximal segment of the tendon to the base of the proximal phalanx; this muscle now functions as an abductor pollicis longus.
- Trim the skin flaps appropriately; fashion the palmar flap so that when sutured it places sufficient tension on the new thumb to hold it in opposition.
- Suture the flaps, but avoid a circumferential closure at the base of the new thumb.
- Apply a pressure dressing of wet cotton and a plaster cast.

POSTOPERATIVE CARE At 3 weeks, the cast is removed and motion therapy is begun. The thumb is appropriately splinted.

BUCK-GRAMCKO POLLICIZATION

Buck-Gramcko reported experience with 100 operations for pollicization of the index finger in children with congenital absence or marked hypoplasia of the thumb. He emphasized a reduction in length of the pollicized digit trapezium. For best results, the index finger has to be rotated initially approximately 160 degrees during the operation so that it is opposite the pulp of the ring finger. This position changes during the suturing of the muscles and the skin so that by the end of the operation there is rotation of approximately 120 degrees. In addition, the pollicized digit is angulated approximately 40 degrees into palmar abduction.

TECHNIQUE 16.18

(BUCK-GRAMCKO)
- Make an S-shaped incision down the radial side of the hand just onto the palmar surface.
- Begin the incision near the base of the index finger on the palmar aspect and end it just proximal to the wrist. Make a slightly curved transverse incision across the base of the index finger on the palmar surface, connecting at right angles to the distal end of the first incision. Connect both ends of the incision on the dorsum of the hand (Fig. 16.30A). Make a third incision on the dorsum of the proximal phalanx of the index finger from the proximal interphalangeal joint extending proximally to end at the incision around the base of the index finger (Fig. 16.30B).
- Through the palmar incision, free the neurovascular bundle between the index and middle fingers by ligating the artery to the radial side of the middle finger.
- Separate the common digital nerve carefully into its component parts for the two adjacent fingers so that no tension is present after the index finger is rotated.
- Sometimes an anomalous neural ring is found around the artery; split this ring carefully so that angulation of the artery after transposition of the finger does not occur. If the radial digital artery to the index finger is absent, it is possible to perform the pollicization on a vascular pedicle of only one artery. On the dorsal side, preserve at least one of the great veins.
- On the dorsum of the hand, sever the tendon of the extensor digitorum communis at the metacarpophalangeal level.
- Detach the interosseous muscles of the index finger from the proximal phalanx and the lateral bands of the dorsal aponeurosis.
- Partially subperiosteally strip the origins of the interosseous muscles from the second metacarpal, being careful to preserve the neurovascular structures.
- Osteotomize and resect the second metacarpal. If the phalanges of the index finger are of normal length, the whole metacarpal is resected with the exception of its head. When the phalanges are relatively short, the base of the metacarpal must be retained to obtain the proper length of the new thumb.
- When the entire metacarpal is resected except for the head, rotate the head as shown in and attach it by sutures to the joint capsule of the carpus and to the carpal bones (Fig. 16.30E), which in young children can be pierced with a sharp needle.
- Rotate the digit 160 degrees to allow opposition (Fig. 16.30F).
- Bony union is not essential, and fibrous fixation of the head is sufficient for good function. When the base of the metacarpal is retained, fix the metacarpal head to its base with one or two Kirschner wires in the previously described position. In attaching the metacarpal head, bring the proximal phalanx into complete hyperextension in relation to the metacarpal head for maximal stability of

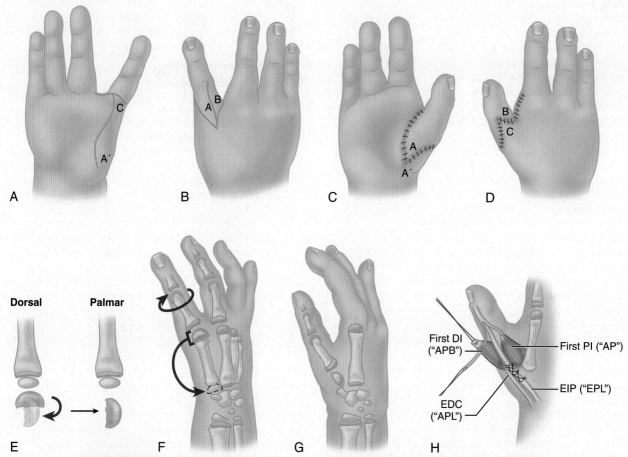

FIGURE 16.30 Pollicization of index finger. **A** and **B,** Palmar and dorsal skin incisions. **C** and **D,** Appearance after wound closure. **E,** Rotation of metacarpal head into flexion to prevent postoperative hyperextension. **F,** Index finger rotated about 160 degrees along long axis to place finger pulp into position of opposition. **G,** Final position of skeleton in about 40 degrees of palmar abduction with metacarpal head secured to metacarpal base or carpus. **H,** Reattachment of tendons to provide control of new thumb. First palmar interosseous *(PI)* functions as adductor pollicis *(AP),* first dorsal interosseous *(DI)* functions as abductor pollicis brevis *(APB),* extensor digitorum communis *(EDC)* functions as abductor pollicis longus *(APL),* and extensor indicis proprius *(EIP)* functions as extensor pollicis longus *(EPL).* **SEE TECHNIQUE 16.18.**

the joint. Unless this is done, hyperextension is likely at the new "carpometacarpal" joint (Fig. 16.30G).

- Suture the proximal end of the detached extensor digitorum communis tendon to the base of the former proximal phalanx (now acting as the first metacarpal) to become the new "abductor pollicis longus."
- Section the extensor indicis proprius tendon, shorten it appropriately, and suture it by end-to-end anastomosis.
- Suture the tendinous insertions of the two interosseous muscles to the lateral bands of the dorsal aponeurosis by weaving the lateral bands through the distal part of the interosseous muscle and turning them back distally to form a loop that is sutured to itself. In this way, the first palmar interosseous becomes an "adductor pollicis" and the first dorsal interosseous becomes an "abductor brevis" (Fig. 16.30H).
- Close the wound by fashioning a dorsal skin flap to close the defect over the proximal phalanx and fashion the rest

of the flaps as necessary for skin closure as in Fig. 16.30C and D.

POSTOPERATIVE CARE The hand is immobilized for 3 weeks, and then careful active motion is begun.

FOUCHER POLLICIZATION

Despite good sensibility, mobility, growth, and integration of pollicized digits, grip and pinch strength reduction (55% and 42% of the uninvolved side, respectively) have prompted technique modifications. Weakness in abduction and adduction as well as the slenderness and cleftlike appearance of the pollicized digit are corrected with the Foucher technique.

■ Outline the incisions on the index finger and palm (Fig. 16.31A). Line *AB,* as depicted in Fig. 16.31A, is situated on the midlateral line and crosses the proximal interphalangeal joint. Line *DE* is on the volar aspect of the index-middle web, and line *EF* is volar to the midlateral line elongating the web incision. Line *F* is more distal than line *A.* Line *GHI* is a longitudinal incision to the volar wrist crease. Begin the dissection volarly to allow refilling of the dorsal veins and simplify the dorsal dissection. Elevate the arteries and veins, noting absence or hypoplasia of the radial digital artery. Preserve the fat around the digital arteries to protect the small vena comitantes. Divide the radial digital artery to the middle finger and be aware of the Hartmann boutonniere deformity (nerve loop around artery). Divide the intermetacarpal ligament and resect the lumbrical.

■ Dissect the first dorsal interosseous muscle from distal to proximal to avoid denervation.

■ Begin the dorsal dissection over the proximal interphalangeal joint and preserve the veins and sensory branches. Expose the extensor mechanism. Longitudinally separate the extensor indicis proprius and extensor indicis communis and extensor digitorum communis tendons along the length of the proximal phalanx to form two separate bands that are sectioned at the proximal phalangeal base.

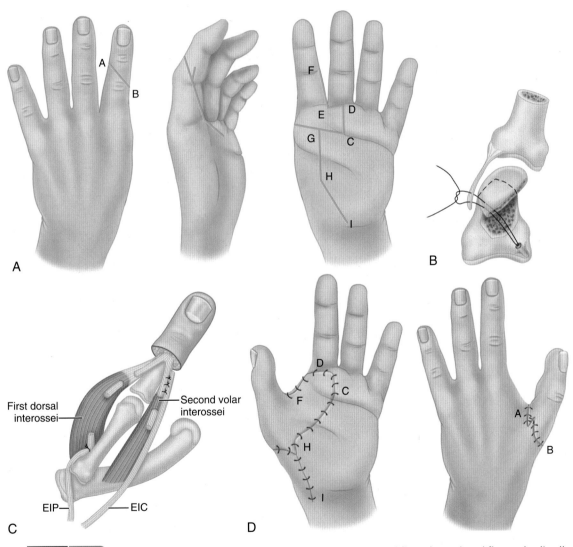

FIGURE 16.31 Foucher index pollicization. **A,** Proposed skin incisions providing a large dorsal flap and a distally based palmar flap, which provide a more weblike fold. **B,** Metacarpal head rotated into flexion and fixed into the metacarpal base with a bone anchor. **C,** New thumb balanced by tendon transfers; adduction is provided by the extensor indicis communis *(EIC),* second volar interosseous muscle (2nd VI), and adductor pollicis (not shown), and abduction is provided by extensor indicis proprius *(EIP)* and first dorsal interosseous muscle (1st DI). **D,** Sutured skin flaps showing weblike space between new thumb and middle finger and circular scar prevention by the radially based Z-plasty.

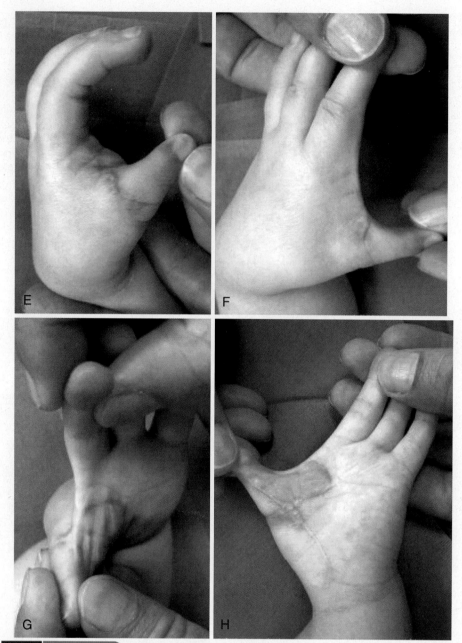

FIGURE 16.31, Cont'd   **E-H,** New thumb at 3 months postoperatively. (**E,** From Foucher G, Medina J, Lorea P, Pivato G: Principalization of pollicization of the index finger in congenital absence of the thumb, *Tech Hand Upper Extr Surg* 9:96, 2005.) **SEE TECHNIQUE 16.19.**

- Separate the metacarpal head from its shaft through the physis, which is destroyed by curettage to prevent overgrowth of the pollicized finger. Dissect the first palmar osseous muscle from the index metacarpal shaft and remove the shaft by sectioning the bone with a palmar slope at its base. Maintain 1 cm of bone at the metacarpal base to preserve the flexor carpi radialis and extensor carpi radialis longus insertions. If present, destroy the pseudoepiphysis at the metacarpal base and open the base like a flower to provide stability for the metacarpal head. Shift the metacarpal head onto the metacarpal base and avoid kinking of the vessels. Rotate the metacarpal head to allow

opposition and fix in flexion to prevent hyperextension of the new carpometacarpal joint (Fig. 16.31B). A suture anchor may facilitate this fixation.
- Next, balance the thumb through tendon transfers (Fig. 16.31C). To provide adduction strength, attach the hypoplastic adductor pollicis, which is often present, to the extensor indicis communis and attach the second palmar interosseous muscles to the distal tendon ulnar slip.
- Abduction and pronation are achieved by transfer of the extensor indicis proprius (through a proximoradial fibrous sling of the first dorsal interosseous muscle) and the first dorsal interosseous muscle to the radial half of the distal

tendon slip over the proximal phalanx. The thumb should rest in 135 degrees of pronation and 45 degrees of palmar abduction.

- Suture the skin, maintaining some tension on the dorsal web fold from the dorsal flap. To prevent circular scarring, make a Z-plasty on the radial aspect of the thumb (Figs. 16.31D, E).

POSTOPERATIVE CARE A fluffy dressing is placed in the new web space, and a drop of superglue maintains contact between the new thumb and middle finger. A dorsal plaster shell is applied, incorporating the elbow with two straps of Elastoplast to prevent escape. No therapy is used, and an opposition splint is used nightly for 2 months. Scar compression may be required if the pollicization is performed early because scar hypertrophy is more common in younger children. At 6 weeks if interphalangeal and metacarpophalangeal joint flexion are limited, a splint is worn for 1 h in the morning and evening until full active flexion is achieved (in 4 to 5 months).

REFERENCES

Barr JS, Chu MW, Thanik V, Sharma S: Pediatric thenar flaps: a modified design, case series and review of the literature, *J Pediatr Surg* 49:1433, 2014.

Borrelli MR, Dupré S, Mediratta S, et al.: Composite grafts for pediatric fingertip amputations: a retrospective case series of 100 patients, *Plast Reconstr Surg Glob Open* 6(6):e1843, 2018.

Chen S-Y, Wang CH, Fu J-P, et al.: Composite grafting for traumatic fingertip amputation in adults: technique reinforcement and experience in 31 digits, *J Trauma* 20:30, 2010.

Del Pinal F, Pennazzato D, Urrutia E: Primary thumb reconstruction in a mutilated hand, *Hand Clin* 32(4):519, 2016.

Fakin RM, Biraima A, Klein H, et al.: Primary functional and aesthetic restoration of the fingernail in distal fingertip amputations with the eponychial flap, *J Hand Surg Eur* 39:499, 2014.

Gil JA, Goodman AD, Harris AP, et al.: Cost-effectiveness of initial revision digit amputation performed in the emergency department versus the operating room, *Hand (NY)*. 1558944718790577, 2018.

Huang Y-C, Liu Y, Chen T-H: Use of homodigital reverse island flaps for distal digital reconstruction, *J Trauma* 68:429, 2010.

Hustedt JW, Chung A, Bohl DD, et al.: Evaluating the effect of comorbidities on the success, risk, and cost of digital replantation, *J Hand Surg Am* 41(12):1145, 2016.

Jones NF, Clune JE: Thumb amputations in children: classification and reconstruction by microsurgical toe transfers, *J Hand Surg Am* pii:S0363-5023(17)32129-9, 2018.

Krauss EM, Lalonde DH: Secondary healing of fingertip amputations: a review, *Hand* 9:282, 2014.

Manske PR: Index pollicisation for thumb deficiency, *Tech Hand Up Extrem Surg* 14(22), 2010.

Mahmoudi E, Huetteman HE, Chung KC: A population based study of replantation after traumatic thumb amputation 2007-2012, *J Hand Surg Am* 42(1):25, 2017.

Mattiassich G, Rittenschober F, Dorninger L, et al.: Long-term outcome following upper extremity replantation after major traumatic amputation, *BMC Musculoskelet Disord* 18(1):77, 2017.

Miller AJ, Rivlin M, Kirkpatrick W, et al.: Fingertip amputation treatment: a survey study, *Am J Orthop* 44(9):E331, 2015.

Morgan EN, Kyle Potter B, Souza JM, et al.: Targeted muscle reinnervation for transradial amputation: description of operative technique, *Tech Hand Up Extrem Surg* 20(4):166, 2016.

Nakanishi A, Kawamura K, Omokawa S, et al.: Predictors of hand dexterity after single-digit replantation, *J Reconstr Microsurg* 2018. [Epub ahead of print].

O'Brien MS, Singh N: Surgical technique utilizing suture-button device for central metacarpal ray, *J Hand Surg Am* 41(8):3247, 2016.

Paige DM, George JA, Kluger DT, et al.: Motor control and sensory feedback enhance prosthesis embodiment and reduce phantom pain after long-term hand amputation, *Front Hum Neurosci* 12:352, 2018.

Panattoni JB, De Ona IR, Ahmed MM: Reconstruction of fingertip injuries: surgical tips and avoiding complications, *J Hand Surg Am* 40(5):1016, 2015.

Pet MA, Morrison SD, Mack JS, et al.: Comparison of patient-reported outcomes after traumatic upper extremity amputation: replantation versus prosthetic rehabilitation, *Injury* 47(12):2783, 2016.

Peterson SL, Peterson EL, Wheatley MJ: Management of fingertip amputations, *J Hand Surg* 39:2093, 2014.

Pierrie SN, Gaston RG, Loeffler BJ: Current concepts in upper-extremity amputation, *J Hand Surg Am* 43(7):657–667, 2018.

Rabarin F, Sain Cast Y, Jeudy J, et al.: Cross-finger flap for reconstruction of fingertip amputations: long-term results, *Orthop Traumatol Surg Res* 102(Suppl 4):S225, 2016.

Salminger S, Roche AD, Sturma A, et al.: Hand transplantation versus hand prosthetics: pros and cons, *Curr Surg Rep* 4:8, 2016.

Shaterian A, Rajaii R, Kanack M, et al.: Predictors of digit survival following replantation: quantitative review and meta-analysis, *J Hand Microsurg* 10(2):66, 2018.

Sindhu K, DeFroda SF, Harris AP, Gil JA: Management of partial fingertip amputation in adults: operative and nonoperative treatment, *Injury* 48(12):2643, 2017.

Solarz MK, Thoder JJ, Rehman S: Management of major traumatic upper extremity amputations, *Orthop Clin North Am* 47(1):127, 2016.

Tatebe M, Urata S, Tanaka K, et al.: Survival rate of limb replantation in different age groups, *J Hand Microsurg* 9(2):92, 2017.

Tessler O, Bartow, Tremblay-Champagne NP, et al.: Long-term health-related quality of life outcomes in digital replantation versus revision amputation, *J Reconstr Microsurg* 33(6):446, 2017.

Tosti R, Eberlin KR: Damage control hand surgery: evaluation and emergency management of the mangled hand, *Hand Clin* 34(1):17, 2018.

Usama S, Kawahara S, Yamaguchi T, Hirase Y: Homodigital artery flap reconstruction for fingertip amputation: a comparative study of the oblique triangular neurovascular advancement flap and the reverse digital artery island flap, *J Hand Surg Eur* 40:291, 2015.

Wilkens SC, Claessen FM, Ogink PT, et al.: Reoperation after combined injury of the index finger: repair versus immediate amputation, *J Hand Surg Am* 41(3):436, 2016.

Yorlets RR, Busa K, Eberlin KR, et al.: Fingertip injuries in children: epidemiology, financial burden, and implications for prevention, *Hand (NY)* 12(4):342, 2017.

Zhu X, Zhu H, Zhang C, Zheng X: Preoperative predictive factors for the survival of replanted digits, *Int Orthop* 41(8):1623, 2017.

The complete list of references is available online at Expert Consult.com.

9.6 Resection or Stabilization of the Medial End of the Clavicle for Old Anterior Sternoclavicular Joint Dislocation, 495

9.7 Stabilization of Old Posterior Sternoclavicular Joint Dislocation (Wang et al.), 496

9.8 Resection of the Lateral End of the Clavicle for Chronic Acromioclavicular Joint Dislocation (Mumford; Gurd), 497

9.9 Reconstruction of the Superior Acromioclavicular Ligament for Chronic Acromioclavicular Joint Dislocation (Neviaser), 498

9.10 Transfer of the Coracoacromial Ligament for Chronic Acromioclavicular Joint Dislocation (Rockwood), 499

9.11 Arthroscopic Transfer of the Coracoacromial Ligament for Chronic Acromioclavicular Joint Dislocation (Boileau et al.), 500

9.12 Open Reduction of Chronic Anterior Shoulder Dislocations (Rowe and Zarins), 505

9.13 Open Reduction of Chronic Posterior Shoulder Dislocation from a Superior Approach (Rowe and Zarins), 506

9.14 Open Reduction of Chronic Posterior Shoulder Dislocation Through an Anteromedial Approach (McLaughlin), 507

9.15 Deltopectoral Approach for Chronic Posterior Shoulder Dislocation (Keppler et al.), 508

9.16 Open Reduction and V-Y Lengthening of Triceps Muscles for Chronic Elbow Dislocation (Speed), 510

10. Peripheral Nerve Injuries

10.1 Epineurial Neurorrhaphy, 536

10.2 Perineurial (Fascicular) Neurorrhaphy, 536

10.3 Interfascicular Nerve Grafting (Millesi, Modified), 537

10.4 Transfer of the Ulnar Nerve Fascicles to Nerve of the Biceps Muscle (Oberlin et al.), 539

10.5 Double Fascicular Transfer from Ulnar and Median Nerves to Nerve of the Brachialis Branches (MacKinnon and Colbert), 540

10.6 Neurotization of the Suprascapular Nerve with the Spinal Accessory Nerve (MacKinnon and Colbert), 541

10.7 Neurotization of the Axillary Nerve with Radial Nerve (MacKinnon and Colbert), 542

10.8 Posterior Approach for Division of the Transverse Scapular Ligament (Swafford and Lichtman), 544

10.9 Approach to the Axillary Nerve, 545

10.10 Approach to the Musculocutaneous Nerve, 546

10.11 Approach to the Radial Nerve, 547

10.12 Approach to the Ulnar Nerve, 550

10.13 Nerve Transfer for Ulnar Nerve Reconstruction (MacKinnon and Novak), 552

10.14 Approach to the Median Nerve, 553

10.15 Approach to the Femoral Nerve, 556

10.16 Approach to the Sciatic Nerve, 558

10.17 Approach to the Common, Superficial, and Deep Peroneal Nerves, 560

10.18 Approach to the Tibial Nerve Deep to the Soleus Muscle, 562

12. Amputations of the Foot

12.1 Terminal Syme Amputation, 588

12.2 Amputation at the Base of the Proximal Phalanx, 588

12.3 Metatarsophalangeal Joint Disarticulation, 591

12.4 Metatarsophalangeal Joint Disarticulation, 591

12.5 First or Fifth Ray Amputation (Border Ray Amputation), 591

12.6 Central Ray Amputation, 592

12.7 Transmetatarsal Amputation, 595

12.8 Chopart Amputation, 599

12.9 Syme Amputation, 601

12.10 Two-Stage Syme Amputation (Wyss et al.; Malone et al.; Wagner), 605

12.11 Boyd Amputation, 605

13. Amputations of the Lower Extremity

13.1 Transtibial Amputation, 610

13.2 Transtibial Amputation (Modified Ertl; Taylor and Poka), 611

13.3 Transtibial Amputation Using Long Posterior Skin Flap (Burgess), 613

13.4 Knee Disarticulation (Batch, Spittler, and McFaddin), 614

13.5 Knee Disarticulation (Mazet and Hennessy), 616

13.6 Knee Disarticulation (Kjøble), 616

13.7 Transfemoral (Above-Knee) Amputation of Nonischemic Limbs, 618

13.8 Transfemoral (Above-Knee) Amputation of Nonischemic Limbs (Gottschalk), 619

14. Amputations of the Hip and Pelvis

14.1 Anatomic Hip Disarticulation (Boyd), 621

14.2 Posterior Flap (Slocum), 623

14.3 Standard Hemipelvectomy, 624

14.4 Anterior Flap Hemipelvectomy, 624

14.5 Conservative Hemipelvectomy, 627

15. Major Amputations of the Upper Extremity

15.1 Amputation at the Wrist, 631

15.2 Disarticulation of the Wrist, 631

15.3 Distal Forearm (Distal Transradial) Amputation, 632

15.4 Proximal Third of Forearm (Proximal Transradial) Amputation, 633

15.5 Disarticulation of the Elbow, 633

15.6 Supracondylar Area, 634

15.7 Amputation Proximal to the Supracondylar Area, 636

15.8 Amputation Through the Surgical Neck of the Humerus, 636

15.9 Disarticulation of the Shoulder, 638

15.10 Anterior Approach (Berger), 640

15.11 Posterior Approach (Littlewood), 641

15.12 Targeted Muscle Reinnervation After Transhumeral Amputation (O'Shaughnessy et al.), 644

16. Amputations of the Hand

16.1 Kutler V-Y or Atasoy Triangular Advancement Flaps (Kutler; Fisher), 652

16.2 Atasoy Triangular Advancement Flaps (Atasoy et al.), 654

16.3 Bipedicle Dorsal Flaps, 655

16.4 Adipofascial Turnover Flap, 656

16.5 Thenar Flap, 656

16.6 Local Neurovascular Island Flap, 657

16.7 Island Pedicle Flap, 657

16.8 Retrograde Island Pedicle Flap, 659

16.9 Ulnar Hypothenar Flap, 659

16.10 Index Ray Amputation, 659

16.11 Transposing the Index Ray (Peacock), 662

16.12 Advancement Pedicle Flap for Thumb Injuries, 664

16.13 Phalangization of Fifth Metacarpal, 666